Musculoskeletal Interventions

Musculoskeletal Interventions
Techniques for Therapeutic Exercise

Editors

Michael L. Voight, DHSc, PT, SCS, OCS, ATC

Professor
School of Physical Therapy
Belmont University
Nashville, Tennessee

Barbara J. Hoogenboom, EdD, PT, SCS, ATC

Associate Professor
Program in Physical Therapy
Grand Valley State University
Grand Rapids, Michigan

William E. Prentice, PhD, PT, ATC

Professor, Coordinator of Sports Medicine Specialization
Department of Exercise and Sport Science
Clinical Professor, Division of Physical Therapy
Department of Medical Allied Professions
Associate Professor, Department of Orthopedics
School of Medicine
University of North Carolina at Chapel Hill
Chapel Hill, North Carolina

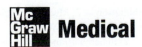

New York Chicago San Francisco Lisbon London Madrid Mexico City
Milan New Delhi San Juan Seoul Singapore Sydney Toronto

Musculoskeletal Interventions: Techniques for Therapeutic Exercise

1 2 3 4 5 6 7 8 9 0   QPD/QPD   0 9 8 7 6

ISBN-13:   978-0-07-145768-2
ISBN-10:   0-07-145768-2

This book was set in Adobe Garamond by TechBooks.
The editors were Michael Brown, Robert Pancotti, and Peter J. Boyle.
The production supervisor was Catherine H. Saggese.
Project management was provided by TechBooks.
The cover designer was Eve Siegel.
Quebecor World/Dubuque was printer and binder.

This book is printed on acid-free paper.

Library of Congress Cataloging-in-Publication Data

Musculoskeletal interventions : techniques for therapeutic exercise / editors, Michael L. Voight,
  Barbara J. Hoogenboom, William E. Prentice.
     p. ; cm.
  Includes index.
  ISBN-13: 978-0-07-145768-2 (alk. paper)
  ISBN-10: 0-07-145768-2 (alk. paper)
  1. Musculoskeletal system—Diseases—Patients—Rehabilitation.   2. Medical rehabilitation.   3. Physical therapy.
  I. Voight, Michael L., 1959-II. Hoogenboom, Barbara J.   III. Prentice, William E.
  [DNLM: 1. Musculoskeletal Diseases—rehabilitation.   2. Rehabilitation—methods. WB 320 M985 2007]
RM701.M872 2007
617.7'062—dc22   2006046607

CONTENTS

CONTRIBUTORS

Jolene L. Bennett, MA, PT, OCS, ATC, CertMDT
Clinical Specialist for Orthopedics and Sports
  Medicine
Spectrum Health Rehabilitation and Sports
  Medicine
Visser Family YMCA
Grandville, Michigan

Jeanine Biese, MEd, OTR, CHT
Assistant Professor
Occupational Therapy Program
Grand Valley State University
Certified Hand Therapist, Rehabilitation
  Professionals
Rockford, Michigan

Turner A. Blackburn, Jr., MEd, PT, ATC
Vice President of Corporate Development
Clemson Sports Medicine and Rehabilitation
Clinic Director, Sports Plus Manchester
Manchester, Georgia

Andrew Bloch, DOM, MSPT, ATC
President
Advanced Body Wellness For Life, Inc.
Miami Beach, Florida

Lee Burton, MS, ATC, CSCS
Assistant Professor and Athletic Training Program
  Director
Averett University
Danville, Virginia

Gray Cook, MSPT, OCS, CSCS
Clinical Director
Orthopedic and Sports Physical Therapy
Danville, Virginia

Mark De Carlo, PT, MHA, SCS, ATC
Methodist Sports Medicine Center
Indianapolis, Indiana

Craig R. Denegar, PhD, PT, ATC
Associate Professor of Orthopaedics and
  Rehabilitation
College of Health and Human Development
Pennsylvania State University
University Park, Pennsylvania

Phillip B. Donley, MS, PT, ATC
Director
Chester County Orthopaedic and Sports Physical
  Therapy
West Chester, Pennsylvania

Todd S. Ellenbecker, DPT, MS, SCS, OCS, CSCS
Clinic Director
Physiotherapy Associates Scottsdale Sports Clinic
Scottsdale, Arizona
National Director of Clinical Research
Physiotherapy Associates
Memphis, Tennessee

Robert Gailey, PhD, PT
Associate Professor
Department of Physical Therapy
University of Miami School of Medicine
Coral Gables, Florida
Health Science Researcher
Miami Veterans Affairs Medical Center
Miami, Florida

John A. Guido, Jr., MHS, PT, SCS, ATC, CSCS
Ochsner Health System
Harahan, Louisiana

Kevin M. Guskiewicz, PhD, ATC
Chairman and Professor
Department of Exercise and Sport Science
University of North Carolina
Chapel Hill, North Carolina

John S. Halle, PT, PhD, ECS
Professor
School of Physical Therapy
Belmont University
Nashville, Tennessee

J. Allen Hardin, PT, MS, SCS, ATC, CSCS

Department of Intercollegiate Athletics
The University of Texas
Austin, Texas

Christopher J. Hirth, MSPT, PT, ATC

Lecturer, Physical Therapist/Athletic Trainer
Department of Exercise and Sport Science
University of North Carolina
Chapel Hill, North Carolina

Barbara J. Hoogenboom, EdD, PT, SCS, ATC

Associate Professor
Program in Physical Therapy
Grand Valley State University
Grand Rapids, Michigan

Daniel N. Hooker, PhD, PT, ATC

Coordinator of Physical Therapy and Athletic
    Training
Division of Sports Medicine
University of North Carolina
Chapel Hill, North Carolina

Stuart L. (Skip) Hunter, PT, ATC

Clemson Sports Medicine
Clemson, South Carolina

Kyle Kiesel, PT, ATC, CSCS

Evansville, Indiana

Nancy E. Lomax, PT

Staff Physical Therapist
Spectrum Health Rehabilitation and Sports
    Medicine Services
Visser Family YMCA
Grandville, Michigan

Ryan McDivitt, ATC

Methodist Sportsmedicine Center
Indianapolis, Indiana

Scott Miller, MS, PT, SCS, CSCS

Sports Medicine Manager
GRSportsCenter Sports Medicine
Grand Rapids, Michigan

Tad E. Pieczynski, PT, MS, CSCS

Assistant Clinic Director
Physiotherapy Associates Scottsdale Sports Clinic
Scottsdale, Arizona

William E. Prentice, PhD, PT, ATC

Professor, Coordinator of Sports Medicine
    Specialization
Department of Exercise and Sport Science
Clinical Professor, Division of Physical Therapy
Department of Medical Allied Professions
Associate Professor, Department of Orthopedics
School of Medicine
University of North Carolina at Chapel Hill
Chapel Hill, North Carolina

T. Kevin Robinson, PT, DSc, OCS

Associate Professor
Physical Therapy Program
Belmont University
Nashville, Tennessee

Anne Marie Schneider, OTR, CHT

Coordinator, Hand Center
Raleigh Orthopaedic and Rehabilitation
    Specialists
Raleigh, North Carolina

Rob Schneider, MSPT, PT, ATC

Physical Therapist
Balance Physical Therapy
Durham, North Carolina

Teresa L. Schuemann, PT, SCS, ATC, CSCS

Director
Skyline Hospital Physical Therapy and Sports
    Rehabilitation Departments
White Salmon, Washington

Patrick D. Sells, DA, ACSM Exercise Specialist®

Assistant Professor, Physical Therapy
Belmont University
Nashville, Tennessee

Michael J. Shoemaker, PT, DPT, GCS

Clinical Specialist for Geriatrics and Pulmonary
Affiliate Faculty
Grand Valley State University Program in Physical
    Therapy
Cook-DeVos Center for Health Sciences
Grand Rapids, Michigan

Robyn K. Smith, MS, PT, SCS

Staff Physical Therapist
Rehab Professionals/GRSportsCenter
Grand Rapids, Michigan

Anna Thatcher, MS, PT, ATC, CSCS
Achieve Orthopaedic and Sports Therapy, P.C.
Phoenix, Arizona

Gregory C. Thomas, DPT, CSCS
PRO Sports Physical Therapy
Scarsdale, New York

Steven R. Tippett, PhD, SCS, ATC
Associate Professor
Department of Physical Therapy and Health
    Science
Bradley University
Peoria, Illinois

Timothy F. Tyler, MSPT, ATC
PRO Sports Physical Therapy
Clinical Research Associate
Nicholas Institute for Sports Medicine and
    Athletic Trauma (NISMAT)
Lenox Hill Hospital
Scarsdale, New York

Michael L. Voight, DHSc, PT, SCS, OCS, ATC
Professor
School of Physical Therapy
Belmont University
Nashville, Tennessee

PREFACE

The art and science of caring for the injured patient or client is constantly changing. The demand for evidence-based practice, expanding options for intervention, and new rehabilitation tools and methods all contribute to the need for textbooks that deal with specific aspects of injury management. Rehabilitation is the primary focus for the physical therapist, but equally important are foundational science, theory, and the expanding service areas of prevention and wellness. This textbook, *Musculoskeletal Interventions: Techniques for Therapeutic Exercise,* builds on and improves on an earlier book edited by Prentice and Voight, *Techniques in Musculoskeletal Rehabilitation.* Chapters contained in the original text that were less applicable to therapeutic exercise (i.e., modalities, pharmacology) were removed to narrow the focus of the current text. This text is intended for the physical therapist interested in gaining more in-depth exposure to the theory and practical application of rehabilitation techniques used for intervention with musculoskeletal injuries and varied pathologies in diverse patient populations.

The purpose of this text is to provide the physical therapist with a comprehensive guide to the systems considerations, design, implementation, and progression of rehabilitation programs for musculoskeletal injuries. It is intended for use in in-depth courses in musculoskeletal rehabilitation that deal with practical application of theory in a clinical setting or as an addition to the library of a practicing physical therapist. The contributing authors have attempted to combine their expertise and knowledge to produce a single text that encompasses many aspects of musculoskeletal rehabilitation.

Organization

The text is divided into five parts, each having a separate theme or purpose. The first part deals with the basic foundations of the rehabilitation process as identified in *The Guide to Physical Therapist Practice.* Chapter 1 begins by addressing the important considerations in designing a rehabilitation program for the patient with a musculoskeletal injury and providing a guide-based overview of the rehabilitative process. Chapter 2 highlights clinical decision making in the context of the patient-client management model. Since it is critical for the physical therapist to understand the importance of the healing process and how it should dictate the course of rehabilitation, Chapter 3 is dedicated to the physiology of healing. Chapter 4, a new addition to this text, gives a detailed account of the neuromuscular scanning examination. This scanning examination is an important skill for the therapist treating primarily musculoskeletal diagnoses and serves an early decision-making tool. Finally, at the end of the first part, Chapter 5, another new addition, presents the concept of algorithms and a template for methodical thinking during the evaluation and treatment selection process.

The second part presents information on the various physiological impairments that may need to be addressed as a part of the rehabilitative process. These chapters include information on impairments due to pain (Chapter 6); posture and function (Chapter 7); muscle performance (Chapter 8); endurance and aerobic capacity (Chapter 9); mobility and range of motion (Chapter 10); and neuromuscular function (Chapter 11). Each chapter also highlights methods for management of the impairment described in the chapter. Physical therapists have many rehabilitation "tools" that they can use to treat a patient with a musculoskeletal injury. How an individual therapist chooses to use these "tools" is often a matter of personal preference. Only rarely does the evidence guide the therapist to the best or the "gold standard" intervention for a given pathology, injury, or postsurgical rehabilitation.

The third part provides an overview of several rehabilitation tools. It provides detailed discussion of how these interventions may be best incorporated into a rehabilitation program to achieve the individualized treatment goals that are established for varied patients and clients with musculoskeletal pathologies. The tools of rehabilitation included in this part are: isokinetics (Chapter 12); plyometric exercise (Chapter 13); open- versus closed-kinetic chain exercise (Chapter 14); proprioceptive neuromuscular facilitation techniques (Chapter 15); joint mobilization and traction techniques (Chapter 16); regaining postural stability and balance (Chapter 17); core stabilization training (Chapter 18); aquatic therapy (Chapter 19); functional movement screening (Chapter 20); functional progressions and functional testing (Chapter 21); orthotics (Chapter 22); designing home exercise programs for home and clinical progressions (Chapter 23); and components of functional exercises (Chapter 24). Of note is the new chapter on functional movement screening, which promotes functional examination and thereby drives functionally-based intervention.

The fourth part of this text goes into detail on specific rehabilitation techniques and interventions (many of which were generally previously described in the third part) applied to the treatment of a wide variety of regional musculoskeletal injuries. This portion of the text is organized by body region and encompasses detailed rehabilitation suggestions for the conditions of the shoulder (Chapter 25); the elbow (Chapter 26); the hand and wrist (Chapter 27); the groin, hip, and thigh (Chapter 28); the knee (Chapter 29); the lower leg (Chapter 30); the ankle and foot (Chapter 31); and the spine (Chapter 32). Each chapter begins with a discussion of the pertinent functional anatomy and biomechanics of that region. It should be noted that the focus of this text is not detailed examination and special test procedures but rather in-depth coverage of rehabilitation interventions. As a result, it is likely that a text such as this will accompany a text on examination and evaluation.

The second portion of each chapter involves in-depth discussion of the pathomechanics, injury mechanisms, rehabilitation concerns, and rehabilitation progressions for specific injuries. An extensive series of photographs that illustrate a wide variety of rehabilitative exercises is presented in each chapter. A new addition to this text is the inclusion of sample rehabilitation guidelines offered by the experts who have written each regional chapter.

The fifth part of the text discusses treatment considerations for specific patient populations: the geriatric patient (Chapter 33); the pediatric patient (Chapter 34); amputees (Chapter 35); and the physically active female (Chapter 36).

Comprehensive Coverage of Research-Based Material

Musculoskeletal Interventions: Techniques for Therapeutic Exercise offers an updated, broad reference and guide for treating musculoskeletal injuries for the physical therapist who creates and administers rehabilitation programs.

Any physical therapist responsible for supervising rehabilitation programs knows that what is currently accepted and "up-to-date" in terms of intervention strategies, machinery, equipment, and rehabilitation protocols changes rapidly. The contributing authors have made a sincere effort to present the most current, evidence-based, comprehensive information on the various aspects of injury rehabilitation. In addition to critical review by the editors, the contents of this text were reviewed by selected physical therapists who are well-respected clinicians, educators, and researchers in this field, to further ensure that the material presented is accurate and current.

Learning Aids

The aids provided in this text to assist the student physical therapist in its use include the following:

Objectives.   These are listed at the beginning of each chapter to identify the concepts presented in the chapter.

Figures and Tables.   Figures and tables included throughout the text have been increased in number and significantly revised in an effort to provide as much visual and graphic demonstration of specific concepts, rehabilitation techniques, and exercises as possible.

Summary.   Each chapter has a summary that outlines the major points presented.

End of Chapter Treatment Guidelines.   Each of the regionally organized chapters (e.g., knee, hip, shoulder) includes a set of guidelines submitted by their authors for state-of-the-art treatment suggestions for common diagnoses.

References.   A comprehensive list of references is presented at the end of each chapter to provide additional information relative to chapter content.

Please tell the author and publisher what you think of this book by sending your comments to pt@mcgraw-hill.com. Put the author and title of the book in the subject line.

ACKNOWLEDGMENTS

The process of preparing the 36 manuscripts for this textbook was a huge undertaking. It was a demanding task that required the dedication of three editors with a vision for producing something better than what existed previously. Each of the three editors brings a unique perspective regarding writing, therapeutic exercise, and the process of rehabilitation. In our diversity we often found consensus and we have this product to show for it.

We would like to thank each of the contributing authors. We asked them to contribute to this text because we have tremendous respect for them personally as well as professionally. These individuals have distinguished themselves as educators, clinicians, and researchers dedicated to the rehabilitation of a wide variety of individuals of all abilities and walks of life. We are exceedingly grateful for their input and willingness to share their ideas in writing and pictures.

Finally, the three of us would like to thank people who have been important to us throughout our careers and during the process of creating and editing this textbook. We thank our many friends and colleagues who have given us professional direction explicitly and implicitly, provided us with mentorship, and taught us the importance of lifelong learning and the necessity of continually seeking answers to questions. These same friends and colleagues constantly keep us laughing, loving life, and enjoying the many facets of the practice of rehabilitation.

Mike would like to give special thanks to several individuals. First to his coeditors and coauthors, Barb and Bill, who put up with countless rewrites and missed deadlines while at the same time constantly changing things—thanks, I owe both of them an extreme debt of gratitude. Secondly, to John Halle and his colleagues at Belmont University. They have provided him the academic freedom and time to pursue this project. They challenge him every day to seek excellence. And lastly, to his close family. To his parents who started him down the right path and gave him educational freedom; to his mentor Tab Blackburn, who has continued to give him professional direction; and finally to his wife Cissy, who has had to pay the price for his passion for excellence while at the same time giving him inspiring wisdom and endless support to help sustain his passion for being an educator.

Barb would like to begin by thanking her great family, Dave, Lindsay, and Matthew, who support her and are patient during projects such as this and throughout all her (crazy) endeavors. You guys keep her going! Second, she thanks her parents, whose dedication to education, excellence, and teaching by example means more every day. Finally, thanks to her outstanding sports physical therapy colleagues and the DPT students at Grand Valley State University, who keep her stretching, learning, and growing every day.

Bill would like to thank his family—Tena, Brian, and Zachary—who make an effort such as this worthwhile. They keep him grounded and help him to maintain his focus in both his personal and his professional life.

Thank you to all—we will forever be indebted.

Michael L. Voight
Barbara J. Hoogenboom
William E. Prentice

PART 1

Foundations of
the Rehabilitation Process

1

CHAPTER 1

Introduction to the Rehabilitation Process: "The Guide to Physical Therapist Practice"

Barbara J. Hoogenboom

OBJECTIVES

After completing this chapter, the therapist should be able to do the following:

- Explain the concepts upon which *The Guide to Physical Therapist Practice* was based.
- Describe the changes that have occurred to the original *Guide to Physical Therapist Practice* since its inception in 1997.
- Explain the four elements of the disablement model as described by Saad Nagi.
- Compare and contrast the disablement model to the medical model of dealing with the effects of disease and injury.
- Identify the components of the examination process as defined by *The Guide*.
- Discuss the decision-making process based upon the examination.
- Describe the three types of intervention as defined by *The Guide* and give examples of each.
- Describe the four categories of preferred practice patterns developed in *The Guide*.
- Describe potential uses of *The Guide* in various settings (clinical, academic, public information, etc.).

Physical therapists play an exciting and vital role in the dynamic health care arena. As a profession, physical therapists contribute in a variety of ways to the health care system. No longer are physical therapists seen only as providers of rehabilitation, but also as participants in the processes of patient education, disease prevention, and promotion of health and wellness. Physical therapists of the twenty-first century must have a united voice with regard to our scope of practice, our models of health care delivery, the types of patients and clients we serve, as well as the types of examination measures and interventions we use to remedy or prevent impairments, functional limitations, and disabilities in our patients and clients. We must be active, knowledgeable educators of the public, other health care providers, third-party payers, and health policy makers as we advocate for the profession of physical therapy.

The Guide to Physical Therapist Practice was first published in the November 1997 issue of *Physical Therapy* as a document to describe the practice of physical therapy.[1] It was developed by consensus of an expert clinician panel chosen from across the United States who represented perspectives from a variety of practice settings. Prior to its publication, the document underwent extensive clinician review and repeated edits. *The Guide* is not a static document, rather it is a "living" document that is intended to grow and change with the profession of physical therapy. Therefore, a revision to the original *Guide* was published in 2001.[2] This evolution represented the culmination of input from the panels, educators, and clinicians and attempted to improve the utility of *The Guide*. Subsequently, in 2003, *The Interactive Guide to Physical Therapist Practice* was released in the form of a CD-ROM that allowed access to the digital version of *The Guide*, search capabilities and cross referencing, as well as an index of tests and measures with hyperlinks to reliability and validity studies and citations.[3]

The Guide was developed in response to a charge from the American Physical Therapy Association's (APTA) House of Delegates in 1992. Part 1 (Chapters 1–3) of *The Guide* was written specifically as a detailed description of the practice of physical therapy. The intended audiences included clinicians, educators, administrators, other health care professionals, policymakers, and third-party payers. When the Commission for Accreditation of Physical Therapist Education (CAPTE) revised its guidelines for accreditation, the language of *The Guide,* Part 1 was adopted.

The Guide is not a cookbook. It provides a framework for physical therapy practice, but does not provide clinical guidelines or protocols for intervention. Clinical guidelines must be developed based upon evidence, whereas the preferred practice patterns contained in *The Guide* are merely patterns considered by *Guide* developers as most commonly used or most appropriate patterns of patient and client intervention.[7] Likewise, there is neither a recommended fee structure in *The Guide* nor any direct connection to current procedural terminology codes. Although some (International Classification of Diseases) ICD-9 codes are listed and referred to in Part 2, they should not be used to code for billing purposes. *The Guide* does not specify the site of care; rather, it uses the *episode of care* concept that crosses all rehabilitation settings related to each episode. *The Guide* also does not address the state-to-state variances in the scope of practice.

DISABLEMENT MODEL

The Guide to Physical Therapist Practice was developed based on the disablement model developed by Saad Nagi in 1969.[5] It was designed to describe the effects of disease and injury at both the personal and societal levels as well as their functional consequences. The disablement model is distinctly different from the classic medical model of disease where the emphasis is on treating the specific diagnosis with pharmacology or surgery. The disablement model emphasizes the functional and health status of individuals, with intervention based on improving these aspects of the patient's condition.[1-3] The model has four elements:

Pathology ↔ Impairment ↔

Functional limitation ↔ Disability

Pathology is the interruption of the normal cellular processes from a biomechanical, physiologic, or anatomic perspective.[1-3] The body often responds to an injury or pathology with a defensive reaction in order to restore the normal state. Examples of this include hemarthrosis in the case of ligament rupture, or the inflammatory process in response to connective tissue damage (tear/stretch). Intervention at this level is generally handled by physicians and is often pharmacologic and/or surgical in nature.

Impairment is any loss or abnormality of physiologic, psychological, or anatomic structure or function at the level of organs and body systems.[1-3] Physical therapists typically measure the signs and symptoms that present in conjunction with an injury, illness, or pathology and identify the subsequent impairments. Physical therapists often intervene trying to attempt correctly identified impairments. Examples of physiologic impairments would be muscle weakness, range-of-motion loss, pain, and abnormal joint play. Anatomic impairments would include structural conditions such as genu recurvatum, scoliosis, femoral anteversion, and alterations in foot alignment.

Functional limitation is a deviation from the normal behavior in performing tasks and activities from that which would be considered traditional or expected for individual.[1-3] Functional limitations are tasks or activities that are not performed in the usual efficient or skilled fashion. Problems with transfers, standing, walking, running, and climbing stairs are all examples of functional limitations.

Disability is the incapacity in performing a broad range of tasks and activities that are usually expected in specific social roles.[1-3] Inability to function as a spouse, student, parent, or worker (in the home or outside of the home) constitutes a disability.

The scope of physical therapist practice overlaps with many portions of the disablement model, as is shown in Figure 1-1.

The disablement process is a two-way continuum affected by intraindividual and extraindividual risk factors (Fig. 1-2).

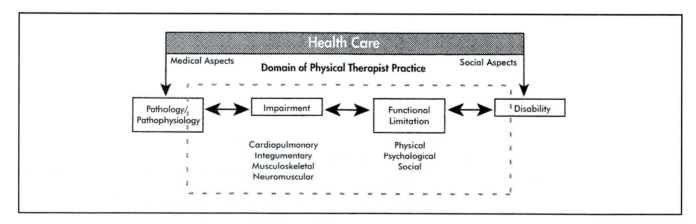

F I G U R E   1 - 1

The scope of physical therapist practice within the continuum of health care services and the context of the disablement model. (Reproduced, with permission, from the APTA, The guide to physical therapist practice, 2nd ed. *Phys Ther* 81(1):9–738, 2001.)

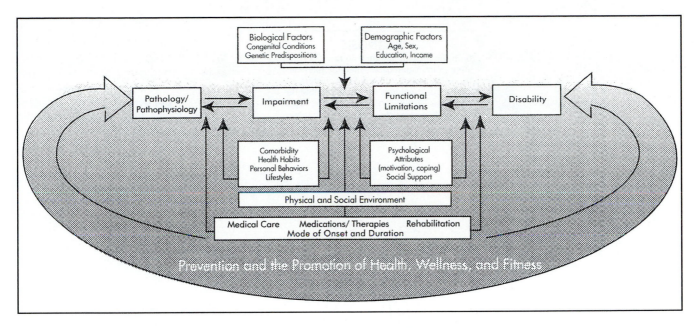

FIGURE 1-2

An expanded disablement model showing interactions among individual and environmental factors, prevention, and the promotion of health, wellness, and fitness. (Reproduced, with permission, from the APTA, The guide to physical therapist practice, 2nd ed. *Phys Ther* 81(1):9–738, 2001.)

Intraindividual factors include habits, lifestyle, behavior, psychosocial characteristics, age and sex, educational level and income, weight, and family history. Extraindividual factors are things like the medical care received, the pharmacologic and other therapies available, the physical environment, and any external supports. The relationship between these aspects will vary between individuals and will ultimately determine the impact of the disease or injury.

Most physical therapists have treated patients who had significant impairments but remained extremely functional. Most have also treated patients who were disabled by what seemed to be minor impairments or functional limitations. Unfortunately, there are few studies in the literature to show a direct cause-and-effect relationship between impairments, functional limitations, and disability.

In addition to the Nagi Model, *The Guide* is also strongly influenced by two additional conceptual frameworks: the integration of prevention and wellness strategies and the patient/client management model. These influential frameworks will be discussed further in subsequent sections or chapters.

OVERVIEW OF *THE GUIDE:* PART 1

The purpose of *The Guide to Physical Therapist Practice* is to improve the quality of physical therapy, promote appropriate use of services, enhance customer satisfaction, and reduce unwarranted variations in physical therapy management. Prevention

and wellness initiatives are also stressed and will help decrease the need for services.[1–3]

Chapter 1 provides a description of "who" physical therapists are and "what" they do. This description includes the various practice settings in which a physical therapist may practice, including some less traditional ones like corporate or industrial health centers and fitness centers. In this chapter, the terms "patients" and "clients" are defined as

- Patient—"Individuals who are the recipients of physical therapy examination, evaluation, diagnosis, prognosis, and intervention and who have a disease, disorder, condition impairment, functional limitation, or disability" (Ref. 2, p. 689)
- Client—"Individuals who engage the services of a physical therapist and who can benefit from the physical therapist's consultation, interventions, professional advice, health promotion, fitness, wellness, or prevention services" (Ref. 2, p. 685). Clients are also businesses, school systems, and others to whom physical therapists provide services.[1–3]

The chapter continues with a discussion of the scope of practice for physical therapists. Physical therapists provide direct services to patients as well as interact with other professionals, provide prevention and wellness services, consult, engage in critical inquiry (research), educate, administrate, and supervise support personnel.

Physical therapy is an integral part of secondary and tertiary rehabilitative care. Chapter 1 of *The Guide* expands on

DIAGNOSIS

Both the process and the end result of evaluating examination data, which the physical therapist organizes into defined clusters, syndromes, or categories to help determine the prognosis (including the plan of care) and the most appropriate intervention strategies.

EVALUATION

A dynamic process in which the physical therapist makes clinical judgments based on data gathered during the examination. This process also may identify possible problems that require consultation with or referral to another provider.

PROGNOSIS
(Including Plan of Care)

Determination of the level of optimal improvement that may be attained through intervention and the amount of time required to reach that level. The plan of care specifies the interventions to be used and their timing and frequency.

EXAMINATION

The process of obtaining a history, performing a systems review, and selecting and administering tests and measures to gather data about the patient/client. The initial examination is a comprehensive screening and specific testing process that leads to a diagnostic classification. The examination process also may identify possible problems that require consultation with or referral to another provider.

INTERVENTION

Purposeful and skilled interaction of the physical therapist with the patient/client and, if appropriate, with other individuals involved in care of the patient/client, using various physical therapy methods and techniques to produce changes in the condition that are consistent with the diagnosis and prognosis. The physical therapist conducts a reexamination to determine changes in patient/client status and to modify or redirect intervention. The decision to reexamine may be based on new clinical findings or on lack of patient/client progress. The process of reexamination also may identify the need for consultation with or referral to another provider.

OUTCOMES

Results of patient/client management, which include the impact of physical therapy interventions in the following domains: pathology/ pathophysiology (disease, disorder, or condition); impairments, functional limitations, and disabilities; risk reduction/prevention; health, wellness, and fitness; societal resources; and patient/client satisfaction.

F I G U R E   1 - 3

The patient/client management model. (Reproduced, with permission, from the APTA, The guide to physical therapist practice, 2nd ed. *Phys Ther* 81(1):9–738, 2001.)

this model with a discussion of the physical therapist's role in primary care and in wellness. The concepts of primary care and wellness involve restoring health, alleviating pain, and preventing the onset of impairments, functional limitations, disabilities, or changes in physical function and health status resulting from injury, disease, or other causes.[1,2] Physical therapists play major roles in secondary and tertiary care of those with conditions of the musculoskeletal, neuromuscular, cardiovascular/pulmonary, and integumentary systems that may have been treated primarily by another practitioner. Often, secondary care is provided in acute care and rehabilitation hospitals as well as outpatient clinics, home health settings, and within school systems.[2,3] Tertiary care is often provided by physical therapists in more specialized, comprehensive, technologically advanced settings in response to another health care practitioners' re-

quest for consultation and specialized services offered by the therapist.[1–3]

The clinical decision-making process presented in *The Guide* comprises the five elements of the patient/client management model (Fig. 1-3): examination, evaluation, diagnosis, prognosis, and intervention. This clinical decision-making model is explored in greater depth in Chapter 2.

The physical therapist begins with a thorough *examination*. There are three components to this:[1–3]

- History—A comprehensive investigation of the current and past health from a variety of sources, including the medical record, the patient, and the patient's caregiver. A complete list of possible types of data is included in this chapter.

- Systems review—A limited examination of the cardiopulmonary, neuromuscular, musculoskeletal, and integumentary systems as a means of screening for other potential health problems. An example of this would be to take a baseline blood pressure and heart rate. Communication ability and educational preferences are also assessed during the systems review.
- Tests and measures—After gathering and analyzing the aforementioned information, specific tests and measures are performed to formulate a diagnosis. An operational definition for each category of tests and measures exists, followed by a three-part description, i.e., general purpose, clinical indications, and specific tests and measures.

There are 24 categories of tests and measures listed alphabetically in *The Guide*. The following is a list of the alphabetically arranged categories of tests and measures:

- Aerobic capacity/endurance
- Anthropometric characteristics
- Arousal, attention, and cognition
- Assistive and adaptive devices
- Circulation
- Cranial and peripheral nerve integrity
- Environmental, home, and work barriers
- Ergonomics and body mechanics
- Gait, locomotion, and balance
- Integumentary integrity
- Joint integrity and mobility
- Motor function
- Muscle performance
- Neuromotor development and sensory integration
- Orthotic, protective, and supportive devices
- Pain
- Posture
- Prosthetic requirements
- Range of motion
- Reflex integrity
- Self-care and home management
- Sensory integrity
- Ventilation and respiration/gas exchange
- Work, community, and leisure integration or reintegration

The following are some relevant examples of tests and measures as well as indications for end data generated by the test/measure:

Anthropometric Characteristics

- Clinical indications—Patient with acute sprained ankle (edema or effusion)
- Tests and measures—Assessment of edema, i.e., palpation/volume/girth measurements
- Data generated—Girth of lower extremity in inches or centimeter

Assistive and Adaptive Devices

- Clinical indications—Patient with total knee replacement (impaired gait, locomotion, and balance)
- Tests and measures—Assessment of safety during use of a cane
- Data generated—Deviations and malfunctions that can be corrected or alleviated using the cane

Environmental, Home, and Work Barriers

- Clinical indications—Patient with osteoporosis (impaired muscle performance)
- Tests and measures—Assessment of current and potential barriers
- Data generated—Adaptations, additions, or modifications that would enhance safety

Ergonomics and Body Mechanics

- Clinical indications—Patient with low back injury (pain)
- Tests and measures—Analysis of preferred postures during performance of tasks and activities
- Data generated—Body alignment during specific job tasks and activities

Joint Integrity and Mobility

- Clinical indications—Patient with glenohumeral adhesive capsulitis (impaired range of motion)
- Tests and measures—Assessment of joint hypermobility and hypomobility
- Data generated—Joint mobility classification and scale

Muscle Performance

- Clinical indications—Patient with urinary incontinence (impaired bladder function)
- Tests and measures—Assessment of pelvic floor musculature
- Data generated—Strength of pelvic floor musculature

Posture

- Clinical indications—Patient with scoliosis (abnormal body alignment)
- Tests and measures—Analysis of resting posture in any position
- Data generated—Alignment and symmetry of body landmarks within segmental planes, while at rest

Prosthetic Requirements

- Clinical indications—Patient with below-the-knee amputation (impaired sensory integrity)

- Tests and measures—Assessment of alignment and fit of the device and inspection of related changes in skin condition
- Data generated—Skin integrity and edema in the residual limb

The interactive CD-ROM version of *The Guide* provides the user with hyperlinks to any available evidence regarding reliability and validity of tests and measures.[3]

The next three steps in the process involve decision making. Using the information gathered through the examination, the physical therapist formulates an *evaluation*. This is the clinical judgement that results from assessing the situation in its entirety from multiple points of view. Factors such as loss of function, social considerations, and health status are taken into consideration when developing a *diagnosis* (cluster of signs and symptoms) and *prognosis* (optimal level of improvement and time to get there), which guides the interventions that are chosen and performed during comprehensive management of the patient.[1]

Intervention describes the skilled interaction of the physical therapist when performing the therapeutic techniques and/or delegating and overseeing services. The goal is to produce a positive change in the condition. Intervention strategies should be constantly evaluated and reevaluated for their effectiveness with goals of remediation of impairments, improvement in functional outcomes, as well as secondary and tertiary prevention and long-term wellness. Continued care is based on the patient's response and progress toward the determined goals.[1–3]

There are three components to the intervention: (1) coordination, communication, and documentation; (2) patient/client-related instruction; and (3) procedural interventions. Management of every patient will include some aspect of the first two intervention components and often one or more procedural interventions. There are nine procedural interventions, listed by level of importance and utilization in the practice of physical therapy:

- Therapeutic exercise
- Functional training in self-care and home management
- Functional training in work, community, and leisure integration or reintegration
- Manual therapy techniques, including mobilization/manipulation
- Prescription, application, and, as appropriate, fabrication of devices and equipment
- Airway clearance techniques
- Integumentary repair and protective techniques
- Electrotherapeutic modalities
- Physical agents and mechanical modalities

Examination findings, the evaluation, diagnosis, and prognosis and any available research evidence should support the choice of intervention. Clinical reasoning will be discussed further in Chapter 5.

Factors that might influence the choice of interventions as well as the prognosis include[1]

- chronicity or severity of current condition,
- level of current impairment,
- functional limitation or disability,
- living environment,
- multisite or multisystem involvement,
- physical function and health status,
- potential discharge destinations,
- preexisting conditions or diseases,
- social supports, and
- stability of condition.

The following are some relevant examples of interventions:

Coordination, Communication, and Focumentation

- Clinical indications—Patient with total knee replacement (discharge destination)
- Anticipated goals—Care is coordinated with patient, family, caregivers, and other health care professionals
- Specific interventions—Discharge planning

Patient/Client-Related Instruction

- Clinical indications—Patient with scoliosis (patient education)
- Anticipated goals—Intensity of care is decreased
- Specific interventions—Written and pictorial instruction

Therapeutic Exercise

- Clinical indications—Patient with below-the-knee amputation (restricted in performing necessary tasks/activities)
- Anticipated goals—Gait, locomotion, and balance are improved
- Specific interventions—Gait and balance training with prosthetic device

Functional Training in Self-Care and Home Management

- Clinical indications—Patient with osteoporosis (restricted in performing self-care and home activities)
- Anticipated goals—Performance and independence of activities of daily living/instrumental activities of daily living increased
- Specific interventions—Self-care and home management task adaptation

Functional Training in Community and Work

- Clinical indications—Patient with low back injury (have a known work-related injury and disability)
- Anticipated goals—Tolerance to positions and activities is increased
- Specific interventions—Ergonomic stressor reduction training

Manual Therapy Techniques

- Clinical indications—Patient with glenohumeral adhesive capsulitis (limited range of motion)
- Anticipated goals—Joint integrity and mobility are improved
- Specific interventions—Joint mobilization and manipulation

Electrotherapeutic Modalities

- Clinical indications—Patient with urinary incontinence (impaired muscle performance)
- Anticipated goals—Ability to perform physical tasks is increased
- Specific interventions—Electrical muscle stimulation and biofeedback

Physical Agents and Mechanical Modalities

- Clinical indications—Patient with acutely sprained ankle (edema or effusion)
- Anticipated goals—Edema or effusion is decreased
- Specific interventions—Cryotherapy, mechanical compression

OVERVIEW OF *THE GUIDE:* PART 2

Part 2 of *The Guide* has four sections, each dedicated to a system: musculoskeletal, neuromuscular, cardiopulmonary, and integumentary. The four chapters in Part 2 are distinguished by a specific graphic that relates to and depicts a structure within the content area. Chapter 4 contains the musculoskeletal patterns, Chapter 5 contains the neuromuscular patterns, Chapter 6 contains the cardiopulmonary patterns, and Chapter 7 contains the integumentary patterns.

The patterns are structured similarly, and each has a diagnostic label based on impairments. The design of each pattern is as follows[1-3]:

- Description of the patient/client diagnostic group (with a list of those patients and diagnoses that would be included and excluded).
- Listing of the likely ICD-9-CM codes.
- Description of the history and systems review section of the examination.
- List of likely tests and measures (based on clinical indications).
- Prognosis with a range of visits expected for an episode of care.
- Anticipated goals for intervention.
- List of likely interventions.
- Outcomes of care.
- Criteria for discharge.
- Primary prevention/risk factor reduction strategies.

The patterns are followed by a glossary of terms, standards of practice, guide for professional conduct and code of ethics, standards of ethical conduct and guide for conduct of the affiliate member, templates for physical therapy documentation, and an example of a patient/client satisfaction questionnaire. At the end, there are two handy indexes, one a numerical and the other an alphabetical index to the patterns and ICD-9 codes.[1-3]

MUSCULOSKELETAL PRACTICE PATTERNS[1-3]

The musculoskeletal panel consisted of nine people with a wide range of experience covering all areas of orthopedic practice. The group, though lively and diverse, all shared a similar philosophy toward physical therapy practice. All were committed to using the patient/client management model as a framework for practice. In an attempt to describe musculoskeletal practice, disorders common to musculoskeletal practice that were treated in a variety of settings were identified. From this list, common interventions were identified. Finally, patterns of disorders emerged, which when grouped because of their similarities would be managed similarly and have comparable outcomes.

The musculoskeletal patterns are impairment based and their titles reflect this. Each has key associations to pathology and medical/surgical diagnoses noted within the descriptive information about the practice pattern. Primary prevention is a significant component to each pattern, because the progression from pathology to impairment, functional limitation, and disability is not inevitable. The first preferred practice pattern, like the first in the other systems' chapters, is a primary prevention pattern. The aim of such a pattern is not intervention for a preexisting condition, impairment, or functional limitation, rather prevention of each of these conditions. The rest of the patterns are for intervention in conditions that fit into the cluster of signs and symptoms that form the movement-based diagnosis. The following is a description of each pattern, the purpose of which is to get a sense of what patients and diagnoses would fall within this category of practice patterns[1-3]:

4A. Primary prevention/risk reduction for skeletal demineralization
- Includes clients with prolonged non-weightbearing state, hormonal changes, steroid use, nutritional deficiency, or those in a known high-risk category (e.g., based on sex, ethnicity, age, lifestyle).
- Patients/clients included in this pattern are in need of primary prevention/risk reduction only and cannot have a primary musculoskeletal pathology.
- Used to design a screening tool and group exercise program or individualized plan.

4B. Impaired posture
- Includes patients with primary spinal or appendicular postural dysfunction due to habit, work, pregnancy, or idiopathic causes.

- Excludes patients with impairments associated with chronic obstructive pulmonary disease, or radicular signs.
- Also excludes patients with recent spinal stabilization surgery.

4C. Impaired muscle performance
- Includes patients with disuse atrophy from systemic disease, prolonged immobilization, and chronic musculoskeletal or neuromuscular dysfunction.
- Also includes patients with pelvic floor muscle dysfunction.
- Excludes patients with amputation, fracture, postmusculoskeletal surgery, specific joint impairments (capsular restrictions or localized inflammation), and muscular pain due to cesarean delivery.

4D. Impaired joint mobility, motor function, muscle performance, and range of motion associated with connective tissue dysfunction
- Include patients with musculotendinous strain and ligamentous sprain.
- Patients may have joint hypermobility, muscle guarding/weakness, and/or swelling.
- Exclude patients with fractures, neurologic dysfunction, open wounds, or radiculopathy.

4E. Impaired joint mobility, motor function, muscle performance, and range of motion associated with localized inflammation
- Include patients with bursitis, tendinitis, synovitis, fasciitis, osteoarthritis, epicondylitis, etc.
- Patients may have edema, muscle weakness, neurovascular/sensory changes, pain, etc.
- Exclude patients with fractures, systemic diseases, open wounds, sepsis, associated surgery, deep vein thrombosis, dislocations, etc.

4F. Impaired joint mobility, motor function, muscle performance, range of motion, and reflex integrity associated with spinal disorders
- Include patients with disk herniation/disease, nerve root compression, stenosis, stable spondylolisthesis, history of spinal surgeries, etc.
- Patients may have altered sensation, weakness, positive neural tension, deep-tendon reflex changes, surgery, etc.
- Exclude patients with fractures, neuromuscular/systemic disease, and SCI.

4G. Impaired joint mobility, motor function, muscle performance, and range of motion associated with fracture
- Include patients with trauma, hormonal changes, steroid use, nutritional deficiency, or those in a known high-risk category (e.g., based on sex, ethnicity, age, lifestyle).
- Exclude patients with flail chest, Paget's disease, and osteogenesis imperfecta.

4H. Impaired joint mobility, motor function, muscle performance, and range of motion associated with joint arthroplasty

- Include patients who have partial or total joint resurfacing of small or large joints.
- Include patients with bone neoplasms, osteoarthritis, rheumatoid arthritis/juvenile rheumatoid arthritis, steroid-induced necrosis, trauma, ankylosing spondylitis, etc.
- Exclude patients with impairments associated with multisite trauma and rheumatoid arthritis with deconditioning (may require classification in additional patterns).

4I. Impaired joint mobility, motor function, muscle performance, and range of motion associated with bony or soft tissue surgery
- Include patients with ligamentous/muscle/tendon repair, open-reduction internal-fixation surgeries, bony debridement/graft, external fixators, soft-tissue/fascial/synovial procedures, etc.
- Exclude patients with amputation, closed head trauma, nonunion fractures, peripheral nerve lesions, total joint replacements, nonhealing wounds, and vascular sequelae (may require additional classification).

4J. Impaired joint mobility, motor function, muscle performance, gait, locomotion, and balance associated with amputation
- Include patients with uni- or bilateral amputation, congenital amputation, residual limb revision due to primary conditions such as diabetes, frostbite, peripheral vascular disease, and trauma.
- Patients may have wound needs, prosthetic needs, gait deviations, and other mobility problems.
- Exclude patients with amputation with respiratory failure and those with open wounds may need classification in additional patterns.

The original *Guide* had areas of musculoskeletal practice not covered by the preferred practice patterns. For instance, there was no pattern dealing with the management of patients with impairments due to upper-extremity amputations. Because *The Guide* is a fluid document and is subject to updating and evolution, the second edition of *The Guide* included amputations of the upper extremity as well as the lower extremity. It is likely that other diagnoses will be added to or placed in different practice patterns on a regular basis as practice evolves and *The Guide* is used by more clinicians.

OVERVIEW OF *THE GUIDE*: PARTS 3 AND 4

When the second edition and revision of *The Guide* was initiated, a task force of expert clinicians and researchers was assembled to identify the vast array of test and measures used in physical therapist examination and to collect the pertinent information on the tests or measure's reliability and validity, as such information could be found in the peer-reviewed literature. Concomitantly, a second task force was convened to identify outcome measures relevant to physical therapist practice and provide similar documentation. The work of both groups was issued on the CD-ROM version of *The Guide* as the *Catalog of Tests and Measures*.[3] These task forces also helped to create the outline of a minimal data set for initial examination and the templates for initial documentation, which can also be found in the second edition of the Guide.

NEXT STEP: USING *THE GUIDE* IN PRACTICE

The Guide is intended for use by physical therapists in all areas of practice. In some types of practice it is used frequently and in others it is not well accepted and virtually ignored. Many orthopedic physical therapists have difficulty in switching their thinking from treatment based upon medical and surgical diagnoses such as anterior cruciate ligament (ACL) tear (nonoperative treatment) or Rotator cuff repair to movement dysfunction-based diagnoses, which are the consequences of such medical and surgical diagnoses. To continue with this illustration, a patient who has sustained an ACL tear is likely to be categorized into practice pattern 4D: "Impaired joint mobility, motor function, muscle performance, and range of motion associated with connective tissue dysfunction." Practice pattern 4D represents a cluster of signs and symptoms that is related to the movement-related dysfunction present in the patient. A patient who has undergone a rotator cuff repair is likely to be categorized into practice pattern 4I: "Impaired joint mobility, motor function, muscle performance, and range of motion associated with bony or soft tissue surgery." Again, the cluster of signs and symptoms, which comprises the name of the practice pattern, summarizes the movement-related consequences of the medical diagnosis or surgery. Note that if the patient with an ACL tear has a reconstructive surgery, he or she may then be categorized in the same practice pattern as the patient who has undergone a rotator cuff repair!

There are several ways that the practice patterns can be useful in both the clinical and the education setting.

The first way to incorporate *The Guide* as a whole is to revise the initial evaluation, progress note, and discharge forms to reflect *Guide* language. A "Guidecizing" form is the quickest way to get clinicians used to using the terminology. From there, *The Guide* can be used for peer review of both routine and difficult or complex patient cases. Compiling data and keeping the APTA informed as to the utility and accuracy of the practice patterns is essential in making *The Guide* a true description of current physical therapy practice.

Another use of *The Guide* and the practice patterns is development of a form to measure various outcomes. This is a great way to assess the efficacy of a variety of interventions. The form can also be used to evaluate the relationships between impairments, functional limitations, and disabilities.

Students in the clinic present another opportunity to use *The Guide*. Many students have been taught using *Guide* terminology and the Nagi and patient/client management models.

Students can have an effect on practicing clinician acceptance of and utilization of *The Guide*. Students could develop a case study or in-service presentation using the patterns. Students can also use the patterns to work through complicated or unfamiliar patient management.

The Guide to Physical Therapist Practice and the practice patterns contained within are excellent tools for teaching in an academic setting. Use of *The Guide* occurs in various courses and applications within physical therapist professional education curricula, in a wide variety of institutions. Besides using Part 1 of *The Guide* to explain the scope of physical therapist practice and the roles of the physical therapist, it provides a framework for patient/client management and describes tests, measures, and interventions. Part 2 can be used as a framework for discussions of patient problems, intervention choices, diagnosis, and prognosis. For instance, patients with rotator cuff tendinitis, bicipital tendinitis, and lateral epicondylitis can all be discussed as part of Pattern 4E: "Impaired joint mobility, motor function, muscle performance, and range of motion associated with localized inflammation." Commonality of examination and intervention procedures can be addressed; additionally, discussion of factors that would relate reasons for a new episode of care or that may modify frequency of visits or duration and episode of care related to a particular body segment may be of instructional value. Finally, the framework of the disablement model is an ideal format for outlining the management of patients and understanding the role of the physical therapist in prevention and wellness.

Case studies can be presented in class identifying the correct classification into practice patterns and using facets of the practice patterns. Written case reports that reflect the language of *The Guide* and it's framework for decision making are becoming commonplace in professional publications.

The impact of *The Guide to Physical Therapist Practice* on the profession of physical therapy is evident. Utilization of *The Guide* will facilitate dialogue and improved understanding of how clinicians classify patients, develop clinical diagnoses, and determine prognoses for common groups of patients and clients. This document will be a part of the professional landscape for many years to come and will continue to influence both the practice of and public understanding of physical therapy in positive ways.

SUMMARY

- *The Guide to Physical Therapist Practice* was published to describe the practice of physical therapy.
- Subsequent revisions have made updates, improvements, and changes in the content of *The Guide*.
- *The Guide* is not a cookbook for provision care, but rather a document to improve the quality of physical therapy services.
- The guide is broken into two components: Part 1 gives a detailed outline as to what the practice of physical therapy

entails. Part 2 describes the preferred practice patterns, i.e., musculoskeletal, neuromuscular, cardiopulmonary, and integumentary.

- The preferred practice patterns are structured with diagnostic labels that are based upon impairments.
- Clinicians should use *The Guide.* Use *The Guide* in different ways and gather data by using it.
- Once you have become familiar with *The Guide,* give feedback to APTA on your use of *The Guide.*

REFERENCES

1. American Physical Therapy Association. The guide to physical therapist practice. *Phys Ther* 77:1163–1650, 1997.

2. American Physical Therapy Association. The guide to physical therapist practice, 2nd ed. *Phys Ther* 81(1):9–738, 2001.

3. American Physical Therapy Association. *The Interactive Guide to Physical Therapist Practice, With Catalog of Tests and Measures.* Version 1.1. Alexandria, VA, American Physical Therapy Association, Released 2003.

4. Jette A. Physical disablement concepts for physical therapy research and practice. *Phys Ther* 74:375–382, 1994.

5. Nagi SZ. *Disability and Rehabilitation.* Columbus, OH, Ohio State University Press, 1969.

6. Pope A, Tarlov A. *Disability in America.* Washington, DC, National Academy Press, 1991.

7. Rothstein JM. On the second edition of the guide. *Phys Ther* 81(1):6–8, 2001.

CHAPTER 2

The Patient/Client Management Model and Clinical Decision Making in Rehabilitation

Barbara J. Hoogenboom

OBJECTIVES

After completing this chapter, the therapist should be able to do the following:

- Understand and discuss the overall process for clinical decision making in rehabilitation.
- Describe the five components of the clinical decision-making model used by *The Guide to Physical Therapist Practice.*
- Describe the sequence of steps in the clinical decision-making process related to evaluation, diagnosis, prognosis and intervention.
- Discuss how the evaluation in the clinical decision-making process leads to determination of the diagnosis.
- Describe the importance of determining the patient prognosis, using clinical decision making.
- Describe the three main types of intervention and the clinical decision making that allows for choices to be made among them.
- Define the components of effective documentation in order to ensure the reproducibility and consistency of patient care.

Good clinical decision making is key to effective patient management. Physical therapists play a critical role in assessing neuromusculoskeletal problems, formulating a comprehensive picture of the problem, and choosing interventions to manage the problem. As more patients enter the medical system through the general practitioner, the patient is often referred to physical therapy without a clear diagnosis, especially those patients with musculoskeletal complaints. Physical therapists are educated in both the technical skills to choose and carry out the examination and intervention procedures and the analytical skills to make the appropriate diagnosis and prognosis.

The physical therapy profession continues to move toward more autonomous practice. The majority of "practice acts" in the United States allow for practice by the physical therapist without referral from a physician. Concurrently, the professional educational level of the physical therapist is changing to the Doctorate in Physical Therapy (DPT) degree. The greater the practitioner autonomy, the more critical effective and efficient clinical decision making becomes. The following case is an example of this need.

Your patient is a 35-year-old female runner who comes to you complaining of mid-back pain for 6 months. The pain disrupts her running in the early morning but not when she runs in the early evening. She tells you she bought a new mattress a month ago, convinced that her old one was "too soft and worn out." No change in symptoms occurred. Ice and heat have not worked either. She called her family physician and asked for a referral to physical therapy. She has not had a physical examination for almost a year and is scheduled for one next month.

Several key issues pertain to this case. The first is that she has had no physician-based medical screening. Second, the symptoms are not consistent with her running, despite the fact that she relates them to this activity. Third, she has tried to manage the pain with simple modalities as well as a change in mattress and nothing has worked. Given these three issues, it is critical that the examination will lead to a valid diagnosis.

While questioning the patient concerning the current condition, she stated that she had not tried anti-inflammatory drugs because they upset her stomach. Further questioning regarding past medical history revealed previous diagnoses of stomach ulcers and acid reflux. The patient stated that she had been off her gastric medication for almost a year. Given this information, the questioning focused on the differential diagnosis of a potential systemic problem (gastric in nature, that will refer pain to the mid back) versus a musculoskeletal issue in the thoracic spine and ribcage.

The patient indicated that she ran in the early morning before eating. In the evening, she would often run a couple of hours after having eaten. She stated that her stress level at work was considerable over the last 6 months and she used running as a way to cope with that. Upon physical examination, the spine range of motion was normal, the ribcage movement was equal and smooth bilaterally, and trunk muscle strength was normal. Her symptoms were nonreplicable, even after running for 15 minutes on the treadmill. She was sent back to the physician with the physical therapy examination findings and diagnosis, which presented the possibility of visceral problems (and lack of musculoskeletal ones) that required physician workup. The physician examined the patient and returned information that an endoscopy revealed a return of her stomach ulcer. Medication was used to manage the condition, and her symptoms promptly disappeared.

Effective and efficient decision making requires approaching a patient problem in a systematic and orderly fashion. Using a standard patient/client management process with all types of patients facilitates valuable learning so that each case decision allows the clinician to add to his or her experiential knowledge base. It also helps make the results of the examination reliable (can be reproduced) and valid (generalizable and examines what is purported to be examined).

Good clinical decision making requires foundation knowledge applied to each patient. The use of anatomic and kinesiologic information is critical to assessing normal and abnormal movement. Understanding both the pathologic and healing processes helps the therapist determine the diagnosis, prognosis, and plan of care.

Theory and base knowledge must be combined with evidence from the research literature for effective and efficient use of resources and achieving optimal outcomes. Sacket et al., in *Evidence Based Medicine*, suggest that evidence-based medicine is a combination of the best research evidence available from basic, applied, and clinical research; the clinical expertise of the practitioner, including skills, knowledge, and experience; and the patient's values, including concerns and expectations.[5] It is each and every clinician's responsibility to stay current with the literature, especially as it relates to their patient populations.

PATIENT/CLIENT MANAGEMENT MODEL

The disablement model is at the core of each clinical decision. As discussed in Chapter 1, the model is a two-way continuum that focuses on the functional outcome of the patient.

Pathology ↔ Impairment ↔
Functional limitation ↔ Disability

Likewise, the disablement model is at the core of the patient/client management model used by *The Guide to Physical Therapist Practice*.[1,2] The patient/client management model described by *The Guide* is very different from the medical model of patient management. The medical model involves performing a history and physical examination, often in combination with invasive tests and measures. This allows the physician to make a diagnosis at the cellular or system level (diagnosis of disease) that generally requires management by pharmacologic agents and/or surgery. The outcomes of medical management are tissue repair and/or "cure" of a condition or disease. Physical therapists rarely use invasive tests and measures and are legally not permitted to do surgery or dispense drugs. Traditionally, physical therapists do not intervene at this level. However, exceptions exist in the musculoskeletal practice area such as the management of simple strains and sprains; inflammatory processes of the muscle, tendon, bursa, capsule, and fascia, and capsular restriction. The tests and measures needed to diagnose and treat these problems are well within the scope of physical therapy practice.

In 1988, Sahrmann used the term "movement dysfunction" in relationship to diagnosis by the physical therapist.[6] Using the terminology of the disablement model, movement dysfunction can be classified as impairment (e.g., muscle weakness) or functional limitation (e.g., balance dysfunction).[1,2] The patient/client management model used in *The Guide* involves a history and physical examination (similar to the medical equivalent) performed with *non*invasive tests and measures, which results in a movement diagnosis which then guides the selection of interventions for managing impairments, functional limitations, and disabilities. The classification of abnormalities involves a movement-related diagnosis of impairment, or the classification or diagnosis of functional limitation. Such diagnoses relate directly to the functional management of the patient, in contrast to medical diagnoses that relate to the management of illness or disease.

The patient/client management model, as illustrated in Figure 1-3, is the clinical decision-making model used in *The Guide to Physical Therapist Practice*.[1,2] The model has five components: examination, evaluation, diagnosis, prognosis, and intervention. The end result of this model is effective outcomes, patient satisfaction, and prevention of future impairments, functional limitations, and disability.

Examination is the first step of the process. It has three parts: the history, systems review, and tests and measures. The examination should be thorough and use all sources, including the patient, family, medical record, and other health care professionals. The history is an account of past and current health status. It is used to identify health risk factors, health needs, and coexisting health problems. An initial diagnosis is also determined based on the information gleaned from the history.

TABLE 2-1

Data Generated from a Patient History

- General demographics
- Social history and social habits
- Occupation/employment
- Growth and development
- Living environment
- History of current condition
- Functional status and activity level
- Medications
- Other tests and measures
- History of current condition
- Medical/surgical history
- Family history
- Health status

The systems review and tests and measures are then used to rule in or out the initial diagnosis. Table 2-1 is the complete list of history categories from *Guide to Physical Therapist Practice*.[1,2]

A systems review is a brief, limited examination designed to gain information concerning the general health of the patient and which systems may need to be managed with the patient. This is a general screening that should be done as a part of every patient's routine examination. It increases the emphasis on managing the whole person. For an autonomous practitioner, this is the key to good patient care. There are five categories: musculoskeletal, neuromuscular, cardiopulmonary, integumentary, and communication. Table 2-2 outlines the specific tests under each category. A more detailed scanning examination for both the upper and lower quarters will be discussed further in Chapter 4.

The systems review portion of the examination is an exercise in clinical decision making which assists in formulating a preliminary diagnosis and prognosis. Hence, the first question that must be addressed by any physical therapist is whether the patient has a diagnosis that is *appropriate* for physical therapy intervention.

The final section of the examination is used to confirm or deny the preliminary diagnosis, redirect the thought process as

TABLE 2-2

The Systems Review

- Musculoskeletal: Gross range of motion, functional strength, and symmetry
- Neuromuscular: General movement patterns
- Cardiopulmonary: Heart rate, blood pressure, respiratory rate, edema
- Integumentary: Skin integrity, color, scar, temperature, height, weight
- Communication/learning ability: Ability to make known, consciousness, orientation, expected emotional/behavioral responses, learning preferences

TABLE 2-3

Tests and Measures

- Aerobic capacity and endurance
- Anthropometric characteristics
- Arousal, attention, and cognition
- Assistive and adaptive devices
- Circulation (arterial, venous, lymphatic)
- Cranial and peripheral nerve integrity
- Environmental, home, work (job/school/play) barriers
- Ergonomics and body mechanics
- Gait, locomotion, and balance
- Integumentary integrity
- Joint integrity and mobility
- Motor function (motor control and learning)
- Muscle performance (strength/power/endurance)
- Neuromotor development/sensory integration
- Orthotic, protective, and supportive devices
- Pain
- Posture
- Prosthetic requirements
- Range of motion (including muscle length)
- Reflex integrity
- Self-care and home management (activities of daily living [ADL]/instrumental activities of daily living [IADL])
- Sensory integrity (including proprioception and kinesthesia)
- Ventilation and respiration
- Work (job/school/play), community, and leisure integration or reintegration

necessary, and move toward a movement-based diagnosis. There are 24 tests and measures listed alphabetically in *Guide to Physical Therapist Practice* (Table 2-3).[1,2] Each test is not performed during an examination, and nor are they appropriate for every patient. The appropriate test and/or measure is chosen based on the results of the history and systems review. For example, the patient is a 21-year-old male college student who comes into the clinic with the complaint of a painful ankle. If he indicates a particular traumatic incident during the history, you would assume that he has a sprained ankle and do anthropometric measurements to assess swelling, joint integrity tests to assess ligamentous integrity, range-of-motion measurement, and gait assessment. If the results of these tests and measures are positive, then a sprained ankle is a reasonable diagnosis. However, if the patient has had no trauma and cannot indicate any activity that would have triggered pain and caused him to seek medical attention, then other diagnoses must be considered. For instance, a history of multiple joint pain and inflammation, and/or a history of recent urinary tract infections and conjunctivitis, may indicate a systemic condition such as Reiter's syndrome or another rheumatic disease. In that case, anthropometric measures, integumentary integrity, joint integrity, range of motion, and gait will all be important to consider before referring back to a physician. A history of an old ankle injury may point toward muscular, ligamentous, structural, or postural issues that must be carefully examined.

The critical thinking and decision making that follows the examination process is known as the evaluation. It is the most important part of the process, because it leads directly to determination of the final diagnosis. Using all the data—including clinical findings, loss of function, social considerations, chronicity of the problem, and patient's overall health status—the clinician formulates an impression. In the case of the 21-year-old college student, the history of an injury followed by the positive ankle swelling, positive anterior drawer test, decreased range of motion, and antalgic gait all would lead the therapist to believe that this patient had sprained his anterior talofibular ligament.

A diagnosis is a label based on a cluster of signs and symptoms. The diagnosis is determined after the collection, organization, and interpretation of information reached through the evaluation process. For the physical therapist, diagnoses are generally movement-related impairments or functional limitations. Sometimes, as in the case of the patient with the ankle sprain, the diagnosis is at the pathology level.

Diagnosis by the physical therapist is the key to good intervention planning. The medical diagnosis is often not useful. For instance, your patient is a 32-year-old female with a referral that states "chondromalacia patella—evaluate and treat." For physical therapists, treatment of a patient with this diagnosis does not mean treating the actual softening of the cartilage, the pathology of chondromalacia patella. Rather, the therapist must explore multiple possible movement dysfunctions that may be causing the chondromalacia patella. Once the key impairment(s) are discovered, the treatment approach will become apparent. Not all patients with chondromalacia patella are treated similarly. If the key impairment is muscle weakness of the quadriceps, then the program emphasizes muscle performance. If the patella is not tracking properly because of structural issues, then patella taping may be in order. The mechanics at the foot should be explored, because excessive subtalar and midtarsal joint pronation during gait can increase the torsional forces on the patella femoral joint, causing pain. Treatment in such a case would be proper footwear and orthoses as needed. Each of these scenarios depicts patients who may have an appropriate medical diagnosis of chondromalacia patella, but all require a more specific movement-related diagnosis to determine the appropriate plan of care.

Prognosis—the predicted optimal level of functional improvement within a time frame—will also help determine intervention strategies. Predicting the level of improvement that may be expected for a patient guides choices regarding the intensity, duration, and style of intervention. The combination of diagnosis and prognosis is used to justify physical therapy management. The prognosis for the patient with an ankle sprain will depend on such things as the degree of sprain and the number of previous ankle sprains.

Intervention is the purposeful and skilled interaction between either the physical therapist or ancillary staff and the

T A B L E   2 - 4

Key Questions for Interventions

- What is the stage of healing: acute, subacute, chronic?
- How long do you have to treat the patient?
- What activities does the patient need to accomplish for function?
- How compliant is the patient?
- How much *skilled* physical therapy is needed?
- What are the issues need to be addressed to prevent recurrence?
- Are there any referrals needed?
- What has worked for other patients with similar problems?
- Are there any precautions?
- What is the skill level of the therapist?

patient, based heavily on the patient's functional needs. Clinical decisions are contingent upon the timely monitoring of the patient's response and progression toward mutually agreed-upon goals. There are a number of issues that guide the type, duration, and intensity of treatment. Table 2-4 outlines key questions that may assist in these decisions. If a patient has a chronic case of subacromial bursitis, it will probably take longer to treat than if the patient presented to physical therapy while in the acute stage, although the latter patient may not tolerate initial aggressive treatment. The patient's activity level should always play a major role in the types of exercises as well as the intensity of treatment. If the patient with chronic subacromial bursitis wants to return to golfing weekly, then exercises mimicking the golf swing and even using the golf clubs are a critical component of the plan of care.

There are three main types of intervention: (1) coordination, communication, and documentation; (2) patient/client-related instruction; and (3) procedural interventions. The first two types are a part of care provided for all patients. Procedural interventions include things such as manual therapy techniques, therapeutic exercise, functional training, and modalities. Table 2-5 lists the procedural interventions as listed in *The Guide* in order of their utilization frequency.[1,2] Choosing procedural interventions is the heart of clinical decision making. The physical therapist is educated in order to treat patients and clients with physiologic, anatomic, and functional impairments. Physical therapy interventions attempt to improve or optimize the functional status of the patient or client. Physical therapists choose and utilize treatment interventions in order to restore function, diminish disability, prevent further sequelae, and promote wellness. The physical therapist chooses, applies, or modifies procedural interventions based upon goals and expected outcomes that have been determined with input from the patient/client. It is important that therapists include patients in goal setting in order to encourage active participation by the patients throughout the rehabilitation process. Some evidence suggests that in many cases therapists do not fully take advantage

TABLE 2-5

Procedural Interventions

- Therapeutic exercise (including aerobic conditioning)
- Functional training in self-care and home management (ADL and IADL)
- Functional training in community and work integration/reintegration (IADL)
- Manual therapy
- Prescription, application, and fabrication of devices and equipment
- Airway clearance techniques
- Integumentary repair and protective techniques
- Electrotherapeutic modalities
- Physical agents and mechanical modalities

of the potential for patient participation in the goal-setting process.[3] The goals and outcomes identified for intervention must be related to specific impairments, functional limitations, or disabilities; may relate to risk reduction, health, wellness, or fitness needs; and must also be measurable and time specific.

Clinical decision making involves not only what interventions to choose but also determining which impairment is most closely related to a functional limitation or disability. Choosing the "correct" impairment for a functional deficit and beginning by treating that impairment is vital for effective, efficient treatment. The therapist may decide to intervene at the functional limitation level, thereby treating an impairment as a part of a functional limitation. For example, a patient with altered gait due to lower extremity weakness can be treated by practicing gait (functional level intervention) or by performing lower extremity strengthening activities (impairment level intervention). Clinical reasoning regarding which procedural interventions to use for intervention is discussed further in Chapter 5 in an algorithmic approach.

The reexamination is performing selected tests and measures to evaluate the patient's progress. It is also used to modify or redirect intervention and may require a change in diagnosis and/or prognosis.

Outcomes relate to the following: functional limitation/disability, patient/client satisfaction, and secondary prevention. Remediation of impairments is important, but the overriding purpose of physical therapy management is *function*. If the patient recovering from adhesive capsulitis cannot return to playing golf, despite an increase in range of motion and joint play, then the outcome (even with an improvement in impairments) may not be considered positive.

DOCUMENTATION

Good documentation is a critical component to the decision-making process. Documentation allows for management of the patient's case and communication with other health care profes-

sionals. Effective note writing also improves the reproducibility and consistency of care, allowing for quality assurance in the clinical setting and providing data for clinical research. Of course, third-party payers demand complete notes for service justification; reimbursement depends upon proper documentation.

Many types of written documentation exist, each with their own structure, function, and focus. As documentation requirements change, so do documentation styles. SOAP notes are one common form of written communication used by many disciplines in a wide variety of medical and health professions. There are four aspects of the SOAP note: *s*ubjective, *o*bjective, *a*ssessment, and *p*lan. Although the terminology differs slightly from the aspects of the patient/client management model used by *The Guide*, SOAP notes still are useful within this framework.

Subjective—The subjective portion of the note provides the reader with information about the patient, including history of present illness, pain behavior, past and current medical history, medications, prior and current function and lifestyle, home life, the patient's goals, and the communication section of the systems review.

Objective—The objective section is where the results of the tests and measures are recorded, including the systems review, observation, and any of the previously described tests and measures, such as range of motion, muscle performance, and aerobic capacity. Information recorded in the "O" section of the note should be recorded in measures and terms that are as objective and reproducible as possible. Any treatment that is performed during the session should be documented in the objective section as well.

Assessment—The assessment statement includes the problem list, short-term goals (anticipated goals), long-term goals (functional outcomes), diagnosis, and prognosis. In the patient/client management model, the term assessment is equivalent to the evaluation, diagnosis, and prognosis. The assessment portion of a note should include an evaluative or summary statement that flows logically from the diagnosis, the factors affecting the diagnosis, and the prognosis (Fig. 2-1).

Plan—The plan section includes coordination and communication of services and referrals that are needed, patient education, a plan for procedural interventions, and outcomes (functional limitations and disabilities, patient satisfaction, and secondary prevention). Discharge planning is also included in this section.

As suggested previously, the SOAP note terminology is easily coordinated with the terminology from *Guide to Physical Therapist Practice*. In the language of *The Guide*, assessment is the same as evaluation and plan is the same as intervention and short-term goals are the same as anticipated goals and long-term goals are the same as outcomes.

This chapter has provided an introduction to the clinical decision-making model using the patient/client management

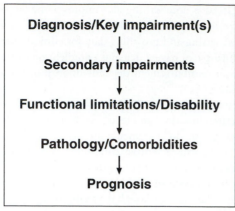

F I G U R E   2 - 1

Evaluative statement for assessment.

model. Clinical decision making will be further discussed in Chapter 4 that covers the scanning examination, and clinical reasoning will be discussed in greater detail in Chapter 5 on algorithms.

SUMMARY

- As physical therapists become autonomous practitioners, it is essential that clinical decision-making skills will be enhanced. Effective decision making requires approaching the problem in a systematic and orderly fashion.
- The patient management model is the clinical decision-making model used in *The Guide to Physical Therapist Practice*. The model has five components: examination, evaluation, diagnosis, prognosis, and intervention.
- The first step in the clinical decision-making process is performing a thorough examination. The examination has three steps: the history, system review, and tests and measures.

- The next step in the clinical decision-making process, the evaluation, is the most important step because it leads directly to determination of the diagnosis.
- A diagnosis is a label based on a cluster of signs and symptoms after the collection of all the relevant data.
- Intervention is the purposeful and skilled interaction based upon the patient's functional needs. There are three main components to intervention: coordination, communication, and documentation; patient/client-related instruction; and procedural interventions.
- A consistent pattern of decision making requires foundation knowledge applied to each patient. The use of anatomic and kinesiologic information is critical to assessing normal and abnormal movement. Understanding both the pathologic and healing process will help to determine the diagnosis, prognosis, and plan of care.
- Successful decision making requires good documentation in order to communicate with other health care professionals and improve the reproducibility and consistency of care.

REFERENCES

1. American Physical Therapy Association. The guide to physical therapist practice. *Phys Ther* 77:1163–1650, 1997.
2. American Physical Therapy Association. The guide to physical therapist practice, 2nd ed. *Phys Ther* 81(1):9–738, 2001.
3. Baker SM, Marshak HH, Rice GT, Zimmerman GJ. Patient participation in physical therapy goal setting. *Phys Ther* 81(5):1118–1126, 2001.
4. Jette AM. Physical disablement concepts for physical therapy research and practice. *Phys Ther* 74:380–386, 1994.
5. Sacket D, Haynes RB, Richardson WS, Strauss SE, Rosenberg W. *Evidence Based Medicine*, 2nd ed. London, Churchill Livingstone, 2000.
6. Sahrmann SA. Diagnosis by the physical therapist. *Phys Ther* 68:1703–1706, 1988.

CHAPTER 3

Understanding and Managing the Healing Process through Rehabilitation

William E. Prentice

OBJECTIVES

After completing this chapter, the therapist should be able to do the following:

- Describe the pathophysiology of the healing process.
- Identify the factors that can impede the healing process.
- Distinguish the four types of tissues in the human body.
- Discuss the etiology and pathology of various musculoskeletal injuries associated with various types of tissues.
- Compare healing processes relative to specific musculoskeletal structures.
- Explain the importance of initial first aid and injury management of these injuries and their impact on the rehabilitation process.
- Discuss the use of various analgesics, anti-inflammatories, and antipyretics in facilitating the healing process during a rehabilitation program.

Injury rehabilitation requires sound knowledge and understanding of the etiology and pathology involved in various musculoskeletal injuries that may occur.[24,84,93] When injury occurs, the therapist is charged with designing, implementing, and supervising the rehabilitation program. Rehabilitation protocols and progressions must be based primarily on the physiologic responses of the tissues to injury and on an understanding of how various tissues heal.[39,46] Thus the therapist must understand the healing process to effectively supervise the rehabilitative process. This chapter discusses the healing process relative to the various musculoskeletal injuries that may be encountered by a therapist.

UNDERSTANDING THE HEALING PROCESS

Rehabilitation programs must be based on the cycle of the healing process (Fig. 3-1). The therapist must have a sound understanding of the sequence of the various phases of the healing process. The physiological responses of the tissues to trauma follow a predictable sequence and time frame.[41] Decisions on how and when to alter and progress a rehabilitation program should be primarily based on recognition of signs and symptoms, as well as on an awareness of the time frames associated with the various phases of healing.[57,72]

The healing process consists of the inflammatory-response phase, the fibroblastic-repair phase, and the maturation-remodeling phase. It must be stressed that although the phases of healing are presented as three separate entities, the healing process is a continuum. Phases of the healing process overlap one another and have no definitive beginning or end points.[73]

Primary Injury

Primary injuries are almost always described as being either chronic or acute in nature, resulting from *macrotraumatic* or *microtraumatic* forces. Injuries classified as macrotraumatic occur as a result of acute trauma and produce immediate pain and disability.

Macrotraumatic injuries include fractures, dislocations, subluxations, sprains, strains, and contusions. Microtraumatic injuries are most often called overuse injuries and result from repetitive overloading or incorrect mechanics associated with reported motion.[59] Microtraumatic injuries include tendinitis, tenosynovitis, bursitis, etc. A *secondary injury* is essentially the

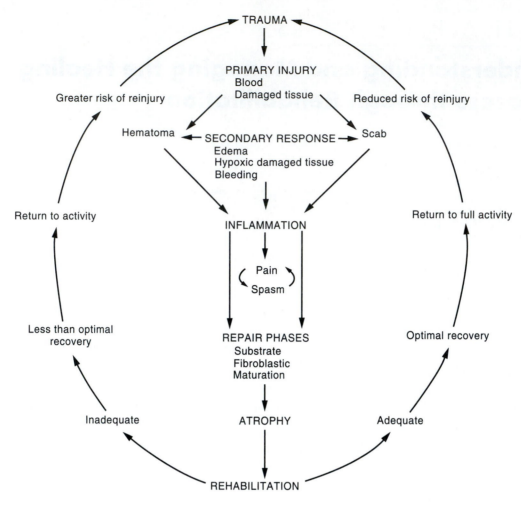

FIGURE 3-1

A cycle of injury. (Reproduced, with permission, from Booher JM, Thibadeau GA. *Athletic Injury Assessment*, 2nd ed. St. Louis, MO, Mosby, 1994.)

inflammatory or hypoxia response that occurs with the primary injury.

Inflammatory-Response Phase

Once a tissue is injured, the process of healing begins immediately[16] (Fig. 3-2A). The destruction of tissue produces direct injury to the cells of the various soft tissues.[35] Cellular injury results in altered metabolism and the liberation of materials that initiate the inflammatory response. It is characterized symptomatically by redness, swelling, tenderness, and increased temperature.[18,54] *This initial inflammatory response is critical to the entire healing process. If this response does not accomplish what it is supposed to or if it does not subside, normal healing cannot take place.*

Inflammation is a process through which *leukocytes* and other *phagocytic cells* and exudates are delivered to the injured tissue. This cellular reaction is generally protective, tending to localize or dispose of injury by-products (e.g., blood and damaged cells) through phagocytosis and thus setting the stage for

repair. Local vascular effects, disturbances of fluid exchange, and migration of leukocytes from the blood to the tissues occur.

VASCULAR REACTION

The vascular reaction involves vascular spasm, formation of a platelet plug, blood coagulation, and growth of fibrous tissue.[77] The immediate response to tissue damage is a vasoconstriction of the vascular walls that lasts for approximately 5–10 minutes. This spasm presses the opposing endothelial linings together to produce a local anemia that is rapidly replaced by hyperemia of the area due to dilation. This increase in blood flow is transitory and gives way to a slowing of the flow in the dilated vessels, which then progresses to stagnation and stasis. The initial effusion of blood and plasma lasts for 24–36 hours.

CHEMICAL MEDIATORS

Three chemical mediators, histamine, leukotaxin, and necrosin, are important in limiting the amount of exudates and thus swelling after injury. Histamine released from the injured mast

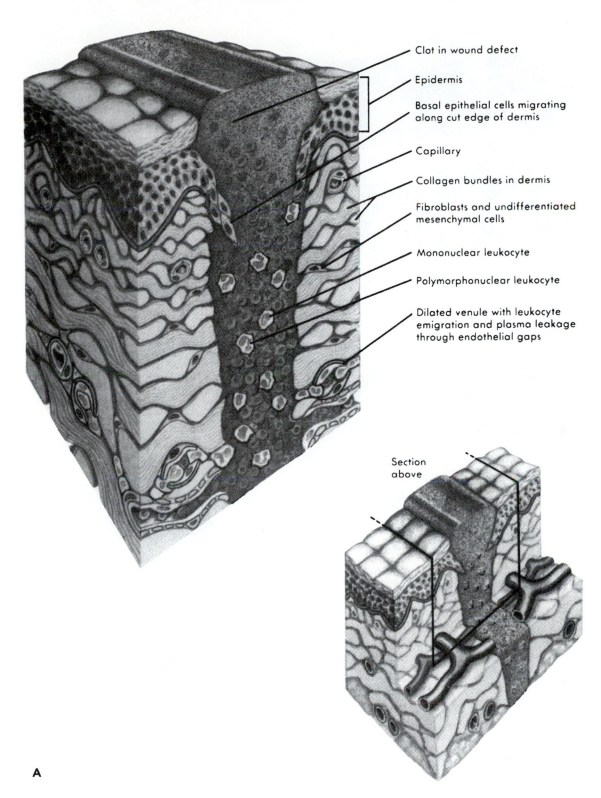

Clot in wound defect

Epidermis

Basal epithelial cells migrating along cut edge of dermis

Capillary

Collagen bundles in dermis

Fibroblasts and undifferentiated mesenchymal cells

Mononuclear leukocyte

Polymorphonuclear leukocyte

Dilated venule with leukocyte emigration and plasma leakage through endothelial gaps

Section above

A

F I G U R E 3 - 2

The healing process. **A,** Inflammatory-response phase; **B,** Fibroblastic-repair phase; **C,** Maturation-remodeling phase. (*Continued*)

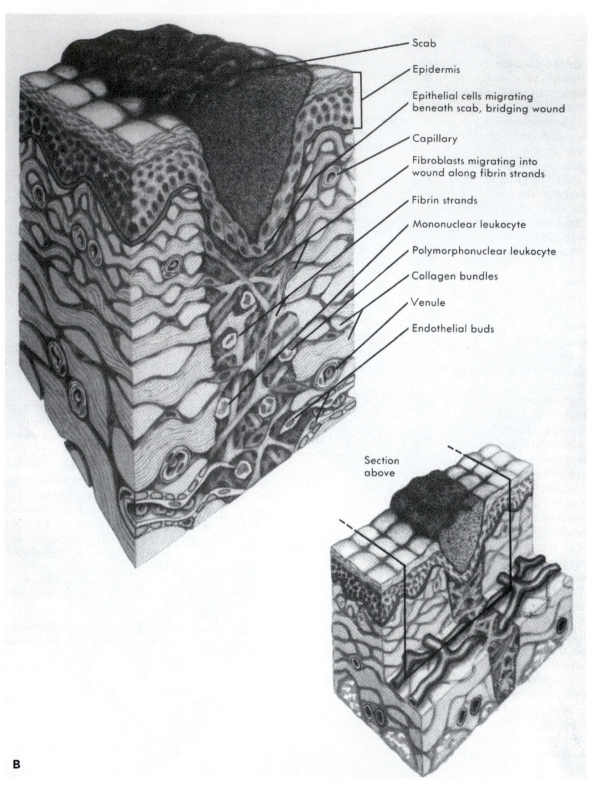

Scab

Epidermis

Epithelial cells migrating beneath scab, bridging wound

Capillary

Fibroblasts migrating into wound along fibrin strands

Fibrin strands

Mononuclear leukocyte

Polymorphonuclear leukocyte

Collagen bundles

Venule

Endothelial buds

Section above

B

F I G U R E   3 - 2

(Continued)

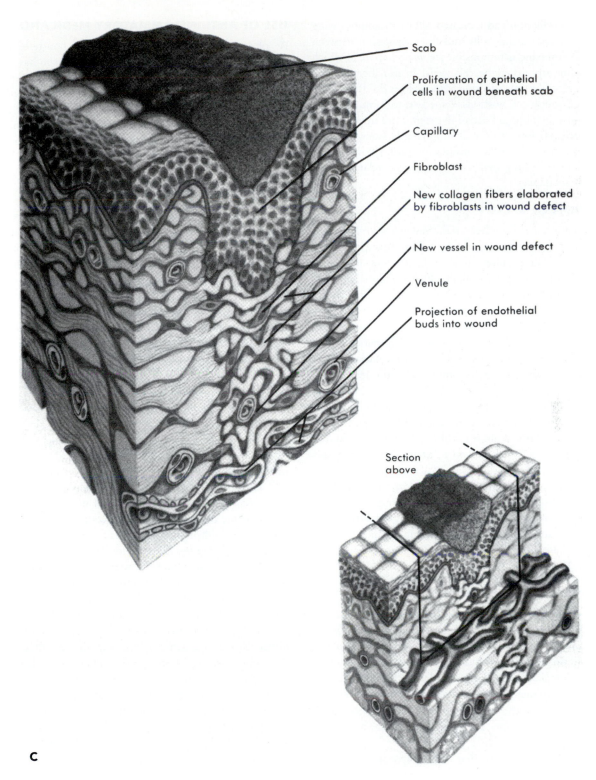

Scab

Proliferation of epithelial cells in wound beneath scab

Capillary

Fibroblast

New collagen fibers elaborated by fibroblasts in wound defect

New vessel in wound defect

Venule

Projection of endothelial buds into wound

Section above

C

FIGURE 3-2

(Continued)

cells causes vasodilation and increased cell permeability, owing to swelling of endothelial cells and then separation between the cells. Leukotaxine is responsible for *margination*, in which leukocytes line up along the cell walls. It also increases cell permeability locally, thus affecting passage of the fluid and white blood cells through cell walls via diapedesis to form exudates. Therefore vasodilation and active hyperemia are important in exudates (plasma) formation and supplying leukocytes to the injured area. Necrosin is responsible for phagocytic activity. The amount of swelling that occurs is directly related to the extent of vessel damage.

FORMATION OF A CLOT

Platelets do not normally adhere to the vascular wall. However, injury to a vessel disrupts the endothelium and exposes the collagen fibers. Platelets adhere to the collagen fibers to create a sticky matrix on the vascular wall, to which additional platelets and leukocytes adhere and eventually form a plug. These plugs obstruct local lymphatic fluid drainage and thus localize the injury response.

The initial event that precipitates clot formation is the conversion of *fibrinogen* to *fibrin*. This transformation occurs because of a cascading effect, beginning with the release of a protein molecule called *thromboplastin* from the damaged cell. Thromboplastin causes *prothrombin* to be changed into *thrombin*, which in turn causes the conversion of fibrinogen into a very sticky fibrin clot that shuts off blood supply to the injured area. Clot formation begins around 12 hours after injury and is completed within 48 hours.

As a result of a combination of these factors, the injured area becomes walled off during the inflammatory stage of healing. The leukocytes phagocytize most of the foreign debris toward the end of the inflammatory phase, setting the stage for the fibroblastic phase. This initial inflammatory response lasts for approximately 2–4 days after initial injury.

CHRONIC INFLAMMATION

A distinction must be made between the acute inflammatory response, as described above, and chronic inflammation. *Chronic inflammation* occurs when the acute inflammatory response does not eliminate the injuring agent and restores tissue to its normal physiological state. Chronic inflammation involves the replacement of leukocytes with *macrophages*, lymphocytes, and *plasma cells*. These cells accumulate in a highly vascularized and innervated loose connective tissue matrix in the area of the injury.[53]

The specific mechanisms that convert an acute inflammatory response to a chronic inflammatory response are to date unknown; however, they seem to be associated with situations that involve overuse or overload with cumulative microtrauma to a particular structure.[28,53] Likewise, there is no specific time frame in which a classification of acute inflammation is changed to chronic inflammation.

It does appear that chronic inflammation is resistant to both physical and pharmacological treatments.[44]

USE OF ANTI-INFLAMMATORY MEDICATIONS

A physician will routinely prescribe nonsteroidal anti-inflammatory drugs (NSAID) for a patient who has sustained an injury.[2] These medications are certainly effective in minimizing pain and swelling associated with inflammation and can enhance return to normal activity. However, there are some concerns that the use of NSAID acutely following injury might actually interfere with inflammation, thus delaying the healing process.

Fibroblastic-Repair Phase

During the fibroblastic phase of healing, proliferative and regenerative activity leading to scar formation and repair of the injured tissue follows the vascular and exudative phenomena of inflammation[41] (Fig. 3-2B). The period of scar formation referred to as *fibroplasia* begins within the first few hours after injury and can last as long as 4–6 weeks. During this period, many of the signs and symptoms associated with the inflammatory response subside. The patient might still indicate some tenderness to touch and will usually complain of pain when particular movements stress the injured structure. As scar formation progresses, complaints of tenderness or pain gradually disappear.[39]

During this phase, growth of endothelial capillary buds into the wound is stimulated by a lack of oxygen, after which the wound is capable of healing aerobically.[18] Along with increased oxygen delivery comes an increase in blood flow, which delivers nutrients essential for tissue regeneration in the area.[18]

The formation of a delicate connective tissue called *granulation tissue* occurs with the breakdown of the fibrin clot. Granulation tissue consists of *fibroblasts*, collagen, and capillaries. It appears as a reddish granular mass of connective tissue that fills in the gaps during the healing process.

As the capillaries continue to grow into the area, fibroblasts accumulate at the wound site, arranging themselves parallel to the capillaries. Fibroblastic cells begin to synthesize an extracellular matrix that contains protein fibers of *collagen* and *elastin*, a ground substance that consists of nonfibrous proteins called proteoglycans, glycosaminoglycans, and fluid. On about day 6 or 7, fibroblasts also begin producing collagen fibers that are deposited in a random fashion throughout the forming scar. As the collagen continues to proliferate, the tensile strength of the wound rapidly increases in proportion to the rate of collagen synthesis. As the tensile strength increases, the number of fibroblasts diminishes, signaling the beginning of the maturation phase.

This normal sequence of events in the repair phase leads to the formation of minimal scar tissue. Occasionally, a persistent inflammatory response and continued release of inflammatory products can promote extended fibroplasia and excessive fibrogenesis, which can lead to irreversible tissue damage.[97] Fibrosis can occur in synovial structures, as with adhesive capsulitis in the shoulder, in extra-articular tissues including tendons and ligaments, in bursa, or in muscle.

Maturation-Remodeling Phase

The maturation-remodeling phase of healing is a long-term process (Fig. 3-2C). This phase features a realignment or remodeling of the collagen fibers that make up scar tissue according to the tensile forces to which that scar is subjected. Ongoing breakdown and synthesis of collagen occur with a steady increase in the tensile strength of the scar matrix. With increased stress and strain, the collagen fibers realign in a position of maximum efficiency parallel to the lines of tension. The tissue gradually assumes normal appearance and function, although a scar is rarely as strong as the normal injured tissue. Usually by the end of approximately 3 weeks, a firm, strong, contracted, nonvascular scar exists. The maturation phase of healing might require several years to be to tally complete.

Role of Progressive Controlled Mobility during the Healing Process

Wolff's law states that bone and soft tissue will respond to the physical demands placed on them, causing them to remodel or realign along lines of tensile force.[101] Therefore it is critical that injured structures be exposed to progressively increasing loads throughout the rehabilitative process.[73]

In animal models, controlled mobilization is superior to immobilization for scar formation, revascularization, muscle regeneration, and reorientation of muscle fibers and tensile properties.[71] However, a brief period of immobilization of the injured tissue during the inflammatory-response phase is recommended and will likely facilitate the process of healing by controlling inflammation, thus reducing clinical symptoms. As healing progresses to the repair phase, controlled activity directed toward return to normal flexibility and strength should be combined with protective support or bracing.[50] Generally, clinical sings and symptoms disappear at the end of this phase.

As the remodeling phase begins, aggressive active range-of-motion and strengthening exercises should be incorporated to facilitate tissue remodeling and realignment. To a great extent, pain will dictate rate of progression. With initial injury, pain is intense; it tends to decrease and eventually subside altogether as healing progresses. Any exacerbation of pain, swelling or other clinical symptoms during or after a particular exercise or activity indicate that the load is too great for the level of tissue repair or remodeling. The therapist must be aware of the time required for the healing process and realize that being overly aggressive can interfere with that process.

Factors That Impede Healing

EXTENT OF INJURY

The nature of the inflammatory response is determined by the extent of the tissue injury. *Microtears* or soft tissue involve only minor damage and are most often associated with overuse. *Macrotears* involve significantly greater destruction of soft tissue and result in clinical symptoms and functional alterations. Macrotears are generally caused by acute trauma.[19]

EDEMA

The increased pressure caused by swelling retards the healing process, causes separation of tissues, inhibits neuromuscular control, produces reflexive neurological changes, and impedes nutrition in the injured part. Edema is best controlled and managed during the initial first-aid management period as described previously.[17]

HEMORRHAGE

Bleeding occurs with even the smallest amount of damage to the capillaries. Bleeding produces the same negative effects on healing as does the accumulation of edema, and its presence produces additional tissue damage and thus exacerbation of the injury.[67]

POOR VASCULAR SUPPLY

Injuries to tissues with a poor vascular supply heal poorly and at a slow rate. This response is likely related to a failure in the initial delivery of phagocytic cells and fibroblasts necessary for scar formation.[67]

SEPARATION OF TISSUE

Mechanical separation of tissue can significantly impact the course of healing. A wound that has smooth edges in good apposition will tend to heal by primary intention with minimal scarring. Conversely, a wound that has jagged, separated edges must heal by secondary intention, with granulation tissue filling the defect and excessive scarring.[76]

MUSCLE SPASM

Muscle spasm causes traction on the torn tissue, separates the two ends, and prevents approximation. Local and generalized ischemia can result from spasm.

ATROPHY

Wasting away of muscle tissue begins immediately with injury. Strengthening and early mobilization of the injured structure retard atrophy.

CORTICOSTEROIDS

Use of corticosteroids in the treatment of inflammation is controversial. Steroid use in the early stages of healing has been demonstrated to inhibit fibroplasia, capillary proliferation, collagen synthesis, and increases in tensile strength of the healing scar. Their use in the later stages of healing and with chronic inflammation is debatable.

KELOIDS AND HYPERTROPHIC SCARS

Keloids occur when the rate of collagen production exceeds the rate of collagen breakdown during the maturation phase of healing. This process leads to hypertrophy of scar tissue, particularly around the periphery of the wound.

INFECTION

The presence of bacteria in the wound can delay healing, causes excessive granulation tissue, and frequently causes large, deformed scars.[12]

HUMIDITY, CLIMATE, AND OXYGEN TENSION

Humidity significantly influences the process of epithelization. Occlusive dressing stimulates the epithelium to migrate twice as fast without crust or scab formation. The formation of a scab occurs with dehydration of the wound and traps wound drainage, which promotes infection. Keeping the wound moist provides an advantage for the necrotic debris to go to the surface and be shed.

Oxygen tension relates to the neovascularization of the wound, which translates into optimal saturation and maximal tensile strength development. Circulation to the wound can be affected by ischemia, venous stasis, hematomas, and vessel trauma.

HEALTH, AGE, AND NUTRITION

The elastic qualities of the skin decrease with aging. Degenerative diseases, such as diabetes and arteriosclerosis, also become a concern of the older patient and can affect wound healing. Nutrition is important for wound healing—in particular, vitamins C (for collagen synthesis and immune system), K (for clotting), and A (for the immune system); zinc (for the enzyme systems) and amino acids play critical roles in the healing process.

PATHOPHYSIOLOGY OF INJURY TO VARIOUS BODY TISSUES

Classification of Body Tissues

There are four types of fundamental tissues in the human body: epithelial, connective, muscular, and nervous[89] (Table 3-1). According to Guyton, all tissues of the body except bone can be defined as soft tissue.[38] Cailliet, however, more technically defines *soft tissue* as the matrix of the human body comprising cellular elements within a ground substance. Furthermore, Cailliet believes that soft tissue is the most common site of functional impairment of the musculoskeletal system.[17] Most musculoskeletal injuries occur to the soft tissues.

Epithelial Tissue

The first fundamental tissue is epithelial tissue (Fig. 3-3). This specific tissue covers all internal and external body surfaces and therefore encompasses structures such as the skin, the outer layer of the internal organs, and the inner lining of the blood vessels and glands. A basic purpose of epithelial tissue is to protect and form structure for other tissues and organs. In addition, this tissue functions in absorption (e.g., in the digestive tract) and secretion (as in glands). A principal physiological characteristic of epithelial tissue is that it contains no blood supply per se,

so it must depend on the process of diffusion for nutrition, oxygenation, and elimination of waste products. Most injuries to this type of tissue are traumatic, including abrasions, lacerations, punctures, and avulsions. Other injuries to this tissue can include infection, inflammation, or disease.

Connective Tissue

The functions of connective tissue in the body are to support, provide a framework, fill space, store fat, help repair tissues, produce blood cells, and protect against infection.[79] Connective tissue consists of various types of cells separated from one another by some type of extracellular matrix. This matrix consists of fibers and ground substance and can be solid, semisolid, or fluid. The primary types of connective tissue cells are macrophages, which function as phagocytes to clean up debris; mast cells, which release chemicals (histamine and heparin) associated with inflammation; and the fibroblasts, which are the principal cells of the connective tissue.

COLLAGEN

Fibroblasts produce collagen and elastin found in varying proportions in different connective tissues. Collagen is a major structural protein that forms strong, flexible, inelastic structures that hold connective tissue together. Collagen enables a tissue to resist mechanical forces and deformation. Elastin, however, produces highly elastic tissues that assist in recovery from deformation. Collagen fibrils are the load-bearing elements of connective tissue. They are arranged to accommodate tensile stress but are not as capable of resisting shear or compressive stress. Consequently the direction of orientation of collagen fibers is along lines of tensile stress.[93]

Collagen has several mechanical and physical properties that allow it to respond to loading and deformation, permitting it to withstand high tensile stress. The mechanical properties of collagen include *elasticity*, which is the capability to recover normal length after elongation; *viscoelasticity*, which allows for a slow return to normal length and shape after deformation; and *plasticity*, which allows for permanent change or deformation. The physical properties include *force relaxation*, which indicates the decrease in the amount of force needed to maintain a tissue at a set amount of displacement or deformation over time; *creep response*, which is the ability of a tissue to deform over time while a constant load is imposed; and *hysteresis*, which is the amount of relaxation a tissue has undergone during deformation and displacement. If the mechanical and physical limitations of connective tissue are exceeded, injury results.[103]

TYPES OF CONNECTIVE TISSUE

There are several types of connective tissue.[42,79,83] *Fibrous connective tissue* is composed of strong collagenous fibers that bind tissues together. There are two types of fibrous connective tissue. *Dense connective tissue* is composed primarily of collagen and is found in tendons, fascia, aponeurosis, ligaments, and joint

TABLE 3-1

Tissues

TISSUE	LOCATION	FUNCTION
EPITHELIAL		
Simple squamous	Alveoli of lungs	Absorption by diffusion of respiratory gases between alveolar air and blood
	Lining of blood and lymphatic vessels	Absorption by diffusion, filtration, and osmosis
Stratified squamous	Surface of lining of mouth and esophagus	Protection
	Surface of skin (epidermis)	
Simple columnar	Surface layer of lining of stomach, intestines, and parts of respiratory tract	Protection, secretion, absorption
Stratified transitional	Urinary bladder	Protection
CONNECTIVE (MOST WIDELY DISTRIBUTED OF ALL TISSUES)		
Areolar	Between other tissues and organs	Connection
Adipose (fat)	Under skin	Protection
	Padding at various points	Insulation, support, reserve food
Dense fibrous	Tendons, ligaments	Flexible but strong connection
Bone	Skeleton	Support, protection
Cartilage	Part of nasal septum, covering articular surfaces of bones, larynx, rings in trachea and bronchi	Firm but flexible support
	Disks between vertebrae	
	External ear	
Blood	Blood vessels	Transportation
MUSCLE		
Skeletal (striated voluntary)	Muscles that attach to bones	Movement of bones
	Eyeball muscles	Eye movements
	Upper third of esophagus	First part of swallowing
Cardiac (striated involuntary)	Wall of heart	Contraction of heart
Visceral (nonstriated involuntary or smooth)	In walls of tubular viscera of digestive, respiratory, and genitourinary tracts	Movement of substances along respective tracts
	In walls of blood vessels and large lymphatic vessels	Changing of diameter of blood vessels
	In ducts of glands	Movement of substances along ducts
	Intrinsic eye muscles (iris and ciliary body)	Changing of diameter of pupils and shape of lens
	Arrector muscles of hairs	Erection of hairs (gooseflesh)
NERVOUS		
	Brain, spinal cord, nerves	Irritability, conduction

capsule. *Tendons* connect muscles to bone. An *aponeurosis* is a thin, sheetlike tendon. A *fascia* is a thin membrane of connective tissue that surrounds individual muscles and tendons or muscle groups. *Ligaments* connect bone to bone. All synovial joints are surrounded by a *joint capsule*, which is a type of connec-

tive tissue similar to a ligament. The orientations of collagen fibers in ligaments and joint capsules are less parallel than in tendons. *Loose connective tissue* forms many types of thin membranes found beneath the skin, between muscles, and between organs. *Adipose tissue* is a specialized form of loose connective

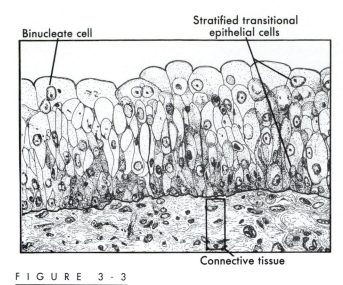

Binucleate cell

Stratified transitional
epithelial cells

Connective tissue

F I G U R E   3 - 3

Epithelial cells exist in several layers.

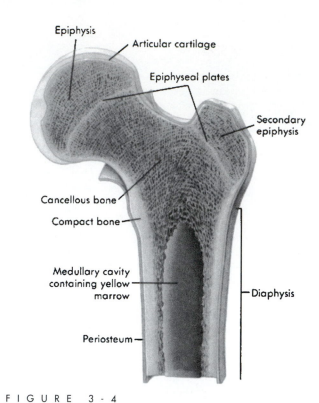

Epiphysis

Articular cartilage

Epiphyseal plates

Secondary
epiphysis

Cancellous bone

Compact bone

Medullary cavity
containing yellow
marrow

Diaphysis

Periosteum

F I G U R E   3 - 4

Structure of bone shown in cross section.

tissue that stores fat, insulates, and acts as a shock absorber. The blood supply to fibrous connective tissue is relatively poor, so healing and repair are slow processes.[83]

Cartilage is a type of rigid connective tissue that provides support and acts as a framework in many structures. It is composed of chondrocyte cells contained in small chambers called lacunae, surrounded completely by an intracellular matrix. The matrix consists of varying ratios of collagen and elastin and a ground substance made of proteoglycans and glycosaminoglycans, which are nonfibrous protein molecules. These proteoglycans act as sponges and trap large quantities of water, which allows cartilage to spring back after being compressed. Cartilage has a poor blood supply, thus healing after injury is very slow. There are three types of cartilage. *Hyaline cartilage* is found on the articulating surfaces of bone and in the soft part of the nose. It contains large quantities of collagen and proteoglycan. *Fibrocartilage* forms the intervertebral disk and menisci located in several joint spaces. It has greater amounts of collagen than proteoglycan and is capable of withstanding a great deal of pressure. *Elastic cartilage* is found in the auricle of the ear and the larynx. It is more flexible than the other types of cartilage and consists of collagen, proteoglycan, and elastin.[79]

Reticular connective tissue is also composed primarily of collagen. It provides the support structure of the walls of various internal organs, including the liver and kidneys.

Elastic connective tissue is composed primarily of elastic fibers. It is found primarily in the walls of blood vessels, airways, and hollow internal organs.

Bone is a type of connective tissue consisting of both living cells and minerals deposited in a matrix (Fig. 3-4). Each bone consists of three major components. The *epiphysis* is an expanded portion at each end of the bone that articulates with another bone. Each articulating surface is covered by an articular, or hyaline, cartilage. The *diaphysis* is the shaft of the

bone. The *epiphyseal* or *growth plate* is the major site of bone growth and elongation. Once bone growth ceases, the plate ossifies and forms the epiphyseal line. With the exception of the articulating surfaces, the bone is completely enclosed by the *periosteum*, a tough, highly vascularized and innervated fibrous tissue.[55]

The two types of bone material are *cancellous*, or spongy, bone and *cortical*, or compact, bone. Cancellous bone contains a series of air spaces referred to as trabeculae, whereas cortical bone is relatively solid. Cortical bone in the diaphysis forms a hollow medullary canal in long bone, which is lined with *endosteum* and filled with bone *marrow*. Bone has rich blood supply that certainly facilitates the healing process after injury. Bone has the functions of support, movement, and protection. Furthermore, bone stores and releases calcium into the bloodstream and manufactures red blood cells.[93]

One additional type of connective tissue in the body is *blood*. Blood is composed of various cells suspended in a fluid intracellular matrix referred to as plasma. Plasma contains red blood cells, white blood cells, and platelets. Although this component does not function in structure, it is essential for the nutrition, cleansing, and physiology of the body.[83]

With connective tissue playing such a major role throughout the human body, it is not surprising that many sport-related injuries involve structures composed of connective tissue. Although tendons are classified as connective tissue, injuries to tendons and tendon healing will be incorporated into the discussion of the musculotendinous unit.

LIGAMENT SPRAINS

A sprain involves damage to a ligament that provides support to a joint. A ligament is a tough, relatively inelastic band of tissue that connects one bone to another. A ligament's primary function is threefold: to provide stability to a joint, to provide control of the position of one articulating bone to another during normal joint motion, and to provide proprioceptive input or a sense of joint position through the function of free nerve endings or mechanoreceptors located within the ligament.

Before discussing injuries to ligaments, a review of joint structure is in order[66] (Fig. 3-5). All *synovial joints* are composed of two or more bones that articulate with one another to allow motion in one or more places. The articulating surfaces of the bone are lined with a very thin, smooth, cartilaginous covering called a hyaline cartilage. All joints are entirely surrounded by a thick, ligamentous joint capsule. The inner surface of this joint capsule is lined by a very thin *synovial membrane* that is highly vascularized and innervated. The synovial membrane produces *synovial fluid*, the functions of which include lubrication, shock absorption, and nutrition of the joint.

Some joints contain a thick fibrocartilage called a *meniscus*. The knee joint, for example, contains two wedge-shaped menisci that deepen the articulation and provide shock absorption in that joint. Finally, the main structural support and joint stability is provided by the ligaments, which may be either thickened portions of a joint capsule or totally separate bands. Ligaments are composed of dense connective tissue arranged in parallel bundles of collagen composed of rows of fibroblasts. Although bundles are arranged in parallel, not all collagen fibers are arranged in parallel.

Ligaments and tendons are very similar in structure. However, ligaments are usually more flattened than tendons, and collagen fibers in ligaments are more compact. The anatomical positioning of the ligaments determines in part what motions a joint can make.

If stress is applied to a joint that forces motion beyond its normal limits or planes of movement, injury to the ligament is likely[34] (Fig. 3-6). The severity of damage to the ligament is classified in many different ways; however, the most commonly used system involves three grades (degrees) of ligamentous sprain:

Grade 1 sprain: There is some stretching or perhaps tearing of the ligamentous fibers, with little or no joint instability. Mild pain, little swelling, and joint stiffness might be apparent.
Grade 2 sprain: There is some tearing and separation of the ligamentous fibers and moderate instability of the joint.

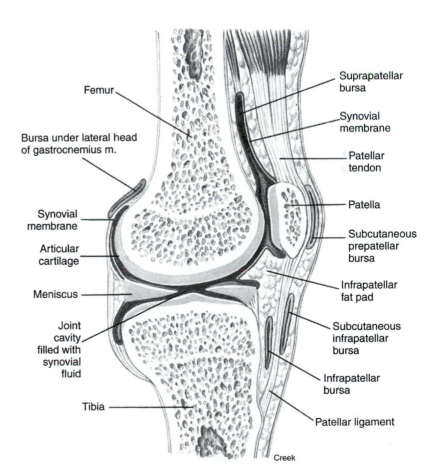

Femur

Bursa under lateral head of gastrocnemius m.

Synovial membrane

Articular cartilage

Meniscus

Joint cavity filled with synovial fluid

Tibia

Suprapatellar bursa

Synovial membrane

Patellar tendon

Patella

Subcutaneous prepatellar bursa

Infrapatellar fat pad

Subcutaneous infrapatellar bursa

Infrapatellar bursa

Patellar ligament

Creek

FIGURE 3-5

Anatomy of a synovial joint.

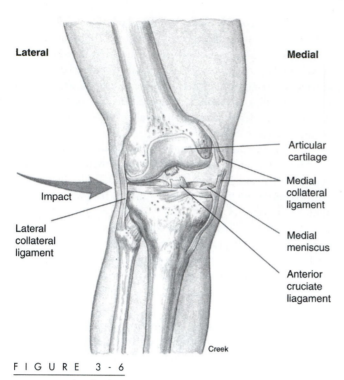

FIGURE 3-6

Example of a ligament sprain in the knee joint.

Moderate to severe pain, swelling, and joint stiffness should be expected.

Grade 3 sprain: There is total rupture of the ligament, manifested primarily by gross instability of the joint. Severe pain might be present initially, followed by little or no pain due to total disruption of nerve fibers. Swelling might be profuse, and thus the joint tends to become very stiff some hours after the injury. A third-degree sprain with marked instability usually requires some form of immobilization lasting several weeks. Frequently the force producing the ligament injury is so great that other ligaments or structures surrounding the joint are also injured. With cases in which there is injury to multiple joint structures, surgical repair reconstruction may be necessary to correct an instability.

Physiology of Ligament Healing

The healing process in the sprained ligament follows the same course of repair as with other vascular tissues. Immediately after injury and for approximately 72 hours there is a loss of blood from damaged vessels and attraction of inflammatory cells into the injured area. If a ligament is sprained outside of a joint capsule (extra-articular ligament), bleeding occurs in a subcutaneous space. If an intra-articular ligament is injured, bleeding occurs inside of the joint capsule until either clotting occurs or the pressure becomes so great that bleeding ceases.

During the next 6 weeks, vascular proliferation with new capillary growth begins to occur along with fibroblastic activity, resulting in the formation of a fibrin clot. It is essential that the torn ends of the ligament be reconnected by bridging of

this clot. Synthesis of collagen and ground substance of proteoglycan as constituents of an intracellular matrix contributes to the proliferation of the scar that bridges between the torn ends of the ligament. This scar initially is soft and viscous but eventually becomes more elastic. Collagen fibers are arranged in a random woven pattern with little organization. Gradually there is a decrease in fibroblastic activity, a decrease in vascularity, and an increase to a maximum in collagen density of the scar.[4] Failure to produce enough scar and failure to reconnect the ligament to the appropriate location on a bone are the two reasons why ligaments are likely to fail.

Over the next several months the scar continues to mature, with the realignment of collagen occurring in response to progressive stresses and strains. The maturation of the scar may require as long as 12 months to complete.[4] The exact length of time required for maturation depends on mechanical factors such as apposition of torn ends and length of the period of immobilization.

FACTORS AFFECTING LIGAMENT HEALING

Surgically repaired extra-articular ligaments have healed with decreased scar formation and are generally stronger than unrepaired ligaments initially, although this strength advantage might not be maintained as time progresses. Unrepaired ligaments heal by fibrous scarring effectively lengthening the ligament and producing some degree of joint instability. With intra-articular ligament tears, the presence of synovial fluid dilutes the hematoma, thus preventing formation of a fibrin clot and spontaneous healing.[42]

Several studies have shown that actively exercised ligaments are stronger than those that are immobilized. Ligaments that are immobilized for periods of several weeks after injury tend to decrease in tensile strength and also exhibit weakening of the insertion of the ligament to bone.[72] Thus it is important to minimize periods of immobilization and progressively stress the injured ligaments while exercising caution relative to biomechanical considerations for specific ligaments.[4,68]

It is not likely that the inherent stability of the joint provided by the ligament before injury will be regained. Thus, to restore stability to the joint, the other structures that surround that joint, primarily muscles and their tendons, must be strengthened. The increased muscle tension provided by resistance training can improve stability of the injured joint.[68,88]

FRACTURES OF BONE

Fractures are extremely common injuries among the athletic population. They can be generally classified as being either open or closed. A closed fracture involves little or no displacement of bones and thus little or no soft-tissue disruption. An open fracture involves enough displacement of the fractured ends that the bone actually disrupts the cutaneous layers and breaks through the skin. Both fractures can be relatively serious if not managed

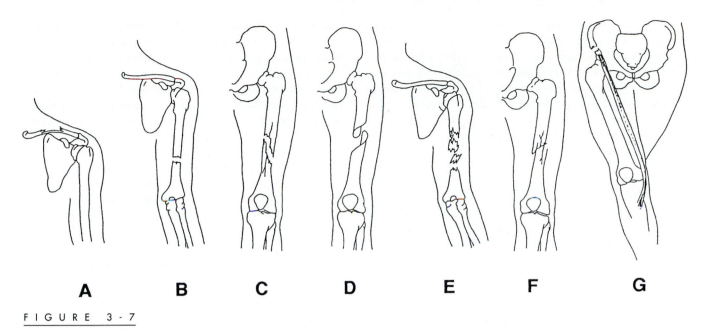

F I G U R E   3 - 7

Fractures of bone. **A,** Greenstick; **B,** Transverse; **C,** Oblique; **D,** Spiral; **E,** Comminuted;
F, Impacted; **G,** Avulsion.

properly, but an increased possibility of infection exists in an open fracture. Fractures may also be considered complete, in which the bone is broken into at least two fragments, or incomplete, where the fracture does not extend completely across the bone.

The varieties of fractures that can occur include greenstick, transverse, oblique, spiral, comminuted, impacted, avulsive, and stress. A *greenstick fracture* (Fig. 3-7A) occurs most often in children whose bones are still growing and have not yet had a chance to calcify and harden. It is called a greenstick fracture because of the resemblance to the splintering that occurs to a tree twig that is bent to the point of breaking. Because the twig is green, it splinters but can be bent without causing an actual break.

A *transverse fracture* (Fig. 3-7B) involves a crack perpendicular to the longitudinal axis of the bone that goes all the way through the bone. Displacement might occur; however, because of the shape of the fractured ends, the surrounding soft tissue (for example, muscles, tendons, and fat) sustains relatively little damage. A *linear fracture* runs parallel to the long axis of a bone and is similar in severity to a transverse fracture.

An *oblique fracture* (Fig. 3-7C) results in a diagonal crack across the bone and two very jagged, pointed ends that, if displaced, can potentially cause a good bit of soft-tissue damage. Oblique and spiral fractures are the two types most likely to result in compound fractures.

A *spiral fracture* (Fig. 3-7D) is similar to an oblique fracture in that the angle of the fracture is diagonal across the bone. In addition, an element of twisting or rotation causes the fracture to spiral along the longitudinal axis of the bone. Spiral fractures used to be fairly common in ski injuries occurring just above the top of the boot when the bindings on the ski failed to release

when the foot was rotated. These injuries are now less common due to improvements in equipment design.

A *comminuted fracture* (Fig. 3-7E) is a serious problem that can require an extremely long time for rehabilitation. In the comminuted fracture, multiple fragments of bone must be surgically repaired and fixed with screws and wires. If a fracture of this type occurs to a weightbearing bone in the leg, a permanent discrepancy in leg length can develop.

In an *impacted fracture* (Fig. 3-7F), one end of the fractured bone is driven up into the other end. As with the comminuted fracture, correcting discrepancies in the length of the extremity can require long periods of intensive rehabilitation.

An *avulsion fracture* (Fig. 3-7G) occurs when a fragment of bone is pulled away at the bony attachment of a muscle, tendon, or ligament. Avulsion fractures are common in the fingers and some of the smaller bones but can also occur in larger bones where tendinous or ligamentous attachments are subjected to a large amount of force.

Perhaps the most common fracture resulting from physical activity is the *stress fracture.* Unlike the other types of fractures that have been discussed, the stress fracture results from overuse or fatigue rather than acute trauma.[49] Common sites for stress fractures include the weightbearing bones of the leg and foot. In either case, repetitive forces transmitted through the bones produce irritations and microfractures at a specific area in the bone. The pain usually begins as a dull ache that becomes progressively more painful day after day. Initially, pain is most severe during activity. However, when a stress fracture actually develops, pain tends to become worse after the activity is stopped.[80]

The biggest problem with a stress fracture is that often it does not show up on an X-ray film until the osteoblasts begin laying down subperiosteal callus or bone, at which point a small white line, or a callus, appears. However, a bone scan might reveal a potential stress fracture in as little as 2 days after onset of symptoms. If a stress fracture is suspected, the patient should, for a minimum of 14 days, stop any activity that produces added stress or fatigue to the area. Stress fractures do not usually require casting but might become normal fractures that must be immobilized if handled incorrectly.[92] If a fracture occurs, it should be managed and rehabilitated by a qualified orthopedist and physical therapist.

Physiology of Bone Healing

Healing of injured bone tissue is similar to soft-tissue healing in that all phases of the healing process can be identified, although bone regeneration capabilities are somewhat limited. However, the functional elements of healing differ significantly from those of soft tissue. Tensile strength of the scar is the single most critical factor in soft-tissue healing, whereas bone has to contend with a number of additional forces, including torsion, bending, and compression.[46] Trauma to bone can vary from contusions of the periosteum to closed, nondisplaced fractures to severely displaced open fractures that also involve significant soft-tissue damage. When a fracture occurs, blood vessels in the bone and the periosteum are damaged, resulting in bleeding and subsequent clot formation (Fig. 3-8). Hemorrhaging from the marrow is contained by the periosteum and the surrounding soft tissue in the region of the fracture. In about 1 week, fibroblasts begin laying down a fibrous collagen network. The fibrin strands within the clot serve as the framework for proliferating vessels. *Chondroblast* cells begin producing fibrocartilage, creating a *callus* between the broken bones. At first, the callus is soft and firm because it is composed primarily of collagenous fibrin. The callus becomes firm and more rubbery as cartilage beings to predominate. Bone-producing cells called *osteoblasts* begin to proliferate and enter the callus, forming cancellous bone trabeculae, which eventually replace the cartilage. Finally the callus crystallizes into bone, at which point remodeling of the bone begins. The callus can be divided into two portions, the external callus located around the periosteum on the outside of the fracture and the internal callus found between the bone fragments. The size of the callus is proportional both to the damage and to the amount of irritation to the fracture site during the healing process. Also during the time *osteoclasts* begin to appear in the area to resorb bone fragments and clean up debris.[42,46,83]

The remodeling process is similar to the growth process of bone in that the fibrous cartilage is gradually replaced by fibrous bone and then by more structurally efficient lamellar bone. Remodeling involves an ongoing process during which osteoblasts lay down new bone and osteoclasts remove and break down bone according to the forces placed upon the healing bone.[62] Wolff's law maintains that a bone will adapt to mechanical stresses and strains by changing size, shape, and structure. Therefore, once the cast is removed, the bone must be subjected to normal stresses and strains so that tensile strength can be regained before the healing process is complete.[36,90]

The time required for bone healing is variable and based on a number of factors, such as severity of the fracture, site of the fracture, extensiveness of the trauma, and age of the patient. Normal periods of immobilization range from as short as 3 weeks for the small bones in the hands and feet to as long as 8 weeks for the long bones of the upper and lower extremities.

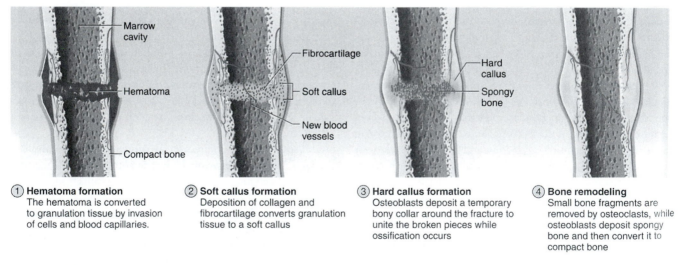

① **Hematoma formation**
The hematoma is converted to granulation tissue by invasion of cells and blood capillaries.

② **Soft callus formation**
Deposition of collagen and fibrocartilage converts granulation tissue to a soft callus

③ **Hard callus formation**
Osteoblasts deposit a temporary bony collar around the fracture to unite the broken pieces while ossification occurs

④ **Bone remodeling**
Small bone fragments are removed by osteoclasts, while osteoblasts deposit spongy bone and then convert it to compact bone

FIGURE   3-8

The healing of a fracture. **1,** Blood vessels are broken at the fracture line; the blood clots and forms a fracture hematoma. **2,** Blood vessels grow into the fracture and a fibrocartilage soft callus forms. **3,** The fibrocartilage becomes ossified and forms a bony callus made of spongy bone. **4,** Osteoclasts remove excess tissue from the bony callus and the bone eventually resembles its original appearance.

In some instances, such as fractures in the four small toes, immobilization might not be required for healing. The healing process is certainly not complete when the splint or cast is removed. Osteoblastic and osteoclastic activity might continue for 2–3 years after severe fractures.[49,62]

CARTILAGE DAMAGE

Osteoarthrosis is a degenerative condition of bone and cartilage in and about the joint. *Arthritis* should be defined as primarily an inflammatory condition with possible secondary destruction.[6] *Arthrosis* is primarily a degenerative process with destruction of cartilage, remodeling of bone, and possible secondary inflammatory components.

Cartilage fibrillates—that is, releases fibers or groups of fibers and ground substance into the joint.[29] Peripheral cartilage that is not exposed to weightbearing or compression–decompression mechanisms is particularly likely to fibrillate. Fibrillation is typically found in the degenerative process associated with poor nutrition or disuses. This process can then extend even to weightbearing areas, with progressive destruction of cartilage proportional to stresses applied on it. When forces are increased, thus increasing stress, osteochondral or subchondral fractures can occur. Concentration of stress on small areas can produce pressures that overwhelm the tissue's capabilities. Typically, lower-limb joints have to handle greater stresses, but their surface area is usually larger than the surface area of upper limbs. The articular cartilage is protected to some extent by the synovial fluid, which acts as a lubricant. It is also protected by the subchondral bone, which responds to stresses in an elastic fashion. It is more compliant than compact bone, and microfractures can be a means of force absorption. Trabeculae might fracture or might be displaced due to pressures applied on the subchondral bone. In compact bone, fracture can be a means of defense to dissipate force. In the joint, forces might be absorbed by joint movement and eccentric contraction of muscles.[27]

In the majority of joints where the surfaces are not congruent, the applied forces tend to concentrate in certain areas, which increase joint degeneration. *Osteophytosis* occurs as a bone attempts to increase its surface area to decrease contact forces. Typically people describe this growth as "bone spurs." *Chondromalacia* is the nonprogressive transformation of cartilage with irregular surfaces and areas of softening. Typically it occurs first in non-weightbearing areas and may progress to areas of excessive stress.[26]

In physically active individuals certain joints maybe more susceptible to a response resembling osteoarthrosis.[70] The proportion of body weight resting on the joint, the pull of musculotendinous unit, and any significant external force applied to the joint are predisposing factors. Altered joint mechanics caused by laxity or previous trauma are also factors that come into play.[45] The intensity of forces can be great, as in the hip, where the previously mentioned factors can produce pressures

or forces 4 times that of body weight and up to 10 times that of body weight on the knee.

Typically, muscle forces generate more stress than body weight itself. Particular injuries are conducive to osteoarthritic changes such as subluxation and dislocation of the patella, osteochondritis dissecans, recurrent synovial effusion, and hemarthrosis. Also, ligamentous injuries can bring about a disruption of proprioceptive mechanisms, loss of adequate joint alignment, and meniscal damage in the knees with removal of the injured meniscus.[40] Other factors that have an impact are loss of full range of motion, poor muscular power and strength, and altered biomechanics of the joint. Spurring and spiking of bone are not synonymous with osteoarthrosis if the joint space is maintained and the cartilage lining is intact. It may simply be an adaptation to the increased stress of physical activity.[29]

Physiology of Cartilage Healing

Cartilage has a relatively limited healing capacity. When chondrocytes are destroyed and the matrix is disrupted, the course of healing is variable, depending on whether damage is to cartilage alone or also to subchondral bone. Injuries to the articular cartilage alone fail to elicit clot formation or a cellular response. For the most part the chondrocytes adjacent to the injury are the only cells that show any signs of proliferation and synthesis of matrix. Thus the defect fails to heal, although the extent of the damage tends to remain the same.[33,58]

If subchondral bone is also affected, inflammatory cells enter the damaged area and formulate granulation tissue. In this case, the healing process proceeds normally, with differentiation of granulation tissue cells into chondrocytes occurring in about 2 weeks. At approximately 2 months, normal collagen has been formed.

Injuries to the knee articular cartilage are extremely common, and until recently methods for treatment did not produce good long-term results. A better understanding of how articular cartilage responds to injury has produced various techniques that hold promise for long-term success.[91] One such technique is autologous chondrocyte implantation, in which a patient's own cartilage cells are harvested, grown ex vivo, and reimplanted in a full-thickness articular surface defect. Results are available with up to 10 years' follow-up, and more than 80 percent of patients have shown improvement with relatively few complications.

INJURIES TO MUSCULOTENDINOUS STRUCTURES

Muscle is often considered to be a type of connective tissue, but here it is treated as the third of the fundamental tissues. The three types of muscles are smooth (involuntary), cardiac, and skeletal (voluntary) muscles. *Smooth muscle* is found with the viscera, where it forms the walls of the internal organs, and within many hollow chambers. *Cardiac muscle* is found only in the heart and is responsible for its contraction. A significant characteristic of the cardiac muscle is that it contracts as a single

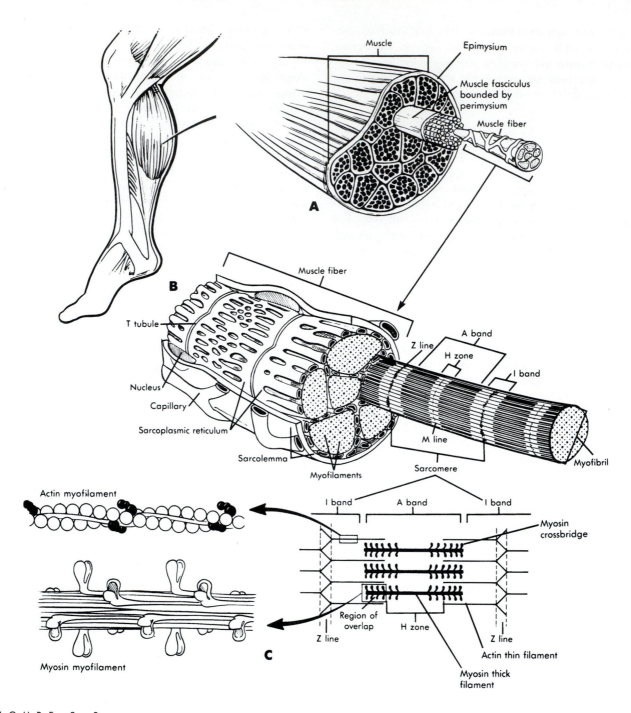

F I G U R E   3 - 9

Parts of a muscle. **A,** Muscle is composed of muscle fasciculi, which can be seen by the unaided eye as striations in the muscle. The fasciculi are composed of bundles of individual muscle fibers (muscle cells). **B,** Each muscle fiber contains myofibrils in which the banding patterns of the sarcomeres are seen. **C,** The myofibrils are composed of actin myofilament and myosin myofilaments, which are formed from thousands of individual actin and myosin molecules.

fiber, unlike smooth and skeletal muscles, which contract as separate units. This characteristic forces the heart to work as a single unit continuously; therefore, if one portion of the muscle should die (as in myocardial infraction), contraction of the heart does not cease.[79]

Skeletal muscle is the striated muscle within the body, responsible for the movement of bony levers (Fig. 3-9). Skeletal muscle consists of two portions: (1) the muscle belly and (2) its tendons, which are collectively referred to as a musculotendinous unit. The muscle belly is composed of separate, parallel elastic fibers called myofibrils. Myofibrils are composed of thousands of small sarcomeres, which are the functional units of the muscle. Sarcomeres contain the contractile elements of the muscle, as well as substantial amount of connective tissue that holds the fibers together. Myofilaments are small contractile elements of protein within the sarcomere. There are two distinct types of myofilaments: thin actin myofilaments and thicker myosin myofilaments. Fingerlike projections, or crossbridges, connect the actin and myosin myofilaments.[83] When a muscle is stimulated to contract, the crossbridges pull the myofilaments closer together, thus shortening the muscle and producing movement at the joint that the muscle crosses.[25]

The *muscle tendon* attaches the muscle directly to the bone. The muscle tendon is composed primarily of collagen fibers and a matrix of proteoglycan, which is produced by the tenocyte cell. The collagen fibers are grouped together into *primary bundles*. Groups of primary bundles join together to form hexagonal-shaped *secondary bundles*. Secondary bundles are held together by intertwined loose connective tissue containing elastin, called the *endotenon*. The entire tendon is surrounded by a connective tissue layer, called the *epitenon*. The outermost layer of the tendon is the *paratenon*, which is a double-layer connective tissue sheath lined on the inside with synovial membrane[56] (Fig. 3-10).

All skeletal muscles exhibit four characteristics: (1) elasticity, the ability to change in length or stretch; (2) extensibility, the ability to shorten and return to normal length; (3) excitability, the ability to respond to stimulation from the nervous system; and (4) contractility, the ability to shorten and contract in response to some neural command.[55]

Skeletal muscles show considerable variation in size and shape. Large muscles generally produce gross motor movements at large joints, such as knee flexion produced by contraction of the large, bulky hamstring muscles. Smaller skeletal muscles, such as the long flexors of the fingers, produce fine motor movements. Muscles producing movements that are powerful in nature are usually thicker and longer, whereas those producing finer movements requiring coordination are thin and relatively shorter. Other muscles may be flat, round, or fan-shaped.[42,83] Muscles may be connected to a bone by a single tendon or by two or three separate tendons at either end. Muscles that have two separate muscle and tendon attachments are called *biceps*, and muscles with three separate muscle and tendon attachments are called *triceps*.

Muscles contract in response to stimulation by the central nervous system. An electrical impulse transmitted from the central nervous system through a single motor nerve to a group of muscle fibers causes a depolarization of those fibers. The motor nerve and the group of muscle fibers that it innervates are collectively referred to as a *motor unit*. An impulse coming form the central nervous system and traveling to a group of fibers through a particular motor nerve causes all the muscle fibers in that motor unit to depolarize and contract. This is referred to as the *all-or-none response* and applies to all skeletal muscles in the body.[42]

Muscle Strains

If a musculotendinous unit is overstretched or forced to contract against too much resistance, exceeding the extensibility limits or the tensile capabilities of the weakest component within the unit, damage can occur to the muscle fibers, at the musculotendinous juncture, in the tendon, or at the tendinous attachment to the bone.[34] Any of these injuries may be referred to as a *strain* (Fig. 3-11). Muscle strains, like ligament sprains, are subject to various classification systems. The following is a simple system of classification of muscle strains:

Grade 1 strain: Some muscle or tendon fibers have been stretched or actually torn. Active motion produces some tenderness and pain. Movement is painful, but full range of motion is usually possible.

Grade 2 strain: Some muscle or tendon fibers have been torn, and active contraction of the muscle is extremely painful. Usually a palpable depression or divot exists somewhere in the muscle belly at the spot where the muscle fibers have been torn. Some swelling might occur because of capillary bleeding.

Grade 3 strain: There is a complete rupture of muscle fibers in the muscle belly, in the area where the muscle becomes tendon, or at the tendinous attachment to the bone. The athlete has significant impairment to, or perhaps total loss of, movement. Pain is intense initially but diminishes quickly because of complete separation of the nerve fibers. Musculotendinous ruptures are most common in the biceps tendon of the upper arm of in the Achilles heelcord in the back of the calf. When either of these tendons rupture, the muscle tends to bunch toward its proximal attachment. With

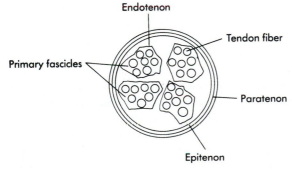

FIGURE 3-10
Structure of a tendon.

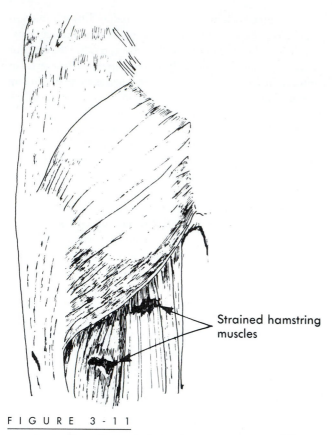

Strained hamstring
muscles

FIGURE 3-11

A muscle strain results in tearing or separation of fibers.

the exception of an Achilles rupture, which is frequently surgically repaired, the majority of third-degree strains are treated conservatively with some period of immobilization.

Physiology of Muscle Healing

Injuries to muscle tissue involve similar processes of healing and repair as discussed for other tissues. Initially there will be hemorrhage and edema followed almost immediately by phagocytosis to clear debris. Within a few days there is a proliferation of ground substance, and fibroblasts begin producing a gel-type matrix that surrounds the connective tissue, leading to fibrosis and scarring. At the same time, myoblastic cells form in the area of injury, which will eventually lead to regeneration or new myofibrils. Thus regeneration of both connective tissue and muscle tissue begins.[13]

Collagen fibers undergo maturation and orient themselves along lines of tensile force according to Wolff's law. Active contraction of the muscle is critical in regaining normal tensile strength.[6,60]

Regardless of the severity of the strain, the time required for rehabilitation is fairly lengthy. In many instances, rehabilitation time for a muscle strain is longer than that for a ligament sprain. These incapacitating muscle strains occur most frequently in the large, force-producing hamstring and quadriceps muscles of the lower extremity. The treatment of hamstring strains requires a

healing period of at least 6–8 weeks and a considerable amount of patience. Attempts to return to activity too soon frequently cause reinjury to the area of the musculotendinous unit that has been strained, and the healing process must begin again.

Tendinitis

Of all the overuse problems associated with physical activity, tendinitis is among the most common.[48] *Tendinitis* is a catchall term that can describe many different pathological conditions or a tendon. It essentially describes any inflammatory response within the tendon without inflammation of the paratenon.[87] *Paratenonitis* involves inflammation of the outer layer of the tendon only and usually occurs when the tendon rubs over a bony prominence. *Tendinosis* describes a tendon that has significant degenerative changes with no clinical or histological signs of an inflammatory response.[20]

In cases of what is most often called *chronic tendinitis*, there is evidence of significant tendon degeneration, loss of normal collagen structure, loss of cellularity in the area, but absolutely no inflammatory cellular response in the tendon.[81] The inflammatory process is an essential part of healing. Inflammation is supposed to be a brief process with an end point after its function in the healing process has been fulfilled. The point or the cause in the pathological process where the acute inflammatory cellular response terminates and the chronic degeneration begins is difficult to determine. As mentioned previously, with chronic tendinitis the cellular response involves a replacement of leukocytes with macrophages and plasma cells.[99]

During muscle activity a tendon must move or slide on other structures around it whenever the muscle contracts. If a particular movement is performed repeatedly, the tendon becomes irritated and inflamed. This inflammation is manifested by pain on movement, swelling, possibly some warmth, and usually crepitus. Crepitus is a crackling sound similar to the sound produced by rolling hair between the fingers by the ear. Crepitus is usually caused by the adherence of the paratenon to the surrounding structures while it slides back and forth. This adhesion is caused primarily by the chemical products of inflammation that accumulate on the irritated tendon.[20]

The key to treating tendinitis is rest. If the repetitive motion causing irritation to the tendon is eliminated, chances are that the inflammatory process will allow the tendon to heal.[65] Unfortunately a patient who is seriously involved with some physical activity might have difficulty in resting for 2 weeks or more while the tendinitis subsides. Anti-inflammatory medications and therapeutic modalities are also helpful in reducing the inflammatory responses. An alternative activity, such as bicycling or swimming, is necessary to maintain fitness levels to a certain degree, while allowing the tendon a chance to heal.[30]

Tendinitis most commonly occurs in the Achilles tendon in the back of the lower leg in runners or in the rotator cuff tendons of the shoulder joint in swimmers or throwers, although it can certainly flare up in any tendon in which overuse and repetitive movements occur.

Tenosynovitis

Tenosynovitis is very similar to tendinitis in that the muscle tendons are involved in inflammation. However, many tendons are subject to an increased amount of friction due to the tightness of the space through which they must move. In these areas of high friction, tendons are usually surrounded by synovial sheaths that reduce friction on movement. If the tendon sliding through a synovial sheath is subjected to overuse, inflammation is likely to occur. The inflammatory process produces by-products that are "stick" and tend to cause the sliding tendon to adhere to the synovial sheath surrounding it.[51]

Symptomatically, tenosynovitis is very similar to tendinitis, with pain on movement, tenderness, swelling, and crepitus. Movement may be more limited with tenosynovitis because the space provided for the tendon and its synovial covering is more limited. Tenosynovitis occurs most commonly in the long flexor tendons of the fingers as they cross over the wrist joint and in the biceps tendon around the shoulder joint. Treatment for tenosynovitis is the same as that for tendinitis. Because both conditions involve inflammation, mild anti-inflammatory drugs, such as aspirin, might be helpful in chronic cases.[51]

Physiology of Tendon Healing

Unlike most soft-tissue healing, tendon injuries pose a particular problem in rehabilitation.[40] The injured tendon requires dense fibrous union of the separated ends and both extensibility and flexibility at the site of attachment. Thus an abundance of collagen is required to achieve good tensile strength. Unfortunately, collagen synthesis can become excessive, resulting in fibrosis, in which adhesions form in surrounding tissues and interfere with the gliding that is essential for smooth motion. Fortunately, over a period of time the scar tissue of the surrounding tissues becomes elongated in its structure because of a breakdown in the cross-links between fibrin units and thus allows the necessary gliding motion. A tendon injury that occurs where the tendon is surrounded by a synovial sheath can be potentially devastating.

A typical time frame for tendon healing would be that during the second week when the healing tendon adheres to the surrounding tissue to form a single mass and during the third week when the tendon separates to varying degrees from the surrounding tissues. However, the tensile strength is not sufficient to permit a strong pull on the tendon for at least 4–5 weeks, the danger being that a strong contraction can pull the tendon ends apart.[85]

INJURY TO NERVE TISSUE

The final fundamental tissue is nerve tissue (Fig. 3-12). This tissue provides sensitivity and communication from the central nervous system (brain and spinal cord) to the muscles, sensory organs, various systems, and the periphery. The basic nerve cell is the neuron. The neuron cell body contains a large

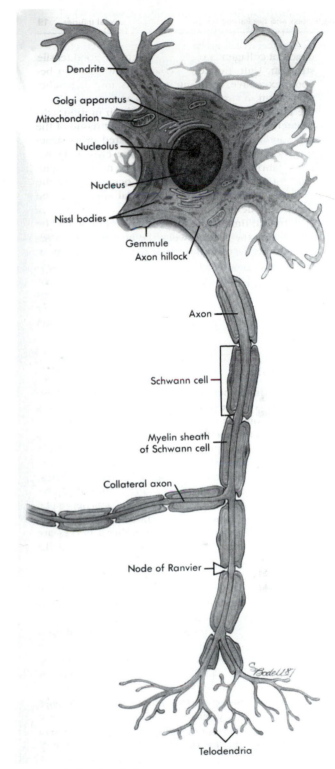

FIGURE 3-12
Structural features of nerve cell.

nucleus and branched extensions called *dendrites*, which respond to neurotransmitter substances released from other nerve cells. From each nerve cell arises a single *axon*, which conducts the nerve impulses. Large axons found in peripheral nerves are enclosed in sheaths composed of *Schwann cells*, which are tightly wound around the axon. A nerve is a bundle of nerve cells held together by some connective tissue, usually a lipid–protein layer called the *myelin sheath*, on the outside of the axon.[93] Neurology is an extremely complex science, and only a brief presentation of its relevance to musculoskeletal injuries is covered here.[16]

Nerve injuries usually involve either contusions or inflammations. More serious injuries involve the crushing of a nerve or complete division (severing). This type of injury can produce lifelong physical disability, such as paraplegia or quadriplegia, and should therefore not be overlooked in any circumstance.

Of critical concern to the therapist is the importance of the nervous system in proprioception and neuromuscular control of movement as an integral part of a rehabilitation program. This will be discussed in great detail in Chapter 11.

Physiology of Nerve Healing

Nerve cell tissue is specialized and cannot regenerate once the nerve cell dies. In an injured peripheral nerve, however, the nerve fiber can regenerate significantly if the injury does not affect the cell body. The proximity of the axonal injury to the cell body can significantly affect the time required for healing. The closer an injury is to the cell body, the more difficult is the regenerative process. In the case of severed nerve, surgical intervention can markedly enhance regeneration.[79]

For regeneration to occur, an optimal environment for healing must exist. When a nerve is cut, several degenerative changes occur that interfere with the neural pathways (Fig. 3-13). Within the first 3–5 days the portion of the axon distal to the cut begins to degenerate and breaks into irregular

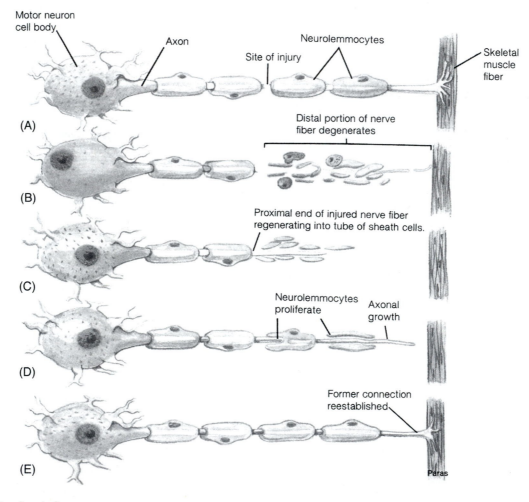

FIGURE 3-13

Neuron regeneration. **A,** If a neuron is severed through a myelinated axon, the proximal portion may survive but **B,** the distal portion will degenerate through phagocytosis. **C–D,** The myelin layer provides a pathway for regeneration of the axon, and **E,** innervation is restored.

segments. There is also a concomitant increase in metabolism and protein production by the nerve cell body to facilitate the regenerative process. The neuron in the cell body contains the genetic material and produces chemicals necessary for maintenance of the axon. These substances cannot be transmitted to the distal part of the axon, and eventually there will be complete degeneration.[83]

In addition, the myelin portion of the Schwann cells around the degenerating axon also degenerates, and the myelin is phagocytized. The Schwann cells divide, forming a column of cells in place of the axon. If the cut ends of the axon contact this column of Schwann cells, the chances are good that an axon may eventually reinnervate distal structures. If the proximal end of the axon does not make contact with the column of Schwann cells, reinnervation will not occur.

The axon proximal to the cut has minimal degeneration initially and then begins the regenerative process with growth from the proximal axon. Bulbous enlargements and several axon sprouts form at the end of the proximal axon. Within about 2 weeks, these sprouts grow across the scar that has developed in the area of the cut and enter the column of Schwann cells. Only one of these sprouts will form the new axon, while the others will degenerate. Once the axon grows through the Schwann cell columns, remaining Schwann cells proliferate along the length of the degenerating fiber and form new myelin around the growing axon, which will eventually reinnervate distal structures.[42]

Regeneration is slow, at a rate of only 3–4 mm/day. Axon regeneration can be obstructed by scar formation due to excessive fibroplasia. Damaged nerves within the central nervous system regenerate very poorly compared to nerves in the peripheral nervous system. Central nervous system axons lack connective tissue sheaths, and the myelin-producing Schwann cells fail to proliferate.[42,83]

ADDITIONAL MUSCULOSKELETAL INJURIES

Dislocations and Subluxations

A dislocation occurs when at least one bone in an articulation is forced out of its normal and proper alignment and stays out until it is either manually or surgically put back into place or reduced.[10] Dislocations most commonly occur in the shoulder joint, elbow, and fingers, but they can occur wherever two bones articulate.[15,64,82]

A subluxation is like a dislocation except that in this situation a bone pops out of its normal articulation but then goes right back into place. Subluxations most commonly occur in the shoulder joint, as well as in the kneecap in females.

Dislocations should never be reduced immediately, regardless of where they occur. The patient should have an X-ray to rule out fractures or other problems before reduction. Inappropriate techniques of reduction might only exacerbate the problem. Return to activity after dislocation or subluxation is largely dependent on the degree of soft-tissue damage.[15]

Bursitis

In many areas, particularly around joints, friction occurs between tendons and bones, skin and bone, or two muscles. Without some mechanism of protection in these high-friction areas, chronic irritation would be likely.[93]

Bursae are essentially pieces of synovial membrane that contain small amounts of synovial fluid. This presence of synovium permits motion of surrounding structures without friction. If excessive movement or perhaps some acute trauma occurs around these bursae, they become irritated and inflamed and begin producing large amounts of synovial fluid. The longer the irritation continues or the more severe the acute trauma, the more fluid is produced. As the fluid continues to accumulate in a limited space, pressure tends to increase and causes irritation of the pain receptors in the area.

Bursitis can be extremely painful and can severely restrict movement, especially if it occurs around a joint. Synovial fluid continues to be produced until the movement or trauma producing the irritation is eliminated.

A bursa that occasionally completely surrounds a tendon to allow more freedom of movement in a tight area is referred to as a *synovial sheath*. Irritation of this synovial sheath may restrict tendon motion.

All joints have many bursae surrounding them. Perhaps the three bursae most commonly irritated as a result of various types of physical activity are the subacromial bursa in the shoulder joint, the olecranon bursa on the tip of the elbow, and the prepatellar bursa on the front surface of the patella. All three of these bursae have produced large amounts of synovial fluid, affecting motion at their respective joints.

Muscle Soreness

Overexertion in strenuous muscular exercise often results in muscular pain. At one time or another almost everyone has experienced muscle soreness, usually resulting from some physical activity to which we are unaccustomed.

There are two types of muscle soreness. The first type of muscle pain is acute and accompanies fatigue. It is transient and occurs during and immediately after exercise. The second type of soreness involves delayed muscle pain that appears approximately 12 hours after injury. It becomes most intense after 24–48 hours and then gradually subsides so that the muscle becomes symptom-free after 3 or 4 days. This second type of pain may best be described as a syndrome of delayed muscle pain, leading to increased muscle tension, edema formation, increased stiffness, and resistance to stretching.[61]

The cause of *delayed-onset muscle soreness* (DOMS) has been debated. Initially it was hypothesized that soreness was due to an excessive buildup of lactic acid in exercised muscles. However, recent evidence has essentially ruled out this theory.[1]

It has also been hypothesized that DOMS is caused by the tonic, localized spasm of motor units, varying in number with the severity of pain. This theory maintains that exercise causes varying degrees of ischemia in the working muscles. This ischemia causes pain, which results in reflex tonic muscle contraction that increases and prolongs the ischemia. Consequently a cycle of increasing severity is begun.[25] As with the lactic acid theory, the spasm theory has also been discounted.

Currently there are two schools of thought relative to the cause of DOMS. DOMS seems to occur from very small tears in the muscle tissue, which seem to be more likely with eccentric or isometric contractions.[1] It is generally believed that the initial damage caused by eccentric exercise is mechanical damage to either the muscular or the connective tissue. Edema accumulation and delays in the rate of glycogen repletion are secondary reactions to mechanical damage.[69]

DOMS might be caused by structural damage to the elastic components of connective tissue at the musculotendinous junction. This damage results in the presence of hydroxyproline, a protein by-product of collagen breakdown, in blood and urine.[19] It has also been documented that structural damage to the muscle fibers results in an increase in blood serum levels of various protein/enzymes, including creatine kinase. This increase indicates that there is likely some damage to the muscle fiber as a result of strenuous exercise.[1]

Muscle soreness can best be prevented by beginning at a moderate level of activity and gradually progressing the intensity of the exercise over time. Treatment of muscle soreness usually also involves some type of stretching activity.[39] As for other conditions discussed in this chapter, ice is important as a treatment for muscle soreness, particularly within the first 48–72 hours.

Contusions

Contusion is synonymous with *bruise*. The mechanism that produces a contusion is a blow from some external object that causes soft tissues (e.g., skin, fat, muscle, ligaments, joint capsule) to be compressed against the hard bone underneath.[100] If the blow is hard enough, capillaries rupture and allow bleeding into the tissues. The bleeding, if superficial enough, causes a bluish-purple discoloration of the skin that persists for several days. The contusion may be very sore to the touch. If damage has occurred to muscle, pain may be elicited on active movement. In most cases the pain ceases within a few days, and discoloration disappears in usually 2–3 weeks.

The major problem with contusions occurs where an area is subjected to repeated blows. If the same area, or more specifically the same muscle, is bruised over and over again, small calcium deposits might begin to accumulate in the injured area. These pieces of calcium might be found between several fibers in the muscle belly, or calcium might form a spur that projects from the underlying bone. These calcium formations, which can significantly impair movement, are referred to as *myositis ossificans*. In some cases myositis ossificans develops from a single trauma.[8]

The key to preventing myositis ossificans from occurring from repeated contusions is protection of the injured area by padding.[8] If the area is properly protected after the first contu-

sion, myositis ossificans might never develop. Protection, along with rest, might allow the calcium to be reabsorbed and eliminate any need for surgical intervention. The two areas that seem to be the most vulnerable to repeated contusions during physical activity are the quadriceps muscle group on the front of the thigh and the biceps muscle on the front of the upper arm.[100] The formation of myositis ossificans in either of these or any other areas can be detected on X-ray films.

MANAGING THE HEALING PROCESS THROUGH REHABILITATION

Rehabilitation exercise progressions can generally be subdivided into three phases, based primarily on the three stages of the healing process: phase 1, the acute phase; phase 2, the repair phase; and phase 3, the remodeling phase. Depending on the type and extent of injury and the individual response to healing, phases will usually overlap. Each phase must include carefully considered goals and a criteria for progressing from one phase to another.[72]

Presurgical Exercise Phase

This phase would apply only to those patients who sustain injuries that require surgery. If surgery can be postponed, exercise may be used as a means to improve its outcome. By allowing the initial inflammatory-response phase to resolve, by maintaining or, in some cases, increasing muscle strength and flexibility, levels of cardiorespiratory fitness, and improving neuromuscular control, the patient may be better prepared to continue the exercise rehabilitative program after surgery.

Phase 1, the Acute Injury Phase

Phase 1 begins immediately when injury occurs and can last as long as day 4 following injury. During this phase, the inflammatory stage of the healing process is attempting to "clean up the mess," thus creating an environment that is conducive to the fibroblastic stage. As indicated in Chapter 1, the primary focus of rehabilitation during this stage is to control swelling and to modulate pain by using the PRICE (protection, restricted activity, ice, compression, and elevation) technique immediately following injury. Ice, compression, and elevation should be used as much as possible during this phase[73] (Fig. 3-14).

Rest of the injured part is critical during this phase. It is widely accepted that early mobility during rehabilitation is essential. However, if the therapist becomes overly aggressive during the first 48 hours following injury, and does not allow the injured part to be rested during the inflammatory stage of healing, the inflammatory process never really gets a chance to accomplish what it is supposed to. Consequently, the length of time required for inflammation might be extended. Therefore, immobility during the first 24–48 hours following injury is necessary to control inflammation.

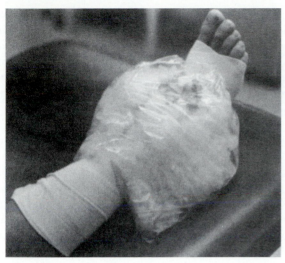

FIGURE 3-14

Musculoskeletal injuries should be treated initially with protection, restricted activity, ice, compression, and elevation.

By day 3 or 4, swelling begins to subside and eventually stops altogether. The injured area may feel warm to the touch, and some discoloration is usually apparent. The injury is still painful to the touch, and some pain is elicited on movement of the injured part.[98] At this point the patient should have already begun active mobility exercises, working through a pain-free range of motion. If the injury involves the lower extremity, the patient should be encouraged to progressively bear more weight.

A physician may choose to have the patient take NSAIDs to help control swelling and inflammation. It is usually helpful to continue this medication throughout the rehabilitative process.[2]

Phase 2, the Repair Phase

Once the inflammatory response has subsided, the repair phase begins. During this stage of the healing process, fibroblastic cells are laying down a matrix of collagen fibers and forming scar tissue. This stage might begin as early as 2 days after the injury and can last for several weeks. At this point, swelling has stopped completely. The injury is still tender to the touch but is not as painful as was during the previous stage. Pain is also less on active and passive motion.[73]

As soon as inflammation is controlled, the therapist should immediately begin to incorporate into the rehabilitation program activities that can maintain levels of cardiorespiratory fitness, restore full range of motion, restore or increase strength, and reestablish neuromuscular control.

As in the acute phase, modalities should be used to control pain and swelling. Cryotherapy should still be used during the early portion of this phase to reduce the likelihood of swelling.

Electrical stimulating currents can help with controlling pain and improving strength and range of motion.[73]

Phase 3, the Remodeling Phase

The remodeling phase is the longest of the three phases and can last for several years, depending on the severity of the injury. The ultimate goal during this maturation stage of the healing process is return to activity. The injury is no longer painful to the touch, although some progressively deceasing pain might still be felt on motion. The collagen fibers must be realigned according to tensile stresses and strains placed upon them during functional exercises.

The focus during this phase should be on regaining functional skills. Functional training involves the repeated performance of movement or skill for the purpose of perfecting that skill. Strengthening exercises should progressively place on the injured structures stresses and strains that would normally be encountered during activity. Plyometric strengthening exercises can be used to improve muscle power and explosiveness.[40] Functional testing should be done to determine specific skill weaknesses that need to be addressed prior to normal activity return.

At this point some type of heating modality is beneficial to the healing process. The deep-heating modalities, ultrasound, or the diathermies should be used to increase circulation to the deeper tissues. Massage and gentle mobilization may also be used to reduce guarding, increase circulation, and reduce pain. Increased blood flow delivers the essential nutrients to the injured area to promote healing, and increased lymphatic flow assists in breakdown and removal of waste products.[73]

USING MEDICATIONS TO EFFECT THE HEALING PROCESS

Medications are most commonly used in rehabilitation for pain relief. Patient is continuously in pain that can be associated with even minor injury.

The over-the-counter nonnarcotic analgesics often used include aspirin (salicylate), acetaminophen, naproxen sodium ketoprofen, and ibuprofen. These belong to the group of drugs called NSAIDs. Aspirin is one of the most commonly used drugs in the world.[78] Because of its easy availability, it is also likely the most misused drug. Aspirin is a derivative of salicylic acid and is used for its analgesic, anti-inflammatory, and antipyretic capabilities.

Analgesia can result from several mechanisms. Aspirin can interfere with the transmission of painful impulses in the thalamus.[78] Soft-tissue injury leads to tissue necrosis. This tissue injury causes the release of arachidonic acid from phospholipid cell walls. Oxygenation of arachidonic acid by cyclooxygenase produces a variety of prostaglandins, thromboxane, and prostacyclin that mediate the subsequent inflammatory reaction.[2] The predominant mechanism of action of aspirin and other NSAIDs is the inhibition of prostaglandin synthesis by blocking the cyclooxygenase pathway.[95] Pain and inflammation are reduced by the blockage of accumulation of proinflammatory prostaglandins in the synovium or cartilage.

Stabilization of the lysosomal membrane also occurs, preventing the efflux of destructive lysosomal enzymes into the joints.[47] Aspirin is the only NSAID that irreversibly inhibits cyclooxygenase; the other NSAIDs provide reversible inhibition. Aspirin can also reduce fever by altering sympathetic outflow from the hypothalamus, which produces increased vasodilation and heat loss through sweating.[22,47] Among the side effects of aspirin usage are gastric distress, heartburn, some nausea, tinnitus, headache, and diarrhea. More serious consequences can develop with prolonged use or high dosages.[3]

Patient should be very cautious about selecting aspirin as a pain reliever, for a number of reasons. Aspirin inhibits aggregation of platelets and thus impairs the clotting mechanism should injury occur.[3] Aspirin's irreversible inhibition of cyclooxygenase, which leads to reduced production of clotting factors, creates a bleeding risk not present with the other NSAIDs.[94] Prolonged bleeding at an injured site will increase the amount of swelling, which has a direct effect on the time required for rehabilitation.

Use of aspirin as an anti-inflammatory medication should be recommended with caution. Other anti-inflammatory medications do not produce many of the undesirable side effects as that of aspirin. Generally prescription anti-inflammatories are considered to be equally effective.

Aspirin sometimes produces gastric discomfort. Buffered aspirin is no less irritating to the stomach than regular aspirin, but enteric-coated tablets resist aspirin breakdown in the stomach and might minimize gastric discomfort. Regardless of the form of aspirin ingested, it should be taken with meals or with large quantities of water (8–10 oz/tablet) to reduce the likelihood of gastric irritation.

Ibuprofen is classified as an NSAID; however, it also has analgesic and antipyretic effects, including the potential for gastric irritation. It does not affect platelet aggregation as aspirin does. Ibuprofen administered at a dose of 200 mg does not require a prescription and at that dosage may be used for analgesia. At a dose of 400 mg, the effects are both analgesic and anti-inflammatory.[9] Dosage forms greater than 200 mg require a prescription. For names and recommended doses of prescription NSAIDs, refer to Table 3-2.

Acetaminophen, like aspirin, has both analgesic and antipyretic effects, but it does not have significant anti-inflammatory capabilities. Acetaminophen is indicated for relief of mild somatic pain and fever reduction through mechanisms similar to those of aspirin.[3]

The primary advantage of acetaminophen is that it does not produce gastritis, irritation, or gastrointestinal bleeding. Likewise, it does not affect platelet aggregation and thus does not increase clotting time after an injury.[75]

For the patient who is not in need of an anti-inflammatory medication but who requires some pain-relieving medication

T A B L E   3 - 2

NSAIDs Frequently Used: Prescription Required

DRUG	DOSAGE RANGE (mg) AND FREQUENCY	MAXIMUM DAILY DOSE (mg)
Aspirin	325–650, every 4 hours	4000
Voltaren	50–75, twice a day	200
Cataflam	50–75, twice a day	200
Dolobid	500–1000, followed by 250–500 mg 2–3 times a day	1500
Nalfon	300–600, 3–4 times a day	3200
Motrin	400–800, 3–4 times a day	3200
Indocin	5–150, a day in 3–4 divided doses	200
Orudis	75, 3 times a day or 50 mg 4 times a day	300
Ponstel	500, followed by 250 mg every 6 hours	1000
Naprosyn	250–500, twice a day	1250
Anaprox	550, followed by 275 mg every 6–8 hours	1375
Feldene	20, per day	20
Clinoril	200, twice a day	400
Tolectin	400, 3–4 times a day	1800
Ansaid	50–100, 2–3 times a day	300
Toradol	10, every 4–6 hours for pain: Not to be used for more than 5 days	40
Lodine	200–400, every 6–8 hours for pain	1200
Relafin	1000, once or twice a day	2000
Myobic	7.5, once per day	15
Daypro	1200, once per day	1800

or an antipyretic, acetaminophen should be the drug of choice. If inflammation is a consideration, physician may elect to use a type of NSAID. Most NSAIDs are prescription medications that, like aspirin, have not only anti-inflammatory but also analgesic and antipyretic effects.[47] They are effective for patients who cannot tolerate aspirin because of associated gastrointestinal distress. Patients who have the aspirin allergy triad of (1) nasal polyps, (2) associated bronchospams/asthma, and (3) history of anaphylaxis should not receive any NSAID. Caution is advised when using NSAIDs in persons who might be subject to dehydration. NSAIDs inhibit prostaglandin synthesis and therefore can compromise the elaboration of prostaglandins within the kidney during salt and/or water deficits. This can lead to ischemia within the kidney.[47,63] Adequate hydration is essential to reduce the risk of renal toxicity in athletes taking NSAIDs.

NSAID anti-inflammatory capabilities are though to be equal to those of aspirin, their advantages being that NSAIDs have fewer side effects and relatively longer duration of action. NSAIDs have analgesic and antipyretic capabilities; the short-acting over-the-counter NSAIDs may be used in cases of mild headache or increased body temperature in place of aspirin or acetaminophen. They can be used to relieve many other mildly to moderately painful somatic conditions like menstrual cramps and soft-tissue injury.[9]

It has been recommended that patients receiving long-acting NSAIDs have monitoring of liver function enzymes during the course of therapy because of case reports of hepatic failure associated with the use of long-acting NSAIDs.[74]

The NSAIDs are used primarily for reducing the pain, stiffness, swelling, redness, and fever associated with localized inflammation, most likely by inhibiting the synthesis of prostaglandins.[9] The therapist must be aware that inflammation is simply a response to some underlying trauma or condition and that the source of irritation must be corrected or eliminated for these anti-inflammatory medications to be effective. Both naproxen and ketoprofen (now available without a prescription) have been shown to provide additional benefit when administered concomitantly with physical therapy.[63]

Muscle spasm and guarding accompany many musculoskeletal injuries. Elimination of this spasm and guarding should facilitate programs of rehabilitation. In many situations, centrally acting oral muscle relaxants are used to reduce spasm and guarding. However, to date the efficacy of using muscle relaxants has not been substantiated, and they do not appear to be superior to analgesics or sedatives in either acute or chronic conditions.[7]

Many analgesics and anti-inflammatory products are available over the counter in combination products (i.e., those containing two or more nonnarcotic analgesics with or without caffeine). Chronic use of analgesics containing aspirin and phenacetin or acetaminophen contributes to the development of papillary necrosis and analgesic-associated nephropathy. The presence of caffeine plays a role in dependency on these products leading to chronic use.

REHABILITATIVE PHILOSOPHY

The rehabilitation philosophy relative to inflammation and healing after injury is to assist the natural process of the body while doing no harm.[53] The course of rehabilitation chosen by the therapist must focus on their knowledge of the healing process and its therapeutic modifiers to guide, direct, and stimulate the structural function and integrity of the injured part. The primary goal should be to have a positive influence on the inflammation and repair process to expedite recovery of function in terms of range of motion, muscular strength and endurance, neuromuscular control, and cardiorespiratory endurance.[29] The therapist must try to minimize the early effects of excessive inflammatory processes including pain modulation, edema control, and reduction of associated muscle spasm, which can produce loss of joint motion and contracture. Finally, the therapist should concentrate on preventing the recurrence of injury by influencing the structural ability of the injured tissue to resist future overloads by incorporating various therapeutic exercises.[53] The subsequent chapters of this book can serve as a guide for the therapist in using the many different rehabilitation tools available.

SUMMARY

- The three phases of the healing process are the inflammatory-response phase, the fibroblastic-repair phase, and the maturation-remodeling phase. These occur in sequence but overlap one another in a continuum.
- Factors that can impede the healing process include edema, hemorrhage, lack of vascular supply, separation of tissue, muscle spasm, atrophy, corticosteroids, hypertrophic scars, infection, climate and humidity, age, health, and nutrition.
- The four fundamental types of tissues in the human body are epithelial, connective, muscle, and nerve tissues.
- Ligament sprains involve stretching or tearing the fibers that provide stability at the joint.
- Fractures can be classified as greenstick, transverse, oblique, spiral, comminuted, impacted, avulsive, or stress.
- Osteoarthritis involves degeneration of the articular cartilage or subchondral bone.
- Muscle strains involve a stretching or tearing of muscle fibers and their tendons and cause impairment to active movement.
- Tendinitis, an inflammation of a muscle tendon that causes pain on movement, usually occurs because of overuse.
- Tenosynovitis is an inflammation of the synovial sheath through which a tendon must slide during motion.
- Dislocations and subluxations involve disruption of the joint capsule and ligamentous structures surrounding the joint.
- Bursitis is an inflammation of the synovial membranes located in areas where friction occurs between various anatomic structures.

- Muscle soreness can be caused by spasm, connective tissue damage, muscle tissue damage, or some combination of these.
- Repeated contusions can lead to the development of myositis ossificans.
- All injuries should be initially managed with rest, ice, compression, and elevation to control swelling and thus reduce the time required for rehabilitation.
- A patient who requires an analgesic for pain relief should be given acetaminophen because aspirin may produce gastric upset and slow clotting time.
- For treating inflammation, NSAIDs are recommended because they do not produce many of the side effects associated with aspirin use.

REFERENCES

1. Allen T. Exercise-induced muscle damage: mechanisms, prevention, and treatment. *Physiother Can* 56(2):67–79, 2004.
2. Almekinders LC. Anti-inflammatory treatment of muscular injuries in sport: an update of recent studies. *Sports Med* 28(6):383–388, 1999.
3. Alper B. Evidence-based medicine. Update: acetaminophen effective in osteoarthritis (NSAIDs more effective). *Clin Adv Nurse Pract* 7(12):98–99, 2004.
4. Arnoczky SP. Physiologic principles of ligament injuries and healing. In: Scott WN, ed. *Ligament and Extensor Mechanism Injuries of the Knee*. St. Louis, MO, Mosby, 1991.
5. Athanasiou KA, Shah AR, Hernandez RJ, LeBaron RG. Basic science of articular cartilage repair. *Clin Sports Med* 20(2):223–247, 2001.
6. Bandy W, Dunleavy K. Adaptability of skeletal muscle: response to increased and decreased use. In: Zachazewski J, Magee D, Quillen W, eds. *Athletic Injuries and Rehabilitation*. Philadelphia, WB Saunders, 1996.
7. Beebe F. A clinical and pharmacologic review of skeletal muscle relaxants for musculoskeletal conditions. *Amer J Ther* 12(2):151–171, 2005.
8. Beiner J. Muscle contusion injury and myositis ossificans traumatica. *Clin Orthop Relat Res* 403S(Suppl):S110–119, 2002.
9. Biederman R. Pharmacology in rehabilitation: nonsteroidal anti-inflammatory agents. *J Orthop Sports Phys Ther* 35(6):356–367, 2005.
10. Bottoni C, Hart L. Recurrent shoulder dislocations after arthroscopic stabilization or nonoperative treatment. *Clin J Sport Med* 13(2):128–129, 2003.
11. Briggs J. Soft and bony tissues—injury, repair and treatment implications. In: Briggs J, ed. *Sports Therapy: Theoretical and Practical Thoughts and Considerations*. Chichester, UK, Corpus, 2001.
12. Booher JM, Thibodeau GA. *Athletic Injury Assessment*, 4th ed. St. Louis, MO, McGraw-Hill, 2000.
13. Brothers A. Basic clinical management of muscle strains and tears: following appropriate treatment, most patients can return to sports activity. *J Musculoskelet Med* 20(6):303–307, 2003.
14. Bryant MW. Wound healing. *CIBA Clin Symp* 29(3):2–36, 1997.
15. Burra G. Acute shoulder and elbow dislocations in the athlete. *Orthop Clin N Am* 33(3):479–495, 2002.
16. Butler D. Nerve structure, function, and physiology. In: Zachazewski J, Magee D, Quillen W, eds. *Athletic Injuries and Rehabilitation*. Philadelphia, WB Saunders, 1996.
17. Cailliet R. *Soft Tissue Pain and Disability*, 3rd ed. Philadelphia, FA Davis, 1996.
18. Carrico TJ, Mehrhof AI, Cohen IK. Biology and wound healing. *Surg Clin N Am* 64(4):721–734, 1984.
19. Clancy W. Tendon trauma and overuse injuries. In: Leadbetter W, Buckwalter J, Gordon S, eds. *Sports-Induced Inflammation*. Park Ridge, IL, American Academy of Orthopaedic Surgeons, 1990.
20. Clarkson PM, Tremblay I. Exercise-induced muscle damage, repair and adaptation in humans. *J Appl Physiol* 65:1–6, 1988.
21. Cox D. Growth factors in wound healing. *J Wound Care* 2(6):339–342, 1993.
22. Curtis J. A group randomized trial to improve safe use of nonsteroidal anti-inflammatory drugs. *Amer J Manag Care* 11(9):537–543, 2005.
23. Curwin S. Tendon injuries, pathophysiology and treatment. In: Zachazewski J, Magee D, Quillen W, eds. *Athletic Injuries and Rehabilitation*. Philadelphia, WB Saunders, 1996.
24. Damjanov I. *Anderson's Pathology*, 10th ed. St. Louis, MO, Mosby, 1996.
25. deVries HA. Quantitative EMG investigation of spasm theory of muscle pain. *Amer J Phys Med* 45:119–134, 1996.
26. Di Domenica F. Physical and rehabilitative approaches in osteoarthritis. *Semin Arthritis Rheum* 34(6; Suppl 2):62–69, 2005.
27. Dieppe P. Pathogenesis and management of pain in osteoarthritis. *Lancet* 365(9463):965–973, 2005.
28. Fantone J. Basic concepts in inflammation. In: Leadbetter W, Buckwalter J, Gordon S, eds. *Sportsinduced Inflammation*. Park Ridge, IL, American Academy of Orthopaedic Surgeons, 1990.
29. Felson D. Osteoarthritis. *Curr Opin Rheumatol* 17(5):624–656, 684–697, 2005.
30. Fitzgerald GK. Considerations for evaluation and treatment of overuse tendon injuries. *Athlet Ther Today* 5(4):14–19, 2000.
31. Frank C. Ligament injuries: pathophysiology and healing. In: Zachazewski J, Magee D, Quillen W, eds. *Athletic Injuries and Rehabilitation*. Philadelphia, WB Saunders, 1996.

32. Frank C, Shrive N, Hiraoka H, Nakamura N, Kaneda Y, Hart D. Optimization of the biology of soft tissue repair. *J Sci Med Sport* 2(3):190–210, 1990.

33. Gelberman R, Goldberg V, An K-N, et al. Soft tissue healing. In: Woo SL-Y, Buckwalter J, eds. *Injury and Repair of Musculoskeletal Soft Tissues.* Park ridge, IL, American Academy of Orthopaedic Surgeons, 1988.

34. Glick JM. Muscle strains: prevention and treatment. *Physician Sports Med* 8(11):73–77, 1980.

35. Goldenberg M. Wound care management: proper protocol differs from athletic trainers' perceptions. *J Athlet Train* 31(1):12–16, 1996.

36. Gradisar IA. Fracture stabilization and healing. In: Gould JA, Davies GJ, eds. *Orthopaedic and Sports Physical Medicine.* St. Louis, MO, Mosby, 1985.

37. Gross A, Cutright D, Bhaskar S, et al. Effectiveness of pulsating water jet lavage in treatment of contaminated crush wounds. *Amer J Surg* 124:73–75, 1972.

38. Guyton AC, Hell J. *Pocket Companion to Textbook of Medical Physiology.* Philadelphia, WB Saunders, 2006.

39. Hart L. Effects of stretching on muscle soreness and risk of injury: a meta-analysis. *Clin J Sport Med* 13(5):321–322, 2003.

40. Henning CE. Semilunar cartilage of the knee: function and pathology. In: Pandolf KB, ed. *Exercise and Sport Science Review.* New York, Macmillan, 1988.

41. Hettinga DL. Inflammatory response of synovial joint structures. In: Gould JA, Davies GJ, eds. *Orthopaedic and Sports Physical Therapy.* St. Louis, MO, Mosby, 1985.

42. Hole J. *Human Anatomy and Physiology.* St. Louis, MO, McGraw-Hill, 1997.

43. Houglum P. Soft tissue healing and its impact on rehabilitation. *J Sport Rehabil* 1(1):19–39, 1992.

44. Hubbel S, Buschbacher R. Tissue injury and healing: using medications, modalities, and exercise to maximize recovery. In: Bushbacher R, Branddom R, eds. *Sports Medicine and Rehabilitation: A Sport Specific Approach.* Philadelphia, Hanley & Belfus, 1994.

45. James CB, Uhl TL. A review of articular cartilage pathology and the use of glucosamine sulfate. *J Athlet Train* 39(4):413–419, 2001.

46. Junge T. Bone healing. *Surg Technol* 34(5):26–29, 2002.

47. Kaplan R. Current status of nonsteroidal anti-inflammatory drugs in physiatry: balancing risks and benefits in pain management. *Amer J Phys Med Rehabil* 84(11):885–894, 2005.

48. Khan KM, Cook JL, Taunton JE, Bonar F. Overuse tendinosis, not tendinitis. Part 1: a new paradigm for a difficult clinical problem. *Physician Sports Med* 28(5): 38–43, 47–48, 2000.

49. Kelly A. Managing stress fractures in athletes. *J Musculoskelet Med* 22(9):463–465, 468–470, 472, 2005.

50. Kibler WB. Concepts in exercise rehabilitation of athletic injury. In: Leadbetter W, Buckwalter J, Gordon S, eds.

51. Kibler W. Current concepts in tendinopathy. *Clin Sports Med* 22(4):xi, xiii, 675–684, 2003.

52. Knight KL. *Cryotherapy in Sport Injury Management.* Champaign, IL, Human Kinetics, 1995.

53. Leadbetter W. Introduction to sports-induced soft-tissue inflammation. In: Leadbetter W, Buckwalter J, Gordon S, eds. *Sports-Induced Inflammation.* Park Ridge, IL, American Academy of Orthopaedic Surgeons, 1990.

54. Leadbetter W, Buckwalter J, Gordon S. *Sports-Induced Inflammation.* Park Ridge, IL, American Academy of Orthopaedic Surgeons, 1990.

55. Loitz-Ramage B, Zernicke R. Bone biology and mechanics. In: Zachazewski J, Magee D, Quillen W, eds. *Athletic Injuries and Rehabilitation.* Philadelphia, WB Saunders, 1996.

56. Maffulli N, Benazzo F. Basic science of tendons. *Sports Med Arthrosc Rev* 8(1):1–5, 2000.

57. Marchesi VT. Inflammation and healing. In: Kissane JM, ed. *Andersons' Pathology*, 9th ed. St. Louis, MO, Mosby, 1996.

58. Martinez-Hernanadez A, Amenta P. Basic concepts in wound healing. In: Leadbetter W, Buckwalter J, Gordon S, eds. *Sports-Induced Inflammation.* Park Ridge, IL, American Academy of Orthopaedic Surgeons, 1990.

59. Matheson G, MacIntyre J, Taunton J. Musculoskeletal injuries associated with physical activity in older adults. *Med Sci Sports Exerc* 21:379–385, 1989.

60. Malone T, Garrett W, Zachewski J. Muscle: deformation, injury and repair. In: Zachazewski J, Magee D, Quillen W, eds. *Athletic Injuries and Rehabilitation.* Philadelphia, WB Saunders, 1996.

61. Malone T, McPhoil T, eds. *Orthopaedic and Sports Physical Therapy.* St. Louis, MO, Mosby, 1997.

62. Mayo Clinic. Fracture healing: what it takes to heal a break. *Mayo Clin Health Lett* 20(2):1–3, 2002.

63. McCormack K, Brune K. Toward defining the analgesic role of non-steroidal anti-inflammatory drugs in the management of acute and soft tissue injuries. *Sports Med* 3:106–117, 1993.

64. Mehta J. Elbow dislocations in adults and children. *Clin Sports Med* 23(4):609–627, 2004.

65. Murrell GAC, Jang D, Lily E, Best T. The effects of immobilization and exercise on tendon healing—abstract. *J Sci Med Sport* 2(1 Suppl):40, 1999.

66. Levangie P, Norkin C. *Joint Structure and Function: A Comprehensive Analysis.* Philadelphia, FA Davis, 2005.

67. Norris S, Provo B, Stotts N. Physiology of wound healing and risk factors that impede the healing process. *AACN Clin Issues Crit Care Nurs* 1(3):545–552, 1990.

68. Ng G. Ligament injury and repair: current concepts. *Hong Kong Physiother J* 20:22–29, 2002.

69. O'Reilly K, Warhol M, Fielding R, et al. Eccentric exercise induced muscle damage impairs muscle glycogen depletion. *J Appl Physiol* 63:252–256, 1987.

70. Panush RS, Brown DG. Exercise and arthritis. *Sports Med* 4:54–64, 1987.

71. Peterson L, Renstrom P. Injuries in musculoskeletal tissues. In: Peterson L, ed. *Sports Injuries: Their Prevention and Treatment*, 3rd ed. Champaign, IL, Human Kinetics, 2001.

72. Prentice W. *Arnheim's Principles of Athletic Training*, 12th ed. St. Louis, MO, McGraw-Hill, 2006.

73. Prentice W.E., ed. *Therapeutic Modalities in Sports Medicine and Athletic Training*. St. Louis, MO, McGraw-Hill, 2003.

74. Purdum P, Shelden S, Boyd J. Oxaprozininduced hepatitis. *Ann Pharmacother* 28:1159–1161, 1994.

75. Rahusen F. Nonsteroidal anti-inflammatory drugs and acetaminophen in the treatment of an acute muscle injury. *Amer J Sports Med* 32(8):1856–1859, 2004.

76. Robbins SL, Cotran RS, Kumar V. *Pathologic Basis of Disease*, 3rd ed. Philadelphia, WB Saunders, 1984.

77. Rywlin AM. Hemopoietic system. In: Kissane JM, ed. *Anderson's Pathology*, 8th ed. St. Louis, MO, Mosby, 1996.

78. Sachs C. Oral analgesics for acute nonspecific pain. *Amer Fam Physician* 71(5):913–918, 847–849, 2005.

79. Saladin K. *Anatomy and Physiology*. New York, McGraw-Hill, 2006.

80. Sanderlin B. Common stress fractures. *Amer Fam Physician* 68(8):1527–1532, 1478–1479, 2003.

81. Sandrey MA. Effects of acute and chronic pathomechanics on the normal histology and biomechanics of tendons: a review. *J Sport Rehabil* 9(4):339–352, 2000.

82. Schenck R. Classification of knee dislocations. *Oper Tech Sports Med* 11(3):193–198, 2003.

83. Seeley R, Stephens T, Tate P. *Anatomy and Physiology*. St. Louis, MO, McGraw-Hill, 2005.

84. Seller RH. *Differential Diagnosis of Common Complaints*. Philadelphia, Elsevier Health Services, 1999.

85. Sharma P. Tendon injury and tendinopathy: healing and repair. *J Bone Joint Surg* 87A(1):187–202, 2005.

86. Shrier I, Stovitz S. Best of the literature. Do anti-inflammatory agents promote muscle healing? *Physician Sports Med* 33(6):12, 2005.

87. Stanish WD, Curwin S, Mandell S. *Tendinitis: Its Etiology and Treatment*. Oxford, Oxford University Press, 2000.

88. Soto-Quijano D. Work-related musculoskeletal disorders of the upper extremity. *Crit Rev Phys Rehabil Med* 17(1):65–82, 2005.

89. Stewart J. *Clinical Anatomy and Physiology*. Miami, FL, MedMaster, 2001.

90. Stone MH. Implications for connective tissue and bone alterations resulting from rest and exercise training. *Med Sci Sports Exerc* 20(5):S162–168, 1988.

91. Terry M, Fincher AL. Postoperative management of articular cartilage repair. *Athlet Ther Today* 5(2):57–58, 2000.

92. Tuan K. Stress fractures in athletes: risk factors, diagnosis, and management. *Orthopedics* 27(6):583–593, 2004.

93. Van de Graaff K. *Human Anatomy*. New York, McGraw-Hill, 2006.

94. Vane J. Inhibition of prostaglandin synthesis as a mechanism of action for aspirin-like drugs. *Nature (New Biol)* 231:232–235, 1971.

95. Vane J. The evolution of nonsteroidal anti-inflammatory drugs and their mechanism of action. *Drugs* 33(1):18–27, 1987.

96. Walker J. Cartilage of human joints and related structures. In: Zachazewski J, Magee D, Quillen W, eds. *Athletic Injuries and Rehabilitation*. Philadelphia, WB Saunders, 1996.

97. Wahl S, Renstrom P. Fibrosis in soft-tissue injuries. In: Leadbetter W, Buckwalter J, Gordon S, eds. *Sports-Induced Inflammation*. Park ridge, IL, American Academy of Orthopaedic Surgeons, 1990.

98. Wells PE, Frampton V, Bowsher D. *Pain Management in Physical Therapy*. Norwalk, CT, Appleton & Lange, 1988.

99. Wilder R. Overuse injuries: tendinopathies, stress fractures, compartment syndrome, and shin splints. *Clin Sports Med* 23(1):55–81, 2004.

100. Wissen WT. An aggressive approach to managing quadriceps contusions. *Athlet Ther Today* 5(1):36–37, 2000.

101. Woo SL-Y, Buckwalter J, eds. *Injury and Repair of Musculoskeletal Soft Tissues*. Park Ridge, IL, American Academy of Orthopaedic Surgeons, 1988.

102. Wroble RR. Articular cartilage injury and autologous chondrocyte implantation: which patients might benefit? *Phys Sports Med* 28(11):43–49, 2000.

103. Zachezewski J. Flexibility for sports. In: Sanders B, ed. *Sports Physical Therapy*. Norwalk, CT, Appleton & Lange, 1990.

CHAPTER 4

The Neuromusculoskeletal Scan Examination

John S. Halle

O B J E C T I V E S

After completing this chapter, the therapist should be able to do the following:

- List and discuss the basic purposes of a scan examination as outlined in this chapter.
- Describe how a scan examination is fundamentally different from an algorithm.
- Discuss the potential role of a prescreening questionnaire in a scan examination.
- Compare and contrast the basic elements of a scan examination to the "five elements of patient/client management," which are described in "The Guide to Physical Therapy Practice."[6]
- List the five elements of the scan examination outlined in this chapter, and summarize the key information that should be obtained from each of those topic areas.
- Describe the vital informational elements derived from each of the following items that are part of the patient history portion of the examination:
  a. Age
  b. Gender
  c. Ethnic makeup
  d. Morphology
  e. Family history
  f. Past medical history
  g. Medications
  h. Mechanism of injury
  i. a.m./p.m. pattern of pain
  j. Nature of pain
  k. Training history
- Within a scan examination, "clearing tests" are typically used. Explain the role and limitations associated with clearing tests.
- Explain what is meant by the terms "Yellow flags" and "Red flags."
- Additionally, when a yellow or red flag finding is identified, discuss the response options available.

PURPOSE OF A SCAN EXAMINATION

Everyone has a concept in their mind about scanning a given situation. When driving and intersections are encountered, a system is employed that examines what is occurring off in the distance, as well as any potential issues that might be coming from the right and left. Attention is also paid to the existence of signs or traffic lights, any obstacles like parked cars or debris in the roadway, and anything out of the ordinary that could signal high risk, such as children playing with a ball. Additionally, in the back of the driver's mind, factors such as the amount of light available due to the time of day, the condition of the road, weather conditions, and the type of vehicle being driven, are all factored into the mix. With this information, the driver is able to successfully scan the intersection and make all needed adjustments to either stop and respond to a potential emergency or pass through this point in space.

The two most important elements that allow the scan described above to work time after time are the employment of a system and experience. When starting to drive, most individuals learn the rules of the road and know to obey traffic lights. When a light turns green, movement into the intersection is started, and on a rare occasion, the car is broadsided. This accident occurs because even though the driver was obeying the rules of the road, the limited system of the typical neophyte drivers does not take the time to additionally check that the other vehicles in their vicinity are also complying with the rules and not trying to push that yellow–red light that they have encountered. This comes with experience and experience takes time and practice.

What does the above have to do with a scan examination performed on a patient? It is a metaphor that illustrates several important points. First, everyone is familiar with the concept of scanning something. A scan is an efficient and relatively quick appraisal of a situation that does not look for every fact, but works extremely hard to identify key facts and insure that all high-risk situations are identified and addressed. Second, the scan is based on a system. Without a system, holes will develop and some of the key facts identified in the first point will be missed. When put in the context of patient care, the potential lack of a system results in less than optimal care, and on occasion, will result in a negative outcome for the patient. In situations like driving, these systems often develop over time with experience and are largely based on visual information. In the realm of patient care, the scan examination is biased to a heavier didactic base that requires the linkage of specific knowledge with pathologies/injuries. While this improves with experience, the system should ideally be very tight from the beginning, for the provision of competent medical care from the first patient seen to the one most recently evaluated. This requires study and a system that is both simple enough to be implemented with all patients examined, and flexible enough that it allows modification based on the region of the body evaluated or on the specific situation. The information gained from this system will be used to develop a working hypothesis regarding what might be underlying cause of the patient's problem. Third, while a quick and nonexhaustive appraisal of the situation, the scan forms the foundational elements for a more detailed examination, either at the initial visit or during a follow-up visit. Fourth, implementation of a scan examination is an efficient way to gain an understanding of the reason that the patient is seeking care. The scan examination provides enough information to develop an excellent grasp of what the patients are seeking and whether or not they have come to the health care provider who is best suited to address the issue. Last, and perhaps most importantly, the scan examination looks for potential pathology that requires referral or immediate care, so that serious or life-threatening pathology is not missed. This key

point goes directly to a point that is often (incorrectly) credited to the Hippocratic oath of "first, do no harm."[23] (While "do no harm" expresses some of the general sentiment of the Hippocratic oath and is a primary goal of all health care providers, the phrase is not included as part of the oath, but rather as part of another writing of Hippocrates[23]). Purposes of the scan examination are summarized as follows:

- Used to develop a working hypothesis (assists with ruling potential causes "in" or "out").
- Is based on a system that is both manageable (simple) and adaptable.
- Provides the basis of why the patient has presented for care.
- Identifies pathologies/problems that require immediate care or referral (a key purpose of the scan examination).

CAVEATS TO CONSIDER WHEN PERFORMING A SCAN EXAMINATION

Prior to getting into the "the specific pieces" that make up the typical scan examination, there are a few caveats that should be addressed. First, while a scan examination is by design quick and efficient, it is not another name for taking shortcuts. Whenever the responsibility for examining patients is accepted, they deserve the health care practitioner's full attention and review in a way that will serve them properly. This leads to the second caveat of having a system that is implemented *every time* a patient is examined. Only with a system will all the basic elements needed to scan the patient be included every time. The system also keeps the practitioner from being myopic; examining only what appears to be obvious. Instead, a system requires that outside possibilities involving other biological systems are reviewed every time an evaluation is performed, and occasionally, this is the truly important information. Third, take notes or use a template while performing the scan examination. Research has shown that health care providers do a better job of accurately summarizing what was observed during the examination if they record information during the examination, and do not try to reconstruct findings from memory at a later time.[81,90,92] If you are basing decisions on your evaluation, then you are obligated to take notes along the way to insure that the summary report is accurate. Fourth, the scan examination is *not* an algorithm. Rather, it is a framework that has specific points that can be applied to a variety of situations. (A discussion of algorithms follows in Chapter 5.) Since it is a framework, it is as adaptable as required and can be used for an upper quarter evaluation, a lower quarter evaluation, or as part of some other requirement. For the purposes of this description, most of the examples provided will be with either upper or lower quarter examinations, since they are the most common application of the scan examination process. Last, physical examination procedures will be used as part of the scan examination that are occasionally called "clearing tests." The basic purpose of these tests is to assist in ruling an area in or out, as a source of the

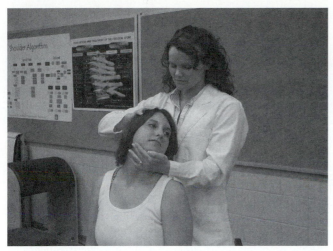

FIGURE 4-1

Example of a Spurling's test (foraminal encroachment test).

patient's problem. An example in the upper quarter screen is a foraminal encroachment test (Spurling's) that is intended to provoke symptoms in patients with a radiculopathy due to an intervertebral foraminal stenosis (see Fig. 4-1, illustrating Spurling's test). A positive foraminal encroachment test suggests that a working hypothesis of cervical radiculopathy is a viable consideration, and further tests should be performed to see if there is any collaborative evidence. Few practitioners have difficulty building on the results of a positive test. Negative findings for a test of this type are often interpreted as "ruling out" the cervical spine as a source of the patient's problem. This is where a caveat or warning needs to be stated. Since no physical exam test has absolute sensitivity or specificity (and many have only fair to good sensitivity and specificity), a negative finding is only one piece of collaborative information that needs to be viewed in light of all the information. Thus, in the presence of a negative foraminal encroachment test, the neck has not been ruled out. Rather, a clear-cut neck problem has not been demonstrated, but the entirety of the information provided by the scan examination will need to be reviewed and patterns or tests that collaborate each other will need to be identified, and applied to the working hypothesis.

CONCEPTUAL SIMILARITIES AND DIFFERENCES BETWEEN A SCAN EXAMINATION AND THE "FIVE ELEMENTS OF PATIENT/CLIENT MANAGEMENT"

Both the scan examination and the elements of patient/client management outlined in the Guide to Physical Therapy Practice[6] (2nd edition, p. 133), are systemic ways of approaching a patient, in an attempt to provide high-quality care. Thus, these two systems are much more similar than they are different. The key difference is that the scan examination is an approach that is typically applied to patients presenting with neuromusculoskeletal complaints, and it is performed as either an upper or lower quarter screen. The Guide to Physical Therapy Practice, on the other hand, has developed the five elements of patient/client management that can be used as a system to approach virtually any type of patient, ranging from a pediatric patient with a permanent neurological condition to a patient with a serious injury to the integument, such as a burn patient. Thus, while the scan examination as outlined here is adaptable beyond the upper and lower quarter, those two regions are the primary focus of scan examinations. In having that focus, the system built will probably have a little more specificity for patients that fall into the neuromusculoskeletal realm, rather than the guide's system that is applicable to all patient categories.

Additionally, small elements of the examination are handled a little differently by each of these approaches. Both systems begin the evaluation with a history and both also consider a wide range of possible reasons for the presenting problem. The scan examination typically has some built-in "systems review" questions that are part of the history, while the guide outlines the systems review as a second step that immediately follows the history. This example of a small difference is largely a semantic one; however, since each is working to accomplish the same task of recognizing the underlying reason for the patient's presentation to insure a pattern of intervention or referral that is based on facts that span each of the major systems: cardiovascular/pulmonary, integumentary, musculoskeletal, and neuromuscular. A second semantic difference is that the scan examination described here will work to identify a specific pathoanatomical dysfunction, while the guide works within movement-based diagnostic categories known as practice patterns.[6] The pathoanatomical approach is the historical way of addressing neuromuscular and musculoskeletal problems within fields like orthopedics and sports medicine. Within those areas, a pathoanatomical focus and description helps facilitate clear communication. Having made that observation, a well-rounded practitioner will be able to articulate the patient's problem with the language associated with either of these two models, depending on the environment. Thus, it could be easily argued that the scan examination to be described below is simply a repackaged version of the five elements of patient/client management model: ([1] examination, [2] evaluation, [3] diagnosis, [4] prognosis, and [5] intervention), which also recognizes that individuals will approach patients in their own unique way with their own individualized system. While making that recognition, the strength of both these approaches is that these are holistic and utilize a system to provide quality patient care.

OVERVIEW OF THE SCAN EXAMINATION

As mentioned previously, two of the features needed for an effective scan examination are that the exam needs to be relatively easy to remember and adaptable. While the labels assigned as memory markers can be anything that makes sense to the examiner, the familiar SOAP (subjective, objective, assessment, and plan), note format will be used here, with one modification. Rather than the traditional SOAP format, a SOAGP (with the "g" representing goals) will be used as the framework for the scan examination. Additionally, since the focus of this chapter is on the examination and not treatment options, the emphasis of this chapter will be on the initial three elements of subjective, objective, and assessment, with only minor coverage of the goals and plans. (Please note that while goals and plans are de-emphasized here, there is no suggestion that these elements are not important. Other chapters of this book address these sections of the entire exam process in greater detail (e.g., see Chapter 23 for additional ideas about treatment plans)).

The basic elements of scan examination model used are the following:

1. Subjective—(History, systems review, yellow and red flags[33]—the patient's basic information and symptoms)
2. Objective—(Evaluative tests and signs elicited from the patient)
3. Assessment—(Refinement of working hypothesis(es) [normally via deductive thinking], into one or more specific problems/dysfunctions, that are supported by collaborative information)
4. Goal—(Based on patient's desires and needs, within the realm of reason—should be stated in terms of both short- and long-term goals)
5. Plan—(Measurable steps designed to accomplish point 4, the goal" listed above).

The above-mentioned elements provide a framework of labels that describe the basic elements of the examination process. The detail for each section is provided below.

Subjective or the Patient History

An old axiom is that "chance (or luck) favors the prepared mind,"[75] which applies strongly to this portion of the examination process. While the patient history might be viewed as a time to ask the patient simply, "why are you here?" a well-done history is foundational to the scan examination. If ranked in a hierarchy, this may be the most important element of the entire examination process for several reasons. It has been said that approximately 80 percent of the information needed to determine what is wrong with a patient can be gleaned from a well-organized history.[40,89] Additionally, this is the primary place in the examination where the evaluator has the opportunity to understand the patient's concerns, identify potential yellow and red flags,[33] and this is the place where a quick systems review is most easily accomplished. Thus, the patient history should be approached with the understanding that the time spent is valuable and there should be a clear purpose to every question asked. An effective patient history will only occur if the evaluator employs a well-organized system and if the evaluator has the didactic background to convert the responses obtained from the

patient into working hypotheses based on the body's physiologic response to some form of abnormal anatomy. For example, if a patient with cervical pain that radiates to the shoulder indicates that the pain is largely relieved when resting the involved forearm on the head, he/she has provided valuable information on a working radiculopathy hypothesis. The abducted position of the shoulder allows the cervical nerve roots to be in a position of relative slack and often decreases the symptoms associated with intervertebral foraminal encroachment. This information can be factored into the findings, if the evaluator is aware of what the patient is telling him/her with the previous description.

The history typically starts with some of the housekeeping information that is needed to paint a picture of the patient. Factors such as the patient's age, gender, and ethnic background are ascertained. These pieces of information are valuable in that specific problems occur either to a much greater frequency or exclusively in individuals of a certain age, gender, or ethnic groups. As an example, a slipped capital femoral epiphysis typically occurs in individuals between 10 and 15 years of age, and is twice as common in males as in females.[88] Thus, both age and gender are key elements that are factored into the prepared mind when considering the presenting patient. Additionally, while getting slightly ahead of the development of this section, these patients will also report that they have thigh or knee pain, which is due to the referral pattern of pain from the femoral head.[88] Thus, the anatomic characteristics of referred pain and the high index of suspicion of the joint above and joint below need to be considered when listening to the patient.

In an effort to keep the subjective portion of the scan examination brief, many if not all of these important background pieces of information can be obtained through a questionnaire that the patient fills out prior to being interviewed. Using a questionnaire has a number of advantages that include the following: (1) provides a built-in system that prevents important information from being overlooked, (2) provides documentation without taking the health care provider's time, (3) utilizes the patients' time while they are waiting to be seen, and (4) a questionnaire is efficient and is a way to accurately collect much more information than typically will be obtained by asking individual questions. It has been shown that in a physical therapy orthopedic setting, the overall percentage of agreement across questionnaire items done as part of a self-administered questionnaire versus a detailed patient–self report by an experienced health care practitioner was 96 percent.[12] In light of the time savings and documentation benefits offered by this type of questionnaire, its use in a clinical setting should be seriously considered (see Table 4-1 for an example of a questionnaire that could be used with men and women—other excellent questionnaires are provided elsewhere[12,58,74]).

Once the basic information on the patient has been obtained, the history turns to the specific reason that the patient has sought care. This phase of the history typically begins with open-ended questions designed to elicit, in the patient's words, what is wrong. Open-ended questions are those that allow the patients to describe in their own terms what the problem is,

TABLE 4-1

Preevaluation Questionnaire, with Special Questions for Women and Men

DATE:
PATIENT'S NAME: DOB: AGE:
DIAGNOSIS: DATE OF ONSET:
PHYSICIAN: THERAPIST

                                                                              PRECAUTIONS:

| *MEDICAL HISTORY* | | **DO NOT COMPLETE: FOR THE THERAPIST** | | |
| HAVE YOU OR ANY IMMEDIATE FAMILY | | RELATION TO | DATE OF | CURRENT |
MEMBER EVER BEEN TOLD YOU HAVE:	CIRCLE ONE:	PATIENT	ONSET	STATUS
Cancer	Yes No			
Diabetes	Yes No			
Hypoglycemia	Yes No			
High blood pressure	Yes No			
Heart disease	Yes No			
Angina or chest pain	Yes No			
Shortness of breath	Yes No			
Stroke	Yes No			
Kidney disease/stones	Yes No			
Urinary tract infection	Yes No			
Allergies	Yes No			
Asthma, hay fever	Yes No			
Rheumatic/scarlet fever	Yes No			
Hepatitis/jaundice	Yes No			
Cirrhosis/liver disease	Yes No			
Polio	Yes No			
Chronic bronchitis	Yes No			
Pneumonia	Yes No			
Emphysema	Yes No			
Migraine headaches	Yes No			
Anemia	Yes No			
Ulcers/stomach problems	Yes No			
Arthritis/gout	Yes No			
Other	Yes No			

Medical testing

1. Are you taking any prescription or over-the-counter medications?   Yes   No
   If yes, please list:
2. Have you had any X-rays or other scans (e.g., MRI, etc.) done recently?   Yes   No
   If yes, when and what were the results?
3. Have you had any laboratory work done recently   Yes   No
   (e.g., urinalysis or blood tests)
   If yes, when and what were the results?
4. Please list any operations that you have had and the approximate date of the surgery(ies):

General health

1. Have you had any recent illnesses within the last 3 weeks   Yes   No
   (e.g., colds, influenza, bladder or kidney infection, other)?
2. Have you noted any lumps or thickening of skin or muscle anywhere on your body?   Yes   No

(Continued)

T A B L E   4 - 1

(Continued)

MEDICAL HISTORY		DO NOT COMPLETE: FOR THE THERAPIST		
HAVE YOU OR ANY IMMEDIATE FAMILY MEMBER EVER BEEN TOLD YOU HAVE:	CIRCLE ONE:	RELATION TO PATIENT	DATE OF ONSET	CURRENT STATUS

3. Do you have any sores that have not healed or any changes in size, shape, or color of a wart or mole? .... Yes No

4. Have you had any unexplained weight loss in the past several months? ... Yes No

5. Do you smoke or chew tobacco? .... Yes No
   If yes, how many packs per day?
   For how many months or years?

6. Do you drink alcohol? .... Yes No
   If yes, how much do you typically drink in the course of a week?

7. Do you consume caffeine? .... Yes No
   If yes, how much in a typical week (to include coffee, tea, chocolate, and soft drinks)?

8. Are you on any special diet prescribed by a physician? .... Yes No

Special questions for women
1. Date of last Pap smear examination:
2. Date of last breast examination by a physician:
3. Do you perform monthly self-breast examinations? .... Yes No
4. Do you take birth control pills or use an intrauterine device? .... Yes No

Special questions for men
1. Do you ever have difficulty with urination (e.g., starting or stopping the flow of urine, or have a very slow flow)? .... Yes No
2. Do you ever have blood in your urine? .... Yes No
3. Do you ever have pain on urination? .... Yes No

Work environment
1. Occupation:
2. Does your job involve:
   a. Prolonged sitting (e.g., desk, computer, truck driver) .... Yes No
   b. Prolonged standing (e.g., equipment operator, sales clerk) .... Yes No
   c. Prolonged walking (e.g., delivery service, etc.) .... Yes No
   d. Frequent and repetitive use of large or small equipment .... Yes No
   e. Prolonged lifting, bending, twisting, climbing, turning .... Yes No
   f. Exposure to chemicals or gases .... Yes No
   g. Other: please describe
3. Do you use any special supports, such as:
   a. Back cushion or neck support .... Yes No
   b. Back brace or corset .... Yes No
   c. Other kind of brace or support for any body part .... Yes No

For the physical therapist
Vital signs:
   Resting heart rate:
   Oral temperature:
   Blood pressure:

(Source: Reproduced from Goodman C, Snyder T. *Differential Diagnosis in Physical Therapy.* Philadelphia, WB Saunders, 1990, pp. 15–17, with permission from Elsevier.)

how they believed it occurred, and how long they have been living with the symptoms that are present. While providing this time for open-ended questions, the clinician may need to work to keep the patient focused on information relevant to the scan examination. Since time is in short supply, the time spent with open-ended questions should not be a time of idle conversation, but a time that paints a picture of the problem. Once that picture has been painted, then it is time for the therapist to begin asking specific questions that are closed-ended and have very brief responses. These questions should all have a specific purpose and potentially reveal something about the patient's underlying problem. For example, asking about what makes the pain (typically what brings a patient into the clinic), better or worst, addresses a basic truism associated with neuromusculoskeletal pathology; via positioning, range of motion, or pressure, a neuromusculoskeletal problem can have the nature of pain changed. If, on the other hand, there is no change in any position or posture, then serious consideration needs to be given to the fact that this problem may lie outside of the scope of a therapist and a referral might be warranted. These probing questions are generally close-ended; they provide the therapist with an opportunity to explore potential yellow or red flags and are used to explore a brief systems review (see Table 4-2 for a description of yellow flags, red flags, and systems review). Effectively performed, this questioning process will be built on a system, permit individualization for each patient seen, and will be accomplished and recorded within 5–10 minutes.

Prior to providing an example of the subjective (history) portion of the examination, it is important to address several other points. These include the following: (1) Recognizing that while the label most frequently used with this section is "subjective," this does not mean that the information provided by a patient is either of less value than that obtained by a physical examination or that the information is even subjective. Rothstein, in an editorial on subjective and objective measures,[82] eloquently describes that measures that are often considered to be entirely subjective, such as pain, can be quantified in a very objective way. Additionally, information that is typically grouped under the heading "subjective," such as age, race, and gender, is not subjective information at all. In fact, these may be examples of the most objective information obtained in the entire examination. Therefore, the occasional tendency to favor information obtained during the physical exam portion (objective) over that obtained from the patient should be resisted. Both sources of information are vital. Part of the art associated with the interpretation of the information collected is to recognize that while differing elements of the total scan examination may be more reliable than others, it is not as simple as elevating the objective portion of the examination over the subjective portion.[82] (2) Recognize that pain or lack of function is what typically brings a patient in to be seen, but that the pain is not the problem. There is an underlying cause of the patient's pain or lack of function. A key purpose of the scan examination is to attempt to identify the underlying cause, and then bring forth a plan that is able to address the problem. Therefore, acknowl-

edge that pain is an important symptom, but do not be led by it. Respect it, and then attempt to determine its underlying cause. Acknowledge it for the patient's validation, but do not focus on it as the hallmark of success of failure associated with the intervention. While more will be said on this later, scenarios can be developed where a patient would have an increased amount of pain in a follow-up visit, yet the therapist could be pleased with the progress. In the treatment of radicular low back pain (LBP) with pain radiating down the gluteal region, posterior thigh, to the popliteal fossa, an intervention might be McKenzie style[63] back extension exercises. On a follow-up visit, the pain might be centralized to only the low back region, with pain in that region as great or greater than what was experienced initially. Yet, due to the centralization of symptoms, this might be considered a positive development and that treatment plan is reinforced and continued. Had the therapist been led only by pain, the increase in pain would have resulted in an abandonment of the approach that was intended to address the underlying cause of the initial pain. (3) When patients provide answers to specific questions, such as "are you experiencing any tingling or decreased sensation," require specificity. To a question like the preceding one, many patients will express something like "I have numbness in my right hand." The follow-up questions that require specificity will focus in on items like (a) which side of the hand is affected (palmar aspect, dorsal aspect, or both), (b) which finger/fingers is/are affected, (c) are the fingertips affected, (d) is the area affected truly numb, or if a pin is stuck in it will you feel it, and (e) is the altered sensation constant or associated with a given time of day or activity? From this type of follow-up that requires very specific responses, the examiner is able to sort out dermatomes, innervation patterns of specific cutaneous nerves, potential polyneuropathies, potential vascular involvement and positioning or temporal events that enhance the symptoms. This will be a level of specificity that the patients are not used to, and will often be met with them having to think about what exactly is involved. Yet, in the hands of an evaluator that has a firm didactic grasp of the pertinent anatomy and pathophysiology, this line of specific questioning will permit the formulation of clear hypotheses that can be directly tested. (4) Require specificity from the patients when they are describing the mechanism of injury. The patients are seeking help and they know prior to making an appointment that the health care provider will want to know "how did this happen?" Since the patients anticipate this, they will think back and try to associate any reasonable temporal event with their current problem. It might be that the individual presenting with LBP recalls that a week before the symptoms developed, he/she was on an amusement park ride. While no discomfort was noted at the time, in thinking back, that was the only event out of the ordinary and the patient therefore attributes their symptoms to this event. While intended to help the evaluator, this information could be counterproductive, since apart from timing, there is nothing that really links this event to this episode of LBP. Specificity in questioning is required to determine if there is a clear mechanism of injury, or if the patient is simply

T A B L E   4 - 2

Definition of Yellow and Red Flags, and *Abridged* List of Yellow and Red Flag Questions

Yellow flags: A yellow flag is metaphorically similar to a yield sign. It indicates a finding that requires some additional attention and follow-up, and *may* warrant a referral to a specialist. (Follow-up questions and the rest of the physical examination will help determine if the finding is manageable in the current environment, or if outside consultation is warranted—common sense and experience assist greatly in sorting out yellow flags). (Very *abridged* list):

Abridged list of yellow-flag findings:

1. Asymmetrical MSRs (old name, DTRs)
2. Present pathological reflexes (e.g., Babinski, Hoffman)
3. Pain of unknown etiology
4. Fatigue
5. Pain that does not fit any dermatomal or cutaneous nerve distribution pattern
6. Pain out of proportion to the findings on physical examination
7. "Give-way weakness" (Patients are not able to provide an accurate status of their underlying condition, secondary to pain or some other limitation)
8. Lump or mass in a region like the wrist (need to determine if new problem is gradually resolving over time, relationship to problem patient is seeking care for, etc.).
9. Asymmetrical joint laxity (need to determine time of injury, other treatment, etc.).
10. Positive findings on special tests (e.g., positive McMurray's test implicating a torn meniscus—if definitive diagnosis required over the short-term, then referral would be warranted).
11. Night pain
12. Significant structural scoliosis (needs to be viewed in light of age of patient and past history with this condition)

Red flags: A red flag is a finding that is clearly outside of the scope of expertise of the therapist, and appropriate care for the patient is dependent on coordination with another health care professional. (While the examination *may* be continued following identifying a red flag, a course of action at the completion of the examination will be to refer the patient. In some cases, the referral could be immediate with care directly coordinated between the therapist and the physician referred to. As was the case with yellow flags, common sense and experience assist greatly in identifying findings that require immediate referral. (Very *abridged* list):

Abridged list of red-flag findings:

1. Loss of bowel or bladder control
2. Fever or chills
3. Dysphagia of unexplained origin
4. Unexplained weight loss
5. Clear and expected changes in vision (e.g., diplopia)
6. Symptoms that are constant and cannot be altered by activity or rest
7. Sudden onset of dizziness or balance problems
8. Sudden weakness or lack of coordination
9. Frequent nausea or vomiting, hemoptysis
10. Night sweats
11. Skin rash of unexplained origin
12. Redness and/or swelling in a joint without any history of injury

trying to be helpful. A clear mechanism of injury assists the examiner. A possible mechanism of injury needs to be viewed as just that, a possible cause of injury with the equally true possibility that the event and this episode of pain are not related. Since pain of unknown etiology is at least a yellow flag, this second type of response needs to be mentally flagged and viewed in light of the other information obtained over the course of the entire scan examination. (5) The information obtained during the subjective portion of the examination will be used to generate a working hypothesis or hypotheses. The danger here is to become too myopic, too fast. While the subjective examination may provide up to 80 percent of the information needed to determine the nature of the patient's problem, it is just part of the scan examination. Use the system developed to stay open-minded and broad so that less obvious or secondary issues are not missed. A metaphor that illustrates this is the instruction that a radiologist provided to neophyte health care providers in how to read X-rays. The radiologist noted that when a radiographic finding is distinct, the eye is drawn to it and unless the individual reading the X-ray is disciplined and is using a system, a less obvious (and often more serious) finding will be missed. Therefore, the radiologist urged that the X-rays should be viewed in a systematic way, to insure that proper attention is paid to all the elements visualized. Likewise, when developing a hypothesis or hypotheses, staying broad and open-minded will best serve the interests of the patients who have entrusted themselves to your care. (See Table 4-3 for an abridged list of questions found as part of the subjective examination.)

EXAMPLE OF QUESTIONS TYPICALLY FOUND AS PART OF THE SUBJECTIVE EXAM OR PATIENT HISTORY

(See Table 4-1 for an example of one questionnaire that could be used as part of the examination.)

1. *Age:* As mentioned previously with a slipped capital femoral epiphysis, there are certain diseases or injuries that are more prevalent in individuals of a given age. Patients reaching the 35–55-year-old age range, for example, are still easily capable of substantial repetitive activity like running the distances associated with marathon training. As a result of the biological changes associated with the loss of cushioning in the heel pad and changes in connective tissue, this group of older joggers tend to have an increased prevalence of plantar fasciitis.[61] These are just two of literally thousands of conditions where age plays a factor that should be considered in the mix of information collected in the scan examination. Proper understanding of lifespan issues requires an excellent didactic background in the pathophysiology associated with disease and injury.

   One other caveat that should be mentioned with age, is the way that this information is obtained. The standard way of asking a question about age is, "how old are you?" While there are times in our lives when we are looking forward to getting older, for someone beyond the young adult stage, this question may imply that their age is the problem. Two ways of obtaining this information in a more neutral way are to use the questionnaire referred to previously that requests the day, month, and year of birth, or ask the same question without any reference to being old, such as, "what is your age?" While a very small point, part of your job as a successful evaluator is to make the patient feel comfortable and not at all defensive. If someone is sensitive about the age, one of these minor changes in approach might help facilitate the conversation.

2. *Gender:* Like age, given diseases or injuries are more common in one gender than the other. The aforementioned slipped capital femoral epiphysis is illustrative of a problem that is much more common in males. Other conditions like rheumatoid arthritis or fibromyalgia are more common in females.[44,54,86] Additionally, there are condi-

tions that are restricted to one gender or the other that often have symptoms suggestive of a neuromuscular complaint. A male over the age of 40 presenting with LBP without a clear mechanism of injury should be questioned about the genitourinary system, specifically about the prostate. This is important because the prostate can refer pain to the low back.[10] Similarly, women of childbearing age presenting with LBP should be questioned about their menstrual cycle, since pregnancy and the alteration in hormonal levels can also be responsible for LBP.[13,87,93] These are but two of potentially thousands of conditions that have a predisposition for one gender over the other. An excellent understanding of pathophysiology (as already discussed) and that of gender is needed by the examiners to successfully evaluate the patients that they see. While a full description of this topic is beyond the scope of this chapter, the interested reader is referred to several excellent texts.[34,37]

3. *Ethnic makeup:* The ethnicity of the patient is also a factor that needs to be considered when examining the individual from a holistic perspective. It should be recognized that like the previously mentioned age and gender, ethnicity can be a factor in the prevalence of the health problem that the patient is seeking assistance with. It is well recognized that there are ethnic differences in the bone mineral content of various races, with Caucasians experiencing higher fracture rates than either Asians or African Americans.[7] Other injury and disease states, such as hypertension and renal disease, are more prevalent in African American populations than among Caucasians.[24,28] While these are but two examples, they illustrate that the genetics associated with the individual are an important factor to keep in mind when considering various hypotheses and the likelihood of a specific problem in the patient that is presenting for care.

   Closely related to ethnic makeup is the issue of culture and socioeconomic factors that can play a role in health and disease. In a recent study examining intimate partner violence in Native American women, it was found that more than half of the women (58.7 percent) receiving care at a tribally operated clinic in southwest Oklahoma reported lifetime physical and/or sexual abuse.[59] Almost as striking as the overall lifetime percentage, was the finding that 30.1 percent of these women reported physical or sexual intimate partner violence in the previous 12 months.[59] These are exceptionally high rates of intimate partner violence and illustrate the need for health care workers to have an understanding of the communities that they serve. This one example serves to drive home the point that the individuals that are served in a health care facility are not simply biological beings that may have a dysfunction of some type, but they are potentially affected by the totality of their day-to-day existence, including lifestyle, genetics, culture, and the morays of the community in which they live.

TABLE 4-3

Abridged List of Questions Found as Part of the Subjective Examination

QUESTION	REASON INFORMATION SOUGHT	EXAMPLE	RED OR YELLOW FLAG
What is your age?	Age specificity present with some diseases	Vertebral body epiphyseal aseptic necrosis (Scheuermann's disease)	—
Sex (typically observed and noted, not asked)?	Sex specificity present with some diseases	Juvenile rheumatoid arthritis	—
Current occupation?	Occupation may relate to either the onset of symptoms or serve as a factor in treatment	Heavy industrial worker versus secretary	—
What problem has caused you to seek medical care?	Identifies the patient's perception and location of the current dysfunction	Trauma versus problem of insidious onset	—
Onset of this problem?	Identifies the length of time current dysfunction has been present	Acute versus chronic condition	—
Any past medical history of similar or related problem? (If so, how was the condition treated and what was the result?)	Provides insight into past history of dysfunction, rehabilitation status, and effectiveness of prior treatment	Recurring rib dysfunction	—
How is your general health? Have you experienced any unexplained weight loss?	Provides insight into other possible problems that may contribute to the current problem	Rheumatoid arthritis, cancer, cardiac problems, etc	*
Any recent infections, fever, or surgery?	Provides information regarding systemic disease that may be related to this problem	Recent history of bladder infection related to low thoracic or lumbar pain	*
What aggravates your symptoms?	The pathomechanics of provoked pain are identified by the patient	Flexion of the cervical spine reproducing upper thoracic pain	—
What relieves your symptoms?	Provides additional insight into pathomechanics and possible treatment approach	Lying on the affected side decreases pain (this is called autospinting and the decrease in pain provided by pressure applied to the involved side may suggest pleuropulmonary involvement).[33] Also, beware of nothing relieving symptoms—suggests nonmechanical problem	*
Is there a specific pattern of pain over a 24-hour period?	Mechanical problems tend to become worse throughout the day and are relieved by rest	Muscle strain aggravated by repetitive use	—
Does the pain ever wake you from a sound sleep? If so, are you able to roll over and go back to sleep?	Provides information about the pattern of pain and alerts the examiner to the possibility of nonmechanical problem	Osteoid osteoma (pattern of night pain, typically relieved by aspirin)[36]	*
What hobbies or recreational pursuits do you engage in?	May relate to onset of symptoms or identify factors that will need to be considered in treatment	Serious rugby player versus avid reader	—
Are you aware of strength or sensory changes?	Provides insight into function of the neuromusculoskeletal system	C5 dermatome identified as area of decreased sensation	—
Any episodes of dizziness or vertigo?	Symptoms may be present with vestibular or vertebral artery problems	Vertebral artery problem	*

(Continued)

(Continued)

QUESTION	REASON INFORMATION SOUGHT	EXAMPLE	RED OR YELLOW FLAG
Current medications?	Relates potentially to both this problem and other medical problems	Steroids—long-term use may be associated with osteoporosis	—
Have X-rays or other special tests been performed? If so, do you know the results?	Provides a more complete picture of what has already been done	X-rays, laboratory work obtained	—
On a scale of 1–10, with 10 representing excruciating pain and 1 representing minimal pain, where would you rate your pain over the past 24 hours?	Provides a pseudoobjective level of the patient's current perception of pain—this can be used to gauge progress at a later point in time	Pain currently at 4:10	—

*Potential yellow or red flags that may suggest additional work-up or referral to an appropriate medical specialist.
(SOURCE: Reproduced from Flynn T. *The Thoracic Spine and Rib Cage*. Newton, MA, Butterworth-Heinemann, 1996, with permission from Elsevier.)

4. *Morphology:* The body type of an individual presenting for an examination is also a factor in the likelihood of developing a given injury or dysfunction. The previously described slipped capital femoral epiphysis also has morphological implications, since it tends to occur more in youngsters who are either tall or thin, or short and obese.[88] This is thought to be due to a potential hormonal imbalance that may be occurring during a period of growth. Here again, there are potentially thousands of conditions that are re-

lated to body type or structural makeup, such as increased incidence of patellofemoral pain in individuals with alignment or range of motion issues.[3,18,55]

This is a broad label and includes less than perfect biomechanics present in many individuals, such as leg length discrepancies, range of motion restrictions, muscle imbalances, in addition to the general body type of the individual. The key point here is that the examiner needs to be aware of the potential role of morphology or biomechanics, make a mental note of any characteristics observed, and follow-up with examination procedures that work to either confirm or reject any working hypotheses generated.

5. *Family history:* Family history, like all of the categories discussed above, is a key factor in performing any scan examination. The old adage, "the apple doesn't fall too far from the tree," is applicable to medical conditions as well as personality traits. An individual with a family history of diabetes is more likely to develop a polyneuropathy secondary to diabetes than an individual without this family history.[17,31] Individuals with parents who have documented Charcot-Marie-Tooth are at risk of inheriting the gene responsible for this mixed motor and sensory neuropathy, and the examiner needs to consider the patient's complaint in light of this information.[11,48] The role of family history, particularly those conditions with known recessive or dominant gene inheritance patterns, needs to be an important piece of information used to generate working hypotheses. Again, to efficiently use this information, the examiners need to have excellent didactic preparation and

T A B L E   4 - 4

Common Upper Motor Neuron/Lower Motor Neuron signs and Symptoms

LOWER MOTOR NEURON (ABRIDGED LIST)	UPPER MOTOR NEURON (ABRIDGED LIST)
Weakness and/or paralysis (flaccid)	Weakness and/or paralysis (spastic)
Hyporeflexia (or areflexia)	Hyperreflexia
Rapid muscle atrophy	No clear muscle atrophy (or slowly developing atrophy that is secondary to disuse)
No pathological reflexes	Pathological reflexes (e.g., Babinski, Hoffman, etc.)
Fasciculations and fibrillations	Altered or loss of voluntary motion

a system where they are able to quickly reference questions that arise. A list of specific conditions associated with family history is beyond the scope of this chapter, and the interested reader is referred to Goodman, Boissonnault, and Fuller.[34]

6. *Past medical history:* The truism of "history tends to repeat itself "[1] is very applicable when evaluating patients. The past medical history will often provide a piece of information that is directly applicable to why the patient that is being evaluated has a current problem. It may be something as straightforward as a history of carpal tunnel syndrome in the right hand, when the patient is now presenting with left hand alterations in sensation and strength. Since there is a significantly increased odds ratio of patients with documented carpal tunnel syndrome (distal median neuropathy) having involvement of the contralateral side,[8,21,43] the information provided may give a vital clue. While the carpal tunnel case is one in which the patients probably also had a high index of suspicion, there are other times when the patients may have not made any linkage between a past medical problem and their current problem. A second example of this is the surgical removal of a lipoma from the dorsal surface of the lower neck. Over time, shoulder pain develops on that side that the patient does not relate to the lipoma resection. An astute examiner will pay particular attention to the manual muscle testing of the upper trunk, since it is not unknown for the spinal accessory nerve to be accidentally resected, resulting in shoulder pain due to an inability of the trapezius muscle to contribute to normal humeroscapular rhythm. Third, the patients may have had this exact problem before, and they may also know what helped them recover from the problem previously. Sage questioning may provide a solution to the problem with which the patient presents.

7. *Medications:* Knowledge of the medications that a person is taking is important for a variety of reasons. The medications give you information that the patient may not have thought was important and did not provide to you, even though asked. For example, patients may not mention that they have any cardiovascular problems, but if you find out that they are on a beta-blocker, a follow-up question can be asked that clarifies the purpose of this medication. With that example, it is also important to know that the range of their heart rate is limited at the upper extreme, so that any exercise prescription developed for the individual would need to take the medication into account. This one example is compounded by the fact that many individuals today are on multiple medications. Prior to performing an evaluation, it is incumbent upon the examiner to take the time to find out both what the patients are taking, and understand why they are taking those medications. (If the examiner in unsure, the Physicians Desk Reference is an excellent course of information on medications.[2])

8. *Mechanism of injury:* In those cases where patients are able to accurately describe how their injury occurred, they can provide the examiner with tremendous insight into what is going on. A simple example is an individuals who underwent an inversion sprain of the ankle and is able to relate that they "rolled over onto the outside of their foot, with resulting ankle pain." Knowledge of the anatomy and the pathophysiology of ankle sprains allows the examiner to speculate (hypothesize) which lateral ligaments of the ankle have been injured, with the most common pattern being the anterior talofibular ligament first, the calcaneofibular ligament second, and the posterior talofibular ligament third. With a good description of the mechanism of injury, each of these structures can be evaluated and the extent of the injury logically deduced.

There may be other cases where the mechanism of injury is not particularly clear to the person, but their description still aids a great deal. The reason that the mechanism may not be clear is that the injury happened too fast. This is often the case in knee injuries on an athletic field, where there was some sudden event such as a collision, with resultant knee pain. The fact that the person heard a "pop" at the time of the injury, and experienced significant knee joint effusion within an hour of the event, however, is very telling. It has been said that with these two pieces of information, the logical deduction that will be correct, the majority of the time is that the individual has sustained an anterior cruciate ligament injury. Therefore, ask questions that will gather all the known information that occurred at or around the time of the injury.

Be aware, that in the patients' desire to assist you by telling you what happened, they may not be truly aware of what occurred. A case that also involves the knee is the individual who sustains a patellar dislocation. It is not unusual for a person who has sustained a dislocation to report that the patella dislocated medially, and then relocated in the trochlear groove. While a medial dislocation is possible, the majority of patellar dislocations occur laterally, since the knee is characterized by valgus.[71,91] The patient may report a dislocation to the inside of the knee because that side of the knee hurts due to the medial retinaculum that has torn to allow the patella to dislocate. The point that this is intended to illustrate is that even though patients believe they know what happened, the injury may occur so fast that their perception is not entirely accurate. Therefore, listen to what the patient has to say and evaluate the information obtained with a critical mind, factoring in what is known about the most common mechanisms of injury to a particular area.

A last point is the aforementioned case of the patients desiring to help identify the cause of their problem. When a clear-cut mechanism of injury is not clear, some individuals will think back to all the events that occurred about the same time as the onset of their symptoms. If this is their "best guess," rather than a known mechanism of injury, then this should probably be treated as an idiopathic cause of their problem. At the very least, pain of unknown origin should be treated as a yellow flag, and in many cases, viewed as a red flag. Thus, just because patients think that they know what caused their pain, the evaluator is still required to critically evaluate this information and give it the range of credibility that it warrants.

9. *A.M./P.M. pattern of pain:* The pattern of pain that the patients describe can be very useful in developing a working hypothesis, since most neuromusculoskeletal dysfunctions can be relieved by position or rest. It would be expected that pain secondary to somatic dysfunction could be both provoked (see later section on provocative tests) and decreased or eliminated by proper positioning and rest. Somatic dysfunction can be defined as impaired or altered function of related components of the somatic (body framework) system; skeletal, arthrodial, and myofascial structures; and related vascular, lymphatic, and neural elements.[14] Thus, the pattern of pain that is typically reported for most neuromusculoskeletal disorders is activity or position dependent and relieved by rest or positioning that removes stress from the affected structure. Pain that cannot be influenced by position or rest, or pain that wakes the patients from a sound sleep and keeps them awake, is at a minimum a yellow flag. An example of this type of pain is an osteoid osteoma, which accounts for 10 to 12 percent of benign bone tumors.[35] Since the pain from this type of a lesion is not directly affected by position, and is a consistent irritation at night when rest should be working to relieve pain, the clinicians have to factor the pattern of pain into their thought process. The majority, if not all patients with a clear pattern of increased pain at night that is not relieved by position, should be referred for additional work-up.

Although the a.m./p.m. pattern of pain should be addressed in an effort to clarify the patient's complaint, there are a couple of other principles that need to be factored into the picture that the patient is telling. First, many conditions have an a.m./p.m. pattern of pain that are not a yellow or red flag, such as early arthritic changes. These patients will often describe that they are stiff (painful) early in the morning, loosen-up as they move around, and then tend to stiffen-up and become painful again toward the end of the day, when they are tired. This pattern of pain is logical, and if it fits with all of the other collaborative information, then it has provided one more confirmation of the patient's presenting problem. Another example of a logical a.m./p.m. pattern of pain is the patient with carpal tunnel syndrome. These patients often describe "tingling in the hand that interrupts sleep"[64] and pain that is partially relieved by shaking their hands back and forth. This pattern of pain is explained by the fact that many individuals assume a curled-up position when they sleep, resulting in a flexed-wrist posture that restricts the needed blood flow to an already compromised median nerve that is passing under the transverse carpal ligament. Again, this pattern of pain is logical, can be explained and even forms the basis

for conservative treatment with a resting night splint, and is not a yellow or red flag.

A second consideration is that the brain tends to stay active, even when the patient is attempting to relax. The typical individuals are constantly on the go throughout the day, with their eyes providing visual information, their ears hearing all that is going on around them, the temperature of the air being constantly assessed, their joints providing them with feedback regarding position, speed, or some other variable, in addition to the challenges and concerns of the day. When trying to relax and go to sleep at night, vision is eliminated with the eyes closed, the environment is normally quiet, temperature is optimally regulated, and joints are not moving. Therefore, the brain that is still receiving afferent input will have a tendency to focus on the incoming information provided, and the reasonably manageable level of pain may appear more pronounced to the patient in the evening. This is often the case with individuals with a shoulder bursitis or other joint inflammation process. This pattern of pain is also logical and fits with the expected characteristics of a patient with a somatic dysfunction. Focused questioning will identify the pattern of pain as keeping with the collaborative evidence gathered in the examination.

It should also be noted that pain that wakes an individual from a sound sleep is not the key element that elevates the a.m./p.m. pattern of pain to a yellow or red flag. The patients described in the preceding paragraph may wake from a sound sleep if they roll over onto the inflamed shoulder. While this wakes them up, they are able to reposition themselves in a way that takes stress off of the shoulder, and fall back to sleep. The key point that elevates the patients to a potential yellow or red flag is when they consistently are awaken in the middle of the night, and once awake they are not able to go back to sleep. This suggests something other than a somatic dysfunction and a work-up by a specialist with the tools to explore systemic conditions, or visceral problems should be considered. When this is coupled with a pattern of pain that is not affected by rest or positioning, then referral is probably warranted.

10. *Nature of pain:* Pain is important, since it is typically what brings the patient into the clinic. Pain can help guide the process, and it needs to be respected when treating a patient. Having said that, a key principle is to not be led by pain (see previous section [point 2, under the subjective examination]). Let pain be one piece of information, but do not have the pain experienced by the patient be the focus of either the examination or the treatment plan.

The nature of the pain can often provide a great deal of information that will help identify a potential problem. Due to the location of receptors in the body and the way that we are physiologically wired, pain due to a superficial structure tends to be more easily located.[25] Pain due to visceral structures is often referred.[65] Regions of the body, such as visceral pleura, are insensitive to pain.[68] Some structures, such as nerves, often have pain that radiates.[85] Pain due to nerve origin may also have descriptive characteristics that help identify a nerve as the structure involved, such as a "bright" or "sharp" pain.[4,42] A full description of the nature of pain is beyond the scope of this chapter, but common characteristics associated with pain have been described elsewhere for the interested reader.[33,36,39,46,58] The key point is that pain can provide valuable clues to what is going on with the patient. Listen to the information provided, know what various descriptions of pain mean, and add this as one piece of the puzzle when assembling the information that will hopefully lead to a collaborative picture of the patient's problem.

11. *Training history:* If the patient is engaged in any athletic, vocational, household repair, or recreational activities that require physical labor, ask about the nature, frequency, duration, and intensity of the activity. Additionally, ask about any changes in the treatment regimen. Individuals presenting for care due to overuse injuries are a significant percentage of the patient population seen. Research has shown that errors in training account for a significant percentage of the injuries that are attributed to overuse problems.[47,49] The most common error associated with the training prescription (activity, frequency, duration, and intensity) is increasing the total volume of the activity too quickly, by ramping up the duration of the activity in too large of increments.

While having unrealistic expectations about how fast mileage or repetitions or sets or some other variable can be added, there are many other training errors that will become evident when listening to a patient's training history. The author once had a patient who complained of knee pain. When asked about what he did recreationally, he indicated that he was a jogger. A follow-up question was asked about his training mileage, and he indicated that he had run 16 miles yesterday. When questioned further about his typical training week, he indicated that over the past three days, he had run 16 miles on each day. Although a well-educated individual (a lawyer), he did not see the need to allow his body a chance to recover from training events that were clearly stressful to his body. When a more balanced training program was developed, his symptoms cleared-up and his performance improved.

Training errors are numerous and a complete list is beyond the scope of this chapter. One final thought, however, is that the potential errors are not restricted to the training prescription variables listed above. An example with running that should be considered in the questioning process is the type and age of the shoes worn. Many recreational joggers will wear their shoes for much longer periods of time than they were designed to be worn. Thus, the shoe has lost all cushioning properties and additional stress is being directly transferred to the jogger. Also, joggers may switch shoes to a new brand and gradually develop symptoms that they do not attribute to the change in shoes.

An important point is to recognize that training errors are common and that the patients will often clearly describe what change has brought on a specific problem, not recognizing the connection between their behavior and the injury.

Bottom line: The above list of 11 items is an abridged list of some of the variables that may be considered in a subjective examination. Each evaluator will build a list over time that suits their style and the typical patient population that they are working with. While the exact items may vary from therapist to therapist, there are several truisms that will be present with everyone. First, as has been stressed repeatedly, there should be a clear system associated with the subjective evaluation, so that key items are not missed. Second, for every question asked, there should be a specific purpose for the question. Use the information provided to categorize symptoms and other information into a workable hypothesis(es). Third, based on this information, the objective portion of the scan examination is planned. Last, know when the information provided indicates that the problem may be outside of the evaluator's area of expertise. "The mark of a true professional is to know the limits of his/her abilities, and to refer, when appropriate."[38]

Objective/Physical Examination

The objective examination builds on the information provided in the subjective/history portion of the scan examination, with modifications designed-in as needed. The objective examination is a fluid process where the examiner can begin to test the hypotheses generated from the responses that the patient provided to the therapist. While a fluid process, it cannot be stressed enough that this evaluation is performed within the context of a system that has key items that should be evaluated with every patient. The system is required to insure that the focus of the examination remains broad (so that some key information is not overlooked), important information is not inadvertently missed, and so that the process of examining the patient is efficient (e.g., not having them change positions back and forth numerous times, etc.).

Metaphorically, for those familiar with golf, this process is a little like approaching a golf course. A skilled golfer approaches the round with a plan (the system). This individual knows where the hazards are, which side of the fairway is optimal to drive to, what regions are out of bounds, and has identified opportunities for either conservative or bold play. While each golf course is different, the basic elements of whatever system used by that individual will be in evidence with every course played. Note that this implies that not all people will utilize the same system when evaluating a golf course, because their unique approach will be based on their particular strengths and weaknesses. This is also true for the objective examination, where the system used by different skilled professionals will not be exactly the same, even though each system will contain virtually all of the same elements. Additionally, as in golf, while the plan (system) reflects that for a par four, there is a drive, a second shot to the green, and a two-putt, that plan will be modified as needed as a person progresses through the round. The art and skill of performing at a high level utilizes a well thought-out plan that can be creatively modified as needed to accomplish the task at hand. In golf, this may mean knowing when to chip back out into the fairway, or when it is appropriate to attempt to blast a shot over trees on a doglegged fairway. In the examination process, this is knowing when to add-on to the framework utilized in the scan examination and follow-up on a lead that will permit a more definitive determination of the patient's problem. The system provides the framework or plan. Based on that information, the evaluator needs to remain flexible and respond to the information provided, both from the subjective (history) and from the physical examination itself. Note that this fluid process is significantly different from following an algorithm that has predetermined sequence of steps that are largely adhered to without a great deal of interpretation. A strong didactic base, coupled with a system and the ability to generate and evaluate multiple hypotheses simultaneously, is needed to perform a competent objective examination.

Although all the information in the paragraph above is accurate, it correctly implies that a skilled evaluator also has experience. So, what about the neophyte therapist starting out with the performance of objective examinations? Three suggestions are the following: (1) Develop a form or series of forms that serve to prompt the evaluation, to insure that no important steps or pieces of information are forgotten. Since each individual approaches the physical examination in his/her own way, individualize this system to fit the style and needs of the person performing the examination. (2) Whenever possible, seek out and develop a relationship with a mentor. Everyone will run into questions or situations that are not clear, where an outside perspective is needed. Develop this type of relationship and ideally have the ability to seek out information on an "as needed" basis, as well as establish a time where regular exchanges and reviews of patients can take place. (3) Have a preplanned system that permits stepping out of the examination room and going to another location to look up information that is needed to complete a thought or review information associated with a particular condition. This may be as simple as stating that "excuse me, I need to follow-up on some patient information—I will be back in a minute." If this allows obtaining information as needed, it will result in both learning and improved care provided for the patient being seen.

RECORD AS YOU GO...

Record as you go during the objective examination process. Research has shown that no one is able to perform a complex examination that includes modifications on the fly, and remember all of the details associated with that examination.[81] It is not a weakness to pause for a few seconds during the evaluation, and jot down any pertinent findings. My preference is to annotate any findings that are not optimal. This includes any subtle limitations of range of motion, any identified areas of less than

perfect sensation, or any other finding associated with any aspect of the physical examination. The advantage of this is that when evaluating most patients, the majority of their findings will be normal. Therefore, by recording all elements that deviate from normal as you go, you are constructing in your mind a complete picture based on all of the data presented. Then, at some later time, such as the end of the entire evaluation process or after the patient has been treated, the therapist is able to sit down and generate a proper record of the visit, with all data (both normal and less than optimal) incorporated into the note.

In addition to being efficient and assisting with reconstructing an accurate picture of the entire evaluation, this process of generating a cursory annotation followed by a formal note has an advantage of reviewing the material twice. An important element of a skilled clinician is the insight provided by reflecting on the findings presented. In the first pass, all potential findings are collected in a serial process and tested against the working hypothesis. When then looking at the entirety of the data at the end of the evaluation, it is not unusual for a paradigm shift in thinking to occur, with a new hypothesis leading to a different conclusion and treatment approach. An accurate evaluation is built upon excellent information and reflection. This will only be accomplished by fastidiously recording as you proceed through the examination.

Two last points are associated with recording the information. First, if you did not record it, from a legal standpoint, you did not do it. Annotation is critical to substantiate your findings and treatment plan. Second, annotate in such a way that the information provided is efficient, useful, and indicates that a thorough evaluation was done. In the preface to *The Four Minute Neurologic Exam*,[32] Stephen Goldberg, MD, makes the observation that "'Neuro WNL' ('the neurological exam is within normal limits') is commonly the last notation on a physical exam report. Regretfully, Dr. Goldberg points out that this often means that virtually no neuro exam took place." The painful joke in some clinical settings is that the acronym WNL is "We never looked." When providing a summary of the findings, provide enough detail on the tests performed that it is clear what was done and what the findings were. While this may take an extra minute or two, it shows attention to detail and the fact that the objective examination was taken seriously. Additionally, it provides any other evaluators that follow with an excellent road map, identifying where that patient's problem was on a given date.

BASIC ELEMENTS OF MOST PHYSICAL EXAMINATIONS

The following is an abridged list of some of the basic elements that should be included in virtually all scanning examinations. Depending on the type of patients that a particular practice sees, this list may not be sufficient and a number of other items should be added. There are several excellent guides that outline many additional examination tests, such as Richard Baxter's *Pocket Guide to Musculoskeletal Assessment*[9] or Mark Dutton's *Orthopaedic Examination, Evaluation, and Intervention*.[22] These references and other pocket guides[41] and texts[60,94] can be used to effectively build upon the scant framework of a "scan examination." As has been described previously, the scan examination is not intended to be a thorough examination, but rather provides a system where a quick evaluation can be performed that at a minimum, identifies that the problem appears to be manageable within the neuromusculoskeletal realm, or that the problem is one that requires referral or immediate attention. From the framework provided by the scan examination, other elements can be added to work toward the desired thorough evaluation, as time permits. At a minimum, the following should be incorporated into the scan examination:

1. *Observation:* The observation begins when walking out to the waiting room to meet the patient. Watch how the patients move from sitting to standing, the contact that they make when shaking hands, and the way that they move back to the examination area. Since everyone responds in a little different way, knowing he/she is being watched, work to carry on a pleasant conversation while surreptitiously paying close attention to the individual's movements. The simple analogy of taking someone's picture when he/she does not know that you are watching provides a much more realistic view than the "posed" state of saying "cheese" to artificially look relaxed. Similarly, if the clinician asks the patients to walk while watching them, their gait may or may not provide the information that you really want. Do as much as you can while the patient is performing normal activities.

    Observation also includes looking at the individuals from a postural perspective, noting any asymmetries in their skeletal frame or musculature. This means that all regions of the body being investigated need to be appropriately exposed, maintaining proper decorum for the patient. Be systematic here also, starting at a location like the malleoli of the ankles, and systematically working up to the head. Look for equal alignment of clear bony landmarks like the fibular heads, greater trochanters, ischial tuberosities, dimples associated with the posterior inferior iliac spines, the iliac crests, etc. Look for folds of the skin that may be present on one side of the trunk but not the other, which could suggest a scoliosis or other issue and are another way to identify a potential structural abnormality. Additionally, look for signs of atrophy, scars, edema, or any other abnormality that provides evidence of a past or current problem. One example of a case where observation can play a key role is the previously mentioned iatrogenic nerve lesion, a transaction of the spinal accessory nerve.[67] During the history, past surgeries may have been asked about, and the patients may relate that nothing has been done to their shoulder, which is the reason they are being seen. By observing a scar over their right upper thorax, a question can be asked about the cause of that scar. The patient relates that "oh, that really was nothing, just a benign lipoma that was removed from the back." If the therapist

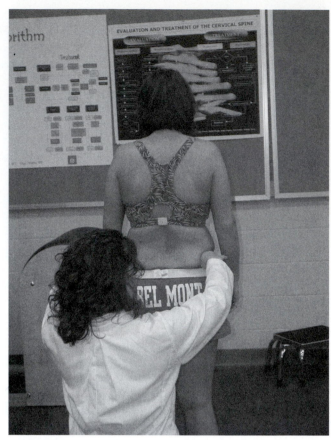

FIGURE   4 - 2

Observation of iliac crest height, looking posterior to anterior.

recognizes that spinal accessory nerve may have been inadvertently transected through this type of minor surgery and that paralysis of the trapezius can cause shoulder pain, a potential linkage between the scar and the patient's problem needs to be explored. The bottom line is that the therapist is required to take the time to adequately observe the patient, through the use of a system, both statically and actively (see Fig. 4-2).

2. *Range of motion:* Since this is a scan examination, the key objective is to see if there are any significant limitations and annotate those. The simplest way to assess this is to have a system that incorporates many motions simultaneously and have the patient actively perform that activity or activities. For example, if the patients are able to reach symmetrically behind and up their backs, reaching the midscapular region with both hands, then they have demonstrated normal or near normal internal rotation and extension of their shoulders (see Fig. 4-3). By reaching up over their heads with their arms (normal flexion), then beginning in this position reaching as far down their backs as they can, to at least the midscapular region, shoulder abduction and external rotation are also assessed. Elbow, wrist, and hand motion will be simultaneously assessed during the upcoming

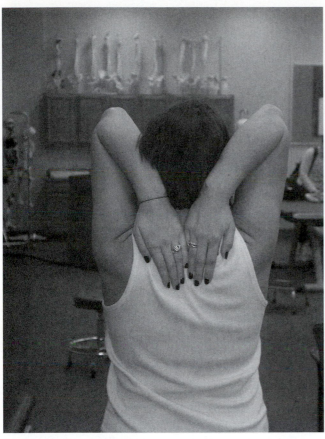

FIGURE 4-3

Scan examination active range of motion assessment of the upper extremities.

strength assessments. If all of the above are normal, then the scan examination can probably proceed to the next element of the evaluators system.

In the case where active range of motion is either not symmetrical or if a clear or subtle range limitation is identified, then the examiner is obligated to both note it and follow-up with a more detailed examination. If weakness happens to the patient's key problem, this may involve an active-assistive approach to ascertain the true range of motion at a given joint. More information may also be obtained by performing passive range of motion, and at the end of the range, providing gentle overpressure. These follow-up procedures can be used to assess the true status of the joint and the surrounding inert and contractile structures.[19] The key purpose of the range of motion portion of the scan examination is to determine if the patient moves normally or not. If movement is not normal, identify the limitation. Then, if time permits, follow-up the basic assessment with more detailed manual procedures to determine the true state of the joint and surrounding structures.

In addition to the extent of the range of motion available, the quality of the motion also needs to be assessed. Did the movement flow smoothly without interruption, or

did the patient grimace with range of motion that started and slowed in a halting fashion? Assess what the patients are attempting to convey through their movement, and work to factor this into the working hypothesis. Work to identify movement patterns that are limited due to weakness and other patterns that are limited due to pain. Through the quality of the motion, the patient will often tell the examiner as much information as is provided through the history or the actual range of motion numbers obtained visually or with a goniometer.

A last point associated with a scan examination is that the range of motion assessment is normally done visually, and not assessed in pure planes as is typically done when recording range of motion with a goniometer. The scan examination's purpose is to identify if movement normal, asymmetrical, or limited, and where this is occurring. Typically, the only time a goniometer would be used during a scan examination is as a type of follow-up, to annotate the previously identified limitation in range of motion.

3. *Strength:* The goal of a scan examination with strength testing is similar to that of range of motion; identify any clear deficiencies or asymmetries. To that end, the typical scan examination does not involve a manual muscle test of all the muscles in a given region, but rather scans the major muscle groups. For the upper extremities, this may involve the following (all of which can be done in a sitting position):

a. Resisted shoulder abduction—tests deltoid group and scapular rotators (see Fig. 4-4).
b. Resisted shoulder flexion—tests shoulder flexors and scapular stabilizers.
c. Resisted protraction—to assess the serratus anterior (see Fig. 4-5).
d. Resisted shoulder internal and external rotation—tests shoulder rotators.

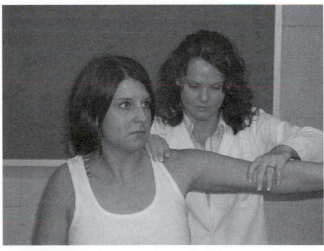

FIGURE 4-4

Manual muscle test of the abductors of the shoulder.

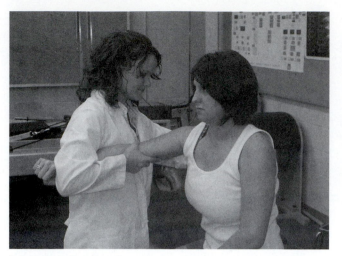

FIGURE 4-5

Manual muscle test of the serratus anterior—insuring that the scapula does not "wing."

e. Resisted elbow flexion and extension—tests muscles of the arm.
f. Resisted elbow supination and pronation—tests supinators and pronators.
g. Resisted wrist extension and flexion—tests forearm muscles.
h. Grip strength—again, assesses extrinsic muscles of the anterior forearm.
i. Resisted finger abduction—tests dorsal interossei and abductors of the thumb and little finger (see Fig. 4-6).
j. Ability to make an "O" with the thumb and index finger and provide normal pressure between the tip of the thumb and the tip of the index finger—tests muscles innervated by the anterior interosseous branch of the median nerve (see Fig. 4-7).
k. Resisted shoulder shrug—assesses the upper trapezius.

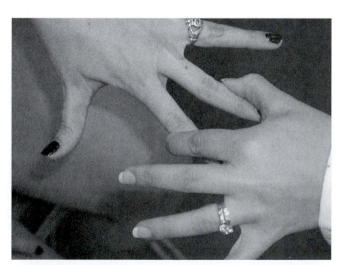

FIGURE 4-6

Manual muscle test of resisted finger abduction.

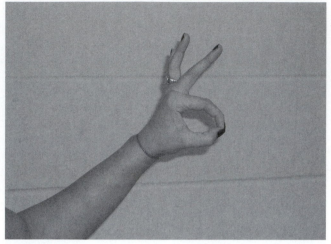

FIGURE 4-7

The "O" sign—assessing for anterior interosseous nerve integrity.

l. May also want to assess resisted neck movements (flexion, extension, rotation, and side bending), if appropriate—depends on the patient's presentation.

These muscle groups are typically tested in a midrange position, since that is where the patient will have near optimal strength as predicted by the length-tension curve.[26,79] The resisted contractions are typically isometric contractions, since they can be performed quickly and provide a reasonable measure of the amount of resistance that the patient is able to generate. There is not really a need to have the patients demonstrate that they can move any particular muscle group through the full range of motion, since this should have already been assessed during the range of motion portion of the scan examination. Additionally, note that the above scheme is working to assess functional muscle groups, rather than individual muscles. If weakness is identified, in addition to annotating that, the clinician is obligated to go back at some point and perform a more in-depth examination. The scan examination provides a good overview of the region under investigation, and the framework upon which a more detailed examination can be built.

A similar scheme as that to the 12 muscle groups outlined above can easily be devised for the lower extremities (see Fig. 4-8). This may proceed in a manner similar to the muscle groups identified above, working down from the hips, or it may involve a combination of muscle group tests and functional tests. For example, it is probably more meaningful to have the patients walk on their toes and then on their heels, than it is to resist plantar flexion or dorsiflexion. This is because the patient's body weight (particularly with toe walking) will provide more resistance than will typically be provided with a group manual muscle test. If there is any issue with toe walking, quantify the potential weakness with the number of unilateral heel raises that the

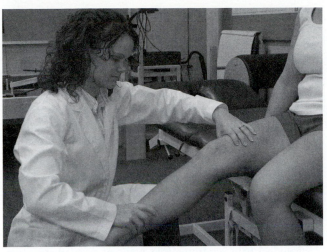

FIGURE   4 - 8

Manual muscle test of the quadriceps—illustrated out of the "closed-packed" position.

patients are able to perform, up to a maximum of 25, that is considered normal.[78] One other functional test that can be used is a deep squat, returning to a standing position. For the young and flexible patients who can easily perform this maneuver, information is provided about the knee extensors and hip extensors. When this is combined with select group muscle tests, a system can be devised that quickly provides a great deal of information on all of the major muscle groups of the lower extremity. Since this is a scan examination, devise a system that is thorough, but avoids needless redundancy. If a functional test is incorporated into the system used with athletic individuals, then drop out a group muscle test that would be redundant (see Fig. 4-9). On the other hand, if the patient is an 80-year-old individual who would typically have difficulty performing a deep squat, have enough flexibility in your system that

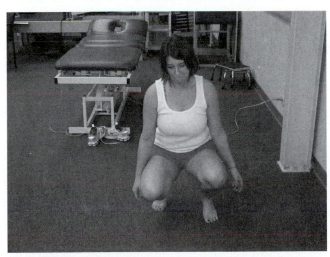

FIGURE   4 - 9

Example of a functional test.

age-appropriate tasks are requested, while still examining all desired muscle groups.

As was the case with an upper quarter scan examination, any identified deficiencies will need to be followed-up at some other time with a more detailed evaluation. At the time of the more detailed follow-up, it is both appropriate and expected that individual manual muscle tests will be performed. There are a number of excellent texts that provide great detail on the correct way to perform manual muscle testing.[20,51,78]

In finishing the overview of this element of the scan examination, the role of pain in scanning the strength of major muscle groups should be addressed. If a patient "yields to pain" during a resisted isometric contraction, then nothing can really be said about the status of the contractile unit (muscle, tendon, and tendon-periosteal insertion.[19]) This is because the strength could be normal, but the patient is yielding because of discomfort. To record the strength as less than normal would then be inaccurate. All that the clinician can really do is annotate that they could not accurately assess the strength of the muscle group in question, because the patient yielded in response to pain. It may be valuable to state the level of resistance provided prior to yielding (e.g., unable to assess patient's true elbow flexion resistance, but patient provided elbow flexion resistance of 4:5, prior to yielding secondary to pain), but that is a personal preference and judgment call. The key point is to recognize that to provide a strength measurement, it needs to be reflective of the patient's best efforts without the overlay of pain or some other factor.

4. *Sensation:* Most of the time if a person has a significant sensory deficit, this typically will be revealed during the history portion of the evaluation. Therefore, insure that the question is asked and listen closely to the patient's response. Additionally, as was outlined previously, require the patient to be precise and identify specific sides of the limb, specific digits, and where any sensory abnormality begins or ends.

While the history will provide significant insight into most sensory issues, the clinician remains obligated to perform, at a minimum, a sensory scan examination of the region in question. To do this, the area to be tested should be exposed, the patient should be relaxed and comfortable, and in keeping with informed consent, should have had the sensory test explained and consented to, prior to the examination. Then, the sensory examination should proceed in a systematic way, usually distal to proximal. The areas assessed should cover all cutaneous peripheral nerves and dermatomes of the region under investigation (see *Clinically Oriented Anatomy*[66] for specific cutaneous nerve fields and dermatomes).

The easiest modality to use for this assessment is light touch, since this can be done with the clinician's fingertips. In the vast majority of cases, due to the initial statement that sensory deficits are usually identified in the history, a scan with light touch is adequate and time efficient. The combination of both a normal history of sensation and normal light touch over a region like the upper extremity in an upper quarter screen provides a strong foundation to move on to the next element in the overall scan examination. Having stated that, the examiner has to recognize that different modalities are carried by different sensory systems. A patient could have a problem like syringomyelia that affects the anterior white commissures at several levels in the spinal cord, disrupting the anterolateral sensory system. In this patient, light touch should be normal, but the modalities of pain and temperature sensation would be altered. Therefore, for this patient who is presenting typically with altered sensation in a region like the shoulders bilaterally ("shawl" or "breastplate" sensory deficit),[83] it is imperative that the clinician additionally perform a "sharp-dull" or some other sensory test that evaluates the modalities carried by the anterolateral system.[30] Again, a scan examination is to provide an overview and is used to identify deficits. If a sensory deficiency is identified by either the history or the light touch scan, then the evaluator is obligated to recognize that additional follow-up may need to be done and that sensation involves several systems that are best evaluated by their unique modalities. Additionally, while typically kept in the back of the clinician's mind, there are also other procedures, such as the extinction phenomena,[73] that may need to be utilized in rare cases where central nervous system involvement is suspected (see *Four Minute Neurological Examination*[32] for additional details).

Sensory testing can add a great deal to the testing of a working hypothesis, if the evaluator has a clear picture of the distributions provided by both dermatomes and cutaneous peripheral nerves. Generally, dermatomes are the extension of problems originating at the root or plexus level, and roughly follow the maps outlined in anatomy atlases like Netter's atlas or Grant's atlas of anatomy.[5,70] Dermatomes also overlap; so if only one root level is affected, there may be no clear sensory involvement, or the area involved would appear smaller than the anatomy atlases typically convey. For dermatomes, it typically requires that at least two levels be affected to have complete sensory loss in a dermatomal distribution. With cutaneous peripheral nerves, however, damage to a given nerve can result in clear sensory loss when only that one nerve has been compromised. For example, if a patient sustained a cut or fracture that severed the superficial radial nerve above the wrist, then a sensory loss would occur in a region on the dorsum of the hand between the thumb and index finger.[66] This loss is unique to this peripheral cutaneous nerve and is in keeping with the more distal site of injury. Since this is a sensory nerve at this point (still has some autonomic motor fibers within the nerve, so it is not a pure sensory nerve[66]), there will not be any distal muscles that can be collaboratively tested. Careful sensory testing will provide collaborative information that can be used with the data

from the rest of the examination to help identify the underlying problem.

An additional point with sensory testing is that the evaluator needs to clearly ascertain the nature of the sensory dysfunction. For some patients, they have normal sensation but may also complain of tingling. Thus, there really is no deficit, but the patient still is identifying a region that does not feel normal. Some patient's will describe distributions that can only be explained by a vascular dysfunction, so in addition to knowing dermatomes and peripheral cutaneous nerves, the evaluator needs to be aware of vascular regions and the manifestations of a less than optimal vascular system. Finally, there will be some patients with a hypesthesia or allodynia associated with their sensory system. These are typically due to conditions like complex regional pain syndrome (old name of sympathetic reflex dystrophy), which affect the sensory system by producing an increase in the perceived sensation. Conditions such as complex regional pain syndrome illustrate the need for the evaluator to have an excellent foundational anatomical and physiological base, understanding the role of autonomic fibers in mixed nerves, in addition to the more frequently considered general sensory afferents. By staying open-minded, collecting the data as it presents, and then working to distill the information within the context of working hypotheses, the evaluating clinician will often be able to use sensation to collaborate the rest of the objective examination.

5. *Palpation:* The history should have provided insight into the region where the patients state that they have pain, if pain is a major factor in their presentation for care. It is the job of the evaluating clinician to know the anatomy of the area well enough that the structures that can be easily palpated are identified and assessed with touch in a systematic way. As has been the case with all elements of the evaluation, the history should have provided the clinician with a set of working hypotheses that need to be distilled down to the one or two most likely involved structures. Additionally, the clinician should have insisted during the history for the patient to identify "the bulls-eye" point of pain. In other words, require through questioning that the individuals provide a specific location where they believe that the pain is emanating from, rather than permitting the patient to simply report that "the shoulder hurts." What is the specific location of the center point of pain? With this information, it is much easier to plan the systematic palpation assessment.

Once the focal point of the palpation assessment has been identified, the planned evaluation should begin away from this point. The reasons for beginning away from this centralized point of pain are the following: (1) It assists in keeping the evaluator from becoming myopic. If the systematic palpation assessment immediately focuses in on the suspected area or structure involved, then it is too easy to stop the assessment as soon as the patient expresses that the therapist's palpation causes pain. If this is done, other potentially involved areas or structures are not investigated and potentially important data are missed. (2) Palpation by its very nature is a provocative test that is meant to reproduce the pain that the patient is seeking to stop. Therefore, as part of the process of performing a sound evaluation and establishing maximum rapport with the patient, it makes sense to not immediately reach out and press on an area that the therapist believes will reproduce pain. Start on structures outside of the key area of interest, and systematically work toward what is believed to be the involved structure. The patient then has the knowledge that the therapist is evaluating numerous structures in the area and that the key goal is not to immediately reproduce pain. When a structure is palpated that is painful, this can be compared to the other structures that have been palpated and questions asked about the nature of the pain produced. For example, firm palpation to the coracoid process in the shoulder is uncomfortable for the normal person. If this is reported as painful, the follow-up questions should assess if this reproduces the pain that has caused the patient to present for care, or if this is simply a structure or area that is uncomfortable when palpated. In an ideal world, the goal of palpation is to identify one structure or one small area that reproduces the same pain that has prompted the patient to seek medical care. (3) Because palpation is expected to be painful, it is probably a good idea to leave the palpation to late in the physical examination. This is closely related to point 2 above, where a key goal is to establish maximum rapport and not immediately reach out and perform procedures that the therapist expects will hurt the patient. Be gentle, explain what is being done, provide a systematic assessment, and work to design the palpation of a region so that it is toward the end of the overall examination and ideally ends with the palpation of the one or two structures that are the primary working hypotheses.

Two final caveats are as follows: (1) When palpating an area, this provides an excellent opportunity for a very close visual inspection of the region. Look for any swelling, potential joint effusion, changes in skin color or texture, atrophy, or evidence of old scars or other sign of injury. If anything out of the ordinary is observed, ask pertinent questions and work those responses into the working hypotheses. Use this time to fully examine the region and make a complete assessment. (2) Understand the potential impact of referred pain and how it may affect the assessment. If pain is referred, there is a good chance that the palpation of a given region will not reproduce the patient's described pain. This is logical, since the real source of the pain is in another region of the body. For example, due to the embryological distribution of root levels associated with the phrenic nerve, an irritation or injury causing pain in the region of the diaphragm may refer pain to the C3 through C5 dermatomes of the neck and shoulder.[65] While this is where the patient is feeling pain, this is not the source

of the pain and palpation will not shed any additional light on the matter. It may be that the key finding from this negative result is to prompt the evaluator to think beyond the one region being investigated and consider referred pain as a key source of the problem. If this is the case, and since referred pain if often associated with visceral structures, an additional question that needs to be asked has to do with the nature of the presenting problem. If it is neuromusculoskeletal, then it may still be within the domain of the therapist performing the evaluation. If it is outside of that sphere, then referral to an appropriate specialist may be the ideal course of treatment. Again, a key element associated with anyone performing scanning examinations is to understand the limits of their skills and professional scope of practice, and utilize other members of the health care team when appropriate.

6. *Provocative tests:* Palpation was potentially a provocative test, since by design the evaluator hopes that he/she is able to put pressure on an involved structure and reproduce the pain that has brought the patient into the clinic. Thus, if the clinician is able to reproduce the patient's exact pain, and if there is an understanding of the structures involved when the pain is reproduced, then the cause of the pain can be understood. In other words, the goal of a provocative test is to reproduce the patient's symptoms in a controlled environment, where the factors that contribute to the generation of pain can be understood.

A classic example of a provocative test is the contractile versus inert tissue test described by Cyriax.[19] In a hypothetical case where a clinician is evaluating shoulder pain and has as working hypotheses a potential subdeltoid bursitis versus a supraspinatus tendonitis, a provocative test can be used to potentially distinguish between these two clinical problems. The provocative test will really involve two elements, one that tests the contractile elements (muscle, tendon, and teno-periosteal elements) and the other that tests the inert structures (a bursa would be an example of an inert structure). For example, with the arm held at the patient's side, the patient is asked to strongly abduct the shoulder while the shoulder is being isometrically stabilized. In the case of a supraspinatus tendonitis, this "contractile" structure will be stressed, causing pain that reproduces the patient's symptoms. Since no movement took place (which is the role of the inert bursa), it would not be expected that this isometric contraction would cause any pain, if the involved structure was the subdeltoid bursa. On the basis of this information gained by a pain-producing (provocative) test, the evaluating clinician can make a judgment regarding the structure most likely involved in this patient.

The flip side of this assessment is to have the patients completely relax their shoulder, putting all of the contractile structures in a state where they are not stressed. Then, the clinician can gently move the shoulder into abduction, through the 50–130° range of motion where a bursa is often irritated.[69] If this causes pain, whereas the previous isometric contraction did not elicit pain, then this finding suggests that the bursa is the involved anatomical structure.

Note five points in the preceding example.

- A test was used to intentionally provoke the patient's symptoms, in an effort to understand what is causing the pain. Both of these tests should not result in a finding of pain reproduction, since they are testing different structures. The more specific a given provocative test is, the better the understanding is of the potential cause of pain when it is reproduced.

- The decision matrix used by the experienced clinician is built upon the collaborative findings of the two preceding tests, as well as any other provocative tests that are felt to be appropriate. No one manual test has perfect sensitivity or specificity. Therefore, in an effort to do the best job identifying the cause of a patient's symptoms, the potential cause of the problem should be looked at through the use of several tests, and the results from each evaluated against the working hypotheses in a collaborative manner.

- There should be clear communication with the patient that some of the testing done may actually create some discomfort, but this is being intentionally done in an effort to better understand the mechanisms involved in creating the problem. If there is clear communication with the patients, and they know ahead of time that while the evaluator is being as gentle as possible they may still experience pain, it is easier for them to tolerate these tests. As has been stated before, this assists with the development of establishing rapport and aids in the informational exchange.

- The clinician needs to know if the pain caused by a provocative test is the same pain that brought the patient into the clinic. For example, if the patient had been describing a radicular pain from the shoulder, down the lateral aspect of the arm, into the ulnar aspect of the forearm, does the provocative test create this type of pain? If the pain created is limited to the base of the neck with no radicular symptoms, then whatever provocative test was used has not provided a great deal of insight into the patient's primary problem. On the other hand, if the test employed did reproduce these symptoms, then the therapist has an increased understanding of the mechanics involved and is in a much better position to design a treatment program to truly treat the problem.

- Understand that when evaluating the neuromusculoskeletal system, most causes of pain can be mechanically provoked. If at the end of the provocative testing there has not been anything that was able to reproduce the patient's symptoms, then the clinician needs to strongly consider that the cause of the pain may not be associated with a neuromusculoskeletal system problem. As was mentioned in the preceding section on pain, this may be a strong indicator that a referral may be warranted.

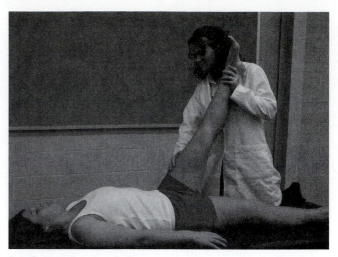

FIGURE 4-10

Example of a straight leg raising test.

There are many provocative tests that can be employed, depending on the region evaluated. The classics are procedures like the foraminal encroachment test[56,62] (Spurling's test—see Fig. 4-1) for potential cervical radiculopathies, the straight leg test[77] for lumbar or sacral nerve root problems (see Fig. 4-10), or the family of thoracic outlet tests[52,72,76] (see Fig. 4-11). The purpose of this chapter is not to list all of these tests, but rather to point out their contribution to the evaluation process. A provocative test that is well understood in terms of the structures involved when it is employed, provides a manual testing procedure that gives the clinician tremendous insight into the mechanism of the patient's problem. When combined with other tests in a collaborative fashion, a strongly defendable hypothesis can be generated that can direct a highly effective treatment program. (For a more complete listing of provocative tests and the mechanisms behind them, see the

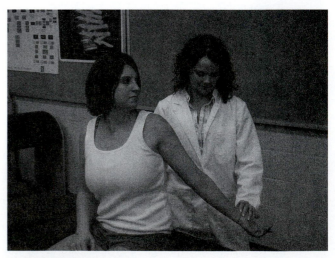

FIGURE 4-11

Example of a thoracic outlet test.

following texts by Dutton et al., Baxter et al., Flynn et al., and others.[9,22,27])

7. *Clearing tests:* A general principle of neuromusculoskeletal assessment is to always evaluate the region (or joint) above and below the primary area of interest. The intent of this principle is to remain broad in the initial evaluation so that areas that often refer pain are not inadvertently missed, and to keep the evaluation from becoming too myopic in its focus. Thus, clearing tests are employed to "clear" a given region as the potential source of the patient's problem, or to clear structures that may potentially create a danger for a patient if a particular procedure is employed later in the evaluation or treatment phase.[80] Two examples are provided below to demonstrate these two uses of clearing tests.

In treating an individual with shoulder pain, the neck should always be examined. It is common for a patient to describe pain in the shoulder or arm that is caused by a nerve root or other impingement in the cervical spine. To clear the neck, one of the tests used is the aforementioned foraminal encroachment test (Spurling's test). This test, through the combination of neck side bending, rotation, and extension, functions to decrease the space provided by the intervertebral foramen (close down the intervertebral space). In the case of an impinged or irritated nerve root, this should irritate the nerve root, reproduce the patient's symptoms, and serve as a type of provocative test. On the other hand, if this procedure does not elicit any discomfort that radiates toward the shoulder, the findings suggest that the neck can be cleared as an obvious source of this patient's shoulder pain. Thus, the negative finding with the Spurling's test, combined with negative findings of any other screening tests used with the cervical spine, work to collectively clear the neck as a likely source of this patient's pain.

Staying with the cervical spine, a second clearing test that is often used in an effort to promote maximum safety for the patient is a vertebral artery test. The combined positioning of the supine patient in an extended, side bent, and rotated position for up to 30 seconds[56] is intended to rule out the vertebral artery as a source of concern should manipulation or other manual procedures be used to treat the cervical spine (see Fig. 4-12). Thus, a positive finding with this test would suggest that the patient had a potential restriction of the vertebral artery and should be referred for additional evaluation. On the other hand, a negative finding (e.g., no nausea, dizziness, diplopia, etc.) is used as a way to clear the vertebral artery and provide the examiner with data that suggest that manipulating the cervical spine should be safe. By employing this vertebral artery test, the therapist is working to promote safety and clear any identifiable potential dangers prior to beginning the treatment program.

While the goals associated with the clearing tests are admirable, the astute evaluator should understand that

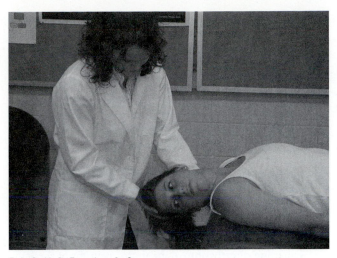

FIGURE 4-12

Vertebral artery test position.

negative findings in the two commonly used clearing tests do not truly clear the neck. An individual can have a cervical radiculopathy in the presence of a negative Spurling's test. Additionally, research has clearly shown that the vertebral artery test is far from specific when attempting to identify patients with vertebral artery restrictions, and a negative finding with this test does not necessarily rule out the possibility of a vertebrobasilar insufficiency or provide a safe environment for cervical manipulation.[15,80] These clearing tests are simply one more bit of collaborative information that should be evaluated within the context of the entire examination. In the presence of negative clearing tests, a region like the cervical spine may drop from being the prime hypothesis being investigated, but the cervical spine still needs to be kept in the back of the examiner's mind as a secondary or tertiary hypothesis. Then, as more data are collected, a considered judgment can be made on the best working hypothesis. There should never be a time, however, where the evaluator dismisses a region like the neck as a potential contributor to the problem at hand, simply because the results of one or two clearing tests were negative.

An additional point that was implied in the section above is that the categorization of tests is not discrete. The Spurling's test mentioned above is both a provocative test and a clearing test. The label designator assigned at any point in time is really the intended use of the test. Regardless of the label assigned, the test remains the same and both types of information (provocative and clearing) are provided when the manual test is employed. The skilled examiner has a well-thought-out system that stays consistent in its key elements and utilizes tests that will provide the data upon which defendable judgments can be made. The labeling of a test may assist with description of one of the purposes of a given test to others, or provide a rationale for assigning tests to particular places in an evaluation scheme, but the potentially multiple uses of a given procedure should be clearly recognized by the evaluator performing these tests.

8. *Muscle stretch reflexes:* Muscle stretch reflexes (MSRs) test the integrity of the segmental level reflex arc, as well as provide information on the central nervous system interacting with the reflex arc. In its simplest form, the MSR consists of a sensory receptor (muscle spindle), an afferent neuron, a synapse, an efferent neuron, and the effector organ of skeletal muscle. When a muscle is abruptly stretched, as is the case when a reflex hammer displaces a tendon, the muscle spindles in the homonymous muscle are stretched and generate an action potential that is conveyed to the spinal cord. This signal brought into the central nervous system is the most common example of a monosynaptic reflex, synapsing directly onto alpha motor neurons of the muscle of origin.[50] This excitatory stimulus typically results in the generation of an action potential down the efferent neuron, creating a contraction in all of the muscle fibers innervated by that particular motor unit. The end result is a visible muscle contraction of the muscle associated with the tendon struck, indicating that the reflex arc is intact (see Fig. 4-13, a simple reflex arc).

The old term of "deep tendon reflex" (DTR) is a misnomer: For years, the reflex arc described above has been known as a deep tendon reflex. While all clinicians need to be aware of the term since it remains in use today, it should also be understood that a better descriptor is MSR. The term MSR is more precise, since it accurately conveys that muscle spindles are the sensory organ activated, since the modality that they are most sensitive to is a change in length.[50] This term also conveys the role that muscle spindles have at the muscle of origin, which is to facilitate the muscle and provide the contraction observed. On the other hand, the old term suggests that the sensory organ of interest resides within the tendon, and the only receptor that would qualify is the Golgi tendon organ. This receptor is not activated by a change in length, but rather by a tension change, which is not significantly affected by a small deflection with a reflex hammer. Additionally, the impact of Golgi tendon activation for the homonymous muscle (muscle of origin) is to inhibit the muscle. This is directly opposite of what is observed when an MSR is evoked. Therefore, in an effort to accurately convey what has been done during the examination, the term MSR should be used, instead of the dated and incorrect term of DTR.

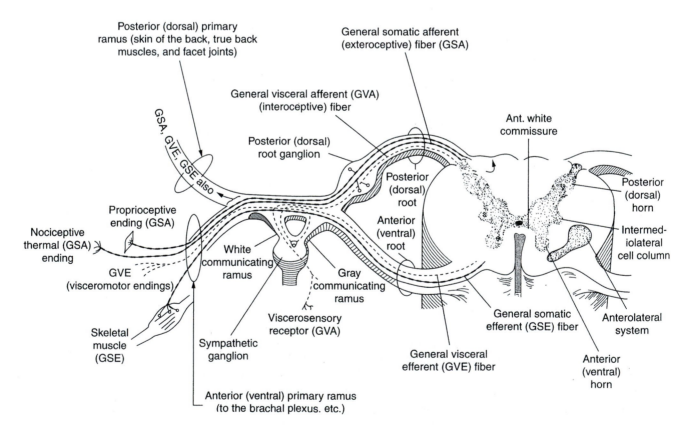

FIGURE 4-13

Typical spinal nerve with reflex arc. (Reproduced, with permission, from Halle J, Greathouse D. In: Prentice WE, ed. *Therapeutic Modalities in Rehabilitation*, 3rd ed. New York, McGraw-Hill, 2005, pp. 201–255.)

While the preceding paragraph identified the key elements involved with eliciting a segmental level reflex, it failed to convey some of the informational richness that can be obtained from this simple test. In any case where the reflexes are not symmetrical, the findings need to be viewed in light of any other collaborative information available. Additionally, in some cases where the reflex findings are symmetrical, but either elevated or depressed, these findings also need to be viewed in light of the other collaborative information. Several illustrative examples will be provided in the paragraphs below to assist in the interpretation of findings associated with the MSRs.

Generally, an asymmetrically depressed or absent reflex is suggestive of pathology that is impacting the reflex arc directly, such as a lower motor neuron (LMN) problem. The converse is generally true for elevated or "brisk" reflexes, which are commonly viewed as indicating that the central nervous system's normal role of integrating reflexes (serving as a governor) has been disrupted. Thus, an asymmetrical brisk reflex is typically indicative of an upper motor neuron (UMN) (premotor neuron) problem.[84] In both of the statements made in this paragraph, the term "asymmetrical" has been used, since it illustrates the important point that not everyone will have the same response to a reflex hammer tapping for a given tendon or muscle belly. Some individuals have bilaterally depressed or even absent reflexes, but these are symmetrical and not restricted to only one of the many MSRs that can be tested. In a similar vein, some individuals have bilaterally brisk reflexes, but this is also relatively uniform throughout all of their reflexes. Therefore, the presence of asymmetrical reflexes suggests pathology and further investigation. Additionally, while the presence of clearly depressed or clearly elevated reflexes can be a normal finding, the astute clinicians must keep this information in the back of their mind and is obligated to investigate further, since this may be a subtle sign of a systemic or symmetrical problem. A few examples are provided below.

Depressed reflexes: In cases where there is complete damage to any element of the reflex arc, such as the afferent or efferent limb, no reflex will be elicited. This would be the case for an individual with a severed peripheral nerve, affecting both the afferent and efferent fibers. Thus, no signal would ever reach the spinal cord, and no efferent signal would consequently be generated. The absence of a reflex, in this case, indicates some type of structural problem that the clinician would need to investigate further. In this simple case, the severed nerve would be accompanied with a host of other findings, such as clear atrophy, sensory loss, and weakness that should make the source of the problem evident (see Table 4-4 for a summary of UMN/LMN signs/symptoms).

A more subtle finding is a depressed, yet intact MSR. This is usually indicative of some type of struc-tural problem that impedes the function of some of the axons within a mixed spinal nerve, with other axons continuing to function normally. A common example of this is the patient with a herniated disk in their lower back. The disk protrusion that compresses the exiting nerve root decrements the function of a percentage of the axons contained within that mixed spinal nerve, so that while the reflex signal is able to be both received via afferents and expressed back to the periphery through efferents, the size of the response is smaller than that found on the unaffected side. In individuals with some type of nerve root compression at the intervertebral foramen, this type of depressed reflex is the expected finding. In severe cases of nerve root impingement, no reflex can be elicited, suggesting that a majority of axons contained within that mixed spinal nerve root are involved.

Note that both the afferent and efferent limb of the reflex arc were included in the discussion of the impact on the reflex arc. While many clinicians view a depressed reflex as being synonymous with an LMN problem, it should be recognized that any condition that affects any element of this arc can result in MSR findings that are not normal. While rare, an individual with tabes dorsalis (tertiary syphilis) will have selective destruction of the dorsal columns of the spinal cord and the neurons that project into the dorsal columns.[29] Since these are the same neurons that bring the afferent action potentials into the spinal cord, the death of these neurons means that the afferent limb of the reflex arc will be disrupted with minimal or absent MSRs, in the presence of completely healthy LMNs. This "artificial" example is provided to illustrate two points. First, any dysfunction within the reflex arc can result in a depressed or absent reflex, so it cannot be considered to be a pure indicator of an LMN problem. Second, in a case like the tabes dorsalis presented, the depression or absence of MSRs will be bilateral and widespread, suggesting that there are other collaborative data available. Thus, the depressed reflex does not stand alone, but is one important piece of the puzzle that is fed into evaluation and compared against the varied working hypotheses that are in play.

Elevated reflexes: In a normally functioning nervous system, the central nervous system (brain and spinal cord) acts as a type of "governor" that helps regulate and control the activity generated by the segmental level reflex. If that normal relationship is disrupted by an insult that affects the central nervous system, then the reflex arc is functionally "released" from this governor. This results in an elevated or brisk reflex, when an MSR is elicited.

In the case of a condition such as a cerebral vascular accident (stroke) affecting one side of the central nervous system, the asymmetrical finding of an elevated MSR on one side would be expected. With a more symmetrical lesion, such as a spinal stenosis narrowing the vertebral foramen (canal) that was affecting the entirety of the spinal cord, bilaterally elevated MSRs would be expected. Both these cases demonstrate that an altered and elevated MSR provides the clinician with information that the central nervous system is not functioning in the expected way with the segmental level reflex arc, and that the peripheral nervous system is probably not the source of this patient's complaint.

The key issue associated with the MSR testing described above is that it provides the clinician with a direct way of assessing the peripheral nervous system, and an indirect way of examining the central nervous system. This type of testing would not really be needed for the clear-cut example of an individual with a severed nerve; the nature of the problem would be obvious. Similarly, this type of testing is not really necessary for the patient who has clearly experienced a cerebral vascular accident, since again, the nature of the problem would be obvious. However, for the typical patient who is seeking an evaluation for a problem that is not directly obvious, having a tool that is able to simultaneously provide information about both the peripheral and central nervous system is invaluable. And, the information provided can often be the key that helps unlock the puzzle. Two examples illustrate this with relatively obscure cases: (1) A patient presents with symmetrically brisk patellar tendon MSRs and Achilles tendon MSRs, while simultaneously having absent MSRs in the upper extremity. This odd finding could result in additional investigation that unfortunately demonstrates that the patient is suffering from amyotrophic lateral sclerosis (Lou Gering's disease), a mixed UMN and LMN pathology; the MSR findings help direct the rest of the examination and referrals. (2) A second patient referred for anterior knee pain, is found to have very brisk patellar tendon MSRs bilaterally. Upon further questioning, the patient also discloses that there have been episodes of fluctuating weakness and diplopia (double vision). Appropriate referral and follow-up testing might reveal that this patient is in the early stages of multiple sclerosis, and the increase in tone of the lower extremity associated with this condition is responsible for the knee pain.

These two rare cases illustrate that a clinician will not find what he/she is not looking for. The only way to guard against missing examples like those provided above is to be systematic and know the anatomy and physiology behind the test being employed. MSRs of the region being examined (e.g., upper extremity or lower extremity) should be a part of every evaluation done, except perhaps the athletic injury that the clin-

TABLE   4-5

Common Muscle Stretch Reflexes

MUSCLE STRETCH REFLEXES (BOLD INDICATES MOST PROMINENT ROOT LEVEL)	
Upper extremity	Lower extremity
Biceps brachii reflex (**C5**, 6)	Patellar tendon reflex (L2-**4**)
Brachioradialis reflex (C5, **6**)	Hamstring reflex (**L5**, S1-2)
Triceps brachii reflex (C6, **7**, 8)	Achilles tendon reflex (L5, **S1**-2)

ician personally witnessed. This information should be noted and factored in as part of the working hypotheses being considered.

Commonly tested MSRs and how they are recorded: In the upper extremity, three MSRs are commonly tested: (1) Biceps brachii (predominantly C5), (2) brachioradialis (predominantly C6), and the triceps brachii (predominantly C7). In the lower extremity, there are two commonly tested MSRs and one less frequently used MSR. The two commonly used reflexes are (1) quadriceps (predominantly L4) and (2) gastrocnemius/soleus (predominantly S1). The less commonly employed Hamstring reflex is predominantly L5. The Hamstring reflex is not used as often because it is much more difficult to elicit and is therefore less reliable and useful. (See Table 4-5 for commonly used reflexes and grading.)

The reflexes are typically graded on a 5-point scale, ranging from zero (0), indicating an absent reflex, to four (4), indicating an extremely brisk reflex.[58] A two (2), is considered normal, with anything above or below that value indicative of a finding that is elevated or depressed to some extent. Again, the key finding is not that a reflex deviates from the 2 level. The key findings are that there is asymmetry between limbs, or the symmetrical but unusual MSR is associated with other collaborative findings revealed during the scan examination.

9. *Pathological reflexes:* Pathological reflex testing is adjunctive to the MSRs described above. For those patients with a UMN problem, it would be expected that a pathological reflex could be elicited. The pathological reflex commonly sought in the lower extremity is the Babinski reflex, which is performed by stroking a blunt object across the sole of the foot, from the lateral side toward the great toe. A "present Babinski" is when this causes the great toe to extend and the other toes to extend and abduct. A response that causes flexion of the great toe and other toes or withdrawal of the foot is a normal response, and is recorded as a "Babinski not present." The more common elicitation of this reflex

that involves stroking the lateral side of the foot progressing to the ball of the foot is really a combination of two pathological reflexes, the Chattock and Babinski.[16] For a more complete description of the technique and findings associated with these two, and other reflexes of the lower extremity (e.g., Oppenheim, Gordon, etc.), the interested reader is referred to the following reference.[16]

The upper limb equivalent to the Babinski is the Hoffman sign (or reflex). This is elicited by having a relaxed and supported hand, and the distal aspect of the middle finger is flipped-up in the direction of the fingernail.[16] In an individual who does not have a UMN lesion, this does not elicit much of a response in the relaxed thumb and index finger of the tested side. In a person with a UMN lesion, the thumb and index finger tend to contract in a motion that draws these two digits toward one another.[16] Since a slight contraction of the thumb and index finger can occur in an individual that has a natural tendency for increased reflexes, it is important to compare one side to the other. If asymmetry is identified, then this present Hoffman's reflex needs to be viewed in light of the other collaborative information and prominently figures into the working hypotheses.

Upper quarter scan examinations should always include testing for the pathological Hoffman sign, and lower quarter scan examinations should always include testing for the pathological Babinski reflex. In addition to this minimal level of screening, there are patient conditions in the upper extremity where a Babinski reflex should also be elicited. In the previously mentioned case of an individual with a vertebral foramen spinal stenosis in the cervical region, with symptoms predominantly affecting the upper extremities, a Babinski reflex should be obtained. If unilateral or bilaterally present Babinski reflexes are demonstrated, this provides a great deal of insight into the location of the primary problem (spinal cord compression in the cervical or upper thoracic region with UMN involvement), and indicates that a referral to a health care provider that can address the base problem is warranted. The bottom line is pathological reflexes should always be performed in the region of interest, and a Babinski or other appropriate lower extremity pathological reflex should additionally be elicited for those upper extremity problems where the working hypotheses involve the spinal cord or other elements of the central nervous system (e.g., the previously mentioned case of multiple sclerosis, etc.).

10. *Special tests:* A scan examination is by definition a systematic and efficient (implies brief) evaluation of a particular area of interest. While the two most common applications of the scan examination are upper and lower quarter screens, the scan examination is adaptable to any particular region of the body, such as examining the knee joint, wrist, or other region of the body. Recognized within this application to a specific joint or region is the need to always consider the joint or region immediately proximal

and distal to that area, since it is common to have referred pain and an initially myopic evaluation does not serve the patient well.

Recognizing that the standard scan examination is by design brief and efficient, there needs to be adequate flexibility built into the design of the scan examination to permit additional investigation and follow-up of an area of particular interest. This is where special tests come into play. In the case of an individual with knee pain and a history that suggests damage to the ligaments and capsule surrounding the joint, or structures associated with the joint such as bursa, further investigation is warranted. The skilled clinician should employ the appropriate tests to help progress to the next stage of the scan examination, which is the assessment. These tests will assist with the revision or refinement of the working hypotheses into one best hypothesis. (The myriad of available special tests is beyond the scope of this chapter, and the interested reader is referred to other sources that provide much more detail on specific tests.[22,34,37,57,60,94])

Final caveat prior to the assessment: The goal of the scan examination up to this point has been to collect data. As the clinician proceeds to the assessment, there is a need to be reflective, reexamine mentally each bit of information to determine how it relates to the variety of working hypotheses in play, and hopefully, distill these data down into one best hypothesis that is consistent with the history and objective findings obtained during the examination. This working hypothesis can be expressed as an anatomical or structural problem, the traditional medical diagnosis, or as a listing of physical therapy diagnoses that demonstrate the functional neuromusculoskeletal problems that can be addressed. In either case, the clinician needs to decide what the problem(s) is/are, and begin to formulate a course of action. This leads to the assessment, discussed next.

Assessment

The assessment will typically be the one hypothesis that is most consistent with all the data collected in the preceding scan examination. In most cases, there is a single explanation that has brought a patient in for care. In rare cases, however, there may be several dysfunctions that are occurring simultaneously, and the astute clinician needs to have a flexible enough system to both look for and allow for this possibility. Once all the data have been reviewed, a decision has to be made on what the problem is; identification of one or more issues is necessary to frame an approach on the best way to address the identified problem. The documentation and communication of the assessment may take one of several forms:

1. One traditional medical diagnosis that provides a pathophysiological structure than can be addressed by the evaluating clinician (an anatomical or structural diagnosis).
2. Two or more medical diagnoses that provide several pathophysiological structures that can be addressed by the evaluating clinician (again, an anatomical or structural diagnosis).

3. A physical therapy diagnosis that demonstrates clear biomechanical or neuromusculoskeletal shortcomings that can be addressed, which is consistent with the patient's presenting problem. These issues may range from muscle weakness, to range of motion limitations, to leg-length discrepancies, to a myriad of other findings that become evident during the scan examination with appropriate special tests for follow-up (the Guide to Physical Therapy Practice language[6]).

4. That a referral to another health care provider is warranted. As has been stressed throughout this chapter, the hallmark of true professionals is knowing the limits of their areas of expertise.[38] A proper referral can be a tremendously valuable service to a patient seeking care.

5. That there is a need to schedule a follow-up appointment to collect additional data and refine the working hypothesis. A reality of life is that there is not infinite time to perform the most detailed and involved evaluation to investigate every possible dysfunction with each patient. The key purpose of the scan examination is to employ a systematic evaluation so as not to miss potential pathology that requires referral or immediate care. A secondary purpose of the examination is to allow the flexibility for a more in-depth examination at a second or third patient visit. This means that if more information is required, recognize this need and build the collection of the data into a subsequent patient visit. The willingness to admit that not all data can or should be collected during the initial visit permits the time for further reflection, mentorship consultation, and consideration of the potential role of other key systems, such as cardiopulmonary, neurological, and integumentary.

The choice of the way to express the assessed findings may be dictated by the environment that the clinician works in, or it may be personal preference. As has been alluded to above, there is a current drive to express physical therapy findings in a form that recognizes that a physical therapy diagnosis (assessment) differs from a medical diagnosis (assessment) (see the Guide to Physical Therapy Practice[6]). Physical therapists cannot typically order tests like X-rays, bone scans, magnetic resonance imaging, or perform arthroscopic explorations, so they do not have the tools to diagnose fractures, stress reactions of bone, torn menisci, or labral tears. Recognizing that this is absolutely true, it is also true that a patient with a clearly positive Lachman's test and pivot shift test to the knee, with a history of hearing "a pop" and experiencing an acute right knee effusion, probably has at a minimum a torn anterior cruciate ligament. These collaborative findings can be expressed in the assessment as a list of the physical therapy limitations associated with this condition.

ASSESSMENT 1

(1) Limited knee joint range of motion of the right knee, (2) knee pain, (3) knee joint effusion, (4) antalgic gait, (5) quadri-

ceps muscle weakness, and (6) altered neuromuscular control; grouped under Preferred Practice Pattern 4D, impaired joint mobility, motor function, muscle performance, and range of motion associated with connective tissue dysfunction. This is the nomenclature associated with the Guide to Physical Therapy Practice.[6] This assessment would probably also result in a referral to a health care professional, like an orthopedic surgeon, for the additional testing needed to make a definitive diagnosis.

A second way of expressing these findings in the assessment would be to provide a probable anatomical cause of the dysfunction, along with a list of the specific items that physical therapy would work to address. An example of this form of assessment with the same patient described above is next discussed.

ASSESSMENT 2

Rule out torn right anterior cruciate ligament.

Physical therapy issues: (1) limited knee joint range of motion, (2) knee pain, (3) knee joint effusion, (4) antalgic gait, (5) quadriceps muscle weakness, and (6) altered neuromuscular control.

Other: Refer to an orthopedic surgeon or other appropriate health care professional for definitive diagnosis.

Neither of these approaches is absolutely correct or incorrect. The first (Assessment 1) follows the basic tenets of the guide,[6] which is the profession's definitive document describing the scope of physical therapy practice.[6] In those settings where this type of description works, it should probably be the approach used, since this is in keeping with the recommendations of the guide.[6] Having recognized the key role and importance of the guide,[6] there are limitations associated with using a list of findings to describe the physical therapy diagnosis. Metaphorically, for those entities for which we have established labels recognized by all parties, it is easier to convey information by using the label than by using a list of descriptors. It is easier to say that there is an elephant in the backyard, than to try to describe a big animal that is gray, wrinkled, possessing a tail, with ears bigger than most animals. While physical therapists cannot examine the genetic code to verify the species of elephant, they are able to identify the basic creature and then convey any specific attributes of that animal that may relate to a specific species. Clearly, great liberty has been taken with the metaphor described above, but it illustrates that physical therapists do not function in a vacuum, but are part of the traditional medical community. Therefore, the communication tends to be much more straightforward with other health professionals when traditional labels like "rule out anterior cruciate ligament tear" are used. These can be stated in a way that demonstrates that this is not a definitive diagnosis, but rather a strong working hypothesis. When supplemented with the list of attributes that the scan examination has identified that can be addressed by physical therapy, then the communication and, if warranted, referral, are clearer for all involved. Therefore, in those settings where the format of Assessment 2 makes sense, it should be considered.

The bottom line of the assessment is to identify, and label, the specific items that should be addressed during the next two phases of the scan examination, the goal and the plan.

Goal

The goal is what the clinician and the patient want to achieve. It is placed in this system in a location that differs from the traditional SOAP note format. The rationale for this transposition of place in the examination process is that the clinicians need to know where they want to go (the goal) prior to developing a plan to get there. Metaphorically, no one would ever look at a map and plan to head out of town on a specific highway, if they had not first determined where they wanted to end up at the completion of the trip. In a similar vein, the clinician, in consultation with the patient, needs to establish one or more goals that meet at least the following minimal list of expectations, if the clinician has determined that the care needed can be provided within his/her scope of practice. These five expectations include that (1) the goals are realistic, (2) the goals meet the patient's expectations, (3) the goals define what will be achieved in the short term, (4) the goals define what will be achieved in the long term, and (5) the goals are measurable. In those occasions where the care or additional evaluation needs to be done by another health care professional, the goal may change to linking the patient with the best health care provider for them.

The initial expectation associated with goals is that they are realistic. To a large degree, this is based on the experience and judgment of the clinician, drawing from the information provided during the scan examination evaluation. It is not realistic to assume that the goal(s) associated with care are to have each patient return to an optimal level of function. A patient encountered by the author early in his career was a gentleman in his early to midseventies, with longstanding diabetes and bilateral above knee amputations. He loved to ride trains, and had been referred for transfer training, general conditioning, and household mobility training. He had been in a wheelchair for over a year, and had new prosthetic limbs. While the scan examination performed on him still utilized the system outlined in this chapter (in terms of history, prepared questions, and a physical examination), the data collected were vital to determining his current physical status, point where a treatment plan should be initiated, and what goals might be sought. While blurring the point of being realistic, with the next paragraph on the patient's expectations, this collected data need to be viewed in light of the wishes of the patient. In this case, back in the late 1970s, the only way to board the steam engine trains that he wanted to ride was to walk up the steps onto the train. Thus, he came to the clinic with an expectation that he would be assisted in learning to walk again, so that he could walk to the train, board it, and ride. Due to his age, level of conditioning, and the extreme energy costs associated with ambulating with the prostheses associated with dual above knee amputations, this was not a realistic goal. The information obtained from the scan examination provided a starting point to begin formulating what was realistic. This led to the next expectation of the goal(s) established, working to meet the patient's expectations.

Serving the patient and working to meet their needs and expectations is really the fundamental reason that health care is provided. To achieve these elements of care, clinicians need to take the time to find out what the patient wants and expects. The information provided by the patient, coupled with the data obtained during the scan examination, allows a merging of the patient's goals with the clinician's therapeutic goals. When combined in this way, the two elements synergistically create a set of goals that are a "force multiplier," in terms of achieving realistic, measurable results. Referring back to the example in the paragraph above, it was not realistic that the patient would be able to walk to the train, climb a short series of stairs, and ambulate to his seat on the train. While that goal was out of reach, this individual appeared capable of transfers, short distance ambulation, and the ability to navigate two or three steps. Following a frank discussion, a mutually agreed upon set of expectations were outlined and agreed to. These provided the basis for short- and long-term goal development, with measurable/objective landmarks. The fact that these goals took the patient's wants and expectations into account created an environment where this individual's motivation and drive are still something that I easily recall nearly 30 years later.

A more common example of the need to take the patient's wants and expectations into account is when dealing with athletes. Athletic patients who are used to training regularly and are injured with some type of overuse problem typically will not settle for a plan that involves rest. Most of these patients want to continue to train, and while they will be polite to the health care professional who recommends rest, they will often leave the office and start the search for another health care provider who understands their particular needs. The clinician who takes the time to find out what the patient wants and expects, should be in a position to educate the patient on what is realistic from the pathophysiological perspective, while also letting the patient know that they are collaboratively working to achieve the patient's goals. This may mean resting the involved structure or limb, while still engaging in "active rest" that allows the patient's conditioning to be maintained by some sort of alternate activity. The bottom line here is that the goals established need to be in line with the patient's expectations to enhance compliance and motivation, yet structured within the framework of what the clinician knows is realistic. This creates an environment where both individuals, the patient and the clinician, are working together as a team for a specific purpose (or outcome).

The mutually established goals should ideally be expressed as both short-term and long-term goals. Metaphorically, no one is comfortable with a global goal like "completing graduate school" or "losing 35 pounds." On the surface, these goals appear so large and unattainable, that it would be extremely easy for the individual working to accomplish the goal to become overwhelmed and discouraged. It makes much more sense to set a series of short-term goals that over time lead to the accomplishment of the global (or long-term) goal. In the case of patient goals, the initial short-term goals set should probably be something that can be accomplished within a few treatment sessions or a time period of a week or less. The goal should be realistic, measurable, and in the direction of the long-term goal. For the clinician to stay engaged in the patient's progress, the short-term goal should ideally be linked with a recheck of some type, so that there is continued dialogue between the two members of this team. This type of exchange and dialogue also permits the necessary adjustments and reestablishment of new sets of short-term goals, on the way to accomplishing the overall goal.

The long-term goal(s) serves as the finish line. The long-term goal is the destination that the patient and provider are trying to reach. This goal(s) is also established initially, so that it is clear what both the patient and health care provider are striving to achieve. In addition to serving as a roadmap and framework for adjusting the short-term goals on the way to achieving the final goal, this gives both members of this rehabilitation team a feel for where they are on this journey. When the long-term goal has been achieved, that is a logical time to discontinue care.

A point that was alluded to in the preceding paragraphs is that all stated goals must be measurable. This is needed both as a way to objectively track progress, and in most cases, because it is required by third party payers. As the expert in this area, work to identify criteria that are reliable, easily obtained, and directly related to the patient's condition. In addition to being measurable, short-term and long-term goals should have clear timelines associated with them. While not all the elements of the classic "behavioral objective" will always be in evidence for each goal stated, they should at least be implied if not explicitly stated. For example, if a short-term goal is to have "10° of additional shoulder flexion in one week," the classic elements of who will do what, by when, and to what extent, are all either stated or implied. In this case, the "who" is the patient, so it does not need to be explicitly stated. The "do what," is achieve an additional 10° of shoulder flexion. The "by when," is reflected in the time specification of one week, and the "to what extent" implies that the clinician will employ a standard assessment methodology and will require proper form (no substitution). Thus, utilization of an objective system of this type allows progress to be tracked and both members of the rehabilitation team to know where they are at in terms of the final goal.

In those cases where the scan examination reveals that either the patient's or the clinician's goals fall outside of the current health care provider's area of expertise, then a referral is indicated. As has been stated previously, the hallmark of a true professional is knowing their own limitations, and referring to other members of the health care team when appropriate.[38] In this case, referral works toward the goal of providing the patient with the best possible care for their particular condition, and it strengthens the entire health care family by having professionals work with each other and draw on specific strengths.

Plan

Once the short- and long-term goals have been identified, then it is a relatively straightforward process to determine how to get there. If the earlier used metaphor of a trip is considered, once the destination is clear, the map can be looked at and the most efficient trip plotted. Extending this metaphor, if there is a specific sight or person that the budding traveler wants to see as part of the trip, that detour can be built into the plan.

From the health care provider's perspective, the basic plan is what should they should do, teach, and recommend to the patient. This will be based on a variety of factors, including but not limited to the clinician's experience level, equipment available, number of visits allowed by third party payers, distance that the patient lives away from the clinic, availability of child care for dependents, and a host of other considerations. Within this context, the health care provider is in a position to specify a treatment program, identify where it will be done (e.g., in the clinic, at home, or in both locations), identify how often items of this treatment program are performed, and any specifics associated with the program such as intensity or cautions. The classic exercise prescription should be in evidence here (see ref. 53), of (1) specificity (what should be done), (2) frequency (how often the activity should be done, or the number of repetitions and sets expected), (3) duration (how long the activity should be performed), and (4) intensity (what level of performance is expected). When this is provided to the patient in a clear manner and with specific expectations, the likelihood of success of the plan increases dramatically. Other elements that also work toward promoting success are to go through the plan with the patient, having them demonstrate any activities that they will be doing at home. Provide a constructive critique and give the patient an opportunity to ask questions and demonstrate understanding, rather than simply verbally acknowledging that they understand. Then, provide the plan in writing, supported with appropriate handouts, videotapes, or other medium that offers a clear reminder when the patient is trying to do these on their own. Additionally, give the patients a specific number or e-mail that they can use if questions arise, and insure that these are addressed at least once a day. (See algorithm section in Chapter 5 for a method of clinical reasoning about intervention.)

A home program should be included in almost all treatment programs, since it provides a number of advantages. First, in today's health care environment, no patient will be authorized to come into the clinic for all of their care. It has to be recognized that whether the treatment is elevation of a swollen limb, ambulation instruction, or some form of therapeutic exercise, the patient will do the majority of this care outside of the clinic's walls. Therefore, utilize this reality and have the program performed whenever it is appropriate, within the patient's normal environment. Second, and perhaps more importantly, there is a need to engage the patients in their own care and make them responsible for the outcome. There is a tendency today to assume that patients will seek care and the health care professional will "fix them." This puts all the responsibility on the health care provider and none on the patient. The reality is that the majority of care will take place outside of the clinic, and the patient needs to be both engaged in that care and take responsibility for seeing that it is enacted. A metaphor used above described the rehabilitation "team," where the health care provider serves as the coach and the patient functions like the player. While the coach may be able to recommend the amount of weight that should be lifted, the specific exercises, warm-ups, etc., it is the job of the player to perform the activities to become stronger, faster, more flexible, etc. The patients must assume the bulk of the responsibility for their care, or it should be understood that most treatment interventions would not be successful. While perhaps a poor metaphor, few would argue that even if a patient arranged and kept regular dental checkups every six months, if they did not brush or floss between those checkups, it would be ludicrous to think that the resulting dental decay and gingivitis was because the dentist had failed them. In a similar vein, the patient must be engaged in his/her own treatment plan, or the chances for optimal success drop logarithmically. (See Chapter 23 for additional ideas about creating treatment plans with specifics.)

Along with the specific elements of the treatment plan, both within and outside of the clinic, there needs to be a clear recheck system. This should specify when the health care provider and the patient will next meet and assess progress, and when a partial or full reassessment will be performed. This gives the patient a concrete vision of when they will have ready access to their health care provider and they can plan for this date with questions and concerns. From the health care provider's perspective, this also allows them to vision out and make plans for those exchanges with the patient. A useful consideration prior to any recheck appointment is for the clinicians to ask themselves three basic questions: (1) What should be done if the patients say that they are better? (2) What should be done if the patients say that there has not been a change in their status? (3) What should be done if the patients indicate that they are worst? Over the course of a week, the practicing clinician will hear all of those responses. Since "luck (chance) favors the prepared mind,"[75] if these options have been thought through in advance, the clinician is not faced with appearing stumped in front of the patient. Rather, the clinician will have thought through potential options and be able to appropriately respond to the vast majority of findings at the time of a recheck. This is somewhat analogous to the skilled chess player who is not concerned only with the next move, but has considered all options associated with the next several moves. Visioning out, considering options, and being in a position to respond to whatever arises during the recheck, works to increase the knowledge base and skill of the clinician. Ultimately, this leads to improved patient care and hopefully, the achievement of the majority of mutually stated goals of the patient and clinician.

With a clear plan and recheck system, care is provided, and a regular evaluation of the patient's status is implemented. Judgments are made, and the cycle of reevaluation, assessment of current short-term goals, and plan modification are performed.

It is hoped that through the use of a system, such as the one outlined here with the scan examination, the care provided will be based on objective information, mutually determined goals, and that the plan will successfully address the patient's neuromusculoskeletal problem.

CONCLUDING THOUGHTS

The key element of any scan examination is a systematically applied evaluation to insure that important information is not inadvertently overlooked. This entails approaching the examination with an open mind that is constantly working to assure that if red or yellow flags are identified, they are annotated and appropriately explored. Both of these features are enacted within the context of an evaluation that is time efficient, while remaining flexible, so that data that point to a given working hypothesis can be explored in more detail where there is the opportunity for additional evidence to either collaborate or refute that hypothesis. The data so obtained provide the framework for the goals and plan to address the patient's presenting condition.

A few concluding thoughts that the novice examiner might find useful are the following: (1) "When hoof-beats are heard, think about horses rather than zebras."[45] What this means is that when data start pointing to several potential hypotheses, the most likely cause is the most commonly occurring hypothesis. If there is another hypothesis that relates to a relatively obscure condition (a zebra), continue to explore the more likely hypothesis first, and in most cases, this will lead to a solution. Having said that, file the alternative hypothesis away, since on a rare occasion, you will see a zebra and do not want to be so myopic that all that is seen is a horse. (2) Do not approach referring a patient to another health care professional as not being successful. All health care professionals have spheres of expertise and all health care providers should ideally be working to insure that the patient is seen by the most appropriate health care provider. As has been stated previously, the hallmark of true professionals is knowing their own limitations.[38] (3) While each health care professional will develop his/her own system, a system should always be used. This has been stressed throughout this chapter because it is that important. The only way that data will be systematically collected, joints above and below the region of interest will be explored, and the possibilities of visceral or referred causes of the patient's problem will be kept within the hypotheses explored, is through a system. Use of a system will assist in not missing key elements and in providing higher quality health care. (4) All the evaluative procedures used (basic scan examination and any follow-up special tests) are based on a strong foundational knowledge of anatomy, histology, biomechanics, physiology, neuroscience, and the other foundational elements needed to understand the workings of the human body. Throughout your career, continue to be a student and work to build upon the knowledge base of the profession and the various interrelationships that exist across all of the basic sciences. This type of curiosity will ultimately work for the patient's advantage by having him/her seen by a highly qualified professional.

SUMMARY

- Use a system to insure that examinations are thorough and reproducible.
- Listen to the patients and their concerns—the history and the information obtained are vital to the evaluation.
- Start broad, with an open mind—let the findings guide your hypotheses.
- Have a rationale for every question asked and every physical examination test performed, so that this information can be translated into useable data.
- Know your areas of expertise and your limitations—a hallmark of a true professional is knowing when to refer (work within the full healthcare team).
- Record as you go throughout the examination to increase accuracy.
- Understand that while "clearing tests" are important, they do *not* truly rule out any region of the body.
- While most dysfunctions are limited to a single problem, be aware that comorbidities are a real possibility.
- Develop a plan that meets both the goals of the patient and that of the rehabilitation professional.
- At the time of goal planning, always consider the following options for the follow-up appointment:
  a. What should be the response if the patient is better?
  b. What should be the response if there is no change in the patient's status?
  c. What should be the response if the patient is worst?

REFERENCES

1. Classic Quotes. Clarence Darrow, 1938, Internet communication.
2. *Physicians Desk Reference.* Montvale, NJ, Thomson, 2005.
3. Aglietti P, Rinonapoli E, Stringa G, et al. Tibial osteotomy for the varus osteoarthritic knee. *Clin Orthop Relat Res* 176:239–251, 1983.
4. Aguggia M. Typical facial neuralgias. *Neurol Sci* 26:s68–70, 2005.
5. Agur A, Dalley A: *Grant's Atlas of Anatomy.* Philadelphia, Lippincott Williams & Wilkins, 2005.
6. American Physical Therapy Association: Guide to Physical Therapist Practice. *Phys Ther* 81:9–746, 2001.
7. Anderson J, Pollitzer W. Ethnic and genetic differences in susceptibility to osteoporotic fractures. *Adv Nutr Res* 9:129–149, 1994.
8. Bahrami M, Rayegani S, Fereidouni M, et al. Prevalence and severity of carpal tunnel syndrome (CTS) during pregnancy. *Electromyogr Clin Neurophysiol* 45:123–125, 2005.
9. Baxter R. *Pocket Guide to Musculoskeletal Assessment,* Philadelphia, WB Saunders, 1998.
10. Benjamin R. Neurologic complications of prostate cancer. *Am Fam Physician* 65:1834–1840, 2002.
11. Bertorini T, Narayanaswami P, Rashed H. Charcot-Marie-Tooth disease (hereditary motor sensory neuropathies) and hereditary sensory and autonomic neuropathies. *Neurologist* 10:327–337, 2004.
12. Boissonnault W, Badke M. Collecting health history information: the accuracy of a patient self-administered questionnaire in an orthopedic outpatient setting. *Phys Ther* 85:531–543, 2005.
13. Borg-Stein J, Dugan S, Gruber J. Musculoskeletal aspects of pregnancy. *Am J Phys Med Rehabil* 84:180–192, 2005.
14. Bourdillon J, Day E, Bookhout M. Examination, general considerations. In: Bourdillon J, Day E, Bookhout M, eds. *Spinal Manipulation,* 5th ed. Boston, Butterworth-Heinemann, 1992, pp. 47–80.
15. Childs J, Flynn T, Fritz J, et al. Screening for vertobrobasilar insufficiency in patients with neck pain: manual therapy decision-making in the presence of uncertainty. *Phys Ther* 35:300–306, 2005.
16. Chusid J. Reflexes. In: Chusid J, ed. *Correlative Neuroanatomy and Functional Neurology,* 16th ed., Chapter 12. Los Altos, CA, Lange Medical Publications, 1976, pp. 206–210.
17. Crook E, Patel S. Diabetic nephropathy in African-American patients. *Curr Diab Rep* 4:455–461, 2004.
18. Crossley K, Cowan S, Bennell K, et al. Patellar taping: is clinical success supported by scientific evidence? *Man Ther* 5:142–150, 2000.
19. Cryrix J. The diagnosis of soft tissue lesions. In: Cyriax J, ed. *Textbook of Orthopaedic Medicine,* 7th ed., Chapter 5. London, Spottiswoode Ballantyne Ltd., 1978, pp. 64–103.
20. Daniels L, Worthingham C. *Muscle Testing: Techniques of Manual Examination.* Philadelphia, WB Saunders, 1986.
21. Diaz J. Carpal tunnel syndrome in female nurse anesthetists versus operating room nurses: prevalence, laterality, and impact of handedness. *Anesth Analg* 93:975–980, 2001.
22. Dutton M. *Orthopaedic Examination, Evaluation and Intervention,* New York, McGraw-Hill, 2004.
23. Everwild. "First, do no harm" is not in the Hippocratic oath, 2005, Internet communication.
24. Falkner B. Insulin resistance in African Americans. *Kidney Int Suppl* 83:S27–S30, 2003.
25. Fields H. Pain from deep tissues and referred pain. In: Fields H, ed. *Pain: Mechanisms and Management.* New York, McGraw-Hill, 1987, pp. 79–98.
26. Fitts R, McDonald K, Schluter J. The determinants of skeletal muscle force and power: their adaptability with changes in activity pattern. *J Biomech* 24:111–122, 1991.

27. Flynn T. *The Thoracic Spine and Rib Cage*. Newton, MA, Butterworth-Heinemann, 1996.

28. Fogo A. Hypertensive risk factors in kidney disease in African Americans. *Kidney Int Suppl* 83:S21, 2003.

29. Gardner E, Kandel E. Touch. In: Kandel E, Schwartz J, Jessell T, eds. *Principles of Neural Science*, 4th ed., Chapter 23. New York, McGraw-Hill, 2000, pp. 451–471.

30. Gardner E, Martin J, Jessell T. The bodily senses. In: Kandel E, Schwartz J, Jessell T, eds. *Principles of Neural Science*, Chapter 22. New York, McGraw-Hill, 2000, pp. 430–450.

31. Gaylor A, Condren M. Type 2 diabetes mellitis in the pediatric population. *Pharmacotherapy* 24:871–878, 2004.

32. Goldberg S. *The Four Minute Neurologic Exam*, Miami, FL, MedMaster, 1992.

33. Goodman C. Red flags: recognizing signs and symptoms. *Phys Ther Mag* 9:55–62, 1993.

34. Goodman C, Boissonnault W, Fuller K. *Pathology: Implications for the Physical Therapist*, Philadelphia, WB Saunders, 2003.

35. Goodman C, Randall T. Musculoskeletal Neoplasms. In: Goodman C, Boissonnault W, Fuller K, eds. *Pathology: Implications for the Physical Therapist*, 2nd ed., Chapter 25. Philadelphia, WB Saunders, 2003, pp. 905–928.

36. Goodman C, Snyder T. Systematic origins of musculoskeletal pain: associated signs and symptoms. In: Goodman C, Snyder T, eds. *Differential Diagnosis in Physical Therapy*. Philadelphia, WB Saunders, 1990, pp. 327–345.

37. Goodman C, Snyder T. *Differential Diagnosis in Physical Therapy*. Philadelphia, WB Saunders, 1995.

38. Goodman C, Snyder T. Introduction to differential screening in physical therapy. In: Goodman C, Snyder T, eds. *Differential Diagnosis in Physical Therapy*, 2nd ed., Chapter 1. Philadelphia, WB Saunders, 1995, pp. 1–23.

39. Goodman C, Snyder T. Oncology. In: Goodman C, Boissonnault W, Fuller K, eds. *Pathology: Implications for the Physical Therapist*, Chapter 8. Philadelphia, WB Saunders, 2003, pp. 236–263.

40. Goodman C, Snyder T. Introduction to the interviewing process. In: Goodman C, Snyder T, eds. *Differential Diagnosis in Physical Therapy*. Philadelphia, WB Saunders, 1990, pp. 7–42.

41. Goodyer P. *Techniques in Musculoskeletal Rehabilitation: Companion Handbook*. New York, McGraw-Hill, 2001.

42. Govind J. Lumbar radicular pain. *Aust Fam Physician* 33:409–412, 2004.

43. Goyal V, Bhatia M, Padma M, et al. Electrophysiological evaluation of 140 hands with carpal tunnel syndrome. *J Assoc Physicians India* 1070–1073, 2001.

44. Gran J. The epidemiology of chronic generalized musculoskeletal pain. *Best Pract Res Clin Rheumatol* 17:547–561, 2003.

45. Greathouse D, Schreck R, Benson C. The United States army physical therapy experience: evaluation and treatment of patients with neuromusculoskeletal disorders. *J Orthop Sports Phys Ther* 19:261–266, 1994.

46. Halle J. Neuromuscular scan examination with selected related topics. In: Flynn T, ed. *The Thoracic Spine and Rib Cage: Musculoskeletal Evaluation and Treatment*, Chapter 7. Boston, Butterworth-Heinemann, 1996, pp. 121–146.

47. Henderson N, Knapik J, Shaffer S, et al. Injuries and injury risk factors among men and women in U.S. Army Combat Medic Advanced individual training. *Mil Med* 165:647–652, 2000.

48. Houlden H, Blake J, Reilly M. Hereditary sensory neuropathies. *Curr Opin Neurol* 17:569–577, 2004.

49. Jones G, Cowan D, Knapik J. Exercise, training and injuries. *Sports Med* 18:202–214, 1994.

50. Kandel E. Nerve cells and behavior. In: Kandel E, Schwartz J, Jessell T, eds. *Principles of Neural Science*, 4th ed., Chapter 2. New York, McGraw-Hill, 2000, pp. 19–35.

51. Kendall F, McCreary E, Provance P. *Muscles: Testing and Function*, Baltimore, MD, Williams & Wilkins, 1993.

52. Koknel T. Thoracic outlet syndrome. *Agri* 17:5–9, 2005.

53. Kramer WJ, Ratamess NA. Fundamentals of resistance training: Progression and exercise prescription. *Med Sci Sports Exerc* 36(4):474–488, 2004.

54. Kvien T. Epidemiology and burden of illness of rheumatoid arthritis. *Pharmacoeconomics* 22:1–12, 2004.

55. Lun V, Meeuwisse W, Stergiou P, et al. Relation between running injury and static lower limb alignment in recreational runners. *Br J Sports Med* 38:576–580, 2004.

56. Magee D. Cervical Spine. In: Magee D, ed. *Orthopedic Physical Assessment*, 4th ed., Chapter 3. Philadelphia, WB Saunders, 2002, pp. 121–182.

57. Magee D. *Orthopedic Physical Assessment*, 4th ed. Philadelphia, WB Saunders, 2002.

58. Magee D. Principles and Concepts. In: Magee D ed. *Orthopedic Physical Assessment*, 4th ed., Chapter 1. Philadelphia, WB Saunders, 2002, pp. 1–66.

59. Malcoe L, Duran B, Montgomery J. Socioeconomic disparities in intimate partner violence against Native American women: a cross-sectional study. *BMC Med* 2:1–14, 2004.

60. Malone T, McPoil T, Nitz A. *Orthopedics and Sports Physical Therapy*. St. Louis, MO, Mosby, 1997.

61. Matheson G, Macintyre J, Taunton J, et al. Musculoskeletal injuries associated with physical activity in older adults. *Med Sci Sports Exerc* 21:379–385, 1989.

62. McClure P. The degenerative cervical spine: pathogenesis and rehabilitation concepts. *J Hand Ther* 13:163–174, 2000.

63. McKenzie R. *Treat Your Own Back*. Minneapolis, MN, Orthopedic Physical Therapy Product, 1997.

64. Michlovitz S. Conservative interventions for carpal tunnel syndrome. *J Orthop Sports Phys Ther* 34:589–600, 2004.

65. Moore K, Dalley A. Abdomen. In: Moore K, Dalley A, eds. *Clinically Oriented Anatomy*, 5th ed., Chapter 2. Philadelphia, Lippincott Williams & Wilkins, 2006, pp. 192–354.

66. Moore K, Dalley A. *Clinically Oriented Anatomy.* Philadelphia, Lippincott Willliams & Wilkins, 2006.

67. Moore K, Dalley A. Neck. In: Moore K, Dalley A, eds. *Clinically Oriented Anatomy,* 5th ed., Chapter 8. Philadelphia, Lippincott Williams & Wilkins, 2006, pp. 1046–1121.

68. Moore K, Dalley A. Thorax. In: Moore K, Dalley A, eds. *Clinically Oriented Anatomy,* 5th ed., Chapter 1. Philadelphia, Lippincott Williams & Wilkins, 2006, pp. 1–191.

69. Moore K, Dalley A. Upper Limb. In: Moore K, Dalley A, eds. *Clinically Oriented Anatomy,* 5th ed., Chapter 6. Philadelphia, Lippincott Williams & Wilkins, 2006, pp. 726–885.

70. Netter F. *Atlas of Human Anatomy.* Teterboro, NJ, Icon Learning Systems, 2003.

71. Norkin C, Levangie P. The knee complex. In: Norkin C, Levangie P, eds. *Joint Structure and Function,* 2nd ed., Chapter 11. Philadelphia, FA Davis, 1992, pp. 337–378.

72. Oates S, Daley R. Thoracic outlet syndrome. *Hand Clin* 12:705–718, 1996.

73. Patten J. The cerebral hemispheres: 1. The lobes of the brain. In: Patten J, ed. *Neurological Differential Diagnosis,* Chapter 8. New York, Springer-Verlag, 1977, pp. 69–85.

74. Pecoraro R, Inui T, Chan M, et al. Validity and reliability of a self-administered health history questionnaire. *Public Health Rep* 94:231–238, 1979.

75. Quote DB. Chance favors the prepared mind, 2005, Internet communication.

76. Rayan G. Thoracic outlet syndrome. *J Shoulder Elbow Surg* 7:440–451, 1998.

77. Rebain R, Baxter G, McDonough S. A systematic review of the passive straight leg raising test as a diagnostic aid for low back pain. *Spine* 27:E388–E395, 2002.

78. Reese N. Techniques of manual muscle testing: lower extremity. In: Reese N, ed. *Muscle and Sensory Testing,* Chapter 4. Philadelphia, WB Saunders, 1999, pp. 234–336.

79. Rhoades R, Tanner G. Skeletal and smooth muscle. In: Rhoades R, Tanner G, eds. *Medical Physiology,* Chapter 9. Boston, Little, Brown and Company, 1995, pp. 165–192.

80. Richter R, Reinking M. How does evidence on the diagnostic accuracy of the vertebral artery test influence teaching of the test in a professional physical therapy education program. *Phys Ther* 85:589–599, 2005.

81. Rose E, Deshikachar A, Schwartz K, et al. Use of a template to improve documentation and coding. *Fam Med* 33:516–521, 2001.

82. Rothstein J. On defining subjective and objective measurements. *Phys Ther* 69:577–579, 1989.

83. Rowland L. Clinical syndromes of the spinal cord and brain stem. In: Kandel E, Schwartz J, Jessell T, eds. *Principles of Neural Science,* 3rd ed., Chapter 46. Norwalk, CT, Appleton & Lange, 1991, pp. 711–730.

84. Rowland L. Diseases of the motor unit. In: Kandel E, Schwartz J, Jessell T, eds. *Principles of Neural Science,* 4th ed., Chapter 35. New York, McGraw-Hill, 2000, pp. 695–712.

85. Saunders D, Saunders R. Evaluation of the spine. In: Saunders D, ed. *Evaluation, Treatment and Prevention of Musculoskeletal Disorders,* 3rd ed. Bloomington, MN, Educational Opportunities, 1993, pp. 33–97.

86. Shaver J. Fibromyalgia syndrome in women. *Nurs Clin North Am* 39:195–204, 2004.

87. Stuge G, Hilde G, Vollestad N. Physical therapy for pregnancy-related low back and pelvic pain: a systematic review. *Acta Obstet Gynecol Scand* 82:989–990, 2003.

88. Tippett S. Considerations with the pediatric patient. In: Prentice W, Voight M, eds. *Techniques in Musculoskeletal Rehabilitation,* Chapter 35. New York, McGraw-Hill, 2001, pp. 697–714.

89. Walton L. The symptoms and signs of disease in the nervous system. In: Walton L, ed. *Essentials of Neurology,* Chapter 1. New York, Churchill Livingstone, 1989, pp. 1–24.

90. Weir C, Hurdle J, Felgar M, et al. Direct text entry in electronic progress notes: an evaluation of input errors. *Methods Inf Med* 42:61–67, 2003.

91. Wilson T, Talwalkar J, Johnson D. Lateral patella dislocation associated with an irreducible posterolateral knee dislocation: literature review. *Orthopedics* 28:459–461, 2005.

92. Wolff A, Bourke J. Reducing medical errors: a practical guide. *Med J Aust* 173:247–251, 2000.

93. Wu W, Meijer O, Uegaki K, et al. Pregnancy-related pelvic girdle pain (PPP), I: terminology, clinical presentation, and prevalence. *Eur Spine J* 13:575–589, 2004.

94. Zachazewski J, Magee D, Quillen W. *Athletic Injuries and Rehabilitation.* Philadelphia, WB Saunders, 1996.

C H A P T E R   5

Clinical Reasoning: An Algorithm-based Approach to Musculoskeletal Rehabilitation

Barbara J. Hoogenboom and Michael L. Voight

O B J E C T I V E S

After completing this chapter, the therapist should be able to do the following:

- Describe the clinical reasoning process.
- Relate clinical reasoning to quality provision of physical therapy, both in terms of diagnosis and selection of interventions.
- Realize that clinical reasoning skill is linked to knowledge and experience.
- Contrast clinical decision processes of experts and novices.
- Relate evidence-based practice to clinical reasoning.
- Describe the algorithmic approach to clinical reasoning for intervention selection.
- Use sample algorithms to examine clinical reasoning for each of the four phases of rehabilitation (acute, intermediate, advanced, and return to function).
- Apply algorithmic thinking to subsequent chapters.

INTRODUCTION

Physical therapists make decisions related to examination, evaluation, diagnosis, prognosis, and intervention on a daily basis. Independent decision making is one of the hallmarks of an autonomous profession, a status for which the profession of physical therapy (PT) is striving.[6] To make reasoned, independent decisions, the physical therapist must use refined, well-developed, clinical reasoning skills. Higgs and Jones have defined clinical reasoning as the practice used by the therapist to *structure* the health care process.[12] Knowledge, clinical data, patient preferences, and professional judgment all play a role in clinical reasoning. Clinical reasoning can also be described as the progression used by practitioners to plan, direct, carry out, and reflect on patient care. Clearly clinical reasoning is not a simple process; rather it is a complex and multifaceted process of analysis and synthesis. Such a process enables therapists to view the client and their rehabilitation with depth and breadth of understanding.

Tacit knowledge combined with accumulated clinical experience contributes to the art of the practice of physical therapy.

Bruning, Schraw, and Ronning describe *schemata* as the complex representations of phenomenon by which individuals receive, store, and organize information.[4] As schemata help therapists to organize and retrieve knowledge, scripts or procedural rules help to guide thinking and organize common occurrences or events. Both of these strategies support effective processing of information by providing efficient mental frameworks for handling complex information.

There are few certainties in patient care. Rather, biological, physiological, and psychological events occur in uncertain, but often in predictable patterns. Every problem solved or decision made by a clinician is probabilistic[11] and involves a combination of hypothesis testing and pattern recognition. Hypothetico-deductive reasoning and early hypothesis generation can occur with a limited data base and is a way to structure the clinical examination and thinking process. A hypothesis is really a clinical impression based on an assumption of causality. By definition, "a hypothesis is a testable idea—a tentative, but best, estimate that only time can prove correct" (Ref. 20, p. 1391). Hence, clinicians apply the clinical reasoning process to the clinical decision-making process for examination and diagnosis as well as selection of interventions.

EXPERT VERSUS NOVICE DECISION MAKING

There is a well-developed body of literature about how experts make decisions.[7,8,11,17] Experienced clinicians use a well-developed collection of clinical experiences for their reasoning, while novice clinicians rely on clear cut patterns and clues. May and Dennis stated: "Experts, when compared with novices in the same field, exhibit a superior structuring of knowledge into clinically relevant patterns that are unlocked by key cues in the decision environment. Patterns stored in memory enable the expert to recognize meaningful relationships and generate likely hypotheses" (Ref. 17, p. 191). In research across many health professions, experts excel within their specific knowledge domains, are able to see relationships, possess enhanced memory (relates to banked experience), are skilled in qualitative analysis, and have well-developed reflection skills.

Likewise, researchers agree that novice decision makers function differently than their expert counterparts.

How do then novices develop into competent decision makers and experts? Although experience is necessary for the contextual problem-solving process used by experts, less is known about the process of how problem-solving expertise is developed.[13] A major distinction that has been described between expert and novice problem solvers is that experts use forward reasoning rather than backward reasoning or hypothetico-deductive reasoning used by novices.[7,8] Forward reasoning is the application of a number of "if/then" rules to a problem to move forward from data to diagnosis or treatment intervention. An algorithmic approach seeks to use a number of "if/then" decisions to assist in problem solving. As previously noted, any problem-solving model that attempts to assist novices and developing clinicians must take into account the knowledge base and organizational skills of the individual. Practitioners with "high knowledge" make more inferences from prior knowledge than novices and intermediate level practioners.[8] Interestingly, experts often seem to do less problem solving than novices because they have a depth and breadth of previously stored solutions to clinical problems that they recall and use.[14] It should be noted, however, that experience alone does not always provide *accurate* solutions to problems or enable clinicians to make efficient, reasoned diagnoses. Although novices tend to solve problems incorrectly or simplistically, experts can also develop patterned thinking and rely too heavily on experience and make premature diagnoses without fully examining subtle possibilities and varied data.

PROBLEM SOLVING, CLINICAL DECISION MAKING, AND THE USE OF EVIDENCE-BASED PRACTICE

Being a good problem solver is not sufficient in this day and age. According to Miller, Nyland, and Wormal, "rehabilitation clinicians must be creative problem solvers who can translate relevant

research into functional interventions" (Ref. 18, p. 453). It is important to remember that in contemporary physical therapy practice, decisions related to clinical practice should be based on the best available evidence whenever possible.

Clinicians should use the literature to determine the best treatment for their patients. Evidence-based practice has been defined as "the conscientious and judicious use of current best evidence in making decisions about the care of individual patients."[21] Implicit in this definition is the need for a method of determining what constitutes the "best" evidence. Before evidence can be integrated into the management of patients, an appraisal of the quality of the evidence must be completed. A major problem in the appraisal process is that of deciding whether the evidence is definitive enough to indicate an effect other than chance. The ability to judge and interpret the evidence for intervention techniques is a skill that must be developed if a clinician wishes to become evidenced based in their practice. Therefore, the ability to interpret and evaluate the evidence becomes an integral part in the clinical decision-making process. The standard for the assessment of the efficacy and value of intervention is the clinical trial. Most desirable is the prospective study which assesses the effect and value of an intervention against those found in a control group, using human subjects.[9] Unfortunately, many of the studies in the literature that address physical therapy topics are not clinical trials, as there is no control to judge efficacy of the intervention and there are no interventions from which to draw comparisons.[3] In addition to a control group, the ideal clinical trial uses a blinded, randomized design, both for subject assignment to groups and assessment of outcomes (Table 5-1). The control can be a current standard practice, a placebo, or no active intervention.[9] Clinicians must constantly remind themselves that without information gathered from controlled clinical trials, they have limited scientific basis for their interventions. Many interventions offered by physical therapists use low levels of evidence or worse, personal testimony for the rationale behind their use. As the profession grows and the evidence base from which physical therapists can glean information increases, the correctness, defensibility, and ultimately the effectiveness of chosen interventions can only increase.

Evidence-based practice is the standard to which physical therapists must strive for direction in clinical decision making and problem solving related to both diagnosis and selection of interventions. Frequent, speedy use of evidence to answer clinical questions, base decisions, or solve problems is mandatory as the profession of PT continues to develop and grow.

CLINICAL REASONING PROCESS

Clinical reasoning is described by Edwards et al. as "a way of thinking and taking action within clinical practice" (Ref. 6, p. 322). Clinical reasoning is often first utilized in the examination process and has both diagnostic and narrative components.[6] The construct known as clinical reasoning has

TABLE 5-1
Levels of Evidence for Research

LEVEL OF EVIDENCE	TYPES OF STUDIES
Level I	• High-quality randomized controlled trials • Systematic review of Level-I randomized controlled trials • Prospective studies (all patients enrolled at the same point in their pathology with >80% follow-up of enrolled patients)
Level II	• Prospective cohort studies • Poor-quality randomized controlled trial (e.g., no blinding, or improper randomization, <80% follow-up) • Systematic review of Level-II studies • Retrospective study • Study of untreated controls from a previous randomized controlled trial
Level III	• Case-control studies • Retrospective cohort studies • Systematic review of Level-III studies
Level IV	• Case series (no, or historical, control group)
Level V	• Expert opinion

Modified from the *J Bone Joint Surg*, instructions for Authors.

also been discussed in Chapter 4 in relationship to the scanning examination. Once again, it is important to note that the clinical reasoning process can not be separated from knowledge. If insufficient knowledge is present, it is likely that diagnoses and decisions based on such knowledge will provide faulty conclusions. In other words, the clinical reasoning process is only as strong and viable as the knowledge base from which the diagnosis or decision is rendered.

Clinical reasoning does not occur in a "clinician induced vacuum." Multiple factors play a role in the clinical reasoning process, not the least of which is the identified problem as it is seen and described by the patient. Narrative reasoning involves the ability to collect and attempt to understand patients' "stories,"[6] experiences, perspectives, contexts, cultural backgrounds, and beliefs. It is important to remember that the patient's personal descriptive traits and characteristics, past experiences and history, comorbidities, life situation, and personal beliefs all strongly affect the process of clinical reasoning. Vital to the process of treatment planning is taking into account the problems as they are *seen by the patient*, named the patient-identified problems (PIPs), as well as the nonpatient identified problems (NPIPs).[19] NPIPs are problems not identified by the patient that may have been preexisting, unknown to a patient, or identified by the therapist or another. Identification of NPIPs are especially important for excellent care as well as a prevention and wellness orientated practice of physical therapy as described in the *Guide to Physical Therapist Practice* (Table 5-2).[1]

The second application of clinical reasoning is during the treatment planning and intervention selection process.

Edwards[6] describes six types of reasoning that comprise decisions made regarding management of patients and clients. These are procedural or intervention reasoning, interactive patient-therapist rapport building reasoning, collaborative patient-therapist reasoning, instructional reasoning, predictive, and ethical reasoning. The prior-listed clinical reasoning strategies are often used in combination. An emergent dialectical model of clinical reasoning has been reported in the literature that includes cognitive and decision-making processes (hypothetico-deductive reasoning), as well as reasoning skills necessary to interact with patients in their individual unique scaffold of experience, personality, and assumptions (narrative or communicative reasoning).[2,6,7,11,12] Although each individual must ultimately construct their own schemata and procedural rules for clinical reasoning, tools exist that may assist practitioners to develop expert skills.

INTRODUCTION TO ALGORITHMS

Algorithms are such tools that assist practitioners to develop expert skills. *Encyclopedia Britannica* defines an algorithm as "systematic procedure that produces—in a finite number of steps—the answer to a question or the solution of a problem."[10] An algorithm provides a graphic, step-by-step procedure for guiding decision making. Alternately, algorithms have been described as decision trees. In the medical fields, algorithms are developed and used for clinical decision making related to the diagnostic process and management of cases. Algorithms can

T A B L E   5 - 2

HOAC II Definitions of Problems

TYPE OF PROBLEM	DEFINITION	EXAMPLES
PIPs	Impairments, functional limitations, and disabilities, easily identified by the patient.	Pain, loss of ROM about a joint, loss of strength, impaired gait, impaired ADLs.
NPIPs	Problems identified by someone other than the patient such as a health care provider, caregiver or family member.	Postural impairments, respiratory dysfunction, general deconditioning, musculoskeletal imbalances.
Anticipated problems	Problems that do not exist at the current time, but may develop related to existing problems (both PIP's and NPIP's). Can be prevented with proper management.	Secondary shortening of muscles due to poor posture or gait deviations.

Data from Rothstein J, Echternach J, Riddle D. *Phys Ther* 83:455–470, 2003.

provide structured care pathways and a systematic approach to the selection of therapeutic interventions. Because algorithms are *not* prescriptive or protocol driven, they allow for clinical decisions and adjustments to be made during the clinical reasoning and decision-making processes. Algorithmic thinking and the associated graphic structure seems to fit the forward reasoning process previously described as being used by experts. An algorithm is simply a decision tree filled with "if/then" decisions related to examination and intervention planning. Rothstein and Echternach[20] described a conceptual scheme for problem solving in physical therapy that they named the *hypothesis-oriented algorithm for clinicians* (HOAC). This algorithm-based scheme was designed to guide the therapist from evaluation to intervention planning with a logical sequence of activities. The HOAC requires the therapist to define goals for patient intervention and determine if they have been met, thereby assisting in clinical decision making. It also requires that the therapist generate hypotheses early in the examination process regarding the underlying cause(s) of functional limitations. Such a strategy is often used by expert physicians and therapists.

The first part of the HOAC is a sequential guide to examination and planning of interventions. The second part of the HOAC is a branching diagram (algorithm) that relates to clinical decisions that must be made throughout the patient care interventions. The HOAC requires that the therapist relate all interventions to hypotheses, thereby forcing justification of all aspects of interventions. Use of such an algorithm-based approach should promote use of suitable, evidence-based interventions and discourage the use of "popular" or routine interventions. In response to changes in the health care system and the practice of physical therapy, the HOAC was revised and became the HOAC II (Figures 5-1 to 5-4).[19] The authors of the HOAC II contend that it links the use of evidence in decision making and documentation of the type and scope of evidence used in the examination and intervention processes.

Such a linkage or connection between evidence and intervention selection and planning is important in the current climate of health care. Physical therapists must justify and provide evidence for selected interventions whenever possible. The HOAC II also provides the physical therapist with a tool for planning and evaluating activities intended for prevention. Like the original HOAC, the second part of the HOAC II is an algorithm that covers intervention, monitoring of intervention effects, and altering the plan of care appropriately to progress toward desired outcomes. Although a detailed discussion of the HOAC and the HOAC II are beyond the scope of this chapter, both are valuable tools that have influenced the current authors thinking about use of algorithms in treatment planning and intervention selection.

HOW TO CONSTRUCT AN ALGORITHM

The process of building a treatment algorithm is not complex. It involves using differently shaped boxes each representing or describing varied aspects of the algorithm. Table 5-3 shows and describes the three differently shaped open forms, as described both by Miller et al.[18] and Rothstein et al.[19] in the HOAC II-Part 2.

There are always two possible choices that arise from the rectangular action/intervention or decision/question box, a "yes" branch and a "no" branch. Based upon the answer to a yes or no decision or question, the next path or trail down the algorithm is chosen. In the Miller et al.[18] scheme the yes or no treatment options for each path must be provided in the algorithm, while in the Rothstein et al.[19] scheme yes or no decisions may lead to another question box or an intervention box. The following algorithm is a generic example of the algorithms that will accompany each chapter and assist the reader in making and describing the many clinical decisions that combine to form a cohesive therapeutic intervention.

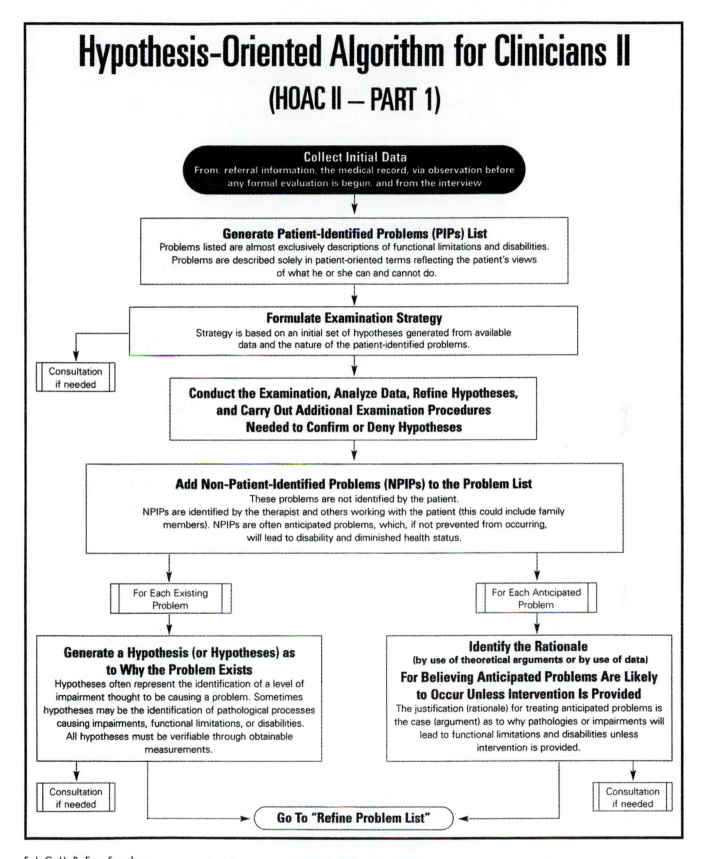

FIGURE 5-1

HOAC II diagram 1—The initial steps of part 1 of the HOAC II. Reproduced, with permission, from the APTA, from Rothstein J, Echternach J, Riddle D. *Phys Ther* 83:455–470, 2003.

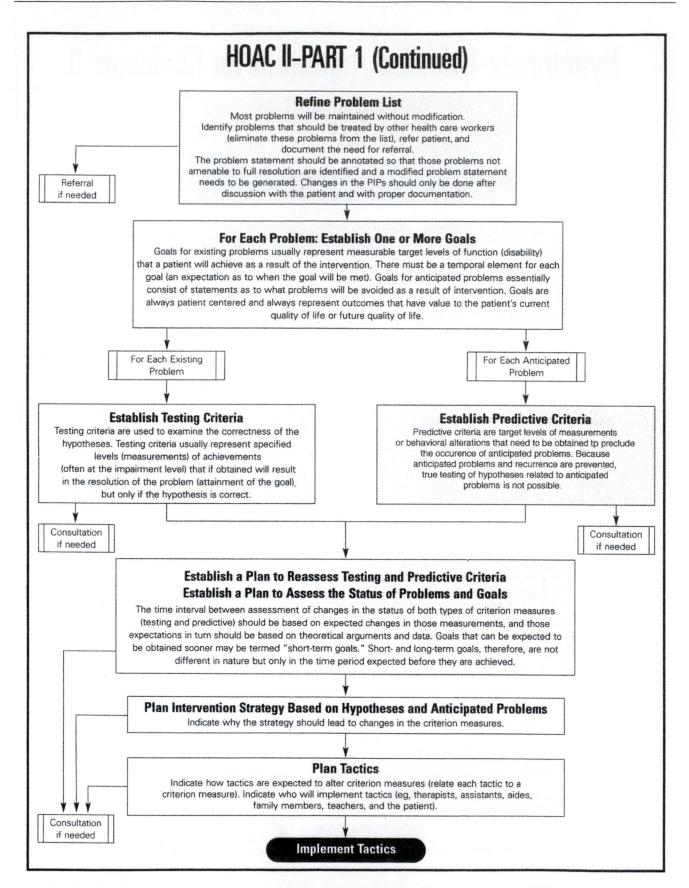

FIGURE 5-2

HOAC II diagram 2—The final steps of Part 1 of the HOAC II. Reproduced, with permission, from the APTA, from Rothstein J, Echternach J, Riddle D. *Phys Ther* 83:455–470, 2003.

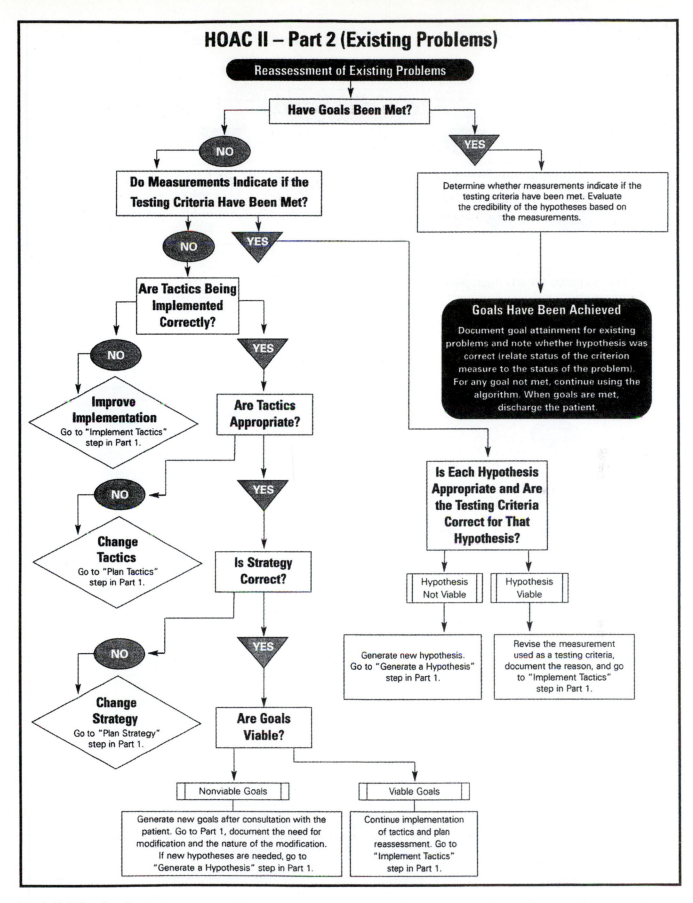

F I G U R E   5 - 3

HOAC II diagram 3—The algorithm for reassessment of existing problems in part 2 of the HOAC II. Reproduced, with permission, from the APTA, from Rothstein J, Echternach J, Riddle D. *Phys Ther* 83:455–470, 2003.

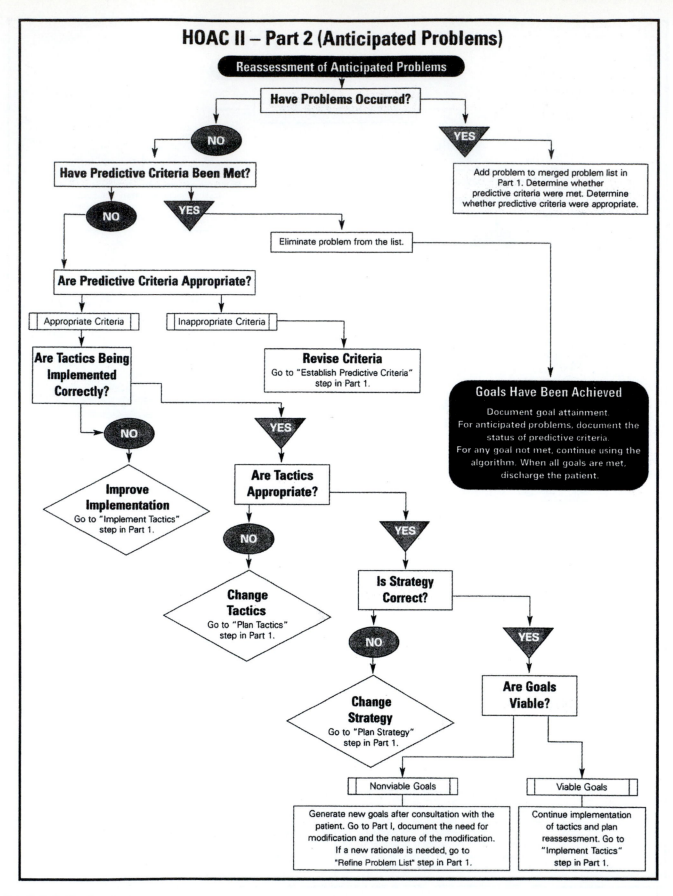

FIGURE 5-4

HOAC II diagram 4—The algorithm for reassessment of anticipated problems in part 2 of the HOAC II. Reproduced, with permission, from the APTA, from Rothstein J, Echternach J, Riddle D. *Phys Ther* 83:455–470, 2003.

TABLE 5-3

Shapes and Descriptions of Algorithm Components

PHYSICAL REPRESENTATION OF ALGORITHM SHAPE	DESCRIPTION OF FORM CONTENTS (MILLER ET AL.[18])	ALTERNATE USE OF FORMS (ROTHSTEIN ET AL.[19,20])
	The oval represents a clinical problem or entity.	The oval represents an assessment of an existing problem.
	The rectangle represents an action to be taken or an intervention to be provided.	The rectangle represents a decision or clinical question.
	The hexagon represents a clinical question that has become apparent which leads to a decision based upon evidence, whenever possible.	The diamond represents interventions, changes in strategy or actions.

Throughout the process of diagnostic reasoning, the identification of the specific anatomical structure or structures causing the impairment or dysfunction prior to the initiation of an intervention remains controversial. Cyriax[5] designed his examination process to selectively stress specific tissues in order to identify the structure involved and its stage of pathology. In contrast, Maitland[15] and McKenzie[16] seldom identify the involved structure, believing that it is not always possible, or even necessary, for the prescription and safe delivery of appropriate therapeutic interventions. Based on the Maitland and McKenzie philosophy, the therapeutic strategy is determined solely from the responses obtained from tissue loading and the effect that loading has on symptoms. Once these responses have been determined, the focus of the intervention is to provide sound

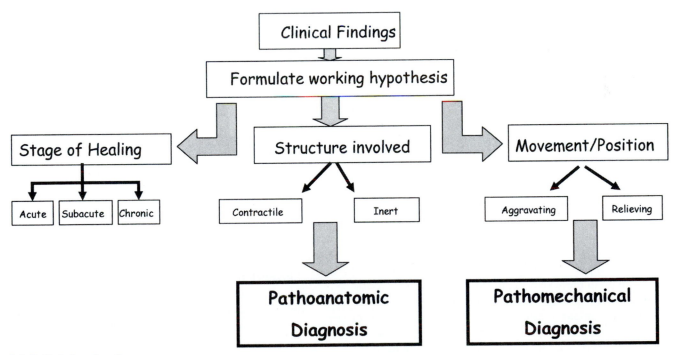

FIGURE 5-5

General evaluation scheme algorithm.

and effective self-management strategies for patients that avoid harmful tissue overloading.[16] Figure 5-5 is an example of an evaluation algorithm.

According to the *Guide to Physical Therapy Practice*, an intervention is "the purposeful and skilled interaction of the physical therapist and the patient/client and, when appropriate, with other individuals involved in the patient/client care, using various physical therapy procedures and techniques to produce changes in the condition consistent with the diagnosis and prognosis."[1] The physical therapy intervention is composed of three interrelated components: communication, coordination, and documentation; patient/client-related instruction; and procedural interventions. As previously discussed in Chapters 1 and 2 of this text, the patient/client management model provides a structure within which interventions are chosen in relationship to a movement-based categorization of signs and symptoms or a movement-based diagnosis (named in a preferred practice pattern).

Choices related to physical therapy procedural interventions are most effectively addressed from a problem-oriented approach, based on the knowledge of anatomy and biomechanics, the evaluation, the patient's functional needs, and on mutually agreed upon goals.[1] Decisions regarding the specific interventions chosen are made in order to most effectively improve the patients' ability to return to the previous level of function. The most successful intervention programs are those that are custom designed from a blend of clinical experience and scientific data (see Chapter 23 for more information on creating exercise programs), with the level of improvement achieved related to goal setting and the attainment of those goals.

INTRODUCTION TO THE FOUR-PHASED APPROACH TO REHABILITATION

A number of principles should guide the intervention through the various stages of healing and return to function. The comprehensive intervention usually follows a four-tiered approach beginning initially in the acute phase and progressing to subacute or intermediate phase, then the advanced phase, and finally, the return to function. Within the four-phased approach, general intervention principles are applied. These are not listed in order of importance, but instead reflect the sequence of application.

Acute Phase (Figure 5-6)

- *Control of pain and inflammation.* Soft tissue injuries are common in the general population and often are a reason for referral to PT. The results of most soft tissue injuries include conditions of pain, inflammation, and edema. Pain serves as the body's protective mechanism, giving an individual cues as to protect the area from additional tissue damage. At the simplest level, the transmission of information relating to pain from the periphery to the central

nervous system (CNS) depends upon integration at three levels: the spinal cord, the brain stem, and forebrain. (Refer Chapter 6 for an in-depth discussion of pain.)

Inflammation and edema occur as a part of the healing process. The inflammatory response is a necessary initial response to an injury. Edema is a subsequent condition that occurs due to the inflammatory response which may inhibit healing and return to function. The goals during this initial phase of intervention for an acute injury therefore are to decrease pain, control inflammation and edema, and protect the damaged structures from further damage, while concurrently attempting to increase the range of motion (ROM) and function. During the acute phase of healing, the principles of PRICE (Protection, rest, ice, compression, and elevation) are recommended. In addition, manual therapy and early motion are introduced to the rehabilitation process. Chapters 10 and 16 provide further information on range of motion and manual techniques, respectively.

The controlled application of a variety of techniques for control of pain, inflammation, and edema can have many therapeutic benefits. These benefits are theoretically achieved through:

- Mechanical stimulation of large-fiber joint afferents of the joint capsule, soft tissue, and other structures that assists in pain reduction,
- Stimulation of endogenous endorphins and enkephalins, which aid in pain reduction,
- Decrease of intra-articular pressure, which aids in pain reduction,
- Mechanical effects, which may improve joint mobility,
- Positive effects on remodeling of local connective tissue,
- Effective gliding of tendons within their sheaths, and
- Increased joint lubrication, important for nourishment of articular cartilage.

- *Application of interventions to provide early motion.* Early motion is important for:

- Reduction of the muscle atrophy that occurs primarily in type I fibers,
- Maintenance of joint function,
- Prevention of ligamentous "creeping,"
- Reduction of the chance of arthrofibrosis or excessive soft tissue scarring, and
- Enhancement of cartilage nutrition and vascularization, crucial for healing.

Research has shown that joint motion is important for healing around a joint and early joint motion stimulates collagen healing in the lines of force, a kind of Wolff's law of ligaments. Early ROM exercises may be performed actively or passively while protecting the healing tissues.

- *Promote and progress tissue healing.* Tissue repair follows a predictable course in response to both internal and

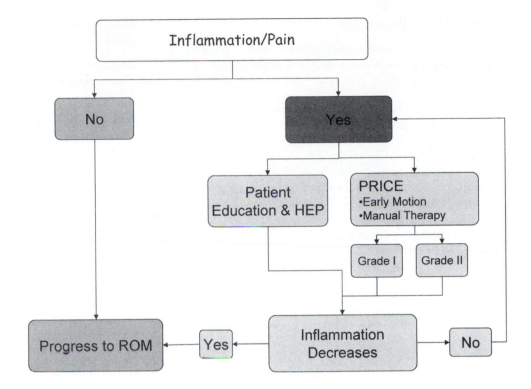

FIGURE 5-6

Inflammation/pain algorithm.

external processes. Physical therapy cannot accelerate the healing process, but with correct intervention choices can ensure that the healing process is not delayed or disrupted and occurs optimally. The support and sequence of tissue repair involves a careful balance between protection and controlled application of functional stresses to the healing tissue.

Clearly, the rehabilitation interventions used to assist during the repair process differ, depending on the degree/extent of the damage, the tissue involved, and stage of healing. Most tissues heal in a predictable manner, with equally predictable markers. These markers inform the clinician as to the stage of the repair that the tissue is in. Awareness of the various stages of healing is essential for determining the intensity of a particular intervention in order for clinician to avoid damaging healing tissues. Decisions to advance or change the rehabilitative process need to be based on the recognition of these signs and symptoms, and on an awareness of the time frames associated with each of the phases. For additional information on the phases of issue healing, refer to Chapter 3.

Intermediate Phase (Figure 5-7)

Therapeutic exercise is the foundation of physical therapy and a primary component of the bulk of interventions. In fact, *The Guide to Physical Therapist Practice* lists therapeutic exercise as one of the three categories of procedural interventions that forms the core of most physical therapy plans of care.[1] Prescribed appropriately, therapeutic exercise can be used to regain,

maintain, and advance a patient's functional status by increasing ROM and mobility (flexibility), muscle performance (strength, power, and endurance), and motor performance (neuromuscular skill).

Therefore, as appropriate, it is the responsibility of the therapist to choose therapeutic interventions and instruct the patient on a supplemental exercise program that

- *Restores full and painfree ROM.* All clinicians would agree that the restoration of, or improvement in, ROM is an important goal of the rehabilitation program. ROM may be viewed as a combination of the amount of joint motion, joint play, and the degree of extensibility of the periarticular and connective tissues that cross the joint, termed flexibility.

Prior to intervention with aggressive ROM exercises, joint play must be normalized in order to prevent complications that are likely to occur if abnormal osteo- and arthro-kinematics during active and passive motion are present. In addition to general information available in Chapters 10 and 16, each regional chapter has specific mobilization techniques included.

A hierarchy exists for ROM during the subacute phase of healing to ensure that any progression is performed in a safe and controlled fashion. The hierarchy for the ROM exercises is as follows

- Passive ROM
- Active-assisted ROM
- Active ROM

Advanced Phase (Figure 5-8)

In this phase of rehabilitation, the therapeutic exercise program must be progressed (both in the clinic and at home), selecting interventions that

- **Restore muscular strength, power, and endurance.** Like ROM, adequate muscular strength, power, and endurance are prerequisites for function. A wide variety of interventions exist that address deficits of muscle performance, and the individual therapist must decide what is the best intervention based upon a variety of patient factors and characteristics. Physical therapists should be experts in selective exercise prescription in order to increase all facets of muscle performance. Chapter 8 provides the foundation for choices of therapeutic interventions for development of muscular strength, power, and endurance.

The hierarchy for the progression of resistive exercises for restoration of muscle performance impairments is

- Single-angle, submaximal isometrics performed in the neutral position
- Multiple angle, submaximal isometrics performed at various angles of the range
- Multiple angle maximal isometrics
- Submaximal, short arc, isotonic exercises
- Submaximal, full ROM isotonic exercise
- Maximal short arc isotonic exercise, progressing to full ROM maximal isotonics
- Open- and closed-kinetic chain exercises in the isotonic mode (refer to Chapter 14 for more details on these topics)

- Isokinetics (refer to Chapter 10 for more details on Isokinetics)

Gentle resistive exercises can be introduced very early in the rehabilitative process. At regular intervals, the clinician should ensure that

- The patient is being compliant with their exercise program at home,
- The patient is aware of the rationale behind the exercise program,
- The patient is performing the exercise program correctly and at the appropriate intensity, and
- The patient's exercise program is being updated and appropriately based on clinical findings and patient response (refer to Chapter 23 for additional suggestions on these points).

Each regional chapter in this text also has many excellent suggestions for specific therapeutic exercises for the advanced phase of rehabilitation where the focus tends to be on muscular performance enhancement.

Return to Function Phase (Figure 5-9)

Assuming proper ROM and muscle performance, the final phase of rehabilitation involves restoration of function. In this phase interventions are chosen, which

- *Restore neuromuscular efficiency and improve the overall fitness and functional outcome of the patient.* Restoration of neuromuscular control and efficiency is vital to the function of the patient. Complete ROM and flexibility about

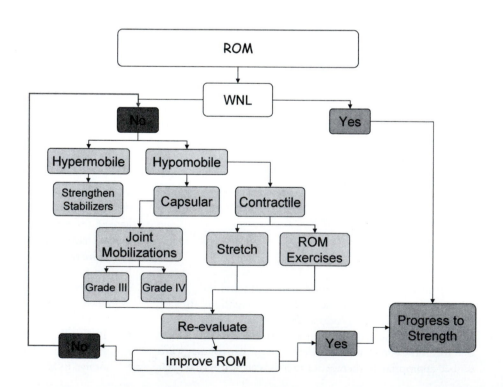

F I G U R E   5 - 7

ROM algorithm.

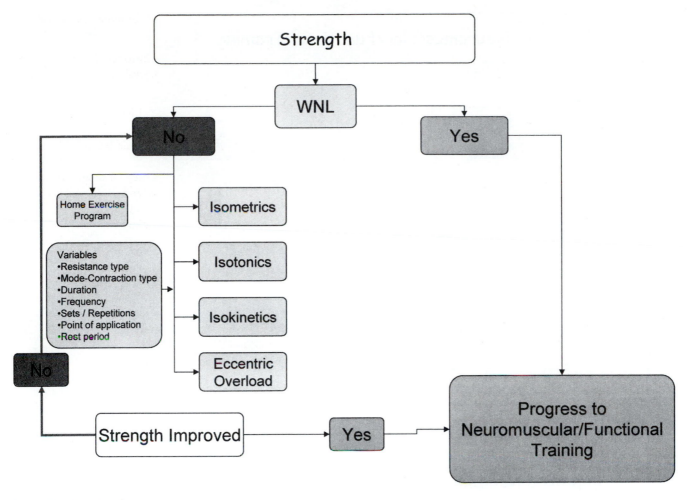

FIGURE 5-8

Muscular strength, power, and endurance algorithm.

a joint is not enough for normal function. Likewise, isolated muscular strengthening in any mode or motion may not be sufficient to provide the motor control and motor performance necessary for the multitude of complex functional tasks in which patients participate. Therefore, the final step of the rehabilitation process is the introduction of activities that challenge neuromuscular function in specific motions, patterns, and tasks, thereby assisting the patient to a return to the highest level of function. Although the restoration of neuromuscular efficiency and control is conceptually viewed as the "last" part of the rehabilitation algorithm, it should be noted that techniques to challenge the neuromuscular control system are present in several previous intervention algorithms. For example, at the most basic level, active ROM challenges the proprioceptive control system. Other exercises that are viewed primarily for strengthening can also have a dual purpose of developing neuromuscular control. Chapter 11 presents a detailed discussion of reactive neuromuscular training, and Chapter 17 presents a comprehensive discussion of techniques to regain postural stability and control. Likewise,

Chapter 13 presents options for plyometric interventions to challenge both muscular performance and neuromuscular control. Additionally, each regional chapter has an excellent variety of advanced, neuromuscular training interventions specific to the region.

SUMMARY

Algorithms are one way to illustrate the process of clinical reasoning. They are a graphic representation of a series of "if/then" decisions that may assist clinicians in developing diagnoses and selecting interventions. They serve to structure the process of clinical reasoning and illustrate the sequential nature of the clinical reasoning process used by therapists with experience and expertise. Finally, because evidence in physical therapy is constantly developing and changing, algorithms should not be viewed as static, rigid, or prescriptive decision-making tools. The clinical reasoning process is a complex, nonlinear process that requires a sufficient knowledge base and application of that knowledge in relation to an ever-changing base of evidence.

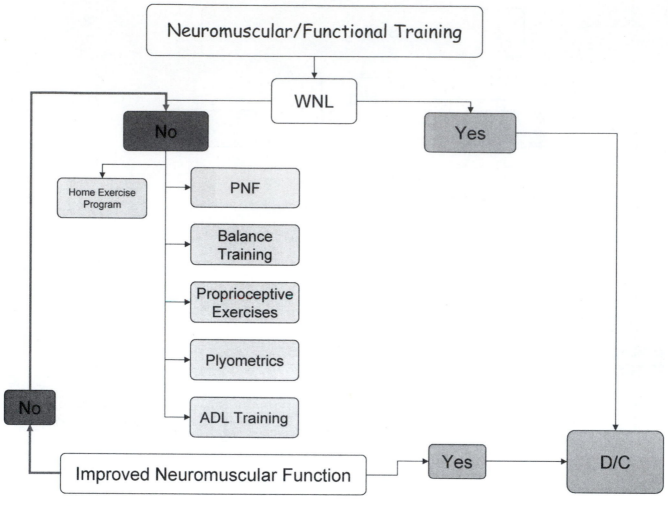

FIGURE 5-9

Neuromuscular efficiency/functional return algorithm.

Summary points are

- The quality of physical therapy provision, both in terms of diagnostic reasoning and selection of interventions, may be impacted by the use of algorithms.
- Clinical reasoning skills are strongly related to experience and develop over a career.
- Clinical decision processes of experts and novices differ. Algorithms may be a tool to enhance the process in novices and progress their skills toward that of experts.
- All clinical reasoning should be an application of evidence-based practice.
- The algorithmic approach to clinical reasoning may be used to guide intervention selection, in broad terms, however, sufficient evidence does not yet exist to allow them to specifically direct clinical intervention decisions.
- Algorithmic thinking can be applied to all subsequent chapters and is useful in the four-phased rehabilitation model which includes

- Acute phase
- Intermediate phase
- Advanced phase
- Return to function

REFERENCES

1. American Physical Therapy Association. The Guide to Physical Therapist Practice, 2nd ed. *Phys Ther* 81(1): 9–738, 2001.
2. Arocha J, Patel V, Patel Y. Hypothesis generation and the coordination of theory and evidence in novice diagnostic reasoning. *Med Decis Making* 13:198–211, 1993.
3. Bloch R. Methodology in clinical back pain trials. Spine 12:430–432, 1987.
4. Bruning R, Schraw G, Ronning R. *Cognitive Psychology,* 3rd ed. Upper Saddle River, NJ, Merrill, 1999.

5. Cyriax J. The diagnosis of soft tissue lesions. In: Cyriax J, ed. Textbook of Orthopaedic Medicine. London, Spottiswoode Ballantyne, 1978.

6. Edwards I, Jones M, Carr J, Baunack-Mayer A, Jensen G. Clinical reasoning strategies in physical therapy. *Phys Ther* 84(4):312–330, 2004.

7. Elstein A, Schwarz A. Evidence base of clinical diagnosis: Clinical problem solving and diagnostic decision making—selective review of the cognitive literature. *BMJ* 324:729–732, 2002.

8. Elstein A, Shulman L, Sprafka S. Medical problem solving: A ten-year retrospective. *Eval Health Professions* 13:5–36, 1990.

9. Friedman LM, Furberg CD, DeMets DL. *Fundamentals of Clinical Trials.* St. Louis, MO, Mosby-Year Books, 1985.

10. http://www.britannica.com/eb/article-9005707?query= algorithm&ct=. Accessed on August 15, 2005.

11. Hack L. Foundations for modalities as procedural interventions: Principles of clinical decision making. *Modalities for Therapeutic Intervention*, 4th ed. Philadelphia, PA, FA Davis, 2005.

12. Higgs J, Jones M. Clinical reasoning in the health professions. In: Higgs J, Jones M, eds. *Clinical Reasoning in the Health Professions*, 2nd ed. Boston, MA, Butterworth-Heinemann, 2000.

13. Jensen G, Shepard K, Gwyer J, Hack L. Attribute dimensions that distinguish master and novice physical therapy clinicians in orthopedic settings. *Phys Ther* 72:711–722, 1992.

14. Kahney H. *Problem Solving: Current Issues.* Buckingham, England, Open University Press, 1993.

15. Maitland GD. Maitland's Vertebral Manipulation, 6th ed. Oxford, Butterworth Heinemann, 2001.

16. McKenzie RA. *The Lumbar Spine: Mechanical Diagnosis and Therapy.* Waikanae, New Zealand, Spinal Publications, 1989.

17. May B, Dennis J. Expert decision making in physical therapy: A survey of practitioners. *Phys Ther* 71:190–216, 1991.

18. Miller T, Nyland J, Wormal W. Therapeutic exercise program design considerations: "Putting it all together." In: Nyland J, ed. *Clinical Decisions in Therapeutic Exercise.* Upper Saddle River, NJ, Pearson Education, Inc., 2006.

19. Rothstein J, Echternach J, Riddle D. The hypothesis-oriented algorithm for clinicians II (HOAC II): A guide for patient management. *Phys Ther* 83:455–470, 2003.

20. Rothstein J, Echternach J. The hypothesis-oriented algorithm for clinicians: A method for evaluation and treatment planning. *Phys Ther* 66:1388–1394, 1986.

21. Sackett DL, Rosenberg WM, Gray JA, et al. Evidence based medicine: What it is and what it isn't. *BMJ* 312:71–72, 1996.

PART 2

Treating Physiologic Impairments During Rehabilitation

Impairment Due to Pain: Managing Pain During the Rehabilitation Process

Craig R. Denegar and Phillip B. Donley

O B J E C T I V E S

After completing this chapter, the therapist should be able to do the following:

- Define pain, its types, and its positive and negative effects.
- Discuss the various techniques for assessing pain.
- Describe the characteristics of sensory receptors.
- Describe how the nervous system relays information about painful stimuli.
- Describe an appropriate neurophysiologic mechanism for pain control for the therapeutic modalities used by therapists.
- Describe how pain perception can be modified by cognitive factors.

UNDERSTANDING PAIN

The International Association for the Study of Pain defines *pain* as "an unpleasant sensory and emotional experience associated with actual or potential tissue damage, or described in terms of such damage."[22] Pain is a subjective sensation with more than one dimension and an abundance of descriptors of its qualities and characteristics. Despite its universality, pain is composed of a variety of human discomforts, rather than being a single entity.[21] The perception of pain can be subjectively modified by past experiences and expectations. Much of what we do to treat patients' pain is to change their perceptions of pain.[4]

Pain does have a purpose. It warns us that there is something wrong and can provoke a withdrawal response to avoid further injury. It also results in muscle spasm and guarding or protection of the injured part. Pain, however, can persist after it is no longer useful. It can become a means of enhancing disability and inhibiting efforts to rehabilitate the patient. Prolonged spasm, which leads to circulatory deficiency, muscle atrophy, disuse habits, and conscious or unconscious guarding, can lead to a severe loss of function.[17] Chronic pain can become a disease state in itself. Often lacking an identifiable cause, chronic pain can totally disable a patient. Research in recent years has led to a better understanding of pain and pain relief. This research also has raised new questions, while leaving many unanswered.

The control of pain is an essential aspect of caring for the injured patient. The therapist has several therapeutic approaches to pain modulation from which to choose.[31] We now have a better understanding of the psychology of pain; however, newer approaches to pain management challenge our understanding of injury and pain. The evolution of the treatment of pain is, however, incomplete. This chapter presents an overview of some theories of pain control that are intended to provide a stimulus for the therapist to develop his or her own rationale for using various techniques of pain modulation in the plan of care for patients they treat. Ideally, it will also interest some in research to establish the physiologic and psychological soundness of the use of a variety of techniques for pain relief and to expand our understanding of pain. Some understanding of what pain is, how it affects us, and how it is perceived is essential for the therapist.

TYPES OF PAIN

Traditionally, pain has been categorized as either *acute* or *chronic*. Acute pain is experienced when tissue damage is impending and after injury has occurred. Pain lasting for more than 6 months is generally classified as chronic.[5] More recently, the term *persistent pain* has been used to differentiate chronic pain that defies intervention from conditions where continuing (persistent) pain is a symptom of a treatable condition.[12,24] There is more research devoted to chronic pain and its treatment, but acute and persistent pain confront the therapist most often.

Referred pain, which also can be either acute or chronic, is pain perceived to be in an area that seems to have little relation to the existing pathology. For example, injury to the spleen often results in pain in the left shoulder. This pattern, known as *Kehr's sign*, is useful for identifying this serious injury and arranging prompt emergency care. Referred pain can outlast the causative events because of altered reflex patterns, continuing mechanical stress on muscles, learned habits of guarding, or the development of hypersensitive areas, called *trigger points*. Irritation of nerves and nerve roots can cause *radiating pain*. Pressure on the lumbar nerve roots associated with a herniated disk or a contusion of the sciatic nerve can result in pain radiating down the lower extremity to the foot.

Deep somatic pain is a type that seems to be *sclerotomic* (associated with a sclerotome, a segment of bone innervated by a spinal segment). There is often a discrepancy between the site of the disorder and the site of the pain.

PAIN ASSESSMENT

Pain is a complex phenomenon that is difficult to evaluate and quantify because it is subjective and influenced by attitudes and beliefs of the therapist and the patient. Quantification is hindered by the fact that pain is a very difficult concept to put into words.[1]

Obtaining an accurate and standardized assessment of pain is problematic. Several tools have been developed. These pain profiles identify the type of pain, quantify the intensity of pain, evaluate the effect of the pain experience on the patient's level of function, and/or assess the psychosocial impact of pain.

The pain profiles are useful. They compel the patient to verbalize the pain and thereby provide an outlet for the patient and provide the therapist a better understanding of the pain experience. They assess the psychosocial response to pain and injury. The pain profile can assist with the evaluation process by improving communication and directing the therapist toward appropriate diagnostic tests. These assessments also assist the therapist in identifying which therapeutic techniques may be effective and when they should be applied. Finally, these profiles provide a standard measure to monitor treatment progress.[12]

Pain Assessment Scales

The following profiles are used in the evaluation of acute and chronic pain associated with illnesses and injuries. Visual analogue scales are quick and simple tests completed by the patient (Fig. 6-1). These scales consist of a line, usually 10 cm in length, the extremes of which are taken to represent the limits of the

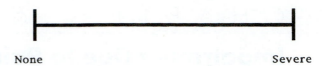

None   Severe

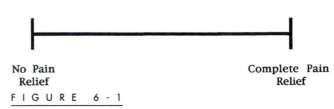

No Pain   Complete Pain
Relief   Relief

FIGURE   6 - 1

Visual analogue scales. (Reproduced, with permission, from Prentice WE. *Therapeutic Modalities for Allied Health Professionals.* New York, McGraw-Hill, 1998.)

pain experience. One end is defined as "No Pain" and the other as "Severe Pain." The patient is asked to mark the line at a point corresponding to the severity of the pain. The distance between "No Pain" and the mark represents pain severity. A similar scale can be used to assess treatment effectiveness by placing "No Pain Relief" at one end of the scale and "Complete Pain Relief" at the other. These scales can be completed daily or more often as pre- and posttreatment assessments.[15]

Pain charts can be used to establish spatial properties of pain. These two-dimensional graphic portrayals are completed by the patient to assess the location of pain and a number of subjective components. Simple line drawings of the body in several postural positions are presented to the patient (Fig. 6-2). The patient draws or colors the pictures in areas which correspond to their pain experience. Different colors are used for different sensations. For example, blue for aching pain, yellow for numbness or tingling, red for burning pain, and green for cramping pain. Descriptions can be added to the form to enhance the communication value. The form could be completed daily.[18]

The McGill Pain Questionnaire (MPQ) is a tool with 78 words that describe pain (Fig. 6-3). These words are grouped into 20 sets, which are divided into 4 categories representing dimensions of the pain experience. Completion of the MPQ can take 20 minutes and is often frustrating for patients who do not speak English well. It is commonly administered to patients with low back pain. When administered every 2 to 4 weeks, it demonstrated changes in status very clearly.[21]

The Activity Pattern Indicators Pain Profile measures patient activity. It is a 64-question, self-report tool that can be used to assess functional impairment associated with pain. The instrument measures the frequency of certain behaviors such as housework, recreation, and social activities.[13]

The most common acute pain profile used in outpatient clinics today is a numeric pain scale. The patient is asked to rate their pain on a scale from 1 to 10, with 10 representing the worst pain they have experienced or could imagine. The question is

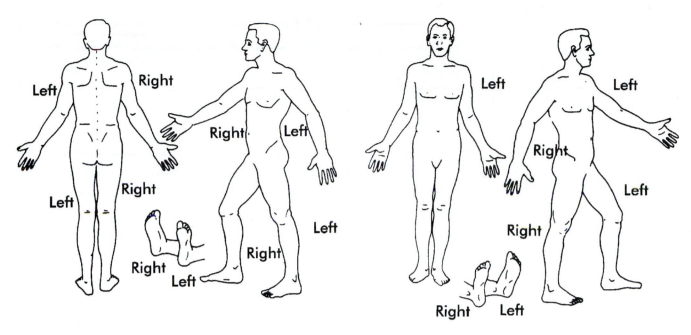

F I G U R E   6 - 2

The pain chart. Use the following instructions: Please use all of the figures to show me exactly where all your pains are, and where they radiate to. Shade or draw with *blue marker*. Only the patient is to fill out this sheet. Please be as precise and detailed as possible. Use *yellow marker* for numbness and tingling. Use *red marker* for burning or hot areas, and *green marker* for cramping. Please remember: blue = pain; yellow = numbness and tingling; red = burning or hot areas; green = cramping. (Reproduced, with permission, from Melzack R. *Pain Measurement and Assessment.* New York, Raven Press, 1983.)

asked before and after treatment. When treatments provide pain relief, patients are asked about the extent and duration of the relief. In addition, the patient may be asked to estimate the portion of the day that they experience pain and about specific activities that increase or decrease their pain. When pain affects sleep, the patient may be asked to estimate the amount of sleep they got in the previous 24 hours. In addition, the amount of medication required for pain can be noted. This information helps the therapist assess changes in pain, select appropriate treatments, and communicate more clearly with the patient about the course of recovery from injury or surgery.

All of these scales help the patient to communicate the severity and duration of his or her pain and appreciate changes that occur. Often in a long recovery, patients lose sight of how much progress has been made in terms of the pain experience and return to functional activities. A review of these pain scales often can serve to reassure the patient, foster a brighter, more positive outlook, and reinforce the commitment to the plan of treatment.

The efficacy of many of the treatments used by therapists has not been fully substantiated. These scales are one source of data that can help therapists identify the most effective approaches to managing common injuries. These assessment tools can also be useful when reviewing a patient's progress with physicians and third-party payors.

TISSUE SENSITIVITY

The structures most sensitive to damaging (noxious) stimuli are: first, the periosteum and joint capsule; second, subchondral bone, tendons, and ligament; third, muscle and cortical bone; and finally, the synovium and articular cartilage. A variety of "silent" fractures produce little or no pain. Different anatomic tissues exhibit varying degrees of sensitivity to pain. Avulsion fractures tend to be quite painful because they tear away the periosteum. Musculoskeletal pain is usually spread over a large area unless it is close to the surface. For example, a hamstring strain usually results in pain over the posterior thigh, whereas an acromioclavicular sprain usually localizes over the joint.

GOALS IN MANAGING PAIN

Regardless of the cause of pain, its reduction is an essential part of treatment. Plan signals the patient to seek assistance and is

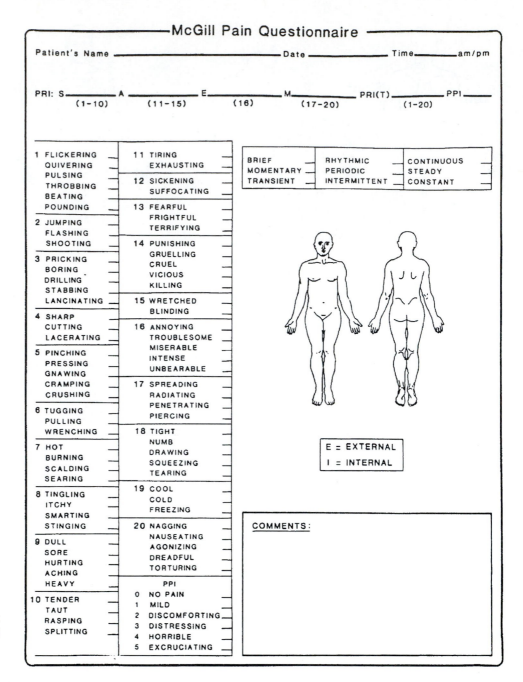

FIGURE 6-3

McGill pain questionnaire. The descriptors fall into four major groups: sensory, 1–10; affective, 11–15; evaluative, 16; and miscellaneous, 17–20. The rank value for each descriptor is based on its position in the word set. The sum of the rank values is the pain rating index (PRI). The present pain intensity (PPI) is based on a scale of 0 to 5. (Reproduced, with permission, from Melzack R. *Pain Measurement and Assessment.* New York, Raven Press, 1983.)

often useful in establishing a diagnosis. Once the injury or illness is diagnosed, pain serves little purpose. Medical or surgical treatment or immobilization is necessary to treat some conditions, but physical therapy and an early return to activity are appropriate following many injuries. The therapist's objectives are to encourage the body to heal through exercise designed to progressively increase functional capacity and to return the patient to work, recreational, and other activities as swiftly and safely as possible. Pain will inhibit therapeutic exercise. The challenge for the therapist is to control acute pain and protect the patient from further injury while encouraging progressive exercise in a supervised environment.

PAIN PERCEPTION AND NEURAL TRANSMISSION

Sensory Receptors

There are several types of sensory receptors in the body, and the therapist should be aware of their existence and the types of stimuli that activate them (Table 6-1). Activation of some of these sense organs with therapeutic agents will decrease the patient's perception of pain. Six different types of receptor nerve endings are commonly described:

1. Meissner's corpuscles are activated by light touch.
2. Pacinian corpuscles respond to deep pressure.

TABLE 6-1

Some Characteristics of Selected Sensory Receptors

TYPE OF SENSORY RECEPTORS	STIMULUS		RECEPTOR	
	GENERAL TERM	SPECIFIC NATURE	TERM	LOCATION
Mechanoreceptors	Pressure	Movement of hair in a hair follicle	Afferent nerve fiber	Base of hair follicles
		Light pressure	Meissner's corpuscle	Skin
		Deep pressure	Pacinian corpuscle	Skin
		Touch	Merkel's touch corpuscle	Skin
Nociceptors	Pain	Distension (stretch)	Free nerve endings	Wall of gastrointestinal tract, pharynx, skin
Proprioceptors	Tension	Distension	Corpuscles of Ruffini	Skin and capsules in joints and ligaments
		Length changes	Muscle spindles	Skeletal muscle
		Tension changes	Golgi tendon organs	Between muscles and tendons
Thermoreceptors	Temperature change	Cold	Krause's end bulbs	Skin
		Heat	Corpuscles of Ruffini	Skin and capsules in joints and ligaments

SOURCE: Previte JJ. *Human Physiology.* New York, McGraw-Hill, 1983.

3. Merkel's corpuscles respond to deep pressure, but more slowly than pacinian corpuscles, and also are activated by hair follicle deflection.
4. Ruffini's corpuscles in the skin are sensitive to touch, tension, and possibly heat; those in the joint capsules and ligaments are sensitive to change in position.
5. Krause's end bulbs are thermoreceptors that react to a decrease in temperature and touch.[26]
6. Pain receptors, called *nociceptors* or *free nerve endings*, are sensitive to extreme mechanical, thermal, or chemical energy.[3] They respond to noxious stimuli, in other words, to impending or actual tissue damage (for example, cuts, burns, sprains, and so on). The term *nociceptive* is from the Latin *nocere*, to damage, and is used to imply pain information. These organs respond to superficial forms of heat and cold, analgesic balms, and massage.

Proprioceptors found in muscles, joint capsules, ligaments, and tendons provide information regarding joint position and muscle tone. The muscle spindles react to changes in length and tension when the muscle is stretched or contracted. The Golgi tendon organs also react to changes in length and tension within the muscle. See Table 6-1 for a more complete listing.

Some sensory receptors respond to phasic activity and produce an impulse when the stimulus is increasing or decreasing, but not during a sustained stimulus. They adapt to a constant stimulus. Meissner's corpuscles and pacinian corpuscles are examples of such receptors.

Tonic receptors produce impulses as long as the stimulus is present. Examples of tonic receptors are muscle spindles, free nerve endings, and Krause's end bulbs. The initial impulse is at a higher frequency than later impulses that occur during sustained stimulation.

Adaptation is the decline in generator potential and the reduction of frequency that occurs with a prolonged stimulus or with frequently repeated stimuli. If some physical agents are used too often or for too long, the receptors can adapt to or accommodate the stimulus and reduce their impulses. The accommodation phenomenon can be observed with the use of superficial hot and cold agents, such as ice packs and hydrocollator packs.

As a stimulus becomes stronger, the number of receptors excited and the frequency of the impulses increase. This provides more electrical activity at the spinal cord level, which may facilitate the effects of some physical agents.

NEURAL TRANSMISSION

Afferent nerve fibers transmit impulses from the sensory receptors toward the brain; whereas *efferent* fibers, such as motor neurons, transmit impulses from the brain toward the periphery. First-order, or primary, afferents transmit the impulses from the sensory receptor to the dorsal horn of the spinal cord (Fig. 6-4). There are four different types of first-order neurons (Table 6-2). Note that A-alpha and A-beta fibers are characterized as being

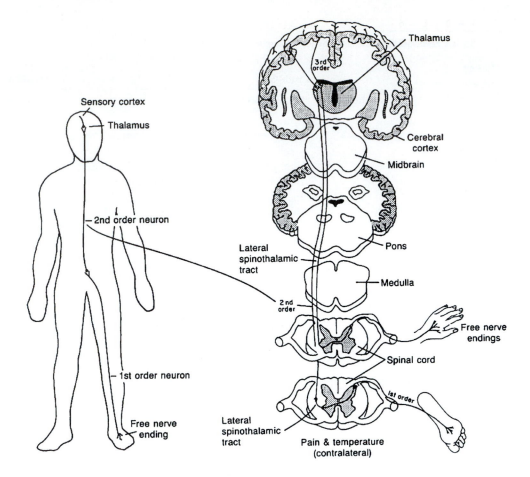

FIGURE 6-4

The lateral spinothalamic tract carries impulses of pain and temperature from the sensory receptors to the cortex. (Reproduced, with permission, from Prentice WE. *Therapeutic Modalities for Allied Health Professionals.* New York, McGraw-Hill, 1998.)

large diameter afferents and A-delta and C fibers as small diameter afferents.

Second-order afferent fibers carry sensory messages from the dorsal horn to the brain. Second-order afferent fibers are categorized as wide dynamic range or nociceptive specific. The wide dynamic range second-order afferents receive input from A-beta, A-delta, and C fibers. These second-order afferents serve relatively large, overlapping receptor fields. The nociceptive specific second-order afferents respond exclusively to noxious stimulation. They receive input only from A-delta and C fibers. These afferents serve smaller receptor fields that do not overlap. All of these neurons synapse with third-order neurons that carry information to various brain centers where the input is integrated, interpreted, and acted upon.

Facilitators and Inhibitors of Synaptic Transmission

For information to pass between neurons, a transmitter substance must be released from one neuron terminal (presynaptic membrane), enter the synaptic cleft, and attach to a receptor site on the next neuron (postsynaptic membrane). In the past, all the activity within the synapse was attributed to neurotransmitters, such as acetylcholine. The neurotransmitters, when released in sufficient quantities, are known to cause depolarization of the postsynaptic neuron. In the absence of the neurotransmitter, no depolarization occurs.

It is now apparent that several compounds that are not true neurotransmitters can facilitate or inhibit synaptic activity. These compounds are classified as biogenic amine transmitters or neuroactive peptides. Serotonin and norepinephrine are examples of biogenic amine transmitters. About two dozen neuroactive peptides have been identified, including *substance P, glutamate, enkephalins,* and β-*endorphin* (BEP).[3]

Serotonin and *enkephalins* are active in descending (efferent) pathways, which block the pain message.[7] Enkephalin is an endogenous (made by the body) opioid that inhibits the depolarization of second-order nociceptive nerve fibers. It is released from interneurons, enkephalin neurons with short axons. The enkephalins are stored in nerve-ending vesicles found in the substantia gelatinosa and several areas of the brain. When released, enkephalin may bind to presynaptic or postsynaptic membranes.[3]

Norepinephrine is a biogenic amine transmitter that is released by the depolarization of some neurons and binds to the postsynaptic membranes. Norepinephrine is found in several areas of the nervous system including a tract that descends from the pons that inhibits synaptic transmission between first-order and second-order nociceptive fibers, thus decreasing pain sensation.[16]

Other endogenous opioids may be active analgesic agents. These neuroactive peptides are released into the central nervous system (CNS) and have an action similar to that of morphine, an

TABLE 6-2

Classification of Afferent Neurons

SIZE	TYPE	GROUP	SUBGROUP	DIAMETER (μm)	CONDUCTION VELOCITY (m/sec)	RECEPTOR	STIMULUS
Large	A α	I	1 a	12–20 (22)	70–120	Proprioceptive mechanoreceptor	Muscle velocity and length change, muscle shortening of rapid speed
	A α	I	1 b				
	A α	II	Muscle	6–12	36–72	Proprioceptive mechanoreceptor	Muscle length information from touch and pacinian corpuscles
	A β	II	Skin			Cutaneous receptors	Touch, vibration, hair receptors
	A δ	III	Muscle	1–5 (6)	6(12)–36(80)	75% mechanoreceptors and thermoreceptors	Temperature change
Small	A δ	III	Skin			25% nociceptors, mechanoreceptors, and thermoreceptors (hot and cold)	Noxious, mechanical, and temperature ($>45°C$, $<10°C$)
	C	IV	Muscle	0.3–1.0	0.4–1.0	50% mechanoreceptors and thermoreceptors	Touch and temperature
	C	IV	Skin			50% nociceptors, 20% mechanoreceptors, and 30% thermoreceptors (hot and cold)	Noxious, mechanical, and temperature ($>45°C$, $<10°C$)

opiate analgesic. There are specific receptors located at strategic sites, called binding sites, to receive these compounds. BEP, a 31-amino acid peptide, and *dynorphin* have potent analgesic effects. These are released within the CNS by mechanisms that are not fully understood at this time.

NOCICEPTION

A nociceptive neuron is one that transmits pain signals. Its cell body is in the dorsal root ganglion near the spinal cord. Approximately 25 percent of the myelinated A-delta and 50 percent of the unmyelinated C fibers contact nociceptors and are considered nociceptive, afferent neurons (Table 6-2). Once a nociceptor is stimulated, it releases a neuropeptide (substance P) that initiates the electrical impulses along the afferent fiber toward the spinal cord. Substance P also serves as a transmitter substance between the first-order afferent fiber and a second-order afferent fiber (Fig. 6-4) at the dorsal horn of the spinal column.

The A-delta and C fibers, which transmit sensations of pain and temperature, have different diameters (A-delta are larger) and different conduction velocities (A-delta are faster). The C

fibers are also connected to more of the nociceptive specific second-order afferents. These differences result in two qualitatively different types of pain, termed fast and slow.[3] Fast pain is brief, well-localized, and well-matched to the stimulus—for example, the initial pain of an unexpected pinprick. Slow pain is an aching, throbbing, or burning sensation that is poorly localized and less specifically related to the stimulus. There is a delay in the perception of slow pain following injury, but the pain will continue long after the noxious stimulus is removed. Fast pain is transmitted over the larger, faster-conducting A-delta afferent neurons and originates from receptors located in the skin. Slow pain is transmitted by the C afferent neurons and originates from both superficial tissue (skin) and deeper tissue (ligaments and muscle).[3]

The various types of afferent fibers follow different courses as they ascend toward the brain. Some A-delta and most C afferent neurons enter the spinal cord through the dorsolateral tract of Lissauer and synapse in marginal zone (lamina 1) or the substantia gelatinosa (lamina 2) with a second-order neuron.[16] Most nociceptive second-order neurons ascend to higher centers along one of three tracts, lateral spinothalamic, spinoreticular, and spinoencephalic, with the remainder ascending along the spinocervical tract or as projections to the cuneate and gracile nuclei of the medulla.[16] Approximately 90 percent of the wide dynamic range second-order afferents terminate in the thalamus.[16] Third-order neurons project to the sensory cortex and numerous other centers in the CNS. These projections allow us to perceive pain. They also permit the integration of past experiences and emotions, which form our response to the pain experience. These connections are also believed to be parts of complex circuits that the therapist may stimulate to manage pain. Most analgesic physical agents are believed to slow or block the impulses ascending along the A-delta and C afferent neuron pathways through direct input into the dorsal horn or through descending mechanisms. These pathways are discussed in more detail in the following section.

NEUROPHYSIOLOGIC EXPLANATIONS OF PAIN CONTROL

The neurophysiologic mechanisms of pain control through stimulation of cutaneous receptors have not been fully explained. Much of what is known and current theory are the result of work involving electroacupuncture and transcutaneous electrical nerve stimulation. The concepts of the analgesic response to cutaneous receptor stimulation presented here were first proposed by Melzack and Wall[20] and Castel.[7] These models essentially present three analgesic mechanisms:

1. Stimulation from ascending A-beta afferents results in the blocking of impulses (pain messages) carried along A-delta and C afferent fibers.
2. Stimulation of descending pathways in the dorsolateral tract of the spinal cord by A-delta and C fiber afferent input results in a blocking of the impulses carried along the A-delta and C afferent fibers.
3. The stimulation of A-delta and C-afferent fibers causes the release of endogenous opioids (BEP) resulting in a prolonged activation of descending analgesic pathways.

These theories or models are not necessarily mutually exclusive. Recent evidence suggests that pain relief may result from combinations of dorsal horn and CNS activity.[2,9]

A decrease in input along nociceptive afferents also results in pain relief. Cooling afferent fibers decreases the rate at which they conduct impulses. Thus, a 20-minute application of cold is effective in relieving pain because of the decrease in activity, rather than an increase in activity along afferent pathways.

Blocking the Pain Impulses with Ascending A-beta Input

Pain modulation due to sensory stimulation and the resultant increase in the impulses in the large diameter (A-beta) afferent fibers was proposed by the gate control theory of pain (Fig. 6-5).[20] Impulses ascending on these fibers stimulate the substantia gelatinosa as they enter the dorsal horn of the spinal cord. Stimulation of the substantia gelatinosa inhibits synaptic

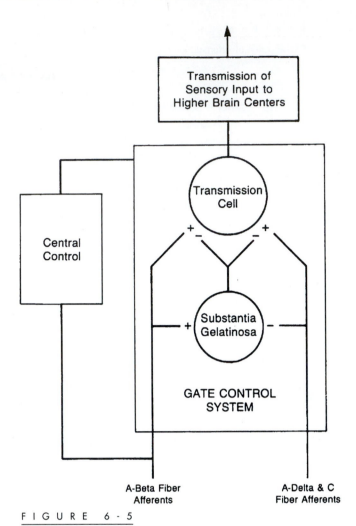

F I G U R E   6 - 5

The gate control system. Increases A-beta input and stimulates the substantia gelatinosa which inhibits the flow of afferent input to sensory centers. (Reproduced, with permission, from Prentice WE. *Therapeutic Modalities for Allied Health Professionals.* New York, McGraw-Hill, 1998.)

transmission in the large and small (A-delta and C fiber) afferent pathways. The "pain message" carried along the smaller diameter fibers is not transmitted to the second-order neurons and never reaches sensory centers. The balance between the input from the small- and large-diameter afferents determines how much of the pain message is blocked or gated.

The concept of sensory stimulation for pain relief, as proposed by the gate control theory, has empirical support. Rubbing a contusion, applying moist heat, or massaging sore muscles decreases the perception of pain. The analgesic response to these treatments is attributed to the increased stimulation of large-diameter afferent fibers.

The gate control theory also proposes that A-delta and C fiber impulses inhibit the substantia gelatinosa, facilitating the perception of pain. The sensation of pain does not diminish rapidly because free nerve endings do not accommodate and

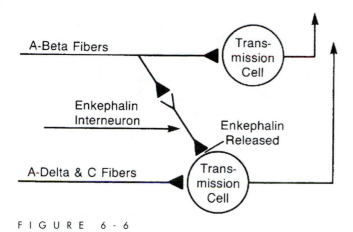

FIGURE 6-6

Presynaptic inhibition of dorsal horn synapse transmission due to A-beta fiber stimulation at enkephalin interneurons. (Reproduced, with permission, from Prentice WE. *Therapeutic Modalities for Allied Health Professionals*. New York, McGraw-Hill, 1998.)

the afferent impulses from them "open the gate" to further pain message transmission.

The discovery and isolation of endogenous opioids in the 1970s led to new theories of pain relief. Castel[7] introduced an endogenous opioid analogue to the gate control theory (Fig. 6-6). This theory proposes increased neural activity in A-alpha and A-beta primary afferent pathways, which triggers a release of enkephalin from enkephalin interneurons found in the dorsal horn. These neuroactive amines inhibit synaptic transmission in the A-delta and C fiber afferent pathways. The end result, as in the gate control theory, is that the pain message is blocked before it reaches sensory levels.

Descending Pain Control Mechanisms

The gate control theory[20] proposed a second analgesic mechanism that involves descending efferent fibers. The central control, originating in higher centers of the CNS, could affect the dorsal horn gating process. Impulses from the thalamus and brain stem (central biasing) are carried into the dorsal horn on efferent fibers in the dorsal or dorsal lateral paths (or tracts). Impulses from the higher centers act to close the gate and block transmission of the pain message at the dorsal horn synapse. Through this system, it was theorized, previous experiences, emotional influences, sensory perception, and other factors could influence the transmission of the pain message and the perception of pain.

Castel[7] offers an endogenous opioid model of descending influence over dorsal horn synapse activity (Fig. 6-7). Stimulation of the *periaqueductal grey* region of the midbrain and the *raphe nucleus* in the pons and medulla by ascending neural input, especially from A-delta and C fiber afferents, and possibly central biasing, activates the descending mechanism. The periaqueductal grey stimulates the raphe nucleus. The raphe nucleus

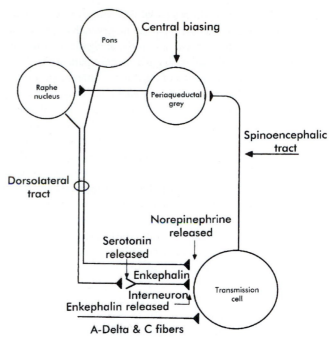

FIGURE 6-7

Stimulation of the periaqueductal grey region of the midbrain and the raphe nucleus in the pons and medulla by ascending neural input, especially from A-delta and C fiber afferents, and possibly central biasing, activates the descending mechanism. (Reproduced, with permission, from Prentice WE. *Therapeutic Modalities for Allied Health Professionals*. New York, McGraw-Hill, 1998.)

in turn sends impulses along serontonergic efferent fibers in the dorsal lateral tract, which synapse with enkephalin interneurons. The interneurons release enkephalin into the dorsal horn, inhibiting the synaptic transmission of impulses to the second-order afferent neurons.

Recently, a second descending, norandrenergic pathway projecting from the pons to the dorsal horn has been identified.[16] The significance of these parallel pathways is not fully understood. It is also not known if these norandrenergic fibers directly inhibit dorsal horn synapses or stimulate the enkephalin interneurons.

This model provides a physiologic explanation for the analgesic response to brief, intense stimulation. The analgesia following accupressure and the use of some transcutaneous electrical nerve simulators (TENS), such as point simulators, is attributed to this descending pain control mechanism.

BEP and Dynorphin

There is evidence that stimulation of the small-diameter afferents (A-delta and C) can stimulate the release of other endogenous opioids.[8,10,19,23–25,27–30] *BEP* and *dynorphin* are neuroactive peptides, with potent analgesic affects. The term endorphin refers to an opiatelike substance produced by the body. The mechanisms regulating the release of BEP and dynorphin have not been fully elucidated. It is apparent, however, that these large endogenous substances play a role in the analgesic response to some forms of stimuli used in the treatment of patients in pain.

One of the main sources of BEP is the anterior pituitary. Here, it shares the prohormone *propiomelanocortin* (POMC) with adrenocorticotropin (ACTH). Prolonged (20–40 minutes) small-diameter afferent fiber stimulation has been thought to trigger the release of BEP from the anterior pituitary gland. Electroacupuncture, and possibly TENS with long-phase durations and low pulse rates (1 to 5 pulses/second), will cause small-diameter afferent fiber depolarization necessary for BEP release. The anterior pituitary gland, however, may not be a source of BEP in low pulse rate, long pulse width TENS-induced analgesia.[11] These results and the recognition that BEP does not readily cross the blood-brain barrier[3] suggesting that if BEP or other endogenous opioids are active analgesic agents within the CNS, they are released from areas within the brain.

The neurons in the hypothalamus that send projections to the PAG and noradrenergic nuclei in the brain stem contain BEP. It is possibly that BEP released from these neurons by stimulation of the hypothalamus is responsible for the analgesic response to the treatments (Fig. 6-8).[6]

Dynorphin, a recently isolated endogenous opioid, is found in the PAG, rostroventral medulla, and the dorsal horn.[16] It has been demonstrated that dynorphin is released during electroacupuncture.[14] Dynorphin may be responsible for suppressing the response to noxious mechanical stimulation.[16]

Summary of Pain Control Mechanisms

The body's pain control mechanisms are probably not mutually exclusive. Rather, analgesia is the result of overlapping processes. It is also important to realize that the theories presented are only models. They are useful in conceptualizing the perception of pain and pain relief. These models will help the therapist understand the effects of therapeutic modalities and form a sound rationale for modality application. As more research is conducted and the mysteries of pain and neurophysiology are solved, new models will emerge. The therapist should adapt these models to fit new developments.

COGNITIVE INFLUENCES

Pain perception and the response to a painful experience can be influenced by a variety of cognitive processes, including anxiety, attention, depression, past pain experiences, and cultural influences. These individual aspects of pain expression are mediated by higher centers in the cortex in ways that are not clearly understood. They can influence both the sensory discriminative and motivational affective dimensions of pain.

Many mental processes modulate the perception of pain through descending systems. Behavior modification, the ex-

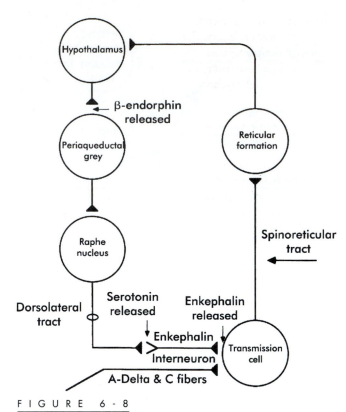

FIGURE 6 - 8

The neurons in the hypothalamus that send projections to the periaqueductal grey and noradrenergic nuclei in the brain stem contain β-endorphin. It is possible that β-endorphin released from these neurons by stimulation of the hypothalamus is responsible for the analgesic response to the treatments. (Reproduced, with permission, from Prentice WE. *Therapeutic Modalities for Allied Health Professionals.* New York, McGraw-Hill, 1998.)

citement of the moment, happiness, positive feelings, focusing (directed attention toward specific stimuli), hypnosis, and suggestion may modulate pain perception. Past experiences, cultural background, personality, motivation to play, aggression, anger, and fear are all factors that could facilitate or inhibit pain perception. Strong central inhibition may mask severe injury for a period of time. At such times, evaluation of the injury is quite difficult. Patients with chronic pain can become very depressed and experience a loss of fitness. They tend to be less active and may have altered appetites and sleep habits. They have a decreased will to work and exercise and often develop a reduced sex drive. They may turn to self-abusive patterns of behavior. Tricyclic drugs are often used to inhibit serotonin depletion for the patient with chronic pain.

Just as pain may be inhibited by central modulation, it may also arise from central origins. Phobias, fear, depression, anger, grief, and hostility are all capable of producing pain in the absence of local pathologic processes. In addition, pain memory, which is associated with old injuries, can result in pain perception and pain response that are out of proportion to a new, often minor, injury. Substance abuse can also alter and confound the perception of pain. Substance abuse may cause the chronic pain patient to become more depressed or may lead to depression and psychosomatic pain.

PAIN MANAGEMENT

How should the therapist approach pain? First, the source of the pain must be identified. Unidentified pain may hide a serious disorder, and treatment of such pain may delay the appropriate treatment of the disorder. Once a diagnosis has been made, several different approaches can provide pain relief. Pain control strategies may include the following:

1. Encourage central biasing through cognitive processes, such as motivation, tension diversion, focusing, relaxation, techniques, positive thinking, thought stopping, and self-control.
2. Minimize the tissue damage through the application of proper first aid and immobilization.
3. Maintain a line of communication with the patient. Let the patient know what to expect following an injury. Pain, swelling, dysfunction, and atrophy will occur following injury. The patient's anxiety over these events will increase his or her perception of pain. Often, a patient who has been told what to expect by someone he or she trusts will be less anxious and suffer less pain.
4. Recognize that all pain, even psychosomatic pain, is very real to the patient.
5. Encourage supervised exercise to encourage blood flow, promote nutrition, increase metabolic activity, and reduce stiffness and guarding, if the activity will not cause further harm to the patient.

The physician may choose to prescribe oral or injectable medications in the treatment of the patient. The most commonly used medications are classified as analgesics, anti-inflammatory agents, or both. The therapist should become familiar with these drugs and should note if the patient is taking any medications. It is also important to work with the referring physician to assure that the patient takes the medications appropriately (see Chapter 23).

When using physical agents, the therapist should match it to each patient's situation. Casts and braces may prevent the application of ice or moist heat; however, TENS electrodes often can be positioned under a cast or brace for pain relief. Following acute injuries, ice may be the therapeutic agent of choice because of the effect of cold on the inflammatory process. There is not one "best" physical agent for pain control. The therapist must select the physical agent that is most appropriate for each patient based on the knowledge of the modalities and professional judgment. In no situation should the therapist apply a physical agent without first developing a clear rationale for the treatment.

In general, physical agents can be used to

1. stimulate large-diameter afferent fibers. This can be done with TENS, massage, and analgesic balms.
2. decrease pain fiber transmission velocity with cold or ultrasound.
3. stimulate small-diameter afferent fibers and descending pain control mechanisms with accupressure, deep massage, or TENS over acupuncture points or trigger points.
4. stimulate a release of BEP or other endogenous opioids through prolonged small-diameter fiber stimulation with TENS.

The goal of most treatment programs is to encourage early pain-free exercise. The physical agents used to control pain do little to promote tissue healing. They should be used to relieve acute pain following injury or surgery or to control pain and other symptoms, such as swelling, to promote progressive exercise. The therapist should not lose sight of the effects of the physical agents or the importance of progressive exercise in restoring the patient's functional ability.

Reducing the perception of pain is as much as art as a science. The therapist's approach to the patient has a great impact on the success of the treatment. The patient will not be convinced of the efficacy and importance of the treatment unless the therapist appears confident about it. The therapist must make the patient a participant rather than a passive spectator in the treatment and rehabilitation process. The therapist is encouraged to keep abreast of the neurophysiology of pain and the physiology of tissue healing to maintain a current scientific basis for selecting treatment approaches and managing the pain experienced by patients.

SUMMARY

- Pain is a response to a noxious stimulus that is subjectively modified by past experiences and expectations.
- Pain is classified as either acute or chronic and can exhibit many different patterns.
- Early reduction of pain in a treatment program will facilitate therapeutic exercise.
- Stimulation of sensory receptors via the therapeutic modalities can modify the patient's perception of pain.
- Four mechanisms of pain control may include:
  - ➤ Decreased transmission of input along nociceptive pathways.
  - ➤ Dorsal horn modulation due to the input from large-diameter afferents through a gate control system, the release of enkephalins, or both.
  - ➤ Descending efferent fiber activation due to the effects of small fiber afferent input on higher centers including the thalamus, raphe nucleus, and periaqueductal grey region.

➤ The central release of endogenous opioids, including BEP, through prolonged small-diameter afferent stimulation.

- Pain perception may be influenced by a variety of cognitive processes mediated by the higher brain centers.
- The selection of a physical agent for controlling pain should be based on current knowledge of neurophysiology and the psychology of pain.
- The application of physical agents for the control of pain should not occur until the diagnosis of the injury has been established.

REFERENCES

1. Addison R. Chronic pain syndrome. *Am J Med* 77:54, 1985.
2. Anderson S, Ericson T, Holmgren E. Electroacupuncture affects pain threshold measured with electrical stimulation of teeth. *Brain* 63:393–396, 1973.
3. Berne R, Levy M. *Physiology*. St. Louis, MO, Mosby, 1988.
4. Bishop B. Pain: Its physiology and rationale for management. *Phys Ther* 60:13–37, 1980.
5. Bonica J. *The Management of Pain*. Philadelphia, PA, Lea & Febiger, 1990.
6. Bowsher D. Central pain mechanisms. In: Wells P, Frampton V, Bowsher D, eds. *Pain Management in Physical Therapy*. Norwalk, CT, Appleton & Lange, 1988.
7. Castel J. *Pain Management Acupuncture and Transcutaneous Electrical Nerve Stimulation Techniques*. Lake Bluff, II, Pain Control Services, 1979.
8. Chapman C, Benedetti C. Analgesia following electrical stimulation: Partial reversal by a narcotic antagonist. *Life Sci* 26:44–48, 1979.
9. Cheng R, Pomeranz B. Electroacupuncture analgesia could be mediated by at least two pain relieving mechanisms: Endorphin and non-endorphin systems. *Lift Sci* 25:1957–1962, 1979.
10. Clement-Jones V, McLaughlin L, Tomlin S. Increased beta-endorphin but not metenkephalin levels in human cerebrospinal fluid after electroacupuncture for recurrent pain. *Lancet* 2:946–948, 1980.
11. Denegar G, Perrin D, Rogol A. Influence of transcutaneous electrical nerve stimulation on pain, range of motion and serum cortisol concentration in females with induced delayed onset muscle soreness. *J Orthop Sports Phys Ther* 11:101–103, 1989.
12. Dickerman J. The use of pain profiles in clinical practice. *Fam Pract Recert* 14:35–44, 1992.
13. Gatchel R. Million behavioral health inventory: Its utility in predicting physical functioning patients with low back pain. *Arch Phys Med Rehabil* 67:878, 1986.
14. Ho W, Wen H. Opioid-like activity in the cerebrospinal fluid of pain patients treated by electroacupuncture. *Neuropharmacology* 28:961–966, 1989.
15. Huskisson E. Visual analogue scales. Pain measurement and assessment. In: Melzack R, ed. *Pain Measurement and Assessment*. New York, Raven Press, 1983, p. 103.
16. Jessell T, Kelly D. Pain and analgesia. In: Kandel E, Schwartz J, Jessell T, eds. *Principles of Neural Science*. Norwalk, CT, Appleton & Lange, 1991, pp. 96–98.
17. Kuland DN. The injured athletes' pain. *Curr Concepts Pain* 1:3–10, 1983.
18. Margoles M. The pain chart: Spatial properties of pain. Pain measurement and assessment. In: Melzack R, ed. *Pain Measurement and Assessment*. New York, Raven Press, 1983, p. 52.
19. Mayer D. Price D, Rafii A. Antagonism of acupuncture analgesia in man by the narcotic antagonist naloxone. *Brain Res* 121:368–372, 1977.
20. Melzack R, Wall P. Pain mechanisms: A new theory. *Science* 150:971–979, 1965.
21. Melzack R. Concepts of pain measurement. In: Melzack R, ed. *Pain Measurement and Assessment*. New York, Raven Press, 1983.
22. Merskey H, Albe Fessard D, Bonica J. Pain terms: A list with definitions and notes on usage. *Pain* 6:249–252, 1979.
23. Pomeranz B, Paley D. Brain opiates at work in acupuncture. *New Scientist* 73:12–13, 1975.
24. Pomeranz B, Chiu D. Naloxone blockade of acupuncture analgesia: Enkephalin implicated. *Life Sci* 19:1757–1762, 1976.
25. Pomeranz B, Paley D. Electro-acupuncture hypoanalgesia is mediated by afferent impulses: An electrophysiological study in mice. *Exp Neurol* 66:398–402, 1979.
26. Previte J. *Human Physiology*. New York, McGraw-Hill, 1983.
27. Salar G, Job I, Mingringo S. Effects of transcutaneous electrotherapy on CSF beta-endorphin content in patients without pain problems. *Pain* 10:169–172, 1981.
28. Sjolund B, Eriksson M. Electroacupuncture and endogenous morphines. *Lancet* 2:1085, 1976.
29. Sjoland B, Eriksson M. Increased cerebrospinal fluid levels of endorphins after electro-acupuncture. *Acta Physiol Scand* 100:382–384, 1977.
30. Wen H, Ho W, Ling N. The influence of electroacupuncture on naloxone: Induces morphine withdrawal—Elevation of immunoassayable beta-endorphin activity in the brain but not in the blood. *Am J Clin Med* 7:237–240, 1979.
31. Willis W, Grossman R. *Medical Neurobiology*, 3rd ed. St. Louis, MO, Mosby, 1981.
32. Wolf S. Neurophysiologic mechanisms in pain modulation: Relevance to TENS. In: Manheimer J, Lampe G, eds. *Clinical Applications of TENS*. Philadelphia, PA, Davis, 1984, pp. 119–126.

CHAPTER 7

Impaired Patterns of Posture and Function

Gray Cook and Kyle Kiesel

O B J E C T I V E S

After completing this chapter, the therapist should be able to do the following:

- Understand the importance of identifying dysfunctional movement patterns.
- Understand the difference between *disability, dysfunction,* and *impairment* as defined.
- Describe why it is important to assess movement patterns in both the loaded and unloaded positions and how this information can be used to guide intervention.
- Discuss the relationship between automatic balance reactions and the fundamental movement patterns of *squatting, lunging,* and *forward bending.*
- Understand the importance of pain provocation during the examination process and appreciate that pain alters motor control.
- Use the information gained from the *Selective Functional Movement Assessment* (SFMA) to select key impairments to assess and design appropriate interventions to normalize dysfunctional movement.

Sahrmann,[20] Kendall,[12] and Janda[11] each have offered perspective regarding human posture and function. They have been instrumental in describing examination of structural as well as functional symmetry. Rehabilitation professionals have progressed from examination of isolated muscles to appreciation of complex movement patterns.

> *There are numerous ways in which slight subtleties in movement patterns contribute to specific muscle weaknesses. The relationship between altered movement patterns and specific muscle weaknesses requires that remediation addresses the changes to the movement pattern; the performance of strengthening exercises alone will not likely affect the timing and manner of recruitment during functional performance.*[20]
>
> Dr. Shirley Sahrmann

CONSIDERING PATTERNS OF MOVEMENT

The human system will migrate toward predictable patterns of movement in response to injury or in the presence of weakness, tightness, or structural abnormality. An isolated approach to either evaluation or treatment will not restore the whole of function.[2] Functional restoration requires a map of dysfunctional patterns and a working knowledge of functional patterns to gain clinical perspective and design an effective treatment strategy. It is the goal of the chapter to outline a system to capture the patterns of posture and function to assist in the deductive process and move toward functional diagnosis. To this end, functional assessment information and movements presently available will be used, but a system will be applied that provides an orderly and selective deductive process with respect to functional movement and its effect on provocation of symptoms.

Several influential contemporaries in physical therapy are guiding the profession toward an ever improving model of normal human function. Expanded knowledge of balance, posture, and functional movement patterns can actually create confusion if not utilized in a systematic manner. James Cyriax, known to many as the father of nonoperative orthopedic medicine was a medical doctor who studied the systematic diagnosis of soft tissue lesions.

> *It is well to remember that the object of the physical examination is to find the movement that elicits the pain of which the patient complains, rather than some*

other nebulous symptom of which he was previously unaware.

Only by sticking to a standard sequence will the physician be sure of leaving nothing out and only by leaving nothing out are true findings feasible. The physician arrives at a diagnosis not from the evidence furnished by one painful movement but by careful detection of a consistent pattern.[4]

Dr. James Cyriax

Dr. James Cyriax created a systematic method for classification of contractile tissue quality based on tension and irritability. This system was used to quickly classify a contractile problem into one of six categories. Once a general classification was assigned, a more detailed examination could be performed including special tests and measures providing increased levels of objectivity and quantifiability. His contribution gave us both a system of deduction and a clinician-friendly template for the development of future clinical tools. It is possible to utilize his template in the functional movement evaluation. Most clinicians agree that a quick and reliable perspective of the problem is paramount to decisions on treatment. Cyriax demonstrated how a small handful of qualitative tests could refine the examination so that more involved quantitative tests could confirm, refine, and rate the identified problem.

The Cyriax model[4] (see Table 7-1) is called selective tension testing. The model makes use of information related to the quality of passive and resisted movement behavior to refine the diagnosis to a soft tissue structure. A review of the Cyriax categories of resisted movements will help lay the framework for a *Selective Functional Movement Assessment*[3] (SFMA).

For the purposes of movement assessment, the first four categories can be utilized. The other two categories are not a part of the SFMA. Using the words functional, dysfunctional, painful, and nonpainful a collection of functional movements that fall into four categories can be described:

1. Functional and nonpainful (FN)
2. Functional and painful (FP)
3. Dysfunctional and nonpainful (DN)
4. Dysfunctional and painful (DP)

T A B L E   7 - 1

Cyriax's Findings for Resisted Movements

1. Strong and painless
2. Strong and painful
3. Weak and painless
4. Weak and painful
5. Painful on repetition
6. All the resisted movements hurt

Data from Cyriax JH, Cyriax PJ. *Illustrated Manual of Orthopedic Medicine*. London, Butterworth's, 1983.

T A B L E   7 - 2

The Functional Orthopedic Examination

- Case review
- History
- SFMA
- Clinical testing (Impairment-based testing)
  - ROM (goniometry)—active/passive
  - Muscle assessment—MMT, Trigger point assessment
  - Joint mobility/stability assessment—glides, end feels, stress testing
  - Palpation
  - Special testing, computer assisted testing, other objective measures
- Trial Intervention

For clarification, the term functional will describe any unlimited or unrestricted movement. Dysfunctional will describe movements that are limited or restricted in some way demonstrating a lack of mobility, stability, or symmetry within a given functional movement. Painful will denote a situation where the selective functional movement reproduces symptoms, increases symptoms, or brings about secondary symptoms that need to be noted. Each time a functional movement is graded in this manner, side notes may be used to help describe the nature and severity of the abnormality identified. This is not the complete evaluation, rather, only the first step in the functional orthopedic examination process which serves to focus the remaining portions of the examination and measures pertinent to the current functional needs of the patient (see Table 7-2).

A FUNCTIONAL PERSPECTIVE TO THE MUSCULOSKELETAL EVALUATION

The bedrock of manual musculoskeletal evaluation is the efficient and effective progression from qualitative screens and tests to quantitative measurement. This logical progression allows the qualitative tests and screens to control the direction of the evaluation while quantitative measurements define and quantify specific information relative to anatomical structure, state of utility, and severity of symptoms. Much like the compass points a traveler toward a destination, the qualitative assessment (SFMA) gives a direction to the problem-solving process used in the musculoskeletal evaluation. Once the traveler is headed in the right direction, then the quantitative data like time, speed, and distance, have relevance. If however the traveler was headed in the wrong direction, then this data is of little use reaching the desired destination. Often the novice clinician will collect a large amount of quantifiable data without ever identifying the nature of the fundamental problem, much like the traveler who might be making excellent time, but in the wrong direction. This fundamental problem is the purpose of this chapter. Information about movement must be collected at three levels:

(a) at the functional level, it reveals disability and is gained by history and observation of daily activities (ADLs); (b) at the fundamental level, it reveals dysfunction and is identified by SFMA; and (c) at the clinical level, we find impairments which are the result of specific clinical testing (quantifiable testing and measurement).

Disability is identified by taking a thorough history outlining how lifestyle activities have been altered or limited by the problem in question. Activities of daily living including work and recreation are included and together constitute functional movement. Disability can be measured with a variety of self-reported questionnaires ranging from generic measures of health such as the SF-36, to disease-specific tools such as the Oswestry low back pain disability questionnaire.[5] Easy to implement, patient-specific tools for disability measurement also exist, such as the patient specific functional scale.[18]

Dysfunction is identified by the clinician's ability to use fundamental movements to demonstrate limitations and/or provoke symptoms. Attempts to identify dysfunction involve an opportunity to relate fundamental movement patterns to the previously gained knowledge regarding functional movement. The SFMA is one way to attempt to identify dysfunction.

Impairments are abnormalities or limitations noted at particular segments of the body. Limitations are measured with respect to strength, range of motion (ROM), irritability, size, shape, and symmetry. This information is compared to normative data and compared bilaterally when appropriate.

THE SELECTIVE FUNCTIONAL MOVEMENT ASSESSMENT

The SFMA should first and foremost identify mobility and stability problems throughout the system. By doing this first, an efficient and effective treatment can be developed to improve or remedy the problem. The evaluation flow chart should start with a case review and history that notes those activities (dynamic) or postures (static) that provoke the symptoms associated with the patient's primary complaint with as much specificity as possible. If a patient reports that most of the symptoms are present with activity and movement, then a clinician is obligated to reproduce some of those movements in various patterns to draw conclusions about functional mobility and stability. However if the patient reports that symptoms are provoked in static postures, like extended standing or extended sitting, then it is equally important to look at the structures that are on stress in these static postures. The history will provide the first indicator for the clinician and direct them to the next series of questions as well as assessment maneuvers. Once it has been established that the patient has a primary complaint associated with a static or dynamic problem (or possibly both), the clinician must then look at functional movement in as many fundamental postures and positions as the patient's current level of symptoms will allow. This is done to create a feedback system to confirm the

functional diagnosis as well as to validate treatment practices. A quick assessment of the patient's available mobility in the upper and lower quarters and the spine is an effective starting point for a functional assessment. An example would be a patient who is asked to forward bend and perform a toe touch within his/her limits of pain, a backward bend, a squat, and perform single-leg stance and note the provocation of symptoms as well as limitations in movement or poor stability in movement. These movements can then be replicated in an unloaded position by having the patient perform a posterior rock in a quadruped, a prone press-up, bilateral knees-to-chest in supine, and single knee-to-chest in supine.

By performing these movements both in loaded and unloaded situations, the clinician can then deduce the interplay between the patient's available mobility and stability. If the first four movements in a loaded position are restricted or limited in some way and/or painful prior to the end ROM, a clue is provided regarding functional movement. However, if these movements when performed on the table (an unloaded situation), do not seem to provoke symptoms or have limitation, then it would seem logical that appropriate joint ROM and muscle flexibility exists to perform them. So, if movements are performed easily in an unloaded situation and *not* in a loaded one, then a stability problem may be the cause of why the patient cannot perform these movements while in a loaded condition. No specific diagnosis has been made but a general scenario is beginning to emerge about this patient. They have the requisite available biomechanical ability to go through the necessary ROM to perform the task, but the neurophysiological response needed for stabilization that creates dynamic alignment and postural support is not available when the functional movement is performed.

The second scenario is a patient who has limitation, restriction, and pain with the first four movements and a similar limitation, restriction, and pain is noted when on the table. This would indicate that in both loaded and unloaded situations the patient demonstrates consistent abnormal biomechanical behavior of one or more joints and therefore would require specific clinical assessment of each joint and muscle complex in question to identify the barriers that restrict movement and are responsible for the provocation of pain. Obviously, these four movements may not be appropriate for all patients but they were used as an example because for almost any situation the interplay between loaded and unloaded conditions can be created and assessed in most musculoskeletal clinical situations. It is important to try such maneuvers prior to specific segmental clinical assessment simply to direct the evaluation in an appropriate and constructive manner. The clinician should always start general and get specific. All too often, inexperienced clinicians are hindered in their ability to capture a functional diagnosis because they are so focused on special tests that serve to confirm a medical diagnosis that they fail to refine, qualify, and quantify the functional parameters of the problem at hand. The therapeutic plan of care needs to be focused on the functional representation with its symptoms and limitations to an activity that is a result and/or cause of the medical diagnosis. Therefore, starting with function and demonstrating through a history whether there is a static or dynamic problem and then whether there is a mobility or stability problem, the clinician can then use clinical tests, special tests, and specific musculoskeletal examination techniques to refine and deduce the structures responsible for the functional limitations.

Specific keys that the clinician should note during musculoskeletal examination when function and posture are initially the primary concern are faulty alignment, loss of spine stability, indicators of tonic holding and/or the absence of cocontraction, provocation of symptoms, functional asymmetries, significant restriction, and agreement or ambiguity between loaded and unloaded functional ROM.

It is important to design a SFMA with simple and fundamental movements so that the natural reactions and responses can be observed. These movements should be viewed loaded and unloaded whenever possible. Examining bilaterally for functional symmetry also assists with refining examination information.

FUNCTIONAL PATTERNS AND POSTURES

The hierarchy of the human balance strategy will often indicate to the clinician the breakdown in functional posture as well as functional movement. Automatic responses are a much more objective indicator of a patient's function than their ability to perform an organized task. As an example, the simple task of maintenance of balance will be described. If a patient is pushed gently from behind, the first and most primary balance strategy would be a quick response to the closed-chain dorsiflexion of the ankles with a concentric contraction of the plantar flexors. However, spine stability, hip stability, and alignment must also be maintained so that a hip hinge does not occur and the body remains upright, rigid, and taut so that the plantar flexors can right the body with a perfectly adjusted contraction. If a greater perturbation is performed with more stress in the form of a forward push, then the patient will use a hip hinge strategy and bend, not at the spine, but at the hip thereby creating an angle between the upper and lower body (controlled hip flexion). Once again, the spine maintains its stability while the extensors of the hip use their concentric force to right the body. This response occurs in the sagittal plane to put some of the body mass behind the foot and some of the body mass in front of the foot thus creating a delicate balance until the body can right itself. A more violent or exaggerated perturbation will bypass the first two strategies and create a step strategy that will significantly widen the base and check the momentum of the body falling forward thus creating balance and protection. These examples may seem like simple balance strategies but when examined using the functional microscope, a squat, a forward bend, and a lunge emerge. The hardest of these to visualize is of course

the squat. How does the dorsiflexion-plantar flexion response in the first balance strategy equate into squat mechanics? This is easily observed if the squat is already a part of your evaluation process. Those individuals who cannot squat without significant limitation or difficulty do not make use of the available closed-chain dorsiflexion at the ankle. Therefore, they start their squat strategy with knee flexion. This knee flexion action places them into a wall squat position where the mass of the body is behind the feet, not a functional squat where the mass of the body is balanced over the feet. Such a position requires significantly elevated activity of the quads and reduced activity of the plantar flexors and hip extensors as control mechanisms. In contrast, using the initially described ankle strategy, the individual who can squat fully starts the squatting process with dorsiflexion as well as core stabilization. They then progress by adding knee flexion and hip flexion and can easily go below parallel while maintaining alignment only because they initiated the squatting motion with trunk stabilization and closed-chain dorsiflexion, the two primary requisite factors in the ankle balance strategy.

Next are forward bending and the hip hinge. Forward bending, when done correctly, should start with a hip hinge (flexion) as well as spine stabilization. The spine should only flex in a segmental manner once all of the available ROM in hip flexion is taken up. Those individuals who have significantly limited forward bending ability or the lack of a toe touch will commonly initiate the motion of forward bending in the thoracic spine, not in the hip. Therefore, they have abandoned the requisite core stabilization and spine stability they need for the maneuver and are trying to perform flexion using segments that should be stable and rigid through the first part of the motion. They make it halfway through the motion using their spinal flexion but then, once the spine is flexed to its limits, they experience significant tension either in the spine or in the hamstrings, both of which serve to protect against any further flexion with faulty mechanics. The assumption that an individual has tight hamstrings with a limited forward bend is based on symptom complaint alone. The hamstrings will almost always be the structure on greatest tension in a forward bend whether it is done correctly or incorrectly simply because that is the muscle that needs to be "set" to pull an individual out of that position. As a side note, the clinical statement that a patient has limited hamstring flexibility should be based not on their subjective complaint but on a functional length assessment of the hamstring muscle group.[12]

Finally, the step strategy for balance is a lunge that involves symmetrical stance followed by single-leg stance, and finally an asymmetrical stance. Spine stability and core stability as well as a balance between the hip ad- and abductors need to exist prior to the step and single-leg stance. The patient also needs to have adequate preparatory muscle activation and stabilization prior to the landing on the opposite leg so that balance can be regained in the presence of a different stance.

When considering these three automatic balance reactions, it should become apparently obvious to the clinician that the squat, dead-lift (weight training version of the forward bend), and lunge are not simply exercises reserved for those wishing to return to sport or athletic competition. They are an integral part of rehabilitation technique with modification as necessary depending on the age and activity level of the patient. Squatting, dead-lifting, and lunging-type exercises are automatically deleted from many rehabilitation activities simply because they are not deemed age appropriate for an elderly individual. However without these three balance strategies, the elderly individual is at greater risk for a fall, dysfunction, or micro-trauma due to substitution and compensation. Instead of appropriately modifying these activities, they have often been deleted from programs at a significant cost to the rehabilitation process. Rehabilitation of the ambulatory human with an orthopedic musculoskeletal problem should follow the same continuum regardless the activity level. The activity level only dictates how far along the continuum the patient progresses.

PROVOCATION OF SYMPTOMS

Finally as we construct a SFMA, we must consider the provocation of symptoms. Unfortunately, a functional orthopedic assessment must involve provocation of symptoms. When the necessity of this fact is explained to the patient in a sensitive and logical manner, it is usually understood and accepted. During the interplay of posture tests to observe movement in transition and movement tests to observe responding posture, provocation of symptoms is usually a resulting fact. Producing these symptoms, however, creates the road map that the clinician will follow to a more specific diagnosis. Once symptoms have been provoked in a functional manner, it is necessary to work backward to more specific breakdowns of the component parts of that functional movement. Inconsistencies observed between symptom provocations that are not the result of symptom magnification may indicate a stability problem, whereas consistent limitation and provocation of symptoms may be indicative of a mobility problem. An example would be standing rotation. With a patient standing, feet planted side-by-side, the patient is asked to rotate as far as possible utilizing all of the segments of the entire body without moving the feet. They are instructed to look over the right shoulder and twist as far as possible and then look over the left shoulder (Fig. 7-29) and twist as far as possible, with the arms held relaxed at the sides. If a consistent production of pain in the left thoracic spine is noted upon standing left rotation, the same maneuver can be repeated in a seated position. The seated position, although similar in rotation, has many differences. Now the hips and lower extremities (LEs) are essentially removed from the movement, and an entirely different posture may be the result of this change in position. If nearly the same provocation of symptoms and limitation is noted at the same degree of left rotation, then an underlying mobility problem somewhere in the spine may be a causative

factor. This mobility problem could be the result of a trigger point, increased muscle tone, reduced muscle tone, joint restriction, faulty alignment, or some combination of the previous. If the same seated rotation does not produce consistent limitation and provocation of symptoms in the same direction at the same degree, then this may be an indicator toward a stability problem. On the other hand, changing position results in a different degree of postural alignment, muscle tone, proprioception, muscle activation, muscle inhibition, and reflex stabilization. The lower body component of this problem must be investigated. Once consistency or inconsistency is observed with respect to movement limitation or provocation of symptoms, continue to look for other instances that support this same behavior. Rule of thumb is *It is not only appropriate but also necessary to use provocation of symptoms in a functional musculoskeletal assessment within reason.* However, the clinician can always control the degree and frequency with which symptoms are provoked and he/she has ample time to prepare and instruct the patient on the maneuvers and the desired effect. Likewise it is important that the examiner pay close attention during the examination to avoid overprovocation. Once the patient starts an active rehabilitation program with manual therapy, therapeutic exercise progression, functional activity, and other treatment maneuvers, it is inappropriate to provoke symptoms (unless for reassessment). Many times, the same clinician who is unwilling to provoke symptoms on the evaluation will have no problem eliciting those same symptoms during the treatment and exercise progression. In the grand scheme of things, it is much more appropriate to provoke symptoms once and then have a strategic plan using therapeutic exercise to correct the situation than to avoid the issue altogether on evaluation only to have it reappear during every therapeutic exercise session.

PAIN AND MOTOR CONTROL

Ultimately, musculoskeletal pain is why the majority of patients seek physical therapy services. The contemporary understanding of pain has moved well beyond the traditional tissue damage model to include the cognitive and behavioral aspects of the entire pain experience.[15–17] It is well accepted that pain alters motor control, although the mechanism of these changes has not been clearly identified. Early work focused on changes in strength and endurance,[1,21] and current research has focused on how pain alters the timing of muscle activation and movement patterns.[6–10,14] The interaction between pain and motor control depends on the motor task.[13] Muscle pain has been shown to cause changes in coordination during functional movements. For example, Zedka et al.[22] studied the lumbar paraspinal muscle response in subjects during natural trunk flexion movements before and after induced pain. This study demonstrated an altered level of paraspinal muscle activity and a 10–40% decrease in ROM during the painful condition.

Interestingly, when hypertonic saline was injected unilaterally, electromyogram changes were seen bilaterally, suggesting that pain alters the entire movement strategy.

The pain adaptation model, as described by Lund et al.,[13] predicts that pain will alter muscle activity depending on a given muscle's role as an agonist or antagonist to control movement for protection. This model is considered the current best explanation of how pain alters motor control[13] and implies that changes are beyond that of previously believed peripheral reflexes. The central nervous system (CNS) response to painful stimuli is complex, but motor changes have consistently been demonstrated and seem to be influenced by higher centers consistent with a change in the transmission of the motor command. Richardson et al.[19] summarize the evidence that pain alters motor control at higher levels of the CNS than previously thought:

Consistent with the identification of changes in motor planning, there is compelling evidence that pain has strong effects at the supraspinal level. Both short-and long-term changes are thought to occur with pain in the activity of the supraspinal structures including the

cortex. One area that has been consistently found to be affected is the anterior cingulated cortex which has long thought to be important in motor responses with its direct projections to motor and supplementary motor areas.

Because evidence suggests that pain alters motor control, assessment of functional movement patterns must take this into consideration. Pain attenuated movement patterns may lead to protective movement and fear of movement, resulting in clinically observed impairments such as decreased ROM, muscle length changes, declines in strength, and ultimately contribute to the resultant disability.

Pain free functional movement for participation in occupation and lifestyle activities is desirable. Many components comprise pain free functional movement. Impairments of each component could potentially alter functional movement resulting in or as a consequence of pain. We identify functional movement patterns through the SFMA[3] and describe key points of assessment for the clinical application. Traditional muscle length, strength, and special tests should be used to help the clinician identify the impairments which are associated with

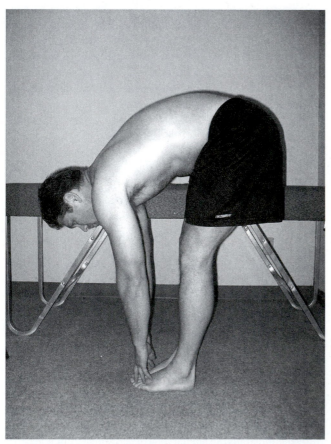

FIGURE 7-1

Forward bending (toe touch maneuver).

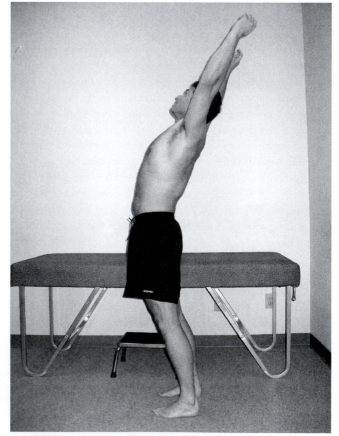

FIGURE 7-2

Backward bending (overhead reaching with spine extension).

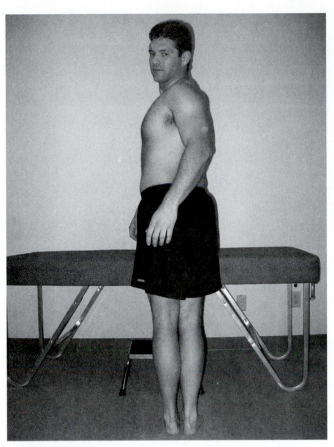

FIGURE 7 - 3

Standing rotation right (head, shoulder, and pelvis motion).

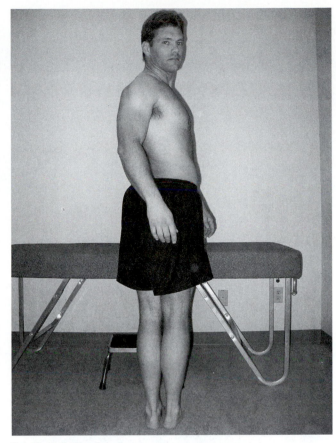

FIGURE 7 - 4

Standing rotation left (head, shoulder, and pelvis motion).

dysfunctional movement. It is important to note that this approach is not a substitute for existing examination and intervention, but a model to efficiently integrate the concepts of posture, muscle balance, and the fundamental patterns of the movement system into contemporary physical therapy practice. It is assumed that the clinician applying this model adheres to accepted indication for manual therapy and therapeutic exercise intervention and has ruled out CNS lesion or a progressing nerve root compression.

What follows is a description of suggested elements of the SFMA, first in seven general categories of functional movement and later in greater detail to better describe the sequence and additional maneuvers contained within the seven general categories of functional movement.

The Selective Functional Movement Assessment

- Forward bending (toe touch maneuver) (Fig. 7-1)
- Backward bending (overhead reaching with spine extension) (Fig. 7-2)
- Standing rotation (head, shoulder, and pelvis rotation) (Figs. 7-3 and 7-4)

- Single leg stance (SLS) (postural muscle response) (Figs. 7-5 and 7-6)
- Deep squatting (heels flat with shoulders flexed) (Fig. 7-7)
- Shoulder pattern extremes (two patterns and two impingement signs) (Figs. 7-8 to 7-11)
- Cervical spine pattern extremes (c-spine movements) (Figs. 7-12 to 7-14)

The first five movements look at a combination of upper quarter, lower quarter, and trunk movements, while the shoulder and cervical assessments look primarily at upper quarter movement quality. Each should be graded with a notation of FN, FP, DN, or DP. All responses other than FN should be broken down to help refine the movement information and direct the clinical testing that will follow. If a movement patter receives FN as a score, move to the next pattern. There is no need for a functional breakdown; however, you may want to re-visit the region on the musculoskeletal examination to further clear the area. When a breakdown is performed, look for consistencies and inconsistencies as well as levels of dysfunction for each movement deduction compared to the original movement pattern and other deductive movements of the same pattern.

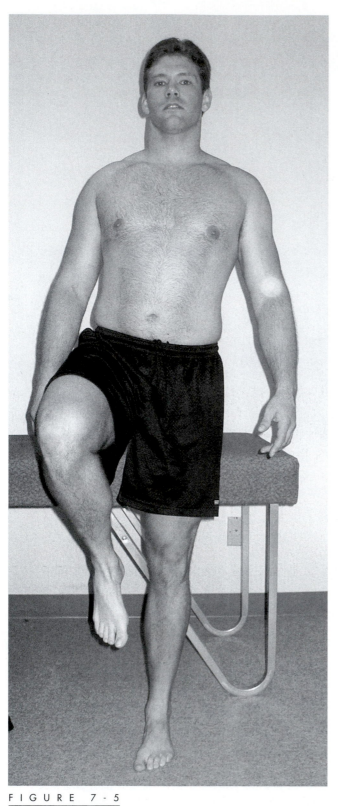

Single limb stance right.

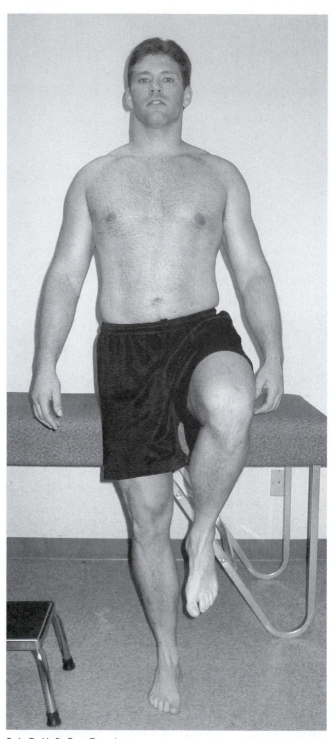

F I G U R E   7 - 6

Single limb stance left.

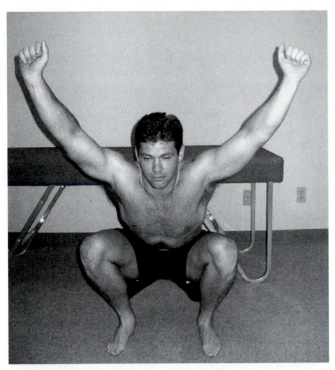

FIGURE 7-7

Deep squatting (heels flat and shoulders flexed).

SELECTIVE FUNCTIONAL MOVEMENT ASSESSMENT BREAKDOWN

Assign each breakdown a grade noting similarities and differences form the original functional movement.

Forward Bending

- Forward bending (Fig. 7-1)
- Left leg on stool, right leg down with right toe touch (Fig. 7-15)
- Repeat, right leg on stool with left leg down with left toe touch
  - This is done to reduce the problem to a symmetrical or asymmetrical dysfunction or pain provocation maneuver.
- Sit and reach (long sitting) (Fig. 7-16)
  - This is done to look at the forward bend maneuver in a nonweight-bearing position.
- Supine active straight leg raise left (Fig. 7-17)
- Supine active straight leg raise right
- Supine passive straight leg raise left (Fig. 7-18)
- Supine passive straight leg raise right
  - This is done to reduce the problem to a symmetrical or asymmetrical dysfunction or pain provocation maneuver in a nonweight-bearing position actively and passively.

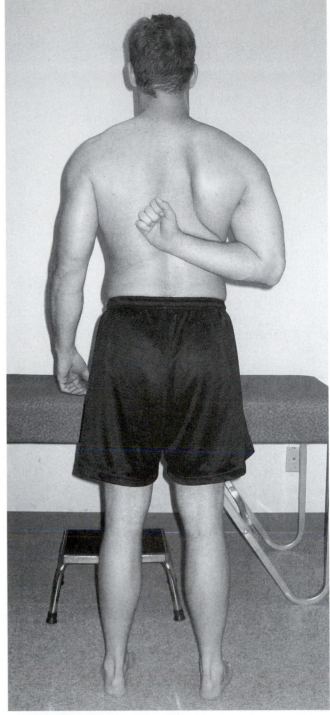

FIGURE 7-8

Shoulder pattern extreme 1 (back scratch).

Backward Bending

- Backward bending with shoulders in maximal flexion (Fig. 7-2)
- Backward bending with left leg on stool (Fig. 7-19)
- Backward bending with right leg on stool

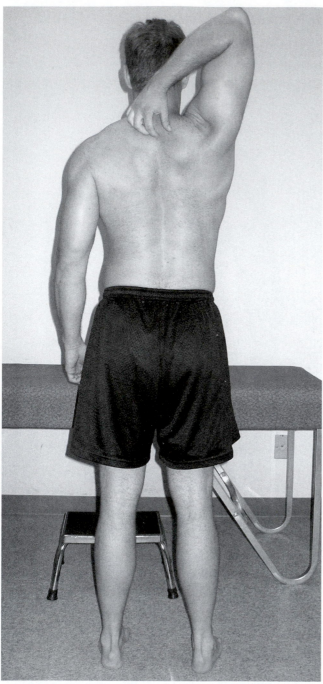

Shoulder pattern extreme 2 (hand behind head).

- This is done to reduce the problem to a symmetrical or asymmetrical dysfunction or pain provocation maneuver.
- Standing hip extension left (Fig. 7-20)
- Standing hip extension right
  - This is done to reduce the problem to a symmetrical or asymmetrical dysfunction or pain provocation maneuver and looks at extension from the bottom up.

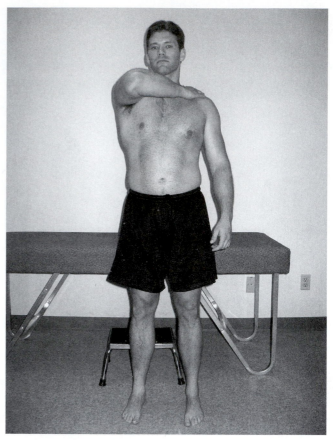

Impingement sign 1 (active horizontal adduction).

- Backward bending with hands on hips (Fig. 7-21)
  - This is done to remove the shoulder joints and musculature from the backward bend maneuver.
- Prone press up (Fig. 7-22)
  - This is done to look at the backward bend maneuver in a nonweight-bearing position.
- Prone active straight leg extension left (Fig. 7-23)
- Prone active straight leg extension right
- Prone passive straight leg extension left (Fig. 7-24)
- Prone passive straight leg extension right
  - This is done to reduce the problem to a symmetrical or asymmetrical dysfunction or pain provocation maneuver in a nonweight-bearing position actively and passively.
- Supine Thomas test left (Fig. 7-25)
- Supine Thomas test right
  - This is done to evaluate the length of the rectus femoris and the hip flexor group on hip extension.
- Supine FABER (simultaneous hip flexon, abduction, and external rotation) test left (Fig. 7-26)
- Supine FABER test right
  - This is done to evaluate the effect of hip flexion, abduction, and external rotation overpressure on the hip and the lumbar spine.

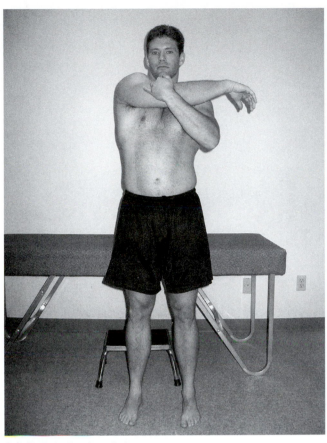

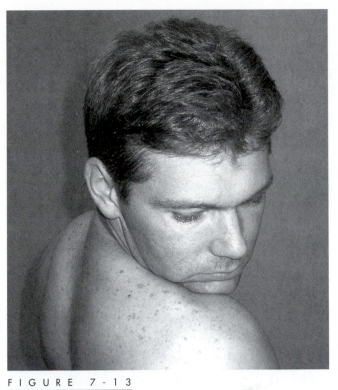

F I G U R E   7 - 1 3

Cervical spine pattern extreme 2 (right rotation).

F I G U R E   7 - 1 1

Impingement sign 2 (passive horizontal adduction).

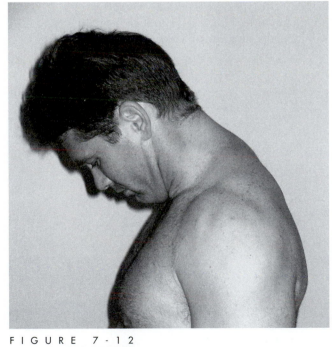

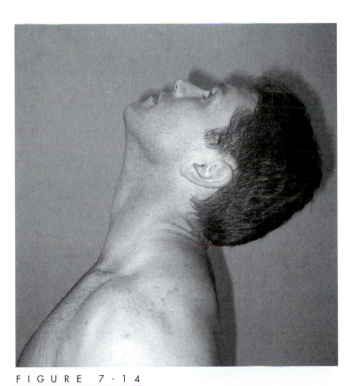

F I G U R E   7 - 1 4

Cervical spine pattern extreme 3 (extension).

F I G U R E   7 - 1 2

Cervical spine pattern extreme 1 (flexion).

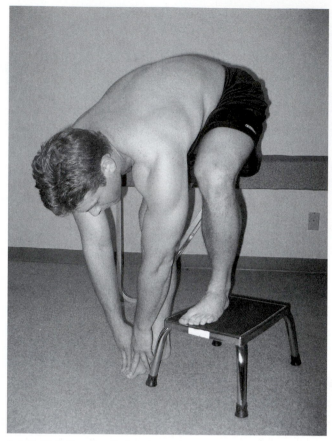

FIGURE 7-15

Left leg on stool, right leg down, with right toe touch.

- Supine latissimus dorsi test left (Fig. 7-27)
- Supine latissimus dorsi test right
  - This is done to evaluate the length of the latissimus dorsi musculature.

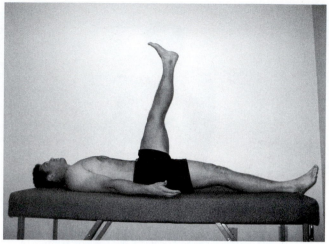

FIGURE 7-17

Supine active straight leg, left.

Standing Rotation

- Standing rotation (Figs. 7-3 and 7-4)
- Standing rotation with the left leg on a stool (Fig. 7-28; **A**, rotation to the left; rotation to the right)
- Standing rotation with the right leg on a stool
  - This is done to reduce the problem to a symmetrical or asymmetrical dysfunction or pain provocation maneuver.
- Seated rotation (Fig. 7-29; **A**, rotation to the left; **B**, rotation to the right)
  - This is done to remove the LE effect on spinal rotation.
- Seated active medial and lateral hip rotation left (Fig. 7-30; **A**, medial rotation; **B**, lateral rotation)
- Seated active medial and lateral hip rotation right
- Seated passive medial and lateral hip rotation right (Fig. 7-31; **A**, medial rotation; **B**, lateral rotation)

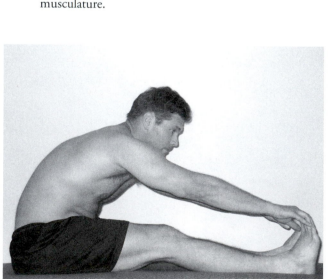

FIGURE 7-16

Sit and reach (long sitting).

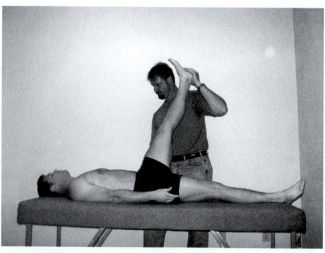

FIGURE 7-18

Supine passive straight leg, left.

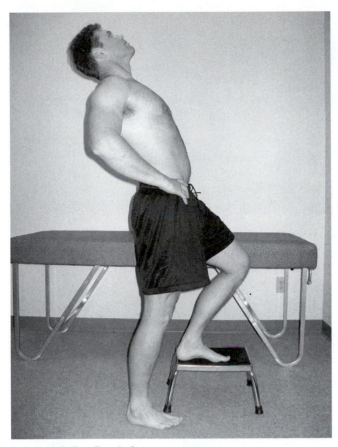

F I G U R E   7 - 1 9

Backward bending with left leg on stool.

- Seated passive medial and lateral hip rotation left
  - This is done to assess the dysfunction or pain provocation maneuver in a nonweight-bearing position actively and passively.
- Seated active medial and lateral tibial rotation left (Fig. 7-32; **A**, medial rotation; **B**, lateral rotation)
- Seated active medial and lateral tibial rotation right
- Seated passive medial and lateral tibial rotation left (Fig. 7-33; **A**, medial rotation; **B**, lateral rotation)
- Seated passive medial and lateral tibial rotation right
  - This is done to assess the dysfunction or pain provocation maneuver in a nonweight-bearing position actively and passively.
- Prone active medial and lateral hip rotation left (Fig. 7-34; **A**, medial rotation; **B**, lateral rotation)
- Prone active medial and lateral hip rotation right
- Prone passive medial lateral hip rotation left (Fig. 7-35; **A**, medial rotation; **B**, lateral rotation)
- Prone passive medial and lateral rotation right
  - This is done to assess the dysfunction or pain provocation maneuver in a nonweight-bearing position actively and passively with hip extended.
- Prone to supine rolling left (Fig. 7-36; **A**, using upper extremities [UEs]; **B**, using LEs)

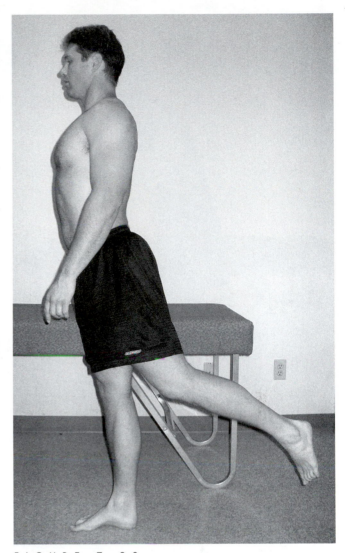

F I G U R E   7 - 2 0

Standing hip extension, left.

- Prone to supine rolling right
- Supine to prone rolling left (Fig. 7-37; **A**, using UEs; **B**, using LEs)
- Supine to prone rolling right
  - When mobility is within functional limits stability can be observed by comparison of left and right rolling. The patient can also be cued to only use the UE or LE for further deduction of movement.
- Quadruped diagonal dynamic stability three repetitions left arm and right leg. Then right arm and left leg (Fig. 7-38)
- Quadruped unilateral dynamic stability three repetitions left arm and left leg. Then right arm and right leg (Fig. 7-39; **A**, both left extremities; **B**, both right extremities)
  - A higher level of stability can be assessed by observing dynamic stability in these two movement patterns with right and left comparisons.

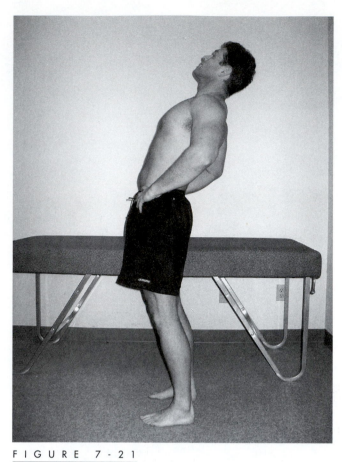

FIGURE 7-21

Backward bending with hands on hips.

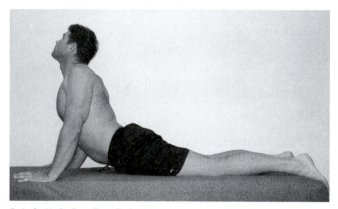

FIGURE 7-22

Prone press up.

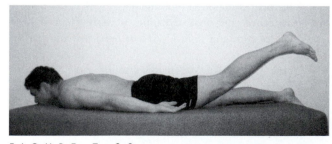

FIGURE 7-23

Prone active straight leg extension, left.

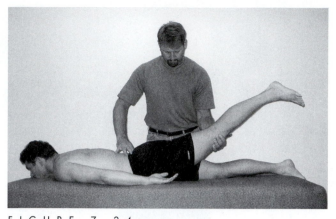

FIGURE 7-24

Prone passive straight leg extension, left.

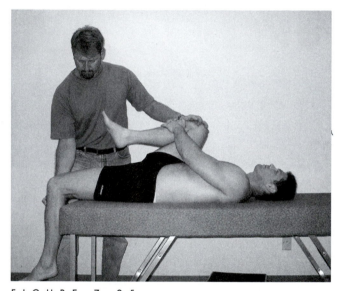

FIGURE 7-25

Supine Thomas test, left.

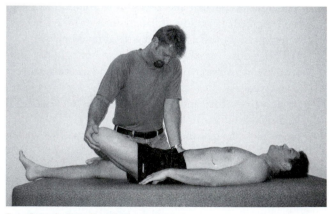

FIGURE 7-26

Supine FABER test, left.

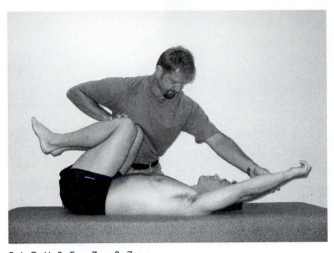

FIGURE 7-27

Supine latissimus dorsi test, left.

Single Leg Stance

- SLS left/right
- Static SLS—bring heel of the left foot to the level of the right knee and hold for 5 seconds (Fig. 7-5)

- Static SLS—bring heel of the right foot to the level of the left knee and hold for 5 seconds (Fig. 7-6)
- Static SLS—extend left hip, and knee and plantar flex ankle and hold for 5 seconds (Fig. 7-40)
- Static SLS—extend right hip, and knee and plantar flex ankle and hold for 5 seconds
  - This is done to reduce the problem to a static balance symmetrical or asymmetrical dysfunction or pain provocation maneuver.
- Dynamic SLS—five swings in the previous flexion/extension pattern with the left leg (Fig. 7-41)
- Dynamic SLS—five swings in the previous flexion/extension pattern with the right leg
  - This is done to reduce the problem to a dynamic balance symmetrical or asymmetrical dysfunction or pain provocation maneuver.

Deep Squatting

- Deep squatting heels flat and shoulders flexed (Fig. 7-7)
  - This is the most extreme squat possible. The upper body requires the spine to extend and the lower body requires the spine to flex. The move requires full mobility of the upper and lower body and dynamic stability of the spine.

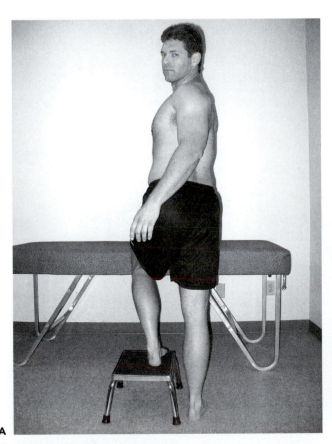
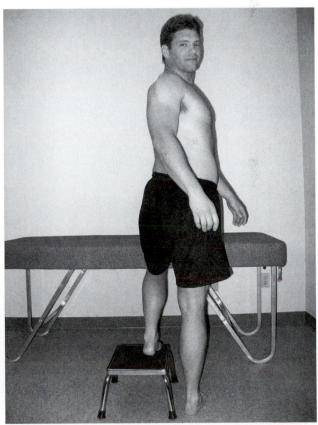

A   B

FIGURE 7-28

A, Standing rotation with left leg on stool, rotation to the left. **B**, Standing rotation with left leg on stool, rotation to the right.

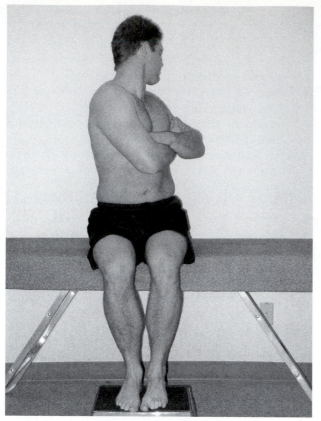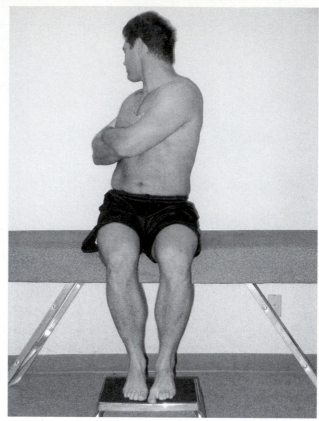

A

B

FIGURE 7-29

A, Seated rotation, left. **B**, Seated rotation, right.

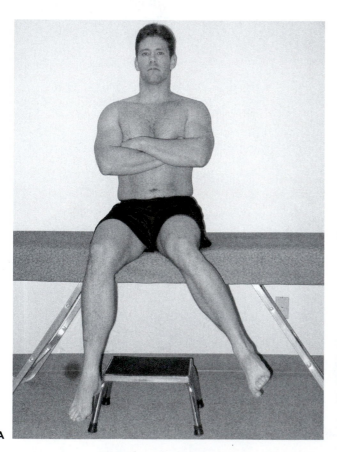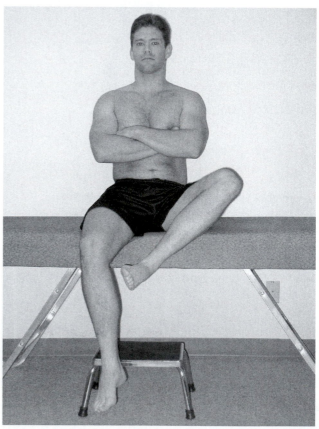

A

B

FIGURE 7-30

A, Seated active hip rotation, left medial. **B**, Seated active hip rotation, left lateral.

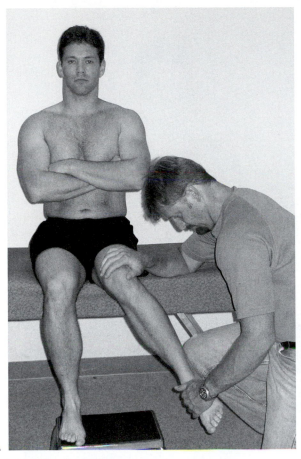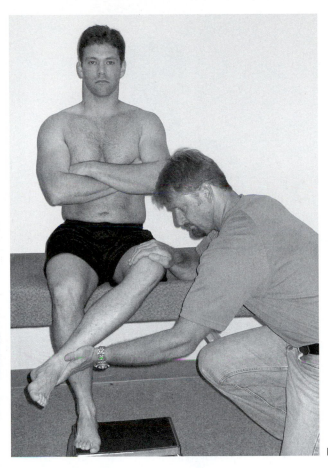

FIGURE 7-31

A, Seated passive hip rotation, left medical. **B**, Seated passive hip rotation, left lateral.

- Deep squat with shoulders at 90° forward flexed (Fig. 7-42)
  - This position lowers the difficulty by moving the hands into a forward position causing an anterior weight shift. It removes the upper body component and reduces the level of dynamic stability needed to perform the squat.
- Deep squat with hand hold (Fig. 7-43)
  - This position allows the evaluator to look at the mobility of the lower body in a squat position without the requirement of dynamic stability.
- Closed-chain dorsiflexion on a stool left and right (Fig. 7-44 depicts left)
- Supine knees to chest tuck maneuver (Fig. 7-45)
- Quadruped posterior rock maneuver (Fig. 7-46)

Shoulder Pattern Extremes

- Movement one (*back scratch*). Left and right (Fig. 7-8)
  - Shoulder—extension/med. rot./add.
  - Elbow—flexion/supination
  - Wrist—flexion/ulnar dev
- Movement two (*back patting*). Left and right (Fig. 7-9)
  - Shoulder—flex./lat. rot./abd.
  - Elbow—extension/sup. flexion./sup.

- Wrist—extension/rad. dev.
- Movement three (*impingement/laxity*). Left and right (Fig. 7-10)
  - Combines flexion with med. rot.
- Movement four (impingement/sprain/degenerative joint disease). Left and right (Fig. 7-11)
  - Acromioclavicular (AC) joint compression test using active followed by passive horizontal adduction

Cervical Spine Pattern Extremes

- Chin to chest (Fig. 7-12)
  - This move indicates a reduced capacity of the short neck flexors and may also indicate reduced occipitalatlanto (OA) mobility.
- Chin to shoulder left and right (Fig. 7-13)
  - This move is a combined pattern that incorporates side-bending and rotation and scapular elevation. Do not allow protraction.
- Face parallel to ceiling (Fig. 7-14)
  - This move looks at the available c-spine extension.
- Supine c-spine flexion with C1–C2 rotation left and right (Fig. 7-47 depicts rotation to the left)

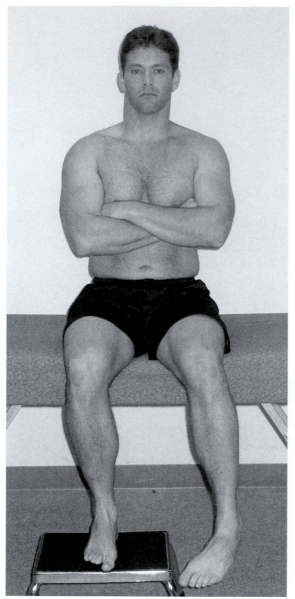
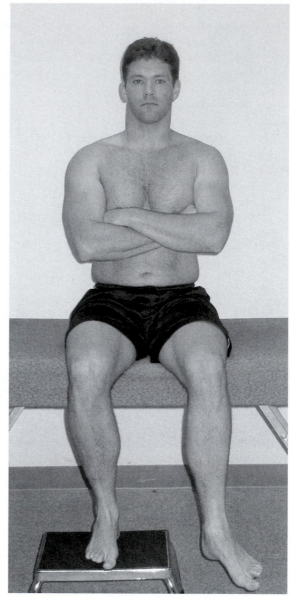

A   **B**

FIGURE   7-32

A, Seated active tibial rotation, left medial. **B**, Seated active tibial rotation, left lateral.

- This move (with the help of the tester) isolates the atlantoaxial (AA) mobility.
- If movement is limited or painful, change the scapular position (retraction, protraction, depression, elevation) and look for consistent or inconsistent responses to the shoulder position changes.

SUMMARY

Pain free functional movement for participation in occupation and lifestyle activities is desirable. Many components comprise pain free functional movement including adequate posture, ROM, muscle performance, motor control, and balance reactions. Impairments of each component could potentially alter functional movement resulting in or as a consequence of pain. In this chapter, we have identified key functional movement patterns through the SFMA[3] and described the critical points of assessment needed for clinical application. Traditional muscle length, strength, and special tests should be used to help the clinician identify the impairments associated with dysfunctional movement. It is important to note that this approach is not a substitute for existing examination and intervention, but a model to efficiently integrate the concepts of posture, muscle balance, and the fundamental patterns of the movement system into contemporary physical therapy practice.

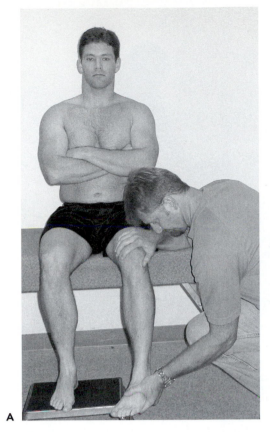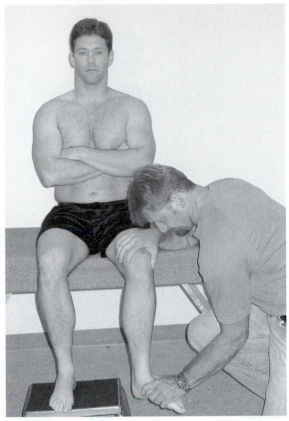

FIGURE 7-33

A, Seated passive tibial rotation, left medial. **B**, Seated passive tibial rotation, left lateral.

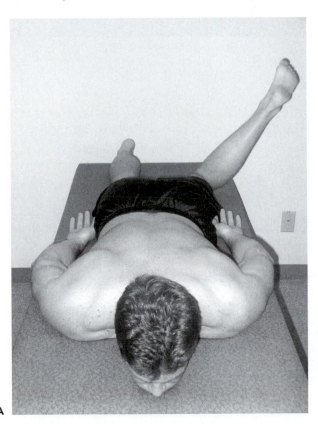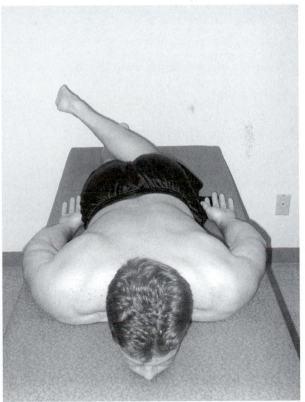

FIGURE 7-34

A, Prone passive hip rotation, left medial. **B**, Prone passive hip rotation, left lateral.

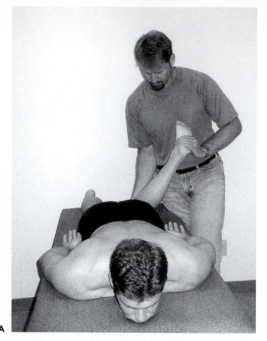
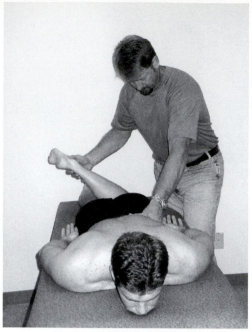

FIGURE 7-35

A, Prone active hip rotation, left medial. **B**, Prone active hip rotation, left lateral.

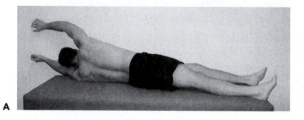
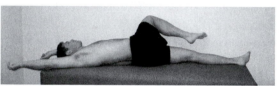

FIGURE 7-36

A, Prone to supine rolling left, using UEs. **B**, Prone to supine rolling left, using LEs.

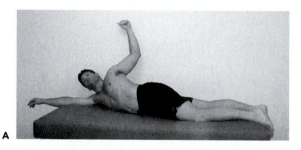
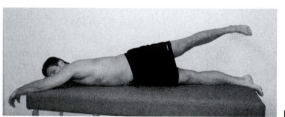

FIGURE 7-37

A, Supine to prone rolling left, using UEs. **B**, Supine to prone rolling left, using LEs.

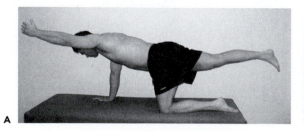
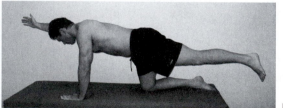

FIGURE 7-38

A, Quadruped diagonal dynamic stability (left UE and right LE). **B**, Quadruped diagonal dynamic stability (right UE and left LE).

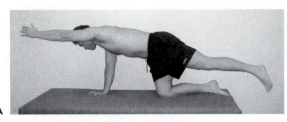
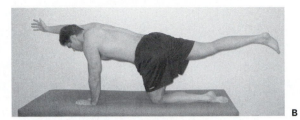

FIGURE 7-39

A, Quadruped unilateral dynamic stability left (left UE and left LE). **B**, Quadruped unilateral dynamic stability right (right UE and right LE).

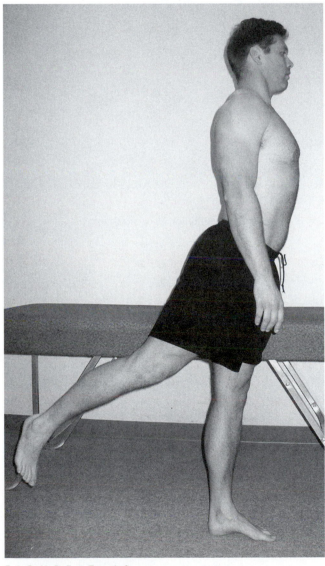

FIGURE 7-40

Static single limb stance left (right hip and knee extension and ankle plantarflexion).

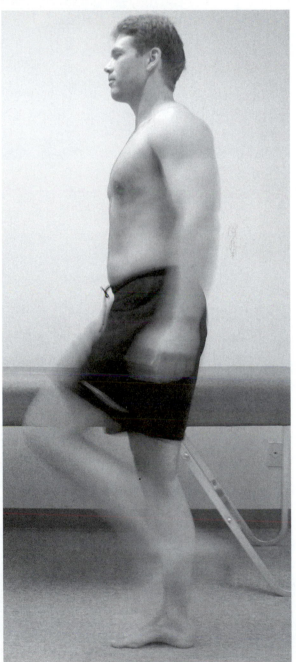

FIGURE 7-41

Dynamic single limb stance (swing through previous flexion and extension patterns).

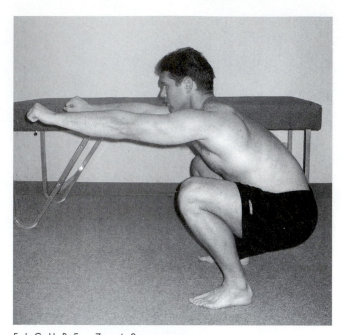

F I G U R E   7 - 4 2

Deep squat with shoulders at 90° flexion.

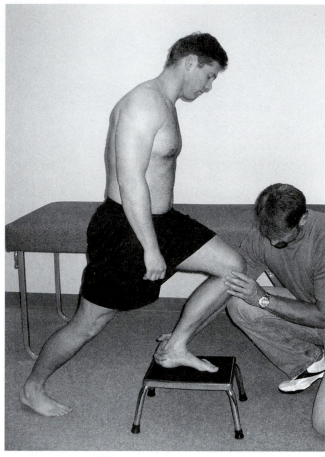

F I G U R E   7 - 4 4

Closed-chain dorsiflexion on a stool, left.

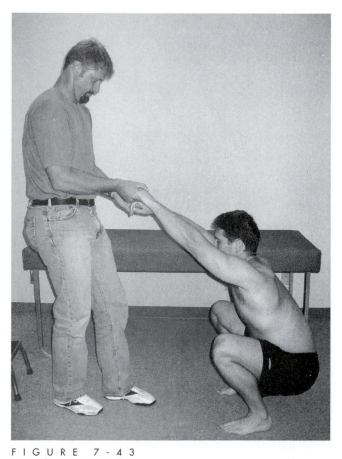

F I G U R E   7 - 4 3

Deep squat with hand hold.

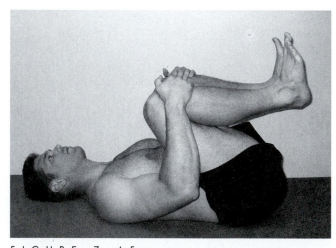

F I G U R E   7 - 4 5

Supine knees to chest, tuck maneuver.

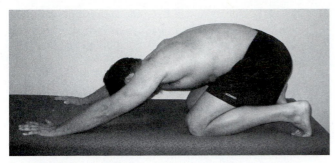

FIGURE 7-46

Quadruped posterior rock maneuver.

- Identifying dysfunctional movement patterns is possible and is important for optimizing human movement.
- Impairments contribute to dysfunctional movement patterns, and over time, dysfunctional movement patterns can progress toward disability.
- It is important to assess movement patterns in both loaded and unloaded positions and draw conclusions about contributory factors based on reproduction of symptoms (Cyriax scheme).
- Information from the functional movement screen must be used to guide intervention choices.

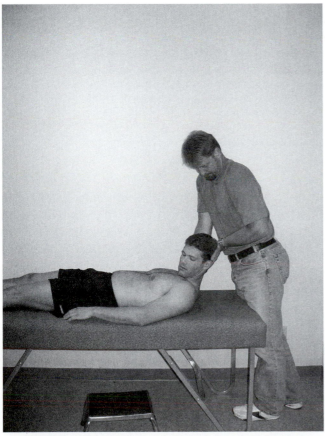

FIGURE 7-47

Supine cervical spine flexion with C1–C2 rotation left.

- Important fundamental movement patterns include *squatting, lunging,* and *forward bending.*
- Pain alters motor control.
- Pain provocation during the examination process, although not optimal, can be important in identification of dysfunctional movement patterns.
- The information gained from the SFMA can be used to select key impairments to examine in greater detail.
- The information from the SFMA can be used to design efficient, appropriate interventions to normalize dysfunctional movement.

REFERENCES

1. Cassisi JE, Robinson ME, O'Conner P, MacMillan M. Trunk strength and lumbar paraspinal muscle activity during isometric exercise in chronic low-back pain patients and controls. *Spine* 18(2):245–251, 1993.
2. Cook EG, Voight M. Essentials of functional exercise. In: Prentice W, ed. *Techniques in Musculoskeletal Rehabilitation.* Chicago, IL, McGraw-Hill, 2001.
3. Cook EG, Kiesel KB. Selective functional movement assessment. *Physical Therapy Course Manual,* Danville, VA, 2004. www.Functionalmovement.com.
4. Cyriax JH, Cyriax PJ. *Illustrated Manual of Orthopedic Medicine.* London, Butterworths, 1983.
5. Fairbanks JC, Couper J, Davies JB. The Oswestry low back pain disability questionnaire. *Physiotherapy* 66:271–273, 1980.
6. Ferreira PH, Ferreira ML, Hodges PW. Changes in recruitment of the abdominal muscles in people with low back pain: Ultrasound measurement of muscle activity. *Spine* 29(22):2560–2566, 2004.
7. Hodges PW. Changes in motor planning of feedforward postural responses of the trunk muscles in low back pain. *Exp Brain Res,* 141(2):261–266, 2001.
8. Hodges PW, Moseley GL, Gabrielsson A, Gandevia SC. Experimental muscle pain changes feedforward postural responses of the trunk muscles. *Exp Brain Res* 151(2):262–2671, 2003.
9. Hodges PW, Richardson CA. Altered trunk muscle recruitment in people with low back pain with upper limb movement at different speeds. *Arch Phys Med Rehabil* 80(9):1005–1012, 1999.
10. Hodges PW, Richardson CA. Delayed postural contraction of transversus abdominis in low back pain associated with movement of the lower limb. *J Spinal Disord* 11(1):46–56, 1998.
11. Janda V, ed. *Movement Patterns in the Pelvic and Hip Region with Special Reference to Pathogenisis of Vertebrogenic Disturbances.* Prague Czechoslovakia, Charles University, 1964.
12. Kendall FP, McCreary EK. *Muscle Testing and Function.* Baltimore, Lippincott Williams & Wilkins, 2004.

13. Lund JP, Donga R, Widmer CG, Stohler CS. The pain-adaptation model: A discussion of the relationship between chronic musculoskeletal pain and motor activity. *Can J Physiol Pharmacol* 69(5):683–694, 1991.

14. Mok NW, Brauer SG, Hodges PW. Hip strategy for balance control in quiet standing is reduced in people with low back pain. *Spine* 29(6):E107–E112, 2004.

15. Moseley GL. A pain neuromatrix approach to patients with chronic pain. *Man Ther* 8(3):130–140, 2003.

16. Moseley GL, Brhyn L, Ilowiecki M, Solstad K, Hodges PW. The threat of predictable and unpredictable pain: differential effects on central nervous system processing? *Aust J Physiother* 49(4):263–267, 2003.

17. Moseley GL, Nicholas MK, Hodges PW. Pain differs from non-painful attention-demanding or stressful tasks in its effect on postural control patterns of trunk muscles. *Exp Brain Res*, 154(1):64–71, 2004.

18. Resnik L, Dobrzykowski E. Guide to outcomes measurement for patients with low back pain syndromes. *J Orthop Sports Phys Ther* 33(6):307–316, 2003; discussion 317–318.

19. Richardson C, Hodges PW, Hides J. Therapeutic exercise for lumbopelvic stabilization. *A Motor Control Approach for the Treatment and Prevention of Low Back Pain*. Edinburgh, Churchill Livingstone, 2004.

20. Sahrmann SA, ed. *Diagnosis and Treatment of Movement Impairment Syndromes*. St. Louis, MO, Mosby, 2002.

21. Shirado O, Kaneda K, Ito T. Trunk-muscle strength during concentric and eccentric contraction: A comparison between healthy subjects and patients with chronic low-back pain. *J Spinal Disord* 5(2):175–182, 1992.

22. Zedka M, Prochazka A, Knight B, Gillard D, Gauthier M. Voluntary and reflex control of human back muscles during induced pain. *J Physiol* 520(Pt 2):591–604, 1999.

Impaired Muscle Performance: Regaining Muscular Strength and Endurance

William E. Prentice

O B J E C T I V E S

After completing this chapter, the therapist should be able to do the following:

- Define muscular strength, endurance, and power and discuss their importance in a program of rehabilitation following injury.
- Discuss the anatomy and physiology of skeletal muscle.
- Discuss the physiology of strength development and factors that determine strength.
- Describe specific methods for improving muscular strength.
- Differentiate between muscle strength and muscle endurance.
- Discuss differences between males and females in terms of strength development.

Following all musculoskeletal injuries, there will be some degree of impairment in muscular strength and endurance. For the therapist supervising a rehabilitation program, regaining, and in many instances improving, levels of strength and endurance are critical for discharging and returning the patient to a functional level following injury.

By definition, *muscular strength* is the ability of a muscle to generate force against some resistance. Maintenance of at least a normal level of strength in a given muscle or muscle group is important for normal healthy living. Muscle weakness or imbalance can result in abnormal movement or gait and can impair normal functional movement. Resistance training plays a critical role in injury rehabilitation.

Muscular strength is closely associated with muscular endurance. *Muscular endurance* is the ability to perform repetitive muscular contractions against some resistance for an extended period of time. As we will see later, as muscular strength increases, there tends to be a corresponding increase in endurance. For the average person in the population, developing muscular endurance is likely more important than developing muscular strength because muscular endurance is probably more critical in carrying out the everyday activities of living. This statement becomes increasingly true with age.

TYPES OF SKELETAL MUSCLE CONTRACTION

Skeletal muscle is capable of three different types of contraction: *isometric contraction*, *concentric contraction*, and *eccentric contraction*. An isometric contraction occurs when the muscle contracts to produce tension but there is no change in muscle length. Considerable force can be generated against some immovable resistance even though no movement occurs. In a concentric contraction the muscle shortens in length while tension increases to overcome or move some resistance. In an eccentric contraction, the resistance is greater than the muscular force being produced, and the muscle lengthens while producing tension. Concentric and eccentric contractions are considered dynamic movements.[56]

Recently, *econcentric contraction*, which combines both a controlled concentric and a concurrent eccentric contraction of the same muscle over two separate joints, has been introduced.[19,30] An econcentric contraction is possible only in muscles that cross at least two joints. An example of an econcentric contraction would be a prone, open-kinetic-chain hamstring curl. The hamstrings contract concentrically to flex the knee, while the hip tends to flex eccentrically, lengthening the hamstring. Rehabilitation exercises have traditionally concentrated on strengthening isolated single-joint motions, despite the fact that the same muscle is functioning at a second joint simultaneously. Therefore it has been recommended that the strengthening program includes exercises that strengthen the muscle in the manner in which it contracts functionally. Traditional strength-training programs have been designed to develop strength in individual muscles, in a single plane of motion. However, because all muscles function concentrically, eccentrically, and isometrically in three planes of motion, a strengthening program should be multiplanar, concentrating on all three types of contraction.[15]

FACTORS THAT DETERMINE LEVELS OF MUSCULAR STRENGTH, ENDURANCE, AND POWER

Size of the Muscle

Muscular strength is proportional to the cross-sectional diameter of the muscle fibers. The greater the cross-sectional diameter or the bigger a particular muscle, the stronger it is, and thus the more force it is capable of generating. The size of a muscle tends to increase in cross-sectional diameter with resistance training. This increase in muscle size is referred to as *hypertrophy*.[42] A decrease in the size of a muscle is referred to as *atrophy*.

Number of Muscle Fibers

Strength is a function of the number and diameter of muscle fibers composing a given muscle. The number of fibers is an inherited characteristic; thus a person with a large number of muscle fibers to begin with has the potential to hypertrophy to a much greater degree than does someone with relatively few fibers.[38]

Neuromuscular Efficiency

Strength is also directly related to the efficiency of the nueromuscular system and the function of the motor unit in producing muscular force.[46] As will be indicated later in this chapter, initial increases in strength during the first 8–10 weeks of a resistance training program can be attributed primarily to increased neuromuscular efficiency.[59] Resistance training will increase neuromuscular efficiency in three ways: there is an increase in the number of motor units being recruited, in the firing rate of each motor unit, and in the synchronization of motor unit firing.[7]

Biomechanical Considerations

Strength in a given muscle is determined not only by the physical properties of the muscle but also by biomechanical factors that dictate how much force can be generated through a system of levers to an external object.[31,38,63]

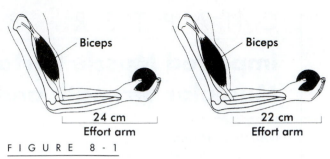

FIGURE 8-1

The position of attachment of the muscle tendon on the lever arm can affect the ability of that muscle to generate force. B should be able to generate greater force than A because the tendon attachment on the lever arm is closer to the resistance.

POSITION OF TENDON ATTACHMENT

If we think of the elbow joint as one of these lever systems, we would have the biceps muscle producing flexion of this joint (Fig. 8-1). The position of attachment of the biceps muscle on the forearm will largely determine how much force this muscle is capable of generating. If there are two athletes, A and B, and A has a biceps attachment that is closer to the fulcrum (the elbow joint) than B's, then A must produce a greater effort with the biceps muscle to hold the weight at a ring angle, because the length of the effort arm will be greater than that for B.

LENGTH–TENSION RELATIONSHIP

The length of a muscle determines the tension that can be generated. By varying the length of a muscle, different tensions can be produced.[31] This length–tension relationship is illustrated in Figure 8-2. At position B in the curve, the interaction of the crossbridges between the actin and myosin myofilaments within the sarcomere is at maximum. Setting a muscle at this particular length will produce the greatest amount of tension. At position A the muscle is shortened, and at position C the muscle is lengthened. In either case the interaction between

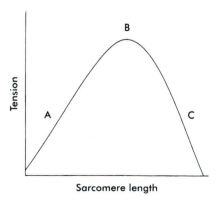

FIGURE 8-2

The length–tension relation of the muscle. Greatest tension is developed at point B, with less tension developed at points A and C.

the actin and myosin myofilaments through the crossbridges is greatly reduced, thus the muscle is not capable of generating significant tension.

Age

The ability to generate muscular force is also related to age.[4] Both men and women seem to be able to increase strength throughout puberty and adolescence, reaching a peak around 20–25 years of age, at which time this ability begins to level off and in some cases decline. After about age 25, a person generally loses an average of 1 percent of his/her maximal remaining strength each year. Thus at age 65, a person would have only about 60 percent of the strength he/she had at age 25.[45] This loss in muscle strength is definitely related to individual levels of physical activity. People who are more active, or perhaps continue to strength-train, considerably decrease this tendency toward declining muscle strength. In addition to retarding this decrease in muscular strength, exercise can also have an effect in slowing the decrease in cardiorespiratory endurance and flexibility, as well as slowing increases in body fat. Thus strength maintenance is important for all individuals regardless of age for achieving total wellness and good health and in rehabilitation after injury.[62]

Overtraining

Overtraining in a physically active patient can have a negative effect on the development of muscular strength. Overtraining is an imbalance between exercise and recovery in which the training program exceeds the body's physiological and psychological limits. Overtraining can result in psychological breakdown (staleness) or physiological breakdown, which can involve musculoskeletal injury, fatigue, or sickness. Engaging in proper and efficient resistance training, eating a proper diet, and getting appropriate rest can all minimize the potential negative effects of overtraining.

Fast-Twitch versus Slow-Twitch Fibers

All fibers in a particular motor unit are either *slow-twitch fibers* or *fast-twitch fibers*. Each kind has distinctive metabolic and contractile capabilities.

SLOW-TWITCH FIBERS

Slow-twitch fibers are also referred to as *type I* or *slow-oxidative* fibers. They are more resistant to fatigue than fast-twitch fibers; however, the time required to generate force is much greater in slow-twitch fibers.[29] Because they are relatively fatigue resistant, slow-twitch fibers are associated primarily with long-duration, aerobic-type activities.

FAST-TWITCH FIBERS

Fast-twitch fibers are capable of producing quick, forceful contractions but have a tendency to fatigue more rapidly than slow-twitch fibers. Fast-twitch fibers are useful in short-term, high-intensity activities, which mainly involve the anaerobic system. Fast-twitch fibers are capable of producing powerful contractions, whereas slow-twitch fibers produce a long-endurance force. There are two subdivisions of fast-twitch fibers. Although both types of fast-twitch fibers are capable of rapid contraction, *type IIa fibers* or *fast-oxidative-glycolytic* fibers are moderately resistant to fatigue, while *type IIb fibers* or *fast-glycolytic* fibers fatigue rapidly and are considered the "true" fast-twitch fibers. Recently, a third group of fast-twitch fibers, *type IIx*, has been identified in animal models. Type IIx fibers are fatigue resistant and are thought to have a maximum power capacity less than that of type IIb but greater than that of type IIa fibers.[45]

RATIO IN MUSCLE

Within a particular muscle are both types of fibers, and the ratio of the two types in an individual muscle varies with each person.[32] Muscles whose primary function is to maintain posture against gravity require more endurance and have a higher percentage of slow-twitch fibers. Muscles that produce powerful, rapid, explosive strength movements tend to have a much higher percentage of fast-twitch fibers.

Because this ratio is genetically determined, it can play a large role in determining ability for a given sport activity. Sprinters and weight lifters, for example, have a large percentage of fast-twitch fibers in relation to slow-twitch fibers.[16] Conversely, marathon runners generally have a higher percentage of slow-twitch fibers. The question of whether fiber types can change as a result of training has to date not been conclusively resolved.[10] However, both types of fibers can improve their metabolic capabilities through specific strength and endurance training.[7]

THE PHYSIOLOGY OF STRENGTH DEVELOPMENT

Muscle Hypertrophy

There is no question that resistance training to improve muscular strength results in an increased size, or hypertrophy, of a muscle. What causes a muscle to hypertrophy? A number of theories have been proposed to explain this increase in muscle size.[22]

First, some evidence exists that there is an *increase in the number of muscle fibers (hyperplasia)* due to fibers splitting in response to training.[39] However, this research has been conducted in animals and should not be generalized to humans. It is generally accepted that the number of fibers is genetically determined and does not seem to increase with training.

Second, it has been hypothesized that because the muscle is working harder in resistance training, more blood is required to supply that muscle with oxygen and other nutrients. Thus it is thought that *the number of capillaries is increased*. This hypothesis is only partially correct; *no new* capillaries are formed

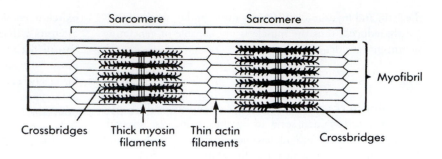

FIGURE   8-3

Muscles contract when an electrical impulse from the central nervous system causes the myofilaments in a muscle fiber to move closer together.

during resistance training; however, a number of dormant capillaries might well become filled with blood to meet this increased demand for blood supply.[45]

A third theory to explain this increase in muscle size seems the most credible. Muscle fibers are composed primarily of small protein filaments, called myofilaments, which are contractile elements in muscle. *Myofilaments* are small contractile elements of protein within the sarcomere. There are two distinct types of myofilaments: thin *actin* myofilaments and thicker *myosin* myofilaments. Fingerlike projections, or crossbridges, connect the actin and myosin myofilaments. When a muscle is stimulated to contract, the crossbridges pull the myofilaments closer together, thus shortening the muscle and producing movement at the joint that the muscle crosses[5] (Fig. 8-3).

These *myofilaments increase in size and number* as a result of resistance training, causing the individual muscle fibers to increase in cross-sectional diameter.[58] This increase is particularly present in men, although women will also see some increase in muscle size. More research is needed to further clarify and determine the specific reasons for muscle hypertorphy.

REVERSIBILITY

If resistance training is discontinued or interrupted, the muscle will atrophy, decreasing in both strength and mass. Adaptations in skeletal muscle that occur in response to resistance training can begin to reverse in as little as 48 hours. It does appear that consistent exercise of a muscle is essential to prevent reversal of the hypertrophy that occurs due to strength training.

Other Physiological Adaptations to Resistance Exercise

In addition to muscle hypertrophy, there are a number of other physiological adaptations to resistance training.[40] The strength of noncontractile structures, including tendons and ligaments, is increased. The mineral content of bone is increased, thus making the bone stronger and more resistant to fracture. Maximal oxygen uptake is improved when resistance training is of sufficient intensity to elicit heart rates at or above training levels. However, it must be emphasized that these increases are minimal and that if increased maximal oxygen uptake is the goal, aerobic exercise rather than resistance training is recommended. There is also an increase in several enzymes important in aerobic and anaerobic metabolism.[3,25,26] All of these adaptations contribute to strength and endurance.

TECHNIQUES OF RESISTANCE TRAINING

There are a number of different techniques of resistance training for strength improvement, including isometric exercise, progressive resistive exercise, isokinetic training, circuit training, and plyometric exercise. Regardless of the specific strength-training technique used, the therapist should integrate functional strengthening activities that involve multiplanar, eccentric, concentric, and isometric contractions.

The Overload Principle

Regardless of which of these techniques is used, one basic principle of reconditioning is extremely important. For a muscle to improve in strength, it must be forced to work at a higher level than it is accustomed to. In other words, the muscle must be overloaded. Without overload the muscle will be able to maintain strength as long as training is continued against a resistance to which the muscle is accustomed, but no additional strength gains will be realized. This maintenance of existing levels of muscular strength may be more important in resistance programs that emphasize muscular endurance rather than strength gains. Many individuals can benefit more in terms of overall health by concentrating on improving muscular endurance. However, to most effectively build muscular strength, resistance training requires a consistent, increasing effort against progressively increasing resistance.[38,56]

Resistive exercise is based primarily on the principles of overload and progression. If these principles are applied, all of the following resistance training techniques will produce improvement of muscular strength over time.

In a rehabilitation setting, progressive overload is limited to some degree by the healing process. If the therapist takes an aggressive approach to rehabilitation, the rate of progression is perhaps best determined by the injured patient's response to a specific exercise. Exacerbation of pain or increased swelling should signal the therapists that their rate of progression is too aggressive.

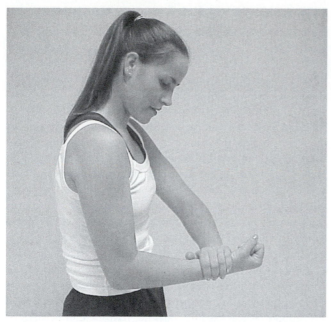

Isometric exercises involve contraction against some immovable resistance.

Isometric Exercise

An *isometric exercise* involves a muscle contraction in which the length of the muscle remains constant while tension develops toward a maximal force against an immovable resistance[6] (Fig. 8-4). An isometric contraction provides stabilization strength that helps maintain normal length–tension and force–couple relationships, which are critical for normal joint arthrokinematics. Isometric exercises are capable of increasing muscular strength.[54] However, strength gains are relatively specific, with as much as a 20 percent overflow to the joint angle at which training is performed. At other angles, the strength curve drops off dramatically because of a lack of motor activity at that angle. Thus, strength is increased at the specific angle of exertion, but there is no corresponding increase in strength at other positions in the range of motion.

Another major disadvantage of these isometric exercises is that they tend to produce a spike in systolic blood pressure that can result in potentially life-threatening cardiovascular accidents.[29] This sharp increase in systolic blood pressure results from a Valsalva maneuver, which increases intrathoracic pressure. To avoid or minimize this effect, it is recommended that breathing be done during the maximal contraction to prevent this increase in pressure.

The use of isometric exercises in injury rehabilitation or reconditioning is widely practiced. There are a number of conditions or ailments resulting from trauma or overuse that must be treated with strengthening exercises. Unfortunately, these problems can be exacerbated with full range-of-motion resistance exercises. It might be more desirable to make use of positional or functional isometric exercises that involve the application of isometric force at multiple angles throughout the range of motion. Functional isometrics should be used until the healing process has progressed to the point that full-range activities can be performed.

During rehabilitation, it is often recommended that a muscle be contracted isometrically for 10 seconds at a time at a frequency of 10 or more contractions per hour. Isometric exercises can also offer significant benefit in a strengthening program.[64]

There are certain instances in which an isometric contraction can greatly enhance a particular movement. For example, one of the exercises in power weight lifting is a squat. A squat is an exercise in which the weight is supported on the shoulders in a standing position. The knees are then flexed, and the weight is lowered to a three-quarter squat position, from which the lifter must stand completely straight once again.

It is not uncommon for there to be one particular angle in the range of motion at which smooth movement is difficult because of insufficient strength. This joint angle is referred to as a sticking point. A power lifter will typically use an isometric contraction against some immovable resistance to increase strength at this sticking point. If strength can be improved at this joint angle, then a smooth, coordinated power lift can be performed through a full range of movement.

Progressive Resistive Exercise

A second technique of resistance training is perhaps the most commonly used and most popular technique for improving muscular strength in a rehabilitation program. *Progressive resistance exercise* uses exercises that strengthen muscles through a contraction that overcomes some fixed resistance such as with dumbbells, barbells, various exercise machines, or resistive elastic tubing. Progressive resistive exercise uses isotonic, or *isodynamic*, contractions in which force is generated while the muscle is changing in length.

CONCENTRIC VERSUS ECCENTRIC CONTRACTIONS

Isotonic contractions can be concentric or eccentric. In performing a bicep curl, to lift the weight from the starting position the biceps muscle must contract and shorten in length. This shortening contraction is referred to as a concentric or positive contraction. If the biceps muscle does not remain contracted when the weight is being lowered, gravity would cause this weight to simply fall back to the starting position. Thus, to control the weight as it is being lowered, the biceps muscle must continue to contract while at the same time gradually lengthening. A contraction in which the muscle is lengthening while still applying force is called an eccentric or negative contraction.

It is possible to generate greater amounts of force against resistance with an eccentric contraction than with a concentric contraction, because eccentric contractions require a much lower level of motor unit activity to achieve a certain force than do concentric contractions. Because fewer motor units are firing to produce a specific force, additional motor units can be recruited to generate increased force. In addition, oxygen use is much lower during eccentric exercise than in comparable concentric exercise. Thus eccentric contractions are less resistant to fatigue than are concentric contractions. The mechanical efficiency of eccentric exercise can be several times higher than that of concentric exercise.[56]

Traditionally, progressive resistive exercise has concentrated primarily on the concentric component without paying much attention to the importance of the eccentric component.[56] The use of eccentric contractions, particularly in rehabilitation of various sport-related injuries, has received considerable emphasis in recent years. Eccentric contractions are critical for deceleration of limb motion, especially during high-velocity dynamic activities.[35] For example, a baseball pitcher relies on an eccentric contraction of the external rotators of the glenohumeral joint to decelerate the humerus, which might be internally rotating at speeds as high as 8000°/second. Certainly, strength deficits or an inability of a muscle to tolerate these eccentric forces can predispose an injury. Thus, in a rehabilitation program the therapist should incorporate eccentric strengthening exercises. Eccentric contractions are possible with all free weights, with the majority of isotonic exercise machines, and with most isokinetic devices. Eccentric contractions are used with plyometric exercise discussed in Chapter 13 and can also be incorporated with functional proprioceptive neuromuscular facilitation (PNF) strengthening patterns discussed in Chapter 15.

In progressive resistive exercise it is essential to incorporate both concentric and eccentric contractions.[33] Research has clearly demonstrated that the muscle should be overloaded and fatigued both concentrically and eccentrically for the greatest strength improvement to occur.[4,22,45] When training specifically for the development of muscular strength, the concentric portion of the exercise should require 1–2 seconds, while the eccentric portion of the lift should require 2–4 seconds. The ratio of the concentric component to the eccentric component should be approximately 1:2. Physiologically the muscle will fatigue much more rapidly concentrically than eccentrically.

FREE WEIGHTS VERSUS EXERCISE MACHINES

Various types of exercise equipment can be used with progressive resistive exercise, including free weights (barbells and dumbbells) or exercise machines such as Cybex, Universal, Paramount, Tough Stuff, Icarian Fitness, King Fitness, Body Solid, Pro-Elite, Life Fitness, Nautilus, BodyCraft, Yukon, Flex, Cam-Bar, GymPros, Nugym, BodyWorks, DP, Soloflex, and Body Master. Dumbbells and barbells require the use of iron plates of varying weights that can be easily changed by adding or subtracting equal amounts of weight to both sides of the bar. The exercise machines for the most part have stacks of weights that are lifted through a series of levers or pulleys. The stack of weights slides up and down on a pair of bars that restrict the movement to only one plane. Weight can be increased or decreased simply by changing the position of a weight key (Fig. 8-5).

There are advantages and disadvantages to free weights and machines. The exercise machines are relatively safe to use in comparison with free weights. For example, a bench press with free weights requires a partner to help lift the weight back onto the support racks if the lifter does not have enough strength to complete the lift; otherwise the weight might be dropped on the chest. With the machines the weight can be easily and safely dropped without fear of injury.

It is also a simple process to increase or decrease the weight by moving a single weight key with the exercise machines, although changes can generally be made only in increments of 10 or 15 pounds. With free weights, iron plates must be added or removed from each side of the barbell.

The biggest disadvantage in using exercise machines is that with few exceptions the design constraints of the machine allow only single-plane motion, limiting or controlling more functional movements that occur in multiple planes simultaneously.

Anyone who has strength-trained using free weights and exercise machines realizes the difference in the amount of weight that can be lifted. Unlike the machines, free weights have no restricted motion and can thus move in many different directions, depending on the forces applied. With free weights, an element of neuromuscular control on the part of the lifter to stabilize the weight and prevent it from moving in any other direction

FIGURE 8-5

Isotonic equipment. **A**, Most exercise machines are isotonic. **B**, Resistance can be easily changed by changing the key in the stack of weights.

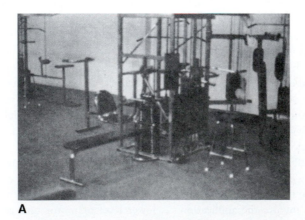

A

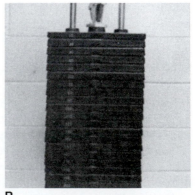

B

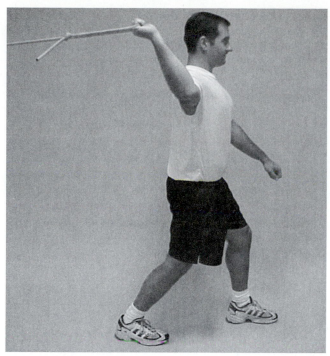

FIGURE 8-6

Strengthening exercises using surgical tubing are widely used in rehabilitation.

than vertical will usually decrease the amount of weight that can be lifted.[66]

SURGICAL TUBING OR THERABAND

Surgical tubing or Theraband, as a means of providing resistance, has been widely used in rehabilitaion (Fig. 8-6). The advantage of exercising with surgical tubing or Theraband is that movement can occur in multiple planes simultaneously. Thus exercise can be done against resistance in more functional movement planes. The use of surgical tubing exercise in plyometrics and PNF strengthening techniques will be discussed in Chapters 13 and 15. Surgical tubing can be used to provide resistance with the majority of the strengthening exercises shown in Chapters 25–32.

Regardless of which type of equipment is used, the same principles of progressive resistive exercise may be applied.

VARIABLE RESISTANCE

One problem often mentioned in relation to progressive resistive exercise reconditioning is that the amount of force necessary to move a weight through a range of motion changes according to the angle of pull of the contracting muscle. It is greatest when the angle of pull is approximately 90°. In addition, once the inertia of the weight has been overcome and momentum has been established, the force required to move the resistance varies according to the force the muscle can produce through the range of motion. Thus it has been argued that a disadvantage of any type of isotonic exercise is that the force required to move the resistance is constantly changing throughout the range of movement. This change in resistance at different points in the range of motion has been labeled *accommodating resistance* or *variable resistance*.

A number of exercise machine manufacturers have attempted to alleviate this problem of changing force capabilities by using a cam in its pulley system (Fig. 8-7). The cam is individually designed for each piece of equipment so that the resistance is variable throughout the movement. The cam

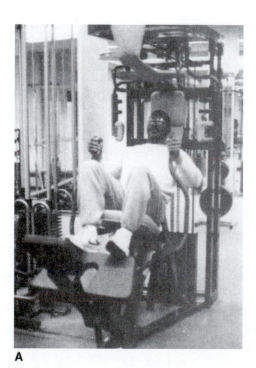
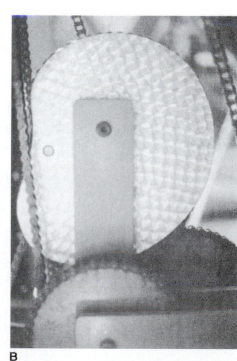

FIGURE 8-7

Exercise machines.
A, Bench-press machine.
B, The cam is designed to equalize resistance throughout the full range of motion.

A   **B**

is intended to alter resistance so that the muscle can handle a greater load, but at the points where the joint angle or muscle length is mechanically disadvantageous, it reduces the resistance to muscle movement. Whether this design does what it claims is debatable.

PROGRESSIVE RESISTIVE EXERCISE TECHNIQUES

Perhaps the single most confusing aspect of progressive resistive exercise is the terminology used to describe specific programs.[32] The following list of terms with their operational definitions may help clarify the confusion:

Repetitions: The number of times a specific movement is repeated

Repetition maximum (RM): The maximum number of repetitions at a given weight

Set: A particular number of repetitions

Intensity: The amount of weight or resistance lifted

Recovery period: The rest interval between sets

Frequency: The number of times an exercise is done in a week's period

RECOMMENDED TECHNIQUES OF RESISTANCE TRAINING

Specific recommendations for techniques of improving muscular strength are controversial among therapists. A considerable amount of research has been done in the area of resistance training relative to (1) the amount of weight to be used, (2) the number of repetitions, (3) the number of sets, and (4) the frequency of training.

A variety of specific programs have been proposed that recommend the optimal amount of weight, number of sets, number of repetitions, and frequency for producing maximal gains in levels of muscular strength. However, regardless of the techniques used, the healing process must dictate the specifics of any strength-training program. Certainly, to improve strength, the muscle must be progressively overloaded. The amount of weight used and the number of repetitions must be sufficient to make the muscle work at higher intensity than it is accustomed to. This factor is the most critical in any resistance training program. The resistance training program must also be designed to ultimately meet the specific competitive needs of the athlete.

Resistance training programs were initially designed by power lifters and body builders. Programs or routines commonly used in training and conditioning include the following:

Single set: One set of 8–12 repetitions of a particular exercise performed at a slow speed.

Tri-sets: A group of three exercises for the same muscle group performed using 2–4 sets of each exercise with no rest in between.

Multiple sets: Two or three warm-up sets with progressively increasing resistance followed by several sets at the same resistance.

Supersets: Either one set of 8–10 repetitions of several exercises for the same muscle group performed one after another, or several sets of 8–10 repetitions of two exercises for the same muscle group with no rest in between.

Pyramids: One set of 8–12 repetitions with light resistance, then an increase in resistance over 4–6 sets until only 1 or 2 repetitions can be performed. The pyramid can also be reversed going from heavy to light resistance.

Split routine: Workouts exercise different muscle groups on successive days. For example, Monday, Wednesday, and Friday might be used for upper body muscles, and Tuesday, Thursday, and Saturday would be used for lower body muscles.

Circuit training: This technique may be useful to the therapist for maintaining or perhaps improving levels of muscular strength or endurance in other parts of the body while the patients allow for healing and reconditioning of an injured body part. Circuit training uses a series of exercise stations, each of which involves weight training, flexibility, calisthenics, or brief aerobic exercises. Circuits can be designed to accomplish many different training goals. With circuit training the patient moves rapidly from one station to the next, performing whatever exercise is to be done at that station within a specified time period. A typical circuit would consist of 8–12 stations, and the entire circuit would be repeated three times.

Circuit training is most definitely an effective technique for improving strength and flexibility. Certainly if the pace or time interval between stations is rapid and if workload is maintained at a high level of intensity with heart rates at or above target training levels, the cardiorespiratory system may benefit from this circuit. However, there is little research evidence that circuit training is very effective in improving cardiorespiratory endurance. It should be, and is most often, used as a technique for developing an improving muscular strength and endurance.[27]

TECHNIQUES OF RESISTANCE TRAINING USED IN REHABILITATION

One of the first widely accepted strength development programs to be used in a rehabilitation program was developed by DeLorme and was based on a repetition maximum of 10 (10 RM).[18] The amount of weight used is what can be lifted exactly 10 times (Table 8-1).

TABLE   8 - 1

DeLorme's Program

SET	AMOUNT OF WEIGHT	REPETITIONS
1	50% of 10 RM	10
2	75% of 10 RM	10
3	100% of 10 RM	10

TABLE 8-2
The Oxford Technique

SET	AMOUNT OF WEIGHT	REPETITIONS
1	100% of 10 RM	10
2	75% of 10 RM	10
3	50% of 10 RM	10

Zinovieff proposed the Oxford technique, which, like De-Lorme's program, was designed to be used in beginning, intermediate, and advanced levels of rehabilitation.[68] The only difference is that the percentage of maximum was reversed in the three sets (Table 8-2). McQueen's technique[48] differentiates between beginning to intermediate and advanced levels, as in shown in Table 8-3.

Sanders' program (Table 8-4) was designed to be used in the advanced stages of rehabilitation and was based on a formula that used a percentage of body weight to determine starting weights.[56] The percentages below represent median starting points for different exercises:

Barbell squat—45 percent of body weight
Barbell bench press—30 percent of body weight
Leg extension—20 percent of body weight
Universal bench press—30 percent of body weight
Universal leg extension—20 percent of body weight
Universal leg curl—10–15 percent of body weight
Universal leg press—50 percent of body weight
Upright rowing—20 percent of body weight

Knight applied the concept of progressive resistive exercise in rehabilitation. His DAPRE (daily adjusted progressive resistive exercise) program (Tables 8-5 and 8-6) allows for individual differences in the rates at which patients progress in their rehabilitation programs.[37]

Berger has proposed a technique that is adjustable within individual limitations (Table 8-7). For any given exercise, the amount of weight selected should be sufficient to allow 6–8 RM in each of the three sets, with a recovery period of 60–90 seconds between sets. Initial selection of a starting weight might require some trial and error to achieve this 6–8 RM range. If at least three sets of 6 RM cannot be completed, the weight is too heavy and should be reduced. If it is possible to do more than three sets of 8 RM, the weight is too light and should be

TABLE 8-3
McQueen's Technique

SETS	AMOUNT OF WEIGHT	REPETITIONS
3 (Beginning/ intermediate)	100% of 10 RM	10
4–5 (Advanced)	100% of 2–3 RM	2–3

TABLE 8-4
Sanders' Program

SETS	AMOUNT OF WEIGHT	REPETITIONS
Total of 4 sets (three times per week)	100% of 5 RM	5
Day 1, 4 sets	100% of 5 RM	5
Day 2, 4 sets	100% of 3 RM	5
Day 3, 1 set	100% of 5 RM	5
2 sets	100% of 3 RM	5
2 sets	100% of 2 RM	5

TABLE 8-5
Knight's DAPRE Program

SET	AMOUNT OF WEIGHT	REPETITIONS
1	50% of RM	10
2	75% of RM	6
3	100% of RM	Maximum
4	Adjusted working weight*	Maximum

*See Table 8-6.

TABLE 8-6
DAPRE Adjusted Working Weight

NUMBER OF REPETITIONS PERFORMED DURING THIRD SET	ADJUSTED WORKING WEIGHT DURING FOURTH SET	NEXT EXERCISE SESSION
0–2	−5–10 lb	−5–10 lb
3–4	−0–5 lb	Same weight
5–6	Same weight	±0–10 lb
7–10	±5–10 lb	±5–15 lb
11	±10–15 lb	±10–20 lb

TABLE 8-7
Berger's Adjustment Technique

SET	AMOUNT OF WEIGHT	REPETITIONS
3	100% of 10 RM	6–8

increased.[8] Progression to heavier weights is then determined by the ability to perform at least 8 RM in each of three sets. When progressing weight, an increase of about 10 percent of the current weight being lifted should still allow at least 6 RM in each of three sets.[9]

For rehabilitation purposes, strengthening exercises should be performed on a daily basis initially, with the amount of weight, number of sets, and number of repetitions governed by the injured athlete's response to the exercise. As the healing process progresses and pain or swelling is no longer an issue, a particular muscle or muscle group should be exercised consistently every other day. At that point the frequency of weight training should be at least three times per week but no more than four times per week. It is common for serious weight lifters to lift every day; however, they exercise different muscle groups on successive days.

It has been suggested that if training is done properly, using both concentric and eccentric contractions, resistance training is necessary only twice each week. However, this schedule has not been sufficiently documented.

The American College of Sports Medicine has prepared a position stand on "Progression models in resistance training for healthy adults," which is summarized in the Appendix.

Isokinetic Exercise

An *isokinetic exercise* involves a muscle contraction in which the length of the muscle is changing while the contraction is performed at a constant velocity.[11] In theory, maximal resis-tance is provided throughout the range of motion by the machine. The resistance provided by the machine will move only at some present speed, regardless of the torque applied to it by the individual. Thus the key to isokinetic exercise is not the resistance but the speed at which resistance can be moved.

Few isokinetic devices are still available commercially (Fig. 8-8). In general, they rely on hydraulic, pneumatic, and mechanical pressure systems to produce this constant velocity of motion. Most isokinetic devices are capable of resisting concentric and eccentric contractions at a fixed speed to exercise a muscle.

ISOKINETICS AS A CONDITIONING TOOL

Isokinetic devices are designed so that regardless of the amount of force applied against a resistance, it can only be moved at a certain speed. That speed will be the same whether maximal force or only half the maximal force is applied. Consequently, in isokinetic training, it is absolutely necessary to exert as much force against the resistance as possible (maximal effort) for maximal strength gains to occur.[11] Maximal effort is one of the major problems with an isokinetic strength-training program.

Anyone who has been involved in a resistance training program knows that on some days it is difficult to find the motivation to work out. Because isokinetic training requires a maximal effort, it is very easy to "cheat" and not go through the workout at a high level of intensity. In a progressive resistive exercise program, the athlete knows how much weight has to be lifted for how many repetitions. Thus isokinetic training is often more effective if a partner system is used, primarily as a

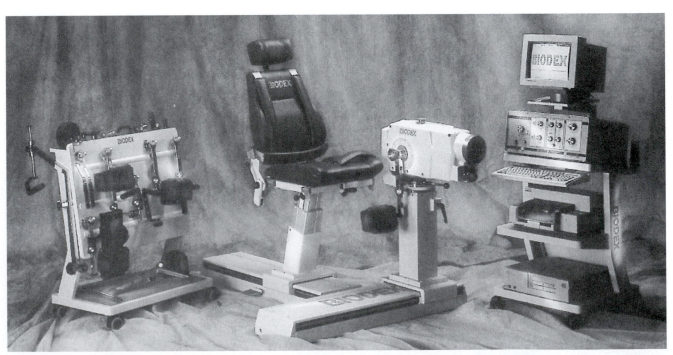

F I G U R E   8 - 8

The Biodex is an isokinetic device that provides resistance at a constant velocity.

means of motivation toward a maximal effort. When isokinetic training is done properly with a maximal effort, it is theoretically possible that maximal strength gains are best achieved through the isokinetic training method in which the velocity and force of the resistance are equal throughout the range of motion. However, there is no conclusive research to support this theory.

Whether this changing force capability is a deterrent to improving the ability to generate force against some resistance is debatable. In real life it does not matter whether the resistance is changing; what is important is that an individual develops enough strength to move objects from one place to another.

Another major disadvantage of using isokinetic devices as a conditioning tool is their cost. With initial purchase costs ranging between $50,000 and $80,000 and the necessity of regular maintenance and software upgrades, the use of an isokinetic device for general conditioning or resistance training is for the most part unrealistic. Thus isokinetic exercises are primarily used as a diagnostic and rehabilitative tool.

ISOKINETICS IN REHABILITATION

Isokinetic strength testing gained a great deal of popularity throughout the 1980s in rehabilitation settings. This trend stems from its providing an objective means of quantifying existing levels of muscular strength and thus becoming useful as a diagnostic tool.[49]

Because the capability exists for training at specific speeds, comparisons have been made regarding the relative advantages of training at fast or slow speeds in a rehabilitation program. The research literature seems to indicate that strength increases from slow-speed training are relatively specific to the velocity used in training. Conversely, training at faster speeds seems to produce a more generalized increase in torque values at all velocities. Minimal hypertrophy was observed only while training at fast speeds, affecting only type II or fast-twitch fibers.[17,52] An increase in neuromuscular efficiency caused by more effective motor unit firing patterns has been demonstrated with slow-speed training.[45]

During the early 1990s, the value of isokinetic devices for quantifying torque values at functional speeds was questioned. This issue, in addition to the theory and use of isokinetic exercise in a rehabilitation setting, will be discussed in detail in Chapter 12.

Plyometric Exercise

Plyometric exercise has also been referred to in the literature as reactive neuromuscular training. It is a technique that is being increasingly incorporated into later stages of the rehabilitation program by the therapist. Plyometric training includes specific exercises that encompass a rapid stretch of a muscle eccentrically, followed immediately by a rapid concentric contraction of that muscle to facilitate and develop a forceful explosive movement over a short period of time.[13,20] The greater the stretch put on the muscle from its resting length immediately before the concentric contraction, the greater the resistance the muscle can overcome. Plyometrics emphasize the speed of the eccentric phase. The rate of stretch is more critical than the magnitude of the stretch. An advantage to using plyometric exercises is that they can help to develop eccentric control in dynamic movements.[43]

Plyometric exercises involve hops, bounds, and depth jumping for the lower extremity and the use of medicine balls and other types of weighted equipment for the upper extremity.[12,14] Depth jumping is an example of a plyometric exercise in which an individual jumps to the ground from a specified height and then quickly jumps again as soon as ground contact is made.[53]

Plyometrics tend to place a great deal of stress on the musculoskeletal system. The learning and perfection of specific jumping skills and other plyometric exercises must be technically correct and specific to one's age, activity, physical, and skill development. Plyometric exercise will be discussed in detail in Chapter 13.

CORE STABILIZATION STRENGTHENING

A dynamic core stabilization training program should be a fundamental component of all comprehensive strengthening as well as injury rehabilitation programs.[34,36] The *core* is defined as the lumbo-pelvic-hip complex. The core is where the center of gravity is located and where all movement begins. There are 29 muscles that have their attachment to the lumbo-pelvic-hip complex.

A core stabilization strengthening program can help to improve dynamic postural control, ensure appropriate muscular balance and joint movement around the lumbo-pelvic-hip complex, allow for the expression of dynamic functional strength, and improve neuromuscular efficiency throughout the entire body. Collectively these factors contribute to optimal acceleration, deceleration, and dynamic stabilization of the entire kinetic chain during functional movements. Core stabilization also provides proximal stability for efficient lower extremity movements. Greater neuromuscular control and stabilization strength will offer a more biomechanically efficient position for the entire kinetic chain, therefore allowing optimal neuromuscular efficiency throughout the kinetic chain. This approach facilitates a balanced muscular functioning of the entire kinetic chain.[15]

Many athletes develop the functional strength, power, neuromuscular control, and muscular endurance in specific muscles to perform functional activities. However, relatively few athletes have developed the muscles required for stabilization. The body's stabilization system has to be functioning optimally to effectively utilize the strength, power, neuromuscular control, and muscular endurance that they have developed in their prime movers. If the extremity muscles are strong and the core is weak, then there will not be enough force created to produce efficient movements. A weak core is a fundamental problem of inefficient movements that leads to injury.[15]

OPEN- VERSUS CLOSED-KINETIC-CHAIN EXERCISES

The concept of the kinetic chain deals with the anatomical functional relationships that exist in the upper and lower extremities. In a weight-bearing position, the lower extremity kinetic chain involves the transmission of forces among the foot, ankle, lower leg, knee, thigh, and hip. In the upper extremity, when the hand is in contact with a weight-bearing surface, forces are transmitted to the wrist, forearm, elbow, upper arm, and shoulder girdle.

An *open kinetic chain* exists when the foot or hand is not in contact with the ground or some other surface. In a *closed kinetic chain*, the foot or hand is weight bearing. Movements of the more proximal anatomical segments are affected by these open- versus closed-kinetic-chain positions. For example, the rotational components of the ankle, knee, and hip reverse direction when changing from open- to closed-kinetic-chain activity. In a closed kinetic chain the forces begin at the ground and work their way up through each joint. Also, in a closed kinetic chain, forces must be absorbed by various tissues and anatomical structures rather than simply dissipating as would occur in an open chain.

In rehabilitation, the use of closed-chain strengthening techniques has become a treatment of choice for many therapists. Most functional activities involve some aspect of weight bearing with the foot in contact with the ground or the hand in a weight-bearing position, so closed-kinetic-chain strengthening activities are more functional than open-chain activities. Therefore rehabilitative exercises should be incorporated that emphasize strengthening of the entire kinetic chain rather than an isolated body segment. Chapter 14 will discuss closed-kinetic-chain activities in detail.

TRAINING FOR MUSCULAR STRENGTH VERSUS MUSCULAR ENDURANCE

Muscular endurance was defined as the ability to perform repeated muscle contractions against resistance for an extended period of time. Most resistance training experts believe that muscular strength and muscular endurance are closely related.[21,50,57] As one improves, there is a tendency for the other to improve also.

It is generally accepted that when resistance training for strength, heavier weights with a lower number of repetitions should be used.[65] Conversely, endurance training uses relatively lighter weights with a greater number of repetitions.

It has been suggested that endurance training should consist of three sets of 10–15 repetitions,[9] using the same criteria for weight selection progression and frequency as recommended for progressive resistive exercise. Thus, suggested training regimens

for muscular strength and endurance are similar in terms of sets and numbers of repetitions.[55] Persons who possess great levels of strength tend to also exhibit greater muscular endurance when asked to perform repeated contractions against resistance.[48]

RESISTANCE TRAINING DIFFERENCES BETWEEN MALES AND FEMALES

The approach to strength training is no different for females than for males. However, some obvious physiological differences exist between the genders.

The average female will not build significant muscle bulk through resistance training. Significant muscle hypertrophy is dependent on the presence of the steroidal hormone *testosterone*. Testosterone is considered a male hormone, although all females posses some level of testosterone in their systems. Women with higher testosterone levels tend to have more masculine characteristics, such as increased facial and body hair, a deeper voice, and the potential to develop a little more muscle bulk.[23,50] For the average female, developing large, bulky muscles through strength training is unlikely, although muscle tone can be improved. Muscle tone basically refers to the firmness of tension of the muscle during a resting state.

The initial stages of a resistance training program are likely to rapidly produce dramatic increases in levels of strength.[1] For a muscle to contract, an impulse must be transmitted from the nervous system to the muscle. Each muscle fiber is innervated by a specific motor unit. By overloading a particular muscle, as in weight training, the muscle is forced to work more efficiently. Efficiency is achieved by getting more motor units to fire, thus causing more muscle fibers to contract, which results in a stronger contraction of the muscle. Consequently, both women and men often see extremely rapid gains in strength when a weight-training program is first begun.[28] In females, these initial strength gains, which can be attributed to improved neuromuscular efficiency, tend to plateau, and minimal improvement in muscular strength is realized during a continuing resistance training program. These initial neuromuscular strength gains are also seen in males, although their strength continues to increase with appropriate training.[1] Again, females who possess higher testosterone levels have the potential to increase their strength further because they are able to develop greater muscle bulk.

Differences in strength levels between males and females are best illustrated when strength is expressed in relation to body weight minus fat. The reduced *strength/body weight ratio* in women is the result of their percentage of body fat. The strength/body weight ratio can be significantly improved through resistance training by decreasing the body fat percentage while increasing lean weight.[45]

The absolute strength differences are considerably reduced when body size and composition are considered. Leg strength can actually be stronger in females than in males, although upper extremity strength is much greater in males.[45]

RESISTANCE TRAINING IN THE ADOLESCENT

The principles of resistance training discussed previously may be applied to adolescents. There are certainly a number of sociological questions regarding the advantages and disadvantages of younger, in particular prepubescent, individuals engaging in rigorous strength-training programs. From a physiological perspective, experts have for years debated the value of strength training in adolescents. Recently, a number of studies have indicated that if properly supervised, adolescents can improve strength, power, endurance, balance, and proprioception; develop a positive body image; improve sport performance; and prevent injuries.[41] A prepubescent child can experience gains in levels of muscle strength without muscle hypertrophy.[51]

A therapist supervising a rehabilitation program for an injured adolescent should certainly incorporate resistive exercise into the program. However, close supervision, proper instruction, and appropriate modification of progression and intensity based on the extent of physical maturation of the individual is critical to the effectiveness of the resistive exercises.[41]

SPECIFIC RESISTIVE EXERCISES USED IN REHABILITATION

Because muscle contractions results in joint movement, the goal of resistance training in a rehabilitation program should be either to regain and perhaps increase the strength of a specific muscle that has been injured or to increase the efficiency of movement about a given joint.[45]

The exercises included throughout Chapters 25–32 show exercises for all motions about a particular joint rather than for each specific muscle. These exercises are demonstrated using free weights (dumbbells or bar weights) and some exercise machines. Other strengthening techniques widely used for injury rehabilitation involving isokinetic exercise, plyometrics, core stability training, closed-kinetic-chain exercises, and PNF strengthening techniques will be discussed in greater detail in subsequent chapters.

SUMMARY

- Muscular strength may be defined as the maximal force that can be generated against resistance by a muscle during a single maximal contraction.
- Muscular endurance is the ability to perform repeated isotonic or isokinetic muscle contractions or to sustain an isometric contraction without undue fatigue.
- Muscular endurance tends to improve with muscular strength, thus training techniques for these two components are similar.
- Muscular strength and endurance are essential components of any rehabilitation program.

- Muscular power involves the speed with which a forceful muscle contraction is performed.
- The ability to generate force is dependent on the physical properties of the muscle, neuromuscular efficiency, as well as the mechanical factors that dictate how much force can be generated through the lever system to an external object.
- Hypertrophy of a muscle is caused by increases in the size and perhaps the number of actin and myosin protein myofilaments, which result in an increased cross-sectional diameter of the muscle.
- The key to improving strength through resistance training is using the principle of overload within the constraints of the healing process.
- Five resistance training techniques that can improve muscular strength are isometric exercise, progressive resistive exercise, isokinetic training, circuit training, and plyometric training.
- Improvements in strength with isometric exercise occur at specific joint angles.
- Progressive resistive exercise is the most common strengthening technique used by the athletic trainer for rehabilitation after injury.
- Circuit training involves a series of exercise stations consisting of resistance training, flexibility, and calisthenic exercises that can be designed to maintain fitness while reconditioning an injured body part.
- Isokinetic training provides resistance to a muscle at a fixed speed.
- Plyometric exercise uses a quick eccentric stretch to facilitate a concentric contraction.
- Closed-kinetic-chain exercises might provide a more functional technique for strengthening of injured muscles and joints in the athletic population.
- Females can significantly increase their strength levels but generally will not build muscle bulk as a result of strength training because of their relative lack of the hormone testosterone.

REFERENCES

1. Akima H, Takahashi H, Kuno SY. Early phase adaptations of muscle use and strength to isokinetic training. *Med Sci Sports Exerc* 31(4):588, 1999.
2. Allerheiligen W. Speed development and plyometric training. In: Baechle T, ed. *Essentials of Strength Training and Conditioning*. Champaign, IL, Human Kinetics, 2000.
3. Always SE, MacDougall D, Sale G, et al. Functional and structural adaptations in skeletal muscle of trained athletes. *J Appl Physiol* 64:1114, 1988.
4. Astrand PO, Rodahl K. *Textbook of Work Physiology*. New York, McGraw-Hill, 1986.
5. Baechle T, ed. *Essentials of Strength Training and Conditioning*. Champaign, IL, Human Kinetics, 2000.

6. Baker D, Wilson G, Carlyon B. Generally vs. specificity: A comparison of dynamic and isometric measures of strength and speed-strength. *Eur J Appl Physiol* 68:350–355, 1994.

7. Bandy W, Lovelace-Chandler V, Bandy B, et al. Adaptation of skeletal muscle to resistance training. *J Orthop Sports Phys Ther* 12(6):248–255, 1990.

8. Berger R. *Conditioning for Men.* Boston, Allyn & Bacon, 1973.

9. Berger R. Effect of varied weight training programs on strength. *Res Q Exerc Sport* 33:168, 1962.

10. Booth F, Thomason D. Molecular and cellular adaptation of muscle in response to exercise: Perspectives of various models. *Physiol Rev* 71:541–585, 1991.

11. Brown LE. *Isokinetics in Human Performance.* Champaign, IL, Human Kinetics, 2000.

12. Chu D. *Jumping into Plyometrics.* Champaign, IL, Human Kinetics, 1998.

13. Chu D. Plyometrics in sports injury rehabilitation and training. *Athlet Ther Today* 4(3):7, 1999.

14. Chu D. *Plyometric Exercise with the Medicine Ball.* Livermore, CA, Bittersweet, 1989.

15. Clark M. *Integrated Training for the New Millennium.* Calabasas, CA, National Academy of Sports Medicine, 2001.

16. Costill D, Daniels J, Evan W, et al. Skeletal muscle enzymes and fiber compositions in male and female track athletes. *J Appl Physiol* 40:149, 1976.

17. Coyle E, Feiring D, Rotkis T, et al. Specificity of power improvements through slow and fast speed isokinetic training. *J Appl Physiol* 51:1437, 1981.

18. DeLorme T, Wilkins A. *Progressive Resistance Exercise.* New York, Appleton-Century-Crofts, 1951.

19. Deudsinger RH. Biomechanics in clinical practice. *Phys Ther* 64:1860–1868, 1984.

20. Duda M. Plyometrics: A legitimate form of power training. *Physician Sports Med* 16:213, 1988.

21. Dudley GA, Fleck SJ. Strength and endurance training: Are they mutually exclusive? (Review) *Sports Med* 4(2):79, 1987.

22. Etheridge G, Thomas T. Physiological and biomedical changes of human skeletal muscle induced by different strength training programs. *Med Sci Sports Exerc* 14:141, 1982.

23. Fahey T. *Basic Weight Training for Men and Women.* Mountain View, CA, Mayfield, 1999.

24. Faulkner J, Green H, White T. Response and adaptation of skeletal muscle to changes in physical activity. In: Bouchard C, Shepard R, Stephens J, eds. *Physical Activity, Fitness, and Health.* Champaign, IL, Human Kinetics, 1994.

25. Fleck SJ, Kramer WJ. Resistance training: Physiological responses and adaptations. *Physician Sports Med* 16:108, 1988.

26. Gettman L, Ward P, Hagan R. A comparison of combined running and weight training with circuit weight training. *Med Sci Sports Exerc* 14:229, 1982.

27. Gettman L. Circuit weight training: A critical review of its physiological benefits. *Physician Sports Med* 9(1):44, 1981.

28. Gravelle BL, Blessing DL. Physiological adaptation in women concurrently training for strength and endurance. *J Strength Cond* 14(1):5, 2000.

29. Graves JE, Pollack M, Jones A, et al. Specificity of limited range of motion variable resistance training. *Med Sci Sports Exerc* 21:84, 1989.

30. Gray GW. Ecocentrics—A theoretical model for muscle function (submitted).

31. Harmen E. The biomechanics of resistance training. In: Baechle T, ed. *Essentials of Strength Training and Conditioning.* Champaign, IL, Human Kinetics, 2000.

32. Hickson R, Hidaka C, Foster C. Skeletal muscle fiber type, resistance training and strength-related performance. *Med Sci Sports Exerc* 26:593–598, 1994.

33. Hortobagyi T, Katch FI. Role of concentric force in limiting improvement in muscular strength. *J Appl Physiol* 68:650, 1990.

34. Jones M, Trowbridge C. Four ways to a safe, effective strength training program. *Athlet Ther Today* 3(2):4, 1998.

35. Kaminski TW, Wabbersen CV, Murphy RM. Concentric versus enhanced eccentric hamstring strength training: Clinical implications. *J Athlet Train* 33(3):216, 1998.

36. King MA. Core stability: Creating a foundation for functional rehabilitation. *Athlet Ther Today* 5(2):6–13, 2000.

37. Knight K. Knee rehabilitation by the DAPRE technique. *Am J Sports Med Phys Fitness* 7:336, 1979.

38. Komi P. *Strength and Power in Sport.* London, Blackwell Scientific, 1992.

39. Kraemer W. General adaptation to resistance and endurance training programs. In: Baechle T, ed. *Essentials of Strength Training and Conditioning.* Champaign, IL, Human Kinetics, 2000.

40. Kraemer WJ, Duncan ND, Volek JS. Resistance training and elite athletes: Adaptations and program considerations. *J Orthop Sports Phys Ther* 28(2):110, 1998.

41. Kraemer WJ, Fleck SJ. *Strength Training for Young Athletes.* Champaign, IL, Human Kinetics, 1993.

42. Kraemer WJ. General adaptations to resistance and endurance training programs. In: Baechle T, ed. *Essentials of Strength Training and Conditioning.* Champaign, IL, Human Kinetics, 2000.

43. Kramer J, Morrow A, Leger A. Changes in rowing ergometer, weight lifting, vertical jump and isokinetic performance in response to standard and standard plus plyometric training programs. *Int J Sports Med* 14(8):440–454, 1993.

44. Mastropaolo J. A test of maximum power theory for strength. *Eur J Appl Physiol* 65:415–420, 1992.

45. McArdle W, Katch F, Katch V. *Exercise Physiology, Energy, Nutrition, and Human Performance.* Philadelphia, Lea & Febiger, 2001.

46. McComas A. Human neuromuscular adaptations that accompany changes in activity. *Med Sci Sports Exerc* 26(12):1498–1509, 1994.

47. McGlynn GH. A reevaluation of isometric training. *J Sports Med Phys Fitness* 12:258, 1972.

48. MacQueen I. Recent advance in the techniques of progressive resistance. *Br Med J* 11:11993, 1954.

49. Nicholas JJ. Isokinetic testing in young nonathletic able-bodied subjects. (Review) *Arch Phys Med Rehabil* 70(3):210, 1989.

50. Nygard CH, Luophaarui T, Suurnakki T, et al. Muscle strength and muscle endurance of middle-aged women and men associated to type, duration and intensity of muscular load at work. *Int Arch Occup Environ Health* 60(4):291, 1998.

51. Ozmun J, Mikesky A, Surburg P. Neuromuscular adaptations following prepubescent strength training. *Med Sci Sports Exerc* 26:514, 1994.

52. Pipes T, Wilmore J. Isokinetic vs. isotonic strength training in adult men. *Med Sci Sports Exerc* 7:262, 1975.

53. Radcliffe JC, Farentinos RC. *High-Powered Plyometrics.* Champaign, IL, Human Kinetics, 1999.

54. Rehfeldt H, Caffiber G, Kramer H, et al. Force, endurance time, and cardiovascular responses in voluntary isometric contractions of different muscle groups. *Biomed Biochem Acta* 48(5–6):S509, 1989.

55. Sale D, MacDougall D. Specificity in strength training: A review for the coach and athlete. *Can J Appl Sports Sci* 6:87, 1981.

56. Sanders M. Weight training and conditioning. In: Sanders B, ed. *Sports Physical Therapy.* Norwalk, CT, Appleton & Lange, 1997.

57. Smith TK. Developing local and general muscular endurance. *Athlet J* 62:42, 1981.

58. Soest A, Bobbert M. The role of muscle properties in control of explosive movements. *Biol Cybern* 69:195–204, 1993.

59. Staron RS, Karapondo DL, Kreamer WJ. Skeletal muscle and adaptations during early phase of heavy resistance training in men and women. *J Appl Physiol* 76:1247–1255, 1994.

60. Stone J. Rehabilitation—speed of movement/muscular power. *Athlet Ther Today* 3(5):10, 1998.

61. Stone J. Rehabilitation—muscular endurance. *Athlet Ther Today* 3(4):21, 1998.

62. Stone M, Fleck S, Triplett N. Health and performance related potential of resistance training. *Sports Med* 11:210–231, 1991.

63. Strauss RH, ed. *Sports Medicine.* Philadelphia, WB Saunders, 1991.

64. Ulmer H, Knierman W, Warlow T, et al. Interindividual variability of isometric endurance with regard to the endurance performance limit for static work. *Biomedical Biochemistry Acta* 48(5–6):S504, 1989.

65. Van Etten L, Verstappen E, Westerterp K. Effect of body building on weight training induced adaptations in body composition and muscular strength. *Med Sci Sports Exerc* 26:515–521, 1994.

66. Weltman A, Stamford B. Strength training: Free weights vs. machines. *Physician and Sports Medicine* 10:197, 1982.

67. Yates JW. Recovery of dynamic muscular endurance. *Eur J Appl Physiol* 56(6):662, 1987.

68. Zinovieff A. Heavy resistance exercise: The Oxford technique. *Br J Physiol Med* 14:129, 1951.

APPENDIX: AMERICAN COLLEGE OF SPORTS MEDICINE[*]

Position Stand

PROGRESSION MODELS IN RESISTANCE TRAINING FOR HEALTHY ADULTS

This pronouncement was written for the American College of Sports Medicine by William J. Kraemer, PhD, FACSM (Chairperson); Kent Adams, PhD; Enzo Cafarelli, PhD, FACSM; Gary A. Dudley, PhD, FACSM; Cathryn Dooly, PhD, FACSM; Matthew S. Feigenbaum, PhD, FACSM; Steven J. Fleck, PhD, FACSM; Barry Franklin, PhD, FACSM; Andrew C. Fry, PhD; Jay R. Hoffman, PhD, FACSM; Robert U. Newton, PhD; Jeffrey Potteiger, PhD, FACSM; Michael H. Stone, PhD; Nicholas A. Ratamess, MS; and Travis Triplett-McBride, PhD.

Summary

American College of Sports Medicine Position Stand on Progression models in resistance training for healthy adults. *Med Sci Sports Exerc* 34(2):364–380, 2002. In order to stimulate further adaptation toward a specific training goal(s), progression in the type of resistance training protocol used is necessary. The optimal characteristics of strength-specific programs include the use of both concentric and eccentric muscle actions and the performance of both single- and multiple-joint exercises. It is also recommended that the strength program sequence exercises to optimize the quality of the exercise intensity (large muscle group exercises before small ones, multiple-joint exercises before single-joint exercises, and higher intensity exercises before lower intensity ones). For initial resistances, it is recommended that loads corresponding to 8–12 RM be used in novice training. For intermediate to advanced training, it is recommended that individuals use a wider loading range, from 1–12 RM in a periodized fashion, with eventual emphasis on heavy loading

---

[*]Data from [*Med Sci Sports Exerc* 34(2):364–380, 2002].

T A B L E   8 A - 1

Summary of Resistance Training Recommendations: An Overview of Different Program Variables Needed for Progression with Different Fitness Levels

	MUSCLE ACTION	SELECTION	ORDER	LOADING	VOLUME	REST INTERVALS	VELOCITY	FREQUENCY
Strength								
Nov.	ECC & CON	SJ & MJ ex.	For Nov., Int., Adv.: Large < small	60–70% of 1 RM	1–3 sets, 8–12 reps	For Nov., Int., Adv.: 2–3 min. for core	S, M	2–3×/week
Int.	ECC & CON	SJ & MJ ex.	MJ < SJ	70–80% of 1 RM	Mult. Sets, 6–12 reps	1–2 min. for others	M	2–4×/week
Adv.	ECC & CON	SJ & MJ ex.—emphasis: MJ	HI < LI	1 RM – PER.	Mult. Sets, 1–12 reps–PER.		US-F	4–6×/week
Hypertrophy								
Nov.	ECC & CON	SJ & MJ ex.	For Nov., Int., Adv.: Large < small	60–70% of 1 RM	1–3 sets, 8–12 reps	1–2 min.	S, M	2–3×/week
Int.	ECC & CON	SJ & MJ ex.	MJ < SJ	70–80% of 1 RM	Mult. Sets, 6–12 reps	1–2 min.	S, M	2–4×/week
Adv.	ECC & CON	SJ & MJ ex.	HI < LI	70–100% of 1 RM with emphasis on 70–85% – PER	Mult. Sets, 1–12 reps with emphasis On 6–12 reps – PER	2–3 min. VH; 1–2 min. – L-MH	S, M, F	4–6×/week
Power								
Nov.	ECC & CON	For Nov., Int., Adv.: Mostly MJ	For Nov., Int., Adv.: Large < small	For Nov., Int., Adv.: Heavy loads (>80%)—strength; Light (30–60%)—velocity—PER	Train for strength	For Nov., Int., Adv.: 2–3 min. for core	M	2–3×/week
Int.	ECC & CON		Most complex < least complex		1–3 sets, 3–6 reps	1–2 min. for others	F	2–4×/week
Adv.	ECC & CON		HI < LI		3–6 sets, 1–6 reps—PER		F	4–6×/week
Endurance								
Nov.	ECC & CON	SJ & MJ ex.	For Nov., Int., Adv.: Variety in sequencing is recommended	50–70% of 1 RM	1–3 sets, 10–15 reps	For Nov., Int., Adv.: 1–2 min for high rep sets	For Nov., Int., Adv.: S—MR	2–3×/week
Int.	ECC & CON	SJ & MJ ex.		50–70% of 1 RM	Mult. Sets, 10–15 reps on more	<1 min for 10–15 reps	M—HR	2–4×/week
Adv.	ECC & CON	SJ & MJ		30–80% of 1 RM—PER	Multi. Sets, 10–25 reps or more—PER			4–6×/week

ECC, eccentric; CON, concentric; Nov., novice; Int., intermediate; Adv., advanced; SJ, single-joint; MJ, multiple-joint; ex., exercises; HI, high intensity; LI, low intensity; 1 RM, 1-repetition maximum; PER, periodized; VH, very heavy; L-MH, light-to-moderately-heavy; S, slow; M, moderate; US, unintentionally slow; F, fast; MR, moderate repetitions; HR, high repetitions; US-F, unintentionally slow to fast.

(1–6 RM) and with at least 3-minutes rest periods between sets performed at a moderate contraction velocity (1–2 seconds concentric; 1–2 seconds eccentric). When training at a specific RM load, it is recommended that 2–10 percent increase in load be applied when the individual can perform the current workload for one to two repetitions over the desired number. The recommendation for training frequency is 2–3 days/week for novice and intermediate training and 4–5 days/week for advanced training. Similar program designs are recommended for hypertrophy training with respect to exercise selection and frequency. For loading, it is recommended the loads corresponding to 1–12 RM be used in periodized fashion, with emphasis on the 6–12 RM zone and with 1–2-minutes rest periods between sets at a moderate velocity. Higher volume, multiple-set programs are recommended for maximizing hypertrophy. Progression in power training entails two general loading strategies: (1) strength training and (2) use of light loads (30–60 percent of 1 RM) performed at a fast contraction velocity with 2–3 minutes of rest between sets for multiple sets per exercise. It is also recommended that emphasis be placed on multiple-joint exercises, especially those involving the total body. For local muscular endurance training, it is recommended that light to moderate loads (40–60 percent of 1 RM) be performed for high repetitions (>15) using short test periods (<90 seconds). In the interpretation of this position stand, as with prior ones, the recommendations should be viewed in context of the individual's target goals, physical capacity, and training status.

Progression of a resistance training program is dependent on the development of appropriate and specific training goals. An overview can be seen in Table 8A-1. It requires the prioritization of training systems to be used during a specific training cycle to achieve desired results. Resistance training progression should be an "individualized" process of exercise prescription using the appropriate equipment, program design, and exercise techniques needed for the safe and effective implementation of a program. Trained and competent strength and conditioning specialists should be involved with this process in order to optimize the safety and design of a training program. Whereas examples and guidelines can be presented, ultimately the good judgment, experience, and educational training of the exercise professionals involved with this process will dictate the amount of training success. Nevertheless, many exercise prescription options are available in the progression of resistance training to attain goals related to health, fitness, and physical performance.

Impaired Endurance: Maintaining Aerobic Capacity and Endurance

Patrick Sells and William E. Prentice

O B J E C T I V E S

After completing this chapter, the therapist should be able to do the following:

- Explain the relationships between heart rate, stroke volume, cardiac output, and rate of oxygen use.
- Describe the function of the heart, blood vessels, and lungs in oxygen transport.
- Describe the oxygen transport system and the concept of maximal rate of oxygen use.
- Describe the principles of continuous and interval training and the potential of each technique for improving aerobic activity.
- Describe the difference between aerobic and anaerobic activity.
- Describe the principles of reversibility and detraining.
- Describe caloric threshold goals associated with various stages of exercise programming.

Although strength and flexibility are commonly regarded as essential components in any injury rehabilitation program, often relatively little consideration is given toward maintaining aerobic capacity and cardiorespiratory endurance. When musculoskeletal injury occurs, the patient is forced to decrease physical activity and levels of cardiorespiratory endurance may decrease rapidly. Thus the therapist must design or substitute alternative activities that allow the individual to maintain existing levels of aerobic capacity during the rehabilitation period. Furthermore, the importance of maintaining and improving functional capacity is becoming increasingly evident regardless of musculoskeletal injury. Recent research has demonstrated a reduction in risk for cardiovascular disease associated in improved levels of aerobic capacity. Sandvik et al.[42] reported mortality rates according to fitness quartiles over 16 years of follow-up. The number of deaths in the least fit portion of the study outnumbered the deaths of the most fit by a margin of 61 deaths to 11 deaths from cardiovascular causes.[42] Myers et al. studied 6213 subjects referred for treadmill testing and concluded that exercise capacity is a more powerful predictor of mortality among men than other established risk factors for cardiovascular disease.[38]

By definition, *cardiorespiratory endurance* is the ability to perform whole-body activities for extended periods of time without undue fatigue.[11,16] The cardiorespiratory system provides a means by which oxygen is supplied to the various tissues of the body. Without oxygen, the cells within the human body cannot possibly function and ultimately death will occur. Thus the cardiorespiratory system is the basic life-support system of the body.[11]

TRAINING EFFECTS ON THE CARDIORESPIRATORY SYSTEM

Basically, transport of oxygen throughout the body involves the coordinated function of four components: heart, blood vessels, blood, and lungs. The improvement of cardiorespiratory endurance through training occurs because of increased capability of each of these four elements in providing necessary oxygen to the working tissues.[48] A basic discussion of the training effects and response to exercise that occur in the heart, blood vessels, blood, and lungs should make it easier to understand why the training techniques discussed later are effective in improving cardiorespiratory endurance.

Adaptation of the Heart to Exercise

The heart is the main pumping mechanism and circulates oxygenated blood throughout the body to the working tissues. The heart receives deoxygenated blood from the venous system

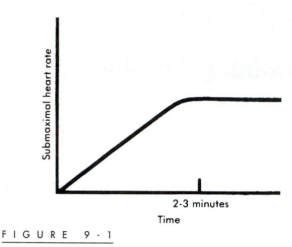

F I G U R E   9 - 1

Plateau heart rate. For the heart rate to plateau at a given level, 2–3 minutes are required.

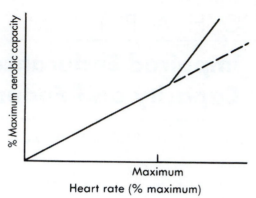

F I G U R E   9 - 2

Maximum heart rate. Maximum heart rate is achieved at about the same time as maximal aerobic capacity.

and then pumps the blood through the pulmonary vessels to the lungs, where carbon dioxide is exchanged for oxygen. The oxygenated blood then returns to the heart, from which it exits through the aorta to the arterial system and is circulated throughout the body, supplying oxygen to the tissues.

HEART RATE

As the body begins to exercise, the working tissues require an increased supply of oxygen (via transport on red blood cells) to meet the increased demand (cardiac output). Increases in heart rate occur as one response to meet the demand. The heart is capable of adapting to this increased demand through several mechanisms. *Heart rate* shows a gradual adaptation to an increased workload by increasing proportionally to the intensity of the exercise and will plateau at a given level after about 2 to 3 minutes (Fig. 9-1). Increases in heart rate produced by exercise are met by a decrease in diastolic filling time. Heart rate parameters change with age, body position, type of exercise, cardiovascular disease, heat and humidity, medications, and blood volume. Conditions that exist in any patient should be taken into consideration when prescribing exercise to improve aerobic endurance. The commonly used equation to predict maximal heart rate (MHR) is 220 – age for healthy men and women. However, the formula has limitations to persons who fall outside the "apparently healthy" classification and should be used with caution. Monitoring heart rate is an indirect method of estimating oxygen consumption.[16] In general, heart rate and oxygen consumption have a linear relationship with exercise intensity. The greater the intensity of the exercise, the higher the heart rate. This relationship is least consistent at very low and very high intensities of exercise (Fig. 9-2). During higher-intensity activities, MHR may be achieved before maximum oxygen consumption, which can continue to rise.[35] Because of these existing relationships, it should become apparent that the rate of oxygen consumption can be estimated by monitoring the heart rate.[13]

STROKE VOLUME

A second mechanism by which the cardiovascular system is able to adapt to increased demands of cardiac output during exercise is to increase *stroke volume* (the volume of blood being pumped out with each beat). Stroke volume is equal to the difference between end diastolic volume and end systolic volume. Tyical values for stroke volume range from 60 to 100 mL per beat at rest and 100 to 120 mL per beat at maximum.[18] Stroke volume will continue to increase only to the point at which diastolic filling time is simply too short to allow adequate filling. This occurs at about 40 to 50 percent of maximal aerobic capacity or at a heart rate of 110 to 120 beats per minute; above this level, increases in the cadiac output are accounted for by increases in heart rate (Fig. 9-3).[12]

CARDIAC OUTPUT

Stroke volume and heart rate collectively determine the volume of blood being pumped through the heart in a given unit of time. Approximately 5 L of blood are pumped through the heart during each minute at rest. This is referred to as the *cardiac*

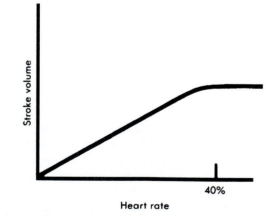

F I G U R E   9 - 3

Stroke volume plateaus. Stroke volume plateaus at about 40 percent of maximal heart rate.

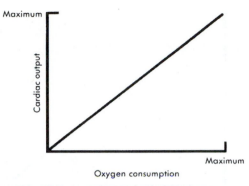

FIGURE 9 - 4

Cardiac output limits maximal aerobic capacity.

output, which indicates how much blood the heart is capable of pumping in exactly 1 minute. Thus cardiac output is the primary determinant of the maximal rate of oxygen consumption possible (Fig. 9-4). During exercise, cardiac output increases to approximately four times that experienced during rest (to about 20 L) in the normal individual and may increase as much as six times in the elite endurance athlete (to about 30 L)

$$Cardiac\ output = Stroke\ volume \times Heart\ rate$$

The aforementioned equation illustrates that any factor that will impact heart rate or stroke volume can either increase or decrease cardiac output. For example, an increase in venous return of blood from working muscle will increase the end diastolic volume. This increased volume will increase stroke volume and, therefore, cardiac output. However, conditions that resist ventricular outflow (high blood pressure) will result in a decrease in cardiac output. Conversely, a condition that would decrease venous return (peripheral artery disease) would decrease stroke volume and attenuate cardiac output.

A commonly reported benefit of aerobic conditioning is a reduced resting heart rate and a reduced heart rate at a standard exercise load. This reduction in heart rate is explained by an increase in stroke volume brought about by increased venous return and to increased contractile conditions in the myocardium. The heart becomes more efficient because it is capable of pumping more blood with each stroke. Because the heat is a muscle, it can hypertrophy, or increase in size and strength due to aerobic exercise, to some extent, but this is in no way a negative effect of training.

Training Effect

$$Increased\ stroke\ volume \times Decreased\ heart\ rate$$
$$= Cardiac\ output$$

During exercise, females tend to have a 5 to 10 percent higher cardiac output than males do at all intensities. This is likely due to a lower concentration of hemoglobin in the female, which is compensated for during exercise by an increased cardiac output.[51]

ADAPTATION IN BLOOD FLOW

The amount of blood flowing to the various organs increases during exercise However, there is a change in overall distribution of cardiac output; the percentage of total cardiac output to the nonessential organs is decreased, whereas it is increased to active skeletal muscle. Volume of blood flow to the heart muscle or myocardium increases substantially during exercise, even though the percentage of total cardiac output supplying the heart muscle remains unchanged. The increase in flow to skeletal muscle is brought about by withdrawal of sympathetic stimulation to arterioles, and vasodilatation is maintained by intrinsic metabolic control.[40] Trained persons have a higher capillary density than their untrained counterparts to better accommodate the increased supply and demand. In skeletal muscle, there is increased formation of blood vessels or capillaries, although it is not clear whether new ones form or dormant ones simply open up and fill with blood.[44]

The total peripheral resistance is the sum of all forces that resist blood flow within the vascular system. Total peripheral resistance decreases during exercise primarily because of vessel vasodilation in the active skeletal muscles.

BLOOD PRESSURE

Blood pressure in the arterial system is determined by the cardiac output in relation to total peripheral resistance to blood flow as follows:

$$BP \sim CO \times TPR,$$

where BP = blood pressure, CO = cardiac output, and TPR = total peripheral resistance.

Blood pressure is created by contraction of the myocardium. Contraction of the ventricles of the heart creates systolic pressure, and relaxation of the heart creates diastolic pressure. Blood pressure is regulated centrally by neural activity on peripheral arterioles and locally by metabolites produced during exercise. During exercise, there is a decrease in total peripheral resistance (via decreased vasoconstriction) and an increase in cardiac output. Systolic pressure increases in proportion to oxygen consumption and cardiac output, while diastolic pressure shows little or no increase.[6] Failure of systolic pressure to increase with increased exercise intensity is considered an abnormal response to exercise and is a general indication to stop an exercise test or session.[1] Blood pressure falls below preexercise levels after exercise and may stay low for several hours. There is general agreement that engaging in consistent aerobic exercise will produce modest reductions in both systolic and diastolic blood pressure at rest as well as during submaximal exercise.[15]

ADAPTATIONS IN THE BLOOD

Oxygen is transported throughout the system bound to *hemoglobin*. Found in red blood cells, hemoglobin is an iron-containing protein that has the capability of easily accepting or giving up molecules of oxygen as needed. Training for improvement of cardiorespiratory endurance produces an increase in total blood volume, with a corresponding increase in the amount of hemoglobin. The concentration of hemoglobin in circulating blood does not change with training; it may actually decrease slightly.

ADAPTATION OF THE LUNGS

As a result of training, pulmonary function is improved in the trained individual relative to the untrained individual. The volume of air that can be inspired in a single maximal ventilation is increased. The diffusing capacity of the lungs is also increased, facilitating the exchange of oxygen and carbon dioxide. Pulmonary resistance to air flow is also decreased.[33]

MAXIMAL AEROBIC CAPACITY

The maximal amount of oxygen that can be used during exercise is referred to as *maximal aerobic capacity* (exercise physiologists refer to this as $\dot{V}O_{2max}$). It is considered to be the best indicator of the level of cardiorespiratory endurance. Maximal aerobic capacity is most often presented in terms of the volume of oxygen used relative to body weight per unit of time (mL $\times$ kg^{-1} $\times$ min^{-1}).[3]

It is common to see aerobic capacity expressed in metabolic equivalents (METs). Resting oxygen consumption is generally considered to be 3.5 mL $\times$ kg^{-1} $\times$ min^{-1} or 1 (MET). Therefore, an exercise intensity of 10 METs is equivalent to a $\dot{V}O_2$ of 35 mL $\times$ kg^{-1} $\times$ min^{-1}. A normal maximal aerobic capacity for most collegiate men and women would fall in the range of 35 to 50 mL $\times$ kg^{-1} $\times$ min$^{-1.35}$.

Rate of Oxygen Consumption

The performance of any activity requires a certain rate of oxygen consumption, which is about the same for all persons, depending on their present level of fitness. Generally, the greater the rate or intensity of the performance of an activity, the greater will be the oxygen consumption. Each person has his/her own maximal rate of oxygen consumption. The person's ability to perform an activity is closely related to the amount of oxygen required by that activity. This ability is limited by the maximal amount of oxygen the person is capable of delivering into the lungs. Fatigue occurs when insufficient oxygen is supplied to muscles. It should be apparent that the greater the percentage of maximal aerobic capacity required during an activity, the less time the activity may be performed (Fig. 9-5).

Three factors determine the maximal rate at which oxygen can be used: (1) external respiration, involving the ventilatory process or pulmonary function; (2) gas transport, which is accomplished by the cardiovascular system (that is, the heart, blood vessels, and blood); and (3) internal respiration, which involves the use of oxygen by the cells to produce energy. Exercise physiologists generally discuss the limiting factors of maximal aerobic capacity based on healthy human subjects in a

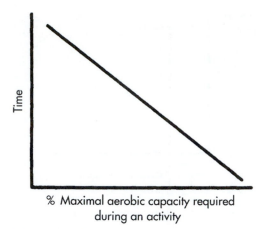

FIGURE 9-5

Maximal aerobic capacity required during activity. The greater the percentage of maximal aerobic capacity required during an activity, the less time that activity can be performed.

controlled environment.[4,27] Under these condtions, research presents agreement that the ability to transport oxygen through the heart, lungs, and blood is the limiting factor to the overall rate of oxygen consumption. This indicates that this is not the ability of the mitochondria to consume oxygen that limits $\dot{V}O_{2max}$. A high maximal aerobic capacity within a person's range indicates that all three systems are working well.

Maximal Aerobic Capacity: An Inherited Characteristic

The maximal rate at which oxygen can be used is a genetically determined characteristic; we inherit a certain range of maximal aerobic capacity, and the more active we are, the higher the existing maximal aerobic capacity will be within that range.[43,50] Therefore, a training program is capable of increasing maximal aerobic capacity to its highest limit within our range.[50]

FAST-TWITCH VERSUS SLOW-TWITCH MUSCLE FIBERS

The range of maximal aerobic capacity inherited is in a large part determined by the metabolic and functional properties of skeletal muscle fibers. As discussed in detail in Chapter 8, there are two distinct types of muscle fibers, *slow-twitch* or *fast-twitch* fibers, each of which has distinctive metabolic as well as contractile capabilities. Because they are relatively fatigue resistant, slow-twitch fibers are associated primarily with long-duration, aerobic-type activities. Fast-twitch fibers are useful in short-term, high-intensity activities, which mainly involve the anaerobic system. In general, if a patient has a high ratio of slow-twitch to fast-twitch muscle fibers, he or she will be able to use oxygen more efficiently and thus will have a higher maximal aerobic capacity.

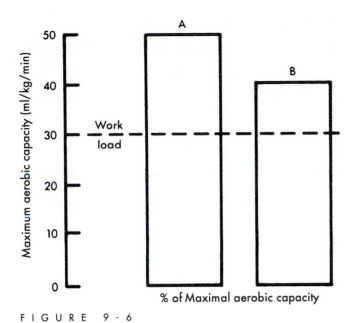

FIGURE 9-6

Patient A should be able to work longer than patient B as a result of a lower percentage use of maximal aerobic capacity.

Cardiorespiratory Endurance and Work Ability

Cardiorespiratory endurance plays a critical role in our ability to carry out normal daily activities.[40] Fatigue is closely related to the percentage of maximal aerobic capacity that a particular workload demands.[49] For example, Figure 9-6 presents two people, A and B. A has maximal aerobic capacity of 50 mL/kg per minute, whereas B has a maximal aerobic capacity of only 40 mL/kg per minute. If both A and B are exercising at the same intensity, then A will be working at a much lower percentage of maximal aerobic capacity than B. Consequently, A should be able to sustain his or her activity over a much longer period of time. Everyday activities may be adversely affected if the ability to use oxygen efficiently is impaired. Thus improvement of cardiorespiratory endurance should be an essential component of any conditioning program and must be included as part of the rehabilitation program for the injured patient.[9]

Regardless the training technique used for the improvement of cardiorespiratory endurance, one principal goal remains the same: *to increase the ability of the cardiorespiratory system to supply a sufficient amount of oxygen to working muscles.* Without oxygen, the body is incapable of producing energy for an extended period of time.

PRODUCING ENERGY FOR EXERCISE

All living systems need to perform a variety of activities such as growing, generating energy, repairing damaged tissues, and eliminating wastes. All of these activities are referred to as metabolic or cellular *metabolism.*

Muscles are metabolically active and must generate energy to move. Energy is produced from the breakdown of certain nutrients from foodstuffs. This energy is stored in a compound called *adenosine triphosphate* (ATP), which is the ultimate usable form of energy for muscular activity. This ATP is produced in the muscle tissue from blood glucose or glycogen. Fats and proteins can also be metabolized to generate ATP. Glucose not needed immediately can be stored as glycogen in the resting muscle and liver. Stored glycogen in the liver can later be converted back to glucose and transferred to the blood to meet the body's energy needs.[7]

It is important to understand that the intensity and duration of exercise selected as an intervention will have implications on the source of "fuel" to engage in the activity. The "fuel" is the ATP needed for muscular contraction. Exercise intensity and duration effect the source or pathway that is used to supply the ATP, i.e., does the ATP come from the breakdown of circulating blood glucose (glycolysis) or from the Krebs cycle and the electron transport chain (oxidative phosphorlization)?

If the combination of duration and intensity is low (40–50 percent of $\dot{V}O_{2max}$), the body relies more heavily on fats stored in adipose tissue to meet its energy needs. The longer the duration of an activity, the greater the amount of fat used, especially during the later stages of endurance events. During rest and submaximal exertion, both fat and carbohydrates are used to provide energy in approximately a 60–40-percent ratio. Carbohydrate must be available to use fat. If glycogen is totally depleted, fat cannot be completely metabolized. Regardless the nutrient source that produces ATP, it is always available in the cell as an immediate energy source. When all available sources of ATP are used, more must be regenerated for muscular contraction to continue.[8,28]

Various sports activities involve specific demands for energy. For example, sprinting and jumping are high-energy-output activities, requiring a relatively large production of energy for a short time. Long-distance running and swimming, on the other hand, are mostly low-energy-output activities per unit of time, requiring energy production for a prolonged time. Other physical activities demand a blend of both high- and low-energy output. These various energy demands can be met by the different processes in which energy can be supplied to the skeletal muscles.[17]

Anaerobic Versus Aerobic Metabolism

Two major energy-generating systems function in muscle tissue: anaerobic and aerobic metabolism. Each of these systems produces ATP.[21] Activities that demand intensive, short-term exercise need ATP that is rapidly available and metabolized to meet energy needs. After a few seconds of intensive exercise, however, the small stores of ATP are used up. The body then utilizes stored glycogen as an energy source. Glycogen can be broken down to supply glucose, which is then metabolized within the muscle cells to generate ATP for muscle contractions.[35]

Glucose can be metabolized to generate small amounts of ATP energy without the need for oxygen. This energy system is referred to as *anaerobic metabolism* (occurring in the absence of oxygen). As exercise continues, the body has to rely on a more complex form of carbohydrate and fat metabolism to generate ATP. This second energy system requires oxygen and is therefore referred to as *aerobic metabolism* (occurring in the presence of oxygen). The aerobic system of producing energy generates considerably more ATP than the anaerobic one.

In most activities, both aerobic and anaerobic systems function simultaneously. The degree to which the two major energy systems are involved is determined by the intensity and duration of the activity.[47] If the intensity of the activity is such that sufficient oxygen can be supplied to meet the demands of working tissues, the activity is considered to be *aerobic.* Conversely, if the activity is of high-enough intensity or the duration is such that there is insufficient oxygen available to meet energy demands, the activity becomes *anaerobic.*[51]

EXCESS POSTEXERCISE OXYGEN CONSUMPTION (OXYGEN DEFICIT)

As the intensity of the exercise increases and insufficient amounts of oxygen are available to the tissues, an oxygen deficit is incurred. Oxygen deficit occurs in the beginning of exercise (within the first 2–3 minutes) when the oxygen demand is greater than the oxygen supplied. It was been hypothesized that this oxygen debt was caused by lactic acid produced during anaerobic activity and this debt must be "paid back" during the postexercise period. However, there is presently a different rationale for this oxygen deficit, which is currently referred to as "excess postexercise oxygen consumption." It is theoretically caused by disturbances in mitochondrial function from an increase in temperature.[35]

TECHNIQUES FOR MAINTAINING CARDIORESPIRATORY ENDURANCE

There are several different training techniques that may be incorporated into a rehabilitation program through which cardiorespiratory endurance can be maintained. Certainly, a primary consideration for the therapist would be whether the injury involves the upper or lower extremity. With injuries that involve the upper extremity, weight-bearing activities can be used, such as walking, running, stair climbing, and modified aerobics. However, if the injury is to the lower extremity, alternative nonweight-bearing activities, such as swimming or stationary cycling, may be necessary. The goal of the therapist is to try to maintain cardiorespiratory endurance throughout the rehabilitation process.

The principles of the training techniques discussed next can be applied with running, cycling, swimming, stair climbing, or any other activity designed to maintain levels of cardiorespiratory fitness.

Continuous Training

Continuous training involves the following considerations:

- The frequency of the activity
- The intensity of the activity
- The type of activity
- The time (duration) of the activity

FREQUENCY OF TRAINING

The American College of Sports Medicine (ACSM) recommends the average person to engage in three to five exercise sessions per week.[1] A competitive athlete should be prepared to train as often as six times per week. Everyone should take off at least 1 day per week to give damaged tissues a chance to repair themselves.

INTENSITY OF TRAINING

The intensity of exercise is also a critical factor, though recommendations regarding training intensities vary.[24] This statement is particularly true in the early stages of training, when the body is forced to make a lot of adjustments to increased workload demands. The ACSM guidelines regarding intensity of exercise recommend the following: 55/65–90 percent of MHR, or 40/50–85 percent of maximum oxygen uptake reserve ($\dot{V}O_2R$) or MHR reserve (HRR). HRR and $\dot{V}O_2R$ are calculated from the difference between resting and maximum heart rate and resting and maximum $\dot{V}O_2$, respectively. To estimate training intensity, a percentage of this value is added to the resting heart rate and/or resting $\dot{V}O_2$ and is expressed as a percentage of HRR or $\dot{V}O_2R$. The lower intensity values, i.e., 40–49 percent of $\dot{V}O_2R$ or HRR and 55–64 percent of MHR, are most applicable to individuals who are quite unfit. These intensities require the therapist to either know the person's maximal values or use a prediction equation to estimate these intensities. A great rule of thumb is to always go with actual data over prediction data when available. There are many limitations to prediction equations. Due to the linear relationship between heart rate, oxygen consumption, and exercise intensity, it becomes a relatively simple process to identify a specific workload (pace) that will make the heart rate plateau at the desired level.[46] By monitoring heart rate, we know whether the pace is too fast or too slow to achieve the desired range of intensity.[31] Prior to selecting an exercise intensity, the therapist should consider several factors. These include current level of fitness, medications, cardiovascular risk profile, individuals likes and dislikes, and patient goals and objectives.[1]

MONITORING HEART RATE   There are several methods to measure heart rate response during exercise. These include, but not limited to, palpation of the heart rate at the radial or carotid artery, pulse oximetry, telemetry (heart rate monitors) or via electrocardiography (ECG). One of the easiest methods is to palpate the radial artery. This assessment can be done by the patient or the therapist. The carotid artery is simple to find, especially during exercise. However, there are pressure receptors located in the carotid artery that, if subjected to hard pressure from the two fingers, will slow down the heart rate, giving a false indication of exactly what the heart rate is. Thus the pulse at the radial artery proves the most accurate measure of heart rate. Regardless of where the heart rate is taken, it should be recorded prior to exercise, during exercise to ensure target intensities and monitored following exercise to ensure recovery. Another factor must be considered when measuring heart rate during exercise. The patient is trying to elevate heart rate to a specific target rate and maintain it at that level during the entire workout.[22] Heart rate can be increased or decreased by speeding up or slowing down the pace. Based on the fact that heart rates will attain a steady state or plateau to a prescribed work rate in 2 to 3 minutes, the therapist should allow sufficient time prior to assessment of heart rate. Thus the patient should be actively engaged in the workout for 2 to 3 minutes before measuring pulse.[53]

There are several formulas that will easily allow the therapist to identify a target training heart rate.[39] Exact determination of MHR involves exercising a patient at a maximal level and monitoring the heart rate using an ECG. This process is difficult outside of a laboratory. However, an approximate estimate of MHR for both males and females in the population is thought to be about 220 beats per minute.[41] MHR is related to age. With aging, MHR decreases.[32] Thus a relatively simple estimate of MHR would be MHR = 220 − age. For a 40-year-old patient, MHR would be about 180 beats per minute (220 − 40 = 180). If you are interested in working at 70 percent of your maximal heart rate, the target heart rate can be calculated by multiplying 0.7 × (220 − age). The intensity range of 70–85 percent of MHR approximates 55–75 percent of $\dot{V}_{O_2max}$. Again using a 40-year-old person as an example, a target heart rate would be 126 beats per minute (0.7 × [220 − 40] = 126).

Another commonly used formula that takes into account your current level of fitness is the Karvonen equation, sometimes referred to as the *heart rate reserve* method.[25,29]

Target training HR = Resting HR + (0.6[Maximum HR − Resting HR])

Resting heart rate generally falls between 60 and 80 beats per minute. A 40-year-old patient with a resting pulse of 70 beats per minute, according to the Karvonen equation, would have a target training heart rate of 136 beats per minute (70 + 0.6[180 − 70] = 136).

Regardless of the formula used, to see minimal improvement in cardiorespiratory endurance, the patient must train with the heart rate elevated to at least 60 percent of its maximal rate.[1,23,30] Exercising at a 70 percent level is considered moderate, because activity can be continued for a long period of time with little discomfort and still produce a training effect.[36] In a trained individual, it is not difficult to sustain a heart rate at the 85 percent level.[14]

TABLE 9-1

Rating of Perceived Exertion

SCALE	VERBAL RATING
6	
7	Very, very light
8	
9	Very light
10	
11	Fairly light
12	
13	Somewhat hard
14	
15	Hard
16	
17	Very hard
18	
19	Very, very hard
20	

Source: Borg GA. Psychophysical basis of perceived exertion. *Med Sci Sports Exerc* 14:377, 1982.

RATING OF PERCEIVED EXERTION Rating of perceived exertion (RPE) can be used in addition to monitoring heart rate to indicate exercise intensity.[5] During exercise, individuals are asked to rate subjectively on a numerical scale from 6 to 20 exactly how they feel relative to their level of exertion (Table 9-1). More intense exercise that requires a higher level of oxygen consumption and energy expenditure is directly related to higher subjective ratings of perceived exertion. Over a period of time, patients can be taught to exercise at a specific RPE that relates directly to more objective measures of exercise intensity.[20,37]

TYPE OF EXERCISE

The type of activity used in continuous training must be aerobic. Aerobic activities are activities that generally involve repetitive, whole-body, large-muscle movements that are rhythmical in nature and use large amounts of oxygen, elevate the heart rate, and maintain it at that level for an extended period of time. Examples of aerobic activities are walking, running, jogging, cycling, swimming, rope skipping, stepping, aerobic dance exercise, rollerblading, and cross-country skiing.

The advantage of these aerobic activities as opposed to more intermittent activities, such as racquetball, squash, basketball, or tennis, is that aerobic activities are easy to regulate in intensity by either speeding up or slowing down the pace.[34] Because we already know that a given intensity of the workload elicits a given heart rate, these aerobic activities allow us to maintain heart rate at a specified or target level. Intermittent activities involve variable speeds and intensities that cause the heart rate to fluctuate considerably. Although these intermittent activities will improve cardiorespiratory endurance, they are much more difficult to monitor in terms of intensity. It is important to point out that any type of activity, from gardening to aerobic exercise, can improve fitness.[39]

TIME (DURATION)

For minimal improvement to occur, the patient must participate in at least 20 minutes of continuous activity with the heart rate elevated to its working level. The ACSM recommends duration of training to be 20–60 minutes of continuous or intermittent (minimum of 10-minutes bouts accumulated throughout the day) aerobic activity. Duration will vary with the intensity of the activity. Lower-intensity activity should be conducted over a longer period of time (30 minutes or more). Patients training at higher levels of intensity should train at least 20 minutes or longer "because of the importance of 'total fitness' and that it is more readily attained with exercise sessions of longer duration and because of the potential hazards and adherence problems associated with high-intensity activity, moderate-intensity activity of longer duration is recommended for adults not training for athletic competition" (see the Appendix).

Generally, the greater the duration of the workout, the greater the improvement in cardiorespiratory endurance.

Interval Training

Unlike continuous training, *interval training* involves activities that are more intermittent. Interval training consists of alternating periods of relatively intense work and active recovery. It allows for performance of much more work at a more intense workload over a longer period of time than if working continuously. We have stated that it is most desirable in continuous training to work at an intensity of about 60 to 80 percent of maximal heart rate. Obviously, sustaining activity at a relatively high intensity over a 20-minute period would be extremely difficult. The advantage of interval training is that it allows work at this 80 percent or higher level for a short period of time followed by an active period of recovery during which you may be working at only 30 to 45 percent of MHR. Thus the intensity of the workout and its duration can be greater than with continuous training.

There are several important considerations in interval training. The training period is the amount of time in which continuous activity is actually being performed, and the recovery period is the time between training periods. A set is a group of combined training and recovery periods, and a repetition is the number of training/recovery periods per set. Training time or distance refers to the rate or distance of the training period. The training/recovery ratio indicates a time ratio for training versus recovery.

An example of interval training would be a patient exercising on a stationary bike. An interval workout would involve 10 repetitions of pedaling at a maximum speed for 20 seconds followed by pedaling at 40 percent of maximum speed for 90 seconds. During this interval training session, heart rate would probably increase to 85–95 percent of maximal level while pedaling at maximum speed and should probably fall to the 35–45 percent level during the recovery period.

Older adults should exercise some caution when using interval training as a method for improving cardiorespiratory endurance. The intensity levels attained during the active periods may be too high and create undue risk for the older adult.

CALORIC THRESHOLDS AND TARGETS

The interplay between the duration, intensity, and frequency of exercise creates a caloric expenditure from exercise sessions. The amount of caloric expenditure is important to a wide range of patients including those interested in weight loss as well as those under very strenuous training regimens. General acceptance exists such that the health benefits and training changes associated with exercise programs are related to the total amount of work (indicated by caloric expenditure) completed during training.[1] These caloric thresholds may be different to elicit improvements in V_{O_2max}, weight loss, or risk of premature chronic disease. The ACSM recommends a range of 150–400 calories of energy expenditure per day in exercise or physical activity. Expenditure of 1000 kcal per week should be the initial goal for those not previously engaged in regular activity. Patients should be moved toward the upper end of the recommendation (300 to 400 kcal per day) to obtain optimal fitness. The estimation of caloric expenditure is easily accomplished using the METs associated with a given activity and the formula[1]:

$$(MET \times 3.5 \times body\ weight\ in\ kg)/200 = kcal/min$$

Numerous charts and tables exist that estimate activities in terms of intensity requirements expressed in METs. If a weekly goal of 1000 kcal is established for a 70-kg person at an intensity of 6 METs, the caloric expenditure would be calculated as follows:

$$(6 \times 3.5 \times 70\ kg)/200 = kcal/min$$

At an exercise intensity of 6 METs, the patient would need to exercise 136 minutes to achieve the 1000 kcal goal. If the patient wants to exercise 4 days each week, 34 minutes of exercise will be required.

The primary goal of weight loss is to consume or burn more calories than are taken in (eaten). The calories used during exercise can be added to the calories cut from the diet to calculate total caloric deficit needed to create weight loss. The aforementioned patient could reduce his/her caloric intake by 400 kcals each day. This will total 2800 kcal that have been restricted from the diet. These calories are then added to the 1000 kcal used for exercise. A pound of fat is equivalent to 3500 kcal. The combination of reduced caloric intake and increased used of kcal for exercise in the example is 3800 kcals, or slightly more than 1 pound of weight loss in 1 week.

COMBINING CONTINUOUS AND INTERVAL TRAINING

As indicated previously, most physical activities involve some combination of aerobic and anaerobic metabolism.[52] Continuous training is generally done at an intensity level that primarily uses the aerobic system. In interval training, the intensity is sufficient to necessitate a greater percentage of anaerobic metabolism.[19] Therefore for the physically active patient, the therapist should incorporate both training techniques into a rehabilitation program to maximize cardiorespiratory fitness.

DETRAINING

Physical training promotes a wide range of physiologic training. These include increased size and number of mitochondria, increased capillary bed density, changes in resting and exercise heart rate, blood pressure, myocardial oxygen consumption, and improved $\dot{V}O_{2max}$ to mention a few. It would seem logical that if the stimulus (exercise) is removed, these changes will dissipate. Long periods of inactivity are associated with the reversal of the aforementioned changes. Improvements may be lost in as little as 12 days to as long as several months to see a complete reversal of changes.

SUMMARY

- The therapist should routinely incorporate activities that will help maintain levels of cardiorespiratory endurance into the rehabilitation program.
- Cardiorespiratory endurance involves the coordinated function of the heart, lungs, blood, and blood vessels to supply sufficient amounts of oxygen to the working tissues.
- The best indicator of how efficiently the cardiorespiratory system functions is the maximal rate at which oxygen can be used by the tissues.
- Heart rate is directly related to the rate of oxygen consumption. It is therefore possible to predict the intensity of the work in terms of a rate of oxygen use by monitoring heart rate.
- Aerobic exercise involves an activity in which the level of intensity and duration is low enough to provide a sufficient amount of oxygen to supply the demands of the working tissues.
- In anaerobic exercise, the intensity of the activity is so high that oxygen is being used more quickly than it can be supplied; thus an oxygen debt is incurred that must be repaid before working tissue can return to its normal resting state.
- Continuous or sustained training for maintenance of cardiorespiratory endurance involves selecting an activity that is aerobic in nature and training at least three times per week for a time period of no less than 20 minutes with the heart rate elevated to at least 60 percent of maximal rate.

- Interval training involves alternating periods of relatively intense work followed by active recovery periods. Interval training allows performance of more work at a relatively higher workload than continuous training.
- Aerobic exercise is a very powerful tool when considering the decreased mortality and morbidity associated with improvements in functional capacity. The therapist with a working knowledge of the principles of exercise prescription and testing are best capable of ensuring the safety and effectiveness of interventions.

REFERENCES

1. Armstrong L, Bubaker P, Whaley M. *ACSM's Guidelines for Exercise Testing and Prescription.* Philadelphia, Lippincott Williams & Wilkins, 2005.
2. Åstrand PO, Rodahl K. *Textbook of Work Physiology.* New York, McGraw-Hill, 1986.
3. Åstrand PO. Åstrand-rhyming nomogram for calculation of aerobic capacity from pulse rate during submaximal work. *J Appl Physiol* 7:218, 1954.
4. Bassett D, Howley E. Limiting factors for maximal oxygen uptake and determinants of endurance performance. *Med Sci Sports Exerc* 32:70–84, 2000.
5. Borg GA. Psychophysical basis of perceived exertion. *Med Sci Sports Exerc* 14:377, 1982.
6. Brooks G, Fahey T, White T. *Exercise Physiology: Human Bioenergetics and Its Applications.* New York, McGraw-Hill, 2004.
7. Brooks G, Mercier J. The balance of carbohydrate and lipid utilization during exercise: The crossover concept. *J App Physiol* 76:2253–2261, 1994.
8. Cerretelli P. Energy sources for muscle contraction. *Sports Med* 13:S106–S110, 1992.
9. Chillag SA. Endurance patients: Physiologic changes and nonorthopedic problems. *South Med J* 79:1264, 1986. Review.
10. Convertino VA. Aerobic fitness, endurance training, and orthostatic intolerance. *Exerc Sport Sci Rev* 15:223, 1987. Review.
11. Cooper KH. *The Aerobics Program for Total Well-Being.* New York, Bantam Books, 1982.
12. Cox M. Exercise training programs and cardiorespiratory adaptation. *Clin Sports Med* 10:19–32, 1991.
13. deVries H. *Physiology of Exercise for Physical Education and Athletics.* Dubuque, IA, illiam C. Brown, 1986.
14. Dicarlo L, Sparling P, Millard-Stafford M. Peak heart rates during maximal running and swimming: Implications for exercise prescription. *Int J Sports Ed* 12:309–312, 1991.
15. Durstein L, Pate R, Branch D. Cardiorespiratory responses to acute exercise. In: American College of Sports Medicine. *Resource Manual for Guidelines for Exercise Testing and Prescription.* Philadelphia, Lea & Febiger, 1993.

16. Fahey T, ed. *Encyclopedia of Sports Medicine and Exercise Physiology.* New York, Garland, 1995.

17. Fox E, Bowers R, Foss M. *The Physiological Basis of Physical Education and Athletics.* Philadelphia, Saunders, 1981.

18. Franklin B. Cardiorespiratory responses to acute exercise. In: American College of Sports Medicine. *Resource Manual for Guidelines for Exercise Testing and Prescription,* 4th ed. Philadelphia, Lippincott Williams & Wilkins, 2001.

19. Gaesser GA, Wilson LA. Effects of continuous and interval training on the parameters of the power–endurance time relationship for high-intensity exercise. *Int J Sports Med* 9:417, 1988.

20. Glass S, Whaley M, Wegner M. A comparison between ratings of percieved exertion among standard protocols and steady state running. *Int J Sports Ed* 12:77–82, 1991.

21. Green J, Patla A. Maximal aerobic power: Neuromuscular and metabolic considerations. *Med Sci Sport Exerc* 24:38–46, 1992.

22. Greer N, Katch F. Validity of palpation recovery pulse rate to estimate exercise heart rate following four intensities of bench step exercise. *Res Q Exerc Sport* 53:340, 1982.

23. Hage P. Exercise guidelines: Which to believe? *Phys Sports Med* 10:23, 1982.

24. Hawley J, Myburgh K, Noakes T. Maximal oxygen consumption: A contemporary perspective. In: Fahey T, ed. *Encyclopedia of Sports Medicine and Exercise Physiology.* New York, Garland, 1995.

25. Hickson RC, Foster C, Pollac M, et al. Reduced training intensities and loss of aerobic power, endurance, and cardiac growth. *J Appl Physiol* 58:492, 1985.

26. Hill A, Long C, Lupton H. Muscular exercise, Lactic acid and the supply and utilization of oxygen. Parts VII–VIII. *Proc Roy Soc B* 97:155–176, 1924.

27. Hill A, Lupton H. Muscular exercise, Lactic acid and the supply and utilization of oxygen. *Q J Med* 16:135–171, 1923.

28. Honig C, Connett R, Gayeski T. O_2 transport and its interaction with metabolism. *Med Sci Sports Exerc* 24:47–53, 1992.

29. Karvonen MJ, Kentala E, Mustala O. The effects of training on heart rate: A longitudinal study. *Ann Med Exp Biol* 35:305, 1957.

30. Koyanagi A, Yamamoto K, Nishijima K. Recommendation for an exercise perscription to prevent coronary heart disease. *Ed Syst* 17:213–217, 1993.

31. Levine G, Balady G. The benefits and risks of exercise testing: The exercise prescription. *Adv Intern Ed* 38:57–79, 1993.

32. Londeree B, Moeschberger M. Effect of age and other factors on maximal heart rate. *Res Q Exerc Sport* 53:297, 1982.

33. MacDougall D, Sale D. Continuous vs. interval training: A review for the patient and coach. *Can J Appl Sport Sci* 6:93, 1981.

34. Marcinik EJ, Hogden K, Mittleman K, et al. Aerobic/calisthenic and aerobic/circuit weight training programs for Navy men: A comparative study. *Med Sci Sports Exerc* 17:482, 1985.

35. McArdle W, Katch F, Katch V. *Exercise Physiology, Energy, Nutrition, and Human Performance.* Philadelphia, Lippincott Williams & Wilkins, 2001.

36. Mead W, Hartwig R. Fitness evaluation and exercise prescription. *Fam Pract* 13:1039, 1981.

37. Monahan T. Perceived exertion: An old exercise tool finds new applications. *Phys Sports Med* 16:174, 1988.

38. Myers J, Praksah M, Froelicher V, Do D, partington S, Atwood J. Exercise capacity and mortality among men referred for exercise testing. *N Engl J Med* 346 (11):793–8041, 2002.

39. Pate R, Pratt M, Blair S. Physical activity and public health: A recommendation from the CDC and ACSM. *JAMA* 273:402–407, 1995.

40. Powers S. Fundamentals of exercise metabolism. In: American College of Sports Medicine. *Resource Manual for Guidelines for Exercise Testing and Prescription.* Philadelphia, Lea & Febiger, 1993.

41. Rowland TW, Green GM. Anaerobic threshold and the determination of training target heart rates in premenarcheal girls. *Pediatr Cardiol* 10:75, 1989.

42. Sandvik L, Erikssen J, Thaulow Er, Erikssen G, Mundal R, Rodahl K. Physical fitness as a predictor of mortality among healthy, middle-aged Norwegian men. *N Engl J Med* 328:533–537.

43. Saltin B, Strange S. Maximal oxygen uptake: Old and new arguments for a cardiovascular limitation. *Med Sci Sports Exerc* 24:30–37, 1992.

44. Smith M, Mitchell J. Cardiorespiratory adaptations to exercise training. In: American College of Sports Medicine. *Resource Manual for Guidelines for Exercise Testing and Prescription.* Philadelphia, Lea & Febiger, 1993.

45. Stachenfeld N, Eskenazi M, Gleim G. Predictive accuracy of criteria used to assess maximal oxygen consumption. *Am Heart J* 123:922–925, 1992.

46. Swain D, Abernathy K, Smith C. Target heart rates for the development of cardiorespiratory fitness. *Med Sci Sports Exerc* 26:112–116, 1994.

47. Vago P, Mercier M, Ramonatxo M, et al. Is ventilatory anaerobic threshold a good index of endurance capacity? *Int J Sports Med* 8:190, 1987.

48. Wagner P. Central and peripheral aspects of oxygen transport and adaptations with exercise. *Sports Med* 11:133–142, 1991.

49. Weltman A, Weltman J, Ruh R, et al. Percentage of maximal heart rate reserve, and $\dot{V}O_2$ peak for determining endurance training intensity in sedentary women. *Int J Sports Med* 10:212, 1989. Review.

50. Weymans M, Reybrouck T. Habitual level of physical activity and cardiorespiratory endurance capacity in children. *Eur J Appl Physiol* 58:803, 1989.

51. Williford H, Scharff-Olson M, Blessing D. Exercise prescription for women: Special considerations. *Sports Ed* 15:299–311, 1993.

52. Wilmore J, Costill D. *Physiology of Sport and Exercise*. Champaign, IL, Human Kinetics, 1994.

53. Zhang Y, Johnson M, Chow N. Effect of exercise testing protocol on parameters of aerobic function. *Med Sci Sports Exerc* 23:625–630, 1991.

APPENDIX

Medicine and Science in Sports and Exercise, Volume 30, Number 6, June 1998.

Position Stand

The Recommended Quantity and Quality of Exercise for Developing and Maintaining Cardiorespiratory and Muscular Fitness and Flexibility in Healthy Adults

This pronouncement was written for the American College of Sports Medicine by Michael L. Pollock, PhD, FACSM (Chairperson), Glenn A. Gaesser, PhD, FACSM (Co-chairperson), Janus D. Butcher, MD, FACSM, Jean-Pierre Després, PhD, Rod K. Dishman, PhD, FACSM, Barry A. Franklin, PhD, FACSM, and Carol Ewing Garber, PhD, FACSM.

Summary

ACSM Position Stand on The Recommended Quantity and Quality of Exercise for Developing and Maintaining Cardiorespiratory and Muscular Fitness and Flexibility in Adults. *Med Sci Sports Exerc* 30(6):975–991, 1998.

The combination of frequency, intensity, and duration of chronic exercise has been found to be effective for producing a training effect. The interaction of these factors provide the overload stimulus. In general, the lower the stimulus the lower the training effect, and the greater the stimulus the greater the effect. As a result of specificity of training and the need for maintaining muscular strength and endurance, and flexibility of the major muscle groups, a well-rounded training program including aerobic and resistance training, and flexibility exercises is recommended. Although age in itself is not a limiting factor to exercise training, a more gradual approach in applying the prescription at older ages seems prudent. It has also been shown that aerobic endurance training of fewer than 2 days per week, at less than 40–50 percent of $\dot{V}O_2R$, and for less than 10 minutes is generally not a sufficient stimulus for developing and maintaining fitness in healthy adults. Even so, many health benefits from physical activity can be achieved at lower intensities of exercise if frequency and duration of training are increased appropriately. In this regard, physical activity can be accumulated through the day in shorter bouts of 10-minute durations.

In the interpretation of this position stand, it must be recognized that the recommendations should be used in the context of participant's needs, goals, and initial abilities. In this regard, a sliding scale as to the amount of time allotted and intensity of effort should be carefully gauged for the cardiorespiratory, muscular strength and endurance, and flexibility components of the program. An appropriate warm-up and cool-down period, which would include flexibility exercises, is also recommended. The important factor is to design a program for the individual to provide the proper amount of physical activity to attain maximal benefit at the lowest risk. Emphasis should be placed on factors that result in permanent lifestyle change and encourage a lifetime of physical activity.

Many people are currently involved in cardiorespiratory fitness and resistance training programs, and efforts to promote participation in all forms of physical activity are being developed and implemented. Thus, the need for guidelines for exercise prescription is apparent. Based on the existing evidence concerning exercise prescription for healthy adults and the need for guidelines, the ACSM makes few recommendations for the quantity and quality of training for developing and maintaining cardiorespiratory fitness, body composition, muscular strength and endurance, and flexibility in the healthy adult.

CARDIORESPIRATORY FITNESS AND BODY COMPOSITION

1. Frequency of training. 3–5 days per week.
2. Intensity of training. 55/65–90 percent of MHR, or 40/50–85 percent of $\dot{V}O_2R$ or HRR. The lower intensity values, i.e., 40–49 percent of $\dot{V}O_2R$ or HRR and 55–64 percent of MHR, are most applicable to individuals who are quite unfit.
3. Duration of training. 20–60 minutes of continuous or intermittent (minimum of 10-minute bouts accumulated throughout the day) aerobic activity. Duration is dependent on the intensity of the activity; thus, lower-intensity activity should be conducted over a longer period of time (30 minutes or more), and, conversely, individuals training at higher levels of intensity should train at least 20 minutes or longer. Because of the importance of "total fitness" and that it is more readily attained with exercise sessions of longer duration and because of the potential hazards and adherence problems associated with high-intensity activity, moderate-intensity activity of longer duration is recommended for adults not training for athletic competition.
4. Mode of activity. Any activity that uses large muscle groups, which can be maintained continuously, and is rhythmical and aerobic in nature, e.g., walking-hiking, running-jogging, cycling-bicycling, cross-country skiing, aerobic dance/group exercise rope skipping, rowing, stair climbing, swimming, skating, and various endurance game activities or some combination thereof.

MUSCULAR STRENGTH AND ENDURANCE, BODY COMPOSITION, AND FLEXIBILITY

1. **Resistance training.** Resistance training should be an integral part of an adult fitness program and of a sufficient intensity to enhance strength, muscular endurance, and maintain fat-free mass. Resistance training should be progressive in nature, individualized, and provide a stimulus to all the major muscle groups. One set of 8–10 exercises that conditions the major muscle groups 2–3 days per week is recommended. Multiple-set regimens may provide greater benefits if time allows. Most persons should complete 8–12 repetitions of each exercise; however, for older and more frail persons (aged approximately 50–60 years and above), 10–15 repetitions may be more appropriate.

2. **Flexibility training.** Flexibility exercises should be incorporated into the overall fitness program sufficient to develop and maintain range of motion. These exercises should stretch the major muscle groups and be performed a minimum of 2–3 days per week. Stretching should include appropriate static and/or dynamic techniques.

CHAPTER 10

Impaired Mobility: Restoring Range of Motion and Improving Flexibility

William E. Prentice

O B J E C T I V E S

After completing this chapter, the therapist should be able to do the following:

- Define flexibility and describe its importance in injury rehabilitation.
- Identify factors that limit flexibility.
- Differentiate between active and passive range of motion.
- Explain the difference between dynamic, static, and proprioceptive neuromuscular facilitation stretching.
- Discuss the neurophysiologic principles of stretching.
- Describe stretching exercises that may be used to improve flexibility at specific joints throughout the body.

When injury occurs, there is almost always some associated loss of the ability to move normally. Loss of motion may be due to pain, swelling, muscle guarding, or spasm; inactivity resulting in shortening of connective tissue and muscle; loss of neuromuscular control; or some combination of these factors. Restoring normal range of motion following injury is one of the primary goals in any rehabilitation program.[90] Thus the therapist must routinely include exercise designed to restore normal range of motion to regain normal function.

Flexibility has been defined as the ability to move a joint or series of joints through a full, nonrestricted, pain-free range of motion.[2,3,26,38,43,65,79] Flexibility is dependent on a combination of (1) joint range of motion, which may be limited by the shape of the articulating surfaces and by capsular and ligamentous structures surrounding that joint, and (2) muscle flexibility, or the ability of the musculotendinous unit to lengthen.[91]

Flexibility involves the ability of the neuromuscular system to allow for efficient movement of a joint through a range of motion.[3,29,48,76,94]

Flexibility can be discussed in relation to movement involving only one joint, such as the knees, or movement involving a whole series of joints, such as the spinal vertebral joints, which must all move together to allow smooth bending or rotation of the trunk. Lack of flexibility in one joint or movement can affect the entire kinetic chain. A person might have good range

of motion in the ankles, knees, hips, back, and one shoulder joint but lack normal movement in the other shoulder joint; this is a problem that needs to be corrected before the person can function normally.[18]

In this chapter we will concentrate primarily on rehabilitative techniques used to increase the length of the musculotendinous unit and its associated fascia, as well as restricted neural tissue. In addition, a discussion of a variety of soft tissue mobilization techniques including myofascial release, strain/counterstrain, positional release therapy (PRT), active release technique, and massage as they relate to improving mobility will be included. Joint mobilization and traction techniques used to address tightness in the joint capsule and surrounding ligaments will be discussed in Chapter 16. Loss of the ability to control movement due to impairment in neuromuscular control will be discussed in Chapter 11.

IMPORTANCE OF FLEXIBILITY TO THE PATIENT

Maintaining a full, nonrestricted range of motion has long been recognized as essential to normal daily living. Lack of flexibility can also create uncoordinated or awkward movement patterns resulting from lost neuromuscular control. In most patients,

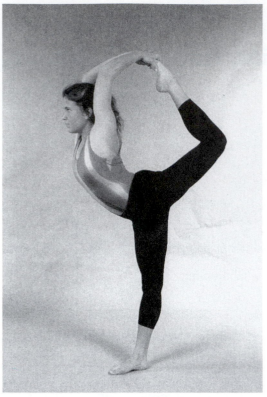

FIGURE   10-1
Some sport activities require superior levels of flexibility.

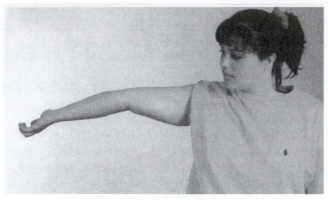

FIGURE   10-2
Excessive joint motion, such as the hyperextended elbow, can predispose a joint to injury.

functional activities require relatively "normal" amounts of flexibility. However some sport activities, such as gymnastics, ballet, diving, and karate require increased flexibility for superior performance (Fig. 10-1).

It has also been generally accepted that flexibility is essential for improving performance in physical activities. However, a review of the evidence-based information in the literature looking at the relationship between flexibility and improved performance is at best conflicting and inconclusive.[93] While many studies done over the years have suggested that stretching improves performance,[11,54,68,100] several recent studies have found that stretching causes decreases in performance parameters such as strength, endurance, power, joint position sense, and reaction times.[9,28,40,55,63,76,83,95,99]

The same can be said when examining the relationship between flexibility and reducing the incidence of injury. While it is generally accepted that good flexibility reduces the likelihood of injury, a true cause-effect relationship has not been clearly established in the literature.[4,17,68,99]

ANATOMIC FACTORS THAT LIMIT FLEXIBILITY

A number of anatomic factors can limit the ability of a joint to move through a full, unrestricted range of motion. *Muscles* and their tendons, along with their surrounding fascial sheaths, are most often responsible for limiting range of motion. When performing stretching exercises to improve flexibility about a particular joint, you are attempting to take advantage of the highly elastic properties of a muscle. Over time it is possible to increase the elasticity, or the length that a given muscle can be stretched. Persons who have a good deal of movement at a particular joint tend to have highly elastic and flexible muscles.

Connective tissue surrounding the joint, such as ligaments on the joint capsule, can be subject to contractures. Ligaments and joint capsules have some elasticity; however, if a joint is immobilized for a period of time, these structures tend to lose some elasticity and actually shorten. This condition is most commonly seen after surgical repair of an unstable joint, but it can also result from long periods of inactivity.

It is also possible for a person to have relatively slack ligaments and joint capsules. These people are generally referred to as being loose-jointed. Examples of this trait would be an elbow or knee that hyperextends beyond 180° (Fig. 10-2). Frequently, there is instability associated with loose-jointedness that can present as great a problem in movement as ligamentous or capsular contractures.

Bony structure can restrict the end point in the range. An elbow that has been fractured through the joint might lay down excess calcium in the joint space, causing the joint to lose its ability to fully extend. However, in many instances we rely on bony prominences to stop movements at normal end points in the range.

Fat can also limit the ability to move through a full range of motion. A person who has a large amount of fat on the abdomen might have severely restricted trunk flexion when asked to bend forward and touch the toes. The fat can act as a wedge between two lever arms, restricting movement wherever it is found.

Skin might also be responsible for limiting movement. For example, a person who has had some type of injury or surgery involving a tearing incision or laceration of the skin, particularly over a joint, will have inelastic scar tissue formed at that site. This scar tissue is incapable of stretching with joint movement.

Over time, skin contractures caused by scarring of ligaments, joint capsules, and musculotendinous units are capable of improving elasticity to varying degrees through stretching. With the exception of bone structure, age, and gender, all the other factors that limit flexibility can be altered to increase range of joint motion.

Neural tissue tightness resulting from acute compression, chronic repetitive microtrauma, muscle imbalances, joint dysfunction, or poor posture can create morphological changes in neural tissues. These changes might include intraneural edema, tissue hypoxia, chemical irritation, or microvascular stasis—all of which could stimulate nociceptors, creating pain. Pain causes muscle guarding and spasm to protect the inflamed neural structures, and this alters normal movement patterns. Eventually neural fibrosis results, which decreases the elasticity of neural tissue and prevents normal movement within surrounding tissues.[19]

ACTIVE AND PASSIVE RANGE OF MOTION

Active range of motion, also called *dynamic flexibility*, refers to the degree to which a joint can be moved by a muscle contraction, usually through the midrange of movement. Dynamic flexibility is not necessarily a good indicator of the stiffness or looseness of a joint, because it applies to the ability to move a joint efficiently, with little resistance to motion.[45]

Passive range of motion, sometimes called *static flexibility*, refers to the degree to which a joint can be passively moved to the end points in the range of motion. No muscle contraction is involved to move a joint through a passive range.

When a muscle actively contracts, it produces a joint movement through a specific range of motion.[76,89] However, if passive pressure is applied to an extremity, it is capable of moving farther in the range of motion. It is essential in sports activities that an extremity be capable of moving through a nonrestricted range of motion.[78]

Passive range of motion is important for injury prevention. There are many situations in physical activity in which a muscle is forced to stretch beyond its normal active limits. If the muscle does not have enough elasticity to compensate for this additional stretch, it is likely that the musculotendinous unit will be injured.

Assessment of Active and Passive Range of Motion

Accurate measurement of active and passive range of joint motion is difficult.[46] Various devices have been designed to accommodate variations in the size of the joints, as well as the complexity of movements in articulations that involve more than one joint.[46] Of these devices, the simplest and most widely used is the *goniometer* (Fig. 10-3).

A goniometer is a large protractor with measurements in degrees. By aligning the individual arms of the goniometer parallel to the longitudinal axis of the two segments involved in

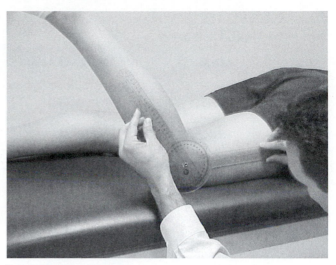

FIGURE 10-3

Measurement of active knee joint flexion using a goniometer.

motion about a specific joint, it is possible to obtain reasonably accurate measurement of range of movement. To enhance reliability standardization of measurement techniques and methods of recording, active and passive ranges of motion are critical in individual clinics where successive measurements might be taken by different athletic trainers to assess progress. Table 10-1 provides a list of what would be considered normal active ranges for movements at various joints.

The goniometer has an important place in a rehabilitation setting, where it is essential to assess improvement in joint flexibility to modify injury rehabilitation programs.

In some clinics a digital inclinometer is used instead of a goniometer. An inclinometer is a more precise measuring instrument with high reliability that has most often been used in research settings. However, digital inclinometers are affordable and can easily be used to accurately measure range of motion of all joints of the body from complex movements of the spine, large joints of the extremities to the small joints of fingers and toes.

STRETCHING TO IMPROVE MOBILITY

The goal of any effective stretching program should be to improve the range of motion at a given articulation by altering the extensibility of the neuromusculotendinous units that produce movement at that joint. It is well documented that exercises that stretch these neuromusculotendinous units and their fascia over time will increase the range of movement possible about a given joint.[39,72]

For many years the efficacy of stretching in improving range of motion has been theoretically attributed to neurophysiologic phenomena involving the stretch reflex. However, a recent study that extensively reviewed the existing literature has suggested

TABLE 10-1

Active Ranges of Joint Motions

JOINT	ACTION	DEGREES OF MOTION
Shoulder	Flexion	0–180°
	Extension	0–50°
	Abduction	0–180°
	Medical rotation	0–90°
	Lateral rotation	0–90°
	Flexion	0–90°
Elbow	Flexion	0–160°
Forearm	Pronation	0–90°
	Supination	0–90°
Wrist	Flexion	0–90°
	Extension	0–70°
	Abduction	0–25°
	Adduction	0–65°
Hip	Flexion	0–125°
	Extension	0–15°
	Abduction	0–45°
	Adduction	0–15°
	Medical rotation	0–45°
	Lateral rotation	0–45°
Knee	Flexion	0–140°
Ankle	Plantarflexion	0–45°
	Dorsiflexion	0–20°
Foot	Inversion	0–30°
	Eversion	0–10°

that improvements in range of motion resulting from stretching must be explained by mechanisms other than the stretch reflex.[17] Studies reviewed indicate that changes in the ability to tolerate stretch and/or the viscoelastic properties of the stretched muscle are possible mechanisms.

NEUROPHYSIOLOGIC BASIS OF STRETCHING

Every muscle in the body contains various types of mechanoreceptors that, when stimulated, inform the central nervous system of what is happening with that muscle. Two of these mechanoreceptors are important in the stretch reflex: the *muscle spindle* and the *Golgi tendon organ*. Both types of receptors are sensitive to changes in muscle length. The Golgi tendon organs are also affected by changes in muscle tension.

When a muscle is stretched, both the muscle spindles and the Golgi tendon organs immediately begin sending a volley of sensory impulses to the spinal cord. Initially impulses coming from the muscle spindles inform the central nervous system that the muscle is being stretched. Impulses return to the muscle

from the spinal cord, causing the muscle to reflexively contract, thus resisting the stretch.[62] The Golgi tendon organs respond to the change in length and the increase in tension by firing off sensory impulses of their own to the spinal cord. If the stretch of the muscle continues for an extended period of time (at least 6 seconds), impulses from the Golgi tendon organs begin to override muscle spindle impulses. The impulses from the Golgi tendon organs, unlike the signals from the muscle spindle, cause a reflex relaxation of the antagonist muscle. This reflex relaxation serves as a protective mechanism that will allow the muscle to stretch through relaxation without exceeding the extensibility limits, which could damage the muscle fibers.[12]

This relaxation of the antagonist muscle during contractions is referred to as *autogenic inhibition.*

In any synergistic muscle group, a contraction of the agonist causes a reflex relaxation in the antagonist muscle, allowing it to stretch and protecting it from injury. This phenomenon is referred to as reciprocal inhibition[82] (see Fig. 15-32 on p. 274).

EFFECTS OF STRETCHING ON THE PHYSICAL AND MECHANICAL PROPERTIES OF MUSCLE

The neurophysiologic mechanisms of both autogenic and reciprocal inhibition result in reflex relaxation with subsequent lengthening of a muscle. Thus the mechanical properties of that muscle that physically allow lengthening to occur are dictated via neural input.

Both muscle and tendon are composed largely of noncontractile collagen and elastin fibers. Collagen enables a tissue to resist mechanical forces and deformation, whereas elastin composes highly elastic tissues that assist in recovery from deformation.[56]

Collagen has several mechanical and physical properties that allow it to respond to loading and deformation, permitting it to withstand high tensile stress.[92] The mechanical properties of collagen include (1) *elasticity*, which is the capability to recover normal length after elongation, (2) *viscoelasticity*, which allows for a slow return to normal length and shape after deformation, and (3) *plasticity*, which allows for permanent change or deformation. The physical properties include (1) *force-relaxation*, which indicates the decrease in the amount of force needed to maintain a tissue at a set amount of displacement or deformation over time, (2) the *creep response*, which is the ability of a tissue to deform over time while a constant load is imposed, and (3) *hysteresis*, which is the amount of relaxation a tissue has undergone during deformation and displacement. If the mechanical and physical limitations of connective tissue are exceeded, it results injury.

Unlike tendon, muscle also has active contractile components which are the actin and myosin myofilaments. Collectively the contractile and noncontractile elements determine the muscle's capability of deforming and recovering from deformation.[101]

Both the contractile and the noncontractile components appear to resist deformation when a muscle is stretched or lengthened. The percentage of their individual contribution to resisting deformation depends on the degree to which the muscle is stretched or deformed and on the velocity of deformation. The noncontractile elements are primarily resistant to the degree of lengthening, while the contractile elements limit high-velocity deformation. The greater the stretch, the more the noncontractile components contribute.[92]

Lengthening of a muscle via stretching allows for viscoelastic and plastic changes to occur in the collagen and elastin fibers. The viscoelastic changes that allow slow deformation with imperfect recovery are not permanent. However, plastic changes, although difficult to achieve, result in residual or permanent change in length due to deformation created by long periods of stretching.

The greater the velocity of deformation, the greater the chance for exceeding that tissue's capability to undergo viscoelastic and plastic change.[101]

EFFECTS OF STRETCHING ON THE KINETIC CHAIN

Joint hypomobility is one of the most frequently treated causes of pain. However, the etiology can usually be traced to faulty posture, muscular imbalances, and abnormal neuromuscular control. Once a particular joint has lost its normal arthrokinematics, the muscles around that joint attempt to minimize the stress at that involved segment. Certain muscles become tight and hypertonic to prevent additional joint translation. If one muscle becomes tight or changes its degree of activation, then synergists, stabilizers, and neutralizers have to compensate, leading to the formation of complex neuromusculoskeletal dysfunctions.

Muscle tightness and hypertonicity have a significant impact on neuromuscular control. Muscle tightness affects the normal length-tension relationships. When one muscle in a force-couple becomes tight or hypertonic, it alters the normal arthrokinematics of the involved joint. This affects the synergistic function of the entire kinetic chain, leading to abnormal joint stress, soft-tissue dysfunction, neural compromise, and vascular/lymphatic stasis. These result in alterations in recruitment strategies and stabilization strength. Such compensations and adaptations affect neuromuscular efficiency throughout the kinetic chain. Decreased neuromuscular control alters the activation sequence or firing order of different muscles involved, and a specific movement is disturbed. Prime movers may be slow to activate, while synergists, stabilizers, and neutralizers substitute and become overactive. When this is the case, new joint stresses will be encountered.[19] For example, if the psoas is tight or hyperactive, then the gluteus maximus will have decreased neural drive. If the gluteus maximus (prime mover during hip extension) has decreased neural drive, then synergists (hamstrings),

stabilizers (erector spinae), and neutralizers (piriformis) substitute and become overactive (synergistic dominance). This creates abnormal joint stress and decreased neuromuscular control during functional movements.

Muscle tightness also causes reciprocal inhibition. Increased muscle spindle activity in a specific muscle will cause decreased neural drive to that muscle's functional antagonist. This alters the normal force-couple activity, which in turn affects the normal arthrokinematics of the involved segment. For example, if a patient has tightness or hypertonicity in the psoas, then the functional antagonist (gluteus maximus) can be inhibited (decreased neural drive), causing decreased neuromuscular control. This in turn leads to *synergistic dominance*—the neuromuscular phenomenon that occurs when synergists compensate for a weak and/or inhibited muscle to maintain force production capabilities.[19] This process alters the normal force-couple relationships, which in turn creates a chain reaction.

IMPORTANCE OF INCREASING MUSCLE TEMPERATURE PRIOR TO STRETCHING

To most effectively stretch a muscle during a program of rehabilitation, intramuscular temperature should be increased prior to stretching.[67] Increasing the temperature has a positive effect on the ability of the collagen and elastin components within the musculotendinous unit to deform. Also, the capability of the Golgi tendon organs to reflexively relax the muscle through autogenic inhibition is enhanced when the muscle is heated. It appears that the optimal temperature of muscle to achieve these beneficial effects is 39°C, or 103°F. This increase in intramuscular temperature can be achieved either through low-intensity warm-up type exercise or through the use of various therapeutic modalities.[41,81] It is recommended that exercise be used as the primary means for increasing intramuscular temperature.

The use of cold prior to stretching has also been recommended. Cold appears to be most useful when there is some muscle guarding associated with delayed-onset muscle soreness.[74]

STRETCHING TECHNIQUES

Stretching techniques for improving flexibility have evolved over the years.[52] The oldest technique for stretching is dynamic stretching (ballistic) which makes use of repetitive bouncing motions. A second technique, known as *static stretching*, involves stretching a muscle to the point of discomfort and then holding it at that point for an extended time. This technique has been used for many years. Another group of stretching techniques known collectively as *proprioceptive neuromuscular facilitation* (PNF) techniques, involving alternating contractions and stretches, has also been recommended.[53,97] Most recently, emphasis has been on the contribution of *stretching myofascial tissue* as well as *stretching tight neural tissue* in enhancing the ability of the neuromuscular system to efficiently control movement through a full range of motion. Researchers have had considerable discussion about which of these techniques is most effective for improving range of motion, and no clear-cut consensus currently exists.[11,30,39,60,72,77]

Agonist Versus Antagonist Muscles

Before discussing the different stretching techniques, it is essential to define the terms *agonist muscle* and *antagonist muscle*. Most joints in the body are capable of more than one movement. The knee joint, for example, is capable of flexion and extension. Contraction of the quadriceps group of muscles on the front of the thigh causes knee extension, whereas contraction of the hamstring muscles on the back of the thigh produces knee flexion.

To achieve knee extension, the quadriceps group contracts while the hamstring muscles relax and stretch. Muscles that work in concert with one another in this manner are called synergistic muscle groups.[8] The muscle that contracts to produce a movement, in this case the quadriceps, is referred to as the agonist muscle. The muscle being stretched in response to contraction of the agonist muscle is called the antagonist muscle.[38] In this example of knee extension, the antagonist muscle would be the hamstring group. Some degree of balance in strength must exist between agonist and antagonist muscle groups. This balance is necessary for normal, smooth, coordinated movement, as well as for reducing the likelihood of muscle strain caused by muscular imbalance. Comprehension of this synergistic muscle action is essential to understanding the various techniques of stretching.

Dynamic Stretching

In dynamic stretching, repetitive contractions of the agonist muscle are used to produce quick stretches of the antagonist muscle.

Over the years, many fitness experts have questioned the safety of the dynamic stretching technique.[44,62] Their concerns have been primarily based on the idea that dynamic stretching creates somewhat uncontrolled forces within the muscle that can exceed the extensibility limits of the muscle fiber, thus producing small microtears within the musculotendinous unit.[33,34,37,66,101] Certainly this might be true in sedentary individuals or perhaps in individuals who have sustained muscle injuries.

However, many physical activities are dynamic and require a repeated dynamic contraction of the agonist muscle. The antagonist contracting eccentrically to decelerate the dynamic stretching of the antagonist muscle before engaging in this type of activity should allow the muscle to gradually adapt to the imposed demands and reduce the likelihood of injury. Because dynamic stretching is more functional, it should be integrated into a reconditioning program during the later stages of healing when appropriate.

A progressive velocity flexibility program has been proposed that takes the patient through a series of stretching exercises where the velocity of the stretch and the range of lengthening are progressively controlled.[73] The stretching exercises progress from slow static stretching, to slow, short, end-range stretching, to slow, full-range stretching, to fast, short, end-range stretching, and to fast, full-range stretching. This program allows the patient to control both the range and the speed with no assistance from a therapist.

Static Stretching

The static stretching technique is another extremely effective and widely used technique of stretching.[48] This technique involves stretching a given antagonist muscle passively by placing it in a maximal position of stretch and holding it there for an extended time. Recommendations for the optimal time for holding this stretched position vary, ranging from as little as 3 seconds to as much as 60 seconds.[45] Several studies have indicated that holding a stretch for 15–30 seconds is the most effective for increasing muscle flexibility.[6,58,61] Stretches lasting longer than 30 seconds seem to be uncomfortable. A static stretch of each muscle should be repeated three or four times. A static stretch can be accomplished by using a contraction of the agonist muscle to place the antagonist muscle in a position of stretch. A passive static stretch requires the use of body weight, assistance from a therapist or partner, or use of a T-bar, primarily for stretching the upper extremity.

Proprioceptive Neuromuscular Facilitation Stretching Techniques

Proprioceptive neuromuscular facilitation techniques were first used by physical therapists for treating patients who had various neuromuscular disorders.[53] More recently, PNF stretching exercises have increasingly been used as a stretching technique for improving flexibility.[24,64,71,73]

There are three different PNF techniques used for stretching: contract-relax, hold-relax techniques, and slow-reversal-hold-relax.[91] All three techniques involve some combination of alternating isometric or isotonic contractions and relaxation of both agonist and antagonist muscles (a 10-second pushing phase followed by a 10-second relaxing phase).

Contract-relax is a stretching technique that moves the body part passively into the agonist pattern. The patient is instructed to push by contracting the antagonist (the muscle that will be stretched) isotonically against the resistance of the therapist. The patient then relaxes the antagonist while the therapist moves the part passively through as much range as possible to the point where limitation is again felt. This contract-relax technique is beneficial when range of motion is limited by muscle tightness.

Hold-relax is very similar to the contract-relax technique. It begins with an isometric contraction of the antagonist (the muscle that will be stretched) against resistance, combined with light pressure from the therapist to produce maximal stretch of the antagonist. This technique is appropriate when there is muscle tension on one side of a joint and may be used with either the agonist or the antagonist.

Slow reversal-hold-relax, also occasionally referred to as the *contract-relax-agonist-contraction* technique, begins with an isotonic contraction of the agonist, which often limits range of motion in the agonist pattern, followed by an isometric contraction of the antagonist (the muscle that will be stretched) during the push phase. During the relax phase, the antagonists are relaxed while the agonists are contracting, causing movement in the direction of the agonist pattern and thus stretching the antagonist. This technique, like the contract-relax and hold-relax, is useful for increasing range of motion when the primary limiting factor is the antagonistic muscle group.

PNF stretching techniques can be used to stretch any muscle in the body.[13,26,27,32,64,66,71,74,77,91] PNF stretching techniques are perhaps best performed with a partner, although they may also be done using a wall as resistance.

Comparing Stretching Techniques

Although all three stretching techniques discussed to this point have been demonstrated to effectively improve flexibility, there is still considerable debate as to which technique produces the greatest increases in range of movement.[7] The dynamic technique is recommended for any one who is involved in dynamic activity, despite its potential for causing muscle soreness in the sedentary physically active individual. In individuals, it is unlikely that dynamic stretching will result in muscle soreness.

Static stretching is perhaps the most widely used technique. It is a simple technique and does not require a partner. A fully nonrestricted range of motion can be attained through static stretching over time.

Much research has been done comparing dynamic and static stretching techniques for the improvement of flexibility. Static and dynamic stretching appear to be equally effective in increasing flexibility, and there is no significant difference between the two.[34] However, much of the literature states that with static stretching there is less danger of exceeding the extensibility limits of the involved joints because the stretch is more controlled. Most of the literature indicates that dynamic stretching is apt to cause muscular soreness, especially in sedentary individuals, whereas static stretching generally does not cause soreness and is commonly used in injury rehabilitation of sore or strained muscles.[33,98] Static stretching is likely a much safer stretching technique, especially for sedentary individuals. However, because many physical activities involve dynamic movement, stretching in a warm-up should begin with static stretching followed by dynamic stretching, which more closely resembles the dynamic activity. PNF stretching techniques are capable of producing dramatic increases in range of motion during one stretching session. Studies comparing static and PNF stretching suggest that PNF stretching is capable of produc-

ing greater improvement in flexibility over an extended training period.[42,43,74] The major disadvantage of PNF stretching is that a partner is usually required to assist with the stretch, although stretching with a therapist or partner can have some motivational advantages.

How long increases in muscle flexibility can be sustained once stretching stops is debatable.[36,84,102] One study indicated that a significant loss of flexibility was evident after only 2 weeks.[102] It was recommended that flexibility can be maintained by engaging in stretching activities at least once a week. However, to see improvement in flexibility, stretching must be done three to five times per week.[35]

SPECIFIC STRETCHING EXERCISES

Chapters 25–32 will include various stretching exercises that may be used to improve flexibility at specific joints or in specific muscle groups throughout the body. The stretching exercises shown in Figure 10-4 provide examples which may be done statically; they may also be done with a partner using a PNF technique. There are many possible variations to each of these exercises.[50] The patient may also perform static stretching exercises using a stability ball (Fig. 10-5). The exercises selected are those that seem to be the most effective for stretching of various muscle groups. Table 10-2 provides a list of guidelines and precautions for stretching.

Stretching Neural Structures

The therapist should be able to differentiate between tightness in the musculotendinous unit and abnormal neural tension. The patient should perform both active and passive multiplanar movements that create tension in the neural structures that are exacerbating pain, limiting range of motion, and increasing neural symptoms, including numbness and tingling.[19] For example, the straight leg raising test not only applies pressure to the sacroiliac joint cell but also may indicate a problem in the sciatic nerve (Fig. 10-6C). Internally rotating and adducting the hip increases the tension on the neural structures in both the greater sciatic notch and the intervertebral foramen. An exacerbation of pain from 30° to 60° indicates some sciatic nerve involvement. If dorsiflexing the ankle with maximum straight leg raising increases the pain, then the pain is likely due to some nerve root (L3-4, S1-3) or sciatic nerve irritation. Figure 10-6 shows the assessment and stretching positions for neural tension in the median, radial, and sciatic nerves as well as the vertebral nerve roots in the spine.

SOFT TISSUE MOBILIZATION TECHNIQUES

Following injury, soft tissue loses some of its ability to tolerate the demands of functional loading. A major part of the management of soft-tissue dysfunction lies in promoting soft-tissue adaptation to restore the tissue's ability to cope with functional

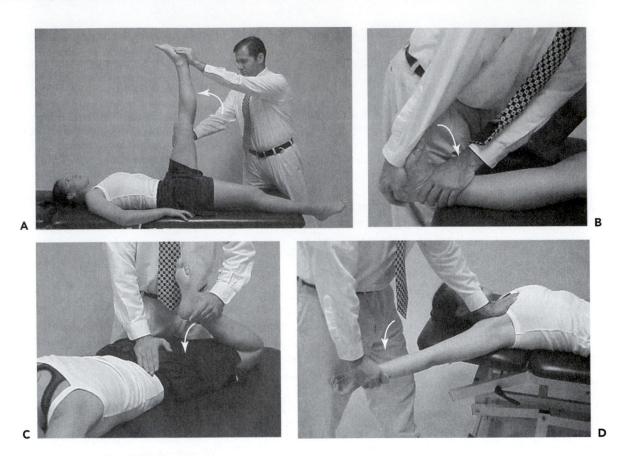

FIGURE 10-4

Examples of stretching exercises that may be done statically or using a PNF technique.
A, hamstrings. **B,** Ankle plantarflexors. **C,** Quadriceps. **D,** Glenohumeral joint extensors.

loading.[49] Specific soft-tissue mobilization involves specific, graded, and progressive application of force using physiologic, accessory, or combined techniques either to promote collagen synthesis, orientation, and bonding in the early stages of the healing process or to promote changes in the viscoelastic response of the tissue in the later stages of healing. Soft-tissue mobilization should be applied in combination with rehabilitation regimes to restore the kinetic control of the tissue.[49]

A variety of manual therapy techniques used in injury rehabilitation could be classified as soft-tissue mobilization.

Myofascial Release Stretching

Myofascial release is a term that refers to a group of techniques used for the purpose of relieving soft tissue from the abnormal grip of tight fascia.[52] It is essentially a form of stretching that has been reported to have significant impact in treating a variety of conditions. Some specialized training is necessary for the therapist to understand specific techniques of myofascial release. It is also essential to have an in-depth understanding of the fascial system.

Fascia is a type of connective tissue that surrounds muscles, tendons, nerves, bones, and organs. It is essentially continuous from head to toe and is interconnected in various sheaths or planes. Fascia is composed primarily of collagen along with some elastic fibers. During movement the fascia must stretch and move freely. If there is damage to the fascia owing to injury, disease, or inflammation, it will not only affect local adjacent structures but may also affect areas far removed from the site of the injury. Thus it may be necessary to release tightness both in the area of injury and in distant areas. It will tend to soften and release in response to gentle pressure over a relatively long period of time.

Myofascial release has also been referred to as soft-tissue mobilization. Soft-tissue mobilization should not be confused with joint mobilization, although it must be emphasized that the two are closely related.[52] Joint mobilization is used to restore normal joint arthrokinematics, and specific rules exist regarding direction of movement and joint position based on the shape of the articulating surfaces (see Chapter 16). Myofascial restrictions are considerably more unpredictable and may occur in many different planes and directions. Myofascial treatment is based on localizing the restriction and moving into the direction of the restriction, regardless of whether that follows the arthrokinematics of a nearby joint. Thus, myofascial manipulation is considerably more subjective and relies heavily

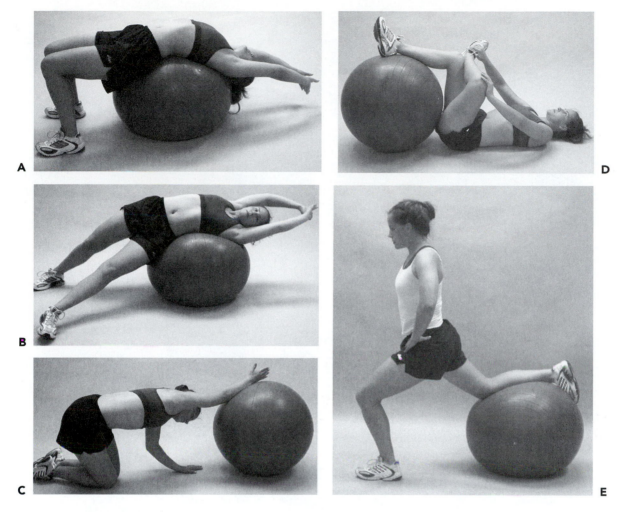

FIGURE 10-5

Static stretching using a stability ball. **A,** Back extension. **B,** Side stretch. **C,** Latissimus dorsi stretch. **D,** Piriformis stretch. **E,** Quadriceps stretch.

TABLE 10-2

Guidelines and Precautions for Sound Stretching Program[85,86]

- Warm up using a slow jog or fast walk before stretching vigorously.
- To increase flexibility, the muscle must be stretched within pain tolerances and tissue healing limitations to attain functional or normal range of motion.
- Stretch only to the point where tightness or resistance to stretch, or perhaps some discomfort, is felt. Stretching should not be painful.[1]
- Increases in range of motion will be specific to whatever muscle or joint is being stretched.
- Exercise caution when stretching muscles that surround painful joints. Pain is an indication that something is wrong and should not be ignored.
- Avoid overstretching the ligaments and capsules that surround joints.
- Exercise caution when stretching the low back and neck. Exercises that compress the vertebrae and their discs can cause damage.
- Stretching from a seated rather than a standing position takes stress off the low back and decreases the chances of back injury.
- Be sure to continue normal breathing during a stretch. Do not hold your breath.
- Static and PNF techniques are most often recommended for individuals who want to improve their range of motion.
- Dynamic stretching should be done only by those who are already flexible or accustomed to stretching, and should be done only after static stretching.

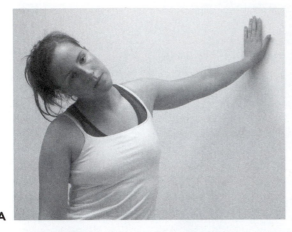
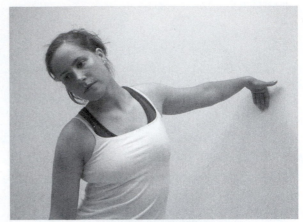
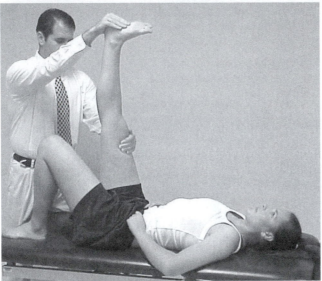
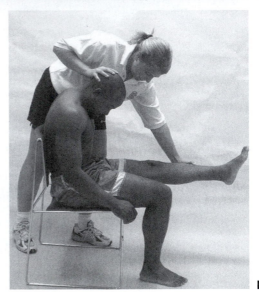

FIGURE 10-6

Neural tension stretches. **A**, Median nerve. **B**, Radial nerve. **C**, Sciatic nerve. **D**, Slump position.

on the experience of the therapist. Myofascial manipulation focuses on large treatment areas, whereas joint mobilization focuses on a specific joint. Releasing myofascial restrictions over a large treatment area can have a significant impact on joint mobility. The progression of the technique is to work from superficial fascial restrictions to deeper restriction. Once more superficial restrictions are released, the deep restrictions can be located and released without causing any damage to superficial tissue. Joint mobilization should follow myofascial release and will likely be more effective once soft-tissue restrictions are eliminated.

As extensibility is improved in the myofascia, elongation and stretching of the musculotendinous unit should be incorporated. In addition, strengthening exercises are recommended to enhance neuromuscular reeducation, which helps promote new, more efficient movement patterns. As freedom of movement improves, postural reeducation may help ensure the maintenance of the less restricted movement patterns.

Generally, acute cases tend to resolve in just a few treatments. The longer a condition has been present, the longer it will take to resolve. Occasionally, dramatic results will occur immediately after treatment. It is usually recommended that treatment be done at least three times per week.

Myofascial release can be done manually by a therapist or by the patient stretching using a bioform foam roller. Figure 10-7 shows examples of stretching using the foam roller.

STRAIN-COUNTERSTRAIN TECHNIQUE

Strain-counterstrain is an approach to decreasing muscle tension and guarding that may be used to normalize muscle function. It is a passive technique that places the body in a position of greatest comfort, thereby relieving pain.[1,51]

In this technique, the therapist locates "tender points" on the patient's body that correspond to areas of dysfunction in

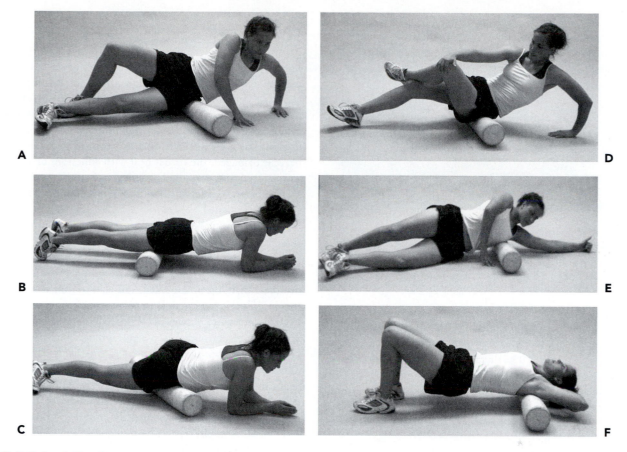

FIGURE 10-7

Myofascial release stretching using a foam roller. **A,** Tensor fascia latae. **B,** Quadriceps.
C, Adductors. **D,** Piriformis. **E,** Teres minor. **F,** Thoracic spine.

specific joints or muscles that are in need of treatment.[88] These tender points are not located in or just beneath the skin, as are many acupuncture points, but instead are deeper in muscle, tendon, ligament, or fascia. They are characterized by tense, tender, edematous spots on the body. They are 1 cm or less in diameter, with the most acute points being 3 mm in diameter, although they may be a few centimeters long within a muscle. There can be multiple points for one specific joint dysfunction. Points might be arranged in a chain, and they are often found in a painless area opposite the site of pain and/or weakness.[51]

The therapist monitors the tension and level of pain elicited by the tender point while moving the patient into a position of ease or comfort. This is accomplished by markedly shortening the muscle.[88] When this position of ease is found, the tender point is no longer tense or tender. When this position is maintained for a minimum of 90 seconds, the tension in the tender point and in the corresponding joint or muscle is reduced or cleared. By slowly returning to a neutral position, the tender point and the corresponding joint or muscle remains pain-free with normal tension. For example, with neck pain and/or tension headaches, the tender point may be found on either the front or back of the athlete's neck and shoulders. The therapist will have the patient lie on his/her back and will gently

and slowly bend the patient's neck until that tender point is no longer tender. After holding that position for 90 seconds, the therapist gently and slowly returns the neck to its resting position. When that tender point is pressed again, the patient should notice a significant decrease in pain there (Fig. 10-8).[88]

The physiologic rationale for the effectiveness of the strain-counterstrain technique can be explained by the stretch reflex.[2] The stretch reflex was discussed in detail in the section "The Neurophysiologic Basis of Stretching." When a muscle is placed in a stretched position, impulses from the muscle spindles create a reflex contraction of the muscle in response to stretch. With strain-counterstrain, the joint or muscle is placed not in a position of stretch but instead in a slack position. Thus muscle spindle input is reduced and the muscle is relaxed, allowing for a decrease in tension and pain.[2]

POSITIONAL RELEASE THERAPY

Positional release therapy is based on the strain-counterstrain technique. The primary difference between the two is the use of a facilitating force (compression) to enhance the effect of the positioning.[15,16]

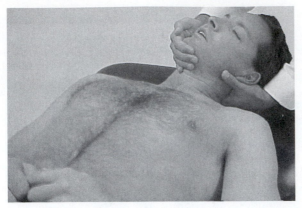

FIGURE   10-8

Strain/counterstrain technique. The body part is placed in a position of comfort for 90 seconds and then slowly moved back to a natural position.

Like strain-counterstrain, PRT is an osteopathic mobilization technique in which the body part is moved into a position of greatest relaxation.[31] The therapist finds the position of greatest comfort and muscle relaxation for each joint with the help of movement tests and diagnostic tender points. Once located, the tender point is maintained with the palpating finger at a subthreshold pressure. The patient is then passively placed in a position that reduces the tension under the palpating finger producing a subjective reduction in tenderness as reported by the patient. This specific position is adjusted throughout the 90-second treatment period. It has been suggested that maintaining contact with the tender point during the treatment period exerts a therapeutic effect.[15,16] This technique is one of the most effective and gentle methods for the treatment of acute and chronic musculoskeletal dysfunction (Fig. 10-9).[80]

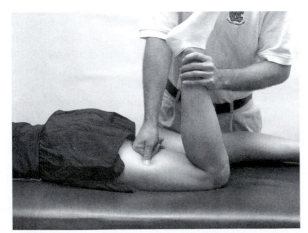

FIGURE   10-9

The positional release technique places the muscle in a position of comfort with the finger or thumb exerting submaximal pressure on a tender point.

ACTIVE RELEASE TECHNIQUE

Active release technique (ART) is a relatively new type of manual therapy that has been developed to correct soft-tissue problems in muscle, tendon, and fascia caused by the formation of fibrotic adhesions that result from acute injury, repetitive or overuse injuries, constant pressure, or tension injuries.[57] When a muscle, tendon, fascia, or ligament is torn (strained or sprained) or a nerve is damaged, the tissues heal with adhesions or scar tissue formation rather than the formation of brand new tissue. Scar tissue is weaker, less elastic, less pliable, and more pain-sensitive than healthy tissue.

These fibrotic adhesions disrupt the normal muscle function, which in turn affects the biomechanics of the joint complex and can lead to pain and dysfunction. ART provides a way to diagnose and treat the underlying causes of cumulative trauma disorders that, left uncorrected, can lead to inflammation, adhesions, fibrosis, and muscle imbalances. All of these can result in weak and tense tissues, decreased circulation, hypoxia, and symptoms of peripheral nerve entrapment, including numbness, tingling, burning, and aching.[59] ART is a deep-tissue technique used for breaking down scar tissue/adhesions and restoring function and movement.[57] In the ART, the therapist first locates through palpation those adhesions in the muscle, tendon, or fascia that are causing the problem. Once these are located, the therapist traps the affected muscle by applying pressure or tension with the thumb or finger over these lesions in the direction of the fibers. Then the patient is asked to actively move the body part such that the musculature is elongated from a shortened position while the therapist continues to apply tension to the lesion (Fig. 10-10). This should be repeated three to five times per treatment session. By breaking up the adhesions, the technique improves the athlete's condition by softening and stretching the scar tissue, resulting in increased range of motion, increased strength, and improved circulation, which optimizes healing. Treatments tend to be uncomfortable during the movement phases as the scar tissue or adhesions tear apart.[57] This is temporary and subsides almost immediately after the treatment. An important part of ART is for the patient to heed the therapist's recommendations regarding activity modification, stretching, and exercise.

MASSAGE

Massage is a mechanical stimulation of the tissues by means of rhythmically applied pressure and stretching (Fig. 10-11).[75] Over the years, many claims have been made relative to the therapeutic benefits of massage, but few are based on well-controlled, well-designed studies. Therapists have used massage to increase flexibility and coordination as well as to increase pain threshold; to decrease neuromuscular excitability in the muscle being massaged; to stimulate circulation, thus improving energy transport to the muscle; to facilitate healing and restore

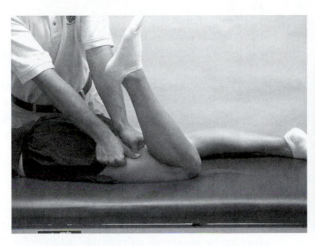
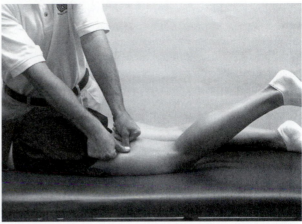

FIGURE 10-10

Active release technique. The muscle is elongated from a shortened position while static pressure is applied to the tender point.

joint mobility; and to remove lactic acid, thus alleviating muscle cramps.[75]

How these effects can be accomplished is determined by the specific approaches used with massage techniques and how they are applied. Generally the effects of massage are either *reflexive* or *mechanical*. The effect of massage on the nervous system will differ greatly according to the method employed, the pressure exerted, and the duration of applications. Through the reflex mechanism, sedation is induced. Slow, gentle, rhythmical, and superficial *effleurage* may relieve tension and soothe, rendering the muscles more relaxed. This indicates an effect on sensory and motor nerves locally and some central nervous system response. The mechanical approach seeks to make mechanical or histological changes in myofascial structures through direct force applied superficially.[75]

Among the massage techniques used by therapists are the following[75]:

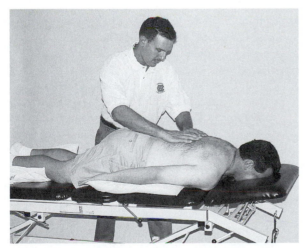

FIGURE 10-11

Massage can be an extremely effective soft-tissue mobilization technique.

1. *Hoffa massage*—the classic form of massage, strokes include effleurage, petrissage, percussion or tapotement, and vibration.
2. *Friction massage*—used to increase the inflammatory response, particularly in case of chronic tendinitis or tenosynovitis.
3. *Acupressure*—massage of acupuncture and trigger points, used to reduce pain and irritation in anatomical areas known to be associated with specific points.
4. *Connective tissue massage*—a stroking technique used on layers of connective tissue, a relatively new form of treatment in this country, primarily affecting circulatory pathologies.
5. *Myofascial release*—used for the purpose of relieving soft tissue from the abnormal grip of tight fascia.
6. *Rolfing*—a system devised to correct inefficient structure by balancing the body within a gravitational field through a technique involving manual soft-tissue manipulation.
7. *Trager*—attempts to establish neuromuscular control so that more normal movement patterns can be routinely performed.

SUMMARY

- Flexibility is the ability of the neuromuscular system to allow for efficient movement of a joint or a series of joints smoothly through a full range of motion.
- Flexibility is specific to a given joint, and the term *good flexibility* implies that there are no joint abnormalities restricting movement.
- Flexibility can be limited by muscles and tendons and their fascia, joint capsules or ligaments, fat, bone structure, skin, or neural tissue.
- *Passive range of motion* refers to the degree to which a joint can be passively moved to the end points in the range of

motion. *Active range of motion* refers to movement through the midrange of motion resulting from active contraction.

- Measurement of joint flexibility is accomplished through the use of a goniometer or an inclinometer.
- An agonist muscle is one that contracts to produce joint motion, while the antagonist muscle is stretched with contraction of the agonist.
- Increases in flexibility can be attributed to neurophysiologic adaptations involving the stretch reflex and associated muscle spindles and Golgi tendon organs, changes in the viscoelastic and plastic properties of muscle, adaptations and changes in the kinetic chain, and alterations in intramuscular temperature.
- Dynamic, static, and PNF techniques have all been used as stretching techniques for improving flexibility.
- Stretching of tight neural structures and myofascial release stretching are also used to reestablish a full range of motion.
- Strain-counterstrain is a passive technique that places a body part in a position of greatest comfort to decrease muscle tension and guarding, and to relieve pain.
- PRT is similar to strain-counterstrain. Pressure is maintained on a tender point with the body part in a position of comfort for 90 seconds.
- ART is a deep-tissue technique used for breaking down scar tissue and adhesions and restoring function and movement.
- Massage is the mechanical stimulation of tissue by means of rhythmically applied pressure and stretching. It allows the therapist, as a health care provider, to help a patient overcome pain and relax through the application of the therapeutic massage techniques.

REFERENCES

1. Alexander KM. Use of strain-counterstrain as an adjunct for treatment of chronic lower abdominal pain. *Phy Ther Case Rep* 2(5):205–208, 1999.
2. Allerheiliger W. Stretching and warm-up. In: Baechle T, ed. *Essentials of strength training and conditioning*. Champaign, IL, Human Kinetics, 2000.
3. Alter M. *The science of flexibility*. Champaign, IL, Human Kinetics, 2004.
4. Andersen JC. Stretching before and after exercise: Effect on muscle soreness and injury risk. *J Athl Train* 40(3):218–220, 2005.
5. Armiger P. Preventing musculotendinous injuries: A focus on flexibility. *Athletic Ther Today* 5(4):20, 2000.
6. Bandy WD, Irion JM. The effect of time of static stretch on the flexibility of the hamstring muscles. *Phys Ther* 74:845–852, 1994.
7. Bandy WD, Irion JM, Briggler M. The effect of static stretch and dynamic range of motion training on the flexibility of the hamstring muscles. *J Orthop Sports Phys Ther* 27(4):295, 1998.
8. Basmajian J. *Therapeutic Exercise*, 4th ed. Baltimore, MD, Lippincott Williams & Wilkins, 1984.

9. Behm DG, Bambury A, Cahill F, Power K. Effect of acute static stretching on force, balance, reaction time, and movement time. *Med Sci Sports Exerc.* 36(8):1397–1402, 2004.
10. Blanke D. Flexibility. In: Mellion, M, ed. *Sports Medicine Secrets*. Philadelphia, PA, Hanley & Belfus, 2002.
11. Boyle P. The effect of static and dynamic stretching on muscle force production. *J Sports Sci* 22(3):273–274, 2004.
12. Burke DG, Culligan CJ, Holt LE. The theoretical basis of proprioceptive neuromuscular facilitation. *J Strength Cond Res* 14(4):496–500, 2000.
13. Carter AM, Kinzey SJ, Chitwood LF, Cole JL. Proprioceptive neuromuscular facilitation decreases muscle activity during the stretch reflex in selected posterior thigh muscles. *J Sport Rehab* 9(4):269–278, 2000.
14. Chaitlow L. *Muscle Energy Techniques*. Philadelphia, PA, Churchill Livingstone, 2001.
15. Chaitlow L. *Positional Release Techniques (Advanced Soft Tissue Techniques)*. Philadelphia, PA, Churchill Livingstone, 2002.
16. Chaitlow L. Positional release techniques in the treatment of muscle and joint dysfunction. *Clin Bull Myofascial Ther* 3(1):25–35, 1998.
17. Chalmers G. Re-examination of the possible role of golgi tendon organ and muscle spindle reflexes in proprioceptive neuromuscular facilitation muscle stretching. *Sports Biomechanics* 3(1):159–183, 2004.
18. Chapman EA, deVries HA, Swezey R. Joint stiffness: Effect of exercise on young and old men. *J Gerontol* 27:218, 1972.
19. Clark M. *Integrated Training for the New Millennium*. Calabasas, CA, National Academy of Sports Medicine, 2001.
20. Condon SA, Hutton RS. Soleus muscle EMG activity and ankle dorsiflexion range of motion from stretching procedures. *Phys Ther* 67:24–30, 1987.
21. Corbin C, Fox K. Flexibility: The forgotten part of fitness. *J Phys Educ* 16(6):191, 1985.
22. Corbin C, Noble L. Flexibility. *J Phys Educ Rec Dance* 51:23, 1980.
23. Corbin C, Noble L. Flexibility: A major component of physical fitness. In Cundiff DE, ed. *ImplemEntation of Health Fitness Exercise Programs*. Reston, VA, American Alliance for Health, Physical Education, Recreation and Dance, 1985.
24. Cornelius W, Jackson A. The effects of cryotherapy and PNF on hip extensor flexibility. *J Athlet Train* 19:183–184, 1984.
25. Cornelius WL, Hagemann RW Jr, Jackson AW. A study on placement of stretching within a workout. *J Sports Med Phys Fitness* 28(3):234, 1988.
26. Cornelius WL. *PNF and Other Flexibility Techniques*. Arlington, VA, Computer Microfilm International. (microfiche; 20 fr.), 1986.

27. Cornelius WL. Two effective flexibility methods. *Athlet Train* 16(1):23, 1981.

28. Cornwell A. The acute effects of passive stretching on active musculotendinous stiffness. *Med Sci Sports Exerc* 29(5), 281, 1997.

29. Couch J. *Runners World Yoga Book*. Mountain View, CA, World, 1982.

30. Cross KM, Worrell TW. Effects of a static stretching program on the incidence of lower extremity musculotendinous strains. *J Athlet Train* 34(1):11, 1999.

31. D' Ambrogio K, Roth G. *Positional Release Therapy: Assessment and Treatment of Musculoskeletal Dysfunction*. St. Louis, Mosby/Year Book, 1996.

32. Decoster L, Cleland J, Altieri C. The effects of hamstring stretching on range of motion: A systematic literature review. *J Orthop Sports Phys Ther* 3(6):377–387, 2005.

33. deVries H. *Physiology of Exercise for Physical Education and Athletics*. Dubuque, IA, Brown, 1986.

34. deVries HA. Evaluation of static stretching procedures for improvement of flexibility. *Res Q* 3:222–229, 1962.

35. De Deyne PG. Application of passive stretch and its implications for muscle fibers. *Phys Ther* 81(2):819–827, 2001.

36. DePino GM, Webright WG, Arnold BL. Duration of maintained hamstring flexibility after cessation of an acute static stretching protocol. *J Athlet Train* 35(1):56, 2000.

37. Entyre BR, Abraham LD. Ache-reflex changes during static stretching and two variations of proprioceptive neuromuscular facilitation techniques. *Electroencephalogr Clin Neurophysiol* 63:174–179, 1986.

38. Entyre BR, Abraham LD. Antagonist muscle activity during stretching: A paradox reassessed. *Med Sci Sports Exerc* 20:285–289, 1988.

39. Entyre BR, Lee EJ. Chronic and acute flexibility of men and women using three different stretching techniques. *Res Q Exerc Sport* 59:222–228, 1988.

40. Fowles JR, Sale DG, MacDougall JD. Reduced strength after passive stretch of the human plantarflexors. *J Appl Physiol* 89(3):1179–1188, 2000.

41. Funk D, Swank AM, Adams KJ, Treolo D. Efficacy of moist heat pack application over static stretching on hamstring flexibility. *J Strength Cond Res* 15(1):123–126, 2001.

42. Godges JJ, MacRae H, Longdon C, et al. The effects of two stretching procedures on hip range of motion and joint economy. *J Orthop Sports Phys Ther* 11:350–357, 1989.

43. Gribble P, Prentice W. Effects of static and hold-relax stretching on hamstring range of motion using the Flex-Ability LE 1000. *J Sport Rehab* 8(3):195, 1999.

44. Hedrick A. Dynamic flexibility training. *Strength Cond J* 22(5):33–38, 2000.

45. Herling J. It's time to add strength training to our fitness programs. *J Phys Educ Program* 79:17, 1981.

46. Holt LE, Pelham TW, Burke DG. Modifications to the standard sit-and-reach flexibility protocol. *J Athlet Train* 34(1):43, 1999.

47. Hubley CL, Kozey JW, Stanish WD. The effects of static stretching exercises and stationary cycling on range of motion at the hip joint. *J Orthop Sports Phys Ther* 6:104–109, 1984.

48. Humphrey LD. Flexibility. *J Phys Educ Rec Dance* 52:41, 1981.

49. Hunter G. Specific soft tissue mobilization in the management of soft tissue dysfunction. *Manual Ther* 3(1):2–11, 1998.

50. Ishii DK. Flexibility strexercises for co-ed groups. *Scholastic Coach* 45:31, 1976.

51. Jones L. *Strain-Counterstrain*. Boise, ID, Jones Strain-CounterStrain, 1995.

52. Keirns M, ed. *Myofascial Release in Sports Medicine*. Champaign, IL, Human Kinetics, 2000.

53. Knott M, Voss P. *Proprioceptive Neuromuscular Facilitation*, 3rd ed. New York, NY, Harper & Row, 1985.

54. Kokkonen JE, Caroline, Nelson, Arnold G. Chronic stretching improves sport specific skills. *Med Sci Sports Exerc* 29(5):67, 1997.

55. Kokkonen JN, Nelson AG, Arnall DA. Acute stretching inhibits strength endurance. *Med Sci Sports Exerc* 35(5):s11, 2001.

56. Kubo K, Kanehisa H, Fukunaga T. Effect of stretching training on the viscoelastic properties of human tendon structures in vivo. *J Appl Physiol* 92(2):595–601, 2002.

57. Leahy M. Improved treatments for carpal tunnel and related syndromes. *Chiropractic Sports Med* 9(1):6, 1995.

58. Lentell G, Hetherington T, Eagan J, et al. The use of thermal agents to influence the effectiveness of a low-load prolonged stretch. *J Orthop Sports Phys Ther* 5:200–207, 1992.

59. Liemohn W. Flexibility and muscular strength. *J Phys Educ Rec Dance* 59(7):37, 1988.

60. Louden KL, Bolier CE, Allison KA, et al. Effects of two stretching methods on the flexibility and retention of flexibility at the ankle joint in runners. *Phys Ther* 65:698, 1985.

61. Madding SW, Wong JG, Hallum A. Effects of duration of passive stretching on hip abduction range of motion. *J Orthop Sports Phys Ther* 8:409–416, 1987.

62. Mann D, Whedon C. Functional stretching: Implementing a dynamic stretching program. *Athletic Ther Today* 6(3):10–13, 2001.

63. Marek S, Cramer J, Fincher L. Acute effects of static and proprioceptive neuromuscular facilitation stretching on muscle strength and power output. *J Athlet Traini* 40(2):94–103, 2005.

64. Markos PD. Ipsilateral and contralateral effects of proprioceptive neuromuscular facilitation techniques on hip motion and electromyographic activity. *Phys Ther* 59: 1366–1373, 1979.

65. McAtee R. *Facilitated Stretching*. Champaign, IL, Human Kinetics, 1999.

66. Moore M, Hutton R. Electromyographic investigation of muscle stretching techniques. *Med Sci Sports Exerc* 12:322–329, 1980.

67. Murphy P. Warming up before stretching advised. *Phys Sports Med* 14(3):45, 1986.

68. Nelson R. An update on flexibility. *Natl Strength Cond Assoc* 27(1),10–16, 2005.

69. Norris C. *Flexibility Principles and Practices*. London, A&C Black, 1995.

70. Power K, Behm D, Cahill F, Carroll M, Young W. An acute bout of static stretching: Effects on force and jumping performance. *Med Sci Sports Exerc* 36(8):1389–1396, 2004.

71. Prentice WE, Kooima E. The use of PNF techniques in rehabilitation of sport-related injury. *Athlet Train* 21(1): 26–31, 1986.

72. Prentice WE. A comparison of static stretching and PNF stretching for improving hip joint flexibility. *J Athlet Train* 18:56–59, 1983.

73. Prentice WE. A review of PNF techniques—implications for athletic rehabilitation and performance. *Forum Medicum* (51):1–13, 1989.

74. Prentice WE. An electromyographic analysis of heat or cold and stretching for inducing muscular relaxation. *J Orthop Sports Phys Ther* 3:133–140, 1982.

75. Prentice W. Sports massage. In: Prentice W, ed. *Therapeutic Modalities in Sports Medicine and Athletic Training*. St. Louis, McGraw-Hill, 2003.

76. Rasch P. *Kinesiology and Applied Anatomy*. Philadelphia, Lea & Febiger, 1989.

77. Sady SP, Wortman M, Blanke D. Flexibility training: Ballistic, static, or proprioceptive neuromuscular facilitation? *Arch Phys Med Rehab* 63:261–263, 1982.

78. Sapega AA, Quedenfeld T, Moyer R, et al. Biophysical factors in range-of-motion exercise. *Phys Sports Med* 9(12):57, 1981.

79. Schilling BK, Stone MH. Stretching: Acute effects on strength and power performance. *Strength Cond J* 22(1): 44, 2000.

80. Schiowitz S. Facilitated positional release. *J Am Osteopath Assoc* 90(2):145–146, 151–55, 1990.

81. Shellock F, Prentice WE. Warm-up and stretching for improved physical performance and prevention of sport related injury. *Sports Med* 2:267–278, 1985.

82. Shindo M, Harayama H, Kondo K, et al. Changes in reciprocal Ia inhibition during voluntary contraction in man. *Exp Brain Res* 53:400–408, 1984.

83. Siatras T, Papadopoulos G, Maeletzi D, Gerodimos V, Kellis P. Static and dynamic acute stretching effect on gymnasts' speed in vaulting. *Ped Ex Sci* 15, 383–391, 2003.

84. Spernoga SG, Uhl TL, Arnold BL, Gansneder BM. Duration of maintained hamstring flexibility after a one-time, modified hold-relax stretching protocol. *J Athlet Train* 36(1):44–48, 2001.

85. St. George F. *The Stretching Handbook: Ten Steps to Muscle Fitness*. Roseville, IL, Simon & Schuster. 1997.

86. Stamford B. A stretching primer. *Physician and Sports Medicine* 22(9):85–86, 1994.

87. Stone J. Myofascial release. *Athlet Ther Today* 5(4):34–35, 2000.

88. Stone J. Strain-counterstrain. *Athlet Ther Today* 5(6):30, 2000.

89. Surburg P. Flexibility/range of motion. In: Winnick JP, ed. *The Brockport Physical Fitness Training Guide*. Champaign, IL, Human Kinetics, 1999.

90. Surburg P. Flexibility training program design. In: Miller P, ed. *Fitness Programming and Physical Disability*. Champaign, IL, Human Kinetics, 1995.

91. Tanigawa MC. Comparison of the hold relax procedure and passive mobilization on increasing muscle length. *Phys Ther* 52:725, 1972.

92. Taylor DC, Brooks DE, Ryan JB. Viscoelastic characteristics of muscle: passive stretching versus muscular contractions. *Med Sci Sports Exerc* 29(12):1619–1624, 1997.

93. Thacker S, Gilchrist J, Stroup D. The impact of stretching on sports injury risk: A systematic review of the literature. *Med Sci Sports Exerc* 36(3):371–378, 2004.

94. Tobias M, Sullivan JP. *Complete Stretching*. New York, NY, Knopf, 1992.

95. Van Hatten B. Passive versus active stretching. *Phys Ther* 85(1):80; author reply 80–81, 2005.

96. van Mechelen P. Prevention of running injuries by warm-up, cool-down, and stretching. *Am J Sports Med* 21(5):711–719, 1993.

97. Voss DE, Lonta MK, Myers GJ. *Proprioceptive Neuromuscular Facilitation: Patterns and Techniques*, 3rd ed. Philadelphia, PA, Lippincott Williams & Wilkins, 1985.

98. Wessel J, Wan A.. Effect of stretching on intensity of delayed-onset muscle soreness. *J Sports Med* 2:83–87, 1984.

99. Winters MV, Blake CG, Trost J. Passive versus active stretching of hip flexor muscles in subjects with limited hip extension: A randomized clinical trial. *Phys Ther* 84(9):800–807, 2004.

100. Worrell T, Smith T, Winegardner J. Effect of hamstring stretching on hamstring muscle performance. *J Orthop Sports Phys Ther* 20(3):154–159, 1994.

101. Zachewski J. Flexibility for sports. In: Sanders b, ed. *Sports Physical Therapy*. Norwalk, CT, Appleton & Lange, 1990.

102. Zebas CJ, Rivera ML. Retention of flexibility in selected joints after cessation of a stretching exercise program. In: Dotson CO, Humphrey JH, eds. *Exercise Physiology: Current Selected Research Topics*. New York, AMS Press, 1985.

CHAPTER 11

Impaired Neuromuscular Control: Reactive Neuromuscular Training

Michael L. Voight and Gray Cook

OBJECTIVES

After completing this chapter, the therapist should be able to do the following:

- Explain why neuromuscular control is important in the rehabilitation process.
- Define and discuss the importance of proprioception in the neuromuscular control process.
- Define and discuss the different levels of central nervous system (CNS) motor control and the neural pathways responsible for the transmission of afferent and efferent information at each level.
- Define and discuss the two motor mechanisms involved with interpreting afferent information and coordinating an efferent response.
- Develop a rehabilitation program that uses various techniques of neuromuscular control exercises.

WHAT IS NEUROMUSCULAR CONTROL AND WHY IS IT IMPORTANT?

The basic goal in rehabilitation is to enhance one's ability to function within the environment and to perform the specific activities of daily living (ADL). The entire rehabilitation process should be focused on improving the functional status of the patient. The concept of functional training is not new. In fact, functional training has been around for many years. It is widely accepted that in order to get better at a specific activity, or to get stronger for an activity, one must practice that specific activity. Therefore, the functional progression for return to ADL can be defined as breaking the specific activities down into a hierarchy and then performing them in a sequence that allows for the acquisition or reacquisition of that skill.

From a historical perspective, the rehabilitation process following injury has focused upon the restoration of muscular strength, endurance, and joint flexibility without any consideration of the role of the neuromuscular mechanism. This is a common error in the rehabilitation process. We cannot assume that clinical programs alone using traditional methods will lead to a safe return to function. Limiting the rehabilitation program to these traditional programs alone often results in an incomplete restoration of ability and quite possibly leads to an increased risk of reinjury.

The overall objective of the functional exercise program is to return the patient to the preinjury level as quickly and as safely as possible. Specific training activities should be designed to restore both dynamic stability about the joint and specific ADL skills. In order to accomplish this objective, a basic tenet of exercise physiology is employed. The SAID (specific adaptations to imposed demands) principle states that the body will adapt to the stress and strain placed upon it.[130] Patients cannot succeed in ADL if they have not been prepared to meet all of the demands of their specific activity.[130] Reactive neuromuscular training (RNT) is not intended to replace traditional rehabilitation but rather to help bridge the gap left by traditional rehabilitation in a complementary fashion via proprioceptive and balance training in order to promote a more functional return to activity.[130] The main objective of the RNT program is to facilitate the unconscious process of interpreting and integrating the peripheral sensations received by the CNS into appropriate motor responses.

TERMINOLOGY: WHAT DO WE REALLY NEED TO KNOW?

Success in skilled performance depends upon how effectively the individual detects, perceives, and uses relevant sensory information. Knowing exactly where our limbs are in space and how much muscular effort is required to perform a particular action is critical for the successful performance in all activities requiring intricate coordination of the various body parts. Fortunately, information about the position and movement of various body parts is available from the peripheral receptors located in and around the articular structures.

About the normal healthy joint, both static and dynamic stabilizers serve to provide support. The role of the capsuloligamentous tissues in the dynamic restraint of the joint has been well established in the literature.[2,3,19,33,45–50,110] Although the primary role of these structures is mechanical in nature by providing structural support and stabilization to the joint, the capsuloligamentous tissues also play an important sensory role by detecting joint position and motion.[33,34,105] Sensory afferent feedback from the receptors in the capsuloligamentous structures projects directly to the reflex and cortical pathways, thereby mediating reactive muscle activity for dynamic restraint.[2,3,33,34,67] The efferent motor response that ensues from the sensory information is called neuromuscular control. Sensory information is sent to the CNS to be processed, and appropriate motor activities are executed.

PHYSIOLOGY OF PROPRIOCEPTION

Although there has been no definitive definition of proprioception, Beard et al. described proprioception as consisting of three similar components: (1) a static awareness of joint position, (2) kinesthetic awareness, and (3) a closed-loop efferent reflex response required for the regulation of muscle tone and activity.[7] From a physiologic perspective, proprioception is a specialized variation of the sensory modality of touch. Specifically defined, proprioception is the cumulative neural input to the CNS from mechanoreceptors in the joint capsules, ligaments, muscles, tendons, and skin.

A rehabilitation program that addresses the need for restoring normal joint stability and proprioception cannot be constructed until one has a total appreciation of both the mechanical and sensory functions of the articular structures.[12] Knowledge of the basic physiology of how these muscular and joint mechanoreceptors work together in the production of smooth controlled coordinated motion is critical in developing a rehabilitation training program. This is because the role of the joint musculature extends beyond absolute strength and the capacity to resist fatigue. Simply restoring mechanical restraints or strengthening the associated muscles neglects the smooth coordinated neuromuscular controlling mechanisms required for joint stability.[12] The complexity of joint motion necessitates synergy and synchrony of muscle firing patterns, thereby permitting proper joint stabilization, especially during sudden changes in joint position, which is common in functional activities. Understanding these relationships and functional implications will allow the clinician greater variability and success in returning patients safely back to their playing environment.

Sherrington first described the term proprioception in the early 1900s when he noted the presence of receptors in the joint capsular structures that were primarily reflexive in nature.[105] Since that time, mechanoreceptors have been morphohistologically identified about the articular structures in both animal and human models. Mechanoreceptors are specialized end organs that function as biological transducers that can convert the mechanical energy of physical deformation (elongation, compression, and pressure) into action nerve potentials yielding proprioceptive information.[45] Although receptor discharge varies according to the intensity of the distortion, mechanoreceptors can also be based upon their discharge rates. Quickly adapting receptors cease discharging shortly after the onset of a stimulus, while slowly adapting receptors continue to discharge while the stimulus is present.[21,33,45] About the healthy joint, quickly adapting receptors are responsible for providing conscious and unconscious kinesthetic sensations in response to joint movement or acceleration, while slowly adapting mechanoreceptors provide continuous feedback and thus proprioceptive information relative to joint position.[21,45,71]

Once stimulated, mechanoreceptors are able to adapt. With constant stimulation, the frequency of the neural impulses decreases. The functional implication is that mechanoreceptors detect change and rates of change, as opposed to steady-state conditions.[104] This input is then analyzed in the CNS for joint position and movement.[139] The status of the articular structures is sent to the CNS so that information regarding static versus dynamic conditions, equilibrium versus disequilibrium, or biomechanical stress and strain relations can be evaluated.[129,130] Once processed and evaluated, this proprioceptive information becomes capable of influencing muscle tone, motor execution programs, and cognitive somatic perceptions or kinesthetic awareness.[92] Proprioceptive information also protects the joint from damage caused by movement exceeding the normal physiologic range of motion and helps to determine the appropriate balance of synergistic and antagonistic forces. All of this information helps to generate a somatosensory image within the CNS. Therefore, the soft tissues surrounding a joint serve a double purpose: they provide biomechanical support to the bony partners making up the joint, keeping them in relative anatomic alignment, and through an extensive afferent neurologic network, they provide valuable proprioceptive information.

Before 1970s, articular receptors in the joint capsule were held primarily responsible for joint proprioception.[104] Since then there has been considerable debate as to whether muscular and articular mechanoreceptors interact. As originally described, the articular mechanoreceptors were located primarily on the parts of the joint capsule that are stretched the most when the joint is moved. This led investigators to believe that these receptors were primarily responsible for perception of joint motion. Skoglund found individual receptors that were active at very specific locations in the range of limb movement (e.g., from 150 to 180° of joint angle for a particular cell).[113] Another cell would fire at a different set of joint angles. By integrating the information, the CNS could "know" where the limb was in space by detecting which receptors were active. The problem with this theory is that several studies have shown that the majority of the capsular receptors only respond at the extremes of the range of motion or during other situations when a strong stimulus is imparted onto the structures such as distraction or compression.[21,43,48,49] Furthermore, other studies have found that the nature of the firing pattern is dependent on whether the movement is active or passive.[14] In addition, the mechanoreceptor firing is dependent on the direction of motion from the joint.[115] The fact that the firing pattern of the joint receptors is dependent on factors other than simple position sense has seriously challenged the thought that the articular mechanoreceptors alone are the means by which the system determines joint position.

A more contemporary viewpoint is that muscle receptors play a more important role in signaling joint position.[25,42] There are two main types of muscle receptors that provide complementary information about the state of the muscles. The muscle spindle is located within the muscle fibers and is most active when the muscle is stretched. The Golgi tendon organ (GTO) is located in the junction between the muscle and the tendon and is most active when the muscle contracts.

Muscle Spindle

The muscle spindle consists of three main components: small muscle fibers called intrafusal fibers that are innervated by the gamma efferent motor neurons, and types Ia and II afferent neurons (Fig. 11-1). The intrafusal fibers are made up of two types, bag and chain fibers, the polar ends of which provide a tension on the central region of the spindle, called the equatorial region. The sensory receptors located here are sensitive to the length of the equatorial region when the spindle is stretched. The major neurologic connection to this sensory region is the Ia afferent fiber, whose output is related to the length of the equatorial region (position information) as well as to the rate of change in length of this region (velocity information). The spin-

dle connects to the alpha motor neurons for the same muscle, providing excitation to the muscle when it is stretched.

There has been a great deal of controversy about what the spindle actually signals to the CNS.[36] A major conceptual problem in the past was that the output of the Ia afferent that presumably signals stretch or velocity is related to two separate factors.[102] First, Ia output is increased by the elongation of the overall muscle via elongation of the spindle as a whole. However, the Ia output is also related to the stretch placed on the equatorial region by the intrafusal fibers by the gamma motor neurons. Therefore, the CNS would have difficulty in interpreting changes in the Ia output as being due to changes in the overall muscle length with a constant gamma motor neuron activity, changes in gamma motor neuron activity with a constant muscle length, or perhaps changes in both.[102] Another problem was presented by Gelfan and Carter, who suggested that there was no strong evidence that the Ia afferent fibers actually sent their information to the primary sensory cortex.[39] Because of these factors, it was widely held that the muscle spindle was not important for the conscious perception of movement or position.

Goodwin et al. were the first to refute this viewpoint.[43] They found as much as 40° of misalignment of arm that had vibration applied to the biceps tendon.[43] The vibration of the tendon produces a small, rapid, alternating stretch and release of the tendon, which affects the muscle spindle and distorts the output of the Ia afferents from the spindles located in the vibrated muscle. The interpretation was that the vibration distorted the Ia information coming from the same muscle, which led to a misperception of the limb's position. Others have found the same results when applying vibration to a muscle tendon.[97,108,109] This information supports the idea that the muscle spindle is important in providing information to the CNS about limb position and velocity of movement.

Golgi Tendon Organ

The GTOs are tiny receptors located in the junction where the muscle "blends into" the tendon. They are ideally located

FIGURE 11-1

The anatomy of muscle receptors: Muscle spindle and Golgi tendon organ. (Reproduced, with permission, from Shumway-Cook A, Woollacott M. Physiology of motor control. In: Shumway-Cook A, Woollacott M, eds. *Motor Control: Theory and Practical Applications.* Baltimore, MD, Williams & Wilkins, 1995, p. 53.)

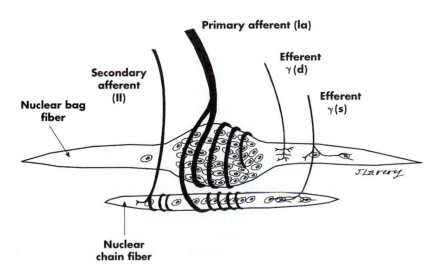

Primary afferent (Ia)

Secondary afferent (II)

Efferent γ(d)

Efferent γ(s)

Nuclear bag fiber

Nuclear chain fiber

to provide information about the tension within the muscles because they lie in series with the muscle force-producing contractile elements. The GTO has been shown to produce an inhibition of the muscle in which it is located when a stretch to the active muscle is produced. The fact that a stretch force near the physiologic limit of the muscle was required to induce the tendon organ to fire led to the speculation that this receptor was primarily a protective receptor that would prevent the muscle from contracting so forcibly that it would rupture the tendon. Houk and Henneman[62] and Stuart et al.[119] have provided a more precise understanding of the sensitivity of the GTOs. Anatomic evidence reveals that each organ is connected to only a small group (3–25) of muscle fibers, not to the entire muscle as had been previously suspected. Therefore, the GTO appears to be in a good position to sense the tensions produced in a limited number of individual motor units, not in the whole muscle. Houk and Henneman determined that the tendon organs could respond to forces of less than 0.1 G.[62] Therefore, the GTOs are very sensitive detectors for active tension in localized portions of a muscle, in addition to having a protective function.

It is most likely that the muscle and joint receptors work complementary to one another in this complex afferent system, with each modifying the function of the other.[15,46] An important concept is that any one of the receptors in isolation from the others is generally ineffective in signaling information about the movements of the body. The reason for this is that the various receptors are often sensitive to a variety of aspects of body motion at the same time. For example, the GTOs probably cannot signal information about movement, because they cannot differentiate between the forces produced in a static contraction and the same forces produced when the limb is moving.[102] Although the spindle is sensitive to muscle length, it is also sensitive to the rate of change in length (velocity) and to the activity in the intrafusal fibers that are known to be active during contractions. Therefore, the spindle confounds information about the position of the limb and the level of contraction of the muscle. The joint receptors are sensitive to joint position, but their output can be affected by the tensions applied and by the direction of movement.

Because both the articular and muscle receptors have well-described cortical connections to substantiate a central role in proprioception, some have suggested that the CNS combines and integrates the information in some way to resolve the ambiguity in the signals produced by any one of the receptors.[102,138] Producing an ensemble of information by combining the various separate sources could enable the generation of less ambiguous information about movement.[36] Therefore, the sensory mechanoreceptors may represent a continuum rather than separate distinct classes of receptor.[105] This concept is further illustrated by research that demonstrated a relationship between the muscle spindle sensory afferent and joint mechanoreceptors.[18] McCloskey has also demonstrated a relationship between the cutaneous afferent and joint mechanoreceptors.[78] These studies suggest a complex role for

the joint mechanoreceptors in smooth, coordinated, and controlled movement.

Neural Pathways

Information generated and encoded by the mechanoreceptors in the muscle tendon units is projected upward via specialized pathways toward the cortex, where it is further analyzed and integrated with other sensory inputs.[99] Proprioceptive information is relayed to the cerebral cortex via one of two major ascending systems, the dorsal column and the spinothalamic tract. Both of these pathways involve three orders of neurons and three synapses in transmitting sensory input from the periphery to the cortex. The primary afferent, which is connected to the peripheral receptor, synapses with a second neuron in the spinal cord or lower brain, depending upon the type of sensation. Before reaching the cerebral cortex, all sensory information passes through an important group of nuclei located in the area of the brain called the *diencephalon*. It is within this group of more than 30 nuclei, collectively called the *thalamus*, that neurophysiologists consider the initial stages of sensory integration and perceptual awareness to begin. Therefore, the second neuron then conveys the information to the thalamus where it synapses with the third and final neuron in the area of the thalamus called the *ventroposterolateral* area. The thalamus achieves these functions by "gating out" irrelevant sensory inputs and directing those that are relevant to an impending or ongoing action toward primary sensory areas within the cortex. The sensory pathways finally terminate in the primary sensory areas located in different regions of the cortex. It is at this point that we become consciously aware of the sensations.

The final perception of what is occurring in the environment around us is achieved after all of these sensations are integrated and then interpreted by the association areas that lie adjacent to the various primary sensory areas associated with the different types of sensory input. With the assistance of memory, objects seen or felt can be interpreted in a meaningful way. The dorsal column plays an important role in motor control because of its speed in transmission. In order for proprioception to play a protective role through reflex muscle splinting, the information must be transmitted and processed rapidly. The heavily myelinated and wide-diameter axons within this system transmit at speeds of 80–100 m/sec. This characteristic facilitates rapid sampling of the environment, which enhances the accuracy of motor actions about to be executed and of those already in progress. By comparison, nociceptor transmission occurs at a rate of about 1 m/sec. Thus proprioceptive information may play a more significant role than pain in the prevention of injuries.

In contrast to the transmission properties associated with the dorsal column system, neurons that make up the spinothalamic tract are small in diameter (some of which are unmyelinated) and conduct slowly (1–40 m/sec). The four spinocerebellar tracts also convey important proprioceptive information from the neuromuscular receptors to the cerebellum. Unlike

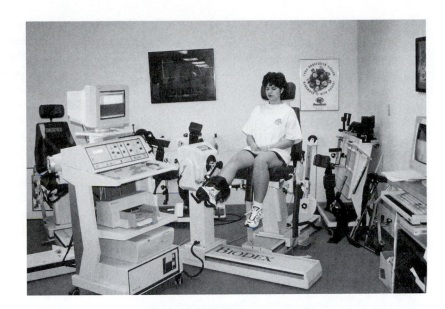

FIGURE 11 - 2

Open-chain proprioceptive testing using the Biodex dynamometer.

the dorsal column, these pathways do not synapse in either the thalamus or cerebral cortex. As a result, the proprioceptive information conveyed by the spinocerebellar tracts does not lead to conscious perceptions of limb position. The afferent sources are believed to contribute to kinesthesia.

ASSESSMENT OF JOINT PROPRIOCEPTION

Assessment of proprioception is valuable for identifying proprioceptive deficits. If deficiencies in proprioception can be clinically diagnosed in a reliable manner, a clinician would know when and if a problem exists and when the problem has been corrected.[130] There are several ways to measure or assess proprioception about a joint. From an anatomic perspective, histological studies can be conducted to identify mechanoreceptors within the specific joint structures. Neurophysiologic testing can assess sensory thresholds and nerve conduction velocities. From a clinical perspective, proprioception can be assessed by measuring the components that make up the proprioceptive mechanism: kinesthesia (perception of motion) and joint position sensibility (perception of joint position).

Measuring either the angle or time threshold to detection of passive motion can assess kinesthetic sensibility. With the subject seated, the patient's limb is mechanically rotated at a slow constant angular velocity (2°/second). With passive motion, the capsuloligamentous structures come under tension and deform the mechanoreceptors located within. The mechanoreceptor deformation is converted into an electrical impulse, which is then processed within the CNS. Patients are instructed to stop the lever arm movement as soon as they perceive motion. Depending on which measurement is used, either the time to detection or degrees of angular displacement is recorded.

Joint position sense is assessed through the reproduction of both active and passive joint repositioning. The examiner places the limb at a preset target angle and holds it there for a

minimum of 10 seconds to allow the patient to mentally process the target angle. Following this, the limb is returned to the starting position. The patient is asked to either actively reproduce or stop the device when passive repositioning of the angle has been achieved (Fig. 11-2). The examiner measures the ability of an individual to accurately reproduce the preset target angle position. The angular displacement is recorded as the error in degrees from the preset target angle. Active angle reproduction measures the ability of both the muscle and capsular receptors while passive repositioning primarily measures the capsular receptors. With both tests of proprioception, the patient is blindfolded during testing to eliminate all visual cueing. In patients with unilateral involvement, the contralateral uninjured limb can serve as an external control for comparison.

The main limitation to current proprioceptive testing is that either time/angle threshold to detection of passive motion does not provide an assessment of the unconscious reflex arc believed to provide dynamic joint stability. The assessment of reflex capabilities is usually performed by measuring the latency of muscular activation to involuntary perturbation through electromyogram (EMG) interpretation of firing patterns of those muscles crossing the respective joint (Fig. 11-3).[132] The ability to quantify the sequence of muscle firing can provide a valuable tool for the assessment of asynchronous neuromuscular activation patterns following injury.[74,140] A delay or lag in the firing time of the dynamic stabilizers about the joint can result in recurrent joint subluxation and joint deterioration.

PROPRIOCEPTION AND MOTOR CONTROL

The efferent response that is produced as the result of the proprioceptive afferent input is termed *neuromuscular control*. In general, there are two motor control mechanisms involved in the interpretation of afferent information and coordinating an efferent response. One of the ways in which motor control is

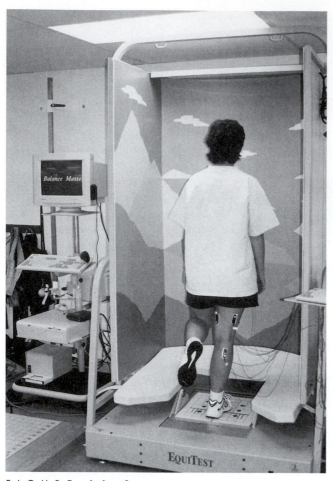

F I G U R E   1 1 - 3

EMG assessment of reflex muscle firing as a result of perturbation on the NeuroCom EquiTest.

achieved relies heavily on the concept that sensory feedback information is used to regulate our movements. This is a more traditional viewpoint of motor control. The closed-loop system of motor control emphasizes the essential role of the reactive or sensory feedback in the planning, execution, and modification of action. The closed-loop systems involve the processing of feedback against a reference of correctness, the determination of error, and a subsequent correction.[102] The feedback mechanism of motor control relies on the numerous reflex pathways in an attempt to continuously adjust ongoing muscle activation.[29,102] The receptors for the feedback supplied to closed-loop systems are the eyes, vestibular apparatus, joint receptors, and muscle receptors. One important point to note about the closed-loop system of feedback motor control is that this loop requires a great deal of time in order for a stimulus to be processed and yield a response. Rapid actions do not provide sufficient time for the system to (1) generate an error, (2) detect the error, (3) determine the correction, (4) initiate the correction, and (5) correct the movement before a rapid movement is completed.[102] The best example of this concept is demonstrated by the left jab of former boxing champion Muhammad Ali. The move-

ment itself was approximately 40 msec, yet visually detecting an aiming error and correcting it during the same movement should require approximately 200 msec.[102] The movement is finished before any correction can begin. Therefore, closed-loop feedback control models seem to have their greatest strength in explaining movements that are very slow in time or that have very high movement accuracy requirements.[102]

In contrast, a more contemporary theory emphasizes the open-loop system, which focuses upon the a priori generation of action plans in anticipation of movement produced by a central executor somewhere in the cerebral cortex.[102] The ability to prepare the muscles prior to movement is called pretuning or feed-forward motor control. The springlike qualities of a muscle can be exploited (through preactivation) by the CNS in anticipation of movements and joint loads. This concept has been termed feed-forward motor control, in which prior sensory feedback (experience) concerning a task is fed forward to preprogram muscle activation patterns.[62] Vision serves an important feed-forward function by preparing the motor system in advance of the actual movement. Preactivated muscles can provide quick compensation for external loads and are critical for dynamic joint stability. Researchers have shown that corrections for rapid changes in body position can occur far more rapidly (30–80 msec) than the closed-loop latencies of 200 msec that have previously been reported.[27,63,69] Therefore, the motor control system operates with a feed-forward mode in order to send some signals "ahead of" the movement that (1) readies the system for the upcoming motor command and/or (2) readies the system for the receipt of some particular kind of feedback information.

Anticipatory muscle activity contributes to the dynamic restraint system in several capacities. By increasing muscle activation levels in anticipation of an external load, the stiffness properties of the entire muscular unit can be increased.[84] Stiffness is one of the measures used to describe the characteristics of elastic materials. It is defined in terms of the amount of tension increase required to increase the length of the object by a certain amount. From a mechanical perspective, muscle stiffness can be defined as the ratio of the change of force to the change in length. If a spring is very stiff, a great deal of tension is needed to increase its length by a given amount; for a less stiff spring, much less tension is required. When a muscle is stretched, the change in tension is instantaneous, just as the change in length of a spring. An increase in tension would offset the perturbation or deforming force and bring the system back to its original position. Research has demonstrated that the muscle spindle is responsible for the maintenance of the muscle stiffness when the muscle is stretched, so that it can still act as a spring in the control of an unexpected perturbation.[60,63,86] Therefore, stiff muscles can resist stretching episodes more effectively, have greater tone, and provide a more effective dynamic restraint to joint displacement. Increased muscle stiffness can improve the stretch sensitivity of the muscle spindle system while at the same time reduce the electromechanical delay required to develop muscle tension.[28,60,80,84] Heightening the stretch sensitivity can improve the reactive capabilities of the muscle by providing additional sensory feedback.[28]

CNS MOTOR CONTROL INTEGRATION

It has already been established that the CNS input provided by the peripheral mechanoreceptors as well as the visual and vestibular receptors is integrated by the CNS to generate a motor response. In addition to the many conscious modifications that can be made while movement is in progress, certain neural connections within the CNS contribute to the modification of movements in progress by providing sensory information at a subconscious level. The influence of some of these reflexive loops is limited to local control of muscle force, but others are capable of influencing force levels in muscle groups quite distant from those originally stimulated. These longer reflex loops are therefore capable of modifying movements to a much larger extent than the shorter reflex loops that are confined to single segments within the spinal cord.

In general, the CNS response falls under three categories or levels of motor control: spinal reflexes, brainstem processing, and cognitive cerebral cortex program planning. The goal of the rehabilitation process is to retrain the altered afferent pathways in order to enhance the neuromuscular control system. To accomplish this goal, the objective of the rehabilitation program should be to hyperstimulate the joint and muscle receptors in order to encourage maximal afferent discharge to the respective CNS levels.[12,71,122,126,127]

First Level of Integration: The M1 Reflex

When faced with an unexpected load, the first reflexive muscle response is a burst of EMG activity that occurs after between 30 and 50 msec. The afferent fibers of the mechanoreceptors synapse with the spinal interneurons and produce a reflexive facilitation or inhibition of the motor neurons.[122,126,131] The monosynaptic stretch reflex or M1 reflex is one of the most rapid reflexes underlying limb control (Fig. 11-4). The latency or time of this response is very short because it involves only one synapse and the information has a relatively short distance to travel. Unfortunately, the muscle response is brief, which does not result in much added contraction of the muscle. The M1 short reflex loop is most often called into play when minute adjustments in muscle length are needed. The stimulus of small muscular stretches occurs during postural sways or when our limbs are subjected to unanticipated loads. Therefore, this mechanism is responsible for regulating motor control of the antagonistic and synergistic patterns of muscle contraction.[99] These adjustments are necessary when misalignment exists between intended muscle length and actual muscle length. This misalignment is most likely to occur in situations where unexpected forces are applied to the limb or the muscle begins to fatigue. In the situation of involuntary and undesirable lengthening of muscles about a joint during conditions of abnormal stress, the short M1 loop

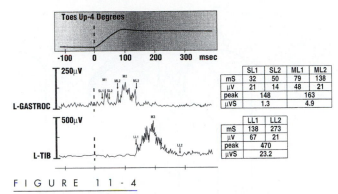

FIGURE 11-4

CNS levels of integration: Short- and long-loop postural reflexes. The components of the evoked postural assessment: (M1) myotatic reflex (SL1, SL2), (M2) segmental (polysynaptic) response (ML1, ML2), and (M3) long-loop response (LL1, LL2) involving the brainstem, cortex, and ascending and descending spinal pathways (SL = short loop, ML = medium loop, LL = long loop). (Reproduced, with permission, from NeuroCom International, Clackamas, OR.)

must provide for reflex muscle splinting in order to prevent injury from occurring. The M1 reflex occurs at an unconscious level and is not affected by outside factors. These responses can occur simultaneously to control limb position and posture. Because they can occur at the same time, are in parallel, are subconscious, and are without cortical interference, they do not require attention and are thus automatic.

There are two important short reflex loops acting in the body: the stretch reflex and the gamma reflex loop. The stretch reflex (Fig. 11-5) is triggered when the length of an extrafusal muscle fiber is altered, causing the sensory endings within the muscle spindle to be mechanically deformed. Once deformed, these sensory endings fire, sending nerve impulses into the spinal cord via an afferent sensory neuron located just outside the spinal cord. The information from the Ia afferent is sent essentially to two places: to the alpha motor neurons in the same muscle and also upward to the various sensory regions in the cerebral cortex. As soon as these impulses reach the spinal cord, they are transferred to alpha motor neurons that innervate the very same muscle that houses the activated muscle spindles. The loop time, or the time from the initial stretch until the extrafusal fibers are increased in their innervation, is about 30–40 msec in humans.[102] Stimulation of the muscle spindle ceases when the muscle contracts, because the spindle fibers, which lie parallel to the extrafusal fibers, return to their original length. It is through the operation of this reflex that we are able to continuously alter muscle tone and/or make subtle adjustments in muscle length during movement. These latter adjustments may be in response to external factors producing unexpected loads or forces on the moving limbs.

For example, consider what happens when an additional load is applied to an already loaded limb being held in a given position in space.[27] The muscles of the limb are set at a given

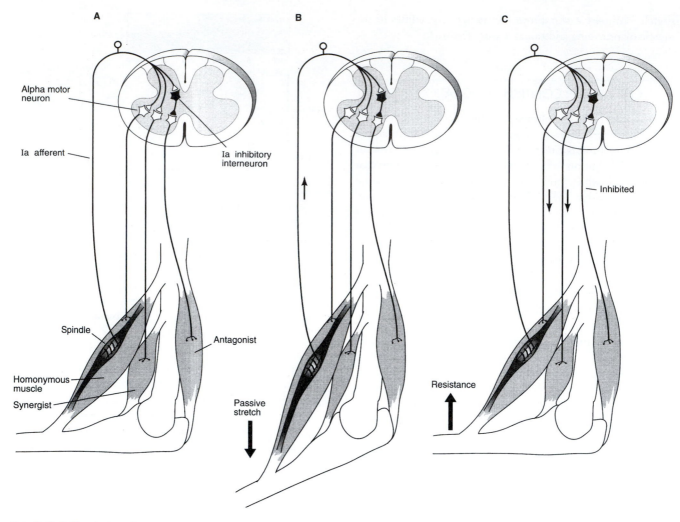

FIGURE   11-5

Excitation of the muscle spindle is responsible for the stretch reflex. **A,** Ia afferent fibers making monosynaptic excitatory connections to alpha motor neurons innervating the same muscle from which they arise and motor neurons innervating synergist muscles. They also inhibit motor neurons to antagonist muscles through an inhibitory interneuron. **B,** When a muscle is stretched, the Ia afferents increase their firing rate. **C,** This leads to contraction of the same muscle and its synergists and relaxation of the antagonist. The reflex therefore tends to counteract the stretch, enhancing the springlike properties of the muscle. (Reproduced, with permission, from Gordon J, Ghez C. Muscle receptors and stretch reflexes. In: Kandel E. et al., eds. *Principles of Neural Science*, 3rd ed. East Norwalk, CT, Appleton & Lange, 1991, p. 576.)

length, and alpha motor neurons are firing in order to maintain the desired limb position in spite of the load and gravity. Now an additional load is added to the end of the limb, causing the muscles to lengthen as the limb drops. This stretching of the extrafusal muscle fibers results in almost simultaneous stretching of the muscle spindle, which then fires and sends signals to the spinal cord and alpha motor neurons that serve the same muscle. The firing rate of these alpha motor neurons is subsequently increased, causing the muscles in the dropping limb to be further contracted, and the limb is restored to its previous position. Visual information to the stimulus of loading would also lead to increased contraction in the falling limb, but initiating the corrective response consciously would involve considerably longer delays because of additional processing at the cortical level.[27] The short-loop M1 stretch reflex response times are possible within 30–50 msec.[58] Visual-based corrections involved corrective delays on the order of 150–200 msec.[58] Given that the rapid correction is required for injury prevention, it is important that these short-loop reflex pathways are available for use.

Muscle spindles also play an important role in the ongoing control and modification of movement by virtue of their involvement in a spinal reflex loop known as the gamma reflex loop. The afferent information from the muscle spindle synapses with both the alpha and gamma motor neurons. The alpha motor neuron sends the information it receives to the muscles involved in the movements. The gamma motor neuron sends the same information back to the muscle spindle, which can be stimulated to begin firing at its polar ends. The independent innervation of the muscle spindle by the gamma motor neuron is thought to be important during muscle contractions when the intrafusal fibers of the spindle would normally be slack. Gamma activation of the spindle results in stretching of the intrafusal fibers even though the extrafusal fibers are contracting. In essence, the gamma system takes up the slack in the spindle caused by muscle contraction, thereby making corrections in minute changes in length of the muscle more quickly.

In the short-loop system of spinal control, the activity of the Ia afferent fibers is determined by two things: (1) The length and the rate of the stretch of the extrafusal muscle fibers. (2) The amount of tension in the intrafusal fibers, which is determined by the firing of the gamma efferent fibers. Both alpha and gamma motor neurons can be controlled by higher motor centers, and they are thought to be "coordinated" in their action by a process termed *alpha–gamma coactivation*.[44,98] Therefore, the output to the main body of the muscle is determined by (1) the level of innervation provided directly from higher centers and (2) the amount of added innervation provided indirectly from the Ia afferent.[102] This helps to explain how an individual can respond quickly to an unexpected event without conscious involvement of the CNS. When an unexpected event or perturbation causes a muscle to stretch, the spindle's sensory receptors are stimulated. The resulting Ia afferent firing causes a stretch reflex that will increase the activity in the main muscle, all within 40 msec. All of this activity occurs at the same level of the spinal cord as did the innervation of the muscle in the first place. Therefore, no high centers were involved in this 40-msec loop.

At this level of motor control, activities to encourage short-loop reflex joint stabilization should dominate.[12,71,110,126] These activities are characterized by sudden alterations in joint position that require reflex muscle stabilization. With sudden alterations or perturbations, both the articular and muscular mechanoreceptors will be stimulated for the production of reflex stabilization. Rhythmic stabilization exercises encourage monosynaptic cocontraction of the musculature, thereby producing a dynamic neuromuscular stabilization.[114] These exercises serve to build a foundation for dynamic stability.

Second Level of Integration: The M2 Reflex

For larger adjustments in limb and overall body position, it is necessary to involve the longer reflex loops that extend beyond single segments within the spinal cord. When the muscle spindle is stretched and the Ia afferent fibers are activated, the information is relayed to the spinal cord, where it synapses with the alpha motor neuron. Additionally, information is sent to higher levels of control, where the Ia information is integrated with other information in the sensory and motor centers in the cerebral cortex to produce a more complete response to the imposed stretch. Approximately 50–80 msec after an unexpected stimulus, there is a second burst of EMG activity (see Fig. 11-4). Because the pathways involved in these neural circuits travel to the more distant subcortical and cortical levels of the CNS to connect with structures such as the motor cortex and cerebellum within the larger projection system, the reflex requires more time or has a longer latency. Therefore, the 80-msec loop time for this activity corresponds not only to the additional distance that the impulses have to travel but also to the multiple synapses that must take place to close the circuit. Both the M1 and M2 responses are responsible for the reflex response that occurs when a tendon is tapped. An example of this occurs when the patellar tendon is tapped with a reflex hammer. The quadriceps muscle is stretched, initiating a reflex response that contracts the quadriceps and produces an involuntary extension of the lower leg.

Even though there is a time lapse for the longer-loop reflexes to take place, there are two important advantages for these reflexes. First, the EMG activity from the long-loop reflex is far stronger than that involved in the monosynaptic stretch reflex. The early short-loop monosynaptic reflex system does not result in much actual increase in force. The long-loop reflex can, however, produce enough force necessary to move the limb/joint back into a more neutral position. Second, because the long-loop reflexes are organized in a higher center, they are more flexible than the monosynaptic reflex. By allowing for the involvement of a few other sources of sensory information during the response, an individual can voluntarily adjust the size or amplitude of the M2 response for a given input to generate a powerful response when the goal is to hold the joint as firmly as possible, or to produce no response if the goal is to release under the increasing load. The ability to regulate this response allows an individual to prepare the limb to conform to different environmental demands.

Therefore, the second level of motor control interaction is at the level of the brainstem.[11,122,130] At this level, afferent mechanoreceptors interact with the vestibular system and visual input from the eyes to control or facilitate postural stability and equilibrium of the body.[12,71,122,127,130] Afferent mechanoreceptor input also works in concert with the muscle spindle complex by inhibiting antagonistic muscle activity under conditions of rapid lengthening and periarticular distortion, both of which accompany postural disruption.[92,126] In conditions of disequilibrium where simultaneous neural input exists, a neural pattern is generated that affects the muscular stabilizers, thereby returning equilibrium to the body's center of gravity.[122] Therefore, balance is influenced by the same peripheral afferent mechanism that mediates joint proprioception and is at least partially dependent upon the individual's inherent ability to integrate joint position sense with neuromuscular control.[120]

INTEGRATION OF BALANCE TRAINING: THE SECOND LEVEL OF MOTOR CONTROL

Both proprioception and balance training have been advocated to restore motor control to the lower extremity. In the clinic, the term "balance" is often used without a clear definition. It is important to remember that proprioception and balance are not the same. Proprioception is a precursor of good balance and adequate function. Balance is the process by which we control the body's center of mass with respect to the base of support, whether it is stationary or moving.

Berg has attempted to define balance in three ways: the ability to maintain a position, the ability to voluntarily move, and the ability to react to a perturbation.[9] All three of these components of balance are important in the maintenance of upright posture. Static balance refers to an individual's ability to maintain a stable antigravity position while at rest by maintaining the center of mass within the available base of support. Dynamic balance involves automatic postural responses to the disruption of the center of mass position. Reactive postural responses are activated to recapture stability when an unexpected force displaces the center of mass.[85]

Postural sway is a commonly used indicator of the integrity of the postural control system. Horak defined postural control as the ability to maintain equilibrium and orientation in the presence of gravity.[57] Researchers measure postural sway as either the maximum or the total excursion of center of pressure while standing on a forceplate. Little change is noted in healthy adults in quiet standing, but the frequency, amplitude, and total area of sway increase with advancing age or when vision or proprioceptive inputs are altered.[32,59,89,91]

In order to maintain balance, the body must make continual adjustments. Most of what is currently known about postural control is based upon stereotypical postural strategies activated in response to anteroposterior perturbation.[57,58,85] Horak and Nashner described several different strategies used to maintain balance.[58] These strategies include the ankle, hip, and stepping strategies. These strategies adjust the body's center of gravity so that the body is maintained within the base of support to prevent the loss of balance or falling. There are several factors that determine which strategy would be the most effective response to postural challenge: speed and intensity of the displacing forces, characteristics of the support surface, and magnitude of the displacement of the center of mass. The automatic postural responses can be categorized as a class of functionally organized long-loop responses that produce muscle activation that brings the body's center of mass into a state of equilibrium.[85] Each of the strategies has reflex, automatic, and volitional components that interact to match the response to the challenge.

Small disturbances in the center of gravity can be compensated by motion at the ankle. The ankle strategy repositions the center of mass after small displacements due to slow-speed perturbations, which usually occur on a large, firm, supporting surface. The oscillations around the ankle joint with normal postural sway are an example of the ankle strategy. Anterior sway of the body is counteracted by gastrocnemius activity, which pulls the body posterior. Conversely, posterior sway of the body is counteracted by contraction of the anterior tibial muscles. If the disturbance in the center of gravity is too great to be counteracted by motion at the ankle, the patient will use a hip or stepping strategy to maintain the center of gravity within the base of support. The hip strategy uses rapid compensatory hip flexion or extension to redistribute the body weight within the available base of support when the center of mass is near the edge of the sway envelope. The hip strategy is usually in response to a moderate or large postural disturbance, especially on an uneven, narrow, or moving surface. The hip strategy is often employed while standing on a bus that is rapidly accelerating. When sudden, large-amplitude forces displace the center of mass beyond the limits of control, a step is used to enlarge the base of support and redefine a new sway envelope. New postural control can then be reestablished. An example of the stepping strategy is the uncoordinated step that often follows a stumble on an unexpected or uneven sidewalk.

The maintenance of balance requires the integration of sensory information from a number of different systems: vision, vestibular, and proprioception. For most healthy adults, the preferred sense for postural control comes from proprioceptive information. Therefore, if proprioception is altered or diminished, balance will also be altered. The functional assessment of the combined peripheral, visual, and vestibular contributions to neuromuscular control can be measured with computerized balance measures of postural stability. The sensory organization test protocol is used to evaluate the relative contribution of vision, vestibular, and proprioceptive input to the control of postural stability when conflicting sensory input occurs.[85] Postural sway is assessed (NeuroCom Smart System) under six increasingly challenging conditions (Fig. 11-6). Baseline sway is recorded in quiet standing with the eyes open. The reliance on vision is evaluated by asking the patient to close the eyes. A significant increase in sway or loss of balance suggests an over-reliance on visual input.[85,107,143] Sensory integration is evaluated when the visual surround moves in concert with sway (sway-referenced vision), creating inaccurate visual input. The patient is then retested on a support surface that moves with sway (sway-referenced support), thereby reducing the quality and availability of proprioceptive input for sensory integration. With the eyes open, vision and vestibular input contribute to the postural responses. With the eyes closed, vestibular input is the primary source of information, because proprioceptive input is altered. The most challenging condition includes sway-referenced vision and sway-referenced support surface.[57,85,107]

Balance activities, both with and without visual input, will enhance motor function at the brainstem level.[11,122] It is important that these activities remain specific to the types of activities or skills that will be required of the athlete upon return to sport.[96] Static balance activities should be used as a precursor to more dynamic skill activity.[96] Static balance skills can be initiated once the individual is able to bear weight on the

Sensory Organization Test (SOT)

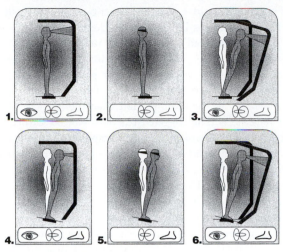

FIGURE 11-6

The sensory organization conditions integrating vestibular, visual, and somatosensory contributions to balance. (Reproduced, with permission, from NeuroCom International, Clackamas, OR.)

lower extremity. The general progression of static balance activities is to progress from bilateral to unilateral and from eyes open to eyes closed.[71,96,122,133,134] With balance training, it is important to remember that sensory systems respond to environmental manipulation. To stimulate or facilitate the proprioceptive system, vision must be disadvantaged. This can be accomplished in several ways: remove vision with either the eyes closed or blindfolded, destabilize vision by demanding hand and eye movements (ball toss) or moving the visual surround, or confuse vision with unstable visual cues that disagree with the proprioceptive and vestibular inputs (sway referencing).

In order to stimulate vision, proprioception must be either destabilized or confused. The logical progression to destabilize proprioception is to progress the balance training from a stable surface to an unstable surface such as a mini-tramp, balance board, or dynamic stabilization trainer.[71,122,130] As joint position changes, dynamic stabilization must occur for the patient to control the unstable surface (Fig. 11-7). Vision can be confused during balance training by having the patient stand on a compliant surface such as a foam mat or using a sway-referenced moving forceplate. Disadvantaging both vision and proprioceptive information can stimulate the vestibular system. This can be accomplished by several different methods. Absent vision with an unstable or compliant surface is achieved with

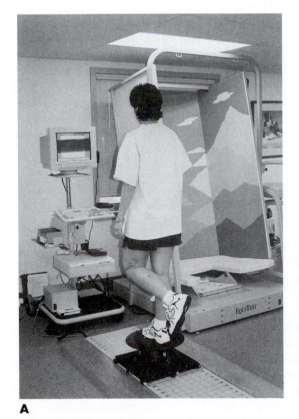

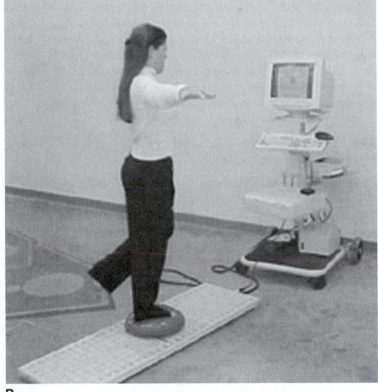

A   **B**

FIGURE 11-7

Unstable surface training on the NeuroCom Balance Master. **A,** Dynamic Stabilization Trainer. **B,** Dynadisc.

eyes-closed training on an unstable surface. Demanding hand and eye movements while on a floor mat or foam pad will destabilize both vision and proprioception. A moving surround with a moving forceplate will confuse both vision and proprioceptive input.

The patients should initially perform the static balance activities while concentrating on the specific task (position sense and neuromuscular control) to facilitate and maximize sensory output. As the task becomes easier, activities to distract the athlete's concentration (catching a ball or performing mental exercises) should be incorporated into the training program. This will help to facilitate the conversion of conscious to unconscious motor programming.[122,130] Balance training exercises should induce joint perturbations in order to facilitate reflex muscle activation.

There have been several studies to assess the effect of lower-quarter injury on standing balance. Usually the balance characteristics of the injured extremity are compared to those of the uninjured extremity. Mizuta et al. measured postural sway in two groups: a functionally stable group and a functionally unstable group, both of which had unilateral anterior cruciate ligament (ACL)-deficient knees.[83] An additional group of individuals was also studied to serve as a control group. When compared to the control group, impairment in standing balance was found in the functionally unstable group but not in the functionally stable group. These results suggest that stabiliometry was a useful tool in the assessment of functional knee stability. Both Friden et al. and Gauffin et al. demonstrated impaired standing balance during unilateral stance in individuals with chronic ACL-deficient knees.[35,38] Following injury to the lower quarter, impaired standing balance may be due to the loss of muscular coordination, which could have resulted from the loss of normal proprioceptive feedback.[4,67]

Third Level of Integration: The Voluntary Reaction—Time Response (M3)

The final response that occurs when an unexpected load is applied to the limb is the voluntary long-loop reaction or M3 response (see Fig. 11-4). Seen as the third burst of EMG activity, it is a powerful and sustained response that brings the limb back into the desired position. The latency of the M3 response is about 120–180 msec, depending upon the task and the circumstances. Information is processed at the cerebral cortex, where the mechanoreceptors interact and influence cognitive awareness of body position and movement in which motor commands are initiated for voluntary movements.[12,92,99,122] It is in this region of the primary sensory cortex that there is a high degree of spatial orientation.

The M3 response is very flexible and can be modified by a host of factors such as verbal instructions or anticipation of the incoming sensory information. The delay in the M3 response makes it sensitive to a number of stimulus alternatives. Therefore, the individual's ability to respond will require some conscious attention. Training at this level of the cerebral cortex

stimulates the conversion of conscious programming to unconscious programming. These responses have often been referred to as triggered reactions. Triggered reactions are prestructured, coordinated reactions in the same or closely related musculature that are "triggered" into action by the mechanoreceptors. The triggered reaction may bypass the information-processing centers because the reaction is stereotyped, predictable, and well practiced. These reactions have latencies from 80 to 180 msec and are far more variable than the latencies of the faster reflexes.[102] The triggered reactions can be learned and can become a more or less automatic response. The individual does not have to spend time processing a response reaction and programming; the reaction is just "triggered off" almost as if it were automatic.[101] Therefore, with training, the speed of the M3 response could be increased in order to produce a more automatic reflex response.

The appreciation of joint position at the highest or cognitive level needs to be included in the RNT program. These types of activities are initiated on the cognitive level and include programming motor commands for voluntary movement. The repetitions of these movements will maximally stimulate the conversion of conscious programming to unconscious programming.[12,71,122,126,127,130] The term for this type of training is the *forced-use paradigm*. By making a task significantly more difficult or asking for multiple tasks, we bombard the CNS with input. The CNS attempts to sort and process this overload information by opening additional neural pathways. When the individual goes back to a basic task of ADL, the task becomes easier. This information can then be stored as a central command and ultimately performed without continuous reference to the conscious mind as a "triggered response."[12,71,122,126,127] As with all training, the single greatest obstacle to motor learning is the conscious mind. We must get the conscious mind out of the act!

COORDINATING THE MUSCLE RESPONSE WITH UNEXPECTED LOADS

The relative roles of these three muscle responses depend upon the duration of the movement. As previously discussed, the quickest action occurring in the body has a movement time of about 40 msec. When this type or action occurs, the M2 response is incapable of completing or modifying the activity once it is initiated. Even the M1 response has only enough time to begin influencing the muscles near the end of the movement. As the movement time increases, there is a greater potential for the M1 and M2 responses to contribute to the intended action. Movements that take a longer time to be completed (>100 msec) will allow both the M1 and M2 responses sufficient time to contribute to all levels of the action. Only when the duration of the movement is 300 msec or longer, is there potential for the M3 long-loop response to be involved in amending the movement. Therefore, for movements that take longer than

300 msec for individuals to complete, closed-loop control is possible at several levels of integration at the same time.

WHY IS RESPONSE TIME IMPORTANT?

When an unexpected load is placed upon a joint, ligamentous damage occurs after between 70 and 90 msec unless an appropriate response ensues.[7,94,140] Therefore, reactive muscle activity must occur with sufficient magnitude in the 40–80-msec time frame after loading begins, in order to protect the capsuloligamentous structures. The closed-loop system of CNS integration may not be fast enough to produce a response to increase muscle stiffness. Simply, there is no time for the system to process the information and process the feedback about the condition. Failure of the dynamic restraint system to control these abnormal forces will expose the static structures to excessive forces. In this case, the open-loop system of anticipation becomes more important in producing the desired response. Preparatory muscle activity in anticipation of joint loading can influence the reactive muscle activation patterns. Anticipatory activation increases the sensitivity of the muscle spindles, thereby allowing the unexpected perturbations to be detected more quickly.[29]

Very quick movements are completed before feedback can be used to produce an action to alter the course of movement. Therefore, if the movement is fast enough, a mechanism like a motor program would have to be used to control the entire action, with the movement being carried out without any feedback. Fortunately, the open-loop control system allows the motor control system to organize an entire action ahead of time. In order for this to occur, previous knowledge of the following needs to be preprogrammed into the primary sensory cortex:

- The particular muscles that are needed to produce an action.
- The order in which these muscles need to be activated.
- The relative forces of the various muscle contractions.
- The relative timing and sequencing of these actions.
- The duration of the respective contractions.

In the open-loop system, movement is organized in advance by a program that sets up some kind of neural mechanism or network that is preprogrammed. A classic example of this occurs in the body as postural adjustments are made before the intended movement. When an individual raises the arm up into forward flexion, the first muscle groups to fire are not even in the shoulder girdle region. The first muscles to contract are those in the lower back and legs (approximately 80 msec before noticeable activity in the shoulder).[8] Since the shoulder muscles are linked to the rest of the body, their contraction affects posture. If no preparatory compensations in posture were made, raising the arm would shift the center of gravity forward, causing a slight loss of balance. The feed-forward motor control system takes care of this potential problem by preprogramming the appropriate postural modification first, rather than requiring the body to make adjustments after the arm begins to move.

Lee has demonstrated that these preparatory postural adjustments are not independent of the arm movement, but rather a part of the total motor pattern.[70] When the arm movements are organized, the motor instructions are preprogrammed to adjust posture first and then move the arm. Therefore, arm movement and postural control are not separate events, but rather different parts of an integrated action that raises the arm while maintaining balance. Lee showed that these EMG preparatory postural adjustments disappear when the individual leans against some type of support prior to raising the arm. The motor control system recognizes that advance preparation of postural control is not needed when the body is supported against the wall.

It is important to remember that most motor tasks are a complex blend of both open- and closed-loop operations. Therefore, both types of control are often at work simultaneously. Both feed-forward and feedback neuromuscular control can enhance dynamic stability if the sensory and motor pathways are frequently stimulated.[71] Each time a signal passes through a sequence of synapses, the synapses become more capable of transmitting the same signal.[50,56] When these pathways are "facilitated" regularly, memory of that signal is created and can be recalled to program future movements.[50,102]

REESTABLISHING PROPRIOCEPTION AND NEUROMUSCULAR CONTROL

Although the concept and value of proprioceptive mechanoreceptors have been documented in the literature, treatment techniques directed at improving their function generally have not been incorporated into the overall rehabilitation program. The neurosensory function of the capsuloligamentous structures has taken a backseat to the mechanical structural role. This is mainly due to the lack of information about how mechanoreceptors contribute to the specific functional activities and how they can be specifically activated.[37,42] Following injury to the capsuloligamentous structures, it is thought that a partial deafferentation of the joint occurs as the mechanoreceptors become disrupted. This partial deafferentation, which is secondary to injury, may be related to either direct or indirect injury. Direct trauma effects would include disruption of the joint capsule or ligaments, whereas posttraumatic joint effusion or hemarthrosis[67] can illustrate indirect effects.

Whether a direct or indirect cause, the resultant partial deafferentation alters the afferent information into the CNS and therefore the resulting reflex pathways to the dynamic stabilizing structures. These pathways are required by both the feed-forward and feedback motor control systems to dynamically stabilize the joint. A disruption in the proprioceptive pathway will result in an alteration of position and kinesthesia.[4,111] Barrack et al. showed an increase in the threshold to detect passive motion in a majority of patients with ACL rupture and functional instability.[4] Corrigan et al., who also found diminished proprioception after ACL rupture, confirmed this finding.[24]

Diminished proprioceptive sensitivity has also been shown to cause giving way or episodes of instability in the ACL-deficient knee.[13] Therefore, injury to the capsuloligamentous structures not only reduces the joint's mechanical stability but also diminishes the capability of the dynamic neuromuscular restraint system. Therefore, any aberration in joint motion and position sense will impact both the feed-forward and feedback neuromuscular control systems. Without adequate anticipatory muscle activity, the static structures may be exposed to insult unless the reactive muscle activity can be initiated to contribute to dynamic restraint.

Deficits in the neuromuscular reflex pathways may have a detrimental effect on the motor control system as a protective mechanism. Diminished sensory feedback can alter the reflex stabilization pathways, thereby causing a latent motor response when faced with unexpected forces or trauma. Beard et al. demonstrated disruption of the protective reflex arc in subjects with ACL deficiency.[7] A significant deficit in reflex activation of the hamstring muscles after a 100 newton anterior shear force in a single-legged closed-chain position was identified, as compared to the contralateral uninjured limb.[7] Beard demonstrated that the latency was directly related to the degree of knee instability; the greater the instability, the greater the latency. Other researchers found similar alterations in the muscle-firing patterns in the ACL-deficient patient.[65,116,140] Solomonow et al. found that a direct stress applied to the ACL resulted in reflex hamstring activity, thereby contributing to the maintenance of joint stability.[116] Although this response was also present in ACL-deficient knees, the reflex was significantly slower.

Although it has been demonstrated that a proprioceptive deficit occurs following knee injury, both kinesthetic awareness and reposition sense can be at least partially restored with surgery and rehabilitation. A number of studies have examined proprioception following ACL reconstruction. Barrett measured proprioception after autogenous graft repair and found that the proprioception was better than that of the average ACL-deficient patient but still significantly worse than the proprioception in the normal knee.[5] Barrett further noted that the patients' satisfaction was more closely correlated with their proprioception than with their clinical score.[5] Harter et al. could not demonstrate a significant difference in the reproduction of passive positioning between the operative and nonoperative knee at an average of 3 years after ACL reconstruction.[53] Kinesthesia has been reported to be restored after surgery as detected by the threshold to the detection of passive motion in the midrange of motion.[4] A longer threshold to the detection of passive motion was observed in the ACL-reconstructed knee compared with the contralateral uninvolved knee when tested at the end range of motion.[4] Lephart et al. found similar results in patients after either arthroscopically assisted patellar tendon autograft or allograft ACL reconstruction.[74] The importance of incorporating a proprioceptive element in any comprehensive rehabilitation program is justified based upon the results of these studies.

The effects of how surgical and nonsurgical interventions may facilitate the restoration of the neurosensory roles is unclear; however, it has been shown that ligamentous retensioning coupled with rehabilitation can restore proprioceptive sensitivity.[72] Since afferent input is altered after joint injury, proprioceptive rehabilitation must focus on restoring proprioceptive sensitivity to retrain these altered afferent pathways and enhance the sensation of joint movement. Restoration may be facilitated by (1) enhancing mechanoreceptor sensitivity, (2) increasing the number of mechanoreceptors stimulated, and (3) enhancing the compensatory sensation from the secondary receptor sites. Research should be directed toward developing new techniques to improve proprioceptive sensitivity.

Methods to improve proprioception after injury or surgery could improve function and decrease the risk for reinjury. Ihara and Nakayama demonstrated a reduction in the neuromuscular lag time with dynamic joint control following a 3-week training period on an unstable board.[65] The maintenance of equilibrium and improvement in reaction to sudden perturbations on the unstable board served to improve the neuromuscular coordination. This phenomenon was first reported by Freeman and Wyke in 1967 when they found that proprioceptive deficits could be reduced with training on an unstable surface.[33] They found that proprioceptive training through stabiliometry, or training on an unstable surface, significantly reduced the episodes of giving way following ankle sprains. Tropp et al. confirmed the work of Freeman by demonstrating that the results of stabiliometry could be improved with coordination training on an unstable board.[124] Hocherman et al. also showed an improvement in the movement amplitude on an unstable board and the weight distribution on the feet found in hemiplegic patients who received training on an unstable board.[55]

Barrett[5] has demonstrated the relationship between proprioception and function. Barrett's study suggests that limb function relies more on proprioceptive input than on strength during activity. Borsa et al. also found a high correlation between diminished kinesthesia with the single-leg hop test.[12] The single-leg hop test was chosen for its integrative measure of neuromuscular control, because a high degree of proprioceptive sensibility and functional ability is required to successfully propel the body forward and land safely on the limb. Giove et al. reported a higher success rate in returning athletes to competitive sports through adequate hamstring rehabilitation.[40] Tibone et al. and Ihara and Nakayama found that simple hamstring strengthening alone was not adequate; it was necessary to obtain voluntary or reflex-level control on knee instability in order to return to functional activities.[65,121] Walla et al. found that 95 percent of patients were able to successfully avoid surgery after ACL injury when they were able to achieve "reflex-level" hamstring control.[136] Ihara and Nakayama found that the reflex arc between stressing the ACL and hamstring contraction could be shortened with training.[65] With the use of unstable boards, the researchers were able to successfully decrease the reaction time. Since afferent input is altered after joint injury, proprioceptive sensitivity to retrain these altered afferent pathways is critical to shorten the time lag of muscular reaction in order to counteract the excessive strain on the passive structures and to guard against injury.

What about Muscle Fatigue?

It has been well established in the literature that muscle fatigue can play a major role in destabilizing a joint.[100,111,117,129] With fatigue, an increase in knee joint laxity has been noted in both males and females.[100,117,118] More importantly, the body's ability to receive and accurately process proprioceptive information is affected by muscular fatigue. There is evidence that exercise to the point of clinical fatigue does have an effect on proprioception.[111,129] Research has demonstrated that the ability to learn or make improvement in joint position sense is severely impaired with muscle fatigue.[75,100] Likewise, muscle fatigue has been shown to alter both kinesthesia and joint position sense.[2,111,129] Skinner et al. showed that the reproduction of passive positioning was significantly diminished following a fatigue protocol.[111] Voight et al. also demonstrated a significant proprioceptive deficit following a fatigue protocol.[129] This suggests that patients who are fatigued may have a change in their proprioceptive abilities and are more prone to injury. Following a lower-quarter isokinetic fatigue protocol, postural sway as measured with EMG and forceplates is also increased following muscular fatigue.[66,129] This suggests that muscular fatigue results in a possible motor control deficit. In addition to disruption balance or postural sway, Nyland et al. also demonstrated on EMG that muscular fatigue affects muscle activity by extending the latency of the muscle firing.[87]

Modifying Afferent/Efferent Characteristics: How Do We Do It?

The mechanoreceptors in and around the respective joints offer information about the change of position, motion, and loading of the joint to the CNS, which in turn stimulates the muscles around the joint to function.[65] If a time lag exists in the neuromuscular reaction, injury may occur. The shorter the time lag, the less stress to the ligaments and other soft-tissue structures about the joint. Therefore, the foundation of neuromuscular control is to facilitate the integration of peripheral sensations relative to joint position and then process this information into an effective efferent motor response. The main objective of the rehabilitation program for neuromuscular control is to develop or reestablish the afferent and efferent characteristics about the joint that are essential for dynamic restraint.[71]

There are several different afferent and efferent characteristics that contribute to the efficient regulation of motor control. As discussed previously, these characteristics include the sensitivity of the mechanoreceptors and facilitation of the afferent neural pathways, enhancing muscle stiffness, and the production of reflex muscle activation. The specific rehabilitation techniques must also take into consideration the levels of CNS integration. For the rehabilitation program to be complete, each of the three levels must be addressed in order to produce dynamic

stability. The plasticity of the neuromuscular system permits rapid adaptations during the rehabilitation program that enhance preparatory and reactive activity.[7,56,65,71,74,141] Specific rehabilitation techniques that produce adaptations that enhance the efficiency of these neuromuscular techniques include balance training, biofeedback training, reflex facilitation through reactive training, and eccentric and high-repetition/low-load exercises.[71]

OBJECTIVES OF NEUROMUSCULAR CONTROL: REACTIVE NEUROMUSCULAR TRAINING

RNT activities are designed both to restore functional stability about the joint and to enhance motor control skills. The RNT program centers around the stimulation of both the peripheral and central reflex pathways to the skeletal muscles. The first objective that should be addressed in the RNT program is the restoration of dynamic stability. Reliable kinesthetic and proprioceptive information provides the foundation on which dynamic stability and motor control are based. It has already been established that altered afferent information into the CNS can alter the feed-forward and feedback motor control systems. Therefore, the first objective of the RNT program is to restore the neurosensory properties of the damaged structures while at the same time enhancing the sensitivity of the secondary peripheral afferents.[74] The restoration of dynamic stability allows for the control of abnormal joint translation during functional activities. In order for this to occur, the reestablishment of dynamic stability is dependent upon the CNS receiving appropriate information from the peripheral receptors. If the information into the system is altered or inappropriate for the stimulus, a bad motor response will ensue.

To facilitate appropriate kinesthetic and proprioceptive information to the CNS, joint reposition exercises should be used to provide a maximal stimulation of the peripheral mechanoreceptors. The use of closed kinetic chain activities creates axial loads that maximally stimulate the articular mechanoreceptors via the increase in compressive forces.[22,45] The use of closed-chain exercises not only enhances joint congruency and neurosensory feedback but also minimizes the shearing stresses about the joint.[128] At the same time, the muscle receptors are facilitated by both the change in length and tension.[22,45] The objective is to induce unanticipated perturbations, thereby stimulating reflex stabilization. The persistent use of these pathways will decease the response time when faced with an unanticipated joint load.[88] In addition to weight-bearing exercises, joint repositioning exercises can be used to enhance the conscious appreciation of proprioception. Rhythmic stabilization exercises can be included early in the RNT program to enhance neuromuscular coordination in response to unexpected joint translation. The intensity of the exercises can be manipulated by increasing either the weight loaded across the joint or the size of the perturbation. The addition of a compressive sleeve, wrap, or taping about the joint can also provide additional proprioceptive information by stimulating the cutaneous mechanoreceptors.[5,71,76,90] Following the restoration of range of motion and strength, dynamic stability can be enhanced with reflex stabilization and basic motor learning exercises.

The second objective of the RNT program is to encourage preparatory agonist–antagonist cocontraction. Efficient coactivation of the musculature restores the normal force couples that are necessary to balance joint forces and increase joint congruency, thereby reducing the loads imparted onto the static structures.[71] The cornerstone of rehabilitation during this phase is postural stability training. Environmental conditions are manipulated to produce a sensory response. Specifically, the three variables of balance that are manipulated include bilateral to unilateral stance, eyes open to eyes closed, and stable to unstable surfaces. The use of unstable surfaces allows the clinician to use positions of compromise in order to produce maximal afferent input into the spinal cord, thereby producing a reflex response. Dynamic coactivation of the muscles about the joint to produce a stabilizing force requires both the feed-forward and feedback motor control systems. In order to facilitate these pathways, the joint must be placed into positions of compromise in order for the patient to develop reactive stabilizing strategies. Although it was once believed that the speed of the stretch reflexes could not be directly enhanced, efforts to do so have been successful in human and animal studies. This has significant implications for reestablishing the reactive capability of the dynamic restraint system. Reducing the electromechanical delay between joint loading and the protective muscle activation can increase dynamic stability. In the controlled clinical environment, positions of vulnerability can be used safely.

Proprioceptive training for functionally unstable joints following injury has been documented in the literature.[65,106,123,125] Tropp et al.[124] and Wester et al.[137] reported that ankle disk training significantly reduced the incidence of ankle sprain. Concerning the mechanism of effects, Tropp et al. suggested that unstable surface training reduced the proprioceptive deficit.[124] Sheth et al. demonstrated changes with healthy adults in the patterns of contractions on the inversion and eversion musculature before and after training on an unstable surface.[106] They concluded that the changes would be supported by the concept of reciprocal Ia inhibition via the mechanoreceptors in the muscles. Konradsen and Ravin also suggested that the afferent input from the calf musculature was responsible for dynamic protection against sudden ankle inversion stress.[68] Pinstaar et al. reported that postural sway was restored after 8 weeks of ankle disk training when carried out 3–5 times a week.[93] Tropp and Odenrick also showed that postural control improved after 6 weeks of training when performed 15 minutes per day.[125] Bernier and Perrin, whose program consisted of balance exercises progressing from simple to complex sessions (3 times a week for 10 minutes), also found that postural sway was improved after 6 weeks of training.[10] Although there were some differences in each of these training programs, the postural control improved after 6–8 weeks of proprioceptive training for participants with functional instability of the ankle.

Once dynamic stability has been achieved, the focus of the RNT program is to restore ADL and sport-specific skills. Exercise and training drills should be incorporated into the program that will refine the physiologic parameters that are required for the return to preinjury levels of function. Emphasis in the RNT program must be placed upon a progression from simple to complex neuromotor patterns that are specific to the demands placed upon the patient during function. The training program should begin with simple activities, such as walking/running, and then progress to highly complex motor skills requiring refined neuromuscular mechanisms including proprioceptive and kinesthetic awareness that provide reflex joint stabilization.

EXERCISE PROGRAM/PROGRESSION

Dynamic reactive neuromuscular control activities should be initiated into the overall rehabilitation program once adequate healing has occurred. The progression to these activities is predicated on the athlete satisfactorily completing the activities that are considered prerequisites for the activity being considered. Keeping this in mind, the progression of activities must be goal-oriented and specific to the tasks that will be expected of the athlete.

The general progression for activities to develop dynamic reactive neuromuscular control is from slow-speed to fast-speed activities, from low-force to high-force activities, and from controlled to uncontrolled activities. Initially these exercises should evoke a balance reaction or weight shift in the lower extremities and ultimately progress to a movement pattern. These reactions can be as simple as a static control with little or no visible movement or as complex as a dynamic plyometric response requiring explosive acceleration, deceleration, or change in direction. The exercises will allow the clinician to challenge the patient using visual and/or proprioceptive input via tubing and other devices (medicine balls, foam rolls, visual obstacles). Although these exercises will improve physiologic parameters, they are specifically designed to facilitate neuromuscular reactions. Therefore, the clinician must be concerned with the kinesthetic input and quality of the movement patterns rather than the particular number of sets and repetitions. Once fatigue occurs, motor control becomes poor and all training effects are lost. Therefore, during the exercise progression, all aspects of normal motor control/movement should be observed. These should include isometric, concentric, and eccentric muscle control; articular loading and unloading; balance control during weight shifting and direction changes; controlled acceleration and deceleration; and demonstration of both conscious and unconscious control.

Phase I: Static Stabilization (Closed-Chain Loading/Unloading)

Phase I involves minimal joint motion and should always follow a complete open-chain exercise program that restores near-full active range of motion. The patient should stand bearing full

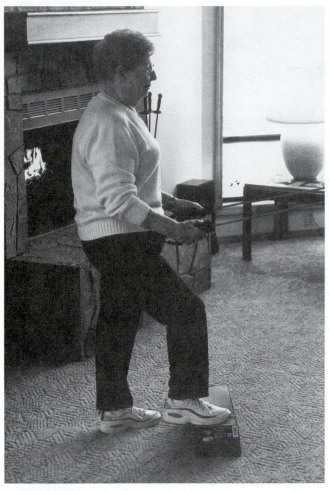

FIGURE 11-8

Static stabilization: Weight shifting technique to enhance transfer onto the left leg.

weight with equal distribution on the affected and unaffected lower extremity. The feet should be positioned approximately shoulder-width apart. Greater emphasis can be placed on the affected lower extremity by having the patient put the unaffected lower extremity on a 6–8-in stool or step bench. This flexes the hip and knee and forces a greater weight shift to the affected side, yet allows the unaffected extremity to assist with balance reactions (Fig. 11-8). The weight-bearing status then progresses to having the unaffected extremity suspended in front or behind the body, forcing a single-leg stance on the affected side (Fig. 11-9). The patient is then asked to continue the single-leg stance while shifting weight to the forefoot and toes by lifting the heel and plantarflexing the ankle. This places the complete responsibility of weight-bearing and balance reactions on the affected lower extremity. This position will also require slight flexion of the hip and knee. Support devices are often helpful and can minimize confusion. When the patient is first asked to progress weight bearing to the forefoot and toes, a heel lift device can be used. A support device can also be used to place the ankle in dorsiflexion, inversion, or eversion to increase kinesthetic input or decrease biomechanical stresses on the hip, knee, and ankle.

At each progression, the clinician may ask that the patient train with eyes closed to decrease the visual input and increase kinesthetic awareness. The clinician may also use an unstable surface with training in this phase to increase the demands on the mechanoreceptor system. The unstable surface will facilitate the reflex pathways mediated by the peripheral efferent receptors. Single or multidirectional rocker devices will assist the progression to the next phase (Fig. 11-10).

The physiologic rationale for this phase of RNT is the use of static compression of the articular structures to produce maximal output of the mechanoreceptors, thereby facilitating isometric contractions of the musculature and providing a dynamic reflex stabilization. The self-generated oscillations will help increase the interplay between visual, mechanoreceptor, and equilibrium reaction. Changes in the isometric muscle tension will assist in the sensitization of the muscle spindle (gamma bias).

The exercise tubing technique used in this phase is called oscillating technique for isometric stabilization (OTIS). The technique can be used to stimulate muscle spindle and mechanoreceptor activity. The exercises involve continuously loaded short-arc movements of one body part, which in turn causes an isometric stabilization reaction of the involved body part. This is accomplished by pulling two pieces of tubing toward the body and returning the tubing to a start position in a smooth rhythmical fashion with increasing speeds. Resistance builds as the tubing is stretched. This forces a transfer of weight in the direction of the tubing. Because the involved body part is only required to react or respond to a simple stimulus, the oscillating stimulus will produce an isometric contraction in the lower extremity that must produce a stabilizing force in the direction opposite to the tubing pull. The purpose of this technique is to quickly involve the proprioceptive system with minimal verbal and visual cueing. Ognibene et al. demonstrated a significant improvement in both single-leg postural stability and reaction time with a 4-week training program using OTIS techniques.[88]

Change in direction—according to anterior, posterior, medial, and lateral weight shifting—will create specific planar demands. Each technique is given a name, which is related to the weight shift produced by the applied tension. The body will then react with an equal and opposite stabilization response. Therefore, the exercise is named for the cause and not the effect. The goal during this phase is static stabilization. Numerous successful repetitions demonstrating stability are required to achieve motor learning and control.

UNIPLANAR EXERCISE

Anterior Weight Shift

The patient faces the tubing and pulls the tubing toward the body using a smooth, comfortable motion. This causes forward weight shift that is stabilized with an isometric counterforce

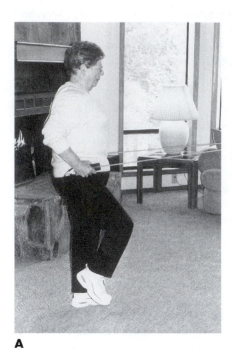

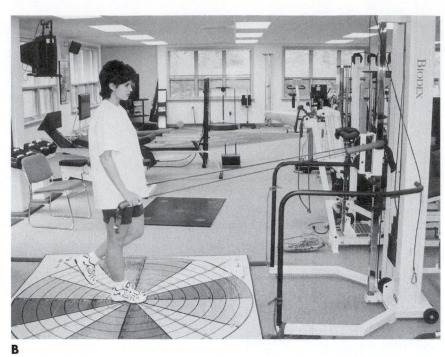

A

B

FIGURE 11-9

Static stabilization: Uniplanar AWS. **A,** Home health setting. **B,** Clinical setting.

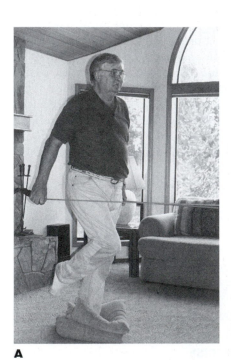

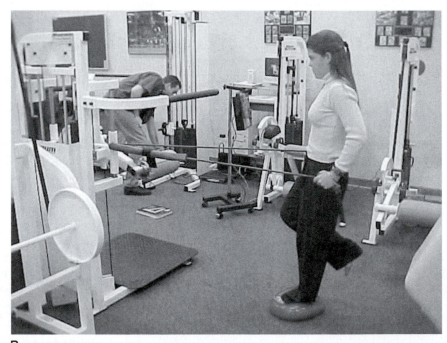

A

B

FIGURE 11-10

Static stabilization: Single-leg stance/unstable surface. **A,** Using pillows in the home
health setting. **B,** Using a Dynadisc in the clinical setting.

consisting of hip extension, knee extension, and ankle plantarflexion. There should be little or no movement noted in the lower extremity. If movement is noted, resistance should be decreased to achieve the desired stability (see Fig. 11-9).

Lateral Weight Shift

The patient stands with the affected side facing the tubing. The tubing is pulled by one hand in front of the body and the other hand behind the body to equalize the force and minimize the rotation. This causes a lateral weight shift (LWS), which is stabilized with an isometric counterforce consisting of hip abduction, knee cocontraction, and ankle eversion.

Medial Weight Shift

The patient stands with the unaffected side facing the tubing. The tubing is pulled in the same fashion as above. This causes a medial weight shift (MWS), which is stabilized with an isometric counterforce consisting of hip adduction, knee cocontraction, and ankle inversion.

Posterior Weight Shift

The patient stands with his/her back to the tubing in the frontal plane. The tubing is pulled to the body from behind, causing a posterior weight shift (PWS), which is stabilized by an isometric counterforce consisting of hip flexion, knee flexion, and ankle dorsiflexion.

MULTIPLANAR EXERCISE

The basic exercise program can be progressed to multiplanar activity by combining the proprioceptive neuromuscular facilitation (PNF) chop and lift patterns of the upper extremities. The chop patterns from the affected and unaffected side will cause a multiplanar stress requiring isometric stabilization. The patient will now be forced to automatically integrate the isometric responses that were developed in the previous uniplanar exercises. The force will be representative of the PNF diagonals of the lower extremities (Fig. 11-11). The lift patterns from the affected to the unaffected side will add multiplanar stress in the opposite direction (Fig. 11-12). Changing the resistance, speed

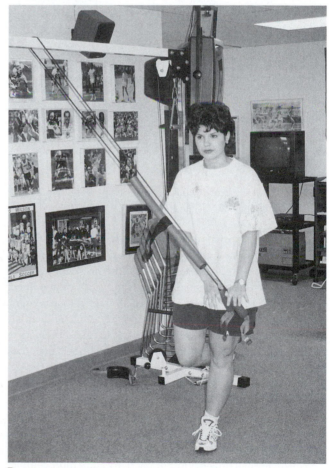

A   **B**

FIGURE 11-11

Static stabilization: Multiplanar PNF chop technique to provide rotational stress. **A,** Home health setting. **B,** Clinical setting.

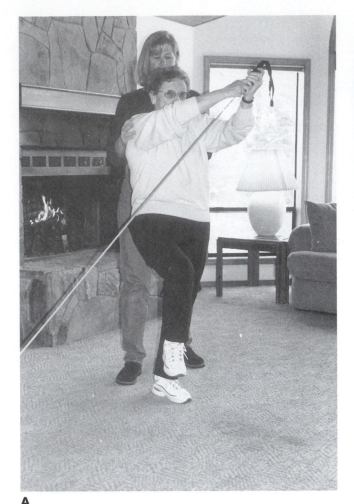

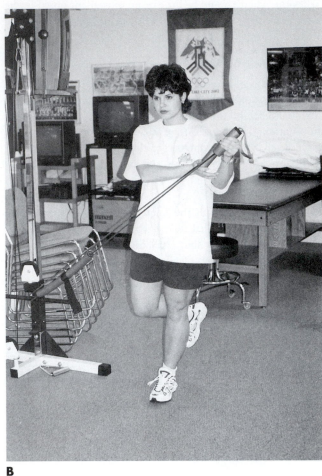

A

B

FIGURE 11-12

Static stabilization: Multiplanar PNF lift technique to provide rotation stress. **A,** Home health setting. **B,** Clinical setting.

of movement, or spatial orientation relative to the resistance can make modifications to the multiplanar exercise. If resistance is increased, the movement speed should be decreased to allow for a strong stabilizing counterforce. If the speed of movement is increased, then resistance should be decreased to allow for a quick counterforce response. By altering the angle of the body in relation to the resistance, the quality of the movement is changed. A greater emphasis can be placed on one component while reducing the emphasis on another component.

TECHNIQUE MODIFICATION

These techniques can also be used with medicine ball exercises. The posture and position are nearly the same, but the medicine ball does not allow for the oscillations provided by the tubing. The medicine ball provides impulse activity and a more complex gradient of loading and unloading (Fig. 11-13). This is referred to as impulse technique for isometric stabilization (ITIS). As described, the patient is positioned to achieve the desired stress. The medicine ball is then used with a rebounding device or

thrown by the clinician. Progression to ball toss while stabilizing on an unstable surface will disrupt concentration, thereby facilitating the conversion to unconscious reflex adaptation.

The elastic tubing and medicine ball techniques are similar in position but differ somewhat in physiologic demands. Therefore, they should be used to complement each other and not replace or substitute the other at random. When performing an ITIS activity with a medicine ball, the force exerted by the exercise device names the weight shift. The tubing will exert a pull and the ball will exert a push; therefore, they will be performed from the opposite sides to achieve the same weight shift.

Phase II: Transitional Stabilization (Conscious Controlled Motion without Impact)

Phase II replaces isometric activity with controlled concentric and eccentric activity progressing through a full range of functional motion. The forces of gravity are coupled with tubing

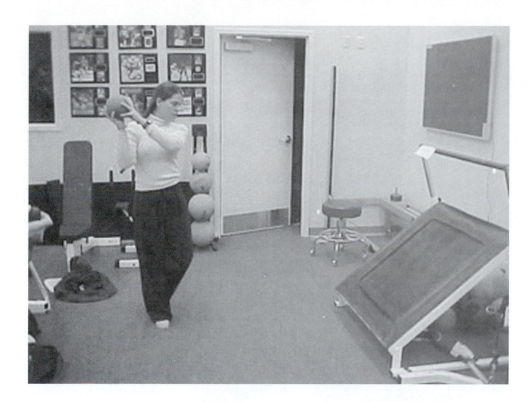

FIGURE 11-13

Static stabilization: ITIS technique in unilateral stance using a plyoball and plyoback for an impulse stimulus.

to simulate stress in both the vertical and horizontal planes. In phase I, gravitational forces statically load the neuromuscular system. Varying degrees of imposed lateral stress via the tubing are used to stimulate isometric stabilization. Phase II requires that the movement occur in the presence of varying degrees of imposed lateral stress. The movement stimulates the mechanoreceptors in two ways: (1) articular movement causes capsular stretch in a given direction at a given speed and (2) the changes in the body position cause loading and unloading of the articular structures and pressure changes in the intracapsular fluid. The exercises in this phase use simple movements such as the squat and lunge. The addition of tubing adds a horizontal stress. Other simple movements such as walking, sidestepping, and the lateral slide board can also be emphasized to stimulate a more efficient and controlled movement.

The physiologic rationales for activities in this phase are the stimulation of dynamic postural responses and facilitation of concentric and eccentric contractions via the compression and translation of the articular structures. This is turn helps to increase muscle stiffness, which has a significant role in producing dynamic stabilization about the joint by resisting and absorbing joint loads.[80,81] Research has established that eccentric loading increases both muscle stiffness and tone.[16,95] Chronic overloading of the musculotendinous unit via eccentric contractions will result in not only connective tissue proliferation but also a desensitization of the GTO and increased muscle spindle activity.[64]

The self-generated movements require dynamic control in the midrange and static control at the end range of motion. Because a change in direction is required at the end ranges of motion, the interplay between visual, mechanoreceptor, and equilibrium reactions continues to increase. The "gamma bias" now responds to changes in both length and tension of the involved musculature.

Assisted techniques can also be used in this phase to progress patients who may find phase II exercise fatiguing or difficult. Assisted exercise is used to reduce the effect of gravity on the body or an extremity to allow for an increase in the quality or quantity of a desired movement. The assisted technique will offset the weight of the body or extremity by a percentage of the total weight. This will allow improved range of motion, a reduction in substitution, minimal eccentric stress, and a reduction in fatigue. The closed-chain tubing program can also benefit from assisted techniques, which allow for a reduction in vertical forces by decreasing relative body weight on one or both lower extremities.

The need for assisted exercise is only transitional in nature. The goal is to progress from unweighted to weight with overloading. The tubing, if used effectively, can also provide an overloading effect by causing exaggerated weight shifting. This overloading will be referred to as resisted techniques (RT) for all closed-chain applications. The two basic exercises used are the squat and the lunge.

SQUAT

The squat is used first because it employs symmetrical movement of the lower extremities. This allows the affected lower extremity to benefit from the visual and proprioceptive feedback from the unaffected lower extremity. The clinician should observe the patient's posture and look for weight shifting, which almost always occurs away from the affected limb. Each joint

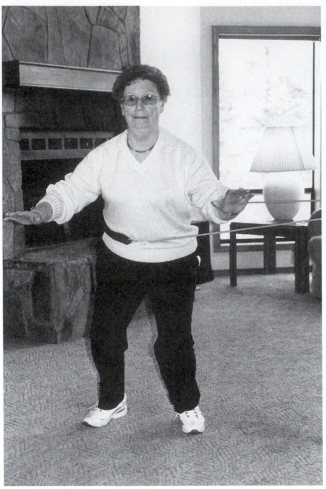

FIGURE 11-14

Transitional stabilization: Resisted squat with an LWS in the home health setting.

can be compared to its unaffected counterpart. In performing the squat, a weight shift may be provided in one of four different directions. The tubing is used to assist, resist, and modify movement patterns. The PWS works to identify closed-chain ankle dorsiflexion. A chair or bench can be used as a range-of-motion block (range-limiting device) when necessary. This minimizes fear and increases safety. The anterior weight shift (AWS) provides an anterior pull that helps facilitate the hip flexion mobility during the descent. Medial and lateral changes may be provided with resistance in order to promote weight bearing on the involved side or decrease weight bearing on the involved side as progression is made (Fig. 11-14). The varying weight shifts may be used to intentionally increase the load or resistance on a particular side for means of strengthening or to facilitate a neuromuscular response on the opposite side. For example, an individual who is reluctant to weight bear on the involved side may be helped in doing so by causing increased weight shift to the uninvolved side. This will create the need to shift weight to the involved side, thus encouraging a joint response to the required stimulus.

Assisted Technique

The patient faces the tubing, which is placed at a descending angle and is attached to a belt. The belt is placed under the buttocks to simulate a swing. A bench is used to allow a proper stopping point. The elastic tension of the tubing is at its greatest when the patient is in the seated position and decreases as the mechanical advantage increases. Therefore, the tension curve of the tubing complements the needs of the patient. The next four exercises follow the assisted squat in difficulty. The tubing is now used to cause weight shifting and demands a small amount of dynamic stability.

Anterior Weight Shift

The patient faces the tubing, which comes from a level halfway between the hips and the knees and attaches to a belt. The belt is worn around the waist and causes an AWS. During the squat movement, the ankles plantarflex as the knees extend.

Posterior Weight Shift

The patient faces away from the tubing at the same level as above and attaches to a belt. The belt is worn around the waist and causes a PWS. This places a greater emphasis on the hip extensors and less emphasis on the knee extensors and plantar flexors.

Medial Weight Shift

The patient stands with the unaffected side toward the tubing at the same level as above. The belt is around the waist and causes an MWS. This places less stress on the affected lower extremity and allows the patient to lean onto the affected lower extremity without incurring excessive stress or loading.

Lateral Weight Shift

The patient stands with the affected side toward the tubing that is at the same level as above. The belt is worn around the waist, which causes a weight shift onto the affected lower extremity. This exercise will place a greater stress on the affected lower extremity, thereby demanding increased balance and control. The exercise simulates a single-leg squat but adds balance and safety by allowing the unaffected extremity to remain on the ground.

LUNGE

The lunge is more specific in that it simulates sports and normal activity. The exercise decreases the base while at the same time producing the need for independent disassociation. The range of motion can be stressed to a slightly higher degree. If the patient is asked to alternate the lunge from the right to the left leg, the clinician can easily compare the quality of the movement between the limbs. When performing the lunge, the patient may often use exaggerated extension movements of the lumbar region to assist weak or uncoordinated hip extension. This substitution is not produced during the squat exercise. Therefore, the lunge must be used not only as an exercise

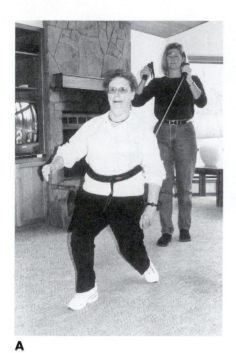
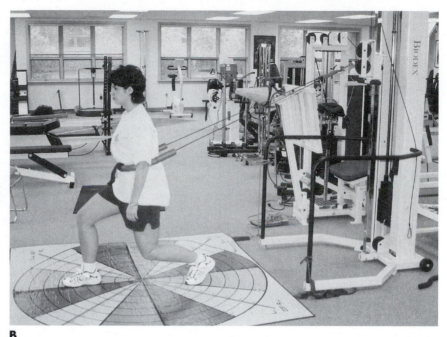

A   **B**

F I G U R E   1 1 - 1 5

Transitional stabilization: Assisted lunge technique. **A,** Home health setting. **B,** Clinical setting.

but also as a part of the functional assessment. The substitution must be addressed by asking the patient to maintain a vertical torso (note that the assisted technique will assist the clinician in minimizing this substitution).

Assisted Technique—Forward Lunge

The patient faces away from the tubing, which descends at a sharp angle (about 60°). This angle parallels the patient's center of gravity, which moves forward and down (Fig. 11-15). This places a stretch on the tubing and assists the patient up from the low point of the lunge position. The ability to perform a lunge with correct technique is often negated due to the inability to support one's body weight. The assisted lunge corrects this by modifying the load required of the patient, thus improving the quality of the movement. The assistance also minimizes eccentric demands for deceleration when lowering and provides balance assistance by helping the patient focus on the center of gravity (anatomically located within the hip and pelvic region). The patient is asked to first alternate the activity to provide kinesthetic feedback. The clinician can then use variations of full and partial motion to stimulate the appropriate control before moving on to the next exercise.

Resisted Technique—Forward Lunge

The patient faces the tubing, which is at an ascending angle from the floor to the level of the waist (Fig. 11-16). The tubing will now increase the eccentric loading on the quadriceps with the deceleration or the downward movement. For the upward movement, the patient is asked to focus on hip extension and

not knee extension. The patient must learn to initiate movement from the hip and not from lumbar hyperextension or excessive knee extension. Initiation of hip extension should automatically stimulate isometric lumbar stabilization along with the appropriate amounts of knee extension and ankle plantarflexion. A foam block is often used to protect the rear knee from flexing beyond 90° and touching the floor. The block can also be made larger to limit range of motion at any point in the lunge.

Resisted Technique—Lateral and Medial Weight Shift

Forward lunges can be performed to stimulate static lateral and medial stabilization during dynamic flexion and extension movements of the lower extremities. The LWS lunge is performed by positioning the patient with the affected lower extremity toward the direction of resistance. The tubing is placed at a level halfway between the waist and the ankle. The patient is then asked to perform a lunge with minimal lateral movement. This movement stimulates static lateral stabilization of the hip, knee, ankle, and foot during dynamic flexion (unloading) and extension (loading). The MWS lunge is performed by positioning the patient with the affected extremity opposite to the resistance. The tubing is attached as described in the LWS. The movement stimulates static medial stabilization of the affected lower extremity in the presence of dynamic flexion and extension.

The lunge techniques teach weight shifting onto the affected lower extremity during lateral body movements. The assisted technique lateral lunge will complement the assisted

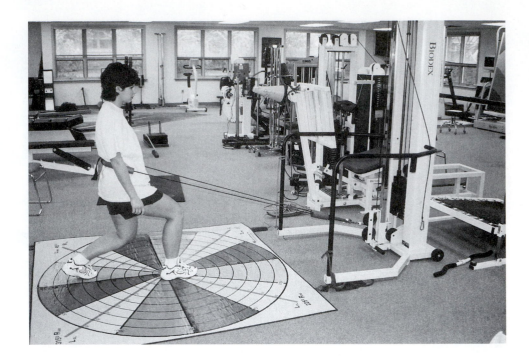

FIGURE   11-16

Transitional stabilization: Resisted forward lunge to facilitate deceleration stress.

technique forward lunge, because it also reduces relative body weight while allowing closed-chain function. The prime mover is the unaffected lower extremity that moves the center of gravity over the affected lower extremity for the sole purpose of visual and proprioceptive input prior to excessive loading. The RT lateral lunge will complement the RT forward lunge, because it also provides an overloading effect on the affected lower extremity. In this exercise, the affected lower extremity is the prime mover, as well as the primary weight-bearing extremity. The affected lower extremity must not only produce the weight shift but also react, respond, and repeat the movement. Sets, repetitions, and resistance for all of the exercises described are selected by the clinician to produce the appropriate reaction without pain or fatigue.

TECHNIQUE MODIFICATION

As in phase I, the medicine ball can be used to add variety and increase stimulation. However, it is used to stimulate control in the beginning, middle, and end ranges of the squat and lunges. The tubing can also be used to create ITIS and OTIS applications to reinforce stability throughout the range of motion.

FUNCTIONAL TESTING

Functional testing provides objective criteria and can help the clinician to justify a progression to phase III or an indication that the patient should continue working in phase II. A single-leg body weight squat or lunge can be performed. The quality and quantity of the repetitions are compared to the unaffected lower extremity and a deficit can be calculated. An isotonic leg press machine can also be used in this manner by setting the weight at the patient's body weight and comparing the repetitions. Open-chain isotonic and isokinetic testing can also be helpful in

identifying problem areas when specificity is needed. Regardless of the mode of testing, it is recommended that the affected lower extremity display 70–80 percent of the capacity demonstrated by the unaffected lower extremity, or no more than a 20–30 percent strength deficit. When the patient has met these criteria, he/she can move safely into phase III.

Phase III: Dynamic Stabilization (Unconscious Control/Loading)

Phase III introduces impact and ballistic exercise to the patient. This movement will produce a stretch-shortening cycle that has been described in plyometric exercises. Plyometric function is not a result of the magnitude of the prestretch, but rather relies on the rate of stretch to produce a more forceful contraction. This is done in two ways.

1.   The stretch reflex is a neuromuscular response to tension produced in the muscle passively. The muscle responds with an immediate contraction to reorient itself to the new position, protect it, and maintain posture. If a voluntary contraction is added in conjunction with this reflex, a more forceful contraction can be produced.
2.   The elastic properties of the tendon allow it to temporarily store energy and release it. When a quick prestretch is followed by a voluntary contraction, the tendon will add to the strength of the contraction by providing force in the direction opposite to the prestretch.

Dynamic training at this level can increase the descending cortical drive to the large motor nerves of the skeletal muscles as well as the small efferent nerves of the muscle spindle.[79] If both the muscle tension and efferent output to the muscle spindles are increased, the stretch sensitivity of the muscle spindle will also be increased, thereby reducing the reflex latency.[64] Both feed-forward and feedback loops are used concurrently to superimpose stretch reflexes on preprogrammed motor activity.

As has been previously discussed, there have been previous studies that have been directed toward reducing muscle reaction times.[7,65,141] Ihara and Nakayama significantly reduced the latency of muscle reaction times with a 3-week training period of unanticipated perturbations via the use of unstable wobble boards.[65] Both Beard et al. and Wojtys et al. found similar results when comparing agility training with traditional strength training.[7,141] Reducing the muscle reaction time in order to produce a protective response following an abnormal joint load will enhance dynamic stability about the joint.

Before the patient is asked to learn any new techniques, he/she is instructed to demonstrate unconscious control by performing various phase II activities while throwing and catching the medicine ball. The squat and lunge exercises are performed with various applications of tubing at the waist level. This activity removes the attention from the lower extremity exercise, thereby stimulating unconscious control. The forces added by throwing and catching the medicine ball stimulate balance reactions needed for the progression to plyometric activities. Simple rope jumping is another transitional exercise that can be used to provide early plyometric information. The double-leg rope jumping is done first. The patient is then asked to perform alternating leg jumping. Rope jumping is effective in building confidence and restoring a plyometric rhythm to movement. Four-way resisted stationary running is an exercise technique used to orient the patient to light plyometric activity.

RESISTED WALKING

Resisted walking uses the same primary components as in gait training. The applied resistance of the tubing, however, allows for a reactive response unavailable in nonresisted activities. For example, a patient may present with a slight Trendelenburg gait associated with a weak gluteus medius. By initiating a program that would incorporate a progression such as that used with the squat, the patient should be able to progress to resisted walking. The addition of resistance permits for increased loading and also brings about the need for improved balance and weight shift.

RESISTED HOPPING

Bilateral hopping should be introduced following adequate training with the jump rope, then followed by increased unilateral training. The use of resistance in the hopping technique is to promote increased resistance in one of four directions. This increased resistance is used to simulate those forces normally seen on the field or court in the return to activity. Introduction of the program should begin with bilateral training and then progress to a unilateral format, which may be accommodated with box drills or diagonal training. At higher levels, implementing cones, hurdles, and/or foam rolls may be used in order to increase the plyometric demands during the hopping drills.

RESISTED RUNNING

Resisted running simply involves jogging or running in place with tubing attached to a belt around the waist. The clinician can analyze the jogging or running activity because it is a stationary drill. The tubing resistance is applied in four different directions, providing simulation of the different forces that the patient will experience as he/she returns to full activity.

1. The PWS run causes a balance reaction that results in an AWS (opposite direction) and simulates the acceleration phase of jogging or running (Fig. 11-17). The patient faces opposite the direction of the tubing resistance and should be encouraged to stay on the toes (for all running exercises). The initial light stepping activity can be progressed to jogging and then running. The most advanced form of the PWS run involves the exaggeration of the hip flexion called "high knees." Exaggeration of hip flexion helps to stimulate a plyometric action in the hip extensors, thus facilitating acceleration. This form of exercise lends itself to slow, controlled endurance conditioning (greater than 3 minutes), or interval training, which depends greatly on the intensity of the resistance, cadence, and rest periods. The interval-training program is most effective and shows the greatest short-term gains. Intervals can be 10 seconds to 1 minute; however, the most common drills are 15–30 seconds in length. The patient is usually allowed a 1–2-minute rest and is required to perform three to five sets. To make sure that the patient is delivering maximum intensity, the clinician should count the number of foot touches (repetitions) that occur during the interval. The clinician needs to only count the touches of the affected lower extremity. The patient is then asked to equal or exceed the amount of foot touches on the next interval (set). This is also extremely effective as a functional test for acceleration. The interval time/repetitions can be recorded and compared to future tests. The clinician should note that the PWS places particular emphasis on the hip flexors and extensors, as well as the plantar flexors of the ankle.

2. The MWS run follows the same progression as the PWS run (from light jogging to high knees) with the resistance now applied medial to the affected lower extremity (which causes an automatic weight shift lateral). Endurance training, interval training, and testing should also be performed for this technique. This technique simulates the forces that the patient will experience when cutting or turning quickly away from the affected side. This drill is the same as in phase I MWS. Although the phase I MWS is static, the same muscles are responsible for dynamic stability. This exercise represents the forces that the patient will encounter when sprinting into a turn on the affected side.

3. The LWS run should follow the same progression as above except that the resistance is now lateral to the affected lower extremity (which causes an automatic MWS). This technique simulates the forces that the patient will experience when cutting or turning quickly toward the affected side.

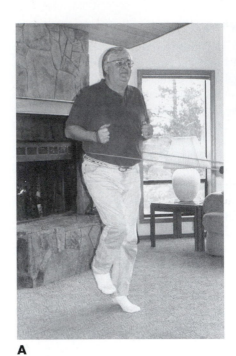 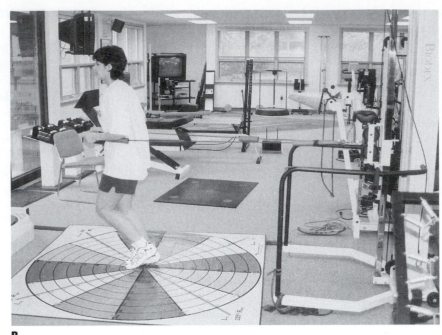

A   **B**

F I G U R E   1 1 - 1 7

Dynamic stabilization—stationary run. **A,** Posterior weight shifting in the home health setting. **B,** Anterior weight shifting in the clinical setting.

When performing the MWS and LWS runs, high knees should be used when working on acceleration. Instructing the patient to perform exaggerated knee flexion or "butt kicks" can emphasize deceleration. The exaggeration of knee flexion places greater plyometric stress on the knee, which has a large amount of eccentric responsibility during deceleration. This exercise represents the forces that the patient will encounter when sprinting into a turn on the unaffected side.

4. The AWS run is probably the most difficult technique to perform correctly and is therefore taught last. The tubing that is set to pull the patient forward stimulates a PWS. This technique simulates deceleration and eccentric loading of the knee extensors. The patient should start with light jogging on the toes and progress to butt kicks. This is a plyometric exercise that incorporates exaggerated knee flexion and extension. This exercise will then serve to assist the patient in developing eccentric/concentric reactions that are required in function. The clinician should note that injuries occur more frequently during deceleration and direction changes than on acceleration or straightforward running. Therefore, AWS training is extremely important to the athlete returning to the court or field.

RESISTED BOUNDING

The bounding exercise is a progression taken from both the hopping and running exercise to increase demands placed on the horizontal component. Therefore, bounding is an exercise technique that will place greater emphasis on the lateral movements. The progression of the bounding exercises will follow the same weight-shifting sequence as the previous running exercise. Side-to-side bounding in a lateral resisted exercise promotes symmetrical balance and endurance required for progression to higher-level strength and power applications. Distraction activities may also be included in the bounding and/or running exercises in order to promote increased upper extremity demands and to detract from visual and/or verbal reference needed on the lower extremity.

It is suggested that the patient be taught how to perform the bounding exercise without the tubing first. A foam roll, cone, or other obstacle can be used to simulate jump height and/or distance. The tubing can then be added to provide the secondary forces to cause anterior, lateral, medial, or posterior weight shifting. Bounding should be taught as a jump from one foot to another. A single lateral bound can be used as a supplementary functional test. Measurements can be taken for a left and right lateral bound. Bounding is only considered valid if the patient can maintain his/her balance when landing. To standardize the bounding exercise, the body height is used for the bound stride and markers can be placed for the left and right foot landings.

1. The AWS lateral combines lateral motion with an automatic PWS or deceleration reaction. It is slightly more demanding than the stationary running exercises because the body weight is driven to a greater distance.

2. The LWS bound causes an excessive lateral plyometric force and will help to develop lateral acceleration and deceleration in the affected lower extremity. This is the most strenuous of the lateral bounding activities because it actually accelerates the body weight onto the affected lower extremity. This is, however, necessary so that the clinician can observe the ability of the affected limb to perform a quick direction change and controlled acceleration/deceleration.

3. The MWS bound is used as an assisted plyometric exercise. The patient works with the total body weight but impact is greatly lowered by reducing both acceleration and deceleration forces. This exercise is an excellent transitional exercise at the end of phase II as well as at the beginning of phase III. It also serves as a warm-up drill providing submaximal stimulation of the proprioceptive system prior to a phase III exercise session.

4. The PWS bound facilitates an anterior lateral push-off of each leg and will stimulate an AWS. This exercise will assist in teaching acceleration and lateral cutting movements.

MULTIDIRECTIONAL DRILLS

Multidirectional drills include jumping (two-foot takeoff followed by a two-foot landing), hopping (one-foot takeoff followed by a landing on the same foot), and bounding (one-foot takeoff followed by an opposite-foot landing). A series of floor markers can be placed in various patterns to simulate functional movements. A weight shift can be produced in any direction by the orientation of the tubing. Obstacles can also be used to make the exercise more complicated.

The jumping exercise can be developed to simulate downhill skiing, while the hopping exercise can be designed to stress single-leg push-off for vertical jumping sports such as basketball and volleyball.

SUMMARY

- There has been increased attention to the development of balance and proprioception in the rehabilitation and reconditioning of athletes following injury. It is believed that injury results in altered somatosensory input that influences neuromuscular control.
- If static and dynamic balance and neuromuscular control are not reestablished following injury, then the patient will be susceptible to recurrent injury and his/her performance may decline.
- The following rules should be employed when designing the RNT program:
  ➤ Make sure that the exercise program is specific to the patient's needs. The most important thing to consider during the rehabilitation of patients is that they should be performing functional activities that simulate their ADL requirements. This rule applies to not only the specific joints involved but also the speed and amplitude of movement required in ADL.
  ➤ Practice does appear to be task specific in both athletes and people who have motor control deficits.[73] As retraining of balance continues, it is best to practice complex skills in their entirety rather than in isolation because the skills will transfer more effectively.[1]
  ➤ Make sure to include a significant amount of "controlled chaos" in the program. Unexpected activities with the ADL are by nature unstable. The more the patient rehearses in this type of environment, the better he/she will react under unrehearsed conditions.
  ➤ Progress from straight plane to multiplane movement patterns. In ADL, movement does not occur along a single joint or plane of movement. Therefore, exercise for the kinetic chain must involve all three planes simultaneously.
  ➤ Begin your loading from the inside out. Load the system first with body weight and then progress to external resistance. The core of the body must be developed before the extremities.
  ➤ Have causative cures as a part of the rehabilitation process. The cause of the injury must eventually become a part of the cure. If rotation and deceleration were the cause of the injury, then use this as a part of the rehabilitation program in preparation for return to activity.
  ➤ Be progressive in nature. Remember to progress from simple to complex. The function progression breaks an activity down into its component parts and then performs them in a sequence that allows for the acquisition or reacquisition of the activity. Basic conditioning and skill acquisition must be acquired before advanced conditioning and skill acquisition.
  ➤ Always ask: Does the program make sense? If it does not make sense, chances are that it is not functional and therefore not optimally effective.
  ➤ Make the rehabilitation program fun. The first three letters of functional are FUN. If it is not fun, then compliance will suffer and so will the results.
  ➤ An organized progression is the key to success. Failing to plan is planning to fail.

REFERENCES

1. Barnett M, Ross D, Schmidt R, Todd B. Motor skills learning and the specificity of training principle. *Res Q Exerc Sport* 44:440–447, 1973.
2. Barrack RL, Lund PJ, Skinner HB. Knee joint proprioception revisited. *J Sport Rehabil* 3:18–42, 1994.
3. Barrack RL, Skinner HB. The sensory function of knee ligaments. In: Daniel D, ed. *Knee Ligaments: Structure, Function, Injury, and Repair*. New York, Raven Press, 1990.

4. Barrack RL, Skinner HB, Buckley SL. Proprioception in the anterior cruciate deficient knee. *Am J Sports Med* 17:1–6, 1989.

5. Barrett DS. Proprioception and function after anterior cruciate reconstruction. *JBJS* 73B:833–837, 1991.

6. Basmajian JV, ed. *Biofeedback: Principles and Practice for Clinicians*. Baltimore, MD, Williams and Wilkins, 1979.

7. Beard DJ, Dodd CF, Trundle HR, et al. Proprioception after rupture of the ACL: An objective indication of the need for surgery? *JBJS* 75B:311, 1993.

8. Bernier JN, Perrin DH. Effect of coordination training on proprioception of the functionally unstable ankle. *J Orthop Sports Phys Ther* 27:264–275, 1998.

9. Belen'kii VY, Gurfinkle VS, Pal'tsev YI. Elements of control of voluntary movements. *Biofizika* 12:135–141, 1967.

10. Berg K. Balance and its measure in the elderly: A review. *Physiother Can* 41:240–246, 1989.

11. Blackburn TA, Voight ML. Single leg stance: Development of a reliable testing procedure. In: *Proceedings of the 12th International Congress of the World Confederation for Physical Therapy*. Alexandria, VA, APTA, 1995.

12. Borsa PA, Lephart SM, Kocher MS, Lephart SP. Functional assessment and rehabilitation of shoulder proprioception for glenohumeral instability. *J Sport Rehabil* 3:84–104, 1994.

13. Borsa PA, Lephart SM, Irrgang JJ, Safran MR, Fu F. The effects of joint position and direction of joint motion on proprioceptive sensibility in anterior cruciate ligament deficient athletes. *Am J Sports Med* 25:336–340, 1997.

14. Boyd IA, Roberts TDM. Proprioceptive discharges from stretch-receptors in the knee joint of the cat. *J Physiol* 122:38–59, 1953.

15. Braxendale RA, Ferrel WR, Wood L. Responses of quadriceps motor units to mechanical stimulation of knee joint receptors in decerebrate cat. *Brain Res* 453:150–156, 1988.

16. Bulbulian R, Bowles DK. The effect of downhill running on motorneuron pool excitability. *J Appl Physiol* 73(3):968–973, 1992.

17. Burgess PR. Signal of kinesthetic information by peripheral sensory receptors. *Ann Rev Neurosci* 5:171, 1982.

18. Cafarelli E, Bigland B. Sensation of static force in muscles of different length. *Exp Neurol* 65:511–525, 1979.

19. Ciccotti MR, Kerlan R, Perry J, Pink M. An electromyographic analysis of the knee during functional activities: I. The normal profile. *Am J Sports Med* 22:645–650, 1994.

20. Ciccotti MR, Kerlan R, Perry J, Pink M. An electromyographic analysis of the knee during functional activities: II. The anterior cruciate ligament—deficient knee and reconstructed profiles. *Am J Sports Med* 22:651–658, 1994.

21. Clark FJ, Burgess PR. Slowly adapting receptors in cat knee joint: Can they signal joint angle? *J Neurophysiol* 38:1448–1463, 1975.

22. Clark FJ, Burgess RC, Chapin JW, Lipscomb WT. Role of intramuscular receptors in the awareness of limb position. *J Neurophysiol* 54:1529–1540, 1985.

23. Cohen H, Keshner E. Current concepts of the vestibular system reviewed: Visual/vestibular interaction and spatial orientation. *Am J Occup Ther* 43:331–338, 1989.

24. Corrigan JP, Cashman WF, Brady MP. Proprioception in the cruciate deficient knee. *JBJS.* 74B:247–250, 1992.

25. Cross MJ, McCloskey DI. Position sense following surgical removal of joints in man. *Brain Res* 55:443–445, 1973.

26. Crutchfield A, Barnes M. *Motor Control and Motor Learning in Rehabilitation*. Atlanta, GA, Stokesville, 1993.

27. Dewhurst DJ. Neuromuscular control system. *IEEE Trans Biomed Eng* 14:167–171, 1965.

28. Dietz VJ, Schmidtbleicher D. Interaction between preactivity and stretch reflex in human triceps bracii during landing from forward falls. *J Physiol* 311:113–125, 1981.

29. Dunn TG, Gillig SE, Ponser ES, Weil N. The learning process in biofeedback: Is it feed-forward or feedback? *Biofeedback Self Regul* 11:143–155, 1986.

30. Ekdhl C, Jarnlo G, Anderson S. Standing balance in healthy subjects. *Scand J Rehabil Med* 21:187–195, 1989.

31. Eklund J. Position sense and state of contraction: The effects of vibration. *J Neurol Neurosurg Psychiatry* 35:606, 1972.

32. Era P, Heikkinen E. Postural sway during standing and unexpected disturbances of balance in random samples of men of different ages. *J Gerontol* 40:287–295, 1985.

33. Freeman MAR, Wyke B. Articular reflexes of the ankle joint. An electromyographic study of normal and abnormal influences of ankle-joint mechanoreceptors upon reflex activity in leg muscles. *Br J Surg* 54:990–1001, 1967.

34. Freeman MAR, Wyke B. Articular contributions to limb reflexes. *Br J Surg* 53:61–69, 1966.

35. Friden T, Zatterstrom R, Lindstand A, Moritz U. Disability in anterior cruciate ligament insufficiency: An analysis of 19 untreated patients. *Acta Orthop Scand* 61:131–135, 1990.

36. Gandevia SC, Burke D. Does the nervous system depend on kinesthetic information to control natural limb movements? *Behav Brain Sci* 15:614–632, 1992.

37. Gandevia SC, McCloskey DI. Joint sense, muscle sense and their contribution as position sense, measured at the distal interphalangeal joint of the middle finger. *J Physiol* 260:387–407, 1976.

38. Gauffin H, Pettersson G, Tegner Y, Tropp H. Function testing in patients with old rupture of the anterior cruciate ligament. *Int J Sports Med* 11:73–77, 1990.

39. Gelfan S, Carter S. Muscle sense in man. *Exp Neurol* 18:469–473, 1967.

40. Giove TP, Miller SJ, Kent BE, Sanford TL, Garrick JG. Non-operative treatment of the torn anterior cruciate ligament. *JBJS* 65A:184–192, 1983.

41. Glaros AG, Hanson K. EMG biofeedback and discriminative muscle control. *Biofeedback Self Regul* 15:135–143, 1990.

42. Glenncross D, Thornton E. Position sense following joint injury. *Am J Sports Med* 21:23–27, 1981.

43. Goodwin GM, McCloskey DI, Matthews PC. The contribution of muscle afferents to kinesthesia shown by vibration induced illusions of movement and by effects of paralyzing joint afferents. *Brain* 95:705–748, 1972.

44. Granit R. *The Basis of Motor Control.* New York, Academic Press, 1970.

45. Grigg P. Peripheral neural mechanisms in proprioception. *J Sport Rehabil* 3:1–17, 1994.

46. Grigg P. Response of joint afferent neurons in cat medial articular nerve to active and passive movements of the knee. *Brain Res* 118:482–485, 1976.

47. Grigg P, Finerman GA, Riley LH. Joint position sense after total hip replacement. *JBJS* 55A:1016–1025, 1973.

48. Grigg P, Hoffman AH. Ruffini mechanoreceptors in isolated joint capsule. Reflexes correlated with strain energy density. *Somatosens Mot Res* 2:149–162, 1984.

49. Grigg P, Hoffman AH. Properties of Ruffini afferents revealed by stress analysis of isolated sections of cats knee capsule. *J Neurophysol* 47:41–54, 1982.

50. Guyton AC. *Textbook of Medical Physiology*, 6th ed. Philadelphia, WB Saunders, 1991.

51. Haddad B. Protection of afferent fibers from the knee joint to the cerebellum of the cat. *Am J Physiol* 172:511–514, 1953.

52. Hagood SM, Solomonow R, Baratta BH, et al. The effect of joint velocity on the contribution of the antagonist musculature to knee stiffness and laxity. *Am J Sports Med* 18:182–187, 1990.

53. Harter RA, Osternig LR, Singer SL, Larsen RL, Jones DC. Long-term evaluation of knee stability and function following surgical reconstruction for anterior cruciate ligament insufficiency. *Am J Sports Med* 16:434–442, 1988.

54. Hellenbrant FA. Motor learning reconsidered: A study of change. In: *Neurophysiologic Approaches to Therapeutic Exercise.* Philadelphia, FA Davis, 1978.

55. Hocherman S, Dickstein R, Pillar T. Platform training and postural stability in hemiplegia. *Arch Phys Med Rehabil* 65:588–592, 1984.

56. Hodgson JA, Roy RR, DeLeon R, et al. Can the mammalian lumbar spinal cord learn a motor task? *Med Sci Sports* 26:1491–1497, 1994.

57. Horak FB. Clinical measurement of postural control in adults. *Phys Ther* 67:1881–1885, 1989.

58. Horak FB, Nashner LM. Central programming of postural movements. Adaptation to altered support surface configurations. *J Neurophysiol* 55:1369–1381, 1986.

59. Horak FB, Shupert CL, Mirka A. Components of postural dyscontrol in the elderly. *Neurobiol Aging* 10:727–738, 1989.

60. Houk JC. Regulation of stiffness by skeletomotor reflexes. *Ann Rev Phys* 41:99–114, 1979.

61. Houk JC, Crago PE, Rymer WZ. Function of the dynamic response in stiffness regulation: A predictive mechanism provided by non-linear feedback. In: Taylor A, Prochazka A, eds. *Muscle Receptors and Feedback.* London, Macmillan, 1981.

62. Houk JC, Henneman E. Responses of Golgi tendon organs to active contractions of the soleus muscle in the cat. *J Neurophysiol* 30:466–481, 1967.

63. Houk JC, Rymer WZ. Neural controls of muscle length and tension. In: Brooks VB, ed. *Handbook of Physiology: Section 1: The Nervous System, Vol. 2: Motor Control.* Bethesda, MD, American Physiological Society, 1981.

64. Hutton RS, Atwater SW. Acute and chronic adaptations of muscle proprioceptors in response to increased use. *Sports Med* 14:406–421, 1992.

65. Ihara H, Nakayama A. Dynamic joint control training for knee ligament injuries. *Am J Sports Med* 14:309–315, 1986.

66. Johnson RB, Howard ME, Cawley PW, Losse GM. Effect of lower extremity muscular fatigue on motor control performance. *Med Sci Sports* 30:1703–1707, 1998.

67. Kennedy JC, Alexander IJ, Hayes KC. Nerve supply to the human knee and its functional importance. *Am J Sports Med* 10:329–335, 1982.

68. Konradsen L, Ravin JB. Prolonged peroneal reaction time in ankle instability. *Int J Sports Med* 12:290–292, 1991.

69. Lee RG, Murphy JT, Tatton WG. Long latency myotatic reflexes in man: Mechanisms, functional significance, and changes in patients with Parkinson's disease or hemiplegia. In: Desmedt J, ed. *Advances in Neurology.* Basel, Karger, 1983.

70. Lee WA. Anticipatory control of postural and task muscles during rapid arm flexion. *J Mot Behav* 12:185–196, 1980.

71. Lephart SM. Reestablishing proprioception, kinesthesia, joint position sense and neuromuscular control in rehabilitation. In: Prentice WE, ed. *Rehabilitation Techniques in Sports Medicine*, 2nd ed. St. Louis, MO, Mosby, 1994.

72. Lephart SM, Henry TJ. Functional rehabilitation for the upper and lower extremity. *Orthop Clin North Am* 26:579–592, 1995.

73. Lephart SM, Kocher MS, Fu FH, et al. Proprioception following ACL reconstruction. *J Sport Rehabil* 1:188–196, 1992.

74. Lephart SM, Pincivero DM, Giraldo JL, Fu F. The role of proprioception in the management and rehabilitation of athletic injuries. *Am J Sports Med* 25:130–137, 1997.

75. Marks R, Quinney HA. Effect of fatiguing maximal isokinetic quadriceps contractions on the ability to estimate knee position. *Percept Mot Skills* 77:1195–1202, 1993.

76. Matsusaka N, Yokoyama S, Tsurusaki T, et al. Effect of ankle disk training combined with tactile stimulation to the leg and foot in functional instability of the ankle. *Am J Sports Med* 29(1):25–30, 2001.

77. Matthews PC. Where does Sherrington's "muscular sense" originate? Muscle, joints, corollary discharges? *Ann Rev Neurosci* 5:189, 1982.

78. McCloskey DI. Kinesthetic sensitivity. *Physiol Rev* 58:763–820, 1978.

79. McComas AJ. Human neuromuscular adaptations that accompany changes in activity. *Med Sci Sports* 26:1498–1509, 1994.

80. McNair PJ, Marshall RN. Landing characteristics in subjects with normal and anterior cruciate ligament deficient knee joints. *Arch Phys Med* 75:584–589, 1994.

81. McNair PJ, Wood GA, Marshall RN. Stiffness of the hamstring muscles and its relationship to function in anterior cruciate deficient individuals. *Clin Biomech* 7:131–173, 1992.

82. Melville-Jones GM, Watt GD. Observations of the control stepping and hopping in man. *J Physiol* 219: 709–727, 1971.

83. Mizuta H, Shiraishi M, Kubota K, Kai K, Takagi K. A stabiliometric technique for the evaluation of functional instability in the anterior cruciate ligament-deficient knee. *Clin J Sports Med* 2:235–239, 1992.

84. Morgan DL. Separation of active and passive components of short-range stiffness of muscle. *Am J Physiol* 32:45–49, 1977.

85. Nashner LM. Sensory, neuromuscular, and biomechanical contributions to human balance. In: Duncan PW, ed. *Balance: Proceedings of the APTA Forum.* Alexandria, VA, APTA, 1986, p. 550.

86. Nichols TR, Houk JC. Improvement of linearity and regulation of stiffness that results from actions of stretch reflex. *J Neurophysiol* 39:119–142, 1976.

87. Nyland JA, Shapiro R, Stine RL, et al. Relationship of fatigued run and rapid stop to ground reaction forces, lower extremity kinematics, and muscle activation. *J Orthop Sports Phys Ther* 20:132–137, 1994.

88. Ognibene J, McMahan K, Harris M, Dutton S, Voight M. Effects of unilateral proprioceptive perturbation training on postural sway and joint reaction times of healthy subjects. In: *Proceedings of National Athletic Training Association Annual Meeting.* Champaign, IL, Human Kinetics, 2000.

89. Palta AE, Winter DA, Frank JS. Identification of age-related changes in the balance control system. In: Duncan PW, ed. *Balance: Proceedings of the APTA Forum.* Alexandria, VA, APTA, 1986.

90. Perlau RC, Frank C, Fick G. The effects of elastic bandages on human knee proprioception in the uninjured population. *Am J Sports Med* 23:251–255, 1995.

91. Peterka RJ, Black OF. Age related changes in human postural control: Sensory organization tests. *J Vestib Res* 1:73–85, 1990.

92. Phillips CG, Powell TS, Wiesendanger M. Protection from low threshold muscle afferents of hand and forearm area 3A of Babson's cortex. *J Physiol* 217:419–446, 1971.

93. Pinstaar A, Brynhildsen J, Tropp H. Postural corrections after standardized perturbations of single limb stance: Effect of training and orthotic devices in patients with ankle instability. *Br J Sports Med* 30:151–155, 1996.

94. Pope MH, Johnson DW, Brown DW, Tighe C. The role of the musculature in injuries to the medial collateral ligament. *JBJS* 61A:398–402, 1972.

95. Pousson M, Hoecke JV, Goubel F. Changes in elastic characteristics of human muscle and induced by eccentric exercise. *J Biomechanics* 23:343–348, 1990.

96. Rine RM, Voight ML, Laporta L, Mancini R. A paradigm to evaluate ankle instability using postural sway measures. *Phys Ther* 74:S72, 1994.

97. Rogers DK, Bendrups AP, Lewis MM. Disturbed proprioception following a period of muscle vibration in humans. *Neurosci Lett* 57:147–152, 1985.

98. Rothwell J. *Control of Human Voluntary Movement,* 2nd ed. London, Chapman & Hall, 1994.

99. Rowinski, MJ. Afferent neurobiology of the joint. In: The role of eccentric exercise. In: *ProClinics.* Shirley, NY, Biodex, 1988.

100. Sakai H, Tanaka S, Kurosawa H, Masujima A. The effect of exercise on anterior knee laxity in female basketball players. *Int J Sports Med* 13:552–554, 1992.

101. Schmidt RA. The acquisition of skill: Some modifications to the perception-action relationship through practice. In: Heuer H, Sanders AF, eds. *Perspectives on Perception and Action.* Hillsdale, NJ, Erlbaum, 1987.

102. Schmidt RA. *Motor Control and Learning.* Champaign, IL, Human Kinetics, 1988.

103. Schulmann D, Godfrey B, Fisher A. Effect of eye movements on dynamic equilibrium. *Phys Ther* 67:1054–1057, 1987.

104. Schulte MJ, Happel LT. Joint innervation in injury. *Clin Sports Med* 9:511–517, 1990.

105. Sherrington CS. *The Interactive Action of the Nervous System.* New Haven, Yale University Press, 1911.

106. Sheth P, Yu B, Laskowski ER, et al. Ankle disk training influences reaction times of selected muscles in a simulated ankle sprain. *Am J Sports Med* 25:538–543, 1997.

107. Shumway-Cook A, Horak FB. Assessing the influence of sensory interaction on balance. *Phys Ther* 66:1548–1550, 1986.

108. Sittig AC, Denier van der Gon JJ, Gielen CM. Different control mechanisms for slow and fast human arm movements. *Neurosci Lett* 22:S128, 1985.

109. Sittig AC, Denier van der Gon JJ, Gielen CM. Separate control of arm position and velocity demonstrated by vibration of muscle tendon in man. *Exp Brain Res* 60:445–453, 1985.

110. Skinner HB, Barrack RL, Cook SD, Haddad RJ. Joint position sense in total knee arthroplasty. *J Orthop Res* 1:276–283, 1984.

111. Skinner HB, Wyatt MP, Hodgdon JA, Conrad DW, Barrack RI. Effect of fatigue on joint position sense of the knee. *J Orthop Res* 4:112–118, 1986.

112. Skoglund CT. Joint receptors and kinesthesia. In: Iggo A, ed. *Handbook of Sensory Physiology.* Berlin, Springer-Verlag, 1973.

113. Skoglund S. Anatomical and physiological studies of the knee joint innervation in the cat. *Acta Physiol Scand Suppl* 36(Suppl 124):1–101, 1956.

114. Small C, Waters CL, Voight ML. Comparison of two methods for measuring hamstring reaction time using the Kin-Com Isokinetic Dynamometer. *J Orthop Sports Phys Ther* 19, 1994.

115. Smith JL. Sensorimotor integration during motor programming. In: Stelmach GE, ed. *Information Processing in Motor Control and Learning.* New York, Academic Press, 1978.

116. Solomonow M, Baratta R, Zhou BH, et al. The synergistic action of the anterior cruciate ligament and thigh muscles in maintaining joint stability. *Am J Sports Med* 15:207–213, 1987.

117. Steiner ME, Brown C, Zarins B, et al. Measurements of anterior–posterior displacement of the knee: A comparison of results with instrumented devices and with clinical examination. *JBJS* 72A:1307–1315, 1990.

118. Stoller DW, Markoff KL, Zager SA, Shoemaker SC. The effect of exercise, ice, and ultrasonography on torsional laxity of the knee. *Clin Orthop* 174:172–180, 1983.

119. Stuart DG, Mosher CG, Gerlack RL, Reinking RM. Mechanical arrangement and transducing properties of Golgi tendon organs. *Exp Brain Res* 14:274–292, 1972.

120. Swanik CB, Lephart SM, Giannantonio FP, Fu F. Reestablishing proprioception and neuromuscular control in the ACL-injured athlete. *J Sport Rehab* 6:183–206, 1997.

121. Tibone JE, Antich TJ, Funton GS, Moynes DR, Perry J. Functional analysis of anterior cruciate ligament instability. *Am J Sports Med* 14:276–284, 1986.

122. Tippett S, Voight ML. *Functional Progressions for Sports Rehabilitation.* Champaign, IL. Human Kinetics, 1995.

123. Tropp H, Askling C, Gillquist J. Prevention of ankle sprains. *Am J Sports Med* 13:259–262, 1985.

124. Tropp H, Ekstrand J, Gillquist J. Factors affecting stabiliometry recordings of single leg stance. *Am J Sports Med* 12:185–188, 1984.

125. Tropp H, Odenrick P. Postural control in single limb stance. *J Orthop Res* 6:833–839, 1988.

126. Voight ML. Proprioceptive concerns in rehabilitation. In: *Proceedings of the 25th FIMS World Congress of Sports Medicine.* Athens, Greece, International Sports Medicine Federation, 1994.

127. Voight ML. Functional exercise training. Presented at the 1990 National Athletic Training Association Annual Conference, Indianapolis, IN, 1990.

128. Voight ML, Bell S, Rhodes D. Instrumented testing of tibial translation during a positive Lachman's test and selected closed-chain activities in anterior cruciate deficient knees. *J Orthop Sports Phys Ther* 15:49, 1992.

129. Voight ML, Blackburn TA, Hardin JA. Effects of muscle fatigue on shoulder proprioception. *J Orthop Sports Phys Ther* 21:348–352, 1996.

130. Voight ML, Cook G, Blackburn TA. Functional lower quarter exercises through RNT. In: Bandy WD, ed. *Current Trends for the Rehabilitation of the Athlete.* Lacrosse, WI, Sports Physical Therapy Section Home Study Course, 1997.

131. Voight ML, Draovitch P. Plyometric training. In: Albert M, ed. *Muscle Training in Sports and Orthopaedics.* New York, Churchill Livingstone, 1991.

132. Voight ML, Nashner LM, Blackburn TA. Neuromuscular function changes with ACL functional brace use: A measure of reflex latencies and lower quarter EMG responses [abstract]. In: *Conference Proceedings,* American Orthopedic Society for Sports Medicine, 1998.

133. Voight ML, Rine RM, Apfel P, et al. The effects of leg dominance and AFO on static and dynamic balance abilities. *Phys Ther* 73(6):S51, 1993.

134. Voight ML, Rine RM, Briese K, Powell C. Comparison of sway in double versus single leg stance in unimpaired adults. *Phys Ther* 73(6):S51, 1993.

135. Voss DE, Ionta MK, Myers BJ. Proprioceptive neuromuscular facilitation: Patterns and Techniques. Philadelphia, Harper & Row, 1985.

136. Walla DJ, Albright JP, McAuley E, Martin V, Eldridge V, El-khoury G. Hamstring control and the unstable anterior cruciate ligament-deficient knee. *Am J Sports Med* 13:34–39, 1985.

137. Wester JU, Jespersen SM, Nielsen KD, et al. Wobble board training after partial sprains of the lateral ligaments

of the ankle: A prospective randomized study. *J Orthop Sports Phys Ther* 23:332–336, 1996.

138. Wetzel MC, Stuart DC. Ensemble characteristics of cat locomotion and its neural control. *Prog Neurobiol* 7:1–98, 1976.

139. Willis WD, Grossman RG. *Medical Neurobiology*, 3rd ed. St Louis, MO, Mosby, 1981.

140. Wojtys E, Huston L. Neuromuscular performance in normal and anterior cruciate ligament-deficient lower extremities. *Am J Sports Med* 22:89–104, 1994.

141. Wojtys E, Huston L, Taylor PD, Bastian SD. Neuromuscular adaptations in isokinetic, isotonic, and agility training programs. *Am J Sports Med* 24(2):187–192, 1996.

142. Woollacott MH. Postural control mechanisms in the young and the old. In: Duncan PW, ed. *Balance: Proceedings of the APTA Forum.* Alexandria, VA, APTA, 1990.

143. Woollacott MH, Shumway-Cook A, Nashner LM. Aging and posture control: Changes in sensory organs and muscular coordination. *Int J Aging Hum Dev* 23:97–114, 1986.

213

CHAPTER 12

Isokinetics in Rehabilitation

Kevin Robinson

OBJECTIVES

After completing this chapter, the therapist should be able to do the following:

- Describe the concept of isokinetic resistance.
- Identify the advantages and disadvantages of isokinetic exercise.
- Describe the testing parameters associated with isokinetic testing and make reasoned choices.
- Interpret the data using a variety of methods (bilateral comparison, torque to body weight, etc.).
- Determine how and when *multijoint systems* are incorporated into the rehabilitation process.
- Apply principles to treatment of a patient with an anterior cruciate ligament reconstruction, lateral ankle sprain, and shoulder instability.
- Become familiar with advancements in isokinetic data presentation.

Although *constant angular devises* have been used to determine muscle function for over 70 years,[44] Hislop and Perrin first described the concept of isokinetics in 1967.[17] The isokinetic concept is based on the principle that the angular velocity of a moving limb can be constantly maintained by changing the force generated by a device to resist the intended movement. Therefore, as the limb accelerates from a resting position to the preset angular velocity, the isokinetic device produces a counterforce equal to the isokinetic speed in order to maintain this preset speed.

Deceleration begins once the muscle's length-tension relationship is reached. The ability of a muscle to generate torque (rotational force) about a joint is a function of a number of physiologic characteristics, including muscle cross-sectional areas, muscle moment arm, motor unit recruitment, and firing frequency.[43] During normal activity, the body must handle the constant acceleration and deceleration forces that occur naturally throughout activities of daily living. Currently, clinicians and researchers have the ability to evaluate how fast a muscle can accelerate to and decelerate from a preset angular velocity.

DEFINITION OF TERMS

A common method used in clinical practice to determine muscle strength is the manual muscle test (MMT).[20] Although the MMT is used clinically, it has been scrutinized because of the inherent limitations.[25] These limitations include inconsistency in grading and method,[9] the potential for subjectivity in reporting,[23] and the fact that the MMT is a static test, not a dynamic one. Because of these limitations, the MMT should not be used exclusively when determining precise isolated muscle impairments or readiness to progress to the next phase in the rehabilitation process.

Although commonly referred to as isokinetic dynamometers (Fig. 12-1), *multijoint systems* (MJSs) are truly multimode dynamometers capable of evaluating isokinetic, isometric, isotonic, and reactive-eccentric methods, and, when needed, can even be used to estimate spasticity in hemiparetic stroke patients.[8] Originally, isokinetics was used primarily as a testing medium. Today, technological advances allow clinicians to advance patients from the acute phases of rehabilitation to the more functional movement patterns faster and safer than ever. To take advantage of the MJS, common terminology must be established.

Isometrics

Popularized as an effective method of muscle strengthening, isometrics have been used throughout the rehabilitation process for decades. Isometric by definition means "same length." Thus, as the muscle contracts, there is no associated lengthening or shortening. Clinically, isometrics are used during the early phases of rehabilitation when motion is limited or painful arcs are noted

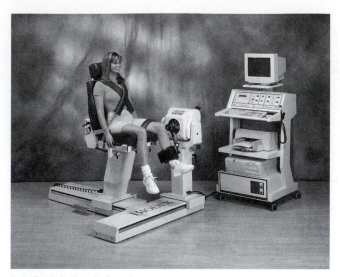

FIGURE 12-1

Biodex system 3 MJSs.

(such as with patellofemoral dysfunction). When initiating isometrics, an important parameter to keep in mind is that of the physiologic overflow. Atha noted that because a 20° physiologic overflow exists with isometric training, patients could rehabilitate within pain-free ranges and still improve strength in the affected ranges.[2] Isometrics can be relatively inexpensive, but without proper supervision patients can overload the healing structure beyond its capabilities. The goal of any rehabilitation program is to strengthen the muscles that surround the joint without overstressing the healing structures. MJSs provide the feedback necessary to safely load the muscle at various points.

Isotonics

In isotonic exercise, mass remains a constant during movement, while the rate of contraction changes. For example, if a person holds a 5-lb weight and performs a knee extension exercise, the weight will not change throughout the range of motion, but the speed of movement is variable. A major drawback to isotonic exercise is that the muscle is maximally loaded at its weakest point in the range of motion. If a weight is placed on the foot and the knee is extended from a flexed position, only the extended position is maximally loaded (the muscle is in a position of active insufficiency) while the rest of the range of motion is "underloaded." Safety is another issue that must be considered when incorporating isotonics into the treatment program. MJSs offer a concentric/concentric isotonic contraction, which can be configured to ensure safe muscular contractions by allowing the clinician to set the range of motion stops so that the patient only works in a pain-free arc of motion. Likewise, the clinician can restrict the amount of force produced, or the amount of work performed by the patient in order to protect from overly aggressive contractions. The MJS constantly monitors the force output throughout the contraction. If the force produced by the

patient suddenly drops, as a result of discomfort for example, then the unit will return the limb back to its starting position.

Isokinetics

Isokinetics is simply defined as "constant velocity." The clinician presets the velocity, not the force, which is applied by the patient. The clinical significance of this mode is that if a patient feels any pain, or when fatigue sets in, the patient will be able to continue the dynamic contraction throughout a full range of motion, but torque production will decrease. Because both isokinetic and isotonic exercise are dynamic, the patient can perform exercises both concentrically (muscle shortens as it contracts) and eccentrically (muscle lengthens as it contracts). Much of the isokinetic research has been completed using concentric contractions, but new research evaluating total neuromuscular performance is approaching. It has been noted that rehabilitation programs incorporating isokinetic exercise are more efficient and effective than programs that do not include isokinetic activity.[29]

TESTING PARAMETERS: WHAT TO LOOK FOR

The data that are collected during isokinetic testing are commonly used to make important decisions on a patient's rehabilitation program. Most commonly, a patient's data are compared bilaterally because this gives a useful comparison of the involved to noninvolved side. Research has shown this to be a reliable method to analyze data because limb dominance has little to no effect. In addition to the bilateral comparison, a patient's data can be compared to a normative or "goal" database. When performing an isokinetic evaluation, Wilk and Arrigo noted 15 parameters for standardized testing (Table 12-1).[39]

Planes of motion. When testing shoulder musculature, the clinician must decide which pattern(s) to test. It is important to

TABLE 12-1

Guidelines for Standardized Isokinetic Testing

1.	Planes of motion to evaluate
2.	Testing position/stabilization
3.	Axis of joint motion
4.	Client education
5.	Active warm-up
6.	Gravity compensation
7.	Rest intervals
8.	Test collateral extremity first
9.	Standardize verbal feedback
10.	Standardize visual feedback
11.	Testing velocities utilized
12.	Test repetitions
13.	System calibration/verification
14.	System level/stabilized
15.	Use semihard end stop

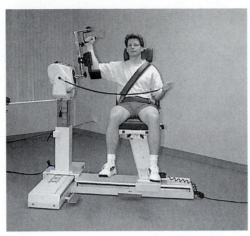

Planes of motion. Testing of the shoulder internal/
external rotators on an overhead athlete should be
performed at a 90°/90° position.

keep in mind the specific motions and actions the patient
will be performing throughout daily function. If the patient
is an overhead athlete, then testing of the shoulder internal
and external rotators should be performed in 90° of shoulder abduction and 90° of elbow flexion (90°/90° position)
(Fig. 12-2). This approximates the normal length–tension
relationships of the overhead athlete.

Position and stabilization. It is extremely important to eliminate
excessive movements above and below the joint being evaluated. Adequate stabilization is a must for accurate data
collection. In addition, the position of the patient with respect to active and passive insufficiency of the muscles being
assessed must also be considered. For example, the sitting
position is often used when testing the quadriceps and
hamstring muscles. However, the sitting position places
the hamstring muscle group at a disadvantage, lengthening that group at both the hip and at the knee. With the
current MJSs, it is now possible to assess the strength of
the hamstring muscle group in a lying position, which not
only eliminates the excessive lengthening of the muscle but
also tests the muscle group in a more functional position.
There is also debate about the best position to test internal
and external shoulder rotation.[22,27] This will be discussed
later in this chapter.

*Align the axis of rotation of the patient with that of the dynamome-
ter.* Wilk noted that this was important for accurate torque
measurements in all joints.[35] Although difficult in joints
that axes are not "fixed" during motion, the manual for the
machine being used has suggestions that should standardize dynamometer axis placement.

Client education. Prior to testing, the patient must understand
exactly what is expected of him/her and what to expect
from the test. How it "feels," what to do, and when to do
it are questions that should be answered prior to testing.

Investigators have noted significant changes in results from
the first testing session to all others.[21]

Active warm-up. The active warm-up should serve two very important purposes. First, it serves to increase core temperature and prepare the muscles for strenuous activity, and,
second, it familiarizes the patient with the testing velocities
being used.

Gravity compensation. When the knee goes from a flexed position to an extended position, gravity works against this
motion. The exact opposite occurs when the patient begins
to flex the knee from full extension (i.e., gravity assists). To
eliminate the effects of gravity, it is suggested that limb
weight be taken and automatically factored into the data.
Most contemporary dynomometers offer this as an automatic feature.

Rest intervals. For the purpose of this chapter, rest intervals deal
with the time between a test set at a specified speed. Touey
et al.[31] noted that 120 seconds was the optimal rest period,
whereas Ariki et al.[1] noted that the optimal rest period was
90 seconds. In either case, it is important to keep in mind
the total amount of time available for testing. If two to
three positions are going to be evaluated, 90–120 seconds
between test speeds greatly increases the time needed to
complete the test.

Testing the uninvolved extremity first. This is an important step
in the familiarization process and greatly reduces potential
apprehension.

Standardization of verbal commands. According to Wilk,[35] verbal commands need to be consistent, encouraging, and
moderate in intensity.

Use (or nonuse) of visual input. It has been noted by researchers
that knowledge of results does not affect mean peak torque.[18] Others, however, have noted an increase in performance during isokinetic testing when knowledge of results
was present.[12,14] For this reason, it is important to choose
one and remain consistent throughout the testing protocol.

Testing velocities. The joint being evaluated will determine exactly what test speeds are suggested (Table 12-2). Much of
the current research dealing with shoulders and knees indicates use of higher velocity testing (180–300°/second)[41] to
accommodate for the high angular velocities encountered
during normal activity. Smaller joints, wrist, ankle, and
forearm are generally tested at slower velocities. However,
it should be noted that no contemporary dynamometer is
capable of testing at the exact velocities encountered during moderate and sport function of the upper and lower
extremities. Currently, testing speeds of 60°, 120°, and
180° per second are commonly used. The use of the slower
speed (60°/second) is to assess strength-generating capabilities for the muscle group, and the use of the higher speeds
(180°/second and above) is to assess the power-generating
abilities. One important clinical consideration is that
the patient needs to be able to achieve the testing speed.
Some patients who have undergone rotator cuff repair or

TABLE   12-2

Suggested Test Speeds

JOINT	PATTERN	ORTHOPEDIC PATIENT	ATHLETE
Knee	Extension/flexion	(60), 180, 300	180, 300, 450
Knee	Tibial external/internal rotation	(60), 60, 120	120, 180, 240
Shoulder	Abduction/adduction	(60), 180, 300	180, 300, 450
Shoulder	Flexion/extension	(60), 180, 300	180, 300, 450
Shoulder	External/internal rotation	(60), 180, 300	180, 300, 450
Shoulder	D1, D2	(60), 180, 300	180, 300, 450
Shoulder	Horizontal abduction/adduction	(60), 180, 300	180, 300, 450
Elbow	Flexion/extension	(60), 180, 300	180, 300
Wrist	Extension/flexion	60, 120	120, 180
Wrist	Radial/ulnar deviation	60, 120	120, 180
Forearm	Supination/pronation	60, 120	120, 180, 240
Ankle	Plantarflexion/dorsiflexion	60, 120	(60), 120, 180
Ankle	Eversion/inversion	60, 120	(60), 120, 180
Hip	Flexion/extension	(120), 180, 300	180, 300, 450
Hip	Abduction/adduction	(120), 180, 300	180, 300, 450
Hip	Internal/external rotation	60, 120	120, 180

Test speeds in parentheses may be approximate, depending on pathology.

who are recovering from a neurological insult (stroke) will not be able to achieve a testing speed of 180° per second on their involved limb.

Number of test repetitions. Davies[10] reported that 10 isokinetic repetitions produced optimal training effects for peak torque to body weight and average power-testing parameters. The important aspect to keep in mind is to ensure consistency of test repetitions. Common testing protocols use three to five repetitions for slow speeds and 10 to 15 repetitions for higher testing speeds. This allows for adequate assessment of strength and power without fatiguing the muscle.

System calibration and verification. According to manufacturer specifications, the isokinetic systems should be calibrated and verified every 30 days,[5] but if the testing is going to be used for legal purposes, the system should be calibrated and verified just prior to testing. Today's calibration/verification procedures are quite simple and take only a moment to complete.

Level installation. When the system is installed, the technician should ensure that the system is level.

Use of a semihard end stop. Once a range of motion is selected, end stops will be created. As the patient moves through the range of motion toward the end stop, the machine will begin to decelerate the limb. This deceleration is caused by the machine's cushion function. A cushion can be adjusted from hard to soft by choosing a numeral, one to nine. A hard cushion offers little to no machine-induced deceleration, whereas a soft cushion yields a greater machine

deceleration. If a large joint is tested (shoulder elevators or back), a softer cushion is recommended. For smaller joints, a harder cushion is recommended. If a harder cushion is selected, it is vital to ensure that "artifact spiking" does not occur (see Fig. 12-3). This occurs when a patient rapidly decelerates into the end range of motion, causing a spike and potentially misrepresenting a peak torque. It is important to understand this concept when choosing a cushion for testing.

The most important concept to remember when testing patients or research participants is to maintain consistency. If the therapist is working in a setting where more than one person

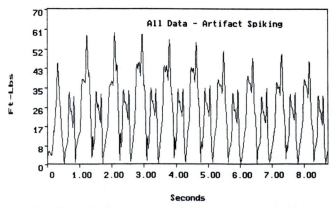

FIGURE   12-3

Artifact spiking caused by dynamometer's hard end stop.

will be testing patients, time should be taken to discuss the previously described parameters and determine exactly how testing will occur.

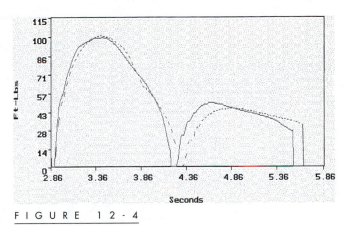

FIGURE 12-4

"Bell-shaped" torque curve.

RELIABILITY OF ISOKINETIC DYNAMOMETERS

There are several published studies that illustrate the reliability of isokinetic dynamometers.[3,11,13] Factors affecting the reliability of test results have been previously discussed in this chapter. Only by eliminating inconsistent variables, the clinician can be assured that the test results are reliable. The important questions that need to be answered are when a test is "nonreliable" and should the patient retest?

A common parameter noted on all reports is the coefficient of variance (CV). The CV is the ratio between the standard deviation and the mean value for a statistical population expressed as a percentage. It is used to objectively determine the reproducibility of test data. A patient with a high CV (25 percent or greater) is not producing a consistent effort. This is not to say that he/she is not trying; it only represents a patient's level of consistency. Pain, lack of understanding, and apprehension all lead to excessive CVs. It is important to evaluate the CV just after the completion of each test speed. If excessive CVs are noticed at a specific speed, a retest can occur after a brief rest period. This saves the evaluator a great deal of time in the long run.

TORQUE CURVE ANALYSIS

Because isokinetic testing evaluates a specific muscle group, the therapist can easily determine the effect this muscle has on the surrounding joint structure. A normal torque curve at slower velocities is said to be "bell shaped" (Fig. 12-4). This is due to

the normal human leverage system and length-tension relationships. When pain is present, this "normal" curve changes in its appearance. For example, if a patient is suffering from a deterioration of the articular surface on the underside of the patella (chondromalacia patella), he/she tends to feel pain throughout the middle of knee range of motion. This pain causes an insufficient quadriceps contraction that leads to a poorly shaped curve (Fig. 12-5). When performing a bilateral comparison, curve analysis can assist with a graphical representation of the involved and uninvolved sides. This can be especially helpful when explaining the results of a test to a patient (Fig. 12-6).

An important parameter in torque curve analysis is the ability for the MJS to store all the collected data. Once the test or training is complete, torque curve analysis can begin. It is important to be able to view all curves from a particular test set. Without the storage of the data points, this would be impossible. There is little published on the ability to diagnose an injury through curve analysis; however, clinicians should combine the curve analysis with their clinical findings to assist

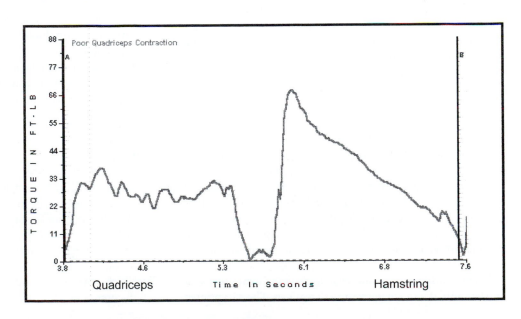

FIGURE 12-5

Poor quadriceps contraction.

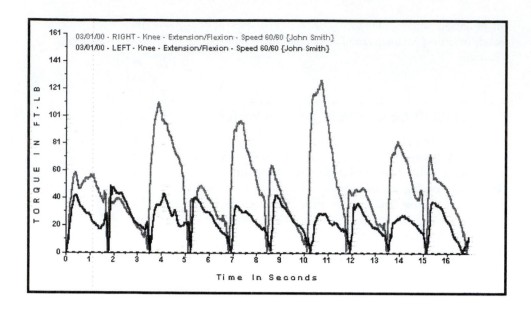

FIGURE 12 - 6

Bilateral overlay.

with the diagnosis. It should be noted, however, that Timm observed a distinct isokinetic torque curve for the impingement syndrome compared with the noninvolved shoulder.[30]

DATA INTERPRETATION

Understanding the data as presented on the isokinetic report is probably one of the most overlooked aspects in the education process. The purpose of the isokinetic test is threefold: first, *find the problem.* Is there an isolated physical impairment that is causing a functional deficit? Does this manifest itself during a concentric or eccentric contraction type? Where in the range of motion is the problem—in the beginning, middle, or end range of motion?

Next, *is the rehabilitation program effective in decreasing this isolated physical impairment?* Clinicians should be able to determine if the treatment program is having a positive or negative effect on patients' progress. Throughout the rehabilitation process, clinicians should be measuring progress objectively to determine if the treatment is effective.

Finally, *has the patient been rehabilitated?* This question goes beyond the realm of isokinetic evaluations only. Although the isokinetic test provides valuable information about the isolated muscle function about a joint, it is just one piece of the total process. To return to function, the patient must also have adequate joint stability. Lower extremity joint stability is comprised of three areas: muscle performance, postural balance, and structural integrity (Fig. 12-7). A deficit in any one of these parameters will lead to inadequate joint stability and, thus, a decrease in function. (Please refer to Chapters 7, 20, and 23 for further information on functional testing and assessment.)

These questions should begin with the patient's first visit and last until the end of the treatment regimen. The data printed

on the reports should be utilized to answer these questions and may include the following:

Peak torque—the highest value of torque developed throughout the range of motion.

Average peak torque—instead of using just one repetition for measuring peak torque, all the repetitions' peak torque are averaged together.

Time to peak torque—a measure of time from the start of the muscular contraction to the point of highest torque development, an indicator of the functional ability to produce torque.

Angle of peak torque—point in the range of motion where peak torque is achieved, a task-specific test of functional ability of a joint. Peak torque usually occurs in a similar point in the range of motion for like speeds and movement patterns.

- Torque at various angles (30° of knee flexion) displays the torque produced for each direction at the preselected position.
- Torque in a certain amount of time (0.20 seconds) displays the time rate torque development, that is, how quickly the patient can achieve a certain level of torque.

Peak torque to body weight—a ratio displayed as a percentage of the maximum torque production to the patient's body weight.

Maximum repetition work—the maximum work (force × distance) produced in a single repetition. This could be a better representation of functional ability (over peak torque) because the muscle must maintain force throughout the range of motion as opposed to force at one instant.

Work to body weight—a ratio displayed as a percentage of the maximum repetition work to the patient's body weight.

Total work—the sum of work for every repetition performed in the bout.

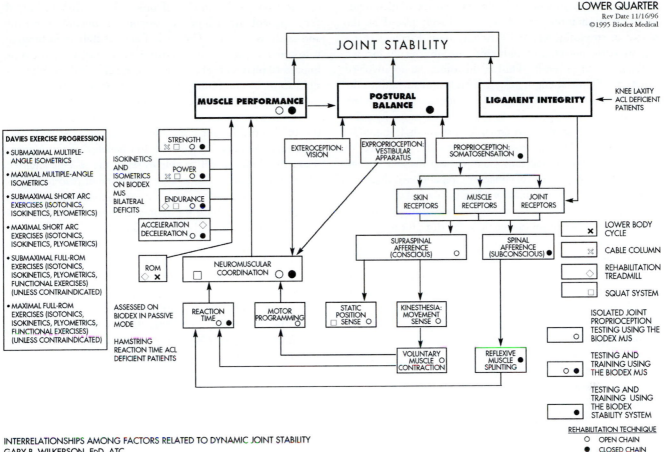

INTERRELATIONSHIPS AMONG FACTORS RELATED TO DYNAMIC JOINT STABILITY
GARY B. WILKERSON, EdD, ATC

FN: 96-205 11/96

FIGURE 12-7

Lower extremity joint stability flowchart.

Work first third, work last third—this is the total work of the first third divided by work in the last third of the test bout.

Average power—the total work divided by the time it takes to perform the work. Power is used to measure muscular efficiency.

Maximum gravity effect on torque—limb weight is measured, then added to torque values when working against gravity and subtracted from torque values when working with gravity.

Acceleration time—the time it takes the limb to accelerate from a resting position to achieve the preset isokinetic velocity. This should not be controlled by the computer but by the patient. The harder and faster the patient contracts, the quicker he/she should achieve isokinetic speed.

Deceleration time—this is the time it takes to go from isokinetic speed back down to 0°/second.

Agonist/antagonist ratio—a ratio between the agonist and antagonist muscle group tested, an important parameter in determining excessive muscular imbalance.

Bilateral and unilateral comparisons—once the test is complete, the clinician must compare the test result to one of two parameters: the noninvolved (uninjured) extremity or a normative (goal) database. In the case of extremity testing, having a noninvolved side to compare to makes the determination of impairment quite easy. Several investigators noted no significant difference between the dominant and nondominant throwing arm in internal and external rotator muscle strength (peak torque).[24,37] Wilk et al. noted that there was no significant difference between the dominant and nondominant throwing arm in abductor muscle strength, but there was a significant difference in adductor strength.[38] Capranica et al. reported no significant difference in force and power values between the dominant and nondominant lower limb.[8] From a shoulder proprioception standpoint, Voight et al. determined that there was no relationship between arm dominance and shoulder proprioception.[32] Thus, it is important to understand that limb dominance does not play a significant role when using bilateral comparisons.

Another parameter to consider is the detraining effect. Once an injury occurs, both the involved and noninvolved extremities begin to lose their strength characteristics. During the rehabilitation process, focus is usually placed on the injured or surgically repaired extremity only. Exercises to regain strength, power, and endurance are unilaterally focused on the involved extremity. During this time, the noninvolved extremity will lose strength as well. This loss of strength to the noninvolved leg makes it difficult to compare bilaterally late in the rehabilitation process. As the involved extremity gains strength, the noninvolved extremity loses strength. It should be noted that some investigators have found a crossover effect of training. Weir et al. noted that when participants were trained unilaterally (three sets of six concentric repetitions), their isometric strength increased at all test angles bilaterally.[34]

Because confusion exists, the use of preseason, preemployment, or preparticipation isokinetic strength tests can serve as an important baseline used for comparison later in the rehabilitation process. Most notably a patient, athlete, or employee would be tested prior to activity or employment. These numbers can be used to determine when the individual has regained normal (preinjury) strength. Objective test data can also be useful when progressing patients through the various phases of rehabilitation.

Another important consideration is the use of normative or goal data. In certain instances, bilateral comparisons are impossible. For example, consider a patient with bilateral injuries or a test of the lumbar spine. In these cases, there is no side-to-side comparison available. To determine if the patient has returned to normal strength levels, it is important to be able to compare to a goal database. The use of normative data is quite popular, but there are many important parameters that need to be noted prior to its use. Is the patient population similar to the one being tested? Are the normative values from athletes, industrial workers, pediatric or geriatric groups, or a sedentary population? Are the data age and gender specific? How were the data collected? Did the participants receive visual feedback? Were there verbal commands? What type of warm-up was used? All of these parameters must be established prior to the inclusion of any normative values.

Because normative values are difficult to use and many reported in the literature are variable, it is the author's opinion that a "goal" database be used only for comparison. These data will provide the clinician only with a general overview of performance. The clinician should not use this information to note normalcy, rather to note when a patient has achieved adequate muscle performance. It should be restated that strength alone is *not* sufficient for determining if a patient is ready to return to activity. For the lower extremity, postural balance and structural integrity should be quantified as well.

TRAINING PARAMETERS AND MODES OF OPERATION

Multijoint or isokinetic systems are capable of much more than isokinetic testing and training. Isometric, isotonic, reactive eccentric, and passive modes of operation all combine to advance patients from injury or surgery to function as quickly and safely as possible. The goal of any rehabilitation program is to progress patients from postinjury or surgery to the more functional phases of rehabilitation as quickly and safely as possible. Only by combining the various modes of operation can the clinician take the fullest advantage of the MJS.

Isometrics can be used early in the rehabilitation process; this mode provides angle-specific contractions and with varying torque outputs. To gain the full benefits of the *isometric mode*, the clinician will be able to select the specific angles of contraction, time of contraction, and time of relaxation. The clinician can also choose which muscle groups (agonist only, antagonist only, or both the agonist and antagonist) to work. Testing can be completed efficiently and is an effective outcome measure.

As discussed previously in this chapter, the MJS allows for a safe progressive isotonic contraction, first beginning with concentric/concentric contractions and progressing to concentric/eccentric or eccentric/concentric contractions. In the *isotonic mode*, the muscle must overcome the torque selected prior to the limb moving in either direction. Because both the agonist and antagonist muscle groups contract concentrically, two different torque limits can be selected. Thus, the agonist torque can be set to a low weight (5 ft/lb) while the antagonist weight higher (100 ft/lb) and vise versa.

As the patient progresses, an isotonic eccentric contraction can be introduced into the rehabilitation program. The clinician has the ability to adjust the concentric and eccentric torque limits as needed as well as the speed of the eccentric contraction. This greatly enhances the clinician's ability to control the movement and maintain a safe rehabilitation environment. Thus, a patient could be asked to lift 10 ft/lb concentrically and lower 30 ft/lb eccentrically at 60°/second. This would be very similar to using two weight stacks on a single piece of exercise equipment.

Another mode of operation is the *reactive eccentric* mode. The reactive eccentric mode allows for an eccentric/eccentric contraction only. To accomplish an eccentric contraction, the clinician sets both the maximum amount of torque the patient can apply and the minimum amount of torque needed to begin the movement. Thus, a window is created for a patient to stay within. If torque levels go too high, the lever arm stops moving. If the torque levels go too low, the lever arm again stops moving. Therefore, for the patient to keep the limb moving the entire time, torque levels must stay between the two limits. This is an excellent way to enhance motor control early in the rehabilitation process.

Aside from the isokinetic mode, the *passive* mode is the most commonly used mode on the MJS. The passive mode is very similar to that of a continual passive motion device in which the clinician sets a range of motion such that the limb will move through without any effort from the patient. This is extremely important in the early phases of the rehabilitation process when the focus is on reducing edema and increasing range of motion. Noyes et al. demonstrated the negative effect of prolonged immobilization on joint surfaces.[26] If a patient is noted to have motion complications, the passive mode can be an excellent tool to restore full range to the joint. The passive mode can also assist with active muscle contractions as well. The clinician can instruct the patient to "kick up" or "pull back" as needed. Thus, concentric, eccentric, and isometric contractions can be accomplished in this one mode. The clinician has the ability to adjust the passive speed, eccentric torque limits, pauses at the end ranges of motion, and range of motion as needed. Therefore, it is important to understand that an MJS is capable of much more than just isokinetic testing. Clinicians should have the ability to adjust the necessary parameters anytime during the rehabilitation process.

CLINICAL CONSIDERATIONS

Prior to the discussion of pathological conditions, it is important to understand the relation of angular velocity to torque outputs. When initiating a treatment regimen, it is important to note the effects of slow angular velocities on the joint as compared to higher velocities (Table 12-3). Because it is important to understand how MJS can be used to treat various pathologies, the following examples give an illustration of exactly where the MJS fits into the rehabilitation process.

Anterior Cruciate Ligament Reconstruction

For the anterior cruciate ligament (ACL)-reconstructed patient (patella tendon graft), begin in the passive mode to regain range of motion. After selecting a safe range to work within, the clinician can incorporate additional modalities (cold, heat, electrotherapy) to assist with the rehabilitation process. While in the passive mode, patients can be instructed to "pull back" or use their hamstrings to begin the strengthening process.

Because the tibia moves posterior in relation to the femur from 90° to 70° degrees of knee flexion, it would be safe to begin submaximal quadriceps contractions. Bouchard et al. noted that maximal isometrics at 70° of knee flexion caused patella fractures in three subjects that were approximately 7, 11, and 12 weeks post-ACL reconstruction.[7] Submaximal quadriceps contractions could begin in the passive mode, but the clini-

cian cannot prevent the patient from excessive concentric force production.

The reactive eccentric mode might provide a safer progression. First, the range of motion should be set to protect excessive anterior tibial translation. Wilk et al. noted that during open-chain knee extension, there was an anterior shear force from 38° to 0° (peaking at 14°) and a posterior shear force from 40° to 101° of knee flexion.[40]

Next, the torque limit for the quadriceps should be set at 20 ft/lb. Yack et al. noted that a 20-lb Lachman evaluation produces less anterior tibial displacement than an open-chain knee extension at 18° of knee flexion.[45] The torque limit for the hamstrings can be set to a greater limit. The patient should be instructed to "pull back" to get the limb to move upward and "kick up" to get the limb to move back into the flexed position. Thus, an eccentric/eccentric contraction sequence occurs. The patient needs to understand that the attachment should always be moving. If the patient applied too much or too little torque, the attachment will stop moving, and this is not the appropriate response.

When the patient is ready to progress to active concentric quadriceps contractions, a few parameters must be kept in mind. If graft strength is in question, set the extension stop below 30° of knee flexion. Next, higher speeds (180–300°/second) should be used early in the rehabilitation process. Finally, raise the tibial pad proximally. All three strategies reduce the stress placed on the healing graft.[36]

Beynnon and Johnson noted that biomechanical studies of healing ACL grafts performed in animals have shown that the graft requires 12 or more months to revascularize and heal and the biomechanical behavior of the graft never returns to normal.[4] During this phase, the patient can progress to the use of the isotonic and isokinetic modes. Begin with concentric/concentric movements (less than 20 ft/lb on the quadriceps) and progress to concentric/eccentric movements. When determining the readiness to return to activity, ensure that adequate muscular strength, power, endurance, acceleration, and deceleration are present and have been assessed by an isokinetic examination. It is equally important that postural balance, neuromuscular control, and functional, structural integrity have also been assessed.

Lateral Ankle Sprain

As with any acute injury, the range of motion needs to be restored. The passive mode can be utilized early in the rehabilitation process. Begin with plantar- and dorsiflexion and progress to inversion and eversion. The Biodex closed-chain (Fig. 12-8) attachment can be a useful tool in this early stage as well. The patient can place the foot in the closed-chain attachment and begin actively loading the joint prior to full weight bearing.

The isometric mode can be used to prevent disuse atrophy. Place the ankle in the neutral position and have the patient perform submaximal contractions without the fear of excessive motion. Next, progress to dynamic strengthening of the

T A B L E   1 2 - 3

Angular Velocity and Torque Outputs

VELOCITY	CONCENTRIC	ECCENTRIC
Slow (30–120°/sec)	High	Low
Moderate (120–270°/sec)	Moderate	Moderate
Fast (300°/sec and above)	Low	High

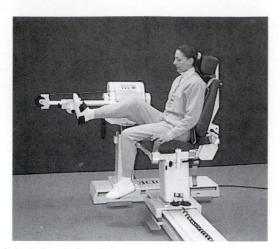

The Biodex closed-chain attachment.

plantar- and dorsiflexors. Begin with slower speed isokinetics (30–60°/second) and progress to faster (120–180°/second) speeds.

When exercising the plantar- and dorsiflexors, remember that the dorsiflexors will fatigue much quicker than the plantarflexors. A simple method to allow for similar fatigue responses is to set the plantarflexor speed slow (60°/second) and the dorsiflexor speed faster (120°/second). Next, progress to concentric/eccentric muscle strengthening. Wilkerson et al. noted that a lateral ankle ligament injury might be associated with an invertor muscle performance deficiency.[42] Again, remember to ensure adequate dynamic functional stability prior to returning to activity via performance of functional tests and screening procedures.

Shoulder Instability/Impingement

Glenohumeral stability is maintained statically by the capsulolabral complex and dynamically by the rotator cuff musculature.[33] The rotator cuff muscles must function synergistically to allow for normal shoulder arthrokinematics. When imbalance or injury occurs, shoulder function diminishes.

An important aspect to consider when testing or training using the isokinetic mode is the position in which the patient is placed. During the initial phases of rehabilitation, the 90° abduction 90° elbow flexed (90°/90°) position should be limited. This is the same position Hoppenfeld describes for the apprehension test and could cause episodes of instability.[19] On the other hand, Rathburn noted that a position placing the humerus against the body could cause a "wringing out" of the supraspinatus tendinous insertion[27] and thus eliminates this position as well. The recommended starting position places the humerus in 20–30° forward flexion and abduction (scapular plane) therefore decreasing the chance of instability and impingement.[22]

According to Wilk et al.,[39] when testing throwers, the 90°/90° seated position closely approximates that of normal throwing motion while ensuring muscle isolation. This position

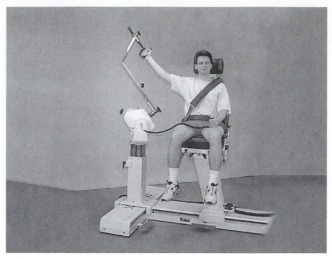

Coactivation of the external rotators in a seated D2 position.

also optimizes the length-tension relationship of the internal and external rotation as they perform the throwing sequence. Based on this information, it is important that clinicians do not overlook the various testing positions. Both the scapular plane and 90°/90° positions have benefits and drawbacks when testing. It is the clinician's responsibility to determine when it

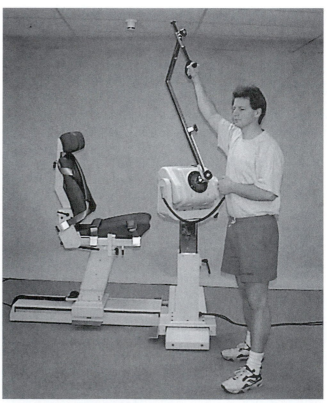

Coactivation of the external rotators in a standing D2 position, incorporating total body movement.

```
Name        : Smith, J.        Clinician     : AB                  Joint          : Knee
ID          : 11999933         Referral      :                    Pattern        : Extension/Flexion
Age         : 30               Cal. Verification: SEP 01, 1999 08:00:00   Treatment      :
Sex         : M                Test Date     : FEB 23, 2000        Involved Side  :
Height (in): 55                Settings      :                    Contraction    : N/A
Weight (lbs): 200              Data Reported : All Data            Mode           :
```

JOINT POSITION SENSE TEST

Test Direction ___ Extension ___

Active Positioning (patient moves limb)

Target Position :   15.0   15.0

		Uninvolved	Involved	Difference
Degrees from Target :	Rep 1 :	2.0	31.0	-29.0
	Rep 2 :	4.0	24.0	-20.0
	Rep 3 :	6.0	31.0	-25.0
	Average :	4.0	28.7	-24.7

Passive Positioning (BIODEX moves limb)

Target Position :   15.0   15.0

		Uninvolved	Involved	Difference
Degrees from Target :	Rep 1 :	9.0	25.0	-16.0
	Rep 2 :	2.0	14.0	-12.0
	Rep 3 :	2.0	15.0	-13.0
	Average :	4.3	18.0	-13.7

Kinesthesia Test: Degrees to Detect Motion

Target Position :   45.0   45.0

		Uninvolved	Involved	Difference
Degrees from Target :	Rep 1 :	10.0	8.0	2.0
	Rep 2 :	13.0	11.0	2.0
	Rep 3 :	8.0	12.0	-4.0
	Average :	10.3	10.3	0

FIGURE 12-11

Biodex proprioception report.

is safe to progress from the scapular plane to the 90°/90° position. Traditionally, when an isokinetic test is performed, "end stops" are placed at 90° external rotation and 0° of internal rotation. Thus, as the patient reaches the end stop the MJS plays a role in the deceleration of the humerus. During normal function when the arm is externally rotating, the internal rotators coactivate to decelerate the humerus. Therefore, the clinician might want to extend the end limit for external rotation beyond 90° to approximately 130° of external rotation and evaluate the patient's ability to decelerate the humerus. The same could be true for the evaluation of the external rotators. This time, have the patient working in a diagonal 2 (D2) position (Fig. 12-9)

seated. Now have the patient concentrically D2 extend toward the body. As the arm passes the horizontal position, the external rotators must contract eccentrically to decelerate the arm. Progress to standing D2 and incorporate a total body movement (Fig. 12-10).

PROPRIOCEPTION

One area of great concern to clinicians is that of proprioception. Proprioception is defined as the cumulative neural input to the central nervous system from specialized nerve endings called mechanoreceptors.[32] When the topic of proprioceptive training comes up, most clinicians think of weight-bearing exercises. This has been an established treatment practice for both the upper and lower extremities. Current research is focusing on proprioception in the non-weightbearing position.[6,16] The three types of proprioceptive tests noted in the literature are passive repositioning, active repositioning, and threshold to detect passive motion.[6,16] Each of these tests can be completed on the MJS. In fact, some systems are even capable of reporting these findings (Fig. 12-11). Unfortunately, no easily accessible, reliable clinical alternative exists for those who do not have MJS.

To complete the passive and active repositioning tests, simply place the patient in the chair and fix the attachment to the limb. Next, blindfold the patient to remove visual feedback. Place the limb at the "target" angle (this is the angle the patient will replicate, 15° of knee flexion or 75° of shoulder external rotation, for example). Return the patient to the starting angle (90° of knee flexion or neutral shoulder rotation). The MJS should be set to the appropriate mode—isokinetic for active repositioning and passive mode (2°/second) for passive repositioning—and testing is now ready to begin. The patient should move (or be moved) toward the target angle and disengage the system when he/she perceives to be there. A record of the exact position (and difference from the target angle) is noted. An average of three test trials is often used in testing. The threshold to detect passive motion works in a similar manner. First, place the patient at the target angle (45° of knee flexion or 45° of shoulder rotation). Place the MJS in the passive mode at 2°/second. Explain to the patient that he/she should disengage the system as soon as any motion is sensed. The MJS will record the exact degrees of movement from the target angle. Although proprioceptive testing is becoming more mainstream, there are limited treatment options available and further research is needed. Lephart noted three things concerning proprioceptive testing: arm dominance is not a factor in the proprioceptive mechanism; functional instability produced diminished sense of proprioception, especially in the functional position of abduction and external rotation; and finally, surgery combined with rehabilitation may restore some, if not all, of the proprioceptive sensibility and may ultimately improve function and prevent the recurrence of symptoms.[6]

ADVANCED TECHNOLOGIES

Recently, a new form of isokinetic evaluation has become commercially available. This new report is designed to reduce the emphasis on "numbers" from an isokinetic evaluation. Isomap is a graphic representation and qualitative analysis of muscle performance (Fig. 12-12). Isomap uses the same isokinetic information necessary to generate a three-speed bilateral report. Instead of the numeric report, a graphical report of neuromuscular performance is generated. The goal of an Isomap evaluation is to identify where in the range of motion, which angular velocities,

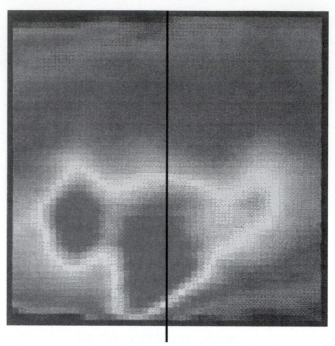

FIGURE   12-12

Isomap is a graphical, rather than numeric, representation and qualitative analysis of muscle performance.

and which muscle groups or contraction types are most effected. By determining this, clinicians can create treatment protocols designed to eliminate the isolated physical impairments.

To understand the Isomap image, one must first break down the map into three different axes: the x axis, y axis, and z axis. On the map (Fig. 12-13), x axis represents the angular velocities selected. The centerline represents no angular velocity. By moving further to the right, the concentric angular velocity increases. To the far left, the eccentric velocity increases. The y axis represents the range of motion covered during the test. The top of the map indicates full extension, and the bottom of the map indicates full flexion. The z axis represents torque output. The greater the torque output, the redder the map gets. Red represents areas of great strength, and blue represents areas of weaker strength. On the "deficit map" the area in red indicates where in the range of motion, at what speeds, and which contraction type the greatest difference occurred between the involved and uninvolved sides. Hence, clinicians now have the opportunity to identify the neuromuscular performance associated with isolated muscle testing. Hiemstra et al. noted that during an Isomap evaluation (five speeds concentric and five speed eccentric) a combined ACL group ($n = 8$ patella tendon) ($n = 16$ hamstring) revealed a global 25.5 percent extensor strength deficit, with eccentric regional (angle and velocity matched) deficits up to 50 percent of control ($n = 30$).[15] Now that Isomap evaluations are commercially available, clinicians and researchers alike can benefit from these technological advances.

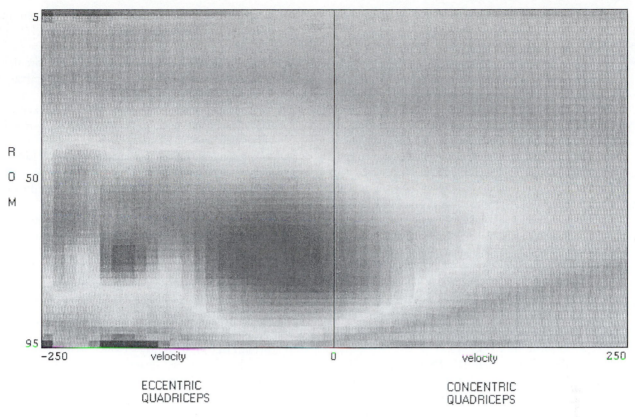

FIGURE 12-13

Isomaps are broken into three different axes—x axis (contraction type/muscle group and speeds), y axis (range of motion), and z axis (torque values).

SUMMARY

- Isokinetic exercise is a movement that occurs at a constant angular velocity with accommodating resistance.
- It is important to be consistent with testing parameters to ensure reliable and valid data.
- Various parameters are defined on the output report. It is best to consider peak torque, total work, and average power when creating a treatment plan.
- MJSs have several modes of operation (isometric, isotonic, reactive eccentric, passive, and isokinetic modes) that can be used throughout the rehabilitation process.
- Slow isokinetic velocities increase compressive and translational forces versus faster isokinetic velocities but are easier for the patient to comprehend.
- There are many ways to interpret the plethora of data that is presented on an isokinetic test. Bilateral comparison is typical if one joint or muscle is uninjured. If no bilateral comparison exists, consider using normative data, torque to body weight values, and agonist/antagonist ratios.
- When treating the ACL-reconstructed patient, remember there is a posterior shear force from 40° to 101° and anterior shear force from 38° to 0° (peaking at 14°).

- When treating shoulder conditions, consider the position in which the internal and external rotators are being exercised and rehabilitated.
- Use slower isokinetic speeds for rehabilitation of smaller joints like the wrist and ankle.
- Prior to return to normal functional activities, ensure that adequate muscle strength, postural stability, and structural integrity have been established, using appropriate objective measures.

REFERENCES

1. Ariki PK, Davies GJ, Siewert MW, et al. Optimum rest interval between isokinetic velocity spectrum rehabilitation speeds. *Phys Ther* 65:735, 1985.
2. Atha J. Strengthening muscle. *Exerc Sport Sci* 9:1–73, 1981.
3. Bemdem MG, Johnson DA. Reliability of the Biodex B-2000. Isokinetic dynamometer and the evaluation of a sport-specific determination for the angle of peak torque during knee extension. *Isokin Exerc Sci* 3:164–168, 1993.
4. Beynnon BD, Johnson RJ. Anterior cruciate ligament

injury rehabilitation in athletes. Biomechanical considerations. *Sports Med* 22:54–64, 1996.

5. *Biodex Advantage Software Manual.* 1994.

6. Borsa PA, Lephart SM, Kocher MS, et al. Functional assessment and rehabilitation of shoulder proprioception for glenohumeral instability. *J Sport Rehabil* 6:327–334, 1997.

7. Bouchard CS, Theriault G, Gauthier JM, et al. Fracture of the patella during rehabilitation of the knee extensor muscles following reconstruction of the anterior cruciate ligament: A brief report. *Clin J Sports Med* 3:126–130, 1993.

8. Capranica L, Cama G, Fanton F, et al. Force and power of preferred and non-preferred leg in young soccer players. *J Sports Med Phys Fitness* 32:358–363, 1992.

9. Daniels L, Worthington C. *Muscle Testing: Techniques of Manual Examination*, 5th ed. Philadelphia, PA, Saunders, 1986.

10. Davies G. *A Compendium of Isokinetic in Clinical Usage*, 3rd ed. Onolaska, WI, S & S Publishers, 1987.

10A. Davies GJ. The need for critical thinking in rehabilitation. *J Sport Rehabil* 4:1–22, 1995.

11. Feiring DC, Ellenbecher TS, Derscheid GL. Test-reliability of the Biodex isokinetic dynamometer. *J Orthop Sports Phys Ther* 23:348–352, 1996.

12. Figoni FI, Morris AF. Effects of knowledge of results on reciprocal isokinetic strength and fatigue. *J Orthop Sports Phys Ther* 6:104–106, 1984.

13. Grabiner MD, Jexiorowski JJ, Divekar AD. Isokinetic measurements of trunk extension and flexion performance collected with the Biodex clinical data station. *J Orthop Sports Phys Ther* 11:590–598, 1990.

14. Hald RD, Bottken EJ. Effects of visual input on maximal and submaximal isokinetic test measurements of normal quadriceps and hamstring. *J Orthop Sports Phys Ther* 9:86, 1987.

15. Hiemstra LA, Webber S, MacDonald PT, et al. Graft site dependent knee strength deficits after patellar tendon and hamstring tendon ACL reconstruction. *Med Sci Sports Exerc* 32(8):1472–1479, 2000.

16. Higgins MJ, Perrin DH. Comparison of weight-bearing and non-weight-bearing conditions on knee joint reposition sense. *J Sport Rehabil* 6:327–334, 1997.

17. Hislop H, Perrin J. The isokinetic concept of exercise. *Phys Ther* 47:114–117, 1967.

18. Hobbel SL, Rose DJ. The relative effectiveness of three forms of visual knowledge of results on peak torque output. *J Orthop Sports Phys Ther* 18(5):601–608, 1993.

19. Hoppenfield S. *Physical Examination of the Spine and Extremities.* Norwalk, CT, Appleton-Century-Crofts, 1976, p. 34.

20. Kendall FD, McCreary EK. *Muscle Testing and Function*, 3rd ed. Baltimore, Lippincott Williams & Wilkins, 1983.

21. Mawdsley RH, Knapik J. Comparison of isokinetic measurements with test repetitions. *Phys Ther* 62:169–172, 1882.

22. Neer CS II. Anterior acromioplasty for the chronic impingement syndrome in the shoulder. A preliminary report. *JBJS* 54A:41–50, 1972.

23. Nelson SG, Duncan PW. Correction of isokinetic and isometric torque readings for the effect of gravity. *Phys Ther* 63:674–676, 1983.

24. Newsham KR, Keith CS, Saunders JE, et al. Isokinetic profile of baseball pitchers' internal/external rotation 180, 300, 450°/second. *Med Sci Sports Exerc* 30:1489–1495, 1998.

25. Nicholas J, Sapega A, Kraus H, et al. Factors influencing manual muscle tests in physical therapy. *J Bone Joint Surg* 60:186, 1978.

26. Noyes FR, Mangine RE, Barber S. Early knee motion after open and arthroscopic anterior cruciate ligament reconstruction. *Am J Sport Med* 15:149–160, 1987.

27. Rathburn JB, McNab I. The microvascular pattern of the rotator cuff. *JBJS* 52B:540–553, 1970.

28. Schmit BD, Dewald J, Zev Rymer W. Variability of the stretch reflex during quantification of spasticity using constant velocity ramp stretches. *Med Rehabil* 81(3): 269–278, 2000.

29. Timm KE. Postsurgical knee rehabilitation: A five year study of four methods and 5,381 patients. *Am J Sports Med* 16:463–468, 1988.

30. Timm KE. The isokinetic torque curve of shoulder instability in high school baseball pitchers. *J Orthop Sports Phys Ther* 11:590–598, 1990.

31. Touey PA, Sforzo GA, McManis BG. Effect of manipulating rest periods on isokinetic muscle performance. *Med Sci Sports Exerc* 26:S170, 1994.

32. Voight ML, Hardin JA, Blackburn TA, et al. The effects of muscle fatigue on and the relationship of arm dominance to shoulder proprioception. *J Orthop Sports Phys Ther* 23:348–352, 1996.

33. Warner JJ, Micheli LS, Arslanian LE, et al. Patterns of flexibility, laxity, and strength in normal shoulder and shoulder with instability and impingement. *Am J Sports Med* 18:366–374, 1990.

34. Weir JP, Housh DJ, Housh TL, et al. The effect of unilateral concentric weight training and detraining on joint angle specificity, cross-training, and bilateral deficits. *J Orthop Sports Phys Ther* 25:264–270, 1997.

35. Wilk KE. *Dynamic Muscle Strength Testing: Instrumented and Non-Instrumented Systems.* New York, Churchill-Livingstone, 1990, pp. 123–150.

36. Wilk KE, Andrews JR. The effects of pad placement and angular velocity on tibial pad placement during isokinetic exercise. *J Orthop Sports Phys Ther* 17:24–30, 1993.

37. Wilk KE, Andrews JR, Arrigo CA. The abductor and

adductor strength characteristics of professional baseball pitchers. *Am J Sports Med* 23:307–311, 1995.

38. Wilk KE, Andrews JR, Arrigo CA, et al. The strength characteristics of internal and external rotator muscles in professional baseball pitchers. *Am J Sports Med* 21:61–66, 1993.

39. Wilk KE, Arrigo CA. Standardized isokinetic testing protocol for the throwing shoulder: The throwers' series. *Isokin Exerc Sci* 1:63–71, 1991.

40. Wilk KE, Escamilla RF, Fleisig GS, et al. A comparison of tibiofemoral joint forces and electromyographic activity during open and closed kinetic chain exercises. *Am J Sports Med* 24:518–527, 1996.

41. Wilk KE, Romaniello WT, Soscia SM, et al. The relationship between subjective knee scores, isokinetic test-

ing, and functional testing in the ACL-reconstructed knee. *J Orthop Sports Phys Ther* 20:60–73, 1994.

42. Wilkerson GB, Pinerola JJ, Caturano RW. Invertor vs. evertor peak torque and power deficiencies associated with lateral ankle injury. *J Orthop Sports Phys Ther* 26:79–87, 1997.

43. Wrigley T, Grant M. Isokinetic dynamometry. *Sports Physiology: Applied Science and Practice.* Edinburgh, Churchill Livingstone, 1995, pp. 259–287.

44. Wyman J. Studies on the relation of work and heat in tortoise muscle. *J Physiol* 61:337–352, 1926.

45. Yack JH, Colline CE, Whieldon TJ. Comparison of closed and open kinetic chain exercise in the anterior cruciate ligament-deficient knee. *Am J Sports Med* 21:49–54, 1993.

Plyometric Exercise in Rehabilitation

Michael L. Voight and Steven R. Tippett

OBJECTIVES

After completing this chapter, the therapist should be able to do the following:

- Describe the mechanical, neurophysiologic, and neuromuscular control mechanisms involved in plyometric training.
- Discuss how biomechanical evaluation, stability, dynamic movement, and flexibility should be assessed before beginning a plyometric program.
- Explain how a plyometric program can be modified by changing intensity, volume, frequency, and recovery.
- Discuss how plyometrics can be integrated into a rehabilitation program.

WHAT IS PLYOMETRIC EXERCISE?

In sports training and rehabilitation of athletic injuries, the concept of specificity has emerged as an important parameter in determining the proper choice and sequence of exercise in a training program. The jumping movement is inherent in numerous sport activities such as basketball, volleyball, gymnastics, and aerobic dancing. Even running is a repeated series of jump-landing cycles. Therefore jump training should be used in the design and implementation of the overall training program.

Peak performance in sport requires technical skill and power. Skill in most activities combines natural athletic ability and learned specialized proficiency in an activity. Success in most activities is dependent upon the speed at which muscular force or power can be generated. Strength and conditioning programs throughout the years have attempted to augment the force production system to maximize the power generation. Because power combines strength and speed, it can be increased by increasing the amount of work or force that is produced by the muscles or by decreasing the amount of time required to produce the force. Although weight training can produce increased gains in strength, the speed of movement is limited. The amount of time required to produce muscular force is an important variable for increasing the power output. A form of training that attempts to combine speed of movement with strength is plyometrics.

The term *plyometric training* is relatively new, but the concept of plyometric training is not. The roots of plyometric training can be traced to Eastern Europe, where it was known simply as jump training. The term *plyometrics* was coined by an American track and field coach, Fred Wilt.[35] The development of the term is confusing. *Plyo-* comes from the Greek word *plythein*, which means "to increase." *Plio* is the Greek word for "more," and *metric* literally means "to measure." Practically, plyometrics is defined as a quick, powerful movement involving prestretching the muscle and activating the stretch-shortening cycle to produce a subsequently stronger concentric contraction. It takes advantage of the length-shortening cycle to increase muscular power.

In the late 1960s and early 1970s when Eastern European countries began to dominate sports requiring power, their training methods became the focus of attention. After the 1972 Olympics, articles began to appear in coaching magazines outlining a strange new system of jumps and bounds that had been used by the Soviets to increase speed. Valery Borzov, the 100-meter gold medalist, credited plyometric exercise for his success. As it turns out, the Eastern European countries were not the originators of plyometrics, just the organizers. This system of hops and jumps has been used by American coaches for years as a method of conditioning. Both rope jumping and bench hops have been used to improve quickness and reaction times. The organization of this training method has been credited to the legendary Soviet jump coach Yuri Verkhoshanski, who during the late 1960s began to tie this method of miscellaneous hops and jumps into an organized training plan.[30]

The main purpose of plyometric training is to heighten the excitability of the nervous system for improved reactive ability of the neuromuscular system.[32] Therefore, any type of exercise that uses the myotatic stretch reflex to produce a more powerful response of the contracting muscle is plyometric in nature. All movement patterns in athletes and in activities of daily living involve repeated stretch-shortening cycles. Picture a jumping athlete preparing to transfer forward energy to upward energy. As the final step is taken before jumping, the loaded leg must stop the forward momentum and change it into an upward direction. As this happens, the muscle undergoes a lengthening eccentric contraction to decelerate the movement and prestretch the muscle. This prestretch energy is then immediately released in an equal and opposite reaction, thereby producing kinetic energy. The neuromuscular system must react quickly to produce the concentric shortening contraction to prevent falling and produce the upward change in direction. Most elite athletes will naturally exhibit this ability with great ease to use stored kinetic energy. Less gifted athletes can train this ability and enhance their production of power. Consequently, specific functional exercise to emphasize this rapid change of direction must be used to prepare patients and athletes for return to activity. Because plyometric exercises train specific movements in a biomechanically accurate manner, the muscles, tendons, and ligaments are all strengthened in a functional manner.

Most of the literature to date on plyometric training has been focused on the lower quarter. Because all movements in athletics involve a repeated series of stretch-shortening cycles, adaptation of the plyometric principles can be used to enhance the specificity of training in other sports or activities that require a maximum amount of muscular force in a minimal amount of time. Whether the athlete is jumping or throwing, the musculature around the involved joints must first stretch and then contract to produce the explosive movement. Because of the muscular demands during the overhead throw, plyometrics have been advocated as a form of conditioning for the overhead throwing athlete.[31,34] Although the principles are similar, different forms of plyometric exercises should be applied to the upper extremity to train the stretch-shortening cycle. Additionally, the intensity of the upper extremity plyometric program is usually less than that of the lower extremity, due to the smaller muscle mass and type of muscle function of the upper extremity compared to the lower extremity.

BIOMECHANICAL AND PHYSIOLOGIC PRINCIPLES OF PLYOMETRIC TRAINING

The goal of plyometric training is to decrease the amount of time required between the yielding eccentric muscle contraction and the initiation of the overcoming concentric contraction. Normal physiologic movement rarely begins from a static starting position but rather is preceded by an eccentric prestretch that

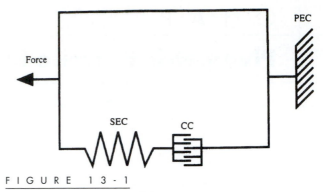

FIGURE 13-1

Three-component model.

loads the muscle and prepares it for the ensuing concentric contraction. The coupling of the eccentric–concentric muscle contraction is known as the stretch-shortening cycle. The physiology of this stretch-shortening cycle can be broken down into two components: proprioceptive reflexes and the elastic properties of muscle fibers. These components work together to produce a response, but they will be discussed separately for the purpose of understanding.

Mechanical Characteristics

The mechanical characteristics of a muscle can best be represented by a three-component model (Fig. 13-1). A contractile component (CC), series elastic component (SEC), and parallel elastic component (PEC) all interact to produce a force output. Although the CC is usually the focal point of motor control, the SEC and PEC also play an important role in providing stability and integrity to the individual fibers when a muscle is lengthened. During this lengthening process, energy is stored within the musculature in the form of kinetic energy.

When a muscle contracts in a concentric fashion, most of the force that is produced comes from the muscle fiber filaments sliding past one another. Force is registered externally by being transferred through the SEC. When eccentric contraction occurs, the muscle lengthens like a spring. With this lengthening, the SEC is also stretched and allowed to contribute to the overall force production. Therefore the total force production is the sum of the force produced by the CC and the stretching of the SEC. An analogy would be the stretching of a rubber band. When a stretch is applied, potential energy is stored and applied as it returns to its original length when the stretch is released.

Significant increases in concentric muscle force production have been documented when immediately preceded by an eccentric contraction.[2,5,9] This increase might be partly due to the storage of elastic energy, because the muscles are able to use the force produced by the SEC. When the muscle contracts in a concentric manner, the elastic energy that is stored in the SEC can be recovered and used to augment the shortening contraction. The ability to use this stored elastic energy is affected by three variables: time, magnitude of stretch, and velocity of stretch.[17] The concentric contraction can be magnified only if the preceding eccentric contraction is of short range and performed quickly without delay.[2,5,9] Bosco and Komi proved this concept experimentally when they compared damped versus undamped jumps.[5] Undamped jumps produced minimal knee flexion upon landing and were followed by an immediate rebound jump. With damped jumps, the knee flexion angle increased significantly. The power output was much higher with the undamped jumps. The increased knee flexion seen in the damped jumps decreased elastic behavior of the muscle, and the potential elastic energy stored in the SEC was lost as heat. Similar investigations produced greater vertical jump height when the movement was preceded by a countermovement as opposed to a static jump.[2,4,6,22]

The type of muscle fiber involved in the contraction can also affect storage of elastic energy. Bosco et al. noted a difference in the recoil of elastic energy in slow-twitch versus fast-twitch muscle fibers.[7] This study indicates that fast-twitch muscle fibers respond to a high-speed, small-amplitude prestretch. The amount of elastic energy used was proportional to the amount stored. When a long, slow stretch is applied to muscle, slow- and fast-twitch fibers exhibit a similar amount of stored elastic energy; however, this stored energy is used to a greater extent with the slow-twitch fibers. This trend would suggest that slow-twitch muscle fibers might be able to use elastic energy more efficiently in ballistic movement characterized by long and slow prestretching in the stretch-shortening cycle.

Neurophysiologic Mechanisms

The proprioceptive stretch reflex is the other mechanism by which force can be produced during the stretch-shortening cycle. Mechanoreceptors located within the muscle provide information about the degree of muscular stretch. This information is transmitted to the central nervous system and becomes capable of influencing muscle tone, motor execution programs, and kinesthetic awareness. The mechanoreceptors that are primarily responsible for the stretch reflex are the Golgi tendon organs and muscle spindles.[24] The muscle spindle is a complex stretch receptor that is located in parallel within the muscle fibers. Sensory information regarding the length of the muscle spindle and the rate of the applied stretch is transmitted to the central nervous system. If the length of the surrounding muscle fibers is less than that of the spindle, the frequency of the nerve impulses from the spindle is reduced. When the muscle spindle becomes stretched, an afferent sensory response is produced and transmitted to the central nervous system. Neurologic impulses are in turn sent back to the muscle, causing a motor response. As the muscle contracts, the stretch on the muscle spindle is relieved, thereby removing the original stimulus. The strength of the muscle spindle response is determined by the rate of stretch.[24] The more rapidly the load is applied to the muscle, the greater the firing frequency of the spindle and resultant reflexive muscle contraction.

The Golgi tendon organ lies within the muscle tendon near the point of attachment of the muscle fiber to the tendon. Unlike the facilitory action of the muscle spindle, the Golgi tendon organ has an inhibitory effect on the muscle by contributing to a tension-limiting reflex. Because the Golgi tendon organs are in series alignment with the contracting muscle fibers, they become activated with tension or stretch within the muscle. Upon activation, sensory impulses are transmitted to the central nervous system. These sensory impulses cause an inhibition of the alpha motor neurons of the contracting muscle and its synergists, thereby limiting the amount of force produced. With a concentric muscle contraction, the activity of the muscle spindle is reduced because the surrounding muscle fibers are shortening. During an eccentric muscle contraction, the muscle stretch reflex generates more tension in the lengthening muscle. When the tension within the muscle reaches a potentially harmful level, the Golgi tendon organ fires, thereby reducing the excitation of the muscle. The muscle spindle and Golgi tendon organ systems oppose each other, and increasing force is produced. The descending neural pathways from the brain help to balance these forces and ultimately control which reflex will dominate.[26]

The degree of muscle fiber elongation is dependent upon three physiologic factors. Fiber length is proportional to the amount of stretching force applied to the muscle. The ultimate elongation or deformation is also dependent upon the absolute strength of the individual muscle fibers. The stronger the tensile strength, the less elongation that will occur. The last factor for elongation is the ability of the muscle spindle to produce a neurophysiologic response. A muscle spindle with a low sensitivity level will result in a difficulty in overcoming the rapid elongation and therefore produce a less powerful response. Plyometric training will assist in enhancing muscular control within the neurologic system.

The increased force production seen during the stretch-shortening cycle is due to the combined effects of the storage of elastic energy and the myotatic reflex activation of the muscle.[2,4,8,9,23,27] The percentage of contribution from each component is unknown.[4] The increased amount of force production is dependent upon the time frame between the eccentric and concentric contractions.[9] This time frame can be defined as the amortization phase.[13] The amortization phase is the electromechanical delay between eccentric and concentric contraction, during which time the muscle must switch from overcoming work to acceleration in the opposite direction. Komi found that the greatest amount of tension developed within the muscle during the stretch-shortening cycle occurred during the phase of muscle lengthening just before the concentric contraction.[21] The conclusion from this study was that increased time in the amortization phase would lead to a decrease in force production.

Physiologic performance can be improved by several mechanisms with plyometric training. Although there has been documented evidence of increased speed of the stretch reflex, the increased intensity of the subsequent muscle contraction might be best attributed to better recruitment of additional motor units.[11] The force–velocity relationship states that the faster a muscle is loaded or lengthened eccentrically, the greater the resultant force output. Eccentric lengthening will also place a load on the elastic components of the muscle fibers. The stretch reflex might also increase the stiffness of the muscular spring by recruiting additional muscle fibers.[11] This additional stiffness might allow the muscular system to use more external stress in the form of elastic recoil.[11]

Another possible mechanism by which plyometric training can increase the force or power output involves the inhibitory effect of the Golgi tendon organs on force production. Because the Golgi tendon organ serves as a tension-limiting reflex, restricting the amount of force that can be produced, the stimulation threshold for the Golgi tendon organ becomes a limiting factor. Bosco and Komi have suggested that plyometric training can desensitize the Golgi tendon organ, thereby raising the level of inhibition.[5] If the level of inhibition is raised, a greater amount of force production and load can be applied to the musculoskeletal system.

Neuromuscular Coordination

The last mechanism in which plyometric training might improve muscular performance centers around neuromuscular coordination (see Chapter 11). The speed of muscular contraction can be limited by neuromuscular coordination. In other words, the body can move only within a set speed range, no matter how strong the muscles are. Training with an explosive prestretch of the muscle can improve the neural efficiency, thereby increasing neuromuscular performance. Plyometric training can promote changes within the neuromuscular system that allow the individual to have better control of the contracting muscle and its synergists, yielding a greater net force even in the absence of morphological adaptation of the muscle. This neural adaptation can increase performance by enhancing the nervous system to become more automatic.

In summary, effective plyometric training relies more on the rate of stretch than on the length of stretch. Emphasis should center on the reduction of the amortization phase. If the amortization phase is slow, the elastic energy is lost as heat and the stretch reflex is not activated. Conversely, the quicker the individual is able to switch from yielding eccentric work to overcoming concentric work, the more powerful the response.

PROGRAM DEVELOPMENT

Specificity is the key concept in any training program. Sport-specific activities should be analyzed and broken down into basic movement patterns. These specific movement patterns should then be stressed in a gradual fashion, based upon individual tolerance to these activities. Development of a plyometric program should begin by establishing an adequate strength base that will allow the body to withstand the large stress that will be placed upon it. A greater strength base will allow for greater force production due to increased muscular cross-sectional area. Additionally, a larger cross-sectional area can contribute to the SEC and subsequently store a greater amount of elastic energy.

Plyometric exercises can be characterized as rapid eccentric loading of the musculoskeletal complex.[11] This type of exercise trains the neuromuscular system by teaching it to more readily accept the increased strength loads.[3] Also, the nervous system is more readily able to react with maximal speed to the lengthening muscle by exploiting the stretch reflex. Plyometric training attempts to fine tune the neuromuscular system, so all training programs should be designed with specificity in mind.[25] This goal will help to ensure that the body is prepared to accept the stress that will be placed upon it during return to function.

Plyometric Prerequisites

BIOMECHANICAL EXAMINATION

Before beginning a plyometric training program, a cursory biomechanical examination and a battery of functional tests should be performed to identify potential contraindications or precautions. Lower-quarter biomechanics should be sound to help ensure a stable base of support and normal force transmission. Biomechanical abnormalities of the lower quarter are not contraindications for plyometrics but can contribute to stress, failure, or overuse injury if not addressed. Before initiating plyometric training, an adequate strength base of the stabilizing musculature must be present. Functional tests are very effective to screen for an adequate strength base before initiating plyometrics. Poor strength in the lower extremities will result in a loss of stability when landing and also increase the amount of stress that is absorbed by the weight-bearing tissues with high-impact forces, which will reduce performance and increase the risk of injury. The Eastern European countries arbitrarily placed a one-repetition maximum in the squat at 1.5–2 times the individual's body weight before initiating lower-quarter plyometrics.[3] If this were to hold true, a 200-lb individual would have to squat 400 lb before beginning plyometrics. Unfortunately, not many individuals would meet this minimal criterion. Clinical and practical experience has demonstrated that plyometrics can be started without that kind of leg strength.[11] A simple functional parameter to use in determining whether an individual is strong enough to initiate a plyometric training program has been advocated by Chu.[10] Power squat testing with a weight equal to 60 percent of the individual's body weight is used. The individual is asked to perform five squat repetitions in 5 seconds. If the individual cannot perform this task, emphasis in the training program should again center on strength training to develop an adequate base.

Because eccentric muscle strength is an important component to plyometric training, it is especially important to ensure that an adequate eccentric strength base is present. Before an individual is allowed to begin a plyometric regimen, a program of closed-chain stability training that focuses on eccentric lower-quarter strength should be initiated. In addition to strengthening in a functional manner, closed-chain weight-bearing exercises also allow the individual to use functional movement patterns. Once cleared to participate in the plyometric program, precautionary safety tips should be adhered to.

TABLE 13-1

TABLE 13-1

Plyometric Static Stability Testing

Single-leg stance—30 sec
  –Eyes open
  –Eyes closed
Single-leg 25% squat—30 sec
  –Eyes open
  –Eyes closed
Single-leg 50% squat—30 sec
  –Eyes open
  –Eyes closed

STABILITY TESTING

Stability testing before initiating plyometric training can be divided into two subcategories: static stability and dynamic movement testing. Static stability testing determines the individual's ability to stabilize and control the body. The muscles of postural support must be strong enough to withstand the stress of explosive training. Static stability testing (Table 13-1) should begin with simple movements of low motor complexity and progress to more difficult high motor skills. The basis for lower-quarter stability centers around single-leg strength. Difficulty can be increased by having the individual close the eyes. The basic static tests are one-leg standing and single-leg quarter squats that are held for 30 seconds. An individual should be able to perform one-leg standing for 30 seconds with eyes open and closed before the initiation of plyometric training. The individual should be observed for shaking or wobbling of the extremity joints. If there is more movement of a weight-bearing joint in one direction than the other, the musculature producing the movement in the opposite direction needs to be assessed for specific weakness. If weakness is determined, the individual's program should be limited and emphasis placed on isolated strengthening of the weak muscles. For dynamic jump exercises to be initiated, there should be no wobbling of the support leg during the quarter knee squats.

After an individual has satisfactorily demonstrated both single-leg static stance and a single-leg quarter squat, more dynamic tests of eccentric capabilities can be initiated. Once an individual has stabilization strength, the concern shifts toward developing and evaluating eccentric strength. The limiting factor in high-intensity, high-volume plyometrics is eccentric capabilities. Eccentric strength can be assessed with stabilization jump tests. If an individual has an excessively long amortization phase or a slow switching from eccentric to concentric contractions, the eccentric strength levels are insufficient.

DYNAMIC MOVEMENT TESTING

Dynamic movement testing will assess the individual's ability to produce explosive, coordinated movement. Vertical or single-leg jumping for distance can be used for the lower quarter.

Researchers have investigated the use of single-leg hop for distance and a determinant for return to play after knee injury. A passing score on their test is 85 percent in regard to symmetry. The involved leg is tested twice, and the average between the two trials is recorded. The noninvolved leg is tested in the same fashion, and then the scores of the noninvolved leg are divided by the scores of the involved leg and multiplied by 100. This provides the symmetry index score. Another functional test that can be used to determine whether an individual is ready for plyometric training is the ability to long jump a distance equal to the individual's height. In the upper quarter, the medicine ball toss is used as a functional assessment.

FLEXIBILITY

Another important prerequisite for plyometric training is general and specific flexibility, because a high amount of stress is applied to the musculoskeletal system. Therefore all plyometric training sessions should begin with a general warm-up and flexibility exercise program. The warm-up should produce mild sweating.[19] The flexibility exercise program should address muscle groups involved in the plyometric program and should include static and short dynamic stretching techniques.[18]

When individuals can demonstrate static and dynamic control of their body weight with single-leg squats, low-intensity in-place plyometrics can be initiated. Plyometric training should consist of low-intensity drills, and should progress slowly in deliberate fashion. As skill and strength foundation increase, moderate-intensity plyometrics can be introduced. Mature athletes with strong weight-training backgrounds can be introduced to ballistic–reactive plyometric exercises of high intensity.[10] Once the individual has been classified as beginner, intermediate, or advanced, the plyometric program can be planned and initiated. Chu has divided lower-quarter plyometric training into six categories (Table 13-2).[11–13]

PLYOMETRIC PROGRAM DESIGN

As with any conditioning program, the plyometric training program can be manipulated through training variables: direction of body movement, weight of the athlete, speed of the execution, external load, intensity, volume, frequency, training age, and recovery.

TABLE 13-2

Chu's Plyometric Categories

In-place jumping
Standing jumps
Multiple-response jumps and hops
In-depth jumping and box drills
Bounding
High-stress sport-specific drills

Direction of Body Movement

Horizontal body movement is less stressful than vertical movement. This is dependent upon the weight of the athlete and the technical proficiency demonstrated during the jumps.

Weight of the Athlete

The heavier the athlete, the greater the training demand placed on the athlete. What might be a low-demand in-place jump for a lightweight athlete might be a high-demand activity for a heavyweight athlete.

Speed of Execution of the Exercise

Increased speed of execution on exercises like single-leg hops or alternate-leg bounding raises the training demand on the individual.

External Load

Adding an external load can significantly raise the training demand. Do not raise the external load to a level that will significantly slow the speed of movement.

Intensity

Intensity can be defined as the amount of effort exerted. With traditional weight lifting, intensity can be modified by changing the amount of weight that is lifted. With plyometric training, intensity can be controlled by the type of exercise that is performed. Double-leg jumping is less stressful than single-leg jumping. As with all functional exercises, the plyometric exercise program should progress from simple to complex activities. Intensity can be further increased by altering the specific exercises. The addition of external weight or raising the height of the step or box will also increase the exercise intensity.

Volume

Volume is the total amount of work that is performed in a single workout session. With weight training, volume would be recorded as the total amount of weight that was lifted (weight times repetitions). Volume of plyometric training is measured by counting the total number of foot contacts. The recommended volume of foot contacts in any one session will vary inversely with the intensity of the exercise. A beginner should start with low-intensity exercise with a volume of approximately 75–100 foot contacts. As ability is increased, the volume is increased to 200–250 foot contacts of low to moderate intensity.

Frequency

Frequency is the number of times an exercise session is performed during a training cycle. With weight training, the frequency of exercise has typically been three times weekly. Unfortunately, research on the frequency of plyometric exercise has not been conducted. Therefore the optimum frequency for increased performance is not known. It has been suggested that 48–72 hours of rest is necessary for full recovery before the next training stimulus.[10] Intensity, however, plays a major role in determining the frequency of training. If an adequate recovery period does not occur, muscle fatigue will result with a corresponding increase in neuromuscular reaction times. The beginner should allow at least 48 hours between training sessions.

Training Age

Training age is the number of years an athlete has been in a formal training program. At younger training ages, the overall training demand should be kept low.

Recovery

Recovery is the rest time used between exercise sets. Manipulation of this variable will depend on whether the goal is to increase power or muscular endurance. Because plyometric training is anaerobic in nature, a longer recovery period should be used to allow restoration of metabolic stores. With power training, a work/rest ratio of 1:3 or 1:4 should be used. This time frame will allow maximal recovery between sets. For endurance training, this work/rest ratio can be shortened to 1:1 or 1:2. Endurance training typically uses circuit training, where the individual moves from one exercise set to another with minimal rest in between.

The beginning plyometric program should emphasize the importance of eccentric versus concentric muscle contractions. The relevance of the stretch-shortening cycle with decreased amortization time should be stressed. Initiation of lower-quarter plyometric training begins with low-intensity in-place and multiple-response jumps. The individual should be instructed in proper exercise technique. The feet should be nearly flat in all landings, and the individual should be encouraged to "touch and go." An analogy would be landing on a hot bed of coals. The goal is to reverse the landing as quickly as possible, spending only a minimal amount of time on the ground.

Success of the plyometric program will depend on how well the training variables are controlled, modified, and manipulated. In general, as the intensity of the exercise is increased, the volume is decreased. The corollary to this is that as volume increases, the intensity is decreased. The overall key to successfully controlling these variables is to be flexible and listen to what the athlete's body is telling you. The body's response to the program will dictate the speed of progression. Whenever in doubt as to the exercise intensity or volume, it is better to underestimate to prevent injury.

Before implementing a plyometric program, the sports therapist should assess the type of athlete who is being rehabilitated and whether plyometrics are suitable for that individual.

TABLE 13-3

Upper-Extremity Plyometric Drills

I. Warm-up drills

Plyoball trunk rotation
Plyoball side bends
Plyoball wood chops
External rotation (ER)/internal rotation (IR) with tubing
Proprioceptive neuromuscular feedback (PNF) D2
   pattern with tubing

II. Throwing movements—standing position

Two-hand chest pass
Two-hand overhead soccer throw
Two-hand side throw overhead
Tubing ER/IR (Both at side and 90° abduction)
Tubing PNF D2 pattern
One-hand baseball throw
One-hand IR side throw
One-hand ER side throw
Plyo push-up (against wall)

III. Throwing movements—seated position

Two-hand overhead soccer throw
Two-hand side-to-side throw
Two-hand chest pass
One-hand baseball throw

IV. Trunk drills

Plyoball sit-ups
Plyoball sit-up and throw
Plyoball back extension
Plyoball long sitting side throws

V. Partner drills

Overhead soccer throw
Plyoball back-to-back twists
Overhead pullover throw
Kneeling side throw
Backward throw
Chest pass throw

VI. Wall drills

Two-hand chest throw
Two-hand overhead soccer throw
Two-hand underhand side-to-side throw
One-hand baseball throw
One-hand wall dribble

VII. Endurance drills

One-hand wall dribble
Around-the-back circles
Figure eight through the legs
Single-arm ball flips

In most cases, plyometrics should be used in the latter phases of rehabilitation, starting in the advanced strengthening phase once the athlete has obtained an appropriate strength base.[31,34] When using plyometric training in the uninjured athlete, the application of plyometric exercise should follow the concept of periodization.[32] The concept of periodization refers to the year-round sequence and progression of strength training, conditioning, and sport-specific skills.[34] There are four specific phases in the year-round periodization model: the competitive season, postseason training, the preparation phase, and the transitional phase.[32] Plyometric exercises should be performed in the latter stages of the preparation phase and during the transitional phase for optimal results and safety. To obtain the benefits of a plyometric program, the athlete should (1) be well conditioned with sufficient strength and endurance, (2) exhibit athletic abilities, (3) exhibit coordination and proprioceptive abilities, and (4) be free of pain from any physical injury or condition.

Remember that the plyometric program is not designed to be an exclusive training program for the athlete. Rather, it should be one part of a well-structured training program that includes strength training, flexibility training, cardiovascular fitness, and sport-specific training for skill enhancement and coordination. By combining the plyometric program with other training techniques, the effects of training are greatly enhanced.

Tables 13-3 and 13-4 suggest upper-extremity and lower-extremity plyometric drills.

GUIDELINES FOR PLYOMETRIC PROGRAMS

The proper execution of the plyometric exercise program must continually be stressed. A sound technical foundation from which higher-intensity work can build should be established. It must be remembered that jumping is a continuous interchange

TABLE 13-4

Lower-Extremity Plyometric Drills

I. Warm-up drills

Double-leg squats
Double-leg leg press
Double-leg squat-jumps
Jumping jacks

II. Entry-level drills—two-legged

Two-legged drills
  Side to side (floor/line)
  Diagonal jumps (floor/four corners)
  Diagonal jumps (four spots)
  Diagonal zig/zag (six spots)
  Plyo leg press
  Plyo leg press (four corners)

III. Intermediate-level drills

Two-legged box jumps
  One-box side jump
  Two-box side jumps
  Two-box side jumps with foam
  Four-box diagonal jumps
  Two-box with rotation
  One-/two-box with catch
  One-/two-box with catch (foam)
Single-leg movements
  Single-leg plyo leg press
  Single-leg side jumps (floor)
  Single-leg side-to-side jumps (floor/four corners)
  Single-leg diagonal jumps (floor/four corners)

IV. Advanced-level drills

Single-leg box jumps
  One-box side jumps
  Two-box side jumps
  Single-leg plyo leg press (four corners)
  Two-box side jumps with foam
  Four-box diagonal jumps
  One-box side jumps with rotation
  Two-box side jumps with rotation
  One-box side jump with catch
  One-box side jump rotation with catch
  Two-box side jump with catch
  Two-box side jump rotation with catch

V. Endurance/agility plyometrics

Side-to-side bounding (20 ft)
Side jump lunges (cone)
Side jump lunges (cone with foam)
Altering rapid step-up (forward)
Lateral step-overs
High stepping (forward)
High stepping (backward)
Depth jump with rebound jump
Depth jump with catch
Jump and catch (plyoball)

between force reduction and force production. This interchange takes place throughout the entire body: ankle, knee, hip, trunk, and arms. The timing and coordination of these body segments yields a positive ground reaction that will result in a high rate of force production.

As the plyometric program is initiated, the individual must be made aware of several guidelines.[32] Any deviation from these guidelines will result in minimal improvement and increased risk for injury. These guidelines include the following:

1. Plyometric training should be specific to the individual goals of the athlete. Activity-specific movement patterns should be trained. These sport-specific skills should be broken down and trained in their smaller components and then rebuilt into a coordinated activity-specific movement pattern.
2. The quality of work is more important than the quantity of work. The intensity of the exercise should be kept at a maximal level.

3. The greater the exercise intensity level, the greater the recovery time.
4. Plyometric training can have its greatest benefit at the conclusion of the normal workout. This pattern will best replicate exercise under a partial to total fatigue environment that is specific to activity. Only low- to medium-stress plyometrics should be used at the conclusion of a workout, because of the increased potential of injury with high-stress drills.
5. When proper technique can no longer be demonstrated, maximum volume has been achieved and the exercise must be stopped. Training improperly or with fatigue can lead to injury.
6. The plyometric training program should be progressive in nature. The volume and intensity can be modified in several ways:

Increase the number of exercises.
Increase the number of repetitions and sets.
Decrease the rest period between sets of exercises.

7. Plyometric training sessions should be conducted no more than three times weekly in the preseason phase of training. During this phase, volume should prevail. During the competitive season, the frequency of plyometric training should be reduced to twice weekly, with the intensity of the exercise becoming more important.

8. Dynamic testing of the individual on a regular basis will provide important progression and motivational feedback.

The key element in the execution of proper technique is the eccentric or landing phase. The shock of landing from a jump is not absorbed exclusively by the foot but rather is a combination of the ankle, knee, and hip joints, all working together to absorb the shock of landing and then transferring the force.

INTEGRATING PLYOMETRICS INTO THE REHABILITATION PROGRAM: CLINICAL CONCERNS

When used judiciously, plyometrics are a valuable asset in the sports rehabilitation program. As previously stated, the majority of lower-quarter sport function occurs in the closed-kinetic chain. Lower-extremity plyometrics are an effective functional closed-chain exercise that can be incorporated into the sports rehabilitation program. According to Davis's law, soft tissue responds to stress imparted upon it to become more resilient along these same lines of stress. As previously mentioned, through the eccentric prestretch, plyometric places added stress on the tendinous portion of the contractile unit. Eccentric loading is beneficial in the management of tendinitis.[33] Through a gradually progressed eccentric loading program, healing tendinous tissue is stressed, yielding an increase in ultimate tensile strength. This eccentric load can be applied through jump-downs (Fig. 13-2).

Clinical plyometrics can be categorized according to the loads applied to the healing tissue. These activities include (1) medial/lateral loading, (2) rotational loading, and (3) shock absorption/deceleration loading. In addition, plyometric drills will be divided into (1) in-place activities (activities that can be performed in essentially the same or small amount of space), (2) dynamic distance drills (activities that occur across a given distance), and (3) depth jumping (jumping down from a predetermined height and performing a variety of activities upon landing). Simple jumping drills (bilateral activities) can be progressed to hopping (unilateral activities).

Medial–Lateral Loading

Virtually all sporting activities involve cutting maneuvers. Inherent to cutting activities is adequate function in the medial and lateral directions. A plyometric program designed to stress the athlete's ability to accept weight on the involved lower extremity and then perform cutting activities off that leg is imperative. Individuals who have suffered sprains to the medial or lateral capsular and ligamentous complex of the ankle and

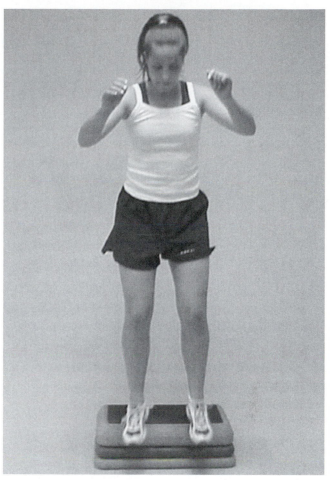

FIGURE   1 3 - 2

Jump-down exercises.

knee, as well as strains of the hip abductor/adductor and ankle invertor/evertor muscles, are candidates for medial–lateral plyometric loading. Medial–lateral loading drills should be implemented following injury to the medial soft tissue around the knee after a valgus stress. By gradually imparting progressive valgus loads, tissue tensile strength is augmented.[36] In the rehabilitation setting, bilateral support drills can be progressed to unilateral valgus loading efforts. Specifically, lateral jumping drills are progressed to lateral hopping activities. However, the medial structures must also be trained to accept greater valgus loads sustained during cutting activities. As a prerequisite to full-speed cutting, lateral bounding drills should be performed (Fig. 13-3). These efforts are progressed to activities that add acceleration, deceleration, and momentum. Lateral sliding activities that require the individual to cover a greater distance can be performed on a slide board. If a slide board is not available, the same movement pattern can be stressed with plyometrics (Fig. 13-4).

IN-PLACE ACTIVITIES

- Lateral bounding (quick step valgus loading)
- Slide bounds

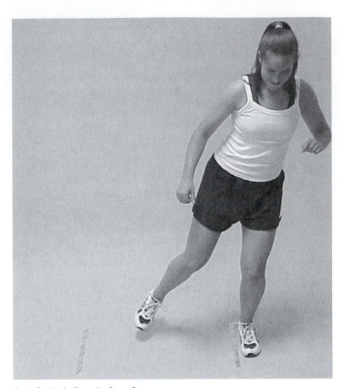

FIGURE 13-3

Lateral bounding drills.

DYNAMIC DISTANCE DRILLS

- Crossovers

Rotational Loading

Because rotation in the knee is controlled by the cruciate ligaments, menisci, and capsule, plyometric activities with a rotational component are instrumental in the rehabilitation program after injury to any of these structures. As previously discussed, care must be taken not to exceed healing time constraints when using plyometric training.

IN-PLACE ACTIVITIES

- Spin jumps

DYNAMIC DISTANCE DRILLS

- Lateral hopping

Shock Absorption (Deceleration Loading)

Perhaps some of the most physically demanding plyometric activities are shock-absorption activities, which place a tremendous amount of stress upon muscle, tendon, and articular cartilage. Therefore, in the final preparation for a return to sports involving repetitive jumping and hopping, shock-absorption drills should be included in the rehabilitation program.

One way to prepare the athlete for shock absorption drills is to gradually maximize the effects of gravity, such as beginning in

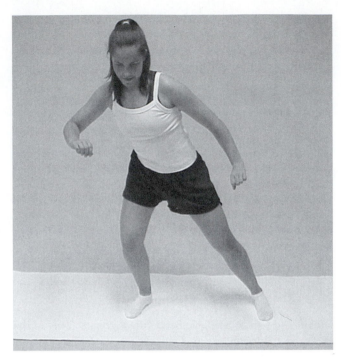

FIGURE 13-4

Lateral sliding activities.

a gravity-minimized position and progressing to performance against gravity. Popular activities to minimize gravity include water activities or assisted efforts through unloading.

IN-PLACE ACTIVITIES

- Cycle jumps
- Five-dot drill

DEPTH JUMPING PREPARATION

- Jump-downs

The activities listed are a good starting point from which to develop a clinical plyometric program. Manipulations of volume, frequency, and intensity can advance the program appropriately. Proper progression is of prime importance when using plyometrics in the rehabilitation program. These progressive activities are reinjuries waiting to happen if the progression does not allow for adequate healing or development of an adequate strength base. A close working relationship fostering open communication and acute observation skills is vital in helping ensure that the program is not overly aggressive.

SUMMARY

- Although the effects of plyometric training are not yet fully understood, it still remains a widely used form of combining strength with speed training to functionally increase power. Although the research is somewhat contradictory, the neurophysiologic concept of plyometric training is on a sound foundation.

- A successful plyometric training program should be carefully designed and implemented after establishing an adequate strength base.
- The effects of this type of high-intensity training can be achieved safely if the individual is supervised by a knowledgeable person who uses common sense and follows the prescribed training regimen.
- The plyometric training program should use a large variety of different exercises, because year-round training often results in boredom and a lack of motivation.
- Program variety can be manipulated with different types of equipment or kinds of movement performed.
- Continued motivation and an organized progression are the keys to successful training.
- Plyometrics are also a valuable asset in the rehabilitation program after a sport injury.
- Used after lower-quarter injury, plyometrics are effective in facilitating joint awareness, strengthening tissue during the healing process, and increasing sport-specific strength and power.
- The most important considerations in the plyometric program are common sense and experience.

REFERENCES

1. Adams T. An investigation of selected plyometric training exercises on muscular leg strength and power. *Track Field Q Rev* 84:36–40, 1984.
2. Asmussen E, Bonde-Peterson F. Storage of elastic energy in skeletal muscles in man. *Acta Physiol Scand* 91:385, 1974.
3. Bielik E, Chu D, Costello F, et al. Roundtable: 1. Practical considerations for utilizing plyometrics. *Natl Strength Cond Assoc J* 8:14, 1986.
4. Bosco C, Komi PV. Muscle elasticity in athletes. In: Komi PV, ed. *Exercise and Sports Biology.* Champaign, IL, Human Kinetics, 1982.
5. Bosco C, Komi PV. Potentiation of the mechanical behavior of the human skeletal muscle through prestretching. *Acta Physiol Scand* 106:467, 1979.
6. Bosco C, Tarkka J, Komi PV. Effect of elastic energy and myoelectric potentiation of triceps surae during stretch-shortening cycle exercise. *Int J Sports Med* 2:137, 1982.
7. Bosco C, Tihanyia J, Komi PV, et al. Store and recoil of elastic energy in slow and fast types of human skeletal muscles. *Acta Physiol Scand* 116:343, 1987.
8. Cavagna GA, Dusman B, Margaria R. Positive work done by a previously stretched muscle. *J Appl Physiol* 24:21, 1968.
9. Cavagna G, Saibene E, Margaria R. Effect of negative work on the amount of positive work performed by an isolated muscle. *J Appl Physiol* 20:157, 1965.
10. Chu D. *Jumping into Plyometrics.* Champaign, IL, Leisure Press, 1992.
11. Chu D. Conditioning/plyometrics. Paper presented at 10th Annual Sports Medicine Team Concept Conference, San Francisco, December 1989.
12. Chu D. Plyometric exercise. *Natl Strength Cond Assoc J* 6:56, 1984.
13. Chu D, Plummer L. The language of plyometrics. *Natl Strength Cond Assoc J* 6:30, 1984.
14. Curwin S, Stannish WD. *Tendinitis: Its Etiology and Treatment.* Lexington, MA, Collamore Press, 1984.
15. Dunsenev CI. Strength training of jumpers. *Track Field Q* 82:4, 1982.
16. Dunsenev CI. Strength training for jumpers. *Sov Sports Rev* 14:2, 1979.
17. Enoka RM. *Neuromechanical Basis of Kinesiology.* Champaign, IL, Human Kinetics, 1989.
18. Javorek I. Plyometrics. *Natl Strength Cond Assoc J* 11:52, 1989.
19. Jensen C. Pertinent facts about warming. *Athlet J* 56:72, 1975.
20. Katchajov S, Gomberaze K, Revson A. Rebound jumps. *Mod Athlet Coach* 14:23, 1976.
21. Komi PV. Physiological and biomechanical correlates of muscle function: Effects of muscle structure and stretch-shortening cycle on force and speed. In: Terjung RL, ed. *Exercise and Sports Sciences Review.* Lexington, MA, Collamore Press, 1984.
22. Komi PV, Bosco C. Utilization of stored elastic energy in leg extensor muscles by men and women. *Med Sci Sports Exerc* 10:261, 1978.
23. Komi PV, Buskirk E. Effects of eccentric and concentric muscle conditioning on tension and electrical activity of human muscle. *Ergonomics* 15:417, 1972.
24. Lundon P. A review of plyometric training. *Natl Strength Cond Assoc* 7:69, 1985.
25. Rach PJ, Grabiner MD, Gregor RJ, et al. *Kinesiology and Applied Anatomy,* 7th ed. Philadelphia, Lea & Febiger, 1989.
26. Rowinski M. *The Role of Eccentric Exercise.* Shirley, NY, Biodex, Pro Clinica, 1988.
27. Thomas DW. Plyometrics—more than the stretch reflex. *Natl Strength Cond Assoc J* 10:49, 1988.
28. Verkhoshanski Y. Are depth jumps useful? *Yessis Rev Sov Phys Educ Sports* 4:74–79, 1969.
29. Verkhoshanski Y. Perspectives in the improvement of speed-strength preparation of jumpers. *Yessis Rev Sov Phys Educ Sports* 4:28–29, 1969.
30. Verkhoshanski Y, Chornonson G. Jump exercises in sprint training. *Track Field Q* 9:1909, 1967.
31. Voight M, Bradley D. Plyometrics. In: Davies GJ, ed. *A Compendium of Isokinetics in Clinical Usage and Rehabilitation Techniques,* 4th ed. Onalaska, WI, S & S, 1994.
32. Voight M, Draovitch P. Plyometrics. In: Albert M, ed. *Eccentric Muscle Training in Sports and Orthopedics.* New York, Churchill Livingstone, 1991.

33. Von Arx F. Power development in the high jump. *Track Tech* 88:2818–2819, 1989.

34. Wilk KE, Voight ML, Keirns MA. Stretch-shortening drills for the upper extremities: Theory and clinical application. *J Orthop Sports Phys Ther* 17:225–239, 1993.

35. Wilt F. Plyometrics—what it is and how it works. *Athlet J* 55b:76, 1975.

36. Woo SL, Inoue M, McGurk-Burleson E, et al. Treatment of the medial collateral ligament injury: Structure and function of canine knees in response to differing treatment regimens. *Am J Sports Med* 15:22–29, 1987.

CHAPTER 14

Open- Versus Closed-Kinetic-Chain Exercise in Rehabilitation

William E. Prentice

OBJECTIVES

After completing this chapter, the therapist should be able to do the following:

- Differentiate between the concepts of an open kinetic chain and a closed kinetic chain.
- Contrast the advantages and disadvantages of using open- versus closed-kinetic-chain exercise.
- Recognize how closed-kinetic-chain exercises can be used to regain neuromuscular control.
- Analyze the biomechanics of closed-kinetic-chain exercise in the lower extremity.
- Compare how both open- and closed-kinetic-chain exercises should be used in rehabilitation of the lower extremity.
- Identify the various closed-kinetic-chain exercises for the lower extremity.
- Examine the biomechanics of closed-kinetic-chain exercises in the upper extremity.
- Explain how closed-kinetic-chain exercises are used in rehabilitation of the upper extremity.
- Recognize the various types of closed-kinetic-chain exercises for the upper extremity.

In recent years, the concept of *closed-kinetic-chain exercise* has received considerable attention as a useful and effective technique of rehabilitation, particularly for injuries involving the lower extremity.[65] The ankle, knee, and hip joints constitute the kinetic chain for the lower extremity. When the distal segment of the lower extremity is stabilized or fixed, as is the case when the foot is weight bearing on the ground, the kinetic chain is said to be closed. Conversely, in an *open kinetic chain*, the distal segment is mobile and not fixed. Traditionally, rehabilitation strengthening protocols have used open-kinetic-chain exercises such as knee flexion and extension on a knee machine.

Closed-kinetic-chain exercises are used more often in rehabilitation of injuries to the lower extremity, but they are also useful in rehabilitation protocols for certain upper-extremity activities. For the most part, the upper extremity functions in an open kinetic chain with the hand moving freely. But there are a number of activities in which the upper extremity functions in a closed kinetic chain.

Despite the recent popularity of closed-kinetic-chain exercises, it must be stressed that both open- and closed-kinetic-chain exercises have their place in the rehabilitative process.[19] This chapter will attempt to clarify the role of both open- and closed-kinetic-chain exercises in that process.

CONCEPT OF THE KINETIC CHAIN

The concept of the kinetic chain was first proposed in the 1970s and initially referred to as the *link system* by mechanical engineers.[55] In this link system, pin joints connect a series of overlapping, rigid segments (Fig. 14-1). If both ends of this system are connected to an immovable frame, there is no movement of either the proximal or the distal end. In this closed link system, each moving body segment receives forces from and transfers forces to adjacent body segments and thus either affects or is affected by the motion of those components.[25] In a closed link system, movement at one joint produces predictable movement at all other joints.[55] In reality, this type of closed link system does not exist in either the upper or the lower extremity. However, when the distal segment in an extremity (that is, the foot or hand) meets resistance or is fixed, muscle recruitment patterns and joint movements are different than when the distal segment moves freely.[55] Thus, two systems—a closed system and an open system—have been proposed.

Whenever the foot or the hand meets resistance or is fixed, as is the case in a closed kinetic chain, movement of the more proximal segments occurs in a predictable pattern. If the foot or

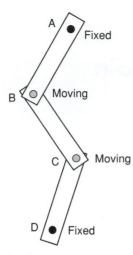

FIGURE 14-1

If both ends of a link system are fixed, movement at one joint produces predictable movement at all other joints.

hand moves freely in space as in an open kinetic chain, movements occurring in other segments within the chain are not necessarily predictable.[11]

To a large extent, the term *closed-kinetic-chain exercise* has come to mean "weight-bearing exercise." However, although all weight-bearing exercises involve some elements of closed-kinetic-chain activities, not all closed-kinetic-chain activities are weight bearing.[54]

Muscle Actions in the Kinetic Chain

Muscle actions that occur during open-kinetic-chain activities are usually reversed during closed-kinetic-chain activities. In open-kinetic-chain exercise, the origin is fixed and muscle contraction produces movement at the insertion. In closed-kinetic-chain exercise, the insertion is fixed and the muscle acts to move the origin. Although this may be important biomechanically, physiologically the muscle can lengthen, shorten, or remain the same length, and thus it makes little difference whether the origin or insertion is moving in terms of the way the muscle contracts.

Concurrent Shift in a Kinetic Chain

The concept of the *concurrent shift* applies to biarticular muscles that have distinctive muscle actions within the kinetic chain during weight-bearing activities. For example, in a closed kinetic chain simultaneous hip and knee extension occur when a person stands from a seated position. To produce this movement, the rectus femoris shortens across the knee while it lengthens across the hip. Conversely, the hamstrings shorten across the hip and simultaneously lengthen across the knee. The resulting concentric and eccentric contractions at opposite ends of the muscle produce the concurrent shift. This type of contraction occurs during functional activities including walking, stair climbing, and jumping and cannot be reproduced by isolated open-kinetic-chain knee flexion and extension exercises.

The concepts of the reversibility of muscle actions and the concurrent shift are hallmarks of closed-kinetic-chain exercises.[54]

ADVANTAGES AND DISADVANTAGES OF OPEN- VERSUS CLOSED-KINETIC-CHAIN EXERCISES

Open- and closed-kinetic-chain exercises offer distinct advantages and disadvantages in the rehabilitation process. The choice to use one or the other depends on the desired treatment goal. Characteristics of closed-kinetic-chain exercises include increased joint compressive forces, increased joint congruency and thus stability, decreased shear forces, decreased acceleration forces, large resistance forces, stimulation of proprioceptors, and enhanced dynamic stability—all of which are associated with weight bearing. Characteristics of open-kinetic-chain exercises include increased acceleration forces, decreased resistance forces, increased distraction and rotational forces, increased deformation of joint and muscle mechanoreceptors, concentric acceleration and eccentric deceleration forces, and promotion of functional activity. These are typical of non-weightbearing activities.[37]

From a biomechanical perspective, it has been suggested that closed-kinetic-chain exercises are safer and produce stresses and forces that are potentially less of a threat to healing structures than open-kinetic-chain exercises.[52] Coactivation or cocontraction of agonist and antagonist muscles must occur during normal movements to provide joint stabilization. Cocontraction, which occurs during closed-kinetic-chain exercise, decreases the shear forces acting on the joint, thus protecting healing soft tissue structures that might otherwise be damaged by open chain exercises.[25] Additionally, weight-bearing activity increases joint compressive forces, further enhancing joint stability.

It has also been suggested that closed-kinetic-chain exercises, particularly those involving the lower extremity, tend to be more functional than open-kinetic-chain exercises because they involve weight-bearing activities.[63] The majority of activities performed in daily living, such as walking, climbing, and rising to a standing position, as well as in most sport activities, involve a closed-kinetic-chain system. Because the foot is usually in contact with the ground, activities that make use of this closed system are said to be more functional. With the exception of a kicking movement, there is no question that closed-kinetic-chain exercises are more activity specific, involving exercise that more closely approximates the desired activity. For example, knee extensor muscle strength in a closed kinetic chain is more closely related to jumping ability than knee extensor strength in a closed kinetic chain.[6] In a clinical setting, specificity of training must be emphasized to maximize carryover to functional activities.[54]

With open-kinetic-chain exercises, motion is usually isolated to a single joint. Open-kinetic-chain activities may include exercises to improve strength or range of motion.[27] They may be applied to a single joint manually, as in proprioceptive neuromuscular facilitation or joint mobilization techniques, or through some external resistance using an exercise machine. Isolation-type exercises typically use a contraction of a specific muscle or group of muscles that produces usually single plane and occasionally multiplanar movement. Isokinetic exercise and testing is usually done in an open kinetic chain and can provide important information relative to the torque production capability of that isolated joint.[4]

When there is some dysfunction associated with injury, the predictable pattern of movement that occurs during closed-kinetic-chain activity might not be possible due to pain, swelling, muscle weakness, or limited range of motion. Thus, movement compensations result that interfere with normal motion and muscle activity. If only closed-kinetic-chain exercise is used, the joints proximal or distal to the injury might not show an existing deficit. Without using open-kinetic-chain exercises that isolate specific joint movements, the deficit might go uncorrected, thus interfering with total rehabilitation.[17] The therapist should use the most appropriate open- or closed-kinetic-chain exercise for the given situation.

Closed-kinetic-chain exercises use varying combinations of isometric, concentric, and eccentric contractions that must occur simultaneously in different muscle groups, creating multiplanar motion at each of the joints within the kinetic chain. Closed-kinetic-chain activities require synchronicity of more complex agonist and antagonist muscle actions.[23]

USING CLOSED-KINETIC-CHAIN EXERCISES TO REGAIN NEUROMUSCULAR CONTROL

In Chapter 11, it was stressed that proprioception, joint position sense, and kinesthesia are critical to the neuromuscular control of body segments within the kinetic chain. To perform a motor skill, muscular forces, occurring at the correct moment and magnitude, interact to move body parts in a coordinated manner.[44] Coordinated movement is controlled by the central nervous system that integrates input from joint and muscle mechanoreceptors acting within the kinetic chain. Smooth coordinated movement requires constant integration of receptor, feedback, and control center information.[44]

In the lower extremity, a functional weight-bearing activity requires muscles and joints to work in synchrony and in synergy with one another. For example, taking a single step requires concentric, eccentric, and isometric muscle contractions to produce supination and pronation in the foot; ankle dorsiflexion and plantarflexion; knee flexion, extension, and rotation; and hip flexion, extension, and rotation. Lack of normal motion secondary to injury in one joint will affect the way another joint or segment moves.[44]

To perform this single step in a coordinated manner, all of the joints and muscles must work together. Thus, exercises that act to integrate, rather than isolate, all of these functioning elements would seem to be the most appropriate. Closed-kinetic-chain exercises, which recruit foot, ankle, knee, and hip muscles in a manner that reproduces normal loading and movement forces in all of the joints within the kinetic chain, are similar to functional mechanics and would appear to be most useful.[44]

Quite often, open-kinetic-chain exercises are used primarily to develop muscular strength while little attention is given to the importance of including exercises that reestablish proprioception and joint position sense.[1] Closed-kinetic-chain activities facilitate the integration of proprioceptive feedback coming from Pacinian corpuscles, Ruffini endings, Golgi-Mazzoni corpuscles, Golgi-tendon organs, and Golgi-ligament endings through the functional use of multijoint and multiplanar movements.[11]

BIOMECHANICS OF OPEN- VERSUS CLOSED-KINETIC-CHAIN ACTIVITIES IN THE LOWER EXTREMITY

Open- and closed-kinetic-chain exercises have different biomechanical effects on the joints of the lower extremity.[16] Walking along with the ability to change direction require coordinated joint motion and a complex series of well-timed muscle activations. Biomechanically, shock absorption, foot flexibility, foot stabilization, acceleration and deceleration, multiplanar motion, and joint stabilization must occur in each of the joints in the lower extremity for normal function.[44] Some understanding of how these biomechanical events occur during both open- and closed-kinetic-chain activities is essential for the athletic trainer.

Foot and Ankle

The foot's function in the support phase of weight bearing during gait is twofold. At heel strike, the foot must act as a shock absorber to the impact or ground reaction forces and then adapt to the uneven surfaces. Subsequently, at push-off, the foot functions as a rigid lever to transmit the explosive force from the lower extremity to the ground.[61]

As the foot becomes weight bearing at heel strike, creating a closed kinetic chain, the subtalar joint moves into a pronated position in which the talus adducts and the plantar flexes while the calcaneous everts. Pronation of the foot unlocks the midtarsal joint and allows the foot to assist in shock absorption. It is important during initial impact to reduce the ground reaction forces and distribute the load evenly on many different anatomical structures throughout the lower-extremity kinetic chain. As pronation occurs at the subtalar joint, there is obligatory internal rotation of the tibia and slight flexion at the knee. The dorsiflexors contract eccentrically to decelerate plantarflexion. In an open kinetic chain, when the foot pronates, the talus is stationary while the foot everts, abducts, and dorsiflexes. The muscles that evert the foot appear to be most active.[61]

The foot changes its function from being a shock absorber to being a rigid lever system as the foot begins to push off the ground. In weight bearing in a closed kinetic chain, supination consists of the talus abducting and dorsiflexing on the calcaneus while the calcaneus inverts on the talus. The tibia externally rotates and produces knee extension. During supination the plantarflexors stabilize the foot, decelerate the tibia, and flex the knee. In an open kinetic chain, supination consists of the calcaneus inverting as the talus adducts and plantarflexes. The foot moves into adduction, plantarflexion, around the stabilized talus.[61] Changes in foot position (i.e., pronation or supination) appear to have little or no effect on the electromyogram (EMG) activity of the vastus medialis or the vastus lateralis.[30]

Knee Joint

It is essential for the therapist to understand forces that occur around the knee joint. Palmitier et al. have proposed a biomechanical model of the lower extremity that quantifies two critical forces at the knee joint (Fig. 14-2).[43] A *shear force* occurs in a posterior direction that would cause the tibia to translate anteriorly if not checked by soft tissue constraints—primarily the anterior cruciate ligament (ACL).[12] The second force is a *compressive force* directed along a longitudinal axis of the tibia. Weight-bearing exercises increase joint compression, which enhances joint stability.

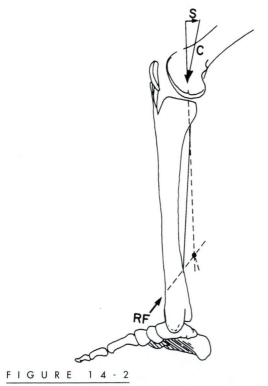

F I G U R E   1 4 - 2

Mathematical model showing shear and compressive force vectors. *S,* shear; *C,* compressive.

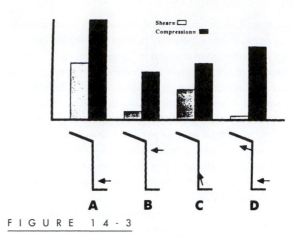

F I G U R E   1 4 - 3

Resistive forces applied in different positions alter the magnitude of the shear and compressive forces. **A,** Resistive force applied distally. **B,** Resistive force applied proximally. **C,** Resistive force applied axially. **D,** Resistive force applied distally with hamstring cocontraction.

In an open-kinetic-chain seated knee joint exercise, as a resistive force is applied to the distal tibia, the shear and compressive forces would be maximized (Fig. 14-3A). When a resistive force is applied more proximally, shear force is significantly reduced, as is the compressive force (Fig. 14-3B). If the resistive force is applied in a more axial direction, the shear force is also smaller (Fig. 14-3C). If a hamstring cocontraction occurs, the shear force is minimized (Fig. 14-3D).

Closed-kinetic-chain exercises induce hamstring contraction by creating a flexion moment at both the hip and the knee, with the contracting hamstrings stabilizing the hip and the quadriceps stabilizing the knee.[58] A *moment* is the product of force and distance from the axis of rotation. Also referred to as torque, it describes the turning effect produced when a force is exerted on the body that is pivoted about some fixed point (Fig. 14-4). Cocontraction of the hamstring muscles helps to counteract the tendency of the quadriceps to cause anterior tibial translation. Cocontraction of the hamstrings is most efficient in reducing shear force when the resistive force is directed in an axial orientation relative to the tibia, as is the case in a weight-bearing exercise.[43] Several studies have shown that cocontraction is useful in stabilizing the knee joint and decreasing shear forces.[29,33,45,53]

The tension in the hamstrings can be further enhanced with slight anterior flexion of the trunk. Trunk flexion moves the center of gravity anteriorly, decreasing the knee flexion moment and thus reducing knee shear force and decreasing patellofemoral compression forces.[42] Closed-kinetic-chain exercises try to minimize the flexion moment at the knee while increasing the flexion moment at the hip.

A flexion moment is also created at the ankle when the resistive force is applied to the bottom of the foot. The soleus stabilizes ankle flexion and creates a knee extension moment, which again helps to neutralize anterior shear force (see Fig. 14-4).

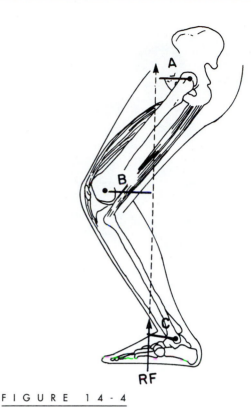

FIGURE 14-4

Closed-kinetic-chain exercises induce hamstring contraction by creating a flexion moment at **A,** Hip, **B,** Knee, **C,** Ankle.

Thus the entire lower-extremity kinetic chain is recruited by applying an axial force at the distal segment.

In an open-kinetic-chain exercise involving seated leg extensions, the resistive force is applied to the distal tibia, creating a flexion moment at the knee only. This negates the effects of a hamstring cocontraction and thus produces maximal shear force at the knee joint. Shear forces created by isometric open-kinetic-chain knee flexion and extension at 30° and 60° of knee flexion are greater than that with closed-kinetic-chain exercises.[38] Decreased anterior tibial displacement during isometric closed-kinetic-chain knee flexion at 30° when measured by knee arthrometry has also been demonstrated.[62]

PATELLOFEMORAL JOINT

The effects of open- versus closed-kinetic-chain exercises on the patellofemoral joint must also be considered. In open-kinetic-chain knee extension exercise, the flexion moment increases as the knee extends from 90° of flexion to full extension, increasing tension in the quadriceps and patellar tendon. Thus the patellofemoral joint reaction forces are increased, with peak force occurring at 36° of joint flexion.[21] As the knee moves toward full extension, the patellofemoral contact area decreases, causing increased contact stress per unit area.[5,31]

In closed-kinetic-chain exercise, the flexion moment increases as the knee flexes, once again causing increased quadriceps and patellar tendon tension and thus an increase in

patellofemoral joint reaction forces. However, the patella has a much larger surface contact area with the femur, and contact stress is minimized.[5,21,31] Closed-kinetic-chain exercises might be better tolerated in the patellofemoral joint because contact stress is minimized.

CLOSED-KINETIC-CHAIN EXERCISES FOR REHABILITATION OF LOWER-EXTREMITY INJURIES

For many years, therapists have made use of open-kinetic-chain exercises for lower-extremity strengthening. This practice has been partly due to design constraints of existing resistive exercise machines. However, the current popularity of closed-kinetic-chain exercises can be attributed primarily to a better understanding of the kinesiology and biomechanics, along with the neuromuscular control factors, involved in rehabilitation of lower-extremity injuries.

For example, the course of rehabilitation after injury to the anterior ACL has changed drastically over the years. (Specific rehabilitation protocols will be discussed in detail in Chapter 29.) Technological advances have created significant improvement in surgical techniques, and this has allowed therapists to change their philosophy of rehabilitation. The current literature provides a great deal of support for accelerated rehabilitation programs that recommend the extensive use of closed-kinetic-chain exercises.[7,13,18,21,39,52,59,66]

Because of the biomechanical and functional advantages of closed-kinetic-chain exercises described earlier, these activities are perhaps best suited to rehabilitation of the ACL.[28] The majority of these studies also indicate that closed-kinetic-chain exercises can be safely incorporated into the rehabilitation protocols very early. Some therapists recommend beginning within the first few days after surgery.

Several different closed-kinetic-chain exercises have gained popularity and have been incorporated into rehabilitation protocols.[34] Among those exercises commonly used are the minisquat, wall slides, lunges, leg press, stair-climbing machines, lateral step-up, terminal knee extension using tubing, and stationary bicycling, slide boards, biomechanical ankle platform system (BAPS) boards, and the Fitter.

Minisquats, Wall Slides, and Lunges

The minisquat (Fig. 14-5) or wall slide (Fig. 14-6) involves simultaneous hip and knee extension and is performed in a 0–40° range.[66] As the hip extends, the rectus femoris contracts eccentrically while the hamstrings contract concentrically. Concurrently, as the knee extends, the hamstrings contract eccentrically while the rectus femoris contracts concentrically. Both concentric and eccentric contractions occur simultaneously at either end of both muscles, producing a concurrent shift contraction. This type of contraction is necessary during weight-bearing activities. It will be elicited with all closed-kinetic-chain exercises and is impossible with isolation exercises.[55]

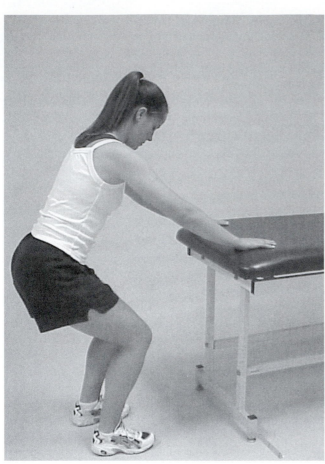

FIGURE   14 - 5

Minisquat performed in 0–40° range.

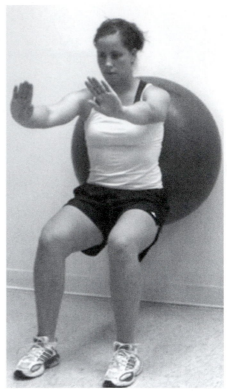

FIGURE   14 - 6

Standing wall slide. A swiss boll may also be used behind the back to facilitate the wall slide.

These concurrent shift contractions minimize the flexion moment at the knee. The eccentric contraction of the hamstrings helps to neutralize the effects of a concentric quadriceps contraction in producing anterior translation of the tibia.[20] Henning et al. found that the half squat produced significantly less anterior shear at the knee than did an open-chain exercise in full extension.[26] A full squat markedly increases the flexion moment at the knee and thus increases anterior shear of the tibia. As mentioned previously, slightly flexing the trunk anteriorly will also increase the hip flexion moment and decrease the knee moment. It appears that increasing the width of the stance in a wall squat has no effect on EMG activity in the quadriceps.[2] However, moving the feet forward does seem to increase activity in the quadriceps as well as the plantarflexors.[9]

Lunges should be used later in a rehabilitation program to facilitate eccentric strengthening of the quadriceps to act as a decelerator (Fig. 14-7).[65] Like the minisquat and wall slide, it facilitates cocontraction of the hamstring muscles.

Leg Press

Theoretically the leg press takes full advantage of the kinetic chain and at the same time provides stability, which decreases strain on the low back.[36] It also allows exercise with resistance lower than body weight and the capability of exercising each leg independently (Fig. 14-8).[43] It has been recommended that leg-press exercises be performed in a 0–60° range of knee flexion.[66]

It has also been recommended that leg-press machines allow full hip extension to take maximum advantage of the kinetic chain. Full hip extension can only be achieved in a supine position. In this position, full hip and knee flexion and extension can occur thus reproducing the concurrent shift and ensuring appropriate hamstring recruitment.[43]

The foot plates should also be designed to move in an arc of motion rather than in a straight line. This movement would facilitate hamstring recruitment by increasing the hip flexion moment and decreasing the knee moment. Foot plates should be fixed perpendicular to the frontal plane of the hip to maximize the knee extension moment created by the soleus.

Stair Climbing

Stair-climbing machines have gained a great deal of popularity, not only as a closed-kinetic-chain exercise device useful in rehabilitation, but also as a means of improving cardiorespiratory endurance (Fig. 14-9). Stair-climbing machines have two basic

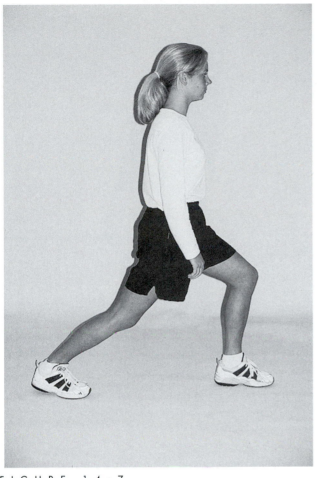

FIGURE 14-7

Lunges are done to strengthen quadriceps eccentrically.

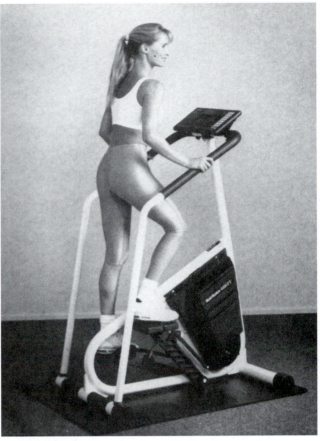

FIGURE 14-9

Stairmaster stepping machine.

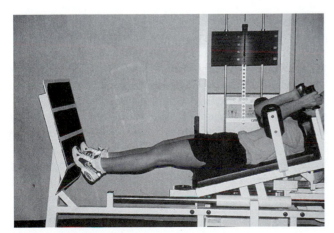

FIGURE 14-8

Leg-press exercise.

designs. One involves a series of rotating steps similar to a department store escalator, while the other uses two foot plates that move up and down to simulate a stepping-type movement. With the latter type of stair climber, also sometimes referred to as a stepping machine, the foot never leaves the foot plate, making it a true closed-kinetic-chain exercise device.

Stair climbing involves many of the same biomechanical principles identified with the leg-press exercise.[51] When exercising on the stair climber, the body should be held erect with only slight trunk flexion, thus maximizing hamstring recruitment through concurrent shift contractions while increasing the hip flexion moment and decreasing the knee flexion moment.

Exercise on a stepping machine produces increased EMG activity in the gastrocnemius. Because the gastrocnemius attaches to the posterior aspect of the femoral condyles, increased activity of this muscle could produce a flexion moment of the femur on the tibia. This motion would cause posterior translation of the femur on the tibia, increasing strain on the ACL. Peak firing of the quadriceps might offset the effects of increased EMG activity in the gastronemius.[15]

Step-Ups

Lateral, forward, and backward step-ups are widely used closed-kinetic-chain exercises (Fig. 14-10). Lateral step-ups seem to be

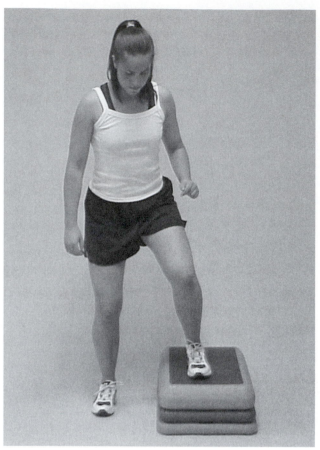

FIGURE   14-10

Lateral step-ups.

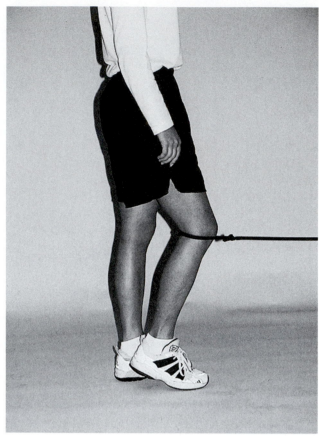

FIGURE   14-11

Terminal knee extensions using surgical tubing resistance.

used more often clinically than forward step-ups. Step height can be adjusted to patient capabilities and generally progresses up to about 8 in. Heights greater than 8 in create a large flexion moment at the knee, increasing anterior shear force and making hamstring cocontraction more difficult.[10,15]

Step-ups elicit significantly greater mean hamstring EMG activity than a stepping machine, whereas the quadriceps are more active during stair climbing.[69] When performing a step-up, the entire body weight must be raised and lowered, whereas on the stepping machine the center of gravity is maintained at a relatively constant height. The lateral step-up can produce increased muscle and joint shear forces compared to stepping exercise.[15] Caution should be exercised by the therapist in using the lateral step-up in cases where minimizing anterior shear forces is essential. Contraction of the hamstrings appears to be of insufficient magnitude to neutralize the shear force produced by the quadriceps.[10] In situations where strengthening of the quadriceps is the goal, the lateral step-up has been recommended as a beneficial exercise.[70] However, lateral stepping exercises have failed to increase isokinetic strength of the quadriceps muscle. It also appears that concentric quadricep contractions produce more EMG activity than eccentric contractions in a lateral step-up.[50]

Terminal Knee Extensions Using Surgical Tubing

It has been reported in numerous studies that the greatest amount of anterior tibial translation occurs between 0° and 30° of flexion during open-kinetic-chain exercise.[22,24,32,41,45,46,66] At one time, therapists avoid open-kinetic-chain terminal knee extension after surgery. Unfortunately, this practice led to quadriceps weakness, flexion contracture, and patellofemoral pain.[48]

Closed-kinetic-chain terminal knee extensions using surgical tubing resistance have created a means of safely strengthening terminal knee extension (Fig. 14-11).[49] Application of resistance anteriorly at the femur produces anterior shear of the femur, which eliminates any anterior translation of the tibia. This type of exercise performed in the 0–30° range also minimizes the knee flexion moment, further reducing anterior shear of the tibia. The use of rubber tubing produces an eccentric contraction of the quadriceps when moving into knee flexion. Weight-bearing terminal knee extensions with tubing increase the EMG activity in the quadriceps.[69]

Stationary Bicycling

The stationary bicycle can be of significant value as a closed-kinetic-chain exercise device (Fig. 14-12).

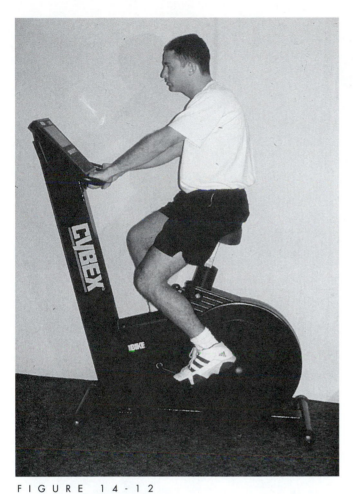

F I G U R E   1 4 - 1 2

Stationary bicycle.

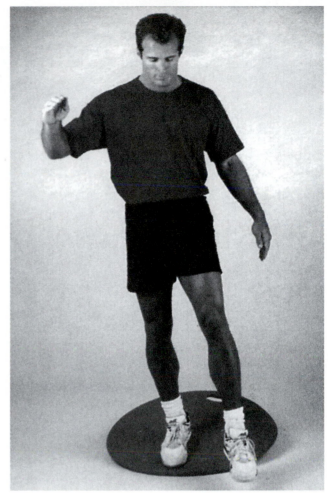

F I G U R E   1 4 - 1 3

BAPS board exercise.

The advantage of stationary bicycling over other closed-kinetic-chain exercises for rehabilitation is that the amount of the weight-bearing force exerted by the injured lower extremity can be adapted within patient limitations. The seat height should be carefully adjusted to minimize the knee flexion moment on the downstroke. However, if the stationary bike is being used to regain range of motion in flexion, the seat height should be adjusted to a lowered position using passive motion of the injured extremity. Toe clips will facilitate hamstring contractions on the upstroke.

BAPS Board and Minitramp

The BAPS board (Fig. 14-13) and minitramp (Fig. 14-14) both provide an unstable base of support that helps to facilitate reestablishing proprioception and joint position sense in addition to strengthening. Working on the BAPS board allows the therapist to provide stress to the lower extremity in a progressive and controlled manner.[11] It allows the patient to work simultaneously on strengthening and range of motion, while trying to regain neuromuscular control and balance. The minitramp may be used to accomplish the same goals, but it can also be used for more advanced plyometric training.

Slide Boards and Fitter

Shifting the body weight from side to side during a more functional activity on either a slide board (Fig. 14-15) or a Fitter (Fig. 14-16) helps to reestablish dynamic control as well improving cardiorespiratory fitness.[11] These motions produce valgus and varus stresses and strains to the joint that are somewhat unique to these two pieces of equipment. Lateral slide exercises have been shown to improve knee extension strength following ACL reconstruction.[8]

BIOMECHANICS OF OPEN- VERSUS CLOSED-KINETIC-CHAIN ACTIVITIES IN THE UPPER EXTREMITY

Although it is true that closed-kinetic-chain exercises are most often used in rehabilitation of lower-extremity injuries, there are many injury situations where closed-kinetic-chain exercises should be incorporated into upper-extremity rehabilitation protocols. Unlike the lower extremity, the upper extremity is most

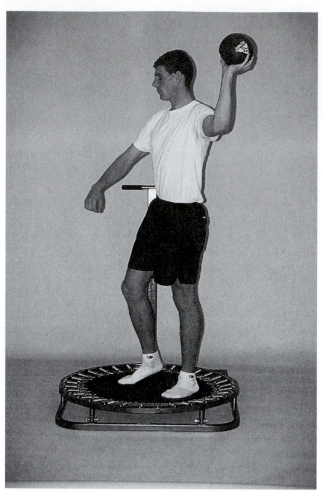

FIGURE 14-14

Minitramp provides an unstable base of support to which other functional plyometric activities may be added.

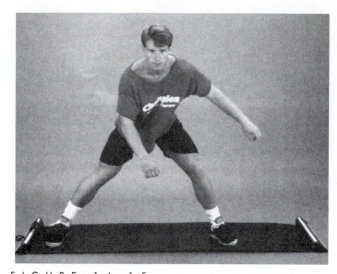

FIGURE 14-15

Slide board training.

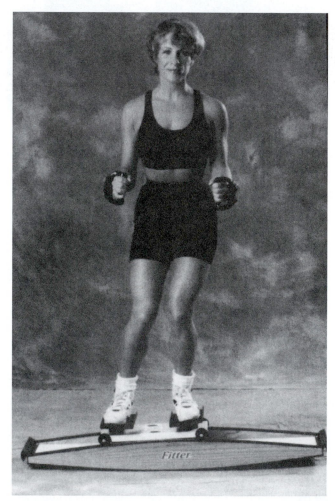

FIGURE 14-16

The Fitter is useful for weight shifting.

functional as an open-kinetic-chain system. Most activities involve movement of the upper extremity in which the hand moves freely. These activities are generally dynamic movements. In these movements, the proximal segments of the kinetic chain are used for stabilization, while the distal segments have a high degree of mobility. Push-ups, chinning exercises, and handstands in gymnastics are all examples of closed-kinetic-chain activities in the upper extremity. In these cases, the hand is stabilized, and muscular contractions around the more proximal segments, the elbow and shoulder, function to raise and lower the body. Still other activities such as swimming and cross-country skiing involve rapid successions of alternating open- and closed-kinetic-chain movements, much in the same way as running does in the lower extremity.[67]

For the most part in rehabilitation, closed-kinetic-chain exercises are used primarily for strengthening and establishing neuromuscular control of those muscles that act to stabilize the shoulder girdle.[60] In particular, the scapular stabilizers and the rotator cuff muscles function at one time or another to control

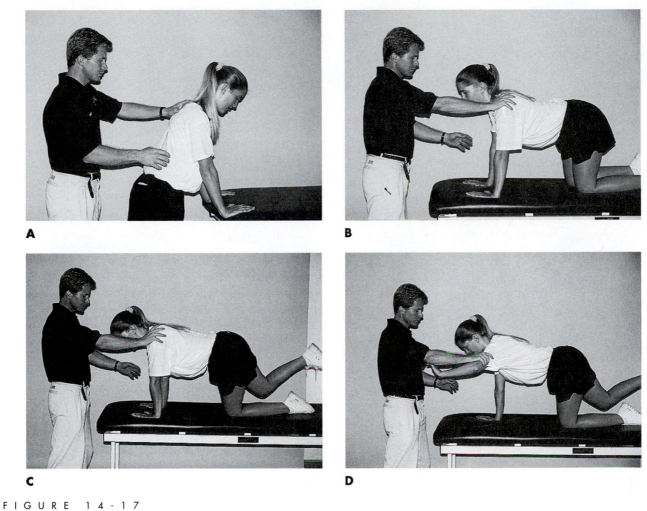

FIGURE 14-17

Weight shifting. **A**, Standing. **B**, Quadruped. **C**, Tripod. **D**, Opposite knee and arm.

movements about the shoulder. It is essential to develop both strength and neuromuscular control in these muscle groups, thus allowing them to provide a stable base for more mobile and dynamic movements that occur in the distal segments.[60]

It must also be emphasized that although traditional upper-extremity rehabilitation programs have concentrated on treating and identifying the involved structures, the body does not operate in isolated segments but instead works as a dynamic unit.[40] More recently rehabilitation programs have integrated closed-kinetic-chain exercises with core stabilization exercises and more functional movement programs. Therapists should recognize the need to address the importance of the legs and trunk as contributors to upper-extremity function and routinely incorporate therapeutic exercises that address the entire kinetic chain.[40]

Shoulder Complex Joint

Closed-kinetic-chain weight-bearing activities can be used to both promote and enhance dynamic joint stability. Most often

closed-kinetic-chain exercises are used with the hand fixed and thus with no motion occurring. The resistance is then applied either axially or rotationally. These exercises produce both joint compression and approximation, which act to enhance muscular cocontraction about the joint producing dynamic stability.[67]

Two essential force couples must be reestablished around the glenohumeral joint: the anterior deltoid along with the infraspinatus and teres minor in the frontal plane, and the subscapularis counterbalanced by the infraspinatus and teres minor in the transverse plane. These opposing muscles act to stabilize the glenohumeral joint by compressing the humeral head within the glenoid via muscular cocontraction.

The scapular muscles function to dynamically position the glenoid relative to the position of the moving humerus, resulting in a normal scapulohumeral rhythm of movement. However, they must also provide a stable base on which the highly mobile humerus can function. If the scapula is hypermobile, the function of the entire upper extremity will be impaired. Thus force couples between the inferior trapezius counterbalanced by the upper trapezius and levator scapula—and the rhomboids and

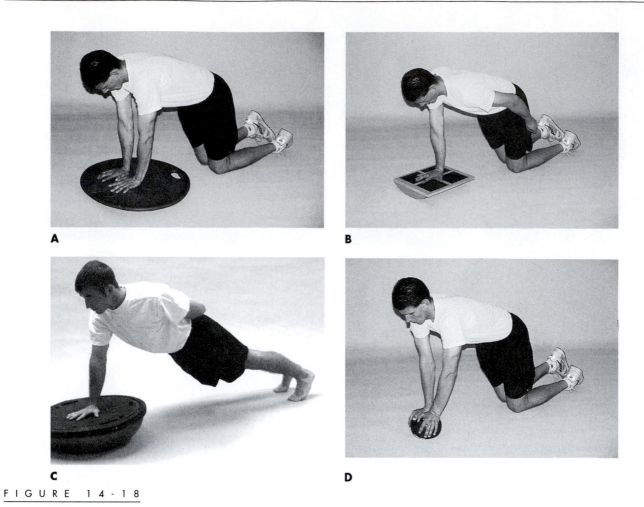

A   **B**

C   **D**

FIGURE 14-18

Weight shifting. **A**, On a BAPS board. **B**, On a wobble board. **C**, Bosu balance trainer.
D, On a Plyboll.

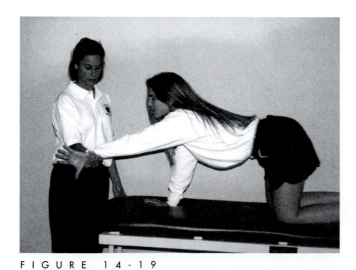

FIGURE 14-19

D2 PNF pattern in a tripod to produce stabilization in the
contralateral support limb.

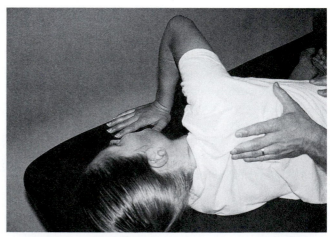

FIGURE 14-20

Rhythmic stabilization for the scapular muscles.

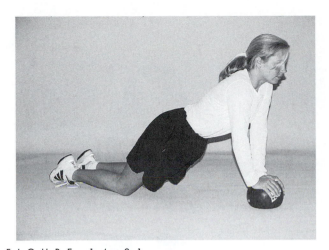

FIGURE 14-21

Push-ups done on a Plyoball.

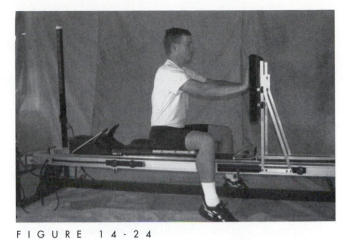

FIGURE 14-24

Push-ups can be done in a variety of positions on a Shuttle 2000.

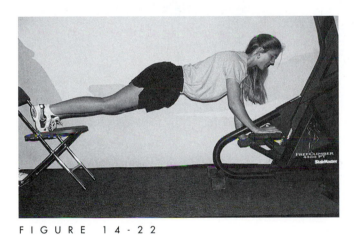

FIGURE 14-22

Push-ups done on a stair climber.

middle trapezius counterbalanced by the serratus anterior—are critical in maintaining scapular stability. Again, closed-kinetic-chain activities done with the hand fixed should be used to enhance scapular stability.[35]

Elbow

The elbow is a hinged joint that is capable of 145° of flexion from a fully extended position. In some cases of joint hyperelasticity, the joint can hyperextend a few degrees beyond neutral. The elbow consists of the humeroulnar, humeroradial, and radioulnar articulations. The concave radial head articulates with the convex surface of the capitellum of the distal humerus and is connected to the proximal ulna via the annular ligament. The proximal radioulnar joint constitutes the forearm, which when working in conjunction with the elbow joint permits approximately 90° of pronation and 80° of supination.

In same activities, the elbow functions in an open kinetic chain. In other activities, the elbow must posses static stability

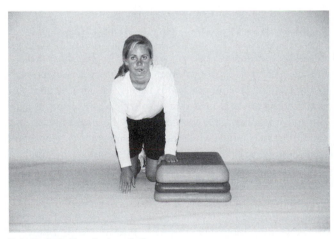

FIGURE 14-23

Single-arm lateral step-ups.

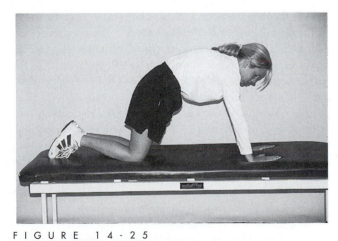

FIGURE 14-25

Push-ups with a plus.

and adequate dynamic strength to be able to transfer force to a hitting implement.

OPEN- AND CLOSED-KINETIC-CHAIN EXERCISES FOR REHABILITATION OF UPPER-EXTREMITY INJURIES

Most typically, closed-kinetic-chain glenohumeral joint exercises are used during the early phases of a rehabilitation program, particularly in the case of an unstable shoulder to promote co-contraction and muscle recruitment, in addition to preventing shutdown of the rotator cuff secondary to pain and/or inflammation.[3] Likewise, closed-kinetic-chain exercise should be used during the late phases of a rehabilitation program to promote muscular endurance of muscles surrounding the glenohumeral and scapulothoracic joints. They may also be used during the later stages of rehabilitation in conjunction with open-kinetic-chain activities to enhance some degree of stability, on which highly dynamic and ballistic motions may be superimposed. At some point during the middle stages of the rehabilitation program, traditional open-kinetic-chain strengthening exercises for the rotator cuff, deltoid, and other glenohumeral and scapular muscles must be incorporated.[27,67]

In the elbow, exercises should also be designed to enhance muscular balance and neuromuscular control of the surrounding agonists and antagonists. Closed-kinetic-chain exercise should be used to improve dynamic stability of the more proximal muscles surrounding the elbow in those activities where the elbow must provide some degree of proximal stability. Open-kinetic-chain exercises for strengthening flexion, extension, pronation, and supination are essential to regain high-velocity dynamic movements of the elbow that are necessary in throwing-type activities.

Weight Shifting

A variety of weight-shifting exercises can be done to assist in facilitating glenohumeral and scapulothoracic dynamic stability through the use of axial compression.[14] Weight shifting can be done in standing, quadruped, tripod, or biped (opposite leg and arm), with weight supported on a stable surface such as the wall or a treatment table (Fig. 14-17**A**–**D**), or on a movable, unstable surface such as a BAPS board, a wobble board, Bosu balance trainer, or a plyoball (Fig. 14-18**A**–**D**). Shifting may be done side to side, forward and backward, or on a diagonal. Hand position may be adjusted from a wide base of support to one hand placed on top of the other to increase difficulty. The patient can adjust the amount of weight being supported as tolerated. The therapist can provide manual force of resistance in a random manner to which the patient must rhythmically stabilize and adapt. A diagonal 2 (D2) proprioceptive neuromuscular facilitation pattern may be used in a tripod to force the contralateral support limb to produce a cocontraction and thus

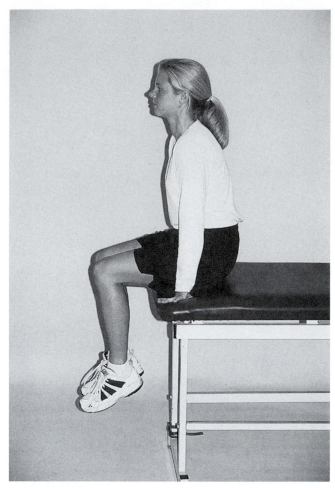

FIGURE 14-26

Press-ups.

stabilization (Fig. 14-19).[67] Rhythmic stabilization can also be used regain neuromuscular control of the scapular muscles with the hand in a closed kinetic chain and random pressure applied to the scapular borders (Fig. 14-20).

Push-Ups, Push-Ups with a Plus, Press-Ups, Step-Ups

Push-ups and/or press-ups are also done to reestablish neuromuscular control. Push-ups done on an unstable surface such as on a plyoball require a good deal of strength in addition to providing an axial load that requires cocontraction of agonist and antagonist force couples around the glenohumeral and scapulothoracic joints, while the distal part of the extremity has some limited movement (Fig. 14-21). A variation of a standard push-up would be to have the patient use reciprocating contractions on a stair climber (Fig. 14-22) or doing single-arm lateral step-ups onto a step (Fig. 14-23). Also, the patient may perform push-ups in a variety of positions, including overhead position on the Shuttle 2000 (Fig. 14-24).[57] Push-ups with a plus are done to strengthen the serratus anterior, which is critical for scapular dynamic stability in overhead activities (Fig. 14-25).

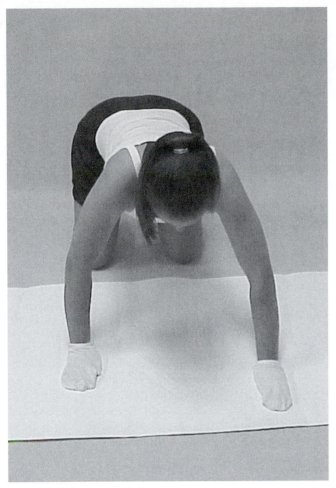

FIGURE 14-27

Slide board strengthening exercise.

Press-ups involve an isometric contraction of the glenohumeral stabilizers (Fig. 14-26).

Slide Board

Upper-extremity closed-kinetic-chain exercises performed on a slide board are useful not only for promoting strength and stability but also for improving muscular endurance.[57,67] In a kneeling position, the patient uses a reciprocating motion, sliding the hands forward and backward, side to side, in a "wax on-wax off" circular pattern, or both hands laterally (Fig. 14-27). It is also possible to do wall slides in a standing position.

SUMMARY

- A closed-kinetic-chain exercise is one in which the distal segment of the extremity is fixed or stabilized. In an open kinetic chain, the distal segment is mobile and not fixed.

- Both open- and closed-kinetic-chain exercises have their place in the rehabilitative process.
- The concepts of the reversibility of muscle actions and the concurrent shift are hallmarks of closed-kinetic-chain exercises.
- Open- and closed-kinetic-chain exercises offer distinct advantages and disadvantages in the rehabilitation process. The choice to use one or the other depends on the desired treatment goal.
- It has been suggested that closed-kinetic-chain exercises are safer due to muscle cocontraction and joint compression, closed-kinetic-chain exercises tend to be more functional, and they facilitate the integration of proprioceptive and joint position sense feedback more effectively than open-kinetic-chain exercises.
- Open- and closed-kinetic-chain exercises have different biomechanical effects on the joints of the lower extremity.
- Closed-kinetic-chain exercises in the lower extremity decrease the shear forces, reducing anterior tibial translation, and increase the compressive forces, which increases stability around the knee joint.
- Minisquat, wall slides, lunges, leg press, stair-climbing machines, lateral step-up, terminal knee extension using tubing, stationary bicycling, slide boards, BAPS boards, and the Fitter are all examples of closed-kinetic-chain activities for the lower extremity.
- Although it is true that closed-kinetic-chain exercises are most often used in rehabilitation of lower-extremity injuries, there are many injury situations where closed-kinetic-chain exercises should be incorporated into upper-extremity rehabilitation protocols.
- Closed-kinetic-chain exercises in the upper extremity are used primarily for strengthening and establishing neuromuscular control of those muscles that act to stabilize the shoulder girdle.
- Closed-kinetic-chain activities, such as push-ups, press-ups, weight shifting, and slide board exercises, are strengthening exercises used primarily for improving shoulder stabilization in the upper extremity.

REFERENCES

1. Andersen S, Terwilliger D, Denegar C. Comparison of open- versus closed-kinetic-chain test positions for measuring joint position sense. *J Sport Rehab* 4(3):165–171, 1995.
2. Anderson R, Courtney C, Carmeli E. EMG analysis of the vastus medialis/vastus lateralis muscles utilizing the unloading narrow and wide-stance squats. *J Sport Rehab* 7(4):236, 1998.
3. Andrews J, Dennison J, Wilk K. The significance of closed-chain kinetic kinetics in upper extremity injuries from a physician's perspective. *J Sport Rehab* 5(1):64–70, 1995.

4. Augustsson J, Esko A, Thornee R, Karlsson J. Weight training of the thigh muscles using closed vs. open kinetic chain exercises: A comparison of performance enhancement. *J Orthop Sports Phys Ther* 27(1):3, 1998.

5. Baratta R, Solomonow M, Zhou B. Muscular coactivation: The role of the antagonist musculature in maintaining knee stability. *Am J Sports Med* 16(2):113–122, 1988.

6. Blackburn JR, Morrissey MC. The relationship between open and closed kinetic chain strength of the lower limb and jumping performance. *J Orthop Sports Phys Ther* 27(6):431, 1988.

7. Blair D, Willis R. Rapid rehabilitation following anterior cruciate ligament reconstruction. *Athlet Train* 26(1):32–43, 1991.

8. Blanpied P, Carroll R, Douglas T, Lyons M. Effectiveness of lateral slide exercise in an anterior cruciate ligament reconstruction rehabilitation home exercise program. *J Orthop Sports Physl Ther* 30(10):602, 2000.

9. Blanpied P. Changes in muscle activation during wall slides and squat-machine exercise. *J Sport Rehab* 8(2):123, 1999.

10. Brask B, Lueke R, Soderberg G. Electromyographic analysis of selected muscles during the lateral step-up. *Phys Ther* 64(3):324–329, 1984.

11. Bunton E, Pitney W, Kane A. The role of limb torque, muscle action and proprioception during closed-kinetic-chain rehabilitation of the lower extremity. *J Athlet Train* 28(1):10–20, 1993.

12. Butler D, Noyes F, Grood E. Ligamentous restraints to anterior-posterior drawer in the human knee: A biomechanical study. *J Bone Joint Surg* 62(A):259–270, 1980.

13. Case J, DePalma B, Zelko R. Knee rehabilitation following anterior cruciate ligament repair/reconstruction: An update. *Athlet Train* 26(1):22–31, 1991.

14. Cipriani D. Open- and closed-chain rehabilitation for the shoulder complex. In: Andrews J, Wilk K, eds. *The Athlete's Shoulder*. New York, NY, Churchill Livingston, 1994.

15. Cook T, Zimmerman C, Lux K, et al. EMG comparison of lateral step-up and stepping machine exercise. *J Orthop Sports Phys Ther* 16(3):108–113, 1992.

16. Cordova ML. Considerations in lower extremity closed kinetic chain exercise: A clinical perspective. *Athlet Ther Today* 6(2):46–50, 2001.

17. Davies G. The need for critical thinking in rehabilitation. *J Sport Rehab* 4(1):1–22, 1995.

18. DeCarlo M, Shelbourne D, McCarroll J, et al. A traditional versus accelerated rehabilitation following ACL reconstruction: A one-year follow-up. *J Orthop Sports Phys Ther* 15(6):309–316, 1992.

19. Ellenbecker TS, Davies GJ. *Closed Kinetic Chain Exercise: A Comprehensive Guide to Multiple-joint Exercise*. Champaign, IL, Human Kinetics, 2001.

20. Escamilla RF. Knee biomechanics of the dynamic squat exercise. *Med Sci Sports Exerc* 33(1):127–141, 2001.

21. Fu F, Woo S, Irrgang J. Current concepts for rehabilitation following anterior cruciate ligament reconstruction. *J Orthop Sports Phys Ther* 15(6):270–278, 1992.

22. Fukubayashi T, Torzilli P, Sherman M. An in-vitro biomechanical evaluation of anterior/posterior motion of the knee: Tibial displacement, rotation, and torque. *J Bone Joint Surg* 64[B]:258–264, 1982.

23. Grahm V, Gehlsen G, Edwards J. Electromyographic evaluation of closed- and open-kinetic-chain knee rehabilitation exercises. *J Athlet Train* 28(1):23–33, 1993.

24. Grood E, Suntag W, Noyes F, et al. Biomechanics of knee extension exercise. *J Bone Joint Surg* 66[A]:725–733, 1984.

25. Harter R. Clinical rationale for closed-kinetic-chain activities in functional testing and rehabilitation of ankle pathologies. *J Sport Rehab* 5(1):13–24, 1995.

26. Henning S, Lench M, Glick K. An in-vivo strain gauge study of elongation of the anterior cruciate ligament. *Am J Sports Med* 13:22–26, 1985.

27. Hillman S. Principles and techniques of open-kinetic-chain rehabilitation: The upper extremity. *Journal of sport Rehabilitation* 3(4): 319–30, 1994.

28. Hooper DM, Morrissey MC, Drechsler W. Open and closed kinetic chain exercises in the early period after anterior cruciate ligament reconstruction: Improvements in level walking, stair ascent, and stair descent. *Am J Sports Med* 29(2):167–174, 2001.

29. Hopkins JT, Ingersoll CD, and Sandrey MA. An electromyographic comparison of 4 closed chain exercises. *J Athlet Train* 34(4):353, 1999.

30. Hung YJ, Gross MT. Effect of foot position on electromyographic activity of the vastus medialis oblique and vastus lateralis during lower-extremity weight bearing activities. *Journal of Orthopaedic and Sports Physical Therapy* 29(2): 93–105, 1999.

31. Hungerford D, Barry M. Biomechanics of the patellofemoral joint. *Clin Orthop* 144:9–15, 1979.

32. Jurist K, Otis V. Anteroposterior tibiofemoral displacements during isometric extension efforts. The roles of external load and knee flexion angle. *Am J Sports Med* 13: 254–258, 1985.

33. Kaland S, Sinkjaer T, Arendt-Neilsen L, et al. Altered timing of hamstring muscle action in anterior cruciate ligament deficient patients. *Am J Sports Med* 18(3):245–248, 1990.

34. Kleiner D, Drudge T, Ricard M. An electromyographic comparison of popular open- and closed-kinetic-chain knee rehabilitation exercises. *J Athlet Train* 29(2):156–157, 1994.

35. Kovaleski JE, Heitman R, Gurchiek L, Tyundle T. Reliability and effects of arm dominance on upper extremity

isokinetic force, work, and power using the closed chain rider system. *J Athlet Train* 34(4):358, 1999.

36. LaFree J, Mozingo A, Worrell T. Comparison of open-kinetic-chain knee and hip extension to closed-kinetic-chain leg press performance. *J Sport Rehab* 3(2):99–107, 1995.

37. Lepart S, Henry T. The physiological basis for open- and closed-kinetic-chain rehabilitation for the upper extremity. *J Sport Rehab* 5(1):71–87, 1995.

38. Lutz G, Stuart M, Franklin H. Rehabilitative techniques for athletes after reconstruction of the anterior cruciate ligament. *Mayo Clin Proc* 65:1322–1329, 1990.

39. Malone T, Garrett W. Commentary and historical perspective of anterior cruciate ligament rehabilitation. *J Orthop Sports Phys Ther* 15(6):265–269, 1992.

40. McMullen J, Uhl TL. A kinetic chain approach for shoulder rehabilitation. *J Ath Train* 35(3): 329.

41. Nisell R, Ericson M, Nemeth G, et al. Tibiofemoral joint forces during isokinetic knee extension. *Am J Sports Med* 17:49–54, 1989.

42. Ohkoshi Y, Yasuda K, Kaneda K, et al. Biomechanical analysis of rehabilitation in the standing position. *Am J Sports Med* 19(6):605–611, 1991.

43. Palmitier R, Kai-Nan A, Scott S, et al. Kinetic- chain exercise in knee rehabilitation. *Sports Med* 11(6):402–413, 1991.

44. Rivera J. Open- versus closed-kinetic-chain rehabilitation of the lower extremity: A functional and biomechanical analysis. *J Sport Rehab* 3(2):154–167, 1994.

45. Renstrom P, Arms S, Stanwyck T, et al. Strain within the anterior cruciate ligament during hamstring and quadriceps activity. *Am J Sports Med* 14:83–87, 1986.

46. Reynolds N, Worrell T, and Perrin D. Effect of lateral step-up exercise protocol on quadriceps isokinetic peak torque values and thigh girth. *J Orthop Sports Phys Ther* 15(3):151–56, 1992.

47. Ross MD, Denegar CR, Winzenried JA. Implementation of open and closed kinetic chain quadriceps strengthening exercises after anterior cruciate ligament reconstruction. *J Strength Cond Res* 15(4):466–473, 2001.

48. Sachs R, Daniel D, Stone M, et al. Patellofemoral problems after anterior cruciate ligament reconstruction. *Am J Sports Med* 17:760–765, 1989.

49. Schulthies SS, Ricard MD, Alexander KJ, Myrer JW. An electromyographic investigation of 4 elastic-tubing closed kinetic chain exercises after anterior cruciate ligament reconstruction. *J Athlet Train* 33(4):328–335, 1998.

50. Selseth A, Dayton M, Cardova M, Ingersoll C, Merrick M. Quadriceps concentric EMG activity is greater than eccentric EMG activity during the lateral step-up exercise. *J Sport Rehab* 9(2):124, 2000.

51. Sheehy P, Burdett RG, Irrgang JJ, VanSwearingen J. An electromyographic study of vastus medialis oblique and vastus lateralis activity while ascending and descending stairs. *J Orthop Sports Phys Ther* 27(6):423–429, 1998.

52. Shellbourne D, Nitz P. Accelerated rehabilitation after anterior cruciate ligament reconstruction. *Am J Sports Med* 18:292–299, 1990.

53. Solomonow M, Barata R, Zhou B, et al. The synergistic action of the anterior cruciate ligament and thigh muscles in maintaining joint stability. *Am J Sports Med* 15:207–213, 1987.

54. Snyder-Mackler L. Scientific rationale and physiological basis for the use of closed-kinetic-chain exercise in the lower extremity. *J Sport Rehab* 5(1): 2–12, 1995.

55. Steindler A. *Kinesiology of the Human Body Under Normal and Pathological Conditions.* Springfield, IL, Charles C. Thomas, 1977.

56. Stiene H, Brosky T, Reinking M. A comparison of closed-kinetic-chain and isokinetic joint isolation exercise in patients with patellofemoral dysfunction. *J Orthop Sports Phys Ther* 24(3):136–141, 1996.

57. Stone J, Lueken J, Partin N. Closed-kinetic-chain rehabilitation of the glenohumeral joint. *J Athlet Train* 28(1):34–37, 1993.

58. Tang SFT, Chen CK, Hsu R, Chou SW, Hong WH, Lew HL. Vastus medialis obliquus and vastus lateralis activity in open and closed kinetic chain exercises in patients with patellofemoral pain syndrome: An electromyographic study. *Arch Phys Med Rehab* 82(10):1441–1445, 2001.

59. Tovin B, Tovin T, Tovin M. Surgical and biomechanical considerations in rehabilitation of patients with intra-articular ACL reconstructions. *J Orthop Sports Phys Ther* 15(6):317–322, 1992.

60. Ubinger ME, Prentice WE, Guskiewicz KM. Effect of closed kinetic chain training on neuromuscular control in the upper extremity. *J Sport Rehab* 8(3):184–194, 1999.

61. Valmassey R. *Clinical Biomechanics of the Lower Extremities.* St. Louis, Mosby, 1996.

62. Voight M, Bell S, Rhodes D. Instrumented testing of tibial translation during a positive Lachman's test and selected closed-chain activities in anterior cruciate deficient knees. *J Orthop Sports Phys Ther* 15:49, 1992.

63. Voight M, Cook G. Clinical application of closed-chain exercise. *J Sport Rehab* 5(1):25–44, 1995.

64. Voight M, Tippett S. *Closed Kinetic Chain.* Paper presented at 41st Annual Clinical Symposium of the National Athletic Trainers Association, Indianapolis, June 12, 1990.

65. Wawrzyniak J, Tracy J, Catizone P. Effect of closed-chain exercise on quadriceps femoris peak torque and functional performance. *J Athlet Train* 31(4):335–345, 1996.

66. Wilk K, Andrew J. Current concepts in the treatment of anterior cruciate ligament disruption. *J Orthop Sports Phys Ther* 15(6):279–293, 1992.

67. Wilk K, Arrigo C, Andrews J. Closed- and open-kinetic-chain exercise for the upper extremity. *J Sport Rehab* 5(1): 88–102, 1995.

68. Willett G, Karst G, Canney E, Gallant D, Wees J. Lower limb EMG activity during selected stepping exercises. *J Sport Rehab* 7(2):102, 1998.

69. Willett G, Paladino J, Barr K, Korta J, Karst G. Medial and lateral quadriceps muscle activity during weight-bearing knee extension exercise. *J Sport Rehab* 7(4):248, 1998.

70. Worrell TW, Crisp E, LaRosa C. Electromyographic reliability and analysis of selected lower extremity muscles during lateral step-up conditions. *J Athlet Train* 33(2):156, 1998.

CHAPTER 15

Proprioceptive Neuromuscular Facilitation Techniques in Rehabilitation

William E. Prentice

OBJECTIVES

After completing this chapter, the therapist should be able to do the following:

- Explain the neurophysiologic basis of *proprioceptive neuromuscular facilitation* (PNF) techniques.
- Discuss the rationale for use of the techniques.
- Identify the basic principles of using PNF in rehabilitation.
- Demonstrate the various PNF strengthening and stretching techniques.
- Describe PNF patterns for the upper and lower extremity, for the upper and lower trunk, and for the neck.
- Discuss the concept of muscle energy technique and explain how it is similar to PNF.

Proprioceptive neuromuscular facilitation (PNF) is an approach to therapeutic exercise based on the principles of functional human anatomy and neurophysiology.[9] It uses proprioceptive, cutaneous, and auditory input to produce functional improvement in motor output and can be a vital element in the rehabilitation process of many conditions and injuries.

The therapeutic techniques of PNF were first used in the treatment of patients with paralysis and various neuromuscular disorders in the 1950s. Originally the PNF techniques were used for strengthening and enhancing neuromuscular control. Since the early 1970s, the PNF techniques have also been used extensively as a technique for increasing flexibility and range of motion.[8,15,28,32,37,45,56,60]

This discussion should guide the therapist using the principles and techniques of PNF as a component of a rehabilitation program.

PNF AS A TECHNIQUE FOR IMPROVING STRENGTH AND ENHANCING NEUROMUSCULAR CONTROL

Original Concepts of Facilitation and Inhibition

Most of the principles underlying modern therapeutic exercise techniques can be attributed to the work of Sherrington,[53] who first defined the concepts of facilitation and inhibition.

According to Sherrington, an impulse traveling down the corticospinal tract or an afferent impulse traveling up from peripheral receptors in the muscle causes an impulse volley, which results in the discharge of a limited number of specific motor neurons, as well as the discharge of additional surrounding (anatomically close) motor neurons in the subliminal fringe area. An impulse causing the recruitment and discharge of additional motor neurons within the subliminal fringe is said to be facilitatory. Any stimulus that causes motor neurons to drop out of the discharge zone and away from the subliminal fringe is said to be inhibitory.[34] Facilitation results in increased excitability, and inhibition results in decreased excitability of motor neurons.[64] Thus the function of weak muscles would be aided by facilitation, and muscle spasticity would be decreased by inhibition.[22]

Sherrington attributed the impulses transmitted from the peripheral stretch receptors via the afferent system as being the strongest influence on the alpha motor neurons.[53] Therefore, the therapist should be able to modify the input from the peripheral receptors and thus influence the excitability of the alpha motor neurons. The discharge of motor neurons can be facilitated by peripheral stimulation, which causes afferent impulses to make contact with excitatory neurons and results in increased muscle tone or strength of voluntary contraction. Motor neurons can also be inhibited by peripheral stimulation, which causes afferent impulses to make contact with inhibitory neurons, resulting in muscle relaxation and allowing for stretching of the muscle.[53] To indicate any technique in which input from peripheral receptors is used to facilitate or inhibit, PNF should be used.[22]

Several different approaches to therapeutic exercise based on the principles of facilitation and inhibition have been proposed. Among these are the Bobath method,[5] Brunnstrom method,[7] Rood method,[49] and the Knott and Voss method,[33] which they called PNF. Although each of these techniques is important and useful, the PNF approach of Knott and Voss probably makes the most explicit use of proprioceptive stimulation.[33]

Rationale for Use

As a positive approach to injury rehabilitation, PNF is aimed at what the patient can do physically within the limitations of the injury. It is perhaps best used to decrease deficiencies in strength, flexibility, and neuromuscular coordination in response to demands that are placed on the neuromuscular system. The emphasis is on selective reeducation of individual motor elements through development of neuromuscular control, joint stability, and coordinated mobility. Each movement is learned and then reinforced through repetition in an appropriately demanding and intense rehabilitative program.[51]

The body tends to respond to the demands placed on it. The principles of PNF attempt to provide a maximal response for increasing strength and neuromuscular control. These principles should be applied with consideration of their appropriateness in achieving a particular goal. It is well accepted that the continued activity during a rehabilitation program is essential for maintaining or improving strength. Therefore an intense program should offer the greatest potential for recovery.[47]

The PNF approach is holistic, integrating sensory, motor, and psychological aspects of a rehabilitation program. It incorporates reflex activities from the spinal levels and upward, either inhibiting or facilitating them as appropriate.

The brain recognizes only gross joint movement and not individual muscle action. Moreover, the strength of a muscle contraction is directly proportional to the activated motor units. Therefore, to increase the strength of a muscle, the maximum number of motor units must be stimulated to strengthen the remaining muscle fibers.[28,33] This "irradiation," or overflow effect, can occur when the stronger muscle groups help the weaker groups in completing a particular movement. This cooperation leads to the rehabilitation goal of return to optimal function.[4,33] The principles of PNF, as discussed in the next section, should be applied to reach that ultimate goal.

Basic Principles of PNF

Margret Knott, in her text on PNF,[33] emphasized the importance of the principles rather than specific techniques in a rehabilitation program. These principles are the basis of PNF that must be superimposed on any specific technique. The principles of PNF are based on sound neurophysiologic and kinesiologic principles and clinical experience.[51] Application of the following principles can help promote a desired response in the patient being treated.

1. The patient must be taught the PNF patterns regarding the sequential movements from starting position to terminal position. The therapist has to keep instructions brief and simple. It is sometimes helpful for the therapist to passively move the patient through the desired movement pattern to demonstrate precisely what is to be done. The patterns should be used along with the techniques to increase the effects of the treatment.

2. When learning the patterns, the patient is often helped by looking at the moving limb. This visual stimulus offers the patient feedback for directional and positional control.

3. Verbal cues are used to coordinate voluntary effort with reflex responses. Commands should be firm and simple. Commands most commonly used with PNF techniques are "Push" and "Pull," which ask for an isotonic contraction; "Hold," which asks for an isometric or stabilizing contraction; and "Relax."

4. Manual contact with appropriate pressure is essential for influencing direction of motion and facilitating a maximal response, because reflex responses are greatly affected by pressure receptors. Manual contact should be firm and confident to give the patient a feeling of security. The manner in which the therapist touches the patient influences their confidence as well as the appropriateness of the motor response or relaxation.[51] A movement response may be facilitated by the hand over the muscle being contracted to facilitate a movement or a stabilizing contraction.

5. Proper mechanics and body positioning of the therapist are essential in applying pressure and resistance. The therapist should stand in a position that is in line with the direction of movement in the diagonal movement pattern. The knees should be bent and close to the patient such that the direction of resistance can easily be applied or altered appropriately throughout the range.

6. The amount of resistance given should facilitate a maximal response that allows smooth, coordinated motion. The appropriate resistance depends to a large extent on the capabilities of the patient. It may also change at different points throughout the range of motion. Maximal resistance may be applied with techniques that use isometric contractions to restrict motion to a specific point; it may also be used in isotonic contractions throughout a full range of movement.

7. Rotational movement is a critical component in all of the PNF patterns because maximal contraction is impossible without it.

8. Normal timing is the sequence of muscle contraction that occurs in any normal motor activity resulting in coordinated movement.[33] The distal movements of the patterns should occur first. The distal movement components should be completed no later than halfway through the total PNF pattern. To accomplish this, appropriate

verbal commands should be timed with manual commands. Normal timing may be used with maximal resistance or without resistance from the athletic trainer.

9. Timing for emphasis is used primarily with isotonic contractions. This principle superimposes maximal resistance, at specific points in the range, upon the patterns of facilitation, allowing overflow or irradiation to the weaker components of a movement pattern. The stronger components are emphasized to facilitate the weaker components of a movement pattern.

10. Specific joints may be facilitated by using traction or approximation. Traction spreads apart the joint articulations, and approximation presses them together. Both techniques stimulate the joint proprioceptors. Traction increases the muscular response, promotes movement, assists isotonic contractions, and is used with most flexion antigravity movements. Traction must be maintained throughout the pattern. Approximation increases the muscular response, promotes stability, assists isometric contractions, and is used most with extension (gravity-assisted) movements. Approximation may be quick or gradual and repeated during a pattern.

11. Giving a quick stretch to the muscle before muscle contraction facilitates a muscle to respond with greater force through the mechanisms of the stretch reflex. It is most effective if all the components of a movement are stretched simultaneously. However, this quick stretch can be contraindicated in many orthopedic conditions because the extensibility limits of a damaged musculotendinous unit or joint structure might be exceeded, exacerbating the injury.

BASIC STRENGTHENING TECHNIQUES

Each of the principles described in previous section should be applied to the specific techniques of PNF. These techniques may be used in a rehabilitation program to strengthen or facilitate a particular agonistic muscle group.[27] The choice of a specific technique depends on the deficits of a particular patient.[44] Specific techniques or combinations of techniques should be selected on the basis of the patient's problem.[3]

The following techniques are most appropriately used for the development of muscular strength, and endurance, as well as for reestablishing neuromuscular control.

Rhythmic initiation. The rhythmic initiation technique involves a progression of initial passive, then active-assistive, followed by active movement against resistance through the agonist pattern. Movement is slow, goes through the available range of motion, and avoids activation of a quick stretch. It is used for patients who are unable to initiate movement and who have a limited range of motion because of increased tone. It may also be used to teach the patient a movement pattern.

Repeated contraction. Repeated contraction is useful when a patient has weakness either at a specific point or throughout the entire range. It is used to correct imbalances that occur within the range by repeating the weakest portion of the total range. The patient moves isotonically against maximal resistance repeatedly until fatigue is evidenced in the weaker components of the motion. When fatigue of the weak components becomes apparent, a stretch at that point in the range should facilitate the weaker muscles and result in a smoother, more coordinated motion. Again, quick stretch may be contraindicated with some musculoskeletal injuries. The amount of resistance to motion given by the therapist should be modified to accommodate the strength of the muscle group. The patient is commanded to push by using the agonist concentrically and eccentrically throughout the range.

Slow reversal. Slow reversal involves an isotonic contraction of the agonist followed immediately by an isotonic contraction of the antagonist. The initial contraction of the agonist muscle group facilitates the succeeding contraction of the antagonist muscles. The slow-reversal technique can be used for developing active range of motion of the agonists and normal reciprocal timing between the antagonists and agonists, which is critical for normal coordinated motion.[46] The patient should be commanded to push against maximal resistance by using the antagonist and then to pull by using the agonist. The initial agonistic push facilitates the succeeding antagonist contraction.

Slow-reversal-hold. Slow-reversal-hold is an isotonic contraction of the agonist followed immediately by an isometric contraction, with a hold command given at the end of each active movement. The direction of the pattern is reversed by using the same sequence of contraction with no relaxation before shifting to the antagonistic pattern. This technique can be especially useful in developing strength at a specific point in the range of motion.

Rhythmic stabilization. Rhythmic stabilization uses an isometric contraction of the agonist, followed by an isometric contraction of the antagonist to produce cocontraction and stability of the two opposing muscle groups. The command given is always "Hold," and movement is resisted in each direction. Rhythmic stabilization results in an increase in the holding power to a point where the position cannot be broken. Holding should emphasize cocontraction of agonists and antagonists.

Treating Specific Problems with PNF Techniques

PNF-strengthening techniques can be useful in a variety of different conditions. To some extent the choice of the most effective technique for a given situation will be dictated by the state of the existing condition and the capabilities and limitations of the individual patient.[62] There are some advantages to using PNF techniques in general.

Relative to strengthening, the PNF techniques are not encumbered by the design constraints of commercial exercise machines, although some of the newer exercise machines have been designed to accommodate triplanar motion and thus will allow for PNF patterned motion.[8] With the PNF patterns, movement can occur in three planes simultaneously thus more closely resembling a functional movement pattern. The amount of resistance applied by the therapist can be easily adjusted and altered at different points through the range of motion to meet patient capabilities. The therapist can choose to concentrate on the strengthening through entire range of motion or through a very specific range. Combinations of several strengthening techniques can be used concurrently within the same PNF pattern.[42] Rhythmic initiation is useful in the early stages of rehabilitation when the patient is having difficulty moving actively through a pain-free arc. Passive movement can allow the patient to maintain a full range while using an active contraction to move through the available pain-free range. Slow reversal should be used to help improve muscular endurance. Slow-reversal-hold is used to correct existing weakness at specific points in the range of motion through isometric strengthening.

Rhythmic stabilization is used to achieve stability and neuromuscular control about a joint.[10] This technique requires co-contraction of opposing muscle groups and is useful in creating a balance in the existing force couples.

PNF Patterns

The PNF patterns are concerned with gross movement as opposed to specific muscle actions. The techniques identified previously can be superimposed on any of the PNF patterns. The techniques of PNF are composed of both rotational and diagonal exercise patterns that are similar to the motions required in most sports and normal daily activities.

The exercise patterns have three component movements: flexion-extension, abduction-adduction, and internal-external rotation. Human movement is patterned and rarely involves straight motion because all muscles are spiral in nature and lie in diagonal directions.

The PNF patterns described by Knott and Voss[33] involve distinct diagonal and rotational movements of the upper extremity, lower extremity, upper trunk, lower trunk, and neck. The exercise pattern is initiated with the muscle groups in the lengthened or stretched position. The muscle group is then contracted, moving the body part through the range of motion to a shortened position.

The upper and lower extremities all have two separate patterns of diagonal movement for each part of the body, which are referred to as the diagonal 1 (D1) and diagonal 2 (D2) patterns. These diagonal patterns are subdivided into D1 moving into flexion, D1 moving into extension, D2 moving into flexion, and D2 moving into extension. Figures 15-1 and 15-2 illustrate the PNF patterns for the upper and lower extremities, respectively. The patterns are named according to the proximal pivots at either the shoulder or the hip (for example, the glenohumeral joint or femoralacetabular joint).

Tables 15-1 and 15-2 describe specific movements in the D1 and D2 patterns for the upper extremities. Figures 15-3 through 15-10 show starting and terminal positions for each of the diagonal patterns in the upper extremity.

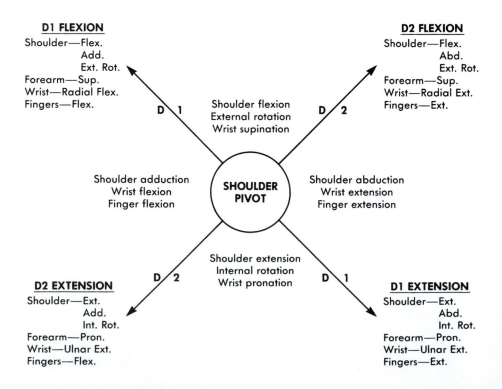

FIGURE 15-1

PNF patterns of the upper extremity.

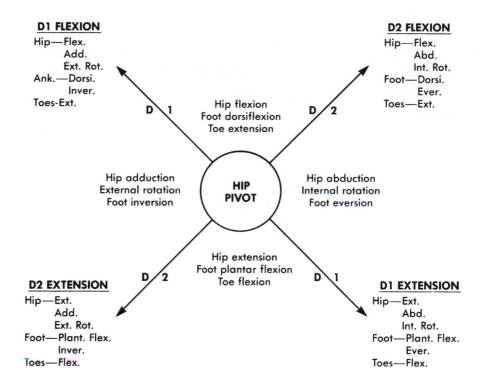

FIGURE 15-2

PNF patterns of the lower extremity.

TABLE 15-1

D1 Upper-Extremity Movement Patterns

BODY PART	MOVING INTO FLEXION		MOVING INTO EXTENSION	
	STARTING POSITION (FIG. 15-3)	TERMINAL POSITION (FIG. 15-4)	STARTING POSITION (FIG. 15-5)	TERMINAL POSITION (FIG. 15-6)
Shoulder	Extended Abducted Internally rotated	Flexed Adducted Externally rotated	Flexed Adducted Externally rotated	Extended Adducted Internally rotated
Scapula	Depressed Retracted Downwardly rotated	Flexed Protracted Upwardly rotated	Elevated Protracted Upwardly rotated	Depressed Retracted Downwardly rotated
Forearm	Pronated	Supinated	Supinated	Pronated
Wrist	Ulnar extended	Radially flexed	Radially flexed	Ulnar extended
Finger and thumb	Extended Abducted	Flexed Adducted	Flexed Adducted	Extended Abducted

Hand position for athletic trainer*	Left and inside of volar surface of hand.
	   Right hand underneath arm in cubital
	   fossa of elbow
			Left hand on back of elbow on humerus.
			   Right hand on dorsum of hand	

Verbal command	Pull		Push	

*For athlete's right arm.

TABLE   15-2

D2 Upper-Extremity Movement Patterns

| BODY PART | MOVING INTO FLEXION | | MOVING INTO EXTENSION | |
	STARTING POSITION (FIG. 15-7)	TERMINAL POSITION (FIG. 15-8)	STARTING POSITION (FIG. 15-9)	TERMINAL POSITION (FIG. 15-10)
Shoulder	Extended Abducted Internally rotated	Flexed Adducted Externally rotated	Flexed Adducted Externally rotated	Extended Adducted Internally rotated
Scapula	Depressed Retracted Downwardly rotated	Flexed Protracted Upwardly rotated	Elevated Protracted Upwardly rotated	Depressed Retracted Downwardly rotated
Forearm	Pronated	Supinated	Supinated	Pronated
Wrist	Ulnar extended	Radially flexed	Radially flexed	Ulnar extended
Finger and thumb	Flexed Abducted	Extended Adducted	Extended Adducted	Flexed Abducted
Hand position for athletic trainer*	Left and on back of humerus. Right hand on dorsum of hand		Left hand on volar surface of humerus. Right hand on cubital fossa of elbow	
Verbal command	Push		Pull	

*For athlete's right arm.

Tables 15-3 and 15-4 describe specific movements in the D1 and D2 patterns for the lower extremities. Figures 15-11 through 15-18 show the starting and terminal positions for each of the diagonal patterns in the lower extremity.

Table 15-5 describes the rotational movement of the upper trunk moving into extension (also called chopping) and mov-ing into flexion (also called lifting). Figure 15-19 and 15-20 show the starting and terminal positions of the upper-extremity chopping pattern moving into flexion to the right. Figures 15-21 and 15-22 show the starting and terminal positions for the upper-extremity lifting pattern moving into extension to the right.

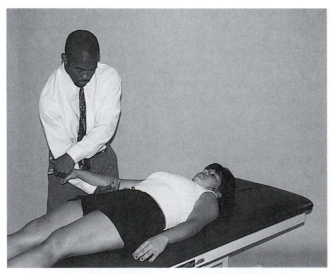

FIGURE   15-3

D1 upper-extremity movement pattern moving into flexion. Starting position.

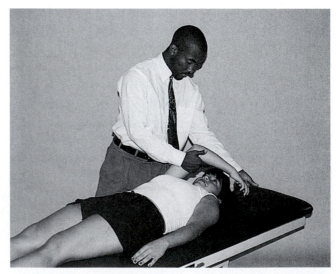

FIGURE   15-4

D1 upper-extremity movement pattern moving into flexion. Terminal position.

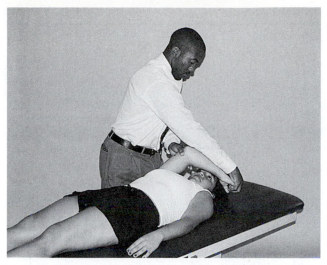

FIGURE 15-5

D1 upper-extremity movement pattern moving into extension. Starting position.

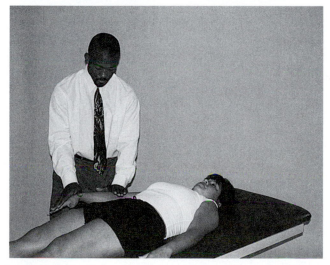

FIGURE 15-6

D1 upper-extremity movement pattern moving into extension. Terminal position.

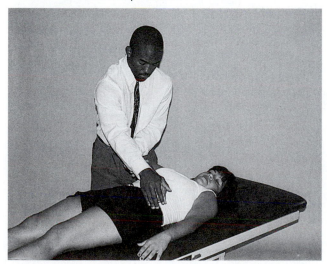

FIGURE 15-7

D2 upper-extremity movement pattern moving into flexion. Starting position.

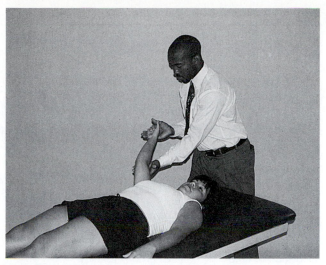

FIGURE 15-8

D2 upper-extremity movement pattern moving into flexion. Terminal position.

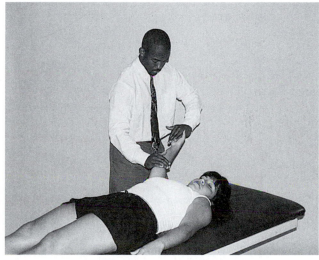

FIGURE 15-9

D2 upper-extremity movement pattern moving into extension. Starting position.

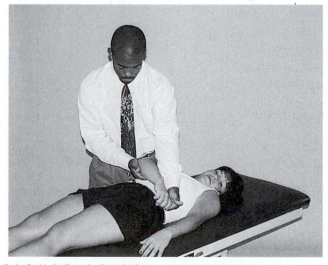

FIGURE 15-10

D2 upper-extremity movement pattern moving into extension. Terminal position.

T A B L E 1 5 - 3

D1 Lower-Extremity Movement Patterns

BODY PART	MOVING INTO FLEXION		MOVING INTO EXTENSION	
	STARTING POSITION (FIG. 15-11)	TERMINAL POSITION (FIG. 15-12)	STARTING POSITION (FIG. 15-13)	TERMINAL POSITION (FIG. 15-14)
Hip	Extended Abducted Internally rotated	Flexed Adducted Externally rotated	Flexed Adducted Externally rotated	Extended Abducted Internally rotated
Knee	Extended	Flexed	Flexed	Extended
Position of tibia	Externally rotated	Internally rotated	Internally rotated	Externally rotated
Ankle and foot	Plantarflexed Everted	Dorsiflexed Inverted	Dorsiflexed Inverted	Plantarflexed Everted
Toes	Flexed	Extended	Extended	Flexed
Hand position for athletic trainer*	Right hand on dorsimedial surface of foot. Left hand on anteromedial thigh near patella		Right hand on lateralplantar surface of foot. Left hand on posteriolateral thigh near popliteal crease	
Verbal command	Pull		Push	

*For athlete's right arm.

T A B L E 1 5 - 4

D2 Lower-Extremity Movement Patterns

BODY PART	MOVING INTO FLEXION		MOVING INTO EXTENSION	
	STARTING POSITION (FIG. 15-15)	TERMINAL POSITION (FIG. 15-16)	STARTING POSITION (FIG. 15-17)	TERMINAL POSITION (FIG. 15-18)
Hip	Extended Adducted Externally rotated	Flexed Abducted Internally rotated	Flexed Abducted Internally rotated	Extended Adducted Externally rotated
Knee	Extended	Flexed	Flexed	Extended
Position of tibia	Externally rotated	Internally rotated	Internally rotated	Externally rotated
Ankle and foot	Plantarflexed Inverted	Dorsiflexed Everted	Dorsiflexed Everted	Plantarflexed Inverted
Toes	Flexed	Extended	Extended	Flexed
Hand position for athletic trainer*	Right hand on dorsilateral surface of foot. Left hand on anterolateral thigh near patella		Right hand on medialplantar surface of foot. Left hand on posteriomedial thigh near popliteal crease	
Verbal command	Pull		Push	

*For athlete's right leg.

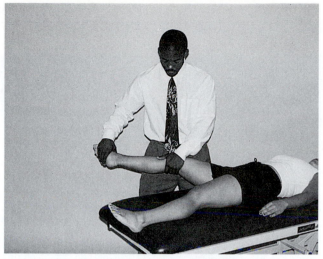

D1 lower-extremity movement pattern moving into flexion. Starting position.

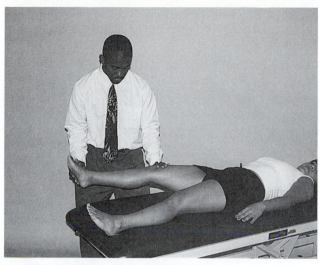

D1 lower-extremity movement pattern moving into extension. Terminal position.

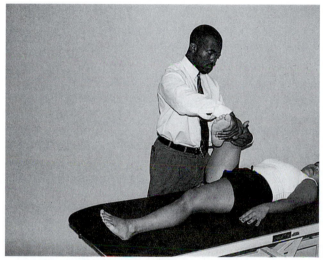

F I G U R E   1 5 - 1 2

D1 lower-extremity movement pattern moving into flexion. Terminal position.

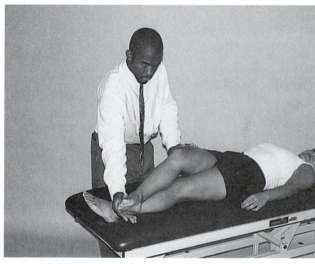

F I G U R E   1 5 - 1 5

D2 lower-extremity movement pattern moving into flexion. Starting position.

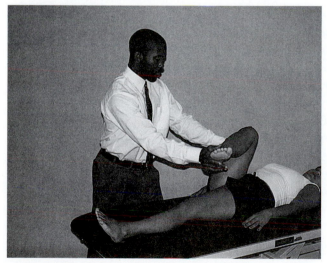

F I G U R E   1 5 - 1 3

D1 lower-extremity movement pattern moving into extension. Starting position.

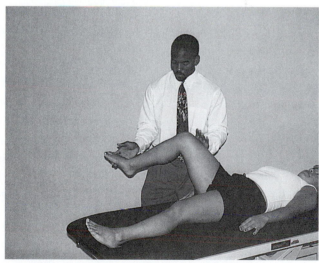

F I G U R E   1 5 - 1 6

D2 lower-extremity movement pattern moving into flexion. Terminal position.

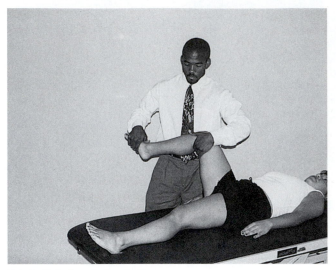

FIGURE 15-17

D2 lower-extremity movement pattern moving into extension. Starting position.

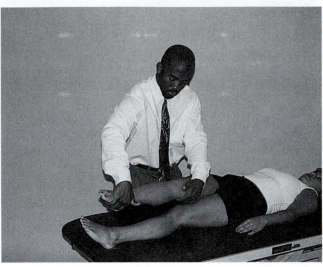

FIGURE 15-18

D2 lower-extremity movement pattern moving into extension. Terminal position.

Table 15-6 describes rotational movement of the lower extremities moving into positions of flexion and extension. Figures 15-23 and 15-24 show the lower-extremity pattern moving into flexion to the left. Figures 15-25 and 15-26 show the lower-extremity pattern moving into extension to the left.

The neck patterns involve simply flexion and rotation to one side (Figs. 15-27 and 15-28) with extension and rotation to the opposite side (Figs. 15-29 and 15-30). The patient should follow the direction of the movement with their eyes.

The principles and techniques of PNF, when used appropriately with specific patterns, can be an extremely effective tool

TABLE 15-5

Upper-Trunk Movement Patterns

BODY PART	MOVING INTO FLEXION (CHOPPING)*		MOVING INTO EXTENSION (LIFTING)*	
	STARTING POSITION (FIG. 15-19)	TERMINAL POSITION (FIG. 15-20)	STARTING POSITION (FIG. 15-21)	TERMINAL POSITION (FIG. 15-22)
Right upper extremity	Flexed Adducted Internally rotated	Extended Abducted Externally rotated	Extended Adducted Internally rotated	Flexed Abducted Externally rotated
Left upper extremity (left hand grasps right forearm)	Flexed Abducted Externally rotated	Extended Adducted Internally rotated	Extended Abducted Externally rotated	Flexed Adducted Internally rotated
Trunk	Rotated and extended to left	Rotated and flexed to right	Rotated and flexed to left	Rotated and extended to right
Head	Rotated and extended to left	Rotated and flexed to right	Rotated and flexed to left	Rotated and extended to right
Hand position of athletic trainer	Left hand on right anterolateral surface of forehead. Right hand on dorsum of right hand		Right hand on dorsum of right hand. Left hand on posteriolateral surface of head	
Verbal command	Pull down		Push up	

*Athlete's rotation is to the right.

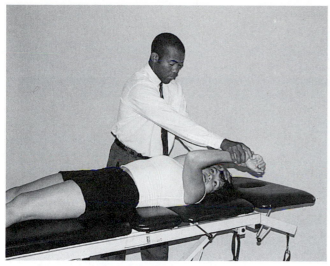

FIGURE 15-19

Upper-trunk pattern moving into extension or chopping. Starting position.

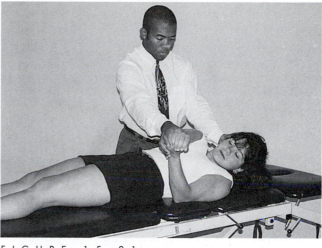

FIGURE 15-21

Upper-trunk pattern moving into flexion or lifting. Starting position.

for rehabilitation of injuries.[54] They can be used to strengthen weak muscles or muscle groups and to improve the neuromuscular control about an injured joint. Specific techniques selected for use should depend on individual patient needs and may be modified accordingly.[13,14]

PNF AS A TECHNIQUE OF STRETCHING FOR IMPROVING RANGE OF MOTION

As indicated previously, PNF techniques can also be used for stretching to increase range of motion.

Evolution of the Theoretical Basis for Using PNF as a Stretching Technique

A review of the current literature seems to indicate that many clinicians feel that the PNF-stretching techniques can be an effective treatment modality for improving flexibility and thus use them regularly in clinical practice.[16,23,43] Over the years, various theories have been proposed to explain the neurological and physical mechanisms through which the PNF techniques improve flexibility.[12] However, to date no consensus agreement exists that embraces a single theoretical explanation.

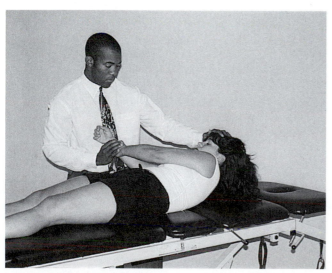

FIGURE 15-20

Upper-trunk pattern moving into extension or chopping. Terminal position.

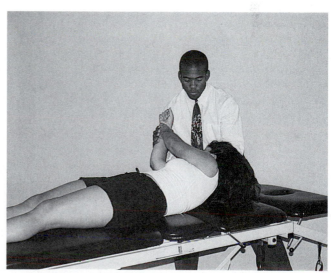

FIGURE 15-22

Upper-trunk pattern moving into flexion or lifting. Terminal position.

T A B L E   1 5 - 6

Lower Trunk Movement Patterns

BODY PART	MOVING INTO FLEXION*		MOVING INTO EXTENSION†	
	STARTING POSITION (FIG. 15-23)	TERMINAL POSITION (FIG. 15-24)	STARTING POSITION (FIG. 15-25)	TERMINAL POSITION (FIG. 15-26)
Right hip	Extended Abducted Externally rotated	Flexed Adducted Internally rotated	Flexed Adducted Internally rotated	Extended Abducted Externally rotated
Left hip	Extended Adducted Internally rotated	Flexed Abducted Externally rotated	Flexed Abducted Externally rotated	Extended Adducted Internally rotated
Ankles	Plantarflexed	Dorsiflexed	Dorsiflexed	Plantarflexed
Toes	Flexed	Extended	Extended	Flexed
Hand position of athletic trainer	Right hand on dorsum of feet. Left hand on anterolateral surface of left knee		Right hand on plantar surface of foot. Left hand on posteriolateral surface of right knee	
Verbal command	Pull up and in		Push down and out	

*Athlete's rotation is to the right.
†Athlete's rotation is to the right in extension.

Neurophysiologic Basis of PNF Stretching

PNF gained popularity as a stretching technique in the 1970s.[37,45,60] The PNF research that has traditionally appeared in the literature since that time has attributed increases in range of motion primarily to neurophysiologic mechanisms involving the stretch reflex.[12] More recent studies have questioned the validity of this theoretical explanation.[1,12,30,31,57] Nevertheless, a brief review of the stretch reflex will serve as a springboard for more currently accepted theories.

The stretch reflex involves two types of receptors: (1) muscle spindles, which are sensitive to a change in length, as well as

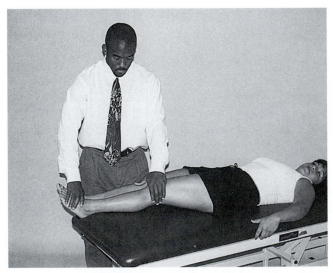

FIGURE   1 5 - 2 3

Lower-trunk pattern moving into flexion to the left. Starting position.

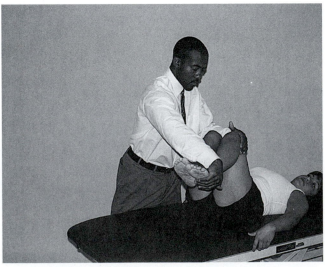

FIGURE   1 5 - 2 4

Lower-trunk pattern moving into flexion to the left. Terminal position.

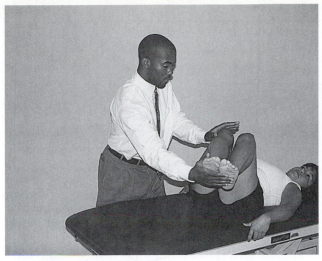

FIGURE 15-25

Lower-trunk pattern moving into extension to the left. Starting position.

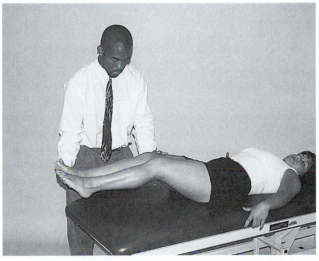

FIGURE 15-26

Lower-trunk pattern moving into extension to the left. Terminal position.

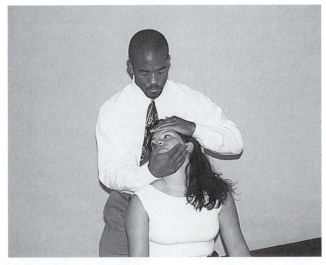

FIGURE 15-27

Neck flexion and rotation to the left. Starting position.

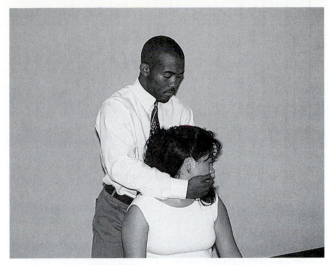

FIGURE 15-28

Neck flexion and rotation to the left. Terminal position.

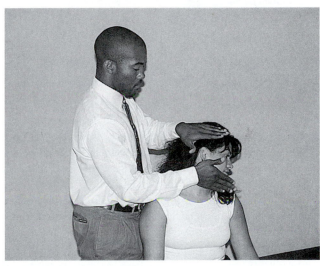

FIGURE 15-29

Neck extension and rotation to the right. Starting position.

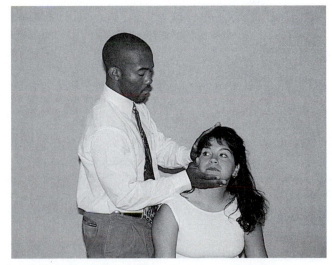

FIGURE 15-30

Neck extension and rotation to the right. Terminal position.

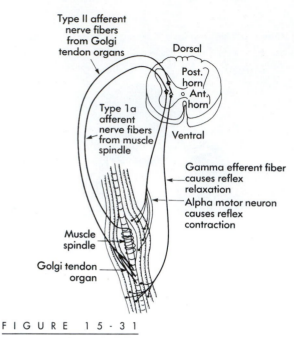

FIGURE 1 5 - 3 1

Diagrammatic representation of the stretch reflex.

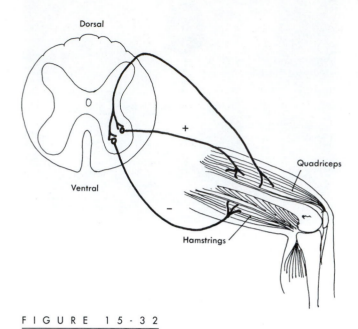

FIGURE 1 5 - 3 2

Diagrammatic representation of reciprocal inhibition.

the rate of change in length of the muscle fiber; and (2) Golgi tendon organs, which detect changes in tension (Fig. 15-31).

Stretching a given muscle causes an increase in the frequency of impulses transmitted to the spinal cord from the muscle spindle along Ia fibers, which in turn produces an increase in the frequency of motor nerve impulses returning to that same muscle, along alphamotor neurons, thus reflexively resisting the stretch. However, the development of excessive tension within the muscle activates the Golgi tendon organs, whose sensory impulses are carried back to the spinal cord along Ib fibers. These impulses have an inhibitory effect on the motor impulses returning to the muscles and cause that muscle to relax.[11]

Two neurophysiologic phenomena have been proposed to explain facilitation and inhibition of the neuromuscular systems. The first, *autogenic inhibition*, is defined as inhibition mediated by afferent fibers from a stretched muscle acting on the alpha motor neurons supplying that muscle, causing it to relax. When a muscle is stretched, motor neurons supplying that muscle receive both excitatory and inhibitory impulses from the receptors. If the stretch is continued for a slightly extended period of time, the inhibitory signals from the Golgi tendon organs eventually override the excitatory impulses and therefore cause relaxation. Because inhibitory motor neurons receive impulses from the Golgi tendon organs while the muscle spindle creates an initial reflex excitation leading to contraction, the Golgi tendon organs apparently send inhibitory impulses that last for the duration of increased tension (resulting from either passive stretch or active contraction) and eventually dominate the weaker impulses from the muscle spindle. This inhibition seems to protect the muscle against injury from reflex contractions resulting from excessive stretch.

A second mechanism, *reciprocal inhibition*, deals with the relationships of the agonist and antagonist muscles (Fig. 15-32.) The muscles that contract to produce joint motion are referred to as agonists, and the resulting movement is called an agonistic pattern. The muscles that stretch to allow the agonist pattern to occur are referred to as antagonists. Movement that occurs directly opposite to the agonist pattern is called the antagonist pattern.

When motor neurons of the agonist muscle receive excitatory impulses from afferent nerves, the motor neurons that supply the antagonist muscles are inhibited by afferent impulses.[4] Thus contraction or extended stretch of the agonist muscle has been said to elicit relaxation or inhibit the antagonist. Likewise, a quick stretch of the antagonist muscle facilitates a contraction of the agonist.

The PNF literature has traditionally asserted that isometric or isotonic submaximal contraction of a target muscle (muscle to be stretched) prior to a passive stretch of that same muscle, or contraction of opposing muscles (agonists) during muscle stretch, produces relaxation of the stretched muscle through activation of the mechanisms of the stretch reflex that include autogenic inhibition and reciprocal inhibition.[12]

However, a number of studies done since the early 1990s have suggested that relaxation following a contraction of a stretched muscle is not due to the inhibition of muscle spindle activity or to subsequent activation of Golgi tendon organs.[1,2,11,12,20,21,27,38,50]

Conclusions are based on the fact that when slowly stretching a muscle to a long length, as in the PNF-stretching techniques, the reflex generated muscle electrical activation from the muscle spindles (as indicated by electromyogram) is very small and clinically insignificant and not likely to effectively resist an applied muscle lengthening force.[12,26,29,35] Furthermore, when a muscle relaxes following an isometric contraction, Golgi tendon organ firing is decreased or even becomes silent.[17,63] Thus, Golgi tendon organs would not be able to inhibit the target muscle in the seconds following contraction when the slow therapeutic stretch would be applied.[12] It is apparent that in general, there is a lack of research-based evidence to support the theory that Golgi tendon organ and muscle spindle reflexes are able to relax target muscles during any of the PNF-stretching techniques.[12] Thus, other mechanisms have been proposed that may explain increases in range of motion with PNF-stretching exercises.

Presynaptic Inhibition

In the PNF-stretching techniques, the contraction and subsequent relaxation of the target muscle is followed by a slow passive stretch of that muscle to a longer length. It has been suggested that lengthening is associated with an increase in presynaptic inhibition of the sensory signal from the muscle spindle.[12,19,24] This occurs with inhibition of the release of a neurotransmitter from the synaptic terminals of the muscle spindle Ia sensory fibers which limits activation in that muscle.

Viscoelastic Changes in Response to Stretching

It has been proposed that viscoelastic changes that occur in a muscle, and not a decrease in muscle activation mediated by Gogi tendon organs, is the mechanism which may explain increases in range of motion associated with the PNF techniques.[8] The viscoelastic properties of collagen in muscle were discussed briefly in Chapter 10. The force that is required to produce a change in length of a muscle is determined by its *elastic stiffness*.[61] Because of the viscous properties of muscle, less force is needed to elongate a muscle if that force is applied slowly rather than rapidly.[61] Also, the force that resists elongation is reduced if the muscle is held at a stretched length over a period of time thus producing *stress relaxation*.[52] As stress relaxation occurs, the muscle will elongate further producing *creep*. These properties have been demonstrated in muscles with no significant electrical activity.[35,36,39]

As the viscoelastic properties within a muscle are changed, during a PNF-stretching procedure, there is an altered perception of stretch and a greater range of motion and greater torque can be achieved before the onset of pain is perceived.[36] This is thought to occur because lengthening interrupts the actin-myosin bonds within the intrafusal fibers of the muscle spindle thus reducing their sensitivity to stretch.[19,25,63]

Stretching Techniques

The following techniques should be used to increase range of motion, relaxation, and inhibition.

Contract-relax is a stretching technique that moves the body part passively into the agonist pattern. The patient is instructed to push by contracting the antagonist (muscle that will

be stretched) isotonically against the resistance of the therapist. The patient then relaxes the antagonist while the therapist moves the part passively through as much range as possible to the point where limitation is again felt. This contract-relax technique is beneficial when range of motion is limited by muscle tightness.

Hold-relax is very similar to the contract-relax technique. It begins with an isometric contraction of the antagonist (muscle that will be stretched) against resistance, followed by a concentric contraction of the agonist muscle combined with light pressure from the therapist to produce maximal stretch of the antagonist. This technique is appropriate when there is muscle tension on one side of a joint and may be used with either the agonist or antagonist.

Slow-reversal-hold-relax technique begins with an isotonic contraction of the agonist, which often limits range of motion in the agonist pattern, followed by an isometric contraction of the antagonist (muscle that will be stretched) during the push phase. During the relax phase, the antagonists are relaxed while the agonists are contracting, causing movement in the direction of the agonist pattern and thus stretching the antagonist. The technique, like the contract-relax and hold-relax, is useful for increasing range of motion when the primary limiting factor is the antagonistic muscle group.

Because a goal of rehabilitation with most injuries is restoration of strength through a full, nonrestricted range of motion, several of these techniques are sometimes combined in sequence to accomplish this goal.[41] Figure 15-33 shows a PNF-stretching technique in which the therapist is stretching an injured patient.

MUSCLE ENERGY TECHNIQUES

Muscle energy is a manual therapy technique, which is a variation of the PNF contract-relax and hold-relax techniques. Like

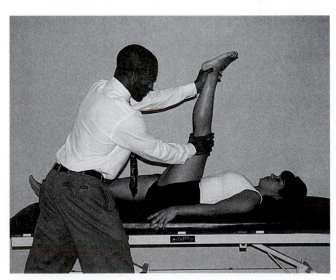

FIGURE 15-33

PNF-stretching technique.

the PNF techniques, the muscle energy techniques are based on the same neurophysiologic mechanisms involving the stretch reflex discussed earlier in this chapter. Muscle energy techniques involve a voluntary contraction of a muscle in a specifically controlled direction at varied levels of intensity against a distinctly executed counterforce applied by the therapist.[28,40,53] The patient provides the corrective *intrinsic* forces and controls the intensity of the muscular contractions while the therapist controls the precision and localization of the procedure.[40] The amount of patient effort can vary from a minimal muscle twitch to a maximal muscle contraction.[28]

Five components are necessary for muscle energy techniques to be effective[28]:

1. Active muscle contraction by the patient
2. A muscle contraction oriented in a specific direction
3. Some patient control of contraction intensity
4. Therapist control of joint position
5. Therapist application of appropriate counterforce

Clinical Applications

It has been proposed that muscles function not only as flexors, extenders, rotators, and side-benders of joints but also as restrictors of joint motion. In situations where the muscle is restricting joint motion, muscle energy techniques use a specific muscle contraction to restore physiologic movement to a joint.[40] Any articulation, whether in the spine or extremities, that can be moved by active muscle contraction can be treated using muscle energy techniques.[40,48]

Muscle energy techniques can be used to accomplish a number of treatment goals[28]:

1. Lengthening of a shortened, contracted, or spastic muscle
2. Strengthening of a weak muscle or muscle group
3. Reduction of localized edema through muscle pumping
4. Mobilization of an articulation with restricted mobility
5. Stretching of fascia

Treatment Techniques

Muscle energy techniques can involve four types of muscle contraction: isometric, concentric isotonic, eccentric isotonic, and *isolytic*. An isolytic contraction involves a concentric contraction by the patient while the therapist applies an external force in the opposite direction, overpowering the contraction and lengthening that muscle.[40]

Isometric and concentric isotonic contractions are most frequently used in treatment.[55] Isometric contractions are most often used in treating hypertonic muscles in the spinal vertebral column, while isotonic contractions are most often used in the extremities. With both types of contraction, the idea is to inhibit antagonistic muscles producing more symmetrical muscle tone and balance.

A concentric contraction can also be used to mobilize a joint against its *motion barrier* if there is motion restriction.

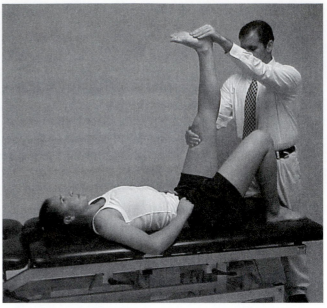

FIGURE   15-34

Isometric muscle energy technique for tightness of the hamstring muscle.

For example, if a knee has a restriction due to tightness in the hamstrings that is limiting full extension, the following isometric muscle energy technique should be used (Fig. 15-34):

1. The patient should lie supine on the treatment table.
2. The therapist stabilizes the knee with one hand and grasps the ankle with the other.
3. The therapist fully extends the knee until an extension barrier is felt.

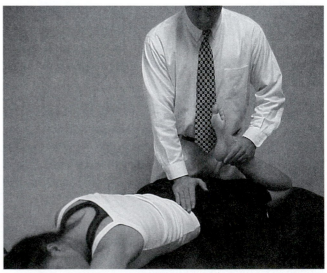

FIGURE   15-35

Position for muscle energy technique for improving weak quadriceps which limits knee extension.

4. The patient is instructed to actively flex the knee using a minimal sustained force.
5. The therapist provides an equal resistant counterforce for 3–7 seconds, after which the patient completely relaxes.
6. The therapist once again extends the knee until a new extension barrier is felt.
7. This is repeated three to five times.

If a strength imbalance exists between the quadriceps and hamstrings, with weak quadriceps limiting knee extension, the following concentric isotonic muscle energy technique may be used (Fig. 15-35):

1. The patient should lie prone on the treatment table.
2. The therapist stabilizes the patient with one hand and grasps the ankle with the other.
3. The therapist fully flexes the knee.
4. The patient instructed to actively extend the knee, using as much force as possible.
5. The therapist provides a resistant counterforce that allows slow knee extension throughout the available range.
6. Once the patient has completely relaxed, the therapist moves the knee back to full flexion and the patient repeats the contraction with additional resistance applied through the full range of extension. This is repeated three to five times with increasing resistance on each repetition.

SUMMARY

- The PNF techniques may be used to increase both strength and range of motion and are based on the neurophysiology of the stretch reflex.
- The motor neurons of the spinal cord always receive a combination of inhibitory and excitatory impulses from the afferent nerves. Whether these motor neurons will be excited or inhibited depends on the ratio of the two types of incoming impulses.
- The PNF techniques emphasize specific principles that may be superimposed on any of the specific techniques.
- The PNF-strengthening techniques include repeated contraction, slow-reversal, slow-reversal-hold, rhythmic stabilization, and rhythmic initiation.
- The PNF-stretching techniques include contract-relax, hold-relax, and slow-reversal-hold-relax.
- The techniques of PNF are rotational and diagonal movements in the upper extremity, lower extremity, upper trunk, and the head and neck.
- Muscle energy techniques involve a voluntary contraction of a muscle in a specifically controlled direction at varied levels of intensity against a distinctly executed counterforce applied by the therapist.

REFERENCES

1. Alter M. *Science of Flexibility*, 2nd ed. Champaign, IL, Human Kinetics, 1996.

2. Anderson B, Burke ER. Scientific, medical, and practical aspects of stretching. *Clin Sports Med* 10:63–86, 1991.

3. Barak T, Rosen E, Sofer R. Mobility: Passive orthopedic manual therapy. In: Gould J, Davies G, eds. *Orthop Sports Phys Ther* St. Louis, Mosby, 1990.

4. Basmajian J. *Therapeutic Exercise*. Baltimore, MD, Lippincott Williams & Wilkins, 1978.

5. Bobath B. The treatment of motor disorders of pyramidal and extrapyramidal tracts by reflex inhibition and by facilitation of movement. *Physiotherapy* 41:146, 1955.

6. Bonnar B, Deivert R, Gould T. The relationship between isometric contraction durations during hold-relax stretching and improvement of hamstring flexibility. *J Sports Med Phys Fitness* 44(3):258–261, 2004.

7. Brunnstrom S. *Movement Therapy in Hemiplegia*. New York, Harper & Row, 1970.

8. Burke DG, Culligan CJ, Holt LE. Equipment designed to stimulate proprioceptive neuromuscular facilitation flexibility training. *Journal of Strength and Conditioning Research* 14(2):135–39, 2000.

9. Burke DG, Culligan CJ, Holt LE. The theoretical basis of proprioceptive neuromuscular facilitation. *J Strength Cond Res* 14(4):496–500, 2000.

10. Burke DG, Holt LE, Rasmussen R. Effects of hot or cold water immersion and modified proprioceptive neuromuscular facilitation flexibility exercise on hamstring length. *J Athlet Train* 36(1):16–19, 2001.

11. Carter AM, Kinzey SJ, Chitwood LE, Cole JL. Proprioceptive neuromuscular facilitation decreases muscle activity during the stretch reflex in selected posterior thigh muscles. *Journal of Sport Rehabilitation* 9(4):269–78, 2000.

12. Chalmers G. Re-examination of the possible role of Golgi tendon organ and muscle spindle reflexes in proprioceptive neuromuscular facilitation muscle stretching. *Sports Biomech* 3(1):159–183, 2004.

13. Cookson J. Orthopedic manual therapy: An overview. II. The spine. *J Am Phys Ther Assoc* 59:259, 1979.

14. Cookson J, Kent B. Orthopedic manual therapy: An overview. I. The extremities. *J Am Phys Ther Assoc* 59:136, 1979.

15. Cornelius, W, Jackson A. The effects of cryotherapy and PNF on hip extension flexibility. *Athlet Train* 19(3):184, 1984.

16. Decicco PV, Fisher MM. The effects of proprioceptive neuromuscular facilitation stretching on shoulder range of motion in overhand athletes. *J Sports Med Phys Fitness* 45(2):183–187, 2005.

17. Edin BB, Vallbo AB. Muscle afferent responses to isometric contractions and relaxations in humans. *J Neurophys* 63:1307–1313, 1990.

18. Engle R, Canner G. Proprioceptive neuromuscular facilitation (PNF) and modified procedures for anterior cruciate ligament (ACL) instability. *J Orthop Sports Phys Ther* 11(6):230–236, 1989.

19. Enoka R. *Neuromechanics of Human Movement*, 3rd ed. Champaign, IL, Human Kinetics, 2002.

20. Enoka RM, Hutton RS, Eldred E. Changes in excitability of tendon tap and Hoffmann reflexes following voluntary contractions *Electroencephalogr Clin Neurophysiol* 48:664–672, 1980.

21. Ferber R, Osternig L, Gravelle D. Effect of PNF stretch techniques on knee flexor muscle EMG activity in older adults. *J Electromyogr Kinesiol* 12:391–397, 2002.

22. Greenman P. *Principles of Manual Medicine*. Baltimore,MD, Lippincott Williams & Wilkins, 1993.

23. Godges JJ, Mattson Bell M, Thorpe D, Shah D. The immediate effects of soft tissue mobilization with proprioceptive neuromuscular facilitation on glenohumeral external rotation and overhead reach. *J Orthop Sports Phys Ther* 33(12):713–718, 2003.

24. Gollhofer A, Schopp A, Rapp W, Stroinik V. Changes in reflex excitability following isometric contraction in humans. *Eur J Appl Physiol Occup Physiol* 77:89–97, 1998.

25. Gregory JE, Mark RF, Morgan DL, Patak A, Polus B, Proske U. Effects of muscle history on the stretch reflex in cat and man. *J Physiol* 424:93–107, 1990.

26. Halbertsma JP, Mulder I, Goeken LN, Eisma WH. Repeated passive stretching: Acute effect on the passive muscle moment and extensibility of short hamstrings. *Arch Phys Med Rehab* 80:407–414, 1999.

27. Holcomb WR. Improved stretching with proprioceptive neuromuscular facilitation. *Strength Cond J* 22(1):59–61, 2000.

28. Hollis M. *Practical Exercise*. Oxford, Blackwell Scientific, 1981.

29. Houk JC, Rymer WZ, Crago PE. Dependence of dynamic response of spindle receptors on muscle length and velocity. *J Neurophysiol* 46:143–166, 1981.

30. Hultborn H. State-dependent modulation of sensory feedback. *J Physiol* 533(Pt 1):5–13, 2001.

31. Jankowska E. Interneuronal relay in spinal pathways from proprioceptors. *Prog Neurobiol* 38:335–378, 1992.

32. Johnson GS. PNF and knee rehabilitation. *J Orthop Sports Phys Ther* 30(7):430–431, 2000.

33. Knott M, Voss D. *Proprioceptive Neuromuscular Facilitation: Patterns and Techniques*. New York, Harper & Row, 1968.

34. Lloyd D. Facilitation and inhibition of spinal motorneurons. *J Neurophysiol* 9:421, 1946.

35. Magnusson SP, Simonsen EB, Aagaard P, Dyhrepoulsen P, McHugh MP, Kjaer M. Mechanical and Physiological Responses to Stretching With and Without Preisometric Contraction in Human Skeletal Muscle. *Arc Phys Med Rehab* 77:373–378, 1996.

36. Magnusson SP, Simonsen EB, Dyhre-Poulsen P, Aagaard P, Mohr T, Kjaer M. Viscoelastic stress relaxation during static stretch in human skeletal muscle in the absence of EMG activitiy. *Scand J Med Sci Sports* 6:323–328, 1996.

37. Markos P. Ipsilateral and contralateral effects of proprioceptive neuromuscular facilitation techniques on hip motion and electromyographic activity. *Phys Ther* 59(11) P:66–73, 1979.

38. McAtee R, Charland J. *Facilitated Stretching*, 2nd ed. Champaign, IL, Human Kinetics, 1999.

39. McHugh MP, Magnusson SP, Gleim GW, Nicholas JA. Viscoelastic stress relaxation in human skeletal muscle. *Med Sci Sports Exerc* 24:1375–1382, 1992.

40. Mitchell F. Elements of muscle energy technique. In: Basmajian J, Nyberg R, eds. *Rational Manual Therapies*. Baltimore, MD, Lippincott Williams & Wilkins, 1993.

41. Osternig L, Robertson R, Troxel R, et al. Differential responses to proprioceptive neuromuscular facilitation stretch techniques. *Med Sci Sports Exerc* 22:106–111, 1990.

42. Osternig L, Robertson R, Troxel R, Hansen P. Muscle activation during proprioceptive neuromuscular facilitation (PNF) stretching techniques . . . stretch-relax (SR), contract-relax (CR) and agonist contract-relax (ACR). *Am J Phys Med* 66(5):298–307, 1987.

43. Padua D, Guskiewicz K, Prentice W. The effect of select shoulder exercises on strength, active angle reproduction, single-arm balance, and functional performance. *J Sport Rehab* 13(1):75–95, 2004.

44. Prentice W. Proprioceptive neuromuscular facilitation [Videotape]. St. Louis, Mosby, 1993.

45. Prentice W. A comparison of static stretching and PNF stretching for improving hip joint flexibility. *Athlet Train* 18(1):56–59, 1983.

46. Prentice W. A manual resistance technique for strengthening tibial rotation. *Athlet Train* 23(3):230–233, 1988.

47. Prentice W, Kooima E. The use of proprioceptive neuromuscular facilitation techniques in the rehabilitation of sport-related injuries. *Athlet Train* 21:26–31, 1986.

48. Roberts BL. Soft tissue manipulation: Neuromuscular and muscle energy techniques. *J Neurosci Nurs* 29(2):123–127, 1997.

49. Rood M. Neurophysiologic reactions as a basis of physical therapy. *Phys Ther Rev* 34:444, 1954.

50. Rowlands A, Marginson V, Lee J. Chronic flexibility gains: effect of isometric contraction duration during proprioceptive neuromuscular facilitation tretching techniques. *Res Q Exerc Sport* 74:47–51, 2003.

51. Saliba V, Johnson G, Wardlaw C. Proprioceptive neuromuscular facilitation. In: Basmajian J, Nyberg R, eds. *Rational Manual Therapies*. Baltimore, MD, Lippincott Williams & Wilkins, 1993.

52. Shrier I. Does stretching help prevent injuries? In: MacAuley D, Best T, eds. *Evidence Based Sports Medicine*. London, BMJ Books, 2002.

53. Sherrington C. *The Integrative Action of the Nervous System*. New Haven, Yale University Press, 1947.

54. Spernoga SG, Uhl TL, Arnold BL, Gansneder BM. Duration of maintained hamstring flexibility after a one-time, modified hold-relax stretching protocol. *J Athlet Train* 36(1):44–48, 2001.

55. Stone J. Muscle energy technique. *Athlet Ther Today* 5(5): 25, 2000.

56. Stone JA. Prevention and rehabilitation: Proprioceptive neuromuscular facilitation. *Athlet Ther Today* 5(1):38–39, 2000.

57. Stuart DG. Reflections of spinal reflexes. *Adv Exp Med Biol* 508:249–257, 2002.

58. Surburg P, Schrader J. Proprioceptive neuromuscular facilitation techniques in sports medicine: A reassessment. *J Athlet Train* 32(1):34–39, 1997.

59. Surberg P. Neuromuscular facilitation techniques in sports medicine. *Phys Ther Rev* 34:444, 1954.

60. Taniqawa M. Comparison of the hold-relax procedure and passive mobilization on increasing muscle length. *Phys Ther* 52(7):725–735, 1972.

61. Taylor DC, Dalton JD, Seaber AV, Garrett WE. Viscoelastic properties of muscle-tendon units. The biomechanical effects of stretching. *Am J Sports Med* 18:300–309, 1990.

62. Worrell T, Smith T, Winegardner J. Effect of hamstring stretching on hamstring muscle performance. *J Orthop Sports Phys Ther* 20(3):154–159, 1994.

63. Wilson LR, Gandevia SC, Burke D. Increased resting discharge of human spindle afferents following voluntary contractions. *J Physiol* 488(Pt 3):833–840, 1995.

64. Zohn D, Mennell J. *Musculoskeletal Pain: Diagnosis and Physical Treatment.* Boston, Little, Brown, 1987.

Joint Mobilization and Traction Techniques in Rehabilitation

William E. Prentice

O B J E C T I V E S

After completing this chapter, the therapist should be able to do the following:

- Differentiate between physiologic movements and accessory motions.
- Discuss joint arthrokinematics.
- Discuss how specific joint positions can enhance the effectiveness of the treatment technique.
- Discuss the basic techniques of joint mobilization.
- Identify Maitland's five oscillation grades.
- Discuss indications and contraindications for mobilization.
- Discuss the use of various traction grades in treating pain and joint hypomobility.
- Explain why traction and mobilization techniques should be used simultaneously.
- Demonstrate specific techniques of mobilization and traction for various joints.

Following injury to a joint, there will almost always be some associated loss of motion. That loss of movement may be attributed to a number of pathologic factors including contracture of inert connective tissue (for example, ligaments and joint capsule), resistance of the contractile tissue or the musculotendinous unit (for example, muscle, tendon, and fascia) to stretch, or some combination of the two.[7,8] If left untreated, the joint will become hypomobile and will eventually begin to show signs of degeneration.[30]

Joint mobilization and traction are manual therapy techniques that are slow, passive movements of articulating surfaces.[33] They are used to regain normal active joint range of motion, restore normal passive motions that occur about a joint, reposition or realign a joint, regain a normal distribution of forces and stresses about a joint, or reduce pain—all of which will collectively improve joint function.[25] Joint mobilization and traction are two extremely effective and widely used techniques in injury rehabilitation.[3]

RELATIONSHIP BETWEEN PHYSIOLOGIC AND ACCESSORY MOTIONS

For the therapist supervising a rehabilitation program, some understanding of the biomechanics of joint movement is essential.

There are basically two types of movements that govern motion about a joint. Perhaps the better known of the two types of movements are the *physiologic movements* that result from either concentric or eccentric active muscle contractions that move a bone or a joint. This type of motion is referred to as *osteokinematic motion*. A bone can move about an axis of rotation, or a joint into flexion, extension, abduction, adduction, and rotation. The second type of motion is *accessory motion*. Accessory motions refer to the manner in which one articulating joint surface moves relative to another. Physiologic movement is voluntary, while accessory movements normally accompany physiologic movement.[2] The two occur simultaneously. Although accessory movements cannot occur independently, they may be produced by some external force. Normal accessory component motions must occur for full-range physiologic movement to take place. If any of the accessory component motions are restricted, normal physiologic cardinal plane movements will not occur.[23,24] A muscle cannot be fully rehabilitated if the joint is not free to move and vice versa.[30]

Traditionally in rehabilitation programs, we have tended to concentrate more on passive physiologic movements without paying much attention to accessory motions. The question is always being asked, "How much flexion or extension is this patient lacking?" Rarely will anyone ask "How much is rolling or gliding restricted?"

It is critical for the therapist to closely evaluate the injured joint to determine whether motion is limited by physiologic movement constraints involving musculotendinous units or by limitation in accessory motion involving the joint capsule and ligaments.[15] If physiologic movement is restricted, the patient should engage in stretching activities designed to improve flexibility. Stretching exercises should be used whenever there is resistance of the contractile or musculotendinous elements to stretch. Stretching techniques are most effective at the end of physiologic range of movement; they are limited to one direction, and they require some element of discomfort if additional range of motion is to be achieved. Stretching techniques make use of long-lever arms to apply stretch to a given muscle.[14] Stretching techniques were discussed in Chapters 10 and 15.

If accessory motion is limited by some restriction of the joint capsule or the ligaments, the therapist should incorporate mobilization techniques into the treatment program. Mobilization techniques should be used whenever there are tight inert or noncontractile articular structures; they can be used effectively at any point in the range of motion, and they can be used in any direction in which movement is restricted. Mobilization techniques use a short-lever arm to stretch ligaments and joint capsules, placing less stress on these structures, and consequently are somewhat safer to use than stretching techniques.[5]

JOINT ARTHROKINEMATICS

Accessory motions are also referred to as *joint arthrokinematics*, which include *spin, roll*, and *glide* (Fig. 16-1).[1,17,19]

Spin occurs around some stationary longitudinal mechanical axis and may be in either a clockwise or counterclockwise direction. An example of spinning is motion of the radial head at the humeroradial joint as occurs in forearm pronation/supination (Fig. 16-1A).

Rolling occurs when a series of points on one articulating surface come in contact with a series of points on another articulating surface. An analogy would be to picture a rocker of a rocking chair rolling on the flat surface of the floor. An anatomic example would be the rounded femoral condyles rolling over a stationary flat tibial plateau (Fig. 16-1B).

Gliding occurs when a specific point on one articulating surface comes in contact with a series of points on another surface. Returning to the rocking chair analogy, the rocker slides across the flat surface of the floor without any rocking at all. Gliding is sometimes referred to as *translation*. Anatomically, gliding or translation would occur during an anterior drawer test at the knee when the flat tibial plateau slides anteriorly relative to the fixed rounded femoral condyles (Fig. 16-1C).

Pure gliding can occur only if the two articulating surfaces are congruent, where either both are flat or both are curved. Since virtually all articulating joint surfaces are incongruent, meaning that one is usually flat while the other is more curved, it is more likely that gliding will occur simultaneously with a rolling motion. Rolling does not occur alone because this would result in compression or perhaps dislocation of the joint.

Although rolling and gliding usually occur together, they are not necessarily in similar proportion, nor are they always in the same direction. If the articulating surfaces are more congruent, more gliding will occur; whereas if they are less congruent, more rolling will occur. Rolling will always occur in the same direction as the physiologic movement. For example, in the knee joint when the foot is fixed on the ground, the femur will always roll in an anterior direction when moving into knee extension and conversely will roll posteriorly when moving into flexion (Fig. 16-2).

The direction of the gliding component of motion is determined by the shape of the articulating surface that is moving. If you consider the shape of two articulating surfaces, one joint surface can be determined to be convex in shape while the other may be considered to be concave in shape. In the knee, the femoral condyles would be considered the convex joint surface, while the tibial plateau would be the concave joint surface. In the glenohumeral joint, the humeral head would be the

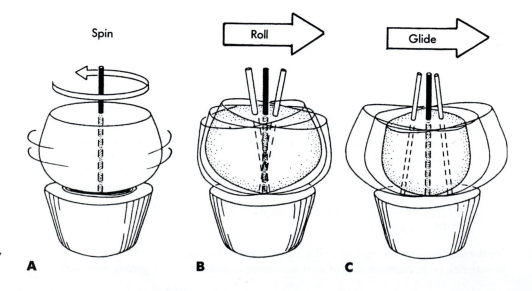

FIGURE 16-1

Joint arthrokinematics. **A,** Spin. **B,** Roll. **C,** Glide.

Spin

Roll

Glide

A   **B**   **C**

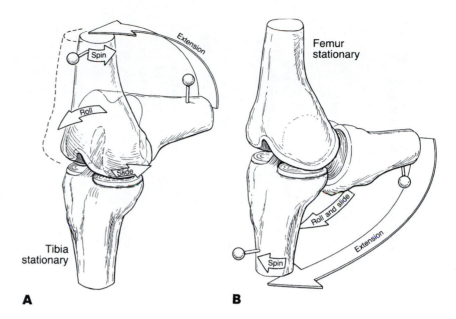

FIGURE 16-2

Convex–concave rule. **A,** Convex moving on concave. **B,** Concave moving on convex.

convex surface, while the glenoid fossa would be the concave surface.

This relationship between the shape of articulating joint surfaces and the direction of gliding is defined by the *convex–concave rule.* If the concave joint surface is moving on a stationary convex surface, gliding will occur in the same direction as the rolling motion. Conversely, if the convex surface is moving on a stationary concave surface, gliding will occur in an opposite direction to rolling. Hypomobile joints are treated by using a gliding technique. Thus it is critical to know the appropriate direction to use for gliding.[9]

JOINT POSITIONS

Each joint in the body has a position in which the joint capsule and the ligaments are most relaxed, allowing for a maximum amount of *joint play.*[4,19] This position is called the *resting position.* It is essential to know specifically where the resting position is, because testing for joint play during an evaluation, and treatment of the hypomobile joint using either mobilization or traction, are usually performed in this position. Table 16-1 summarizes the appropriate resting positions for many of the major joints.

Placing the joint capsule in the resting position allows the joint to assume a *loose-packed position* in which the articulating joint surfaces are maximally separated. A *close-packed position* is one in which there is maximal contact of the articulating surfaces of bones with the capsule and ligaments tight or tense. In a loose-packed position, the joint will exhibit the greatest amount of joint play, while the close-packed position allows for no joint play. Thus the loose-packed position is most appropriate for mobilization and traction (Fig. 16-3).

Both mobilization and traction techniques use a translational movement of one joint surface relative to the other. This translation may be either perpendicular or parallel to the *treatment plane.* The treatment plane falls perpendicular to, or at a right angle to, a line running from the axis of rotation in the convex surface to the center of the concave articular surface (Fig. 16-4).[17,19] Thus the treatment plane lies within the concave surface. If the convex segment moves, the treatment plane remains fixed. However, the treatment plane will move along with the concave segment. Mobilization techniques use glides that translate one articulating surface along a line parallel with the treatment plane. Traction techniques translate one of the articulating surfaces in a perpendicular direction to the treatment plane. Both techniques use a loose-packed joint position.[17]

JOINT MOBILIZATION TECHNIQUES

The techniques of joint mobilization are used to improve joint mobility or to decrease joint pain by restoring accessory movements to the joint and thus allowing full, nonrestricted, pain-free range of motion.[25,34]

Mobilization techniques may be used to attain a variety of either mechanical or neurophysiologic treatment goals: reducing pain; decreasing muscle guarding; stretching or lengthening tissue surrounding a joint, in particular capsular and ligamentous tissue; reflexogenic effects that either inhibit or facilitate muscle tone or stretch reflex; and proprioceptive effects to improve postural and kinesthetic awareness.[1,12,24,28,30]

Movement throughout a range of motion can be quantified with various measurement techniques. Physiologic movement is measured with a goniometer and composes the major portion of the range. Accessory motion is thought of in millimeters, although precise measurement is difficult.

Accessory movements may be hypomobile, normal, or hypermobile.[6] Each joint has a range-of-motion continuum with an anatomic limit (AL) to motion that is determined by

T A B L E   1 6 - 1

Shape, Resting Position, and Treatment Planes of Various Joints

JOINT	CONVEX SURFACE	CONCAVE SURFACE	RESTING POSITION (LOOSE-PACKED)	CLOSE-PACKED POSITION	TREATMENT PLANE
Sternoclavicular	Clavicle^a	Sternum^a	Anatomic position	Horizontal	In sternum
Acromioclavicular	Clavicle	Acromion	Anatomic position, in horizontal plane at 60° to sagittal plane	Adduction	In acromion
Glenohumeral	Humerus	Glenoid	Shoulder abducted 55°, horizontally adducted 30°, rotated so that forearm is in horizontal plane	Abduction and lateral rotation	In glenoid fossa in scapular plane
Humeroradial	Humerus	Radius	Elbow extended, forearm supinated	Flexion and forearm production	In radial head perpendicular to long axis of radius
Humeroulnar	Humerus	Ulna	Elbow flexed 70°, forearm supinated 10°	Full extension and forearm supination	In olecranon fossa, 45° to long axis of ulna
Radioulnar (proximal)	Radius	Ulna	Elbow flexed 70°, forearm supinated 35°	Full extension and forearm supination	In radial notch of ulna, parallel to long axis of ulna
Radioulnar (distal)	Ulna	Radius	Supinated 10°	Extension	In radius, parallel to long axis of radius
Radiocarpal	Proximal carpal bones	Radius	Line through radius and third metacarpal	Extension	In radius, perpendicular to long axis of radius
Metacarpophalangeal	Metacarpal	Proximal phalanx	Slight flexion	Full flexion	In proximal phalanx
Interphalangeal	Proximal phalanx	Distal phalanx	Slight flexion	Extension	In proximal phalanx
Hip	Femur	Acetabulum	Hip flexed 30°, abducted 30°, slight external rotation	Extension and medial rotation	In acetabulum
Tibiofemoral	Femur	Tibia	Flexed 25°	Full extension	On surface of tibial plateau
Patellofemoral	Patella	Femur	Knee in full extension	Full flexion	Along femoral groove
Talocrural	Talus	Mortise	Plantarflexed 10°	Dorsiflexion	In the mortise in anterior/posterior direction
Subtalar	Calcaneous	Talus	Subtalar neutral between inversion/eversion	Supination	In talus, parallel to foot surface
Intertarsal	Proximal articulating surface	Distal articulating surface	Foot relaxed	Supination	In distal segment
Metatarsophalangeal	Tarsal bone	Proximal phalanx	Slight extension	Full flexion	In proximal phalanx
Interphalangeal	Proximal phalanx	Distal phalanx	Slight flexion	Extension	In distal phalanx

^aIn the sternoclavicular joint the clavicle surface is convex in a superior/inferior direction and concave in an anterior/posterior direction.

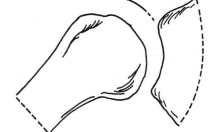
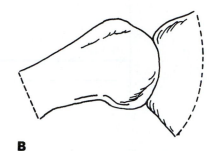

FIGURE 16-3

Joint capsule resting position.
A, Loose-packed position. **B,**
Close-packed position.

A   **B**

both bony arrangement and surrounding sort tissue (Fig. 16-5). In a hypomobile joint, motion stops at some point referred to as a pathologic point of limitation (PL), short of the anatomic limit caused by pain, spasm, or tissue resistance. A hypermobile joint moves beyond its anatomic limit because of laxity of the surrounding structures. A hypomobile joint should respond well to techniques of mobilization and traction. A hypermobile joint should be treated with strengthening exercises, stability exercises, and if indicated, taping, splinting, or bracing.[29,30]

In a hypomobile joint, as mobilization techniques are used in the range-of-motion restriction, some deformation of soft-tissue capsular or ligamentous structures occurs. If a tissue is stretched only into its elastic range, no permanent structural changes will occur. However, if that tissue is stretched into its plastic range, permanent structural changes will occur. Thus, mobilization and traction can be used to stretch tissue and break adhesions. If used inappropriately, they can also damage tissue and cause sprains of the joint.[30]

Treatment techniques designed to improve accessory movement are generally slow, small-amplitude movements, the amplitude being the distance that the joint is moved passively within its total range. Mobilization techniques use these small-amplitude oscillating motions that glide or slide one of the articulating joint surfaces in an appropriate direction within a specific part of the range.[22]

Maitland has described various grades of oscillation for joint mobilization. The amplitude of each oscillation grade falls within the range-of-motion continuum between some beginning point (BP) and the AL.[23,24] Figure 16-5 shows the various grades of oscillation that are used in a joint with some limitation of motion. As the severity of the movement restriction increases, the PL will move to the left, away from the AL. However, the relationships that exist among the five grades in terms of their positions within the range of motion remain the same. The five mobilization grades are defined as follows:

- Grade I. A small-amplitude movement at the beginning of the range of movement. Used when pain and spasm limit movement early in the range of motion.[37]

- Grade II. A large-amplitude movement within the midrange of movement. Used when spasm limits movement sooner with a quick oscillation than with a slow one, or when slowly increasing pain restricts movement halfway into the range.

- Grade III. A large-amplitude movement up to the PL in the range of movement. Used when pain and resistance from spasm, inert tissue tension, or tissue compression limit movement near the end of the range.

- Grade IV. A small-amplitude movement at the very end of the range of movement. Used when resistance limits movement in the absence of pain and spasm.

- Grade V. A small-amplitude, quick thrust delivered at the end of the range of movement, usually accompanied by a popping sound, which is called a manipulation. Used when minimal resistance limits the end of the range. Manipulation is most effectively accomplished by the velocity of the thrust rather than by the force of the thrust.[21] Most authorities agree that manipulation should be used only by individuals trained specifically in these techniques, because a great deal of skill and judgment is necessary for safe and effective treatment.[32]

Joint mobilization uses these oscillating gliding motions of one articulating joint surface in whatever direction is appropriate for the existing restriction. The appropriate direction for these oscillating glides is determined by the convex–concave

Glide

Traction

Treatment plane

90°

FIGURE 16-4

Treatment plane. The treatment plane is perpendicular to a line drawn from the axis of rotation to the center of the articulating surface of the concave segment.

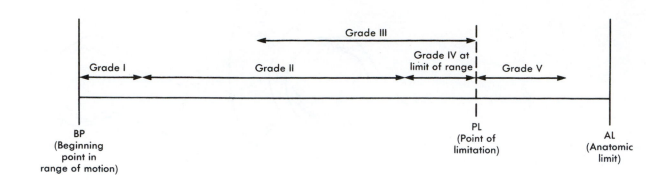

FIGURE 16-5

Maitland's five grades of motion.

rule, described previously. When the concave surface is stationary and the convex surface is mobilized, a glide of the convex segment should be in the direction opposite to the restriction of joint movement (Fig. 16-6A).[17,19,35] If the convex articular surface is stationary and the concave surface is mobilized, gliding of the concave segment should be in the same direction as the restriction of joint movement (Fig. 16-6B). For example, the glenohumeral joint would be considered to be a convex joint with the convex humeral head moving on the concave glenoid. If shoulder abduction is restricted, the humerus should be glided in an inferior direction relative to the glenoid to alleviate the motion restriction. When mobilizing the knee joint, the concave tibia should be glided anteriorly in cases where knee extension is restricted. If mobilization in the appropriate direction exacerbates complaints of pain or stiffness, the therapist should apply the technique in the opposite direction until the patient can tolerate the appropriate direction.[35]

Typical mobilization of a joint may involve a series of three to six sets of oscillations lasting between 20 and 60 seconds each, with one to three oscillations per second.[23,24]

Indications for Mobilization

In Maitland's system, grades I and II are used primarily for treatment of pain and grades III and IV are used for treating stiffness. Pain must be treated first and stiffness second.[24] Painful conditions should be treated on a daily basis. The purpose of the small-amplitude oscillations is to stimulate mechanoreceptors within the joint that can limit the transmission of pain perception at the spinal cord or brainstem levels.

Joints that are stiff or hypomobile and have restricted movement should be treated three to four times per week on alternating days with active motion exercise. The therapist must continuously reevaluate the joint to determine appropriate progression from one oscillation grade to another.

Indications for specific mobilization grades are relatively straightforward. If the patient complains of pain before the therapist can apply any resistance to movement, it is too early, and all mobilization techniques should be avoided. If pain is elicited when resistance to motion is applied, mobilization using grades I, II, and III is appropriate. If resistance can be applied before pain is elicited, mobilization can be progressed to grade IV. Mobilization should be done with both the patient and the therapist positioned in a comfortable and relaxed manner. The therapist should mobilize one joint at a time. The joint should be stabilized as near one articulating surface as possible, while moving the other segment with a firm, confident grasp.

Contraindications for Mobilization

Techniques of mobilization and manipulation should not be used haphazardly. These techniques should generally not be

FIGURE 16-6

Gliding motions. **A,** Glides of the convex segment should be in the direction opposite to the restriction. **B,** Glides of the concave segment should be in the direction of the restriction.

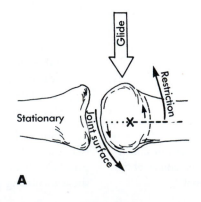

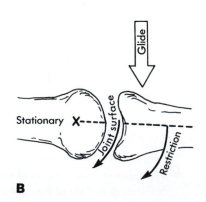

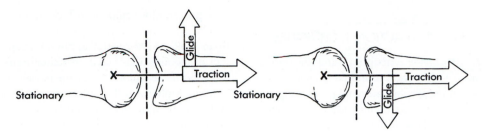

F I G U R E 1 6 - 7

Traction versus glides. Traction should be perpendicular to the treatment plane, while glides are parallel to the treatment plane.

used in cases of inflammatory arthritis, malignancy, bone disease, neurologic involvement, bone fracture, congenital bone deformities, and vascular disorders of the vertebral artery. Again, manipulation should be performed only by those therapists specifically trained in the procedure, because some special knowledge and judgment are required for effective treatment.[24]

JOINT TRACTION TECHNIQUES

Traction refers to a technique involving pulling on one articulating segment to produce some separation of the two joint surfaces. While mobilization glides are done parallel to the treatment plane, traction is performed perpendicular to the treatment plane (see Fig. 16-7). Like mobilization techniques, traction may be used either to decrease pain or to reduce joint hypomobility.[38]

Kaltenborn has proposed a system using traction combined with mobilization as a means of reducing pain or mobilizing hypomobile joints.[14] As discussed earlier, all joints have a certain amount of joint play or looseness. Kaltenborn referred to this looseness as *slack*. Some degree of slack is necessary for normal joint motion. Kaltenborn's three traction grades are defined as follows.[17] (Fig. 16-8):

- Grade I traction (loosen). Traction that neutralizes pressure in the joint without actual separation of the joint surfaces. The purpose is to produce pain relief by reducing the com-

pressive forces of articular surfaces during mobilization and is used with all mobilization grades.
- Grade II traction (tighten or "take up the slack"). Traction that effectively separates the articulating surfaces and takes up the slack or eliminates play in the joint capsule. Grade II is used in initial treatment to determine joint sensitivity.
- Grade III traction (stretch). Traction that involves actual stretching of the soft tissue surrounding the joint to increase mobility in a hypomobile joint.

Grade I traction should be used in the initial treatment to reduce the chance of a painful reaction. It is recommended that 10-second intermittent grades I and II traction be used, distracting the joint surfaces up to a grade III traction and then releasing distraction until the joint returns to its resting position.[16]

Kaltenborn emphasizes that grade III traction should be used in conjunction with mobilization glides to treat joint hypomobility (Fig. 16-8).[17] Grade III traction stretches the joint capsule and increases the space between the articulating surfaces, placing the joint in a loose-packed position. Applying grades III and IV oscillations within the patient's pain limitations should maximally improve joint mobility (Fig. 16-9).[16]

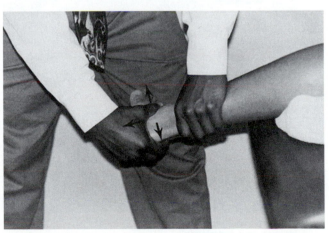

F I G U R E 1 6 - 9

Traction and mobilization. Traction and mobilization should be used together.

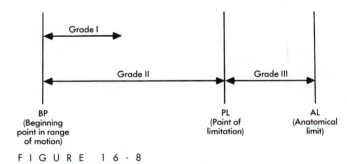

F I G U R E 1 6 - 8

Kaltenborn's grades of traction.

MOBILIZATION AND TRACTION TECHNIQUES

Figures 16-10 to 16-73 provide descriptions and illustrations of various mobilization and traction techniques. These figures should be used to determine appropriate hand positioning, stabilization (S), and the correct direction for gliding (G), traction (T), and/or rotation (R). The information presented in this chapter should be used as a reference base for appropriately incorporating joint mobilization and traction techniques into the rehabilitation program.

Mulligan Joint Mobilization Technique

Brian Mulligan, an Australian physiotherapist proposed a concept of mobilizations based on Kaltenborn's principles. While Kaltenborn's technique relies on passive accessory mobilization, the Mulligan technique combines passive accessory joint mobilization applied by a therapist with active physiological movement by the patient for the purpose of correcting positional faults and returning the patient to normal pain-free function.[18,27] It is a noninvasive and comfortable intervention, and has applications for the spine and the extremities. Mulligan's

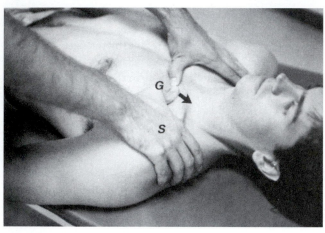

FIGURE 16-10

Posterior and superior clavicular glides. When posterior or superior clavicular glides are done at the sternoclavicular joint, use the thumbs to glide the clavicle. Posterior glides are used to increase clavicular retraction, and superior glides increase clavicular retraction and clavicular depression.

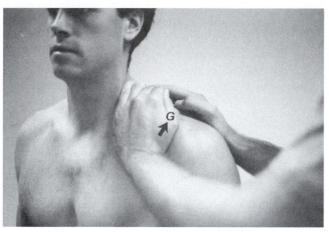

FIGURE 16-12

Posterior clavicular glides. Posterior clavicular glides done at the acromioclavicular (AC) joint apply posterior pressure on the clavicle while stabilizing the scapula with the opposite hand. They increase mobility of the AC joint.

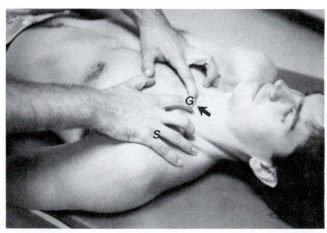

FIGURE 16-11

Inferior clavicular glides. Inferior clavicular glides at the sternoclavicular joint use the index fingers to mobilize the clavicle, which increases clavicular elevation.

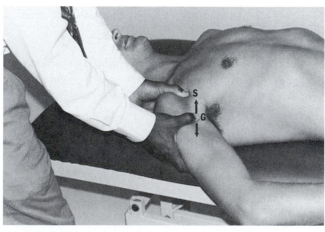

FIGURE 16-13

Anterior/posterior glenohumeral glides. Anterior/posterior glenohumeral glides are done with one hand stabilizing the scapula and the other gliding the humeral head. They initiate motion in the painful shoulder.

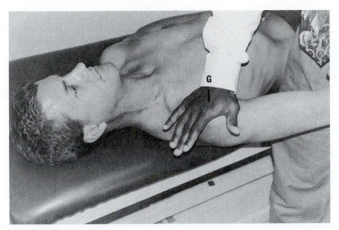

F I G U R E   1 6 - 1 4

Posterior humeral glides. Posterior humeral glides use one hand to stabilize the humerus at the elbow and the other to glide the humeral head. They increase flexion and medial rotation.

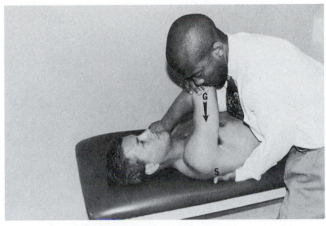

F I G U R E   1 6 - 1 6

Posterior humeral glides. Posterior humeral glides may also be done with the shoulder at 90°. With the patient in supine position, one hand stabilizes the scapula underneath, while the patient's elbow is secured at the therapist's shoulder. Glides are directed downward through the humerus. They increase horizontal adduction.

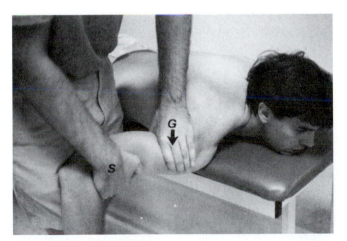

F I G U R E   1 6 - 1 5

Anterior humeral glides. In anterior humeral glides the patient is prone. One hand stabilizes the humerus at the elbow, and the other glides the humeral head. They increase extension and lateral rotation.

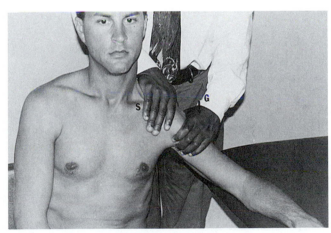

F I G U R E   1 6 - 1 7

Inferior humeral glides. For inferior humeral glides the patient is in the sitting position with the elbow resting on the treatment table. One hand stabilizes the scapula, and the other glides the humeral head inferiorly. These glides increase shoulder abduction.

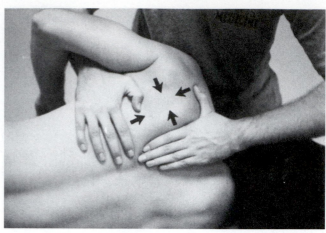

F I G U R E   1 6 - 1 8

Lateral glenohumeral joint traction. Lateral glenohumeral joint traction is used for initial testing of joint mobility and for decreasing pain. One hand stabilizes the elbow while the other applies lateral traction at the upper humerus.

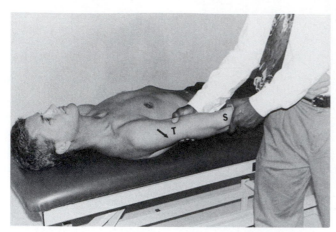

F I G U R E   1 6 - 2 0

General scapular glides. General scapular glides may be done in all directions, applying pressure at either the medial, inferior, lateral, or superior border of the scapula. Scapular glides increase general scapulothoracic mobility.

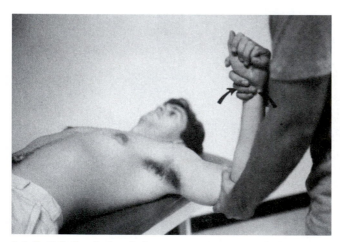

F I G U R E   1 6 - 1 9

Medial and lateral rotation oscillations. Medial and lateral rotation oscillations with the shoulder abducted at 90° can increase medial and lateral rotation in a progressive manner according to patient's tolerance.

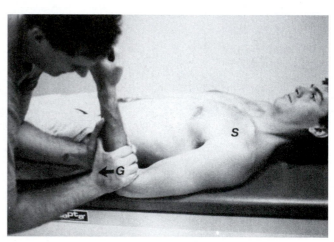

F I G U R E   1 6 - 2 1

Inferior humeroulnar glides. Inferior humeroulnar glides increase elbow flexion and extension. They are performed using the body weight to stabilize proximally with the hand grasping the ulna and gliding inferiorly.

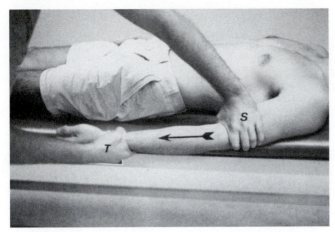

FIGURE 16-22

Humeroradial inferior glides. Humeroradial inferior glides increase the joint space and improve flexion and extension. One hand stabilizes the humerus above the elbow while the other grasps the distal forearm and glides the radius inferiorly.

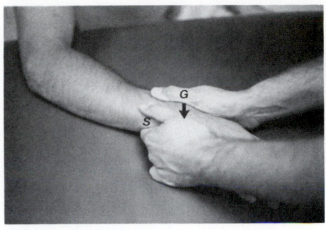

FIGURE 16-24

Distal anterior/posterior radial glides. Distal anterior/posterior radial glides are done with one hand stabilizing the ulna and the other gliding the radius. These glides increase pronation.

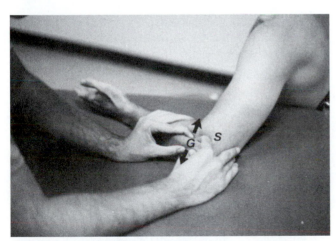

FIGURE 16-23

Proximal anterior/posterior radial glides. Proximal anterior/posterior radial glides use the thumbs and index fingers to glide the radial head. Anterior glides increase flexion, while posterior glides increase extension.

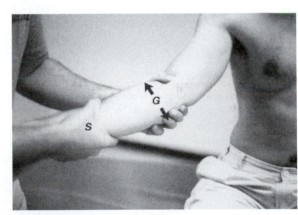

FIGURE 16-25

Medial and lateral ulnar oscillations. Medial and lateral ulnar oscillations increase flexion and extension. Valgus and varus forces are used with a short-lever arm.

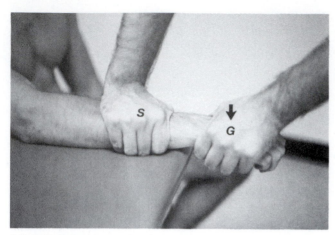

FIGURE 16-26

Radiocarpal joint anterior glides. Radiocarpal joint anterior glides increase wrist extension.

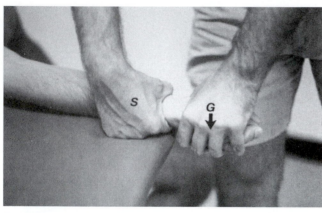

FIGURE 16-27

Radiocarpal joint posterior glides. Radiocarpal joint posterior glides increase wrist flexion.

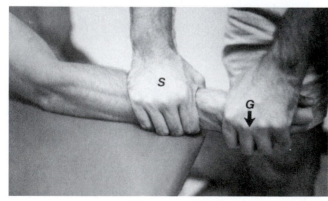

FIGURE 16-28

Radiocarpal joint ulnar glides. Radiocarpal joint ulnar glides increase radial deviation.

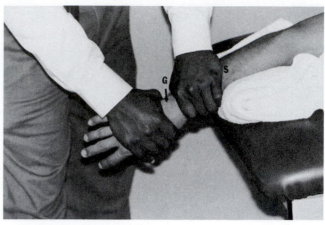

FIGURE 16-29

Radiocarpal joint radial glides. Radiocarpal joint radial glides increase ulnar deviation.

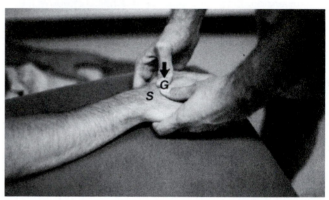

FIGURE 16-30

Carpometacarpal joint anterior/posterior glides. Carpometacarpal joint anterior/posterior glides increase mobility of the hand.

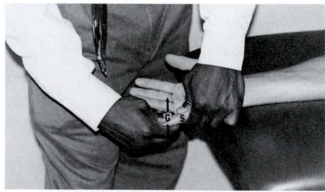

FIGURE 16-31

Metacarpophalangeal (MP) joint anterior/posterior glides. In MP joint anterior or posterior glides, the proximal segment, in this case the metacarpal, is stabilized and the distal segment is mobilized. Anterior glides increase flexion of the MP joint. Posterior glides increase extension.

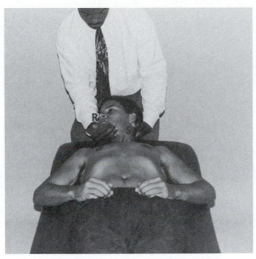

F I G U R E   1 6 - 3 2

Cervical vertebrae rotation oscillations. Cervical vertebrae rotation oscillations are done with one hand supporting the weight of the head and the other rotating the head in the direction of the restriction. These oscillations treat pain or stiffness when there is some resistance in the same direction as the rotation.

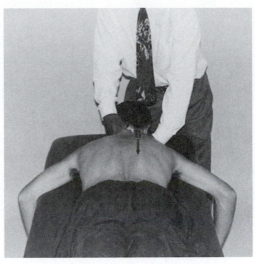

F I G U R E   1 6 - 3 4

Unilateral cervical facet anterior/posterior glides. Unilateral cervical facet anterior/posterior glides are done using pressure from the thumbs over individual facets. They increase rotation or flexion of the neck toward the side where the technique is used.

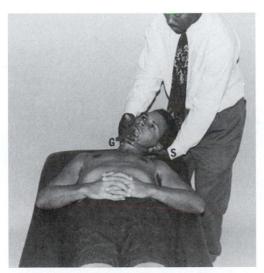

F I G U R E   1 6 - 3 3

Cervical vertebrae sidebending. Cervical vertebrae sidebending may be used to treat pain or stiffness with resistance when sidebending the neck.

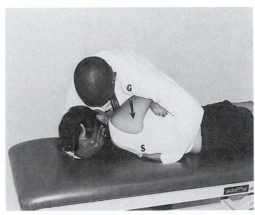

F I G U R E   1 6 - 3 5

Thoracic vertebral facet rotations. Thoracic vertebral facet rotations are accomplished with one hand underneath the patient providing stabilization, and the weight of the body pressing downward through the rib cage to rotate an individual thoracic vertebra. Rotation of the thoracic vertebra is minimal, and most of the movement with this mobilization involves the rib facet joint.

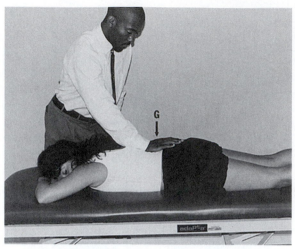

FIGURE 16-36

Anterior/posterior lumbar vertebral glides. In the lumbar region, anterior/posterior lumbar vertebral glides may be accomplished at individual segments using pressure on the spinous process through the pisiform in the hand. These decrease pain or increase mobility of individual lumbar vertebrae.

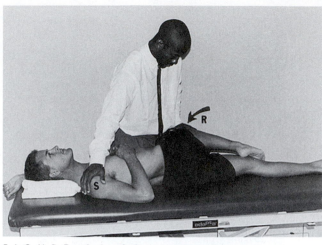

FIGURE 16-38

Lumbar vertebral rotations. Lumbar vertebral rotations decrease pain and increase mobility in lumbar vertebrae. These rotations should be done in a sidelying position.

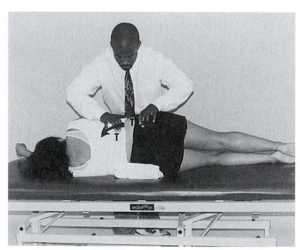

FIGURE 16-37

Lumbar lateral distraction. Lumbar lateral distraction increases the space between transverse processes and increases the opening of the intervertebral foramen. This position is achieved by lying over a support, flexing the patient's upper knee to a point where there is gapping in the appropriate spinal segment, then rotating the upper trunk to place the segment in a close-packed position. Then finger and forearm pressure are used to separate individual spaces. This pressure is used for reducing pain in the lumbar vertebrae associated with some compression of a spinal nerve.

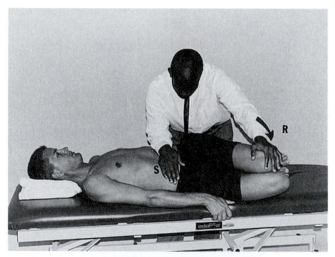

FIGURE 16-39

Lateral lumbar rotations. Lateral lumbar rotations may be done with the patient in supine position. In this position, one hand must stabilize the upper trunk, while the other produces rotation.

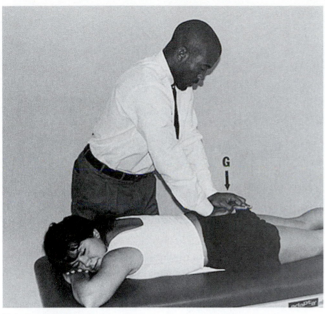

FIGURE 16-40

Anterior sacral glides. Anterior sacral glides decrease pain and reduce muscle guarding around the sacroiliac joint.

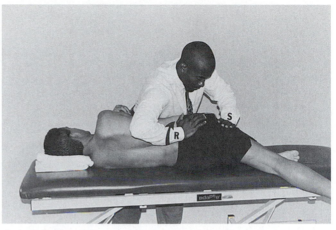

FIGURE 16-42

Anterior innominate rotation. An anterior innominate rotation in a sidelying position is accomplished by extending the leg on the affected side, and then stabilizing with one hand on the front of the thigh while the other applies pressure anteriorly over the posterosuperior iliac spine to produce an anterior rotation. This technique will correct a unilateral posterior rotation.

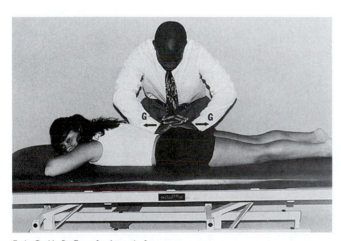

FIGURE 16-41

Superior/inferior sacral glides. Superior/inferior sacral glides decrease pain and reduce muscle guarding around the sacroiliac joint.

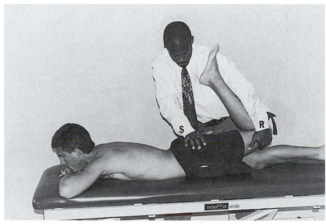

FIGURE 16-43

Anterior innominate rotation. An anterior innominate rotation may also be accomplished by extending the hip, applying upward force on the upper thigh, and stabilizing over the posterosuperior iliac spine. This technique is once again used to correct a posterior unilateral innominate rotation.

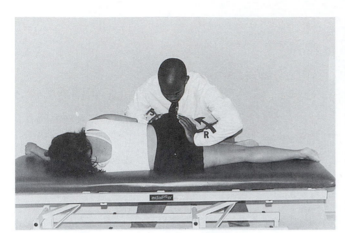

FIGURE   16-44

Posterior innominate rotation. A posterior innominate rotation with the patient in sidelying position is done by flexing the hip, stabilizing the anterosuperior iliac spine, and applying pressure to the ischium in an anterior direction.

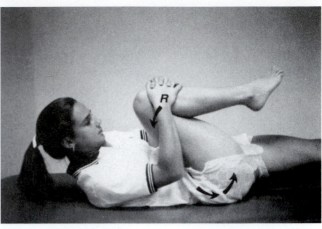

FIGURE   16-46

Posterior innominate rotation self-mobilization (supine). Posterior innominate rotation may be easily accomplished using self-mobilization. In a supine position, the patient grasps behind the flexed knee and gently rocks the innominate in a posterior direction.

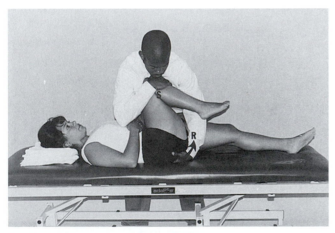

FIGURE   16-45

Posterior innominate rotation. Another posterior innominate rotation with the hip flexed at 90° stabilizes the knee and rotates the innominate anteriorly through upward pressure on the ischium.

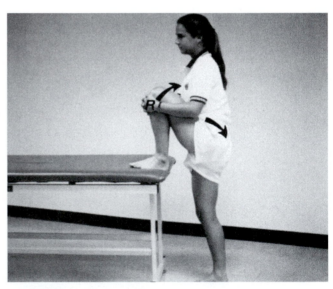

FIGURE   16-47

Posterior rotation self-mobilization (standing). In a standing position, the patient can perform a posterior rotation self-mobilization by pulling on the knee and rocking forward.

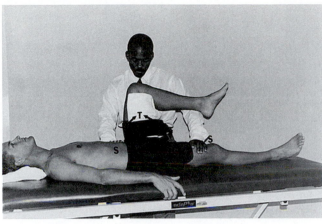

FIGURE 16-48

Lateral hip traction. Because the hip is a very strong, stable joint, it may be necessary to use body weight to produce effective joint mobilization or traction. An example of this would be in lateral hip traction. One strap should be used to secure the patient to the treatment table. A second strap is secured around the patient's thigh and around the therapist's hips. Lateral traction is applied to the femur by leaning back away from the patient. This technique is used to reduce pain and increase hip mobility.

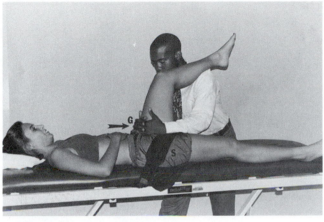

FIGURE 16-50

Inferior femoral glides. Inferior femoral glides at 90° of hip flexion may also be used to increase abduction and flexion.

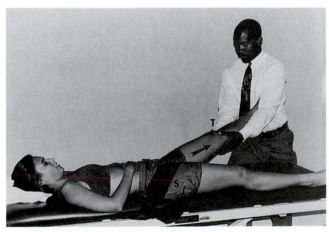

FIGURE 16-49

Femoral traction. Femoral traction with the hip at 0° reduces pain and increases hip mobility. Inferior femoral glides in this position should be used to increase flexion and abduction.

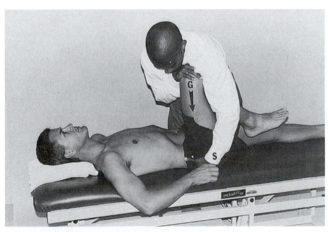

FIGURE 16-51

Posterior femoral glides. With the patient supine, a posterior femoral glide can be done by stabilizing underneath the pelvis and using the body weight applied through the femur to glide posteriorly. Posterior glides are used to increase hip flexion.

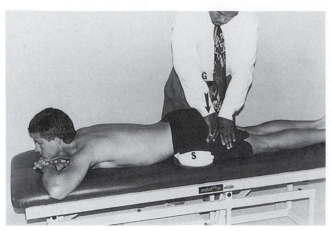

FIGURE 16-52

Anterior femoral glides. Anterior femoral glides increase extension and are accomplished by using same support to stabilize under the pelvis and applying an anterior glide posteriorly on the femur.

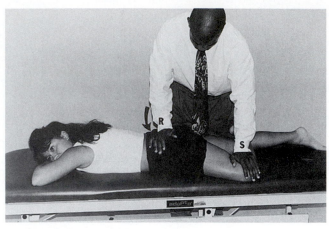

FIGURE 16-54

Lateral femoral rotation. Lateral femoral rotation is done by stabilizing a bent knee in the figure-4 position and applying rotational force to the ischium. This technique increases lateral femoral rotation.

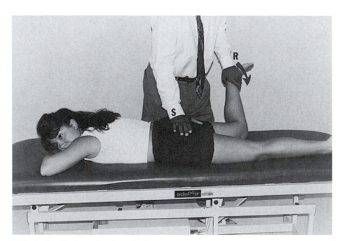

FIGURE 16-53

Medial femoral rotations. Medial femoral rotations may be used for increasing medial rotation and are done by stabilizing the opposite innominate while internally rotating the hip through the flexed knee.

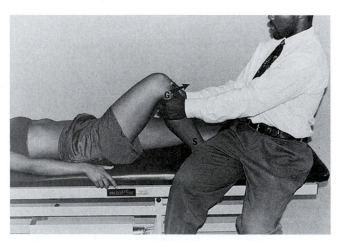

FIGURE 16-55

Anterior tibial glides. Anterior tibial glides are appropriate for the patient lacking full extension. Anterior glides should be done in prone position with the femur stabilized. Pressure is applied to the posterior tibia to glide anteriorly.

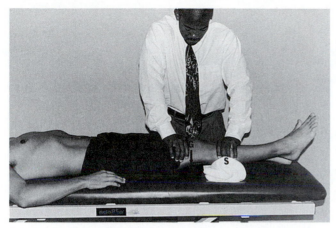

F I G U R E   1 6 - 5 6

Posterior femoral glides. Posterior femoral glides are appropriate for the patient lacking full extension. Posterior femoral glides should be done in supine position with the tibia stabilized. Pressure is applied to the anterior femur to glide posteriorly.

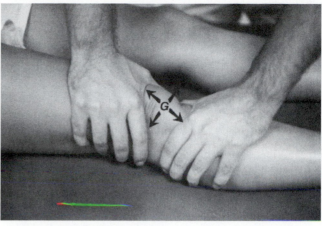

F I G U R E   1 6 - 5 8

Patellar glides. Superior patellar glides increase knee extension. Inferior glides increase knee flexion. Medial glides stretch the lateral retinaculum. Lateral glides stretch tight medial structures.

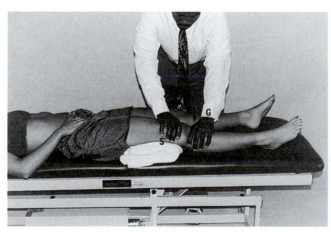

F I G U R E   1 6 - 5 7

Posterior tibial glides. Posterior tibial glides increase flexion. With the patient in supine position, stabilize the femur, and glide the tibia posteriorly.

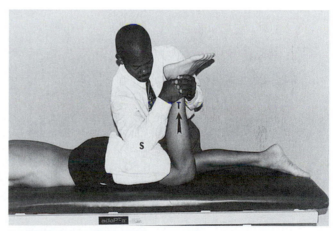

F I G U R E   1 6 - 5 9

Tibiofemoral joint traction. Tibiofemoral joint traction reduces pain and hypomobility. It may be done with the patient prone and the knee flexed at 90°. The elbow should stabilize the thigh while traction is applied through the tibia.

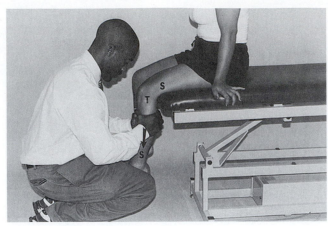

FIGURE 16-60

Alternative techniques for tibiofemoral joint traction. In very large individuals an alternative technique for tibiofemoral joint traction uses body weight of the sports therapist to distract the joint once again for reducing pain and hypomobility.

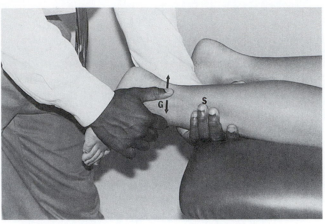

FIGURE 16-62

Distal anterior and posterior fibular glides. Anterior and posterior glides of the fibula may be done distally. The tibia should be stabilized, and the fibular malleolus is mobilized in an anterior or posterior direction.

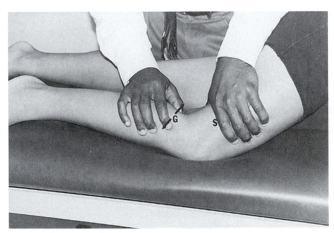

FIGURE 16-61

Proximal anterior and posterior glides of the fibula. Anterior and posterior glides of the fibula may be done proximally. They increase mobility of the fibular head and reduce pain. The femur should be stabilized. With the knee slightly flexed, grasp the head of the femur, and glide it both anteriorly and posteriorly.

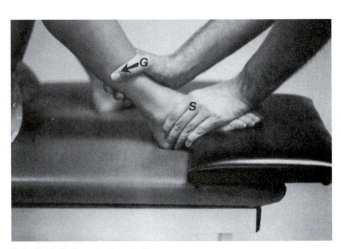

FIGURE 16-63

Posterior tibial glides. Posterior tibial glides increase plantarflexion. The foot should be stabilized, and pressure on the anterior tibia produces a posterior glide.

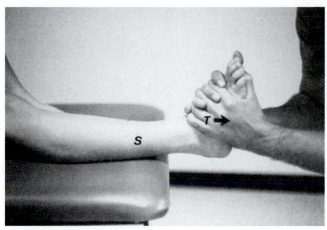

FIGURE 16-64

Talocrural joint traction. Talocrural joint traction is performed using the patient's body weight to stabilize the lower leg and applying traction to the midtarsal portion of the foot. Traction reduces pain and increases dorsiflexion and plantarflexion.

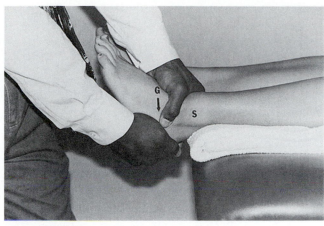

FIGURE 16-66

Posterior talar glides. Posterior talar glides may be used for increasing dorsiflexion. With the patient supine, the tibia is stabilized on the table, and pressure is applied to the anterior aspect of the talus to glide it posteriorly.

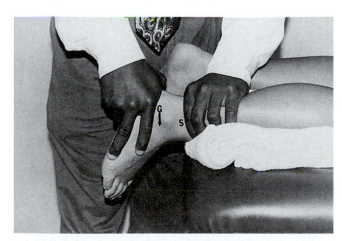

FIGURE 16-65

Anterior talar glides. Plantarflexion may also be increased by using an anterior talar glide. With the patient prone, the tibia is stabilized on the table, and pressure is applied to the posterior aspect of the talus to glide it anteriorly.

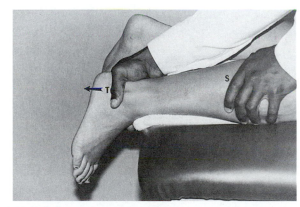

FIGURE 16-67

Subtalar joint traction. Subtalar joint traction reduces pain and increases inversion and eversion. The lower leg is stabilized on the table, and traction is applied by grasping the posterior aspect of the calcaneus.

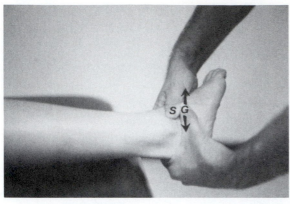

F I G U R E   1 6 - 6 8

Subtalar joint medial and lateral glides. Subtalar joint medial and lateral glides increase eversion and inversion. The talus must be stabilized while the calcaneus is mobilized medially to increase inversion and laterally to increase eversion.

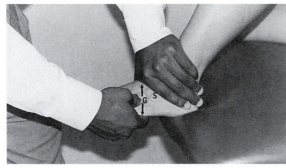

F I G U R E   1 6 - 6 9

Anterior/posterior calcaneocuboid glides. Anterior/ posterior calcaneocuboid glides may be used for increasing adduction and abduction. The calcaneus should be stabilized while the cuboid is mobilized.

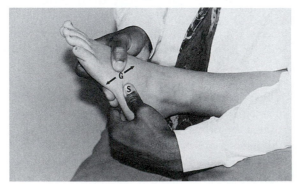

F I G U R E   1 6 - 7 0

Anterior/posterior cuboidmetatarsal glides. Anterior/ posterior cuboidmetatarsal glides are done with one hand stabilizing the cuboid and the other gliding the base of the fifth metatarsal. They are used for increasing mobility of the fifth metatarsal.

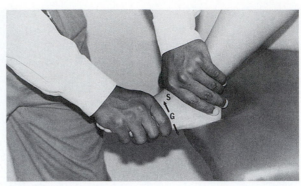

F I G U R E   1 6 - 7 1

Anterior/posterior carpometacarpal glides. Anterior/ posterior carpometacarpal glides decrease hypomobility of the metacarpals.

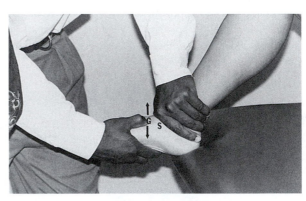

F I G U R E   1 6 - 7 2

Anterior/posterior talonavicular glides. Anterior/ posterior talonavicular glides also increase adduction and abduction. One hand stabilizes the talus while the other mobilizes the navicular bone.

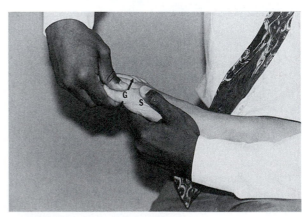

F I G U R E   1 6 - 7 3

Anterior/posterior metacarpophalangeal glides. With anterior/posterior metacarpophalangeal glides, the anterior glides increase extension, and posterior glides increase flexion. Mobilizations are accomplished by isolating individual segments.

concept uses what are referred to as either *mobilizations with movement* (MWMs) for treating the extremities, or *sustained natural apophyseal glides* (SNAGs) for treating problems in the spine.[36] Instead of the therapist using oscillations or thrusting techniques, the patient moves in a specific direction as the therapist guides the restricted body part. MWMs and SANGs have the potential to quickly restore functional movements in joints, even after many years of restriction.[27]

Principles of Treatment

A basic premise of the Mulligan technique for a therapist choosing to make use of MWMs in the extremities or SNAGs in the spine is to never cause pain to the patient.[10] During assessment the therapist should look for specific signs, which may include a loss of joint movement, pain associated with movement, or pain associated with specific functional activities.[13] A passive accessory joint mobilization is applied following the principles of Kaltenborn discussed earlier in this chapter (i.e., parallel or perpendicular to the joint plane). The therapist must continuously monitor the patient's reaction to ensure that no pain is recreated during this mobilization. The therapist experiments with various combinations of parallel or perpendicular glides until the appropriate treatment plane and grade of movement are discovered, which together significantly improve range of motion, and/or significantly decrease or better yet, eliminate altogether the original pain. Failure to improve range of motion or decrease pain indicates that the therapist has not found the correct contact point, treatment plane, grade, or direction of mobilization. The patient then actively repeats the restricted and/or painful motion or activity while the therapist continues to maintain the appropriate accessory glide. Further increases in range of motion or decreases in pain may be expected during a treatment session that typically involves three sets of 10 repetitions. Additional gains may be realized through the application of pain-free, passive overpressure at the end of available range.[20]

An example of MWM might be in a patient with restricted ankle dorsiflexion. The patient is standing on a treatment table with the therapist manually stabilizing the foot. A nonelastic belt passes around both the distal leg of the patient and the waist of the therapist who applies a sustained anterior glide of the tibia by leaning backward away from the patient. The patient then performs a slow dorsiflexion movement until the first onset of pain or end of range. Once this end point is reached, the position is sustained for 10 seconds. The patient then relaxes and returns to the standing position followed by release of the anteroposterior glide, and then followed by a 20-second rest period.[27]

SUMMARY

- Mobilization and traction techniques increase joint mobility or decrease pain by restoring accessory movements to the joint.

- Physiologic movements result from an active muscle contraction that moves an extremity through traditional cardinal planes.
- Accessory motions refer to the manner in which one articulating joint surface moves relative to another.
- Normal accessory component motions must occur for full-range physiologic movement to take place.
- Accessory motions are also referred to as joint arthrokinematics, which include spin, roll, and glide.
- The convex–concave rule states that if the concave joint surface is moving on the stationary convex surface, gliding will occur in the same direction as the rolling motion. Conversely, if the convex surface is moving on a stationary concave surface, gliding will occur in an opposite direction to rolling.
- The resting position is one in which the joint capsule and the ligaments are most relaxed, allowing for a maximum amount of joint play.
- The treatment plane falls perpendicular to a line running from the axis of rotation in the convex surface to the center of the concave articular surface.
- Maitland has proposed a series of five graded movements or oscillations in the range of motion to treat pain and stiffness.
- Kaltenborn uses three grades of traction to reduce pain and stiffness.
- Kaltenborn emphasizes that traction should be used in conjunction with mobilization glides to treat joint hypomobility.
- Mulligan's technique combines passive accessory movement with active physiological movement to improve range of motion or minimize pain.

REFERENCES

1. Barak T, Rosen E, Sofer R. Mobility: Passive orthopedic manual therapy. In: Gould J, Davies G, eds. *Orthopedic and Sports Physical Therapy*. St. Louis, MO, Mosby, 1990.
2. Basmajian J, Banerjee S. *Clinical Decision Making in Rehabilitation: Efficacy and Outcomes*. Philadelphia, Churchill-Livingstone, 1996.
3. Boissonnault W, Bryan J, Fox KS. Joint manipulation curricula in physical therapist professional degree programs. *J Orthop Sports Phys Ther* 34(4):171–181, 2004.
4. Conroy DE, Hayes KW. The effect of joint mobilization as a component of comprehensive treatment for primary shoulder impingement syndrome. *J Orthop Sports Phys Ther* 28(1):3–14, 1998.
5. Cookson J. Orthopedic manual therapy: An overview: II. The spine. *J Am Phys Ther Assoc* 59:259, 1979.
6. Cookson J, Kent B. Orthopedic manual therapy: An overview: I. The extremities. *J Am Phys Ther Assoc* 59:136, 1979.
7. Cyriax J. *Cyriax's Illustrated Manual of Orthopaedic Medicine*. London, Butterworth, 1996.

8. Donatelli R, Owens-Burkhart H. Effects of immobilization on the extensibility of periarticular connective tissue. *J Orthop Sports Phys Ther* 3:67, 1981.

9. Edmond S. *Joint Mobilization and Manipulation: Extremity and Spinal Techniques.* Philadelphia, Elsevier Health Sciences, 2006.

10. Exelby L. The Mulligan concept: Its application in the management of spinal conditions. *Man Ther* 7(2):64–70, 2002.

11. Green T, Refshauge K, Crosbie J, Adams R. A randomized controlled trial of a passive accessory joint mobilization on acute ankle inversion sprains. *Phys Ther* 81(4):984–994, 2001.

12. Grimsby O. *Fundamentals of Manual Therapy: A Course Workbook.* Vagsbygd, Norway, Sorlandets Fysikalske Institutt, 1981.

13. Hall T. Effects of the Mulligan traction straight leg raise technique on range of movement. *J Man Manipulative Ther* 9(3):128–133, 2001.

14. Hollis M. *Practical Exercise.* Oxford, Blackwell Scientific, 1999.

15. Hsu AT, Ho L, Chang JH, Chang GL, Hedman T. Characterization of tissue resistance during a dorsally directed translational mobilization of the glenohumeral joint. *Arch Phys Med Rehabil* 83(3):360–366, 2002.

16. Kaltenborn F. *Manual Mobilization of the Joints, Vol. II: The Spine.* Minneapolis, MN, Orthopedic Physical Therapy Products, 2003.

17. Kaltenborn F, Morgan D, Evjenth O. *Manual Mobilization of the Joints, Vol. I: The Extremities.* Minneapolis, MN, Orthopedic Physical Therapy Products, 2002.

18. Kavanagh J. Is there a positional fault at the inferior tibiofibular joint in patients with acute or chronic ankle sprains compared to normals? *Man Ther* 4(1):19–24, 1999.

19. Kisner C, Colby L. *Therapeutic Exercise: Foundations and Techniques.* Philadelphia, FA Davis, 2002.

20. MacConaill M, Basmajian J. *Muscles and Movements: A Basis for Kinesiology.* Baltimore, Williams & Wilkins, 1977.

21. Maigne R. *Orthopedic Medicine.* Springfield, IL, Charles C Thomas, 1976.

22. Macintyre J. Passive joint mobilization for acute ankle inversion sprains. *Clin J Sport Med* 12(1):54, 2002.

23. Maitland G. *Extremity Manipulation.* London, Butterworth, 1991.

24. Maitland G. *Vertebral Manipulation.* Philadelphia, Elsevier Health Science, 2005.

25. Mangus B, Hoffman L, Hoffman M. Basic principles of extremity joint mobilization using a Kaltenborn approach. *J Sport Rehabil* 11(4):235–250, 2002.

26. Mennell J. *The Musculoskeletal System: Differential Diagnosis from Symptoms and Physical Signs.* New York, Aspen, 1991.

27. Mulligans Concept Available at: www.bmulligan.com/about/concept.htm.

28. Paris S. *The Spine: Course Notebook.* Atlanta, Institute Press, 1979.

29. Paris S. Mobilization of the spine. *Phys Ther* 59:988, 1979.

30. Saunders D. *Evaluation, Treatment and Prevention of Musculoskeletal Disorders.* Saunder Group Inc., 2004.

31. Schiotz E, Cyriax J. *Manipulation Past and Present.* London, Heinemann, 1978.

32. Stoddard A. *Manual of Osteopathic Practice.* London, Hutchinson Ross, 1980.

33. Stone JA. Joint mobilization. *Athlet Ther Today* 4(6):59–60, 1998.

34. Taniqawa M. Comparison of the hold-relax procedure and passive mobilization on increasing muscle length. *Phys Ther* 52(7):725–735, 1972.

35. Wadsworth C. *Manual Examination and Treatment of the Spine and Extremities.* Baltimore, William & Wilkins, 1988.

36. Wilson E. The Mulligan concept: NAGS, SNAGS and mobilizations with movement. *J Bodywork Mov Ther* 5(2) 81–89, 2001.

37. Zohn D, Mennell J. *Musculoskeletal Pain: Diagnosis and Physical Treatment.* Boston, Little, Brown and Company, 1987.

38. Zusman M. Reappraisal of a proposed neurophysiological mechanism for the relief of joint pain with passive joint movements. *Physiother Pract* 1:61–70, 1985.

SUGGESTED READINGS

Bukowski E. Assessing joint mobility. *Clin Manage* 11:48–56, 1991.

Cibulka M, Rose S, Delitto A. Hamstring muscle strain treated by mobilizing the sacroiliac joint. *Phys Ther* 66:1220–1223, 1986.

Cochrane C. Joint mobilization principles: Considerations for use in the child with central nervous system dysfunction. *Phys Ther* 67:1105–1109, 1987.

Don Tigny R. Measuring PSIS movement. *Clin Manage* 10:43–44, 1990.

Eiff M, Smith A, Smith G. Early mobilization versus immobilization in the treatment of lateral ankle sprains. *Am J Sports Med* 22:83–88, 1994.

Gibson H, Ross J, Allen J. The effect of mobilization on forward bending range. *J Man Manipulative Ther* 1:142–147. 1993.

Gratton P. Early active mobilization after flexor tendon repairs. *J Hand Ther* 6:285–289, 1993.

Harris S, Lundgren B. Joint mobilization for children with central nervous system disorders: Indications and precautions. *Phys Ther* 71:890–896, 1991.

Lee M, Latimer J, Maher C. Manipulation: Investigation of a proposed mechanism. *Clin Biomech* 8:302–306, 1993.

Lee R, Evans J. Towards a better understanding of spinal posteroanterior mobilisation. *Physiotherapy* 80:68–73, 1994.

Levin S. Early mobilization speeds recovery. *Phys Sports Med* 21:70–74, 1993.

Maitland G. Treatment of the glenohumeral joint by passive movement. *Physiotherapy* 69:3–7, 1983.

May E. Controlled mobilization after flexor tendon repair in the hand: Techniques, methods and results. *Aust Occup Ther J* 41:143, 1994.

McCollam R, Benson C. Effects of postero-anterior mobilization on lumbar extension and flexion. *J Man Manipulative Ther* 1:134–141, 1993.

Mulligan B. Extremity joint mobilisations combined with movements. *N Z J Physiother* 20:28–29, 1992.

Mulligan B. Mobilisations with movement (MWM's). *J Man Manipulative Ther* 1:154–156, 1993.

Nield S, Davis K, Latimer J. The effect of manipulation on the range of movement at the ankle joint. *Scand J Rehabil Med* 25:161–166, 1993.

Ottenbacher K, Difabio R. Efficacy of spinal manipulation/mobilization therapy: A meta-analysis. *Spine* 10:833–837, 1985.

Petersen P, Sites S, Grossman I. Clinical evidence for the utilisation and efficacy of upper extremity mobilisation. *Br J Occup Ther* 55:112–116, 1992.

Prentice W. Techniques of manual therapy for the knee. *J Sport Rehabil* 1:249–257, 1992.

Quillen W, Halle J, Rouillier L. Manual therapy: Mobilization of the motion-restricted shoulder. *J Sport Rehabil* 1:237–248, 1992.

Randall T, Portney L, Harris B. Effects of joint mobilization on joint stiffness and active motion of the metacarpal-phalangeal joint. *J Orthop Sports Phys Ther* 16:30–36, 1992.

Schoensee S, Jensen G, Nicholson G. The effect of mobilization on cervical headaches. *J Orthop Sports Phys Ther* 21:184–196, 1995.

Smith R, Sebastian B, Gajdosik R. Effect of sacroiliac joint mobilization on the standing position of the pelvis in healthy men. *J Orthop Sports Phys Ther* 10:77–84, 1988.

Stuberg W. Manual therapy in pediatrics: Some considerations. *PT—Mag Phys Ther* 1:54–56, 1993.

Taylor N, Bennell K. The effectiveness of passive joint mobilisation on the return of active wrist extension following Colles' fracture: A clinical trial. *N Z J Physiother* 22:24–28, 1994.

Wilson F. Manual therapy versus traditional exercises in mobilisation of the ankle post-ankle fracture: A pilot study. *NZJ Physiother* 19:11–16, 1991.

Wise P. Mobilisation technique improves neural mobility. *Aust J Physiother* 40:51–54, 1994.

Zito M. Joint mobilization: Stretch specificity using a distraction. *J Orthop Sports Phys Ther* 23:65, 1996.

CHAPTER 17

Regaining Postural Stability and Balance

Kevin M. Guskiewicz

OBJECTIVES

After completing this chapter, the therapist should be able to do the following:

- Define and explain the roles of the three sensory modalities responsible for maintaining balance.
- Explain how movement strategies along the closed kinetic chain help maintain the center of gravity in a safe and stable area.
- Differentiate between subjective and objective balance assessment.
- Differentiate between static and dynamic balance assessment.
- Evaluate the effect that injury to the ankle, knee, and head has on balance and postural equilibrium.
- Identify the goals of each phase of balance training, and how to progress the patient through each phase.
- State the differences among static, semidynamic, and dynamic balance-training exercises.

Although maintaining balance while standing may appear to be a rather simple motor skill for normal individuals, this feat cannot be taken for granted in patients with musculoskeletal dysfunction. Muscular weakness, proprioceptive deficit, and range-of-motion (ROM) deficits may challenge a person's ability to maintain the center of gravity (COG) within the body's base of support, or in other words, cause him/her to lose the balance. Balance is the single most important element dictating movement strategies within the closed kinetic chain. Acquisition of effective strategies for maintaining balance is therefore essential for athletic performance. Although balance is often thought of as a static process, it is actually a highly integrative dynamic process involving multiple neurological pathways. Though *balance* is the more commonly used term, *postural equilibrium* is a broader term that involves the alignment of joint segments in an effort to maintain the COG within an optimal range of the maximum limits of stability (LOS), which will be discussed later.

Despite being classified at the end of the continuum of goals associated with therapeutic exercise,[47] maintenance of balance is a vital component in the rehabilitation of joint injuries, which should not be overlooked. Traditionally, orthopedic rehabilitation has placed the emphasis on isolated joint mechanics such as improving ROM and flexibility, and increasing muscle strength

and endurance, rather than on afferent information obtained by the joint(s) to be processed by the postural control system. However, research in the area of proprioception and kinesthesia has emphasized the need to train the joint's neural system.[48–52] Joint position sense, proprioception, and kinesthesia are vital to all functional movements requiring balance. Current rehabilitation protocols should therefore focus on a combination of open- and closed-kinetic-chain exercises. The necessity for a combination of open- and closed-kinetic-chain exercises can be seen during gait (walking or running), as the foot and ankle prepare for hell strike (open chain) and prepare to control the body's COG during midstance and toe-off (closed chain). This chapter focuses on the postural control system, various balance-training techniques, and technological advancements that are enabling therapists to assess and treat balance deficits in a variety of patients.

THE POSTURAL CONTROL SYSTEM

The therapist must first have an understanding of the postural control system and its various components. The postural control system utilizes complex processes involving both sensory

FIGURE 17-1

Dynamic equilibrium.
(Reproduced, with
permission, from Allison L,
Fuller K, Hedenberg R, et al.
*Contemporary Management
of Balance deficits.*
Clackamas, OR, NeuroCom
International, 1994.)

| Determination of body position | → | Choice of body movement |

Compare, select, and combine senses

Select and adjust muscle contractile pattern

| Vision | Vestibular | Somatosensation |

| Ankle muscles | Thigh muscles | Trunk muscles | Neck muscles |

Environmental interaction ← Generation of body movement

and motor components. Maintenance of postural equilibrium includes sensory detection of body motions, integration of sensorimotor information within the central nervous system (CNS), and execution of appropriate musculoskeletal responses. Most daily activities, such as walking, climbing stairs, reaching, or throwing a ball, require static foot placement with controlled balance shifts, especially if a favorable outcome is to be attained. So, balance should be considered both a dynamic and a static process. The successful accomplishment of static and dynamic balance is based on the interaction between body and environment.[46] The complexity of this dynamic process can be seen in Figure 17-1. From a clinical perspective, separating the

sensory and motor processes of balance means that a person may have impaired balance for one or both of the following two reasons: (1) the position of the COG relative to the base of support is not accurately sensed and (2) the automatic movements required to bring the COG to a balanced position are not timely or effectively coordinated.[64]

The position of the body in relation to gravity and its surroundings is sensed by combining visual, vestibular, and somatosensory inputs. Balance movements also involve motions of the ankle, knee, and hip joints, which are controlled by the coordinated actions along the kinetic chain (Fig. 17-2). These processes are all vital for producing fluid movements.

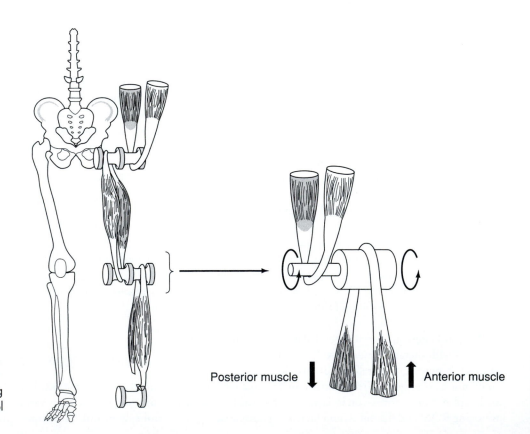

FIGURE 17-2

Paired relationships
between major postural
musculatures that execute
coordinated actions along
the kinetic chain to control
the center of gravity.

Posterior muscle ↓   ↑ Anterior muscle

CONTROL OF BALANCE

The human body is a very tall structure balanced on a relatively small base, and its COG is quite high, being just above the pelvis.[80] Many factors enter into the task of controlling balance within the base of support. Balance control involves a complex network of neural connections and centers that are related by peripheral and central feedback mechanisms.[36]

The postural control system operates as a feedback control circuit between the brain and the musculoskeletal system. The sources of afferent information supplied to the postural control system collectively come from visual, vestibular, and somatosensory inputs. The involvement of the CNS in maintaining upright posture can be divided into two components. The first component, *sensory organization,* involves those processes that determine the timing, direction, and amplitude of corrective postural actions based upon information obtained from the vestibular, visual, and somatosensory (proprioceptive) inputs.[60] Despite the availability of multiple sensory inputs, the CNS generally relies on only one sense at a time for orientation information. For healthy adults, the preferred sense for balance control comes from somatosensory information (i.e., feet in contact with the support surface and detection of joint movement).[39,60] In considering orthopedic injuries, the somatosensory system is of most importance and will be the focus of this chapter.

The second component, *muscle coordination,* is the collection of processes that determine the temporal sequencing and distribution of contractile activity among the muscles of the legs and trunk that generate supportive reactions for maintaining balance. Research suggests that balance deficiencies in people with neurological problems can result from inappropriate interaction among the three sensory inputs that provide orientation information to the postural control system. A patient may be inappropriately dependent on one sense for situations presenting intersensory conflict.[60,73]

From a clinical perspective, stabilization of upright posture requires the integration of afferent information from the three senses, which work in combination and are all critical to the execution of coordinated postural corrections. Impairment of one component is usually compensated for by the remaining two. Often one of the systems provides faulty or inadequate information about different surfaces and/or changes in visual acuity and/or peripheral vision. In this case it is crucial that one of the other senses provides accurate and adequate information so that balance can be maintained. For example, when somatosensory conflict is present, as when the individual is standing on a moving platform or a compliant foam surface, balance is significantly decreased when the eyes are closed rather than open.

Somatosensory inputs provide information concerning the orientation of body parts to one another and to the support surface.[22,64] *Vision* measures the orientation of the eyes and head in relation to surrounding objects and plays an important role in the maintenance of balance. On a stable surface, closing the eyes should cause only minimal increases in postural sway in healthy subjects. However, if somatosensory input is disrupted due to ligamentous injury, closing the eyes will increase sway significantly.[13,17,39,40,64] The *vestibular* apparatus supplies information that measures gravitational, linear, and angular accelerations of the head in relation to inertial space. It does not, however, provide orientation information in relation to external objects, and therefore plays only a minor role in the maintenance of balance when the visual and somatosensory systems are providing accurate information.[64]

SOMATOSENSATION AS IT RELATES TO BALANCE

The terms *somatosensation, proprioception, kinesthesia,* and *balance* are often used interchangeably. Somatosensation is the more global term used to denote the proprioceptive mechanisms related to postural control and can accurately be used synonymously with the other terms. Somatosensation is therefore best defined as a specialized variation of the sensory modality of touch that encompasses the sensation of joint movement (kinesthesia) and joint position (joint position sense).[48,52] As previously discussed, balance refers to the ability to maintain the body's COG within the base of support provided by the feet. Somatosensation and balance work closely, as the postural control system utilizes sensory information related to movement and posture from peripheral sensory receptors (e.g., muscle spindles, Golgi tendon organ (GTO), joint afferents, cutaneous receptors). So the question remains, how does proprioception influence postural equilibrium and balance?

Somatosensory input is received from mechanoreceptors, but it is unclear whether the tactile senses, the muscle spindles, or the GTOs are more responsible for controlling balance. Nashner[59] concluded, after using electromyography (EMG) responses following platform perturbations, that other pathways had to be involved in the responses they recorded because the latencies were longer than those normally associated with a classic myotatic reflex. The stretch-related reflex is the earliest mechanism for increasing the activation level of muscles about a joint following an externally imposed rotation of the joint. Rotation of the ankles is the most probable stimulus of the myotatic reflex that occurs in many persons. It appears to be the first useful phase of activity in the leg muscles after a change in erect posture.[59] The myotatic reflex can be seen when perturbations of gait or posture automatically evoke functionally directed responses in the leg muscles to compensate for imbalance or increased postural sway.[15,59] Muscle spindles sense a stretching of the agonist, thus sending information along its afferent fibers to the spinal cord. There the information is transferred to alpha and gamma motor neurons that carry information back to the muscle fibers and muscle spindle, respectively, and contract the muscle to prevent or control additional postural sway.[15]

Postural sway was assessed on a platform moving into a "toes-up" and "toes-down" position, and a stretch reflex was found in the triceps surae after a sudden ramp displacement into the toes-up position.[14] A medium latency response (103–118 ms) was observed in the stretched muscle, followed by a delayed response of the antagonistic anterior tibialis muscle (108–124 ms). The investigators also blocked afferent proprioceptive information in an attempt to study the role of proprioceptive information from the legs for the maintenance of upright posture. These results suggested that proprioceptive information from pressure and/or joint receptors of the foot (ischemia applied at ankle) plays an important role in postural stabilization during low frequencies of movement, but is of minor importance for the compensation of rapid displacements. The experiment also included a "visual" component, as subjects were tested with eyes closed and then with eyes open. Results suggested that when subjects were tested with eyes open, visual information compensated for the loss of proprioceptive input.

Another study[15] used compensatory EMG responses during impulsive disturbance of the limbs during stance on a treadmill to describe the myotatic reflex. Results revealed that during backward movement of the treadmill, ankle dorsiflexion caused the COG to be shifted anteriorly, thus evoking a stretch reflex in the gastrocnemius muscle, followed by weak anterior tibialis activation. In another trial, the movement was reversed (plantar flexion), thus shifting the COG posteriorly and evoking a stretch reflex of the anterior tibialis muscle. Both of these studies suggest that stretch reflex responses help control the body's COG, and that the vestibular system is unlikely to be directly involved in the generation of the necessary responses.

Elimination of all sensory information from the feet and ankles revealed that proprioceptors in the leg muscles (gastrocnemius and tibialis anterior) were capable of providing sufficient sensory information for stable standing.[21] Researchers speculated that group I or group II muscle spindle afferents and group Ib afferents from GTOs were the probable sources of this proprioceptive information. The study demonstrated that normal subjects can stand in a stable manner when receptors in the leg muscles are the only source of information about postural sway.

Other studies[5,40] have examined the role of somatosensory information by altering or limiting somatosensory input through the use of platform-sway referencing or foam platforms. These studies reported that subjects still responded with well-coordinated movements but the movements were often either ineffective or inefficient for the environmental context in which they were used.

BALANCE AS IT RELATES TO THE CLOSED KINETIC CHAIN

Balance is the process of maintaining the COG within the body's base of support. The human body is a very tall structure balanced on a relatively small base, and its COG is quite high, being just above the pelvis.[80] Many factors enter into the task of controlling balance within this designated area. One component often overlooked is the role balance plays within the *kinetic chain*. Ongoing debates as to how the kinetic chain should be defined and whether open- or closed-kinetic-chain exercises are best have caused many therapists to lose sight of what is most important. An understanding of the postural control system and the theory of the kinetic (segmental) chain about the lower extremity helps conceptualize the role of the chain in maintaining balance. Within the kinetic chain, each moving segment transmits forces to every other segment along the chain, and its motions are influenced by forces transmitted from other segments (see Chapter 14).[11] The act of maintaining equilibrium or balance is associated with the closed kinetic chain, as the distal segment (foot) is fixed beneath the base of support.

The coordination of automatic postural movements during the act of balancing is not determined solely by the muscles acting directly about the joint. Leg and trunk muscles exert indirect forces on neighboring joints through the inertial interaction forces among body segments.[61,62] A combination of one or more strategies (ankle, knee, hip) is used to coordinate movement of the COG back to a stable or balanced position when a person's balance is disrupted by an external perturbation. Injury to any one of the joints or corresponding muscles along the kinetic chain can result in a loss of appropriate feedback for maintaining balance.

BALANCE DISRUPTION

Let us say, for example, that an individual stumbles at the bottom of a staircase, causing him/her to land in an unexpected position, therefore compromising his/her normal balance. To prevent itself from falling, the body must correct itself by returning the COG to a position within safer LOS. Afferent mechanoreceptor inputs from the hip, knee, and ankle joints are responsible for initiating automatic postural responses through the use of one of three possible movement strategies.

Selection of Movement Strategies

Three principle joint systems (ankles, knees, and hips) are located between the base of support and the COG. This allows for a wide variety of postures that can be assumed while the COG is still positioned above the base of support. As described by Nashner,[64] motions about a given joint are controlled by the combined actions of at least one pair of muscles working in opposition. When forces exerted by pairs of opposing muscle about a joint (e.g., anterior tibialis and gastrocnemius/soleus) are combined, the effect is to resist rotation of the joint relative to a resting position. The degree to which the joint resists rotation is called joint stiffness. The resting position and the stiffness of the joint are altered independently by changing the activation levels of one or both muscle groups.[41,64] Joint resting position and joint stiffness are by themselves an inadequate basis for controlling postural movements, and it is theorized that the myotatic stretch reflex is the earliest mechanism for increasing the activation level of the muscles of a joint following an externally imposed rotation of the joint.[64]

When a person's balance is disrupted by an external perturbation, movement strategies involving joints of the lower extremity coordinate movement of the COG back to a balanced position. Three strategies (ankle, hip, stepping) have been identified along a continuum.[39] In general, the relative effectiveness of ankle, hip, and stepping strategies in repositioning the COG over the base of support depends on the configuration of the base of support, the COG alignment in relation to the LOS, and the speed of the postural movement.[39,40]

The *ankle strategy* shifts the COG while maintaining the placement of the feet by rotating the body as a rigid mass about the ankle joints. This is achieved by contracting either the gastrocnemius or the anterior tibialis muscles to generate torque about the ankle joints. Anterior sway of the body is counteracted by gastrocnemius activity, which pulls the body posteriorly. Conversely, posterior sway of the body is counteracted by contraction of the tibialis anterior. Thus, the importance of these muscles should not be underestimated when designing the rehabilitation program. The ankle strategy is most effective in executing relatively slow COG movements when the base of support is firm and the COG is well within the LOS perimeter. The ankle strategy is also believed to be effective in maintaining a static posture with the COG offset from the center. The thigh and lower-trunk muscles contract and thereby resist the destabilization of these proximal joints due to the indirect effects of the ankle muscles on the proximal joints (Table 17-1). Under normal sensory conditions, activation of ankle musculature is almost exclusively selected to maintain equilibrium. However, there are subtle differences associated with loss of somatosensation and with vestibular dysfunction in terms of postural control strategies. Persons with somatosensory loss appear to rely on their hip musculature to retain their COG while experiencing forward or backward perturbation or with different support surface lengths.[22]

If the ankle strategy is not capable of controlling excessive sway, the *hip strategy* is available to help control motion of the COG through the initiation of large and rapid motions at the hip joints with antiphase rotation of the ankles. This is most effective when the COG is located near the LOS perimeter, and when the LOS boundaries are contracted by a narrowed base of support. Finally, when the COG is displaced beyond the LOS, a step or stumble (*stepping strategy*) is the only strategy that can be used to prevent a fall.[62,64]

It is proposed that LOS and COG alignment are altered in individuals exhibiting a musculoskeletal abnormality such as an ankle or knee sprain. For example, weakness of ligaments following acute or chronic sprain about these joints is likely to reduce ROM, therefore shrinking the LOS and placing the person at greater risk for a fall with a relatively smaller sway envelope.[62] Pintsaar et al.[71] revealed that impaired function is related to a change from ankle synergy toward hip synergy for postural adjustments among patients with functional ankle instability. This finding, which is consistent with previous results reported by Tropp et al.,[78] suggests that sensory proprioceptive function for the injured athletes is affected.

ASSESSMENT OF BALANCE

Several methods of balance assessment have been proposed for clinical use. Many of the techniques have been criticized for

TABLE 17-1

Function Anatomy of Muscles Involved in Balance Movements

| JOINT | EXTENSION | | FLEXION | |
	ANATOMIC	FUNCTION	ANATOMIC	FUNCTION
Hip	Paraspinals	Paraspinals	Abdominal	Abdominals
	Hamstrings	Hamstrings	Quadriceps	Quadriceps
		Tibialis		Gastrocnemius
Knee	Quadriceps	Paraspinals	Hamstrings	Abdominals
		Quadriceps	Gastrocnemius	Hamstrings
		Gastrocnemius		Tibialis
Ankle	Gastrocnemius	Abdominals	Tibialis	Paraspinals
		Quadriceps		Hamstrings
		Gastrocnemius		Tibialis

Adapted from Nashner LM. Physiology of Balance. In: Jacobson G, Newman C, Kartush J, eds. *Handbook of Balance Function and Testing.* St. Louis, MO, Mosby, 1993, pp. 261–279.

offering only a subjective ("qualitative") measurement of balance rather than an objective ("quantitative") measure.

Subjective Assessment

Prior to the mid 1980s, there were very few methods for systematic and controlled assessment of balance. The assessment of static balance in patients has traditionally been performed through the use of the standing Romberg test. This test is performed standing with feet together, arms at the side, and eyes closed. Normally a person can stand motionless in this position, but the tendency to sway or fall to one side is considered a positive Romberg's sign indicating a loss of proprioception.[8] The Romberg test has, however, been criticized for its lack of sensitivity and objectivity. It is considered to be a rather qualitative assessment of static balance because a considerable amount of stress is required to make the subject sway enough for an observer to characterize the sway.[44]

The use of a quantifiable clinical test battery called the Balance Error Scoring System (BESS) is recommended over the standard Romberg test. Three different stances (double, single, and tandem) are completed twice, once while on a firm surface and once while on a piece of medium-density foam (balance pad by Airex is recommended) for a total of six trials (Fig. 17-3). Patients are asked to assume the required stance by placing their hands on the iliac crests, and upon eye closure the 20-second test begins. During the single-leg stances, subjects are asked to maintain the contralateral limb in 20°–30° of hip flexion and 40°–50° of knee flexion. Additionally, the patients are asked to stand quietly and as motionless as possible in the stance

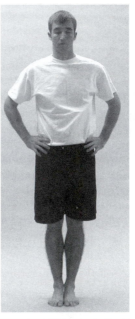
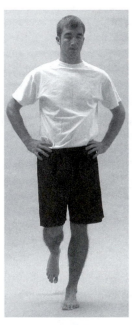
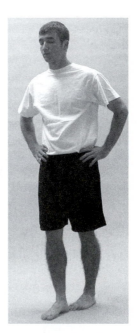
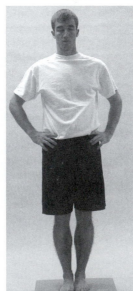
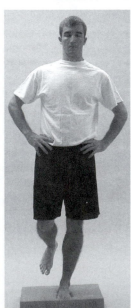
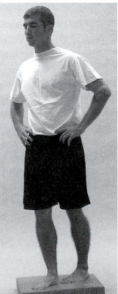

FIGURE 17 - 3

Stance positions for Balance Error Scoring System. **A,** Double-leg, firm surface. **B,** Single-leg, firm surface. **C,** Tandem, firm surface. **D,** Double-leg, foam surface. **E,** Single-leg, foam surface. **F,** Tandem, foam surface.

TABLE 17-2

Balance Error Scoring System

ERRORS
Hands lifted off iliac crests
Opening eyes
Step, stumble, or fall
Moving hip into more than 30° of flexion or abduction
Lifting forefoot or heel
Remaining out of testing position for more than 5 seconds

The BESS score is calculated by adding one error point for each error or any combination of errors occurring during one movement. Error scores from each of the six trials are added for a total BESS score, and higher scores represent poor balance.

TABLE 17-3

High-Technology Balance Assessment Systems

STATIC SYSTEMS	DYNAMIC SYSTEMS
Chattecx Balance System	Biodex Stability System
EquiTest	Chattecx Balance System
Forceplate	EquiTest
Pro Balance Master	EquiTest with EMG
Smart Balance Master	Forceplate
	Kinesthetic Ability Trainer
	Pro Balance Master
	Smart Balance Master

position, keeping their hands on the iliac crests and eyes closed. The single-limb stance tests are performed on the nondominant foot. This same foot is placed toward the rear on the tandem stances. Subjects are told that upon losing their balance, they are to make any necessary adjustments and return to the testing position as quickly as possible. Performance is scored by adding one error point for each error committed (Table 17-2). Trials are considered to be incomplete if the patient is unable to sustain the stance position for longer than 5 seconds during the entire 20-second testing period. These trials are assigned a standard maximum error score of 10. Balance test results during injury recovery are best utilized when compared to baseline measurements, and clinicians working with patients on a regular basis should attempt to obtain baseline measurements when possible.

Semidynamic and dynamic balance assessment can be performed through functional reach tests, timed agility tests such as the figure-eight test,[16,20,82] carioca or hop test,[42,82] Bass test for Dynamic Balance,[79] timed "T-Band kicks," and timed balance-beam walking with the eyes open or closed. The objective in most of these tests is to decrease the size of the base of support, in an attempt to determine the patient's ability to control upright posture while moving. Many of these tests have been criticized for failing to quantify balance adequately, as they merely report how long a particular posture is maintained, angular displacement, or the distance covered after walking.[6,22,48,64] At any rate, they can often provide the therapist with valuable information about a patient's function and/or ability to return to play.

Objective Assessment

Advancements in technology have provided the medical community with commercially available balance systems (Table 17-3) for quantitatively assessing and training static and dynamic balance. These systems provide easy, practical, and cost-effective methods of quantitatively assessing and training functional balance through analysis of postural stability. Thus, the potential exists to assess injured patients and (1) identify possible abnormalities that might be associated with injury,

(2) isolate various systems that are affected, and (3) develop recovery curves based on quantitative measures for determining readiness to return to activity.

Most manufacturers use computer-interfaced forceplate technology consisting of a flat, rigid surface supported on three or more points by independent force-measuring devices. As the patient stands on the forceplate surface, the position of the center of vertical forces exerted on the forceplate over time is calculated (Fig. 17-4). Movements of the center of vertical force provide an indirect measure of postural sway activity.[63] The Kistler

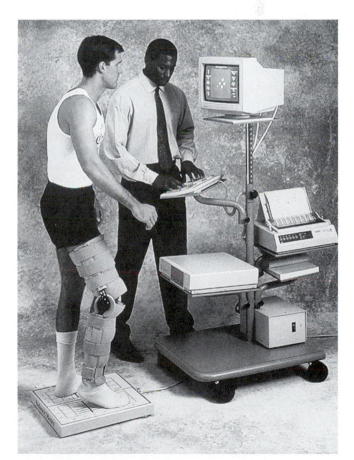

FIGURE 17-4

Athlete training on the Balance Master.

and, more recently, Bertec forceplates are used for much of the work in the area of postural stability and balance.[6,18,28,54,57] Manufacturers such as Chattecx Corporation (Hixson, TN) and NeuroCom International, Inc. (Clackamas, OR) have also developed systems with expanded diagnostic and training capabilities that make interpretation of results easier for athletic trainers. Therapists must be aware that the manufacturers often use conflicting terminology to describe various balance parameters: therapists should consult frequently with the manufacturer to ensure that there is a clear understanding of the measure being taken. These inconsistencies have created confusion in the literature, because what some manufacturers classify as *dynamic balance*, others claim is really *static balance*. Our classification system (see the section "Balance Training") will, we hope, clear up some of the confusion and allow for a more consistent labeling of the numerous balance-related exercises.

Force platforms ideally evaluate three aspects of postural control: steadiness, symmetry, and dynamic stability. *Steadiness* is the ability to keep the body as motionless as possible. This is a measure of postural sway. *Symmetry* is the ability to distribute weight evenly between the two feet in an upright stance. This is a measure of center of pressure (COP), center of balance (COB), or center of force (COF), depending which testing system you are using. Although inconsistent with our classification system, *dynamic stability* is often defined as the ability to transfer the vertical projection of the COG around a stationary supporting base.[28] This is often referred to as a measure of one's perception of "safe" LOS, as the goal is to lean or reach as far as possible without losing one's balance. Some manufacturers measure dynamic stability by assessing a person's postural response to external perturbations from a moving platform in one of four directions: tilting toes up, tilting toes down, shifting medial–lateral (M-L), and shifting anterior–posterior (A-P). Platform perturbation on some systems is unpredictable and determined by the positioning and sway movement of the subject. In such cases, a person's reaction response can be determined (Fig. 17-5). Other systems have a more predictable sinusoidal waveform, which remains constant regardless of subject positioning (Fig. 17-6).

Many of these force platform systems measure the vertical ground reaction force and provide a means of computing the COP. The COP represents the center of the distribution of the total force applied to the supporting surface. The COP is calculated from horizontal movement and vertical force data generated by triaxial force platforms. COB, in the case of the Chattecx Balance System, is the point between the feet where the ball and heel of each foot has 25 percent of the body weight. This point is referred to as the relative weight positioning over the four load cells as measured only by vertical forces. The center of vertical force, on NeuroCom's EquiTest, is the center of the vertical force exerted by the feet against the support surface. In any case (COP, COB, COF), the total force applied to the force platform fluctuates because it includes both body weight and the inertial effects of the slightest movement of the body that occur even when one attempts to stand motionless. The

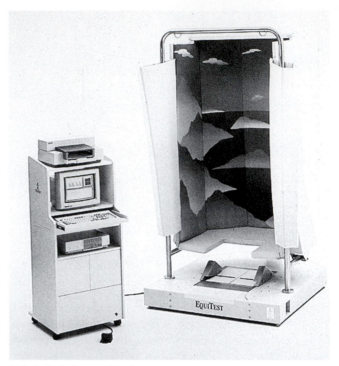

F I G U R E   1 7 - 5

EquiTest.

movement of these force-based reference points is theorized to vary according to the movement of the body's COG and the distribution of muscle forces required to control posture. Ideally, healthy clients should maintain their COP very near the A-P and M-L midlines.

Once the COP, COB, or COF is calculated, several other balance parameters can be attained. Deviation from this point in any direction represents a person's postural sway. Postural sway can be measured in various ways, depending on which system is being used. Mean displacement, length of sway path, length of sway area, amplitude, frequency, and direction with respect to the COP can be calculated on most systems. An equilibrium score, comparing the angular difference between the calculated maximum anterior to posterior COG displacements to a theoretical maximum displacement, is unique to NeuroCom International's EquiTest. Sway index, representing the degree of scatter of data about the COB, is unique to the Chattecx Balance System.

Forceplate technology allows for quantitative analysis and understanding of a subject's postural instability. These systems are fully integrated with hardware/software systems for quickly and quantitatively assessing and rehabilitating balance disorders. Most manufacturers allow for both static and dynamic balance assessment in either double- or single-leg stances, with eyes open or eyes closed. NeuroCom's EquiTest System is equipped with a moving visual surround (wall) that allows for the most sophisticated technology available for isolating and assessing sensory modality interaction.

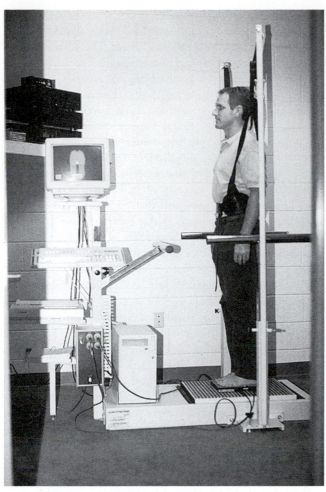

FIGURE 17-6

Chattecx Balance System.

Long forceplates have been developed by some manufacturers in an attempt to combat criticism that balance assessment is not functional. Inclusion of the long forceplate (Fig. 17-7) adds a vast array of dynamic balance exercises for training, such as walking, step-up-and-over, side and crossover steps, hopping, leaping, and lunging. These activities can be practiced and perfected through the use of the computer's visual feedback.

Biodex Medical Systems (Shirley, NY) manufactures a dynamic multiaxial tilting platform that offers computer-generated data similar to those of a forceplate system. The Biodex Stability System (Fig. 17-8) utilizes a dynamic multiaxial platform that allows up to 20° of deflection in any direction. It is theorized that this degree of deflection is sufficient to stress the joint mechanoreceptors that provide proprioceptive feedback (at end ranges of motion) necessary for balance control. Therapists can therefore assess deficits in dynamic muscular control of posture relative to joint pathology. The patient's ability to control the platform's angle of tilt is quantified as a variance from center, as well as degrees of deflection over time, at various stability levels. A large variance is indicative of poor muscle response. Exercises performed on a multiaxial unstable system

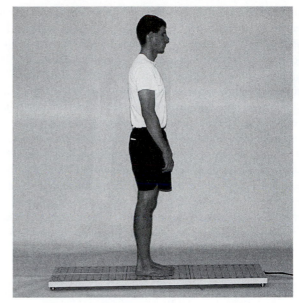

FIGURE 17-7

Balance Master with accessory 5-ft forceplate.

such as the Biodex are similar to those of the Biomechanical Ankle Platform System (BAPS board) and are especially effective for regaining proprioception and balance following injury to the ankle joint.

INJURY AND BALANCE

It has long been theorized that failure of stretched or damaged ligaments to provide adequate neural feedback in an

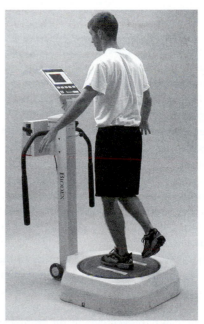

FIGURE 17-8

Biodex Stability System.

injured extremity may contribute to decreased proprioceptive mechanisms necessary for maintenance of proper balance. Research has revealed these impairments in individuals with ankle injury[24,32,72] and anterior cruciate ligament (ACL) injury.[4,69] The lack of proprioceptive feedback resulting from such injuries might allow excessive or inappropriate loading of a joint. Furthermore, although the presence of a capsular lesion might interfere with the transmission of afferent impulses from the joint, a more important effect might be alteration of the afferent neural code that is conveyed to the CNS.[84] Decreased reflex excitation of motor neurons can result form either or both of the following events: (a) a decrease in proprioceptive input to the CNS and (b) an increase in the activation of inhibitory interneurons within the spinal cord. All of these factors may lead to progressive degeneration of the joint and continued deficits in joint dynamics, balance, and coordination.

Ankle Injuries

Joint proprioceptors are believed to be damaged during injury to the lateral ligaments of the ankle because joint receptor fibers possess less tensile strength than the ligament fibers. Damage to the joint receptors is believed to cause joint deafferentation, which diminishes the supply of messages from the injured joint up the afferent pathway, disrupting proprioceptive function.[25] Freeman et al.[25] were the first to report a decrease in the frequency of functional instability following ankle sprains when coordination exercises were performed as part of rehabilitation. The term *articular deafferentation* was introduced to designate the mechanism they believed to be the cause of functional instability of the ankle. This finding led to the inclusion of balance training in ankle rehabilitation programs.

Since 1965, Freeman[24] has theorized that if ankle injuries cause partial deafferentation and functional instability, a person's postural sway would be altered due to a proprioception deficit. Some studies[76,77] have not supported Freeman's theory, but other, more recent studies using high-tech equipment (forceplate, kinesthesiometer, etc.) have revealed balance deficits in ankles following acute sprians[26,32,70] and/or in ankles with chronic instabilities.[10,23,27,71]

Differences were identified between injured and uninjured ankles in 14 ankle-injured subjects using a computerized strain gauge forceplate.[26] Four of five possible postural sway parameters (standard deviation of the mean COP dispersion, mean sway amplitude, average speed, and number of sway amplitudes exceeding 5 and 10 mm) taken in the frontal plane from a single-leg stance position were reported to discriminate between injured and noninjured ankles. The authors reported that the application of an ankle brace eliminated the differences between injury status when tested on each parameter, therefore improving balance performance. More importantly this study suggests that the stabilometry technique of selectively analyzing postural sway movements in the frontal plane, where the diameter of the supporting area is smallest, leads to higher sensitivity. Because difficulties of maintaining balance after a

ligament lesion involves the subtalar axis, it is proposed that increased sway movements of the different body segments would be found primarily in the frontal plane. The authors speculated that this could explain nonsignificant findings of earlier stabilometry studies[76,77] involving injured ankles.

Orthotic intervention and postural sway was studied in 13 subjects with acute inversion ankle sprains and 12 uninjured subjects under two treatment conditions (orthotic, nonorthotic) and four platform movements (stable, inversion/ eversion, plantarflexion/dorsiflexion, medial/lateral perturbations).[32] Results revealed that ankle-injured subjects swayed more than uninjured subjects when assessed in a single-leg test. The analysis also revealed that custom-fit orthotics can restrict undesirable motion at the foot and ankle, and enhance joint mechanoreceptors to detect perturbations and provide structural support for detecting and controlling postural sway in ankle-injured subjects. A similar study[70] reported improvements in static balance for injured subjects while wearing custom-made orthotics.

Studies involving subjects with chronic ankle instabilities[10,23,27] indicate that individuals with a history of inversion ankle sprain are less stable in a single-limb stance on the involved leg as compared to the uninvolved leg and/or noninjured subjects. Significant differences between injured and uninjured subjects for sway amplitude but not for sway frequency, using a standard forceplate, were revealed.[10] The effect of stance perturbation on frontal plane postural control was tested in three groups of subjects: a control group (no previous ankle injury), a functional ankle instability and 8-week training program group, and a mechanical instability without functional instability group (without shoe, with shoe, with brace and shoe).[71] The authors reported a relative change from ankle to hip synergy at medially directed translations of the support surface on the NeuroCom EquiTest. The impairment was restored after 8 weeks of ankle disk training. The effect of a shoe and brace did not exceed the effect of the shoe alone. Impaired ankle function was shown to be related to coordination, as subjects changed from ankle toward hip strategies for postural adjustments.

Similarly, researchers[38] reported that lateral ankle joint anesthesia did not alter postural sway or passive joint position sense, but did affect the COB position (similar to COP) during both static and dynamic testing. This suggests the presence of an adaptive mechanism to compensate for the loss of afferent stimuli from the region of the lateral ankle ligaments.[38] Subjects tended to shift their COB medially during dynamic balance testing and slightly laterally during static balance testing. The authors speculated that COB shifting may provide additional proprioceptive input form cutaneous receptors in the sole of the foot or stretch receptors in the peroneal muscle tendon unit, which therefore prevents increased postural sway.

Increased postural sway frequency and latencies are parameters thought to be indicative of impaired ankle joint proprioception.[14,72] Cornwall et al.[10] and Pintsaar et al.,[71] however, found no differences between chronically injured subjects and control subjects on these measures. This raises the question whether postural sway is in fact caused by a proprioceptive deficit. Increased postural sway amplitudes in the absence of sway frequencies might suggest that chronically injured subjects recover their ankle joint proprioception over time. Thus, more research is warranted for investigating loss of joint proprioception and postural sway frequency.[10]

In summary, results of studies involving both chronic and acute ankle sprains suggest that increased postural sway and/or balance instability might be due not to a single factor but to disruption of both neurological and biomechanical factors at the ankle joint. Loss of balance could result from abnormal or altered biomechanical alignment of the body, thus affecting the transmission of somatosensory information from the ankle joint. It is possible that observed postural sway amplitudes following injury result form joint instability along the kinetic chain, rather than from deafferentation. Thus, the orthotic intervention[32,65,66] may have provided more optimal joint alignment.

Knee Injuries

Ligamentous injury to the knee has been proven to impair subjects' ability to accurately detect position.[2–4,48,51,52] The general consensus among numerous investigators performing proprioceptive testing is that a clinical proprioception deficit occurs in most patients after an ACL rupture who have functional instability and that this deficit seems to persist to some degree after an ACL reconstruction.[2] Because of the relationships between proprioception (somatosensation) and balance, it has been suggested that the patient's ability to balance on the ACL-injured leg may also be decerased.[4,69]

Studies have evaluated the effects of ACL ruptures on standing balance using forceplate technology; although some studies have revealed balance deficits,[26,56] others have not.[19,37] Thus, there appear to be conflicting results from these studies, depending on which parameters are measured. Mizuta et al.[56] found significant differences in postural sway when measuring COP and sway distance area between 11 functionally stable and 15 functionally unstable subjects who had unilateral ACL-deficient knees. Faculjak et al.,[19] however, found no differences in postural stability between 8 ACL-deficient subjects and 10 normal subjects when measuring average latency and response strength on an EquiTest System.

Several potential reasons for this discrepancy exist. First, it has been suggested that there might be a link between static balance and isometric strength of the musculature at the ankle and knee. Isometric muscle strength could therefore compensate for any somatosensory deficit present in the involved knee during a closed-chain static balance test. Second, many studies fail to discriminate between *functionally unstable* ACL-deficient knees and knees that were not functionally unstable. This presents a design flaw, especially considering that functionally stable knees would most likely provide adequate balance despite ligamentous pathology. Another suggested reason

for not seeing differences between injured knees and uninjured knees on static balance measures could be explained by the role that joint mechanoreceptors play. Neurophysiologic studies[29,30,45,48] have revealed that joint mechanoreceptors provide enhanced kinesthetic awareness in the near-terminal ROM or extremes of motion. Therefore, it could be speculated that if the maximum LOS are never reached during a static balance test, damaged mechanoreceptors (muscle or joint) might not even become a factor. Dynamic balance tests or functional hop tests that involve dynamic balance could challenge the postural control system (ankle strategies are taken over by hip and/or stepping strategies), requiring more mechanoreceptor input. These tests would most likely discriminate between functionally unstable ACL-deficient knees and normal knees.

Head Injury

Neurological status following mild head injury has been assessed using balance as a criterion variable. Physicians have long evaluated head injuries with the Romberg tests of sensory modality function to test "balance." This is an easy and effective sideline test; however, the literature suggests there is more to posture control than just balance and sensory modality,[59,60,65,69,74] especially when assessing people with head injury.[31,34,35] The postural control system, which is responsible for linking brain-to-body communication, is often affected as a result of mild head injury. Several studies have identified postural stability deficits in patients up to 3 days postinjury using commercially available balance systems.[31,34,35] It appears that this deficit is related to a sensory interaction problem in which the injured athlete fails to use the visual system effectively. This research suggests that objective balance assessment can be used for establishing recovery curves for making return to functional activity decision in concussed patients. Rehabilitation of concussed patients using balance techniques has yet to be studied.

BALANCE TRAINING

Developing a rehabilitation program that includes exercises for improving balance and postural equilibrium is vital for a successful return to competition from a lower-extremity injury. Whether the patient has sustained a quadriceps strain or an ankle sprain, the injury has caused a disruption at some point between the body's COG and base of support. This is likely to have caused compensatory weight shifts and gait changes along the kinetic chain that have resulted in balance deficits. These deficits may be detected through the use of functional assessment tests and/or computerized instrumentation for assessing balance. Having the advanced technology available to quantify balance deficits is an amenity but not a necessity. Imagination and creativity are often the best tools available to therapists with limited resources who are trying to design balance-training protocols.

Because virtually all functional activities involve closed-chain lower-extremity function, functional rehabilitation should be performed in the closed kinetic chain. However, ROM, movement speed, and additional resistance may be more easily controlled in the open chain initially. Therefore, adequate, safe function in an open chain may be the first step in the rehabilitation process, but should not be the focus of the rehabilitation plan. The therapist should attempt to progress the patient to functional closed-chain exercises quickly and safely. Depending on severity of injury, this could be as early as 1 day postinjury.

Because there are close relationships between somatosensation, kinesthesia, and balance, many of the exercises proposed for kinesthetic training indirectly enhance balance. Several methods of regaining balance have been proposed in the literature and are included in the most current rehabilitation protocols for ankle[43,75,84] and knee injury.[12,42,53,74,83]

A variety of activities can be used to improve balance, but the therapist should consider five general rules before beginning:

- The exercises must be safe yet challenging.
- Stress multiple planes of motion.
- Incorporate a multisensory approach.
- Begin with static, bilateral, and stable surfaces and progress to dynamic, unilateral, and unstable surfaces.
- Progress toward activity-specific exercises.

There are several ways in which the therapist can meet these goals. Balance exercises should be performed in an open area, where the patient will not be injured in the event of a fall. It is best to perform exercises with an assistive device within arm's reach (e.g., chair, railing, table, wall), especially during the initial phase of rehabilitation. When considering exercise duration for balance exercises, the therapist can use either sets and repetitions or a time-based protocol. The patient can perform two or three sets of 15 repetitions and progress to 30 repetitions as tolerated, or perform 10 of the exercises for a 15-second period and progress to 30-second period later in the program.

Classification of Balance Exercises

Static balance is when the COG is maintained over a fixed base of support (unilateral or bilateral) while standing on a stable surface. Examples of static exercises are a single-leg, double-leg, or tandem-stance Romberg task. *Semidynamic* balance involves one of two possible activities: The person maintains his/her COG over a fixed base of support while standing on a moving surface (Chattecx Balance System or EquiTest) or unstable surface (Biodex Stability System, BAPS, medium-density foam, or minitramp); or the person transfers his/her COG over a fixed base of support to selected ranges and/or directions within the LOS while standing on a stable surface (Balance Master's LOS, functional reach tests, minisquats, or T-Band kicks). *Dynamic* balance involves the maintenance of the COG within the LOS over a moving base of support (feet), usually while on a stable surface. These tasks require the use of a stepping strategy. The base of support is always changing its position, forcing the

COG to be adjusted with each movement. Examples of dynamic exercises are walking on a balance beam, step-up-and-over, or bounding. *Functional* balance tasks are the same as dynamic tasks with the inclusion of sport-specific tasks such as throwing and catching.

PHASE 1

The progression of activities during phase 1 should include nonballistic types of drills. Training for static balance can be initiated once the patient is able to bear weight on the extremity. The patient should first be asked to perform bilateral 20-second Romberg tests on a variety of surfaces, beginning with a hard/firm surface (see Fig. 17-3A) and followed by more challenging surfaces (Figs. 17-9 and 17-10). Once a comfort zone is established, the patient should be progressed to performing unilateral balance tasks on both the involved and the uninvolved extremities on a variety of surfaces. The purpose of the different surfaces is to safely challenge the injured patient, while keeping the patient motivated to rehabilitate the injured extremity.

The therapist should make comparisons from these tests to determine the patient's ability to balance bilaterally and unilaterally. It should be noted that even though this is termed static balance, the patient does not remain perfectly motionless. To maintain static balance, the patient must make many small corrections at the ankle, hip, trunk arms, or head (see "Selection of Movement Strategies"). A patient who is having difficulties performing these activities should not be progressed to the next surface. Repetitions of modified Romberg tests can be performed by first using the arms as a counterbalance and then attempting the activity without using the arms. Static balance activities should be used as a precursor to more dynamic

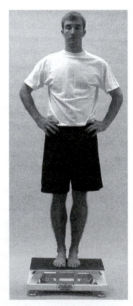

FIGURE 17-9

Bilateral stance on Tremor Box, which tremors along the horizontal plane in the A-P, M-L, and diagonal directions.

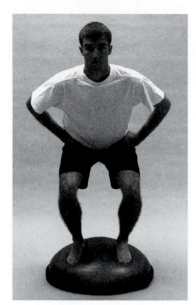

FIGURE 17-10

Bilateral stance on Bosu Balance Trainer—bubble side up.

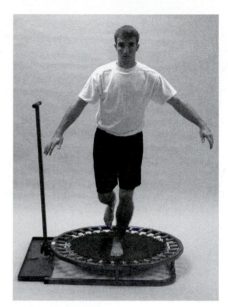

FIGURE 17-11

Unilateral stance on minitramp.

activities. The general progression of these exercises should be from bilateral to unilateral, with eyes open to eyes closed. The exercises should attempt to eliminate or alter the various sensory information (visual, vestibular, and somatosensory) in order to challenge the other systems. In most orthopedic rehabilitation situations, this is going to involve eye closure and changes in the support surface, so the somatosensory system can be overloaded or stressed. This principle is similar to the overload principle in therapeutic exercise. Research suggests that balance activities, both with and without visual input, will enhance motor function at the brainstem level.[7,75] However, as the patient becomes more efficient at performing activities involving static balance, eye closure is recommended so that only the somatosensory system is left to control balance.

As improvement occurs on a firm surface, single-leg static balance drills should progress to an unstable surface such as foam (see Fig. 17-3E), minitramp (Fig. 17-11), rocker board on foam (Fig. 17-12), rocker board on hard surface (Fig. 17-13), Bosu Balance Trainer with flat side up (Fig. 17-14), Bosu Balance Trainer with bubble side up (Fig. 17-15), or BAPS board (Fig. 17-16). Additionally, the therapist can introduce light shoulder, back, or chest taps to challenge the patient's ability to maintain balance (Fig. 17-17). Finally, the use of multiaxial devices such as the Biodex Stability System on a relatively easy level can be initiated during the later part of phase 1. These exercises increase awareness of the location of the COG under a challenged condition, thereby helping to increase ankle strength in the closed kinetic chain. Such training can also increase sensitivity of the muscle spindle and thereby increase proprioceptive input to the spinal cord, which may provide compensation for altered joint afference.[48]

Although static and semidynamic balance exercises may not be very functional, they are the first step toward regaining proprioceptive awareness, reflex stabilization, and postural orientation. The patient should attempt to assume a functional stance while performing static balance drills. Training in different positions places a variety of demands on the musculotendinous structures about the ankle, knee, and hip joints.

PHASE 2

Phase 2 should be considered the transition phase from static to more dynamic balance activities. Dynamic balance will be

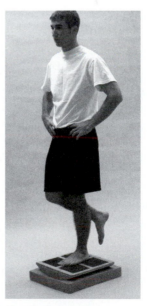

FIGURE 17-12

Unilateral stance on rocker board and foam.

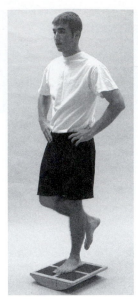

FIGURE 17·13

Unilateral stance on rocker board.

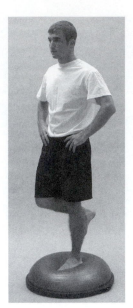

FIGURE 17·15

Unilateral stance on Bosu Balance Trainer — bubble side up.

especially important for patients who perform activities such as running, jumping, and cutting, which encompass about 95 percent of all athletes. Such activities require the patients to repetitively lose and gain balance to perform their sport without falling or becoming injured.[43] Dynamic balance activities should be incorporated into the rehabilitation program only once sufficient healing has occurred and the patient has adequate ROM, muscle strength, and endurance. This could be as early as a few days postinjury in the case of a grade 1

ankle sprain, or as late as 6 weeks postsurgery in the case of an anterior cruciate reconstruction. Before the therapist progresses the patient to challenging dynamic and activity-specific balance drills, several semidynamic (intermediate) exercises should be introduced.

These semidynamic balance drills involve displacement or perturbation of the COG away from the base of support. The patient is challenged to return and or steady the COG above the base of support throughout several repetitions of the exercise.

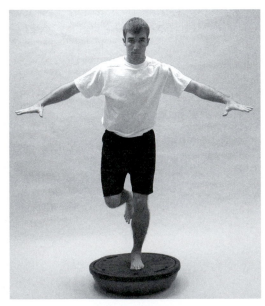

FIGURE 17·14

Unilateral stance on Bosu Balance Trainer—flat side up.

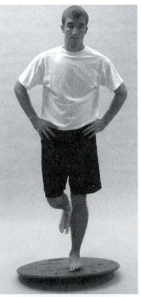

FIGURE 17·16

Unilateral stance on BAPS board.

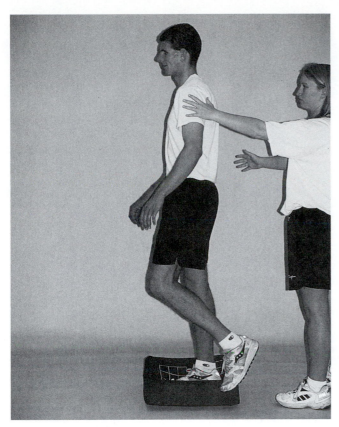

FIGURE 17-17

Athletic trainer causing perturbations using shoulder taps.

Some of these exercises involve a bilateral stance, some involve a unilateral stance, while others involve transferring weight from one extremity to the other.

The bilateral-stance balance drills include the minisquat, which is performed with the feet shoulder-width apart and the COG centered over a stable base of support. The trunk should be positioned upright over the legs as the patient slowly flexes the hips and knees into a partial squat—approximately 60° of knee flexion (Fig. 17-18). The patient then returns to the starting position and repeats the task several times. Once ROM, strength, and stability have improved, the patient can progress to full squats, which approach 90° of knee flexion. These should be performed in front of a mirror so that the patients can observe the amount of stability on their return to the extended position. A large Physioball can also be used to perform sit-to-stand activities (Fig. 17-19). Once the patient reaches a comfort zone, the balance squat exercise can be performed on more challenging surfaces such as the Bosu (Fig. 17-20) or Dynadisc (Fig. 17-21). Other rotational maneuvers and weight-shifting exercises can be conducted to assist the patient in controlling his/her COG during semidynamic movements (Figs. 17-22 to 17-25). These exercises are important in the rehabilitation of ankle, knee, and hip injuries, as they help improve weight transfer, COG sway velocity, and left/right weight symmetry. They can be performed in an attempt to challenge A-P stability or M-L stability.

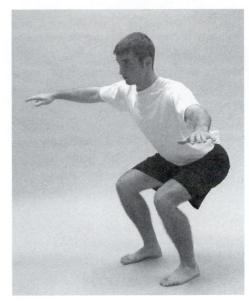

FIGURE 17-18

Minisquat.

The therapist has a variety of options for unilateral semi-dynamic balance exercises. Unilateral minisquats are a good starting point. These can be performed while holding on to a chair or support rail with the uninvolved knee flexed to 45°. The patient should emphasize controlled hip and knee flexion, followed by a smooth return to the starting position on the involved extremity. Once this skill is mastered, the patient can progress to more dynamic exercises, such as a step-up. Step-ups can be performed either in the sagittal plane (forward step-up) or in the transverse plane (lateral step-up). These drills should begin with the heel of the uninvolved extremity on the floor.

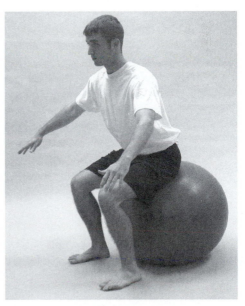

FIGURE 17-19

Sit-to-stand using Physioball.

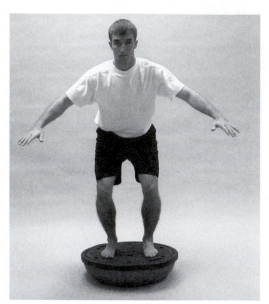

F I G U R E   1 7 - 2 0

Squat on Bosu Balance Trainer—flat side up.

Using a 2 count, the patient should shift body weight toward
the involved side and use the involved extremity to slowly raise
the body onto the step.[75] The involved knee should not be
"locked" into full extension. Instead, the knee should be positioned in approximately 5° of flexion, while balancing on the
step for 3 seconds. Following the 3 count, the body weight
should be shifted toward the uninvolved side and lowered to
the heel of the uninvolved side (Figs. 17-26 and 17-27). *Step-
up-and-over* activities are similar to step-ups but involve more
dynamic transfer of the COG. These should be performed by
having the patient either both ascend and descend using the
involved extremity (Fig. 17-28) or ascend with the involved extremity and descend with the uninvolved extremity, forcing the
involved leg to support the body on the descend (Fig. 17-29).

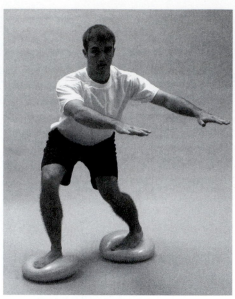

F I G U R E   1 7 - 2 2

Bilateral stance rotation on Dynadisc.

The therapist can also introduce the patient to more challenging static tests during this phase. For example, the very
popular TheraBand kicks (T-Band kicks or steamboats) are excellent for improving balance. TheraBand kicks are performed
with an elastic material (attached to the ankle of the uninvolved leg) serving as a resistance against a relatively fast kicking motion. The patient's balance on the involved extremity
is challenged by perturbations caused by the kicking motion
of the uninvolved leg (Fig. 17-30). Four sets of these exercises should be performed, one for each of four possible

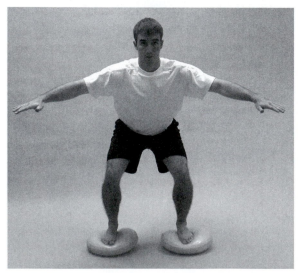

F I G U R E   1 7 - 2 1

Squat on Dynadisc.

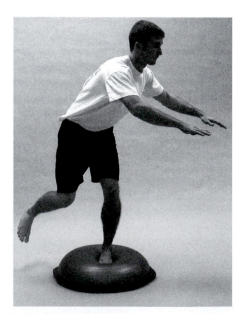

F I G U R E   1 7 - 2 3

Unilateral stance rotation on Bosu Balance
Trainer—bubble side up.

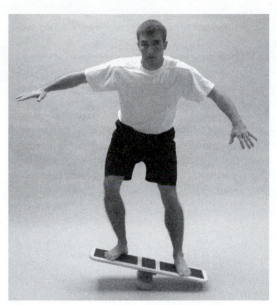

FIGURE 17-24

Bilateral stance on Extreme Balance Board.

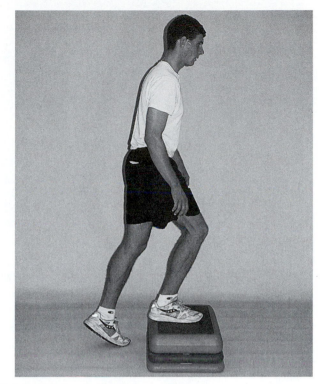

FIGURE 17-26

Forward step-up.

kicking motions: hip flexion, hip extension, hip abduction, and hip adduction. T-Band kicks can also be performed on foam or a minitramp if additional somatosensory challenges are desired.[74] Another good exercise to introduce prior to advancing to phase 3 is a balance beam walk, which can be performed against resistance to further challenge the athlete (Fig. 17-31).

The Balance Shoes (Orthopedic Physical Therapy Products, Minneapolis, MN) are another excellent tool for improving the strength of lower-extremity musculature and—ultimately—improving balance. The shoes allow

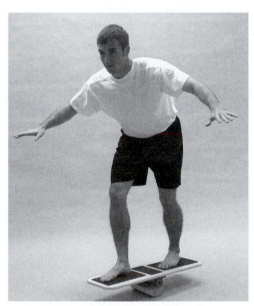

FIGURE 17-25

Tandem stance on Extreme Balance Board.

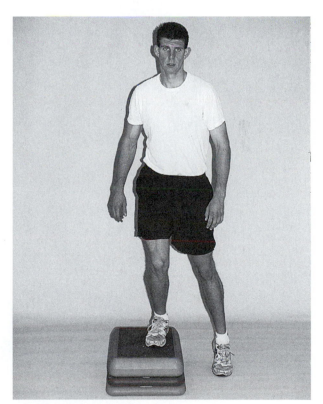

FIGURE 17-27

Lateral step-up.

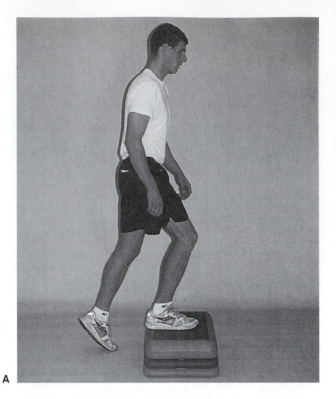
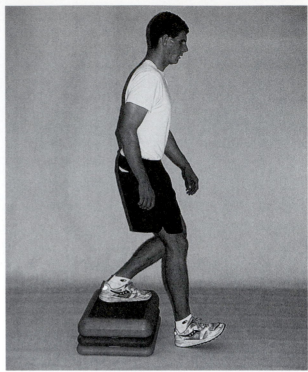

FIGURE 17-28

Step up and over. **A,** Ascending on the uninvolved extremity. **B,** Descending on the involved extremity.

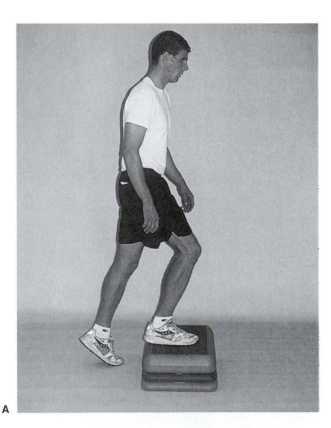
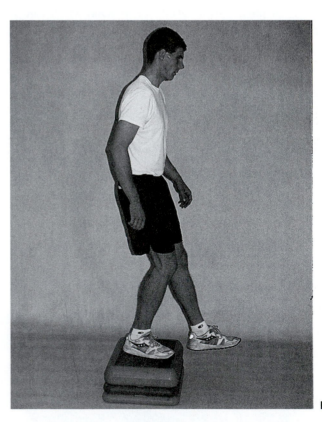

FIGURE 17-29

Step up and over. **A,** Ascending on the involved extremity. **B,** Descending on the uninvolved extremity.

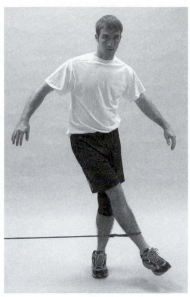

FIGURE 17-30

TheraBand kicks.

lower-extremity balance and strengthening exercises to be performed in a functional, closed-kinetic-chain manner. The shoes consist of a cork sandal with a rubber sole, and a rubber hemisphere similar in consistency to a lacrosse ball positioned under the midsole (see Fig. 30-28). The design of the sandals essentially creates an individualized perturbation device for each limb that can be utilized in any number of functional activities, ranging from static single-leg stance to dynamic gait activities performed in multiple directions (forward walking, sidestepping, carioca walking, etc.).

Clinical use of the Balance Shoes has resulted in a number of successful clinical outcomes from a subjective standpoint, including treatment of ankle sprains and chronic instability, anterior tibial compartment syndrome, lower-leg fractures, and a number of other orthopedic problems, as well as enhancement of core stability. Research has revealed that training in the Balance Shoes results in reduced rear foot motion and improved postural stability in excessive pronators,[55] and that functional activities in the Balance Shoes increase gluteal muscle activity.[9,58]

PHASE 3

Once the patient can successfully complete the semidynamic exercises presented in phase 2, he/she should be ready to perform more dynamic and functional types of exercises. The general progression for activities to develop dynamic balance and control is from slow-speed to fast-speed activities, from low-force to high-force activities, and from controlled to uncontrolled activities.[43] In other words, the patient should be working toward activity specific drills. These exercises will likely be different depending on specific functional activities. Therapists need to use their imagination to develop the best protocols for their patients.

Bilateral jumping drills are a good place to begin once the patient has reached phase 3. These can be performed either

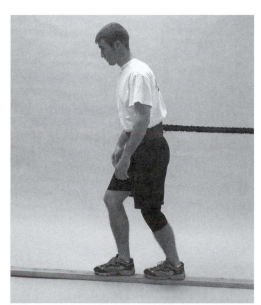

FIGURE 17-31

Balance beam walk against resistance.

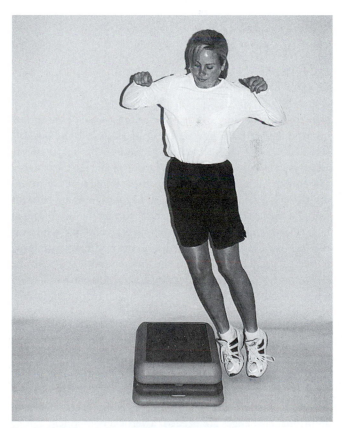

FIGURE 17-32

Bilateral hops.

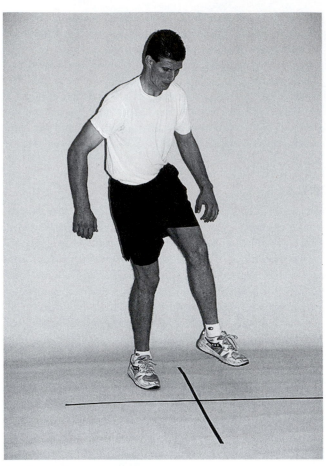

FIGURE   1 7 - 3 3

Diagonal hops.

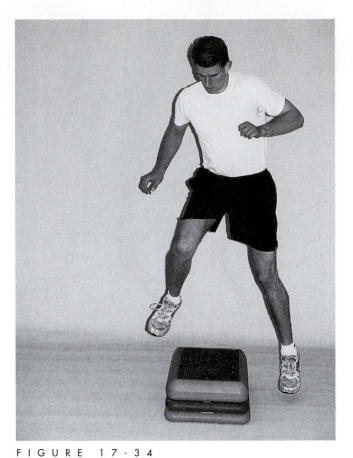

FIGURE   1 7 - 3 4

Lateral jumps over box.

front to back or side to side. The patient should concentrate on landing on each side of the line as quickly as possible (Fig. 17-32).[74,75] As the patient progresses through these exercises, eye closure can be used to further challenge the patient's somatosensation. After mastering these straight-plane jumping patterns, the patient can begin diagonal jumping patterns through the use of a cross on the floor formed by two pieces of tape (Fig. 17-33). The intersecting lines create four quadrants that can be numbered and used to perform different jumping sequences, such as 1-3-2-4 for the first set and 1-4-2-3 for the second set.[74,75] A larger grid can be designed to allow for longer sequences and longer jumps, both of which require additional strength, endurance, and balance control.

Bilateral dynamic balance exercises should progress to unilateral dynamic balance exercises as quickly as possible during phase 3. At this stage of the rehabilitation, pain and fatigue should be less prominent factors. All jumping drills performed bilaterally should now be performed unilaterally, by practicing first on the uninvolved extremity (Fig. 17-33). If additional challenges are needed, a vertical component can be added by having the patient jump over an object, such as a box (Fig. 17-34).

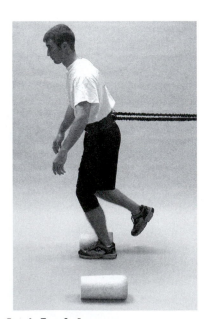

FIGURE   1 7 - 3 5

Lateral bounding.

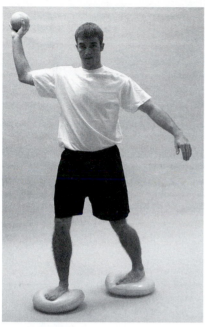

FIGURE 17-36

Control dynamic balance while throwing ball while balancing on Dynadisc.

Tubing can be added to dynamic unilateral training exercises. The patient can perform stationary running against the tube's resistance, followed by lateral and diagonal bounding exercises. Diagonal bounding, which involves jumping from one foot to the other, places greater emphasis on lateral movements. It is recommended that the patient first learn the bounding exer-

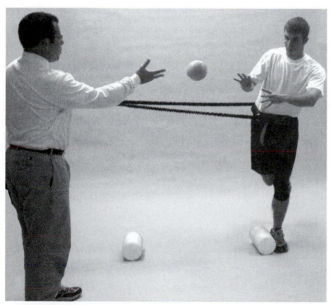

FIGURE 17-37

Control dynamic balance while throwing and catching a ball during lateral bounding.

cise without tubing, and then attempt the exercise with tubing. A foam roll, towel, or other obstacle can be used to increase jump height and/or distance (Fig. 17-35).[81] The final step in trying to improve dynamic balance may involve incorporating functional activities. At this stage of the rehabilitation program, the patient should be able to safely concentrate on the functional activity (catching and throwing), while subconsciously controlling dynamic balance (Figs. 17-36 and 17-37).

CLINICAL VALUE OF HIGH-TECH TRAINING AND ASSESSMENT

One benefit of using the commercially available balance systems is that not only can deficits be detected, but progress can also be charted quantitatively using the computer-generated results. For example, NeuroCom's Balance Master (with long forceplate) is capable of assessing a patient's ability to perform coordinated movements. The system, equipped with a 5-ft-long force platform, is capable of identifying specific components underlying performance of several functional tasks. Exercises are also available on the system that help to improve the deficits.[66]

Results of a step-up-and-over test are presented in Fig. 17-38. The components analyzed in this particular task are (1) the *lift-up index*, which quantifies the maximum lifting (concentric) force exerted by the leading leg and is expressed as a percentage of the person's weight, (2) *movement time*, or the number of seconds required to complete the task, beginning with initial weight shift to the nonstepping leg and ending with impact of the lagging leg onto the surface, and (3) the *impact index*, which quantifies the maximum vertical impact force (percentage of body weight) as the lagging leg lands on the surface.[66]

Research on the clinical applicability of these measures has revealed interesting results. Preliminary observations from two studies in progress suggest that deficits in impact control are a common feature of patients with ACL injuries, even when strength and ROM of the involved knee are within normal limits. Several other performance assessments are available on this system, including *sit to stand, walk test, step and quick turn, forward lunge, weight bearing/squat, and rhythmic weight shift*.

SUMMARY

- There are very close relationships among proprioception, kinesthesia, and balance.
- The most common form of proprioception training involves unilateral balance drills on challenging surfaces.
- Exercises performed on foam or multiaxial devices are good precursors for more dynamic balance exercises such as lunges, lateral bounding, and unilateral hopping drills.

Name:	Doe, John J	Diagnosis:	ACL Tear L Knee	File:	HBM1.QBM
ID:	ATID00001	Operator ID:	Jodi Bower	Date:	03/06/97
DOB:	11/22/55	Referred by:	Dr. Tom Merkle	Time:	6:35:06 PM
Height:	5'11"	Comments:	DOI: 7/4/96; DOS: 7/6/96		

STEP UP/OVER TEXT (8 inch curb)

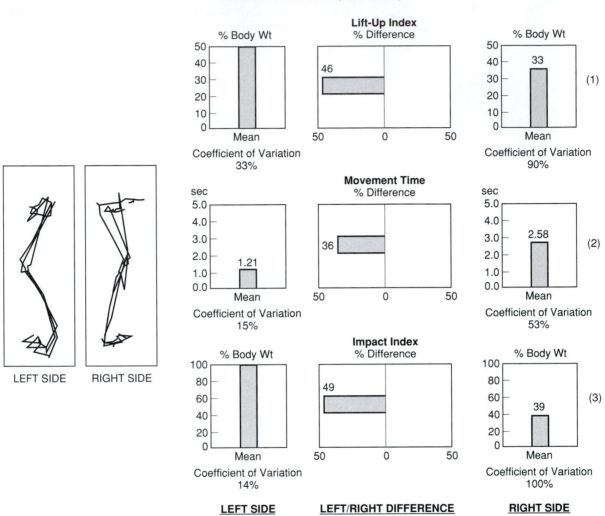

LEFT SIDE   RIGHT SIDE

LEFT SIDE   **LEFT/RIGHT DIFFERENCE**   **RIGHT SIDE**

FIGURE 17-38

Results from a step-up-and-over protocol on the NeuroCom New Balance Master's long forceplate. (Balance Master Version 6.0 and NeuroCom are registered trademarks of NeuroCom International Inc.)

- The goal of any rehabilitation program should be to move safely through a progression of balance exercises (phase 1 through phase 3).
- The use of commercially manufactured balance systems adds a nice feature to balance training and assessment, allowing the therapist to quantify progress.
- With a little creativity, the therapist can design low-cost, yet very effective exercises for regaining balance.

REFERENCES

1. Balogun JA, Adesinasi CO, Marzouk DK. The effects of a wobble board exercise training program on static balance performance and strength of lower extremity muscle. *Physiother Can* 44:23–30, 1992.

2. Barrack RL, Lund P, Skinner H. Knee joint proprioception revisited. *J Sport Rehabil* 3:18–42, 1994.

3. Barrack RL, Skinner HB, Buckley SL. Proprioception in the anterior cruciate deficient knee. *Am J Sports Med* 17: 1–6, 1989.

4. Barrett D. Proprioception and function after anterior cruciate reconstruction. *J Bone Joint Surg Br* 73:833–837, 1991.

5. Black F, Wall C, Nashner L. Effect of visual and support surface orientations upon postural control in vestibular deficient subjects. *Acta Otolaryngol* 95:199–210, 1983.

6. Black O, Wall C, Rockette H, Kitch R. Normal subject postural sway during the Romberg test. *Am J Otolaryngol* 3(5):309–318, 1982.

7. Blackburn T, Voight M. Single leg stance: Development of a reliable testing procedure. In: *Proceedings of the 12th International Congress of the World Confederation for Physical Therapy*, 1995.

8. Booher J, Thibodeau G. *Athletic Injury Assessment.* St. Louis, MO, Mosby, 1995.

9. Bullock-Saxton JE, Janda V, Bullock ME. Reflex activation of gluteal muscle in walking. *Spine* 18(6):704–708, 1993.

10. Cornwall M, Murrell P. Postural sway following inversion sprain of the ankle. *J Am Podiatr Med Assoc* 81:243–247, 1991.

11. Davies G. The need for critical thinking in rehabilitation. *J Sport Rehabil* 4(1):1–22, 1995.

12. DeCarlo M, Klootwyk T, Shelbourne K. ACL surgery and accelerated rehabilitation: Revisited. *J Sport Rehabil* 6(2):144–156, 1997.

13. Diener H, Dichgans J, Guschlbauer B, et al. Role of visual and static vestibular influences on dynamic posture control. *Hum Neurobiol* 5:105–113, 1986.

14. Diener H, Dichgans J, Guschlbauer B, Mau H. The significance of proprioception on postural stabilization as assessed by ischemia. *Brain Res* 296:103–109, 1984.

15. Dietz V, Horstmann G, Berger W. Significance of proprioceptive mechanisms in the regulation of stance. *Prog Brain Res* 80:4119–4123, 1989.

16. Donahoe B, Turner D, Worrell T. The use of functional reach as a measurement of balance in healthy boys and girls ages 5–15. *Phys Ther* 73(6):S71, 1993.

17. Dornan J, Fernie G, Holliday P. Visual input: Its importance in the control of postural sway. *Arch Phys Med Rehabil* 59:586–591, 1978.

18. Ekdahl C, Jarnlo G, Anderson S. Standing balance in healthy subjects: Evaluation of a quantitative test battery on a force platform. *Scand J Rehabil Med* 21:187–195, 1989.

19. Faculjak P, Firoozbakhshsh K, Wausher D, McGuire M. Balance characteristics of normal and anterior cruciate ligament deficient knees. *Phys Ther* 73:S22, 1993.

20. Fisher A, Wietlisbach S, Wilberger J. Adult performance on three tests of equilibrium. *Am J Occup Ther* 42(1):30–35, 1988.

21. Fitzpatrick R, Rogers DK, McCloskey DI. Stable human standing with lower-limb muscle afferents providing the only sensory input. *J Physiol* 480(2):395–403, 1994.

22. Flores A. Objective measures of standing balance. *Neurol Rep Am Phys Ther Assoc* 16(1):17–21, 1992.

23. Forkin DM, Koczur C, Battle R, Newton RA. Evaluation of kinesthetic deficits indicative of balance control in gymnasts with unilateral chronic ankle sprains. *J Orthop Sports Phys Ther* 23(4):245–250, 1996.

24. Freeman M. Instability of the foot after injuries to the lateral ligament of the ankle. *J Bone Joint Surg* 47B:678–685, 1965.

25. Freeman M, Dean M, Hanham I. The etiology and prevention of functional instability of the foot. *J Bone Joint Surg* 47B:669–677, 1965.

26. Friden T, Zatterstrom R, Lindstrand A, Moritz U. A stabilometric technique for evaluation of lower limb instabilities. *Am J Sports Med* 17(1):118–122, 1989.

27. Garn SN, Newton RA. Kinesthetic awareness in subjects with multiple ankle sprains. *Phys Ther* 68:1667–1671, 1988.

28. Goldie P, Bach T, Evans O. Force platform measures for evaluating postural control: Reliability and validity. *Arch Phys Med Rehabil* 70:510–517, 1989.

29. Grigg P. Mechanical factors influencing response of joint afferent neurons from cat knee. *J Neurophysiol* 38:1473–1484, 1975.

30. Grigg P. Response of joint afferent neurons in cat medial articular nerve to active and passive movements of the knee. *Brain Res* 118:482–485, 1976.

31. Guskiewicz KM, Perrin DH, Gansneder B. Effect of mild head injury on postural stability. *J Athlet Train* 31(4):300–306, 1996.

32. Guskiewicz KM, Perrin DH. Effect of orthotics on postural sway following inversion ankle sprain. *J Orthop Sports Phys Ther* 23(5):326–331, 1996.

33. Guskiewicz KM, Perrin DH. Research and clinical applications of assessing balance. *J Sport Rehabil* 5:45–63, 1996.

34. Guskiewicz KM, Ross SE, Marshall SW. Postural stability and neuropsychological deficits following concussion in collegiate athlete. *J Athlet Train* 36(3):263–273, 2001.

35. Guskiewicz KM, Riemann BL, Riemann DH, Nashner LM. Alternative approaches to the assessment of mild head injury in athletes. *Med Sci Sports Exerc* 29(7):S213–S221, 1997.

36. Guyton A. *Textbook of Medical Physiology*, 8th ed. Philadelphia, WB Saunders, 1991.

37. Harrison E, Duenkel N, Dunlop R, Russell G. Evaluation of single-leg standing following anterior cruciate ligament surgery and rehabilitation. *Phys Ther* 74(3):245–252, 1994.

38. Hertel JN, Guskiewicz KM, Kahler DM, Perrin DH. Effect of lateral ankle joint anesthesia on center of balance,

postural sway and joint position sense. *J Sport Rehabil* 5:111–119, 1996.

39. Horak FB, Nashner LM, Diener HC. Postural strategies associated with somatosensory and vestibular loss. *Exp Brain Res* 82:167–177, 1990.

40. Horak F, Nashner L. Central programming of postural movements: Adaptation to altered support surface configurations. *J Neurophysiol* 55:1369–1381, 1986.

41. Houk J. Regulation of stiffness by skeleto-motor reflexes. *Ann Rev Physiol* 41:99–114, 1979.

42. Irrgang J, Harner C. Recent advances in ACL rehabilitation: Clinical factors. *J Sport Rehabil* 6(2):111–124, 1997.

43. Irrgang J, Whitney S, Cox E. Balance and proprioceptive training for rehabilitation of the lower extremity. *J Sport Rehabil* 3:68–83, 1994.

44. Jansen E, Larsen R, Mogens B. Quantitative Romberg's test: Measurement and computer calculations of postural stability. *Acta Neurol Scand* 66:93–99, 1982.

45. Johansson H, Alexander IJ, Hayes KC. Nerve supply of the human knee and its functional importance. *Am J Sports Med* 10:329–335, 1982.

46. Kauffman TL, Nashner LM, Allison LK. Balance is a critical parameter in orthopedic rehabilitation. *Orthop Phys Ther Clin North Am* 6(1):43–78, 1997.

47. Kisner C, Colby LA. *Therapeutic Exercise: Foundations and Techniques*, 3rd ed. Philadelphia, FA Davis, 1996.

48. Lephart SM. Re-establishing proprioception, kinesthesia, joint position sense, and neuromuscular control in rehabilitation. In: Prentice WE, ed. *Rehabilitation Techniques in Sports*, 2nd ed. St. Louis, MO, Mosby, 1993, pp. 118–137.

49. Lephart SM, Henry TJ. Functional rehabilitation for the upper and lower extremity. *Orthop Clin North Am* 26(3):579–592, 1993.

50. Lephart SM, Kocher MS. The role of exercise in the prevention of shoulder disorders. In: Matsen FA, Fu FH, Hawkins RJ, eds. *The Shoulder: A Balance of Mobility and Stability*. Rosemont, IL, American Academy of Orthopaedic Surgeons, 1993, pp. 597–620.

51. Lephart SM, Kocher MS, Fu FH, et al. Proprioception following ACL reconstruction. *J Sport Rehabil* 1:186–196, 1992.

52. Lephart SM, Pincivero D, Giraldo J, Fu F. The role of proprioception in the management and rehabilitation of athletic injuries. *Am J Sports Med* 25:130–137, 1997.

53. Mangine R, Kremchek T. Evaluation-based protocol of the anterior cruciate ligament. *J Sport Rehabil* 6(2):157–181, 1997.

54. Mauritz K, Dichgans J, Hufschmidt A. Quantitative analysis of stance in late cortical cerebellar atrophy of the anterior lobe and other forms of cerebellar ataxia. *Brain* 102:461–482, 1979.

55. Mitchell TB, Guskiewicz KM, Hirth CJ, et al. Effects of training in exercise sandals on 2-D rearfoot motion and postural sway in abnormal pronators. Undergraduate honors thesis, University of North Carolina, Chapel Hill, NC, 2000.

56. Mizuta H, Shiraishi M, Kubota K, Kai K, Takagi K. A stabilometric technique for evaluation of functional instability in the anterior cruciate ligament deficient knee. *Clin J Sports Med* 2:235–239, 1992.

57. Murray M, Seireg A, Sepic S. Normal postural stability: Qualitative assessment. *J Bone Joint Surg* 57A(4):510–516, 1975.

58. Myers RL, Padna DA, Prentice WE, et al. Electromyographic analysis of the gluteal musculature during closed chain exercise. Master's thesis, University of North Carolina, Chapel Hill, NC, 2002.

59. Nashner L. Adapting reflexes controlling the human posture. *Exp Brain Res* 26:59–72, 1976.

60. Nashner L. Adaptation of human movement to altered environments. *Trends Neurosci* 5:358–361, 1982.

61. Nashner L. A functional approach to understanding spasticity. In: Struppler A, Weindl A, eds. *Electromyography and Evoked Potentials*. Berlin, Springer-Verlag, 1985, pp. 22–29.

62. Nashner L. Sensory, neuromuscular and biomechanical contributions to human balance. In: Duncan P, ed. *Balance: Proceedings of the APTA Forum*, June 13–15, 1989. Alexandria, VA, American Physical Therapy Association, 1989, pp. 5–12.

63. Nashner L. Computerized dynamic posturography. In: Jacobson G, Newman C, Kartush J, eds. *Handbook of Balance Function and Testing*. St. Louis, MO, Mosby, 1993, pp. 280–307.

64. Nashner L. Practical biomechanics and physiology of balance. In: Jacobson G, Newman C, Kartush J, eds. *Handbook of Balance Function and Testing*. St. Louis, MO, Mosby, 1993, pp. 261–279.

65. Nashner L, Black F, Wall C, III. Adaptation to altered support and visual conditions during stance: Patients with vestibular deficits. *J Neurosci* 2(5):536–544, 1982.

66. NeuroCom International, Inc. *The Objective Quantification of Daily Life Tasks: The NEW Balance Master 6.0* [manual]. Clackamas, OR, 1997.

67. Newton R. Review of tests of standing balance abilities. *Brain Inj* 3:335–343, 1992.

68. Norre M. Sensory interaction testing in platform posturography. *J Laryngol Otolaryngol* 107:496–501, 1993.

69. Noyes F, Barber S, Mangine R. Abnormal lower limb symmetry determined by function hop test after anterior cruciate ligament rupture. *Am J Sports Med* 19(5):516–518, 1991.

70. Orteza L, Vogelbach W, Denegar C. The effect of molded and unmolded orthotics on balance and pain while jogging following inversion ankle sprain. *J Athlet Train* 27(1):80–84, 1992.

71. Pintsaar A, Brynhildsen J, Tropp H. Postural corrections after standardized perturbations of single limp stance:

Effect of training and orthotic devices in patients with ankle instability. *Br J Sports Med* 30:151–155, 1996.

72. Shambers GM. Influence of the fusimotor system on stance and volitional movement in normal man. *Am J Phys Med* 48:225–227, 1969.

73. Shumway-Cook A, Horak F. Assessing the influence of sensory interaction on balance. *Phys Ther* 66(10):1548–1550, 1986.

74. Swanik CB, Lephart SM, Giannantonio FP, Fu FH. Reestablishing proprioception and neuromuscular control in the ACL-injured athlete. *J Sport Rehabil* 6(2):182–206, 1997.

75. Tippett S, Voight M. *Functional Progression for Sports Rehabilitation.* Champaign, IL, Human Kinetics, 1995.

76. Tropp H, Ekstrand J, Gillquist J. Factors affecting stabilometry recordings of single limb stance. *Am J Sports Med* 12:185–188, 1984.

77. Tropp H, Ekstrand J, Gillquist J. Stabilometry in functional instability of the ankle and its value in predicting injury. *Med Sci Sports Exerc* 16:64–66, 1984.

78. Tropp H, Odenrick P. Postural control in single limb stance. *J Orthop Res* 6:833–839, 1988.

79. Trulock SC. A comparison of static, dynamic and functional methods of objective balance assessment. Master's thesis, University of North Carolina, Chapel Hill, NC, 1996.

80. Vander A, Sherman J, Luciano D. *Human Physiology: The Mechanisms of Body Function*, 5th ed. New York, McGraw-Hill, 1990.

81. Voight M, Cook G. Clinical application of closed kinetic chain exercise. *J Sport Rehabil* 5(1):25–44, 1996.

82. Whitney S. Clinical and high tech alternatives to assessing postural sway in athletes. Paper presented at the annual meeting of the National Athletic Trainers' Association, Dallas, TX, June 11, 1994.

83. Wilk K, Zheng N, Fleisig G, Andrews J, Clancy W. Kinetic chain exercise: Implications for the anterior cruciate ligament patient. *J Sport Rehabil* 6(2):125–143, 1997.

84. Wilkerson G, Nitz J. Dynamic ankle stability: Mechanical and neuromuscular interrelationships. *J Sport Rehabil* 3:43–57, 1994.

CHAPTER 18

Core Stabilization Training in Rehabilitation

Barbara J. Hoogenboom and Jolene L. Bennett

OBJECTIVES

After completing this chapter, the therapist should be able to do the following:

- Describe the functional approach to kinetic chain rehabilitation.
- Define the concept of the core.
- Discuss the anatomic relationships between the muscular components of the core.
- Explain how the core functions to maintain postural alignment and dynamic postural equilibrium during functional activities.
- Describe procedures for assessing the core.
- Discuss the rationale for core stabilization training and relate to efficient functional performance of activities.
- Discuss the guidelines for core stabilization training.
- Identify appropriate exercises for core stabilization training and their progressions.

To stay on the cutting edge of research, science, and practical application, the clinician needs to follow a comprehensive, systematic, and integrated functional approach when rehabilitating a patient. To develop a comprehensive rehabilitation program, the clinician must fully understand the functional kinetic chain. In order to understand the kinetic chain, the clinician must first understand the definition of function. *Function* is integrated, multiplanar movement that requires acceleration, deceleration, and stabilization.[28,31,55] Functional kinetic chain rehabilitation is a comprehensive approach that strives to improve all components necessary to allow a patient to return to a high level of function. The clinician must understand that the kinetic chain operates as an integrated functional unit. Functional kinetic chain rehabilitation must therefore address each link in the kinetic chain and strive to develop functional strength and neuromuscular efficiency. Functional strength is the ability of the neuromuscular system to reduce force, produce force, and dynamically stabilize the kinetic chain during functional movements in a smooth and coordinated fashion.[1] Neuromuscular efficiency is the ability of the central nervous system (CNS) to allow agonists, antagonists, synergists, stabilizers, and neutralizers to work efficiently and interdependently during dynamic kinetic chain activities.[1]

Traditionally, rehabilitation has focused on isolated absolute strength gains, in isolated muscles, using single planes of motion. However, all functional activities are naturally multiplanar and require a blend of acceleration, deceleration, and dynamic stabilization.[27,31,55] Movement may appear to be one plane dominant, but the other planes need to be dynamically stabilized to allow for optimal neuromuscular efficiency.[1] Understanding that functional movements require a highly complex, integrated system allows the clinician to make a paradigm shift. The paradigm shift focuses on training the entire kinetic chain using all planes of movement and establishing high levels of functional strength and neuromuscular efficiency.[15,57,61,64,78,88] The paradigm shift dictates that we train to allow force reduction, force production, and dynamic stabilization to occur efficiently during all kinetic chain activities.[12,28].

A dynamic, core stabilization training program is an important component of all comprehensive functional rehabilitation programs.[10,13,22,23,28,31,55] A core stabilization program will improve dynamic postural control, ensure appropriate muscular balance, and affect joint arthrokinematics around the lumbo-pelvic-hip complex. A carefully crafted core stabilization program will allow for the expression of dynamic functional strength and improve neuromuscular efficiency throughout the entire kinetic chain.[1,11,16,28,29,31,51,61,64–66,88,89]

WHAT IS THE CORE?

The *core* is defined as the lumbo-pelvic-hip complex.[1,28] The core is where our center of gravity is located and where all movement begins.[33,34,78,79] There are 29 muscles that have an attachment to the lumbo-pelvic-hip complex.[7,8,28,80] An efficient core allows for maintenance of the normal length-tension relationship of functional agonists and antagonists, which allows for the maintenance of the normal force-couple relationships in the lumbo-pelvic-hip complex. Maintaining the normal length-tension relationships and force-couple relationships allows for the maintenance of optimal arthrokinematics in the lumbo-pelvic-hip complex during functional kinetic-chain movements.[88,89,96] This provides optimal neuromuscular efficiency in the entire kinetic chain, allowing for optimal acceleration, deceleration, and dynamic stabilization of the entire kinetic chain during functional movements. It also provides proximal stability for efficient lower-extremity and upper extremity movements.[1,28,33,34,43,55,78,79,88,89]

The core operates as an integrated functional unit, whereby the entire kinetic chain works synergistically to produce force, reduce force, and dynamically stabilize against abnormal force.[1] In an efficient state, each structural component distributes weight, absorbs force, and transfers ground reaction forces.[1] This integrated, interdependent system needs to be trained appropriately to allow it to function efficiently during dynamic kinetic-chain activities.

Core stabilization exercise programs have been labeled many different terms some of which include dynamic lumbar stabilization, neutral spine control, muscular fusion, and lumbopelvic stabilization. The authors of this chapter use the terms "butt and gut" to educate their patients, colleagues, and health care students. This catchy phrase illustrates the importance of the entire abdominal and pelvic region working together to provide functional stability and efficient movement.

CORE STABILIZATION TRAINING CONCEPTS

Many individuals develop the functional strength, power, neuromuscular control, and muscular endurance in specific muscles that enable them to perform functional activities.[1,28,46,55] However, few people develop the muscles required for spinal stabilization.[43,46,47] The body's stabilization system has to be functioning optimally to effectively use the strength, power, neuromuscular control, and muscular endurance developed in the prime movers. If the extremity muscles are strong and the core is weak, then there will not be enough trunk stabilization created to produce efficient upper extremity movements. A weak core is a fundamental problem of many inefficient movements that leads to injury.[43,46,47,55]

The core musculature is an integral component of the protective mechanism that relieves the spine of deleterious forces inherent during functional activities.[14] A core stabilization training program is designed to help an individual gain strength, neuromuscular control, power, and muscle endurance of the lumbo-pelvic-hip complex. This approach facilitates a balanced muscular functioning of the entire kinetic chain.[1] Greater neuromuscular control and stabilization strength will offer a more biomechanically efficient position for the entire kinetic chain therefore allowing optimal neuromuscular efficiency throughout the kinetic chain.

Neuromuscular efficiency is established by the appropriate combination of postural alignment (static/dynamic) and stability strength, which allows the body to decelerate gravity, ground reaction forces, and momentum at the right joint, in the right plane, and at the right time.[12,31,54] If the neuromuscular system is not efficient, it will be unable to respond to the demands placed on it during functional activities.[1] As the efficiency of the neuromuscular system decreases, the ability of the kinetic chain to maintain appropriate forces and dynamic stabilization decreases significantly. This decreased neuromuscular efficiency leads to compensation and substitution patterns, as well as poor posture during functional activities.[29,88,89] Such poor posture leads to increased mechanical stress on the contractile and non-contractile tissue, leading to repetitive microtrauma, abnormal biomechanics, and injury.[16,29,62,63]

REVIEW OF FUNCTIONAL ANATOMY

To fully understand functional core stabilization training and rehabilitation, the clinician must fully understand functional anatomy, lumbo-pelvic-hip complex stabilization mechanisms, and normal force-couple relationships.[4,7,8,80]

A review of the key lumbo-pelvic-hip complex musculature will allow the clinician to understand functional anatomy and therefore develop a comprehensive kinetic-chain rehabilitation program. The key lumbar spine muscles include the transversospinalis group, erector spinae, quadratus lumborum, and latissimus dorsi (Fig. 18-1). The key abdominal muscles include the rectus abdominus, external oblique, internal oblique, and transversus abdominus (TA) (Fig. 18-2). The key hip musculature includes the gluteus maximus, gluteus medius, and psoas (Fig. 18-3).

The transversospinalis group includes the rotatores, interspinales, intertransversarii, semispinalis, and multifidus. These muscles are small and have a poor mechanical advantage for contributing to motion.[27,80] They contain primarily type I muscle fibers and are therefore designed mainly for stabilization.[27,80] Researchers[80] have found that the transversospinalis muscle group contains two to six times the number of muscle spindles found in larger muscles. Therefore, it has been established

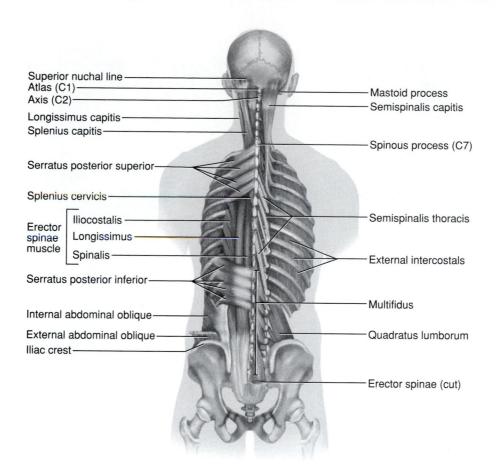

FIGURE 18-1

Spinal muscles.

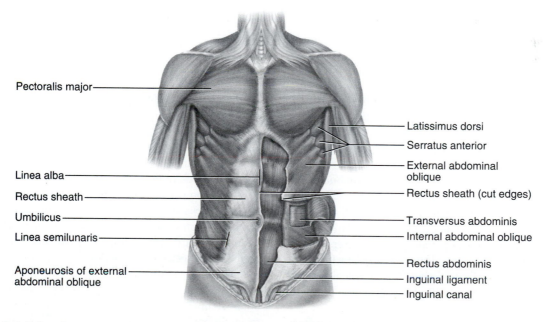

FIGURE 18-2

Abdominal muscles.

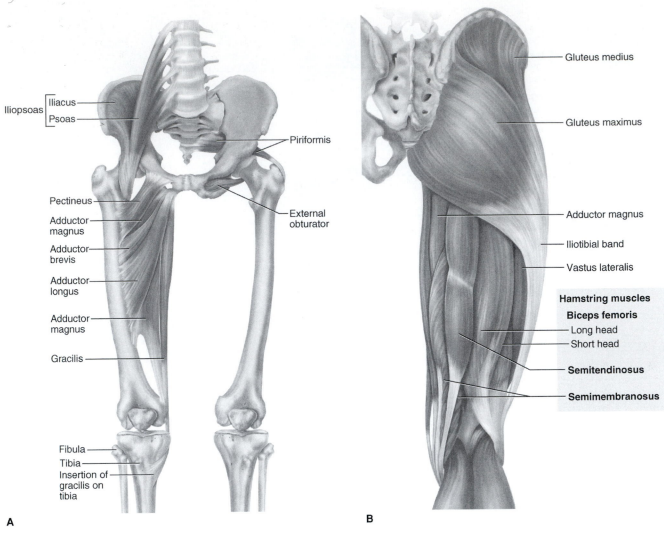

FIGURE 18-3

Hip muscles.

that this group is primarily responsible for providing the CNS with proprioceptive information.[80] This group is also responsible for inter- or intrasegmental stabilization and segmental eccentric deceleration of flexion and rotation of the spinal unit during functional movements.[4,80] The transversospinalis group is constantly put under a variety of compressive and tensile forces during functional movements and therefore needs to be trained adequately to allow dynamic postural stabilization and optimal neuromuscular efficiency of the entire kinetic chain.[80] The multifidus is the most important of the transversospinalis muscles. It has the ability to provide intrasegmental stabilization to the lumbar spine in all positions.[27,97] Wilke et al.[97] found increased segmental stiffness at L4-L5 with activation of the multifidus.

Additional key back muscles include the erector spinae, quadratus lumborum, and the latissimus dorsi. The erector spinae muscle group functions to provide dynamic interseg-

mental stabilization and eccentric deceleration of trunk flexion and rotation during kinetic-chain activities.[80] The quadratus lumborum muscle functions primarily as a frontal plane stabilizer that works synergistically with the gluteus medius and tensor fascia lata. The latissimus dorsi has the largest moment arm of all back muscles and therefore has the greatest effect on the lumbo-pelvic-hip complex. The latissimus dorsi is the bridge between the upper extremity and the lumbo-pelvic-hip complex. Any functional upper-extremity kinetic-chain rehabilitation pay particular attention to the latissimus and its function on the lumbo-pelvic-hip complex.[80]

The abdominals are made up of four muscles: rectus abdominus, external oblique, internal oblique, and TA.[80] The abdominals operate as an integrated functional unit, which helps maintain optimal spinal kinematics.[4,7,8,80] When working efficiently, the abdominals offer sagittal, frontal, and transversus plane stabilization by controlling forces that reach the lumbo-pelvic-hip complex.[80] The rectus abdominus eccentrically decelerates trunk extension and lateral flexion, as well as providing dynamic stabilization during functional movements. The external obliques work concentrically to produce contralateral rotation and ipsilateral lateral flexion, and work eccentrically to decelerate trunk extension, rotation, and lateral flexion during functional movements.[80] The internal oblique works concentrically to produce ipsilateral rotation and lateral flexion and works eccentrically to decelerate extension, rotation, and lateral flexion. The internal oblique attaches to the posterior layer of the thoracolumbar fascia. Contraction of the internal oblique creates a lateral tension force on the thoracolumbar fascia, which creates intrinsic translational and rotational stabilization of the spinal unit.[34,43] The TA is probably the most important of the abdominal muscles. The TA functions to increase intra-abdominal pressure (IAP), provide dynamic stabilization against rotational and translational stress in the lumbar spine, and provide optimal neuromuscular efficiency to the entire lumbo-pelvic-hip complex.[43,46–48,58] Research has demonstrated that the TA works in a feed-forward mechanism.[43] Researchers have demonstrated that contraction of the TA precedes the initiation of limb movement and all other abdominal muscles, regardless of the direction of reactive forces.[26,43] Cresswell et al.[25,26] demonstrated that like the multifidus, the TA is active during all trunk movements, suggesting that this muscle has an important role in dynamic stabilization.[46]

Key hip muscles include the psoas, gluteus medius, gluteus maximus, and hamstrings.[7,8,80] The psoas produces hip flexion and external rotation in the open chain position. The psoas produces hip flexion, lumbar extension, lateral flexion, and rotation in the closed-chain position. The psoas eccentrically decelerates hip extension and internal rotation, as well as trunk extension, lateral flexion, and rotation. The psoas works synergistically with the superficial erector spinae and creates an anterior shear force at L4-L5.[80] The deep erector spinae, multifidus, and deep abdominal wall (transversus, internal oblique, and external oblique)[80] counteract this force. It is extremely common for clients to develop tightness in their psoas. A tight psoas increases the anterior shear force and compressive force at the L4-L5 junction.[80] A tight psoas also causes reciprocal inhibition of the gluteus maximus, multifidus, deep erector spinae, internal oblique, and TA. This leads to extensor mechanism dysfunction during functional movement patterns.[51,61,63,65,66,80,89] Lack of lumbo-pelvic-hip complex stabilization prevents appropriate movement sequencing and leads to synergistic dominance by the hamstrings and superficial erector spinae during hip extension. This complex movement dysfunction also decreases the ability of the gluteus maximus to decelerate femoral internal rotation during heel strike, which predisposes an individual with a knee ligament injury to abnormal forces and repetitive microtrauma.[14,19,51,65,66]

The gluteus medius functions as the primary frontal plane stabilizer of the pelvis and lower extremity during functional movements.[80] During closed-chain movements, the gluteus medius decelerates femoral adduction and internal rotation.[80] A weak gluteus medius increases frontal and transversus plane stress at the patellofemoral joint and the tibiofemoral joint.[80] A weak gluteus medius leads to synergistic dominance of the tensor fascia latae and the quadratus lumborum.[19,51,53] This leads to tightness in the iliotibial band and the lumbar spine. This will affect the normal biomechanics of the lumbo-pelvic-hip complex and the tibiofemoral joint as well as the patellofemoral joint. Research by Beckman and Buchanan[9] has demonstrated decreased electromyogram (EMG) activity of the gluteus medius following an ankle sprain. Clinicians must address the altered hip muscle recruitment patterns or accept this recruitment pattern as an injury-adaptive strategy and thus accept the unknown long-term consequences of premature muscle activation and synergistic dominance.[9,29]

The gluteus maximus functions concentrically in the open chain to accelerate hip extension and external rotation. It functions eccentrically to decelerate hip flexion and femoral internal rotation.[80] It also functions through the Iliotibial band to decelerate tibial internal rotation.[80] The gluteus maximus is a major dynamic stabilizer of the sacroiliac (SI) joint. It has the greatest capacity to provide increased compressive forces at the SI joint secondary to its anatomic attachment at the sacrotuberous ligament.[80] It has been demonstrated by Bullock-Saxton[15,16] that the EMG activity of the gluteus maximus is decreased following an ankle sprain. Lack of proper gluteus maximus activity during functional activities leads to pelvic instability and decreased neuromuscular control. This can eventually lead to the development of muscle imbalances, poor movement patterns, and injury.

The hamstrings work concentrically to flex the knee, extend the hip, and rotate the tibia. They work eccentrically to decelerate knee extension, hip flexion, and tibial rotation. The hamstrings work synergistically with the anterior cruciate ligament.[80] All of the muscles mentioned play an integral role in the kinetic chain by providing dynamic stabilization and optimal neuromuscular control of the entire lumbo-pelvic-hip complex. These muscles have been reviewed so the clinician realizes that muscles not only produce force (concentric contractions) in one plane of motion, but also reduce force (eccentric contractions) and provide dynamic stabilization in all planes of movement during functional activities. When isolated, these muscles do not effectively achieve stabilization of the lumbo-pelvic-hip complex. It is the synergistic, interdependent functioning of the entire lumbo-pelvic-hip complex that enhances the stability and neuromuscular control throughout the entire kinetic chain.

TA AND MULTIFIDUS ROLE IN CORE STABILIZATION

The TA muscle is the deepest of the abdominal muscles and plays a primary role in trunk stability. The horizontal orientation of its fibers has a limited ability to produce torque to the spine necessary for flexion or extension movement although it has been shown to be an active trunk rotator.[81] The TA is a primary trunk stabilizer via modulation of IAP, tension through the thoracolumbar fascia and compression of the SI joints.[25,91] For many decades, IAP was believed to be an important contributor to spinal control by the pressure within the abdominal cavity putting force on the diaphragm superiorly and pelvic floor inferiorly to extend the trunk.[6,35,73] It was hypothesized that the IAP would provide an extensor moment and thus reduce the muscular force required by the trunk extensors and decrease the compressive load on the lumbar spine.[95] Recent research by Hodges et al.[42] utilized electrical stimulation applied to the phrenic nerve of humans to produce an involuntary increase in IAP without abdominal or extensor muscle activity. IAP was increased by the contraction of the diaphragm, pelvic floor muscles, and the TA with no flexor moment noted. It has been demonstrated through research that IAP may directly increase spinal stiffness.[45] Hodges et al.[42] used a tetanic contraction of the diaphragm to produce IAP which resulted in increased stiffness in the spine. Bilateral contraction of the TA assists in IAP and thus enhances spinal stiffness.

The role of the thoracolumbar fascia in trunk stability has also been discussed in the literature, and it has been theorized that the contraction of the TA could produce an extensor torque via the horizontal pull of the TA via its extensive attachment into the thoracolumbar fascia.[34] Recently, this theory was tested by Tesh et al.[93] by placing tension on the thoracolumbar fascia of cadavers. No approximation of the spinous processes or trunk extension movement was noted although a small amount of compression on the spine was noted. This small amount of compression may play a role in the control of intervertebral shear forces. Hodges et al.[42] electrically stimulated contraction of the TA in pigs and demonstrated that when tension was developed in the thoracolumbar fascia, without an associated increase in IAP, there was no significant effect on the intervertebral stiffness. In the next step of that same research study, the thorocolumbar fascial attachments were cut and an increase in IAP decreased the spinal stiffness. This demonstrates that the thoracolumbar fascia and IAP work in concert to enhance trunk stability.[42] Trunk stability is also dependent on the joints caudal to the lumbar spine. The SI joint is the connection between the lumbar spine and the pelvic region, which ultimately connects the trunk to the lower extremities. The SI joint is dependent on the compressive force between the sacrum and ilia. The horizontal direction and anterior attachment on the ilium of the TA produces the compressive force necessary for spinal stability. Richardson et al.[84] utilized ultrasound to detect movement of the sacrum and ilium while having subjects voluntarily contract their transverse abdominals. They demonstrated that a voluntary contraction of the TA reduced the laxity of the SI joint. This study also pointed out that this reduction in joint laxity of the SI joint was greater than that during a bracing contraction. The researchers did note that they were unable to

exclude changes in activity in other muscles such as the pelvic floor, which may have reduced the laxity via counternutation of the sacrum.[84] The aforementioned research findings illustrate that the TA plays an important role in maintaining trunk stability by interacting with IAP, thoracolumbar fascia tension, and compressing the SI joints via muscular attachments.

The multifidi are the most medial of the posterior trunk muscles, and they cover the lumbar zygapophyseal joints except for the ventral surfaces.[81] The multifidi are primary stabilizers and when the trunk is moving from flexion to extension. The multifidi contribute only 20 percent of the total lumbar extensor moment, while the lumbar erector spinae contribute 30 percent, and the thoracic erector spinae function as the predominant torque generator at 50 percent of the extension moment arm.[56] The multifidus, lumbar, and thoracic erector spinae muscles have a high percentage of type I fibers and are postural control muscles similar to the TA.[56] The multifidus has been shown to be active during all antigravity activities including static tasks, such as standing, and dynamic tasks, such as walking.[97]

Clinical observation and experimental evidence confirm that when the TA contracts, the multifidi are also activated.[81] A girdlelike cylinder of muscular support is produced due to the coactivation of the TA, multifidus, and the thick thoracolumbar fascial system. EMG evidence suggests that the TA and internal obliques contract in anticipation of movement of the upper and lower extremities, often referred to as the feed forward mechanism. This feed forward mechanism gives the TA and multifidus muscular girdle a unique ability to stabilize the spine regardless of the direction of limb movements.[44,45] Figure 18-4 illustrates this "hooplike" connection between the TA and multifidus and its function as a deep ring of muscular stability.

As noted previously, the pelvic floor muscles play an important role in the development of IAP and thus enhance trunk stability. It has also been demonstrated that the pelvic floor is active during repetitive arm movement tasks independent on the direction of movement.[49] Sapsford et al.[90] discovered that maximal contractions of the pelvic floor was associated with activity of all abdominal muscles and submaximal contraction of the pelvic floor muscles was associated with a more isolated contraction of the TA. In this same study it was also determined that the specificity of the response was better when the lumbar spine and pelvis were in a neutral position.[90] Clinically this information is helpful in guiding the patient in the process of TA contraction by instructing them to perform a submaximal pelvic floor isometric hold. Another interesting fact to note is that men and women with incontinence have almost a double the incidence of low back pain than people without incontinence issues.[30] In summary, the lumbopelvic region may be visualized as a cylinder with the inferior wall being the pelvic floor, the superior wall being the diaphragm, the posterior wall being the multifidus, and the transversus abdominal muscles forming the anterior and lateral walls. All walls of the cylinder must be activated and taut for optimal

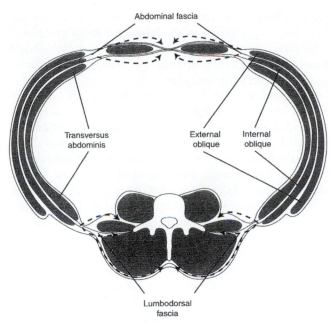

FIGURE 18-4

Hoop like ring of stability. (Reproduced, with permission, from McGill S. *Low Back Disorders*. Champaign, IL, Human Kinetics, 2002, p. 81.)

trunk stabilization to occur with all static and dynamic activities (see Fig. 18-5).

POSTURAL CONSIDERATIONS

The core functions to maintain postural alignment and dynamic postural equilibrium during functional activities. Optimal alignment of each body part is a cornerstone to a functional training and rehabilitation program. Optimal posture and alignment will allow for maximal neuromuscular efficiency because the normal length-tension relationship, force-couple relationship, and arthrokinematics will be maintained during functional movement patterns.[14,28,29,50,51,53,55,58,62,64,88,89] If one segment in the kinetic chain is out of alignment, it will create predictable patterns of dysfunction throughout the entire kinetic chain. These predictable patterns of dysfunction are referred to as *serial distortion patterns*.[28] Serial distortion patterns represent the state in which the body's structural integrity is compromised because segments in the kinetic chain are out of alignment. This leads to abnormal distorting forces being placed on the segments in the kinetic chain that are above and below the dysfunctional segment.[14,28,29,55] To avoid serial distortion patterns and the chain reaction that one misaligned segment creates, we must emphasize stable positions to maintain the structural integrity of the entire kinetic chain.[16,28,55,65,66] A comprehensive core stabilization program will prevent the development of serial distortion patterns and

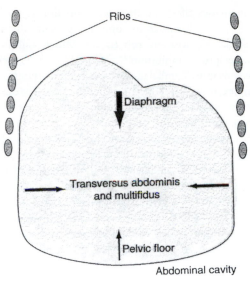

FIGURE 18-5

Lumbopelvic cylinder. (Reproduced, with permission, from Richardson C, Jull G, Hodges P, Hides J. *Therapeutic Exercise for Spinal Segemental Stabilzation In Low Back Pain*. Philadelphia, PA, Churchill Livingstone, 1999, p. 95.)

provide optimal dynamic postural control during functional movements.

MUSCULAR IMBALANCES

An optimally functioning core helps to prevent the development of muscle imbalances and synergistic dominance. The human movement system is a well-orchestrated system of interrelated and interdependent components.[16,61] The functional interaction of each component in the human movement system allows for optimal neuromuscular efficiency. Alterations in joint arthrokinematics, muscular balance, and neuromuscular control affect the optimal functioning of the entire kinetic chain.[16,88,89] Dysfunction of the kinetic chain is rarely an isolated event. Typically a pathology of the kinetic chain is part of a chain reaction involving some key links in the kinetic chain and numerous compensations and adaptations that develop.[61] The interplay of many muscles about a joint is responsible for the coordinated control of movement. If the core is weak, normal arthrokinematics are altered. Changes in normal length-tension and force-couple relationships, in turn affect neuromuscular control. If one muscle becomes weak, tight, or changes its degree of activation, then synergists, stabilizers, and neutralizers have to compensate.[16,29,61,64–66,88,89] Muscle tightness has a significant impact on the kinetic chain. Muscle tightness affects the normal length-tension relationship.[89] This impacts the normal force-couple relationship. When one muscle in a force couple becomes tight, it changes the normal arthrokinematics of two articular partners.[14,61,89] Altered arthrokinematics affect the synergistic function of the kinetic chain.[14,29,61,89] This leads to abnormal pressure distribution over articular surfaces and soft tissues. Muscle tightness also leads to reciprocal inhibition.[14,29,50–53,61,92,96] Therefore, if one develops muscle imbalances throughout the lumbo-pelvic-hip complex, it can affect the entire kinetic chain. For example, a tight psoas causes reciprocal inhibition of the gluteus maximus, TA, internal oblique, and multifidus.[47,51,53,77,80] This muscle imbalance pattern may decrease normal lumbo-pelvic-hip stability. Specific substitution patterns develop to compensate for the lack of stabilization, including tightness in the iliotibial band.[29] This muscle imbalance pattern will lead to increased frontal and transverse plane stress at the knee. Dr. Vladamir Janda has proposed a syndrome named the "crossed pelvis syndrome" in which a weak abdominal wall and weak gluteals are counterbalanced with tight hamstrings and hip flexors.[51] A strong core with optimal neuromuscular efficiency can help to prevent the development of muscle imbalances. Therefore, a comprehensive core stabilization training program should be an integral component of all rehabilitation programs. A strong, efficient core provides the stable base upon which the extremities can function with maximal precision and effectiveness. It is important to remember that the spine, pelvis, and hips must be positioned in proper alignment with proper activation of all muscles during any core strengthening exercise. No one muscle works in isolation, thus attention should be paid to the position and activity of all muscles during open- and closed-chain exercises.

NEUROMUSCULAR CONSIDERATIONS

A strong and stable core can improve optimal neuromuscular efficiency throughout the entire kinetic chain by helping to improve dynamic postural control.[37,43,47,57,83,88,89] A number of authors have demonstrated kinetic-chain imbalances in individuals with altered neuromuscular control.[9,14–16,43,46–48,50–54,61–66,76,77,83,88] Research has demonstrated that people with low back pain have an abnormal neuromotor response of the trunk stabilizers accompanying limb movement, significantly greater postural sway and decreased limits of stability.[46,47,77] Research has also demonstrated that approximately 70 percent of patients suffer from recurrent episodes of back pain. Furthermore, it has been demonstrated that individuals have decreased dynamic postural stability in the proximal stabilizers of the lumbo-pelvic-hip complex following lower-extremity ligamentous injuries,[9,14–16] and that joint and ligamentous injury can lead to decreased muscle activity.[29,92,96] Joint and ligament injury can lead to joint effusion, which in turn leads to muscle inhibition. This leads to altered neuromuscular control in other segments of the kinetic chain secondary to altered proprioception and kinesthesia.[9,16] Therefore, when an individual with a knee ligament injury has joint effusion, all of the muscles that

cross the knee can be inhibited. Several muscles that cross the knee joint are attached to the lumbo-pelvic-hip complex.[80] Therefore, a comprehensive rehabilitation approach should focus on reestablishing optimal core function in order to positively affect peripheral joints.

Research has also demonstrated that muscles can be inhibited from an arthrokinetic reflex.[14,61,92,96] This is referred to as athrogenic muscle inhibition. Arthrokinetic reflexes are mediated by joint receptor activity. If an individual has abnormal arthrokinematics, the muscles that move the joint will be inhibited. For example, if an individual has a sacral torsion, the multifidus and the gluteus medius can be inhibited.[41] This will lead to abnormal movement in the kinetic chain. The tensor fascia latae will become synergistically dominant and the primary frontal plane stabilizer.[80] This can lead to tightness in the iliotibial band. This can also decrease the frontal and transverse plane control at the knee. Furthermore, if the multifidus is inhibited,[41] the erector spinae and the psoas become facilitated. This will further inhibit the lower abdominals (internal oblique and TA) and the gluteus maximus.[43,46] This also decreases frontal and transverse plane stability at the knee. As previously mentioned, an efficient core will improve neuromuscular efficiency of the entire kinetic chain by providing dynamic stabilization of the lumbo-pelvic-hip complex and therefore improve pelvofemoral biomechanics. This is yet another reason that all rehabilitation programs should include a comprehensive core stabilization training program.

ASSESSMENT OF THE CORE

Before a comprehensive core stabilization program is implemented, an individual must undergo a comprehensive assessment to determine muscle imbalances, arthrokinematic deficits, core strength, core muscle endurance, core neuromuscular control, core power, and overall function of the lower-extremity kinetic chain. Assessment tools include activity-based tests that are performed in the clinical setting, EMG with surface or indwelling electrodes, and technologically advanced testing and training techniques using real-time ultrasound. Real-time ultrasound has been used extensively in research settings and has been proven to be a reliable tool in evaluating the activation patterns of various abdominal muscles.[38,94] Real-time ultrasound, although not currently readily available in clinical settings, is a great asset in the laboratory setting. Perhaps, the future will allow for more use of real-time ultrasound in clinical practice.

It has been previously stated that muscle imbalances and arthrokinematic deficits can cause abnormal movement patterns to develop throughout the entire kinetic chain. It is therefore extremely important to thoroughly assess each individual with a kinetic-chain dysfunction for muscle imbalances and arthrokinematic deficits. It is recommended that the interested reader use the reference list to explain

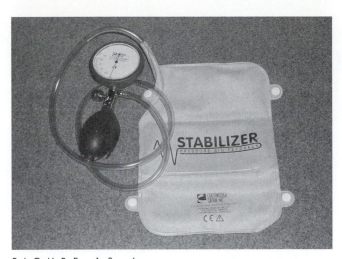

FIGURE   18-6

Stabilizer® pressure feedback unit.

a comprehensive muscle imbalance assessment procedure thoroughly.[1,14,19,22,23,28,48,52,54,55,64,88,89,96]

Core strength can be assessed by using the straight leg-lowering test (Fig. 18-4).[3,48,58,76,88,89] The individual is placed supine. A pressure biofeedback device called the Stabilizer® (see Fig. 18-6) is placed under the lumbar spine at approximately L4-L5. The cuff pressure is raised to 40 mm Hg. The individual's legs are maintained in full extension while flexing the hips to 90°. The individual is instructed to perform a drawing-in maneuver (pull belly button to spine) and then flatten the back maximally into the table and pressure cuff. The individual is instructed to lower the legs toward the table while maintaining the back flat. The test is over when the pressure in the cuff decreases. The hip angle is then measured with a goniometer to determine the angle (see Fig. 18-7). Using the Kendall[59] rating scale, this test gives you a basic idea how strong the lower abdominal muscle groups (rectus abdominus and external obliques) are

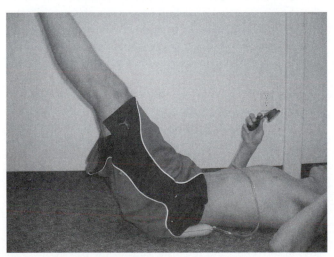

FIGURE   18-7

Abdominal strength assessed using leg-lowering test.

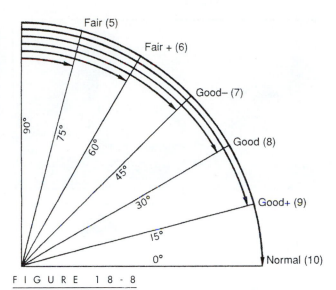

FIGURE   18-8

Key to muscle grading. See numerical equivalents for word symbols used in grading. (Reproduced, with permission, from Kendall FP, McCreary EK, Provance PG, Rodgers MM, Romani WA. *Muscles Testing and Function*, 5th ed. Baltimore, MD, Lippincott Williams & Wilkins, 2005: p. 155.)

(see Fig. 18-8 for a general guideline of Kendall strength measures). Using the pressure feedback device ensures that there is no compensation with the lumbar extensors or large hip flexors to stabilize the long lever arm of the legs.

As noted previously in this chapter, decreased core muscular endurance has been implicated in patients with low back pain. Biering-Sorensen[11] demonstrated that decreased trunk extensor endurance predicts those who are at greater risk of low back pain. McGill et al.[70] also demonstrated that the balance of endurance among the trunk extensors, flexors, and lateral trunk muscles may better discriminate between people with and without low back pain. These endurance tests developed by McGill[70] have shown to have high reliability coefficients and are easy test to administer in the clinical setting.

Testing for the trunk flexors begins with the subject in a sit-up type posture with their back resting on a box that is angled at 60° from the floor. Both knees and hips are flexed to 90°, the arms folded across the chest, and toes secured under an external support (see Fig. 18-9). The test is measured in seconds, and the stopwatch is started when the box is pulled back 10 cm (4 in). The person holds the isometric posture as long as possible, and the test time is finished when any part of the subjects' back touches the box.[70]

The lateral trunk muscle endurance test is performed with the person lying in the full side-bridge position (see Fig. 18-10). Legs are extended, and the top foot is placed in front of the lower foot for support. Subjects support themselves on one elbow and their feet while lifting their hips off the floor to create a straight line over their body length. The uninvolved arm is held across the chest with the hand placed on the

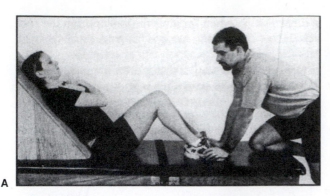

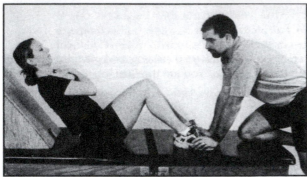

FIGURE   18-9

Flexor endurance test. (Reproduced, with permission, from McGill S. *Low Back Disorders*. Champaign, IL, Human Kinetics, 2002, p. 226.)

opposite shoulder. The test is timed in seconds from the point when the hips are off the ground and the body is in a straight line until the person loses the straight back posture and the hip returns to the ground.[70] The trunk extensors are tested in the "Biering-Sorensen position" with the upper body unsupported out over the end of a plinth table and the pelvis, knees, and hips secured (see Fig. 18-11.) The upper limbs are held across the chest with the hands resting on the opposite shoulders. The test time is the time the trunk remains in a straight horizontal plane.[70]

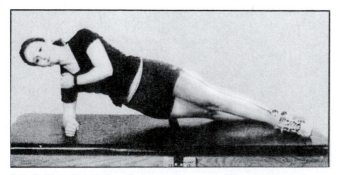

FIGURE   18-10

Lateral muscular test. (Reproduced, with permission, from McGill S. *Low Back Disorders*, Champaign, IL, Human Kinetics, 2002, p. 225.)

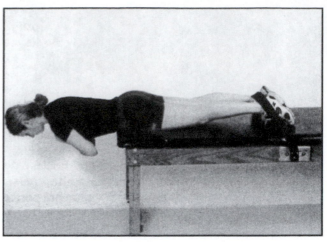

FIGURE   18-11

Back extensors test lateral muscular test. (Reproduced, with permission, from McGill S. *Low Back Disorders*. Champaign, IL, Human Kinetics, 2002, p. 226.)

McGill and colleagues have collected normative data for the aforementioned endurance tests (see Table 18-1 for mean times in seconds and ratios normalized to the extensor endurance test score for normal subjects with the mean age of 21; $n = 92$ men and $n = 137$ women). Note that women had greater trunk extensor endurance than the men. McGill et al. performed these three endurance tests on a group of men with and without low back pain history. All subjects were free of back pain at the time of testing (see Table 18-2 for details). Comparison of Table 18-1 and 18-2 shows that there is a difference in endurance ratios when subjects have a history of low back pain, even when the symptoms have been resolved for greater than 6 months. The extensor endurance is diminished relative to both the flexors and the lateral musculature in subjects with a history of low back pain.[71] McGill has developed the following endurance ratios to determine if imbalances exist (Table 18-3). This data is a general guideline for the clinician to reference but more research is needed to draw strong conclusions about endurance ratios and injury prevalence. Likewise, the normative data must be used with caution because the average age is 21.[70]

Neuromuscular control of the deep core muscles, TA, and multifidi are evaluated with the quality of movement emphasized rather than quanity of muscular strength or endurance time. Unfortunately, no objectifiable manual muscle test exists for either of these important muscles/muscle groups. In order to attempt to objectively examine these groups, Hides et al.[40] have developed prone and supine tests to evaluate the muscular coordination of the TA and multifidus. The first test for the TA is performed in the prone position with the Stabilizer pressure biofeedback unit placed under the abdomen with the navel in the center and the distal edge of the pad in line with the right and left anterior superior iliac spines. The pressure pad is inflated to 70 mm Hg. It is important to instruct the

TABLE 18-1

Mean Endurance Times (Seconds) and Ratios Normalized to the Extensor Endurance Test Score[69]

TEST	MEN MEAN	SD	WOMEN MEAN	SD	ALL MEAN	SD
Extension test	161	61	185	60	173	62
Flexion test	136	66	134	81	134	76
Right lateral test	95	32	75	32	83	33
Left lateral test	99	37	78	32	86	36
Flexion/extension ratio	0.84		0.72		0.77	
Right lateral/left lateral ratio	0.96		0.96		0.96	
Right lateral/extension ratio	0.58		0.40		0.48	
Left lateral/extension ratio	0.61		0.42		0.50	

Mean age 21 years (men = 92; women = 137). SD = standard deviation.

patient to relax their abdomen fully prior to the start of the test. The patient is then instructed to take a relaxed breath in and out and then, without breathing in, draw the abdomen in toward the spine without taking a breath (see Fig. 18-12). The patient is asked to hold this contraction for a minimum of 10 seconds with a slow and controlled release. Optimal performance, indicating proper neuromuscular control of the TA, would be a 4–10-mm Hg reduction in the pressure with no pelvic or spinal movement noted. It is important to monitor pelvic and lower extremity positioning as the patient may compensate by putting pressure through their legs or tilting their pelvis to elevate the lower abdomen rather than isolating the TA contraction.

Testing for the TA is also performed in the supine position and relies on palpation and visualization of the lower abdomen. Instructions to the patient remain the same as the prone test and the clinician palpates for bilateral TA contraction just medially and inferiorly to the anterior superior iliac spines and lateral to the rectus abdominus (see Fig. 18-13). The Stabilizer pad may also be placed under the lower lumbar region to monitor if compensation occurs with pelvis. The pressure reading should remain the same throughout the test. If the pressure reading changes, this indicates that the patient is tilting his/her pelvis anteriorly (pressure decreases) or posteriorly (pressure increases) in an attempt to flatten his/her lower abdomen. The patient is asked to hold this contraction for a minimum of 10 seconds

TABLE 18-2

Mean Endurance Times (Seconds) Comparing Normal Workers With Those Who Have Had Back Disorders[69]

TEST	NO BACK DISORDERS MEAN (SEC)	SD	HISTORY BACK DISORDERS MEAN (SEC)	SD
Extension	103	35	90	49
Flexion	66	23	84	45
Right lateral test	54	21	58	23
Left lateral test	54	22	65	27
Flexion/extension ratio	0.71		1.15	
Right lateral/left lateral ratio	1.05		0.93	
Right lateral/extension ratio	0.57		0.97	
Left lateral/extension ratio	0.58		1.03	

Men, mean age = 34 years (n = 24 have never had back troubles, n = 26 lost work due to low back disorders) from same workplace. Note that all men were asymptomatic at time of testing.
SD = standard deviation.

TABLE 18-3

Endurance Test Ratio Discrepancies That May Suggest Trunk Muscular Endurance Imbalances[69]

Right lateral test/left lateral test endurance	>0.05
Flexion/extension endurance	>1.0
Lateral test (either side)/ extensor endurance	>0.75

with a slow and controlled release. With a correct contraction of the TA, the clinician feels a slowly developing deep tension in the lower abdominal wall. Incorrect activation of the TA would be evident when the internal oblique dominates and this is detected when a rapid development of tension is palpated or the abdominal wall is pushed out rather than drawn in.

The neuromuscular control of the multifidi are examined with the patient in the prone position and the clinician palpating the level of the multifidus for muscular activation. The patient is instructed to breath in and then out and to hold the breath out while swelling out the muscles under the clinician's fingers. The patient is then asked to hold the contraction while resuming a normal breathing pattern for a minimum of 10 seconds. The clinician palpates the multifidus for symmetrical activation and slow development of muscular activation. This sequence is repeated at the multiple segments in the lumbar spine (see Fig. 18-14). Compensation patterns may include anterior or posterior pelvic tilting or elevation of the rib cage in an attempt to swell out the multifidus.

A proper and thorough evaluation of the core muscles will lead the clinician in developing a proper core stabilization program. It is imperative that neuromuscular control of the TA and multifidus precedes all other stabilization exercises. These muscles provide the foundation from which all the other care muscles work.

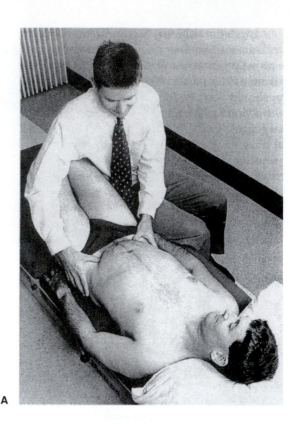

A

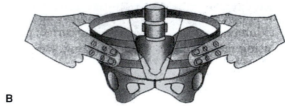

B

FIGURE 18-13

Supine transverse abdominal test. (Reproduced, with Permission, from Richardson C, Hodges P, Hides J. *Therapeutic Exercise for Lumbopelvic Stabilization*, 2nd ed. Philadelphia, PA, Churchill Livingstone, 2004, p. 192.)

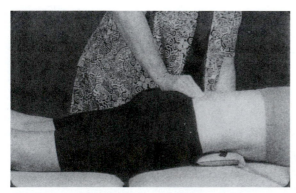

FIGURE 18-12

Prone transverse abdominal test. (Reproduced, with permission, from Richardson C, Hodges P, Hides J. *Therapeutic Exercise for Lumbopelvic Stabilization*, 2nd ed. Philadelphia, PA, Churchill Livingstone, 2004, p. 186.)

SCIENTIFIC RATIONALE FOR CORE STABILIZATION TRAINING

Most individuals train their core stabilizers inadequately compared to other muscle groups.[1] Although adequate strength, power, muscle endurance, and neuromuscular control are important for lumbo-pelvic-hip stabilization, performing exercises incorrectly or that are too advanced is detrimental. Several authors have found decreased firing of the TA, internal oblique, multifidus, and deep erector spinae in individuals with chronic low back pain.[43,46–48,77,82] Performing core training with inhibition of these key stabilizers leads to the development of muscle imbalances and inefficient neuromuscular control in the

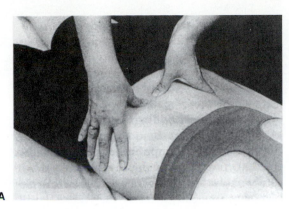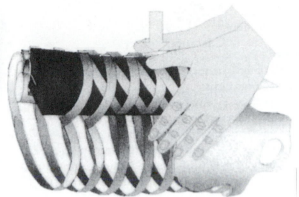

FIGURE 18-14

Prone multifidus test. (Reproduced, with permission, from Richardson C, Hodges P, Hides J. *Therapeutic Exercise for Lumbopelvic Stabilization*, 2nd ed. Philadelphia, PA, Churchill Livingstone, 2004, p. 196.)

kinetic chain. It has been demonstrated that abdominal training without proper pelvic stabilization increases intradiscal pressure and compressive forces in the lumbar spine.[3,10,43,46-48,74,75] Furthermore, it has been demonstrated that hyperextension training without proper pelvic stabilization can increase intradiscal pressure to dangerous levels, cause buckling of the ligamentum flavum, and lead to narrowing of the intervertebral foramen.[3,10,75]

Research has also demonstrated decreased stabilization endurance in individuals with chronic low back pain.[10,18,33,34] The core stabilizers are primarily type I slow-twitch muscle fibers.[33,34,78,79] These muscles respond best to time under tension. Time under tension is a method of contraction that lasts for 6–20 seconds and emphasizes hypercontractions at end ranges of motion. This method improves intramuscular coordination, which improves static and dynamic stabilization. To get the appropriate training stimulus, you must prescribe the appropriate speed of movement for all aspects of exercises.[22,23] Core strength endurance must be trained appropriately to allow an individual to maintain dynamic postural control for prolonged periods of time.[3]

Research has demonstrated decreased cross-sectional area of the multifidus in subjects with low back pain and that there was not spontaneous recovery of the multifidus following resolution of symptoms.[41] It has also been demonstrated that the traditional curl up increases intradiscal pressure and increases compressive forces at L2-L3.[3,10,74,75]

Additional research has demonstrated increased EMG activity and pelvic stabilization when an abdominal drawing-in maneuver was performed prior to initiating core training.[3,10,13,22,36,37,48,72,76,83] Also, maintaining the cervical spine in a neutral position during core training will improve posture, muscle balance, and stabilization. If the head protracts during movement, then the sternocleidomastoid is preferentially recruited. This increases the compressive forces at C0-C1 vertebral junction. This can also lead to pelvic insta-

bility and muscle imbalances secondary to the pelvo-occular reflex. This reflex is important to maintain the eyes level.[62,63] If the sternocleidomastoid muscle is hyperactive and extends the upper cervical spine, then the pelvis will rotate anteriorly to realign the eyes. This can lead to muscle imbalances and decreased pelvic stabilization.[62,63]

GUIDELINES FOR CORE STABILIZATION TRAINING

As discussed previously, prior to performing a comprehensive core stabilization program, each individual must undergo a comprehensive evaluation. All muscle imbalances and arthrokinematic deficits need to be corrected prior to initiating an aggressive core-training program.

A comprehensive core stabilization training program should be systematic, progressive, and functional. The rehabilitation program should emphasize the entire muscle contraction spectrum, focusing on force production (concentric contractions), force reduction (eccentric contractions), and dynamic stabilization (isometric contractions). The core stabilization program should begin in the most challenging environment the individual can control. A progressive continuum of function should be followed to systematically progress the individual. The program should be manipulated regularly by changing any of the following variables: plane of motion, range of motion, loading parameters (physioball, medicine ball, Bodyblade®, power sports trainer, weight vest, dumbbell, tubing), body position, amount of control, speed of execution, amount of feedback, duration (sets, reps, tempo, time under tension), and frequency.[1,10,12,13,16,21-24,28,31,32,36,48,54,55,57,60,64,67-69,75,76,88,89] (Please refer to Tables 18-4 to 18-8.)

T A B L E   1 8 - 4

Program Variation

1. Plane of motion
2. Range of motion
3. Loading parameter
4. Body position
5. Speed of movement
6. Amount of control
7. Duration
8. Frequency

Specific Core Stabilization Guidelines

When designing a functional core stabilization training program, the clinician should create a proprioceptively enriched environment and select the appropriate exercises to elicit a maximal training response. The exercises must be safe and challenging, stress multiple planes, incorporate a multisensory environment, be derived from fundamental movement skills, and be activity specific.

The clinician should follow a progressive functional continuum to allow optimal adaptations.[28,31,36,55] The following are key concepts for proper exercise progression: slow to fast, simple to complex, known to unknown, low force to high force, eyes open to eyes closed, static to dynamic, and correct execution to increased reps/sets/intensity.[21,22,28,31,36,55]

The goal of core stabilization should be to develop optimal levels of functional strength and dynamic stabilization.[1,10] Neural adaptations become the focus of the program instead of striving for absolute strength gains.[14,28,52,76] Increasing proprioceptive demand by utilizing a multisensory, multimodal (tubing, Bodyblade, physioball, medicine ball, power sports trainer, weight vest, cobra belt, dumbbell) environment becomes more important than increasing the external resistance. The concept of quality before quantity is stressed. Core stabilization training is specifically designed to improve core stabilization and neuromuscular efficiency. You must be concerned with the sensory information that is stimulating your CNS. If you train with poor technique and neuromuscular control, then you develop poor motor patterns and stabilization.[28,55] The focus of your program must be on function. To determine if your program is functional, answer the following questions: Is it dynamic?

T A B L E   1 8 - 5

Exercise Selection

1. Safe
2. Challenging
3. Stress multiple planes
4. Proprioceptively enriched
5. Activity specific

T A B L E   1 8 - 6

Exercise Progression

1. Slow to fast
2. Simple to complex
3. Stable to unstable
4. Low force to high force
5. General to specific
6. Correct execution to increased intensity

Is it multiplanar? Is it multidimensional? Is it proprioceptively challenging? Is it systematic? Is it progressive? Is it based on functional anatomy and science? Is it activity specific?[28,31,55]

CORE STABILIZATION TRAINING PROGRAM

As noted in the previous section, the training program must progress in a scientific, systematic pattern with the ultimate goal of training the trunk stabilizers to be active in all phases of functional tasks. These tasks may include simple static postures, such as standing or sitting, and progress to very complex tasks, such as high-intensity athletic skills. Patient education is the key to a successful exercise program. The patient must be able to visualize the muscle activation patterns desired and have a high level of body awareness allowing them to activate their core muscles with the proper positioning, neuromuscular control, and level of force generation needed for each individual task. All of these items vary from a simple task of picking up a sock from the floor to a professional baseball pitcher throwing a 95 mph fastball.

Muscular activation of the deep core stabilizers (TA and multifidus) coordinated with normal breathing patterns is the foundation for all core exercises. The authors of this chapter state to their patients that this is "home base" and all exercises must start with this concept first. Varying opinions[69,81] about the activation of the abdominal muscles during activities exist in the exercise science world. McGill[69] is a proponent of the abdominal bracing technique where the patient is advised to stiffen or activate both the trunk flexors and extensors maximally to prevent spinal movement. They use the training technique of demonstrating this bracing pattern at the elbow joint. They

T A B L E   1 8 - 7

Guidelines for a Functional Core Stabilization Program

1. Is it dynamic?
2. Is it multiplanar?
3. Is it proprioceptively enriched?
4. Is it systematic?
5. Is it progressive?
6. Is it activity-specific?

TABLE 18-8

Teaching Cues for Activation of Core Muscles

VERBAL CUES
1. Draw navel back toward spine without moving your spine or tilting your pelvis.
2. Make your waist narrow.
3. Pull your abdomen away from your waistband of your pants.
4. Draw lower abdomen in while simulating zipping up a tight pair of pants.
5. You must continue breathing normal while contracting lower abdominals.
6. Pelvic floor tightening.
   a. Women: contract pelvic floor so you do not leak urine.
   b. Men: draw up scrotum as if you are walking in waist deep cold water.

PHYSICAL CUES
1. Use of mirror for visual feedback.
2. Put your hands on your waist like you are mad—draw abdomen away from fingertips while still breathing normally.
3. Tactile facilitation.
   a. Use of tape on skin for cutaneous feedback.
   b. String tied snuggly around waist.
4. EMG biofeedback unit.
5. Electrical muscular stimulation.
6. Isometric contraction and holding of pelvic floor and hip adductors

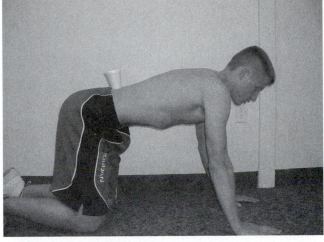

FIGURE 18-16

Quadriped transverse abdominal drawing in maneuver.

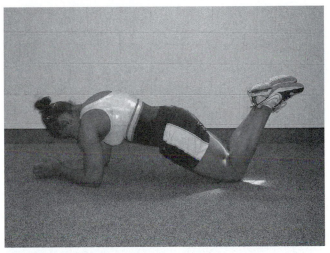

FIGURE 18-17

Front plank $^1/_2$.

ask the patient to stiffen their elbow joint by simultaneously activating their elbow flexors and extensors and resisting an external force that attempts to flex their elbow. Once the patient has mastered that concept, they apply the same principles to the trunk. These authors find this concept to be too rigid for

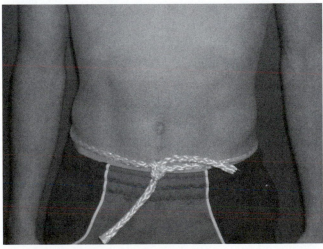

FIGURE 18-15

Power position.

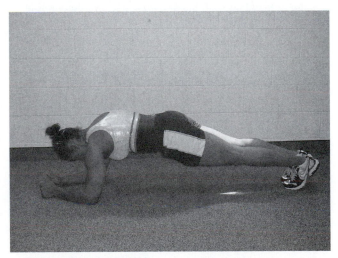

FIGURE 18-18

Front plank full.

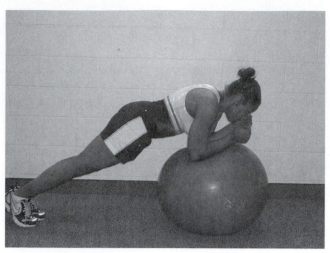

F I G U R E   1 8 - 1 9

Front full plank with upper extremities unstable on ball.

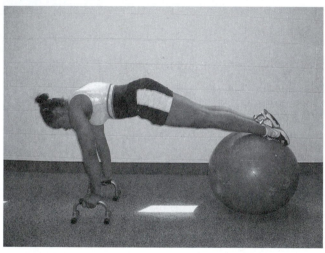

F I G U R E   1 8 - 2 0

Front full plank with lower extremities unstable on ball.

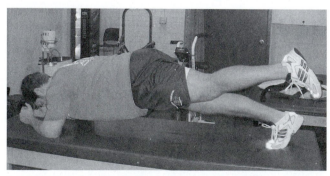

F I G U R E   1 8 - 2 1

Front plank with narrow base of support.

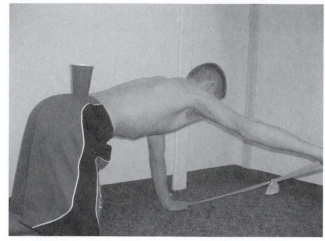

F I G U R E   1 8 - 2 2

Quadriped with resistance to upper extremity.

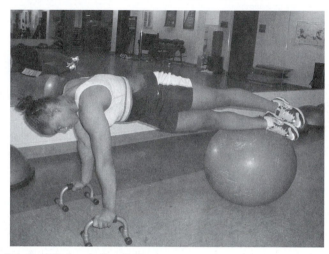

F I G U R E   1 8 - 2 3

Plank on ball with trunk rotation.

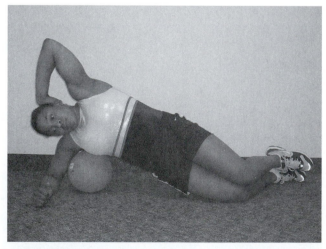

F I G U R E   1 8 - 2 4

Side plank $1/2$. Note that ball is under axilla to unload stresses on shoulder and cervical region.

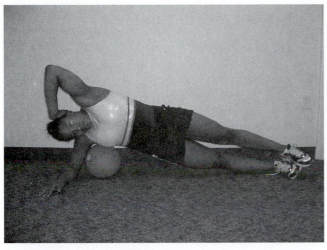

FIGURE 18-25

Side plank full with ball to unload shoulder.

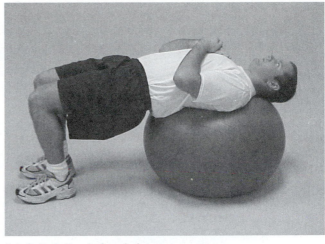

FIGURE 18-28

Trunk bridge unstable trunk.

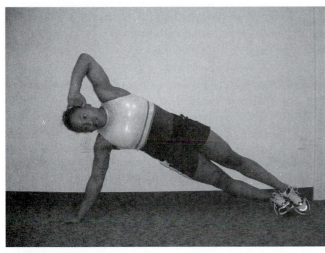

FIGURE 18-26

Side plank full: Single arm stabilization.

our patients to follow through with for all tasks especially complex tasks that require high speed, multidirectional movements. Richardson et al.[81] teach the abdominal hollowing technique where the navel is drawn back toward the spine without spinal movement occurring. It should be noted that Richardson et al. do not ask their patients to do a maximal contraction but desire a submaximal, steady development of muscle activation. The authors of this chapter have used a teaching technique that incorporates submaximal abdominal hollowing and moderate bracing of the trunk. While standing in front of a mirror, the patients are asked to put their hands on their iliac crests so their fingers rest anteriorly on their transverse abdominals and internal obliques. A good way to state this to the patient is "put your hands on your hips like you are mad." The patient is then instructed to draw their navel back toward their spine without moving their trunk or body while continuing to breathe normally. A good verbal cue is to "make your waist narrow like you

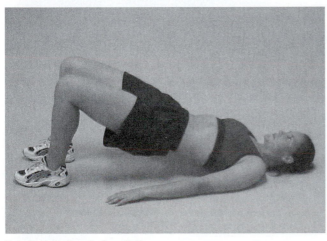

FIGURE 18-27

Trunk bridge stable.

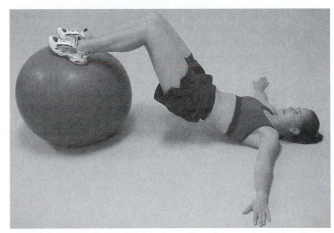

FIGURE 18-29

Trunk bridge unstable legs.

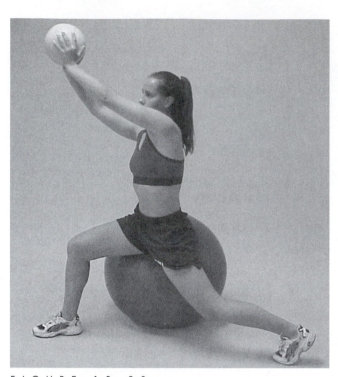

FIGURE 18-30
Stability ball PNF with a power ball.

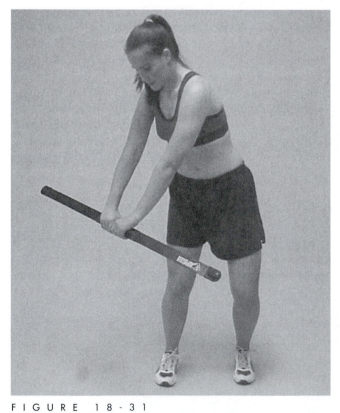

FIGURE 18-31
Closed chain PNF with body blade.

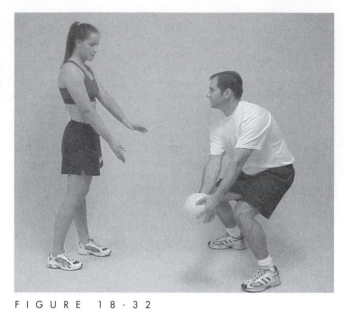

FIGURE 18-32
Closed chain medicine ball toss and catch with eccentric/concentric trunk rotation.

are putting on a tight pair of jeans," without sucking in your breath. While in that position the patient is also instructed to not let anyone "push them around" or push them off balance. This helps incorporate the total body bracing technique and the use of the upper and lower extremities to facilitate total body stabilization. When the patient has correctly activated the core muscles, a string is tied snuggly around the patient's waist to act as tactile feedback (Fig. 18-15). This string can remain in place throughout the exercise progression, and it gives the patient feedback when they have lost TA and multifidus control. The authors call this "the power position" or "home base" and use these key words when teaching the progression of all core

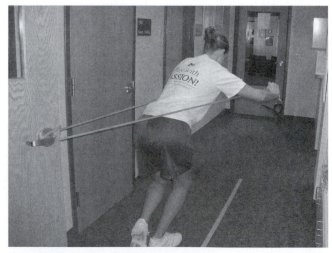

FIGURE 18-33
Closed chain single leg stance with resisted shoulder movements.

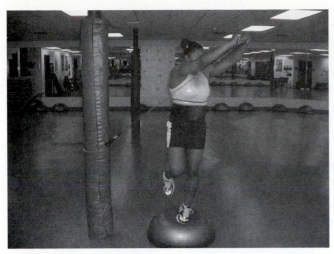

FIGURE   18-34

Closed chain unstable base and single leg stance with resisted trunk rotation.

exercises (see Table 18-8 for other teaching cues for proper muscular activation of core muscles). It should be stressed that proper muscular activation cannot be achieved if the patient is holding the breath.

Once neuromuscular control of the TA and multifidus is accomplished in the prone and supine positions as described in the assessment section of this chapter, progression of exercises into other positions can take place. Quadriped is a good starting position for the patient to learn and enhance their power position. Placing a glass of water on the lumbosacral region facilitates the patient keeping their body steady and minimizing trunk movement. The patient is instructed to keep the trunk straight like a tabletop and then draw the stomach up toward the spine (activating the TA and multifidus) while maintaining the normal breathing pattern. This position is held for minimum 10 seconds and progressed in time to up to 30–60 seconds working on endurance of these trunk muscles. The patient is advised to release the contraction slowly in an

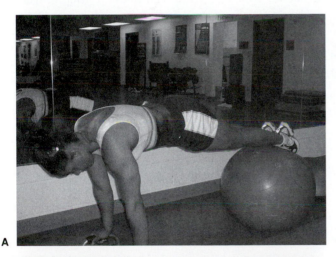

A

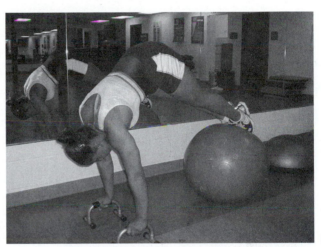

B

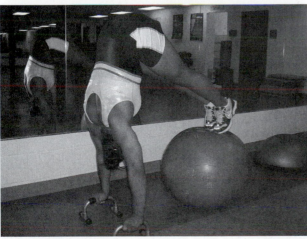

C

FIGURE   18-35

Pike ups: Moving legs on unstable surface of ball into trunk flexion and then return to starting position with slow eccentric control and no lumbar lordosis. (**A**) Start position. (**B**) Midrange. (**C**) End position.

eccentric manner and no spinal movement should occur during this release phase (Fig. 18-16). When this position is mastered by the patient and the clinician feels that the patient is ready to be progressed in intensity of exercise, the ½ front plank is attempted (Fig. 18-17). Difficulty is increased by making the trunk lever arm longer thus putting more resistance on the core muscles. The same principles apply for the ½ front plank as for the quadriped position. The progression is then to the full front plank (see Fig. 18-18) for front plank progression series. Alternatives to add to the quadriped and plank positions would be making the base of support unstable using things such as a ball, foam, or wobble boards. These items can be placed at either end of the kinetic chain, the feet, or the upper chest (see Figs. 18-19 and 18-20). The base of support can also be made less stable by making it narrower by taking away a point of stability, for example an arm or leg support (Fig. 18-21). External resistance may also be applied to the arm or leg, and this external load can be held in a static position or moved dynamically such as in a proprioceptive neuromuscular facilitation (PNF) pattern with the upper extremities (Fig. 18-

22). Adding trunk rotation is a progression from the front plank position and adds difficulty to the exercise (see Fig. 18-23). All of these tasks may be more proprioceptively challenging by using unstable bases of support, or taking away visual input, by asking patient to perform the exercises with their eyes closed (see Table 18-6 for pattern of exercise progression that can be followed for any exercise position).

Another position used to train the core muscles is the side plank position. This position is the same position as used to test the endurance of the lateral trunk muscles noted in the assessment section of this chapter. The basic side plank starts with a shortened lever arm (knees are flexed to 90°) and a ball under the axilla area to relieve some pressure on the shoulder and cervical region (Fig. 18-24). If the patient is very weak in his/her upper extremities, the ball will facilitate his/her ability to perform this sequence of side planks and minimize chances of upper quarter muscular strain or injury. The patient is instructed that he/she must keep his/her power position activated during all positions. The progression of difficulty is similar to the front plank noted previously. Progress from a ½ side plank to full side plank (Figs. 18-25 and 18-26). Placing a larger ball under the forearm of the supporting arm while in the full side plank position can also change the stability of the base of support. Placing a smaller ball under the feet in the full side plank is a very difficult position to maintain and should be only used for the advanced patient who has excellent core control. Trunk bridging in supine can progress from a stable base to an unstable base by placing a ball at the scapular region or beneath the feet (Figs. 18-27 to 18-29).

Exercises are progressed from open- to closed-chain positions and the same principles of progression apply for closed chain. Start with the power position and stable base with static hold positions working on core muscular endurance and then progress to unstable surfaces, external forces that provide balance pertubations such as ball tossing and catching,

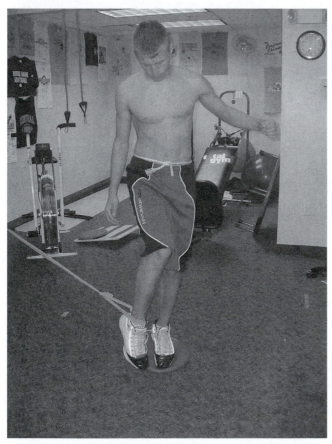

FIGURE 18-36

Functional core strengthening: Soccer kick with lower extremity resistance and unstable base. Emphasis on core stability and power position throughout the full kicking motion.

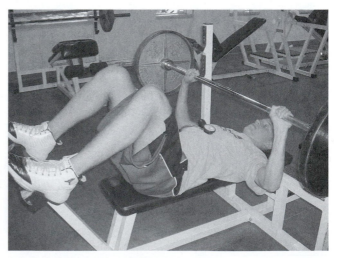

FIGURE 18-37

Core stabilization while performing bench press.

Bodyblade®, or elastic band dynamic movements (Figs. 18-30 to 18-35). The final progression of the closed chain position is to progress exercises to the specific functional tasks required by each individual patient (see Fig. 18-36). This can vary from work tasks such as climbing ladders and repeated lifting and loading of heavy boxes to sport-specific tasks such as performing a double axel in figure skating. The clinician should thoroughly evaluate the needs of each patient and use those specific positions to train the neuromuscular control and endurance of all the core muscles with specific attention placed on the TA and multifidus.

It should also be noted that the power position should not be abandoned when the patient is performing other exercises such as weight, lifting, walking, or other aerobic tasks such as step aerobics, aqua aerobics, or running (see Figs. 18-37 and 18-38 for examples how the Stabilizer is used to train the power position with such tasks as the bench press and squatting for weight lifting). The authors also use a headlamp to educate the patient on core stabilization when walking or running. The patient is instructed to keep the beam of light focused on a spot on the wall in front of the treadmill with minimal movement of the beam of light allowed (Fig. 18-39). The patient is also advised to listen to their stride cadence while walking or running

on the treadmill and make the cadence symmetrical and quiet thus minimizing the impact forces from the foot extending up the kinetic chain. This technique requires the lower extremities to eccentrically absorb the forces of gravity with walking or running and thus activates all muscles of the lower extremities and core in an eccentric functional manner.

The Roman back extension device is a common tool used for lumbar extension strengthening. It is important to instruct the patient that the power position must be maintained at all times and the trunk should remain in a straight plane throughout the entire pattern of movement. The hamstrings and gluteal muscles should initiate the trunk extension moment when moving from a flexed position to the neutral position. Lumbar extension or lordosis at the lumbar vertebral level should not occur. Hyperextension of the lumbar spine is not encouraged with this exercise (Fig. 18-40). This type of exercise should only be used if the patient has excellent core control and understands the power position and can maintain this stable position during the exercise. Another form of hyperextension commonly prescribed in the clinical setting is the "superman" exercise, where the patient is prone and then actively extends both upper extremities and lower extremities simultaneously (see Fig. 18-41). This position has been determined to place up to 6000 N (about 1400 lb) of

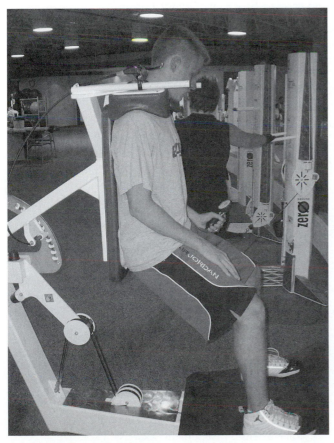

FIGURE 18-38

Core stabilization while squat lifting.

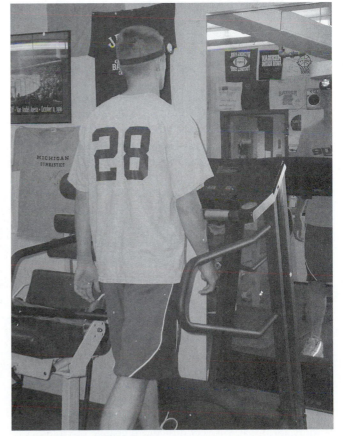

FIGURE 18-39

Core stabilization with walking.

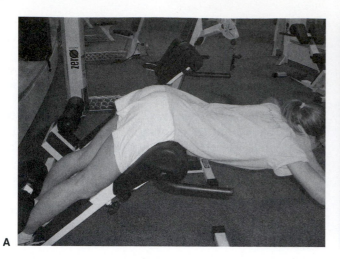
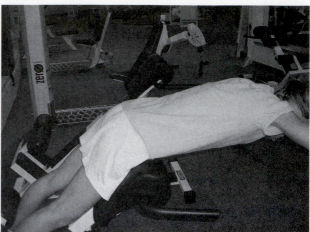

A   B

FIGURE 18-40

Trunk extension using Roman chair. (**A**) Incorrect position—noted lumbar lordosis. (**B**) Correct position—note trunk straight line position.

force on a hyperextended spine.[17] This exercise is not advised for any patient including elite level athletes.

What about the traditional sit-up, partial sit-up, or crunch, and their role in core stability and strengthening? Axler and McGill[5] studied the forces applied to the spine with various trunk flexion exercises and determined that the traditional sit-up imposed approximately 3300 N (730 lb) of compression on the spine. Excessive compression on the spine was also evident with the partial sit-ups, sit-ups with legs straight and bent, and various other trunk flexion positions. The National Institute of Occupational Safety and Health (NIOSH) has set the safe limit for low back compression at 3300 N in workers and repetitive loading above this level is linked with higher injury rates in workers. So why do clinicians and other health care professionals instruct their patients in these types of flexion-biased exercises? The authors of this chapter use this research evidence to instruct their patients as to why sit-ups are ill-advised, potentially injurious, and an inefficient method of core strengthening. When the patient is asked why they do sit-ups, most of them respond with the statement "because we want to have a flat stomach and sit-ups are supposed to help prevent low back injuries." In actuality, sit-ups produce the direct opposite effects. Sit-ups put an excessive amount of compression on the spine, so, rather than injury prevention they may play a causative role in low back pain. When a sit-up is performed, the abdomen actually becomes more prominent, rather than becoming flat. Of greatest importance, activation of the rectus abdominus that occurs during curls and sit-ups is counterproductive to activation of the important deep core muscles: the TA and internal obliques. The deep horizontal muscles are the muscles that produce the flat stomach and narrow waist that is desired by all patients. The authors agree that it is very difficult to change the mindset of the layperson who is heavily influenced by popular media, fads,

and miracle equipment. The authors have found that once the patients are educated on the basic science of core strengthening and they experience different and effective exercise positions, they will be much more compliant with their exercise program and never go back to the "dreaded sit-up."

In summary, the core strengthening program must always start with the foundational neuromuscular control of the TA and multifidus, performed in power position. Abdominal strength is *not* the key, rather, it is abdominal endurance within a stabilized trunk that enhances function and may prevent or minimize injury. The trunk must be dynamic and able to move in multiple directions at various speeds, yet have internal stability that provides a strong base of support in order to support

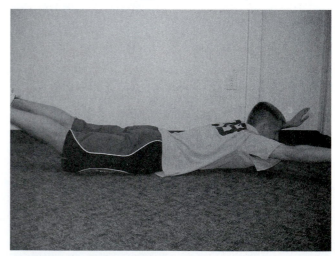

FIGURE 18-41

Trunk extension "superman" exercise: Excessive compressive force on spine and not a recommended exercise.

functional mobility and extremity function. The clinician is only limited by his/her own imagination in the development of core stabilization exercises. If the power position is maintained throughout the exercise sequence and the exercise is individualized to the needs of a patient, then it is an appropriate exercise! The key is to integrate individual exercises into functional patterns and simulate the demands of simple tasks and progress to the highest level of skill needed by each individual patient.

SUMMARY

- Functional kinetic-chain rehabilitation must address each link in the kinetic chain and strive to develop functional strength and neuromuscular efficiency.
- A core stabilization program should be an integral component for all individuals participating in a closed kinetic-chain rehabilitation program.
- A core stabilization training program will allow an individual to gain optimal neuromuscular control of the lumbo-pelvic-hip complex and allow the individual with a kinetic-chain dysfunction to return to activity more quickly and safely.
- The important core muscles do not function as prime movers, rather they function as stabilizers.
- There are some clinical methods of measuring the function of the TA and multifidus function.
- Real-time ultrasound is an effective research tool for assessment of core stabilizers.
- The Stabilizer is a useful adjunct to examination and training of the core.
- Many possibilities exist for core training progressions. Progression is achieved by changing position, lever arms, resistance, and stability of surfaces.
- Trunk flexion activities such as the curl and sit-up are not only unnecessary but also may cause injury.

REFERENCES

1. Aaron G. The use of stabilization training in the rehabilitation of the athlete. *Sports Physical Therapy Home Study Course*. LaCrosse, WI, Sports Physical Therapy Section of the American Physical Therapy Association, 1996.
2. Aruin AS, Latash ML. Directional specificity of postural muscles in feed-forward postural reactions during fast voluntary arm movements. *Exp Brain Res* 103:323–332, 1995.
3. Ashmen KJ, Swanik CB, Lephart SM. Strength and flexibility characteristics of athletes with chronic low back pain. *J Sports Rehab* 5:275–286, 1996.
4. Aspden RM. Review of the functional anatomy of the spinal ligaments and the erector spinae muscles. *Clin Anat* 5:372–387, 1992.
5. Axler CT, McGill SM. Low back loads over a variety of abdominal exercises: Searching for the safest abdominal challenge. *Med Sci Sports Exerc* 29:804–810, 1997.
6. Bartelink DL. The role of intra-abdominal pressure in relieving the pressure on the lumbar vertebral discs. *J Bone Joint Surg* 39B:718–725, 1957.
7. Basmajian J. *Muscles Alive: Their Functions Revealed by EMG*, 5th ed. Baltimore, MD, Lippincott Williams & Wilkins, 1985.
8. Basmajian J. *Muscles Alive*. Baltimore, MD, Lippincott Williams & Wilkins, 1974.
9. Beckman SM, Buchanan TS. Ankle inversion and hypermobility: Effect on hip and ankle muscle electromyography onset latency. *Arch Phys Med Rehabil* 76:1138–1143, 1995.
10. Beim G, Giraldo JL, Pincivero DM, et al. Abdominal strengthening exercises: A comparative EMG study. *J Sports Rehab* 6:11–20, 1997.
11. Biering-Sorenson F. Physical measurements as risk indicators for low-back trouble over a one-year period. *Spine* 9:106–119, 1984.
12. Blievernicht J. *Balance*. Course manual. Chicago. San Diego, CA, IDEA Health and Fitness Association, 1996.
13. Bittenham D, Brittenham G. *Stronger Abs and Back*. Champaign, IL, Human Kinetics, 1997.
14. Bullock-Saxton JE. *Muscles and Joint: Inter-relationships With Pain and Movement Dysfunction*. Course manual. 1997.
15. Bullock-Saxton JE. Local sensation changes and altered hip muscle function following severe ankle sprain. *Phys Ther* 74:17–23, 1994.
16. Bullock-Saxton JE, Janda V, Bullock M. Reflex activation of gluteal muscles in walking: An approach to restoration of muscle function for patients with low back pain. *Spine* 18:704–708, 1993.
17. Callaghan JP, Gunning JL, McGill SM. Relationship between lumbar spine load and muscle activity during extensor exercises. *Phys Ther* 78(1):8–18, 1978.
18. Calliet R. *Low Back Pain Syndrome*. Oxford, Blackwell, 1962.
19. Chaitow L. *Muscle Energy Techniques*. New York, Churchill Livingstone, 1997.
20. Chek P. *Dynamic Medicine Ball Training*. Correspondence course. La Jolla, CA, Paul Chek Seminars, 1996.
21. Chek P. *Swiss Ball Training*. Correspondence course. La Jolla, CA, Paul Chek Seminars, 1996.
22. Chek P. *Scientific Back Training*. Correspondence course. La Jolla, CA, Paul Chek Seminars, 1994.
23. Chek P. *Scientific Abdominal Training*. Correspondence course. La Jolla, CA, Paul Chek Seminars, 1992.
24. Creager C. Therapeutic exercise using foam rollers. *Executive Physical Therapy*. Berthoud, CO, Executive Physical Therapy, 1996.
25. Cresswell AG, Grundstrom H, Thorstensson A. Observations on intra-abdominal pressure and patterns of

abdominal intra-muscular activity in man. *Acta Physiol Scand* 144:409–418, 1992.

26. Cresswell AG, Oddson L, Thorstensson A. The influence of sudden perturbations on trunk muscle activity and intra-abdominal pressure while standing. *Exp Brain Res* 98:336–341, 1994.

27. Crisco J, Panjabi MM. The intersegmental and multisegmental muscles of the lumbar spine. *Spine* 16:793–799, 1991.

28. Dominguez RH. *Total Body Training.* East Dundee, II, Moving Force Systems, 1982.

29. Edgerton VR, Wolf S, Roy RR. Theoreical basis for patterning EMG amplitudes to assess muscle dysfunction. *Med Sci Sports Exerc* 28:744–751, 1996.

30. Finkelstein MM. Medical conditions, medications, and urinary incontinence. Analysis of a population-based survey. *Canadian Family Physician* 48:96–101, 2002.

31. Gambetta V. *Building the Complete Athlete.* Course manual. Chicago. Sarasota, FL, Gambetta Sports Training Systems, 1996.

32. Gambetta V. *The Complete Guide to Medicine Ball Training.* Sarasota, FL, Optimum Sports Training, 1991.

33. Gracovetsky S, Farfan H. The optimum spine. *Spine* 11:543–573, 1986.

34. Gracovetsky S, Farfan H, Heuller C. The abdominal mechanism. *Spine* 10:317–324, 1985.

35. Grillner S, Nilsson J, Thorstensson A. Intra-abdominal pressure changes during natural movements in man. *Acta Physiologica Scandinavica* 103:275–283, 1978.

36. Gustavsen R, Streeck R. *Training Therapy: Prophylaxis and Rehabilitation.* New York, Thieme, 1993.

37. Hall T, David A, Geere J, Salvenson K. Relative recruitment of the abdominal muscles during three levels of exertion during abdominal hollowing. *Manipulative Physiotherapists Association of Australia.* Melbourne, Australia, Australian Physiotherapy Association, 1995.

38. Henry SM, Westervelt KC. The use of real-time ultrasound feedback in teaching abdominal hollowing exercises to healthy subjects. *J Orthop Sports Phys Ther* 35:338—345, 2005.

39. Hides J. Paraspinal mechanism and support of the lumbar spine. In: Richardson C, Hodges P, Hides J. *Therapeutic Exercise for Lumbopelvic Stabilization,* 2nd ed. Philadelphia, PA, Churchill Livingstone, 2004.

40. Hides J, Richardson C, Hodges P. Local segmental control. In: Richardson C, Hodges P, Hides J. *Therapeutic Exercise for Lumbopelvic Stabilization.* 2nd ed. Philadelphia, PA, Churchill Livingstone, 2004.

41. Hides JA, Stokes MJ, Saide M, et al. Evidence of lumbar multifidus wasting ipsilateral to symptoms in subjects with acute/subacute low back pain. *Spine* 19:165–177, 1994.

42. Hodges P, Kaigle-Holm A, Holm S, et al. Intervertebral stiffness of the spine is increased by evoked contraction of transversus abdominis and the diaphragm: In vivo porcine studies. *Spine* 28:2594–2601, 2003.

43. Hodges PW, Richardson CA. Contraction of the abdominal muscles associated with movement of the lower limb. *Phys Ther* 77:132, 1997.

44. Hodges PW, Richardson CA. Delayed postural contraction of tranverse abdominis in low back pain associated with movement of the lower limb. *J Spinal Disord* 1:46–56, 1998.

45. Hodges PW, Richardson CA. Feedforward contraction of transverse abdominis is not influenced by the direction of arm movement. *Exp Brain Res* 114:362–370, 1997.

46. Hodges PW, Richardson CA. Inefficient muscular stabilization of the lumbar spine associated with low back pain. *Spine* 21:2640–2650, 1996.

47. Hodges PW, Richardson CA. Neuromotor dysfunction of the trunk musculature in low back pain patients. In: *Proceedings of the International Congress of the World Confederation of Physical Therapists,* Washington, DC, 1995.

48. Hodges PW, Richardson CA, Jull G. Evaluation of the relationship between laboratory and clinical tests of transverse abdominus function. *Physiother Res Int* 1:30–40, 1996.

49. Hodges PW, Sapsford RR, Pengel HM. Feedforward activity of the pelvic floor muscles precedes rapid upper limb movements. In: *Proceedings of the 7th International Physiotherapy Congress,* Sydney, Australia, 2002.

50. Janda V. Physical therapy of the cervical and thoracic spine. In: Grant R, ed. *Physical Therapy of the Cervical and Thoracic Spine.* New York, Churchill Livingstone, 1988.

51. Janda V. Muscle weakness and inhibition in back pain syndromes. In: Grieve GP. *Modern Manual Therapy of the Vertebral Column.* New York, Churchill Livingstone, 1986.

52. Janda V. *Muscle Function Testing.* London, Butterworths, 1983.

53. Janda V. Muscles, central nervous system regulation and back problems. In: Korr IM, ed. *Neurobiologic Mechanisms in Manipulative Therapy.* New York, Plenum, 1978.

54. Janda V, Vavrova M. *Sensory Motor Stimulation* (video). Brisbane, Body Control Systems, 1990.

55. Jesse J. *Hidden Causes of Injury, Prevention, and Correction for Running Athletes.* Pasadena, Athletic Press, 1977.

56. Jorgensson A. The iliopsoas muscle and the lumbar spine. *Australian Physiotherapy* 39:125–132, 1993.

57. Jull G, Richardson CA, Comerford M. Strategies for the initial activation of dynamic lumbar stabilization. In: *Proceedings of Manipulative Physiotherapists Association of Australia,* Australia, 1991.

58. Jull G, Richardson CA, Hamilton C, et al. *Towards the Validation of a Clinical Test for the Deep Abdominal Muscles in Back Pain Patients.* Australia, Manipulative Physiotherapists Association of Australia, 1995.

59. Kendall FP. *Muscles Testing and Function,* 5th ed. Baltimore, MD, Lippincott Williams & Wilkins, 2005.

60. Kennedy B. An Australian program for management of back problems. *Physiotherapy* 66:108–111, 1980.

61. Lewit K. Muscular and articular factors in movement restriction. *Man Med* 1:83–85, 1998.

62. Lewit K. *Manipulative Therapy in the Rehabilitation of the Locomotor System.* London, Butterworths, 1985.

63. Lewit K. Myofascial pain: Relief by post-isometric relaxation. *Arch Phys Med Rehabil* 65:452, 1984.

64. Liebenson CL. *Rehabilitation of the Spine.* Baltimore, MD, Lippincott Williams & Wilkins, 1996.

65. Liebenson CL. Active muscle relaxation techniques. Part I. Basic principles and methods. *J Manipulative Physiol Ther* 12:446–454, 1989.

66. Liebenson CL. Active muscle relaxation techniques. Part II: Clinical application. *J Manipulative Physiol Ther* 13(1): 2–6, 1990.

67. Mayer TG, Gatchel RJ. *Functional Restoration for Spinal Disorders: The Sports Medicine Approach.* Philadelphia, PA, Lea & Febiger, 1988.

68. Mayer-Posner J. *Swiss Ball Applications for Orthopedic and Sports Medicine.* Denver, Ball Dynamics International, 1995.

69. McGill S. *Ultimate Back Fitness and Performance.* Waterloo, Wabuno Publishers, 2004.

70. McGill SM, Childs A, Liebenson C. Endurance times for stabilization exercises: Clinical targets for testing and training from a normal database. *Arch Phys Med Rehab* 80:941–944, 1999.

71. McGill SM, Grenier S, Bluhm M, et al. Previous history of LBP with work loss is related to lingering effects in biomechanical physiological, personal, and psychosocial characteristics. *Ergonomics* 46(7):731–746, 2003.

72. Miller MI, Medeiros JM. Recruitment of the internal oblique and transverse abdominus muscles on the eccentric phase of the curl-up. *Phys Ther* 67:1213–1217, 1987.

73. Morris JM, Benner F, Lucas DB. An electromyographic study of the intrinsic muscles of the back in man. *J Anat* 96:509–520, 1962.

74. Nachemson A. The load on the lumbar discs in different positions of the body. *Clin Orthop* 45:107–122, 1966.

75. Norris CM. Abdominal muscle training in sports. *Br J Sports Med* 27:19–27, 1993.

76. O'Sullivan PE, Twomey L, Allison G. *Evaluation of Specific Stabilizing Exercises in the Treatment of Chronic Low Back Pain with Radiological Diagnosis of Spondylolisthesis.* Australia, Manipulative Physiotherapists Association of Australia, 1995.

77. O'Sullivan PE, Twomey L, Allison G, et al. Altered patterns of abdominal muscle activation in patients with chronic low back pain. *Aust J Physiother* 43:91–98, 1997.

78. Panjabi MM. The stabilizing system of the spine. Part I: Function, dysfunction, adaptation, and enhancement. *J Spinal Disord* 5:383–389, 1992.

79. Panjabi MM, Tech D, White AA. Basic biomechanics of the spine. *Neurosurgery* 7:76–93, 1980.

80. Porterfield JA, DeRosa C. *Mechanical Low Back Pain: Perspectives in Functional Anatomy.* Philadelphia, PA, Saunders, 1991.

81. Richardson C, Hodges P, Hides J. *Therapeutic Exercise for Lumbopelvic Stabilization-Second Edition.* Philadelphia, PA, Churchill Livingstone, 2004.

82. Richardson CA, Jull G. Muscle control—pain control. What exercises would you prescribe? *Manual Med* 1:2–10, 1996.

83. Richardson CA, Jull G, Toppenberg R, Comerford M. Techniques for active lumbar stabilization for spinal protection. *Aust J Physiother* 38:105–112, 1992.

84. Richardson CA, Snijders CJ, Hides JA, Damen L, Pas MS, Storm J. The relation between the transversus abdominis muscles, sacroiliac joint mechanics, and low back pain. *Spine* 27:399–405, 2002.

85. Robinson R. The new back school prescription: Stabilization training. Part I. *Occupational Med* 7:17–31, 1992.

86. Saal JA. The new back school prescription: Stabilization training. Part II. *Occupational Med* 7:33–42, 1993.

87. Saal JA. Nonoperative treatment of herniated disc: An outcome study. *Spine* 14:431–437, 1989.

88. Sahrmann S. *Diagnosis and Treatment of Movement Impairment Syndromes.* Philadelphia, PA, Elsevier Publishing, 2001.

89. Sahrmann S. Posture and muscle imbalance: Faulty lumbo-pelvic alignment and associated musculolskeletal pain syndromes. *Orthop Div Rev—Can Phys Ther* 12:13–20, 1992.

90. Sapsford RR, Hodges PW, Richardson CA, Cooper DH, Markwell SJ, Jull GA. Co-activation of the abdominal and pelvic floor muscles during voluntary exercises. *Neurourol Urodyn* 20:31–42, 2001.

91. Snijders CJ, Vleeming A, Stoekart R, Mens JMA, Kleinrensink GJ. Biomechanical modeling of sacroiliac joint stability in different postures. *Spine: State Art Rev* 9:419–432, 1995.

92. Stokes M, Young A. The contribution of reflex inhibition to arthrogenous muscle weakness. *Clin Sci* 67:7–14, 1984.

93. Tesh KM, Shaw Dunn J, Evans JH. The abdominal muscles and vertebral stability. *Spine* 12:501–508, 1987.

94. Teyhen DS, Miltenberger CE, Deiters HM, et al. The use of ultrasound imaging of the abdominal drawing-in maneuver in subjects with low back pain. *J Orthop Sports Phys Ther* 35:346–355, 2005.

95. Thomson KD. On the bending moment capability of the pressurized abdominal cavity during human lifting activity. *Ergonomics* 31:817–828, 1988.

96. Warmerdam ALA. *Arthrokinetic Therapy: Manual Therapy to Improve Muscle and Joint Functioning.* Continuing education course, Marshfield, WI. Port Moody, British Columbia, Canada, Arthrokinetic Therapy and Publishing, 1996.

97. Wilke HJ, Wolf S, Claes LE. Stability increase of the lumbar spine with different muscle groups: A biomechanical in vitro study. *Spine* 20:192–198, 1995.

CHAPTER 19

Aquatic Therapy in Rehabilitation

Barbara J. Hoogenboom and Nancy E. Lomax

OBJECTIVES

After completing this chapter, the therapist should be able to do the following:

- Explain the principles of buoyancy and specific gravity and the role they have in the aquatic environment.
- Identify and describe the three major resistive forces at work in the aquatic environment.
- Apply the principles of buoyancy and resistive forces to exercise prescription and progression.
- Contrast the advantages and disadvantages of aquatic therapy in relation to traditional land-based exercise.
- Identify and describe techniques of aquatic therapy for the upper extremity, lower extremity, and trunk.
- Select and utilize various types of equipment for aquatic therapy.
- Incorporate functional, work- and sport-specific movements and exercises performed in the aquatic environment into rehabilitation.
- Understand and describe the necessity for transition from the aquatic environment to the land environment.

In recent years, widespread interest has developed in the area of aquatic therapy. It has rapidly become a popular rehabilitation technique for treatment of a variety of patient/client populations. This newfound interest has sparked numerous research efforts to evaluate the effectiveness of aquatic therapy as a therapeutic intervention. Current research shows aquatic therapy to be beneficial in the treatment of everything from orthopedic injuries to spinal cord damage, chronic pain, cerebral palsy, multiple sclerosis, and many other conditions, making it useful in a variety of settings.[24,31] It is also gaining acceptance as a preventative maintenance tool to facilitate overall fitness, cross-training, and sport-specific skills for healthy athletes (Fig. 19-1).[27,28] General conditioning, strength, and a wide variety of movement skills can all be enhanced by aquatic therapy.[16,40,45]

Water healing techniques have been traced back through history as early as 2400 BC but it was not until the late nineteenth century that more traditional types of aquatic therapy came into existence.[3,20] The development of the Hubbard tank in 1820 sparked the initiation of present-day therapeutic use of water by allowing aquatic therapy to be conducted in a highly controlled clinical setting.[7] Loeman and Roen took this a step farther in 1824 and stimulated interest in actual pool or what we now call aquatic therapy. Only recently, however, has water come into its own as a therapeutic exercise medium.[34]

Aquatic therapy is believed to be beneficial because it decreases joint compression forces. The perception of weightlessness experienced in the water assists in decreasing pain and eliminating or drastically reducing the body's protective muscular spasm and pain that can carry over into the patient's daily functional activities.[45,47] The primary goal of aquatic therapy is to teach the patient/client how to use water as a modality for improving movement, strength, and fitness.[2,45] Then, along with other therapeutic modalities and treatments, aquatic therapy can become one link in the patient/client's recovery chain.[1]

PHYSICAL PROPERTIES AND RESISTIVE FORCES

The therapist must understand several physical properties of the water before designing an aquatic therapy program. Land

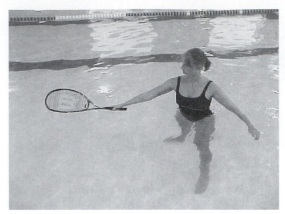

FIGURE 19-1

Example of sport-specific training in the aquatic environment.

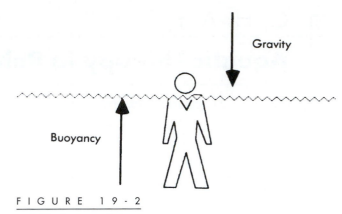

FIGURE 19-2

The buoyant force.

exercise cannot always be converted to aquatic exercise, because buoyancy rather than gravity is the major force governing movement. A thorough understanding of buoyancy, specific gravity, the resistive forces of the water, and their relationships must be the groundwork of any therapeutic aquatic program. The program must be individualized to the patient/client's particular injury/condition and activity level if it is to be successful.

Buoyancy

Buoyancy is one of the primary forces involved in aquatic therapy. All objects, on land or in the water, are subjected to the downward pull of the earth's gravity. In the water, however, this force is counteracted to some degree by the upward buoyant force. According to Archimedes' Principle, any object submerged or floating in water is buoyed upward by a counterforce that helps support the submerged object against the downward pull of gravity. In other words, the buoyant force assists motion toward the water's surface and resists motions away form the surface.[21,45] Because of this buoyant force, a person entering the water experiences an apparent loss of weight.[14] The weight loss experienced is nearly equal to the weight of the liquid that is displaced when the object enters the water (Fig. 19-2).

For example, a 100-lb individual, when almost completely submerged, displaces a volume of water that weighs nearly 95 lb; therefore that person feels as though she/he weighs less than 5 lb. This sensation occurs because, when partially submerged, the individual only bears the weight of the part of the body that is above the water. With immersion to the level of the seventh cervical vertebra, both males and females only bear approximately 6–10 percent of their total body weight (TBW). The percentages increase to 25–31 percent TBW for females and 30–37 percent TBW for males at the xiphisternal level and 40–51 percent TBW for females and 50–56 percent TBW for males at the anterosuperior iliac spine (ASIS) level (Table 19-1).[22] The percentages differ slightly for males and females due to the differences in their centers of gravity. Males carry a higher percentage of their weight in the upper body, whereas females carry a higher percentage of their weight in the lower body. The center of gravity on land corresponds with a center of buoyancy in the water.[34] Variations of build and body type only minimally effect weight-bearing values. Due to the decreased percentage of weight bearing offered by the buoyant force, each joint that is below the water is decompressed or unweighted. This allows ambulation and vigorous exercise to be performed with little impact and drastically reduced friction between joint articular surfaces.

Through careful use of Archimedes' Principle, a gradual increase in the percentage of weight bearing can be undertaken. Initially, the patient/client would begin non-weightbearing in the deep end of the pool. A wet vest or similar buoyancy device might be used to help the patient/client remain afloat for the desired exercises (Fig. 19-3). Other commercial equipment available for the use in the aquatic environment will be discussed in the upcoming section "Facilities and Equipment."

Specific Gravity

Buoyancy is partially dependent on body weight. However, the weight of different parts of the body is not constant. Therefore, the buoyant values of different body parts will vary. Buoyant values can be determined by several factors. The ratio of bone weight to muscle weight, the amount and distribution of fat, and the depth and expansion of the chest all play a role. Together, these factors determine the specific gravity of the

TABLE 19-1

Weight-Bearing Percentages

BODY LEVEL	PERCENTAGE OF WEIGHT BEARING	
	MALE	FEMALE
C7	8	8
Xiphisternal	28	35
ASIS	47	54

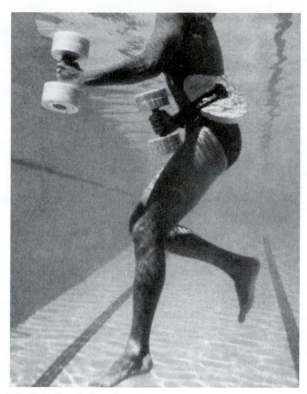

FIGURE   19-3

Deep-water running.

individual body part. On the average, humans have a specific gravity slightly less than that of water. Any object with a specific gravity less than that of water will float. An object with a specific gravity greater than that of water will sink. However, as with buoyant values, the specific gravity of all body parts is not uniform. Therefore, even with a total-body specific gravity of less than the specific gravity of water, the individual might not float horizontally in the water. Additionally, the lungs, when filled with air, can further decrease the specific gravity of the chest area. This allows the head and chest to float higher in the water than the heavier, denser extremities. Many athletes tend to have a low percentage body fat (specific gravity greater than water) and are "sinkers." Therefore, compensation with flotation devices at the extremities and trunk might be necessary for some athletes.[4,45]

Resistive Forces

Water has 12 times the resistance of air.[42] Therefore, when an object moves in the water, several resistive forces are at work that must be considered. Forces must be considered for both their potential benefits and precautions. These forces include the cohesive force, the bow force, and the drag force.

COHESIVE FORCE

There is a slight but easily overcome cohesive force that runs in a parallel direction to the water surface. This resistance is formed by the water molecules loosely binding together, creat-

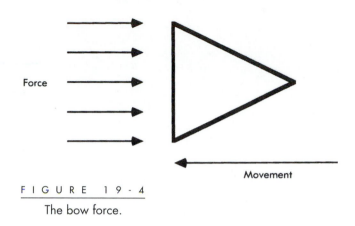

FIGURE   19-4

The bow force.

ing a surface tension. Surface tension can be seen in still water, because the water remains motionless with the cohesive force intact unless disturbed.

BOW FORCE

A second force is the bow force, or the force that is generated at the front of the object during movement. When the object moves, the bow force causes an increase in the water pressure at the front of the object and a decrease in the water pressure at the rear of the object. This pressure change causes a movement of water from the high-pressure area at the front to the low-pressure area behind the object. As the water enters the low-pressure area, it swirls in to the low-pressure zone and forms eddies, or small whirlpool turbulences.[13] These eddies impede flow by creating a backward force, or drag force (Fig. 19-4).

DRAG FORCE

This third force, the fluid drag force, is very important in aquatic therapy. The bow force, and therefore also the drag force, on an object can be controlled by changing the shape of the object or the speed of its movement (Fig. 19-5).

Frictional resistance can be decreased by making the object more streamlined. This change minimizes the surface area at the

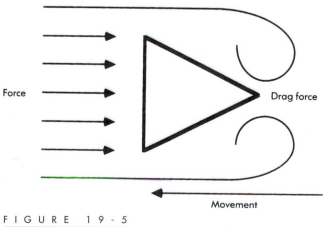

FIGURE   19-5

Drag force.

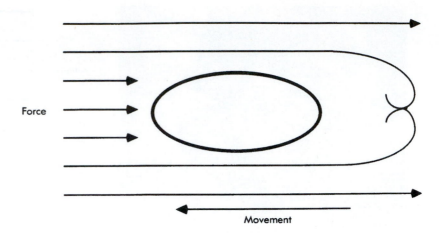

FIGURE   19-6

Streamlined movement. This creates less drag force and less turbulence.

front of the object. Less surface area causes less bow force and less of a change in pressure between the front and rear of the object, resulting in less drag force. In a streamlined flow, the resistance is proportional to the velocity of the object. When working with a patient/client with generalized weakness, consideration of the aquatic environment is necessary. Increased activity occurring around the patient/client and turbulence of the water will make walking a challenging activity (Fig. 19-6).

On the other hand, if the object is not streamlined, a turbulent situation (also referred to as pressure or form drag) exists. In a turbulent situation, drag is a function of the velocity squared. Therefore by increasing the speed of movement two times, the resistance the object must overcome is increased four times.[14] This provides a method to increase resistance progressively during aquatic rehabilitation. Considerable turbulence can be generated when the speed of movement is increased, causing muscles to work harder to keep the movement going. Another method to increase resistance is to change directions of movement, creating increased drag. Finally, by simply changing the shape of a limb through the addition of rehabilitation equipment that increases surface area, the therapist can modify the patient/client's workout intensity to match strength increases (Fig. 19-7).

Drag force must also be considered when portions of a limb or joint must be protected after injury or surgery. For example, when working with a patient/client with an acutely injured medial collateral ligament, or anterior crucial ligament of the knee, resistance must not be placed distal to the knee, due to the increased torque that occurs due to drag forces.

Quantification of resistive forces that occur during aquatic exercise has been a challenge. Pöyhönen et al. examined knee flexion and extension in the aquatic environment using an anatomic model in barefoot and hydroboot-wearing conditions. They found that the highest drag forces and drag coefficients occurred during early extension from a flexed position (150°–140° of flexion) while wearing the hydroboot (making the foot less streamlined), and that faster velocity was associated with higher drag forces.[38]

Once therapy has progressed, the patient/client could be moved to neck-deep water to begin light-weightbearing. Gradual increases in the percentage of weight bearing are accomplished by systematically moving the patient/client to shallower water. Even when in waist-deep water, both male and female patients/clients are only bearing approximately 50 percent of their TBW. By placing a sinkable bench or chair in the shallow water, step-ups can be initiated under partial-weightbearing

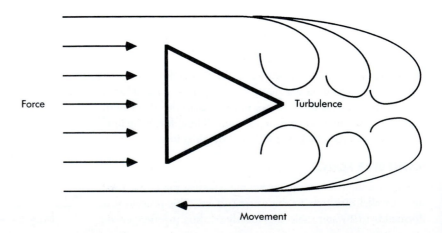

FIGURE   19-7

Turbulent flow.

TABLE 19-2

Indications and Benefits of Aquatic Therapy

INDICATIONS FOR USE OF AQUATIC THERAPY	ILLUSTRATION OF BENEFITS
Swelling/peripheral edema	Assist in edema control, decrease pain, increase mobility as edema decreases
Decreased range of motion	Earlier initiation of rehabilitation, controlled active movements
Decreased strength	Strength progression from assisted to resisted to functional; gradual increase in exercise intensity
Decreased balance, proprioception, coordination	Earlier return to function in supported, forgiving environment, slower movements
Weight-bearing restrictions	Can partially or completely unweight the lower extremities; regulate weight-bearing progressions
Cardiovascular deconditioning or potential deconditioning due to inability to train	Gradual increase of exercise intensity, alternative training environment for lower weight bearing
Gait deviations	Slower movements, easier assessment, and modification of gait
Difficulty or pain with land interventions	Increased support, decreased weight bearing, assistance due to buoyancy, more relaxed environment

Reproduced from Irion JM. Aquatic therapy. In: Bandy WD, Sanders B, eds. *Therapeutic Exercise: Techniques for Intervention*. Baltimore, Lippincott, Williams & Wilkins, 2001; Sova R. *Aquatic Activities Handbook*. Boston, Jones & Bartlett, 1993; and Thein JM, Thein Brody L. Aquatic-based rehabilitation and training for the elite athlete. *Orthop Sports Phys Ther* 27(1):32–41, 1998.

conditions long before the patient/client is capable of performing the same exercise in full-weightbearing on land. Thus the advantages of low-weightbearing are coupled with the proprioceptive benefits of closed-kinetic-chain exercise, making aquatic therapy an excellent functional rehabilitation activity.

ADVANTAGES AND BENEFITS OF AQUATIC REHABILITATION

The addition of an aquatic therapy program can offer many advantages to a patient or patient/client's therapy (Table 19-2).[18,45] The buoyancy of the water allows active exercise while providing a sense of security and causing little discomfort.[43] Utilizing a combination of the water's buoyancy, resistance, and warmth, the patient/client can typically achieve more in the aquatic environment than is possible on land.[28] Early in the rehabilitation process, aquatic therapy is useful in restoring range of motion and flexibility. As normal function is restored, resistance training and sport specific activities can be added.

Following an injury, the aquatic experience provides a medium where early motions can be performed in a supportive environment. The slow motion effect of moving through water provides extra time to control movement, which allows the patient/client to experience multiple movement errors without severe consequences.[41] This is especially helpful in lower-extremity injuries where balance and proprioception are impaired. Geigle et al. demonstrated a positive relationship between use of a supplemental aquatic therapy program and unilateral tests of balance when treating athletes with inversion ankle sprains.[18] The increased amount of time to react and correct movement errors, combined with a medium in which the fear of falling is removed, assists the patient's ability to regain proprioception.

Turbulence functions as a destabilizer and as a tactile sensory stimulus. The stimulation from the turbulence generated during movement provides feedback and perturbation challenge that aids in the return of proprioception and balance. There is also an often-overlooked benefit of edema reduction due to hydrostatic pressure. This would benefit pain reduction and increase range of motion.

By understanding buoyancy and utilizing its principles, the aquatic environment can provide a gradual transition from non-weightbearing to full-weightbearing land exercises. This gradual increase in percentage of weight bearing helps provide a return to smooth coordinated movements that are pain-free. By utilizing the buoyancy force to decrease apparent weight and joint compressive forces, locomotor activities can begin much earlier following an injury to the lower extremity. This provides an enormous advantage to the athletic population. The ability to work out hard without fear of reinjury provides a psychological boost to the athlete. This helps keep motivation high and can help speed the athlete's return to normal function.[28] Psychologically, aquatic therapy increases confidence, because the patient or patient/client experiences increased success at locomotor, stretching, or strengthening activities while in the water. Tension and anxiety are decreased, and the patient/client's morale increases, as does post exercise vigor.[13,14,34]

Muscular strengthening and reeducation can also be accomplished through aquatic therapy.[36,45] Progressive resistance exercises can be increased in extremely small increments by using combinations of different resistive forces. The intensity of exercise can be controlled by manipulating the flow of the water (turbulence), the body's position, or through the addition of exercise equipment. This allows individuals with minimal muscle contraction capabilities to do work and see improvement. The aquatic environment can also provide a challenging resistive workout to an athlete nearing full recovery.[45] Additionally, water serves as an accommodating resistance medium. This allows the muscles to be maximally stressed through the full range of motion available. One drawback to this, however, is that strength gains depend largely on the effort exerted by the patient/client, which is not easily quantified.

In another study, Pöyhönen et al.[38] studied the biomechanical and hydrodynamic characteristics of the therapeutic exercise of knee flexion and extension using kinematic and electromyographic analyses in flowing and still water. They found that the flowing properties of water modified the agonist/antagonist neuromuscular function of the quadriceps and hamstrings in terms of early reduction of quadriceps activity and concurrent increased activation of the hamstrings. They also found that flowing water (turbulence) causes additional resistance when moving the limb opposite the flow. They concluded that when prescribing aquatic exercise, the turbulence of the water must be considered in terms of both resistance and alterations of neuromuscular recruitment of muscles.

Strength gains through aquatic exercise are also brought about by the increased energy needs of the body working in an aquatic environment. Studies have shown that aquatic exercise requires higher energy expenditure than the same exercise performed on land.[9,13,14,45] The patient/client not only has to perform the activity but must also maintain a level of buoyancy and overcome the resistive forces of the water. For example, the energy cost for water running is four times greater than the energy cost for running the same distance on land.[13,14,26]

A simulated run in either shallow or deep water assisted by a tether or flotation devices can be an effective means of alternate fitness training (cross-training) for the injured athlete. It should be noted that a study of shallow-water running (xiphoid level) and deep-water running (using an aqua jogger), at the same rate of perceived exertion, found a significant difference of 10 beats per minute in heart rate, with shallow-water running demonstrating a greater heart rate. The authors of this study point out that aquatic rehabilitation professionals should not prescribe shallow-water working heart rates from heart rates values obtained during deep-water exercise.[40] All patients and patients/clients should be instructed in how to accurately monitor their heart rate while exercising in water, whether deep or shallow.[9]

Not only does the patient or patient/client benefit from early intervention, but aquatic exercise also helps prevent cardiorespiratory deconditioning through alterations in cardiovascular dynamics as a result of hydrostatic forces.[6,23,44] The heart actually functions more efficiently in the water than on land. Hydrostatic pressure enhances venous return, leading to a greater stroke volume and a reduction in the heart rate needed to maintain cardiac output.[46] There is also a decrease in ventilations and an increase in central blood volume. This means that the injured athlete can maintain a near-normal maximal aerobic capacity with aquatic exercise.[15,32] Due to the hydrostatic effects on heart efficiency, it has been suggested that an environment-specific exercise prescription is necessary.[27,44,48] Some research suggests the use of perceived exertion as an acceptable method for controlling exercise intensity. Other research suggests the use of target heart rate values as with land exercise, but compensates for the hydrostatic changes by setting the target range 10 percent lower than that would be expected for land exercise.[42,45] (Fig. 19-8). Regardless of the method used, the keys to successful use of aquatic therapy are supervision and monitoring of the patient or patient/client during activity and good communication between patient/client and therapist.

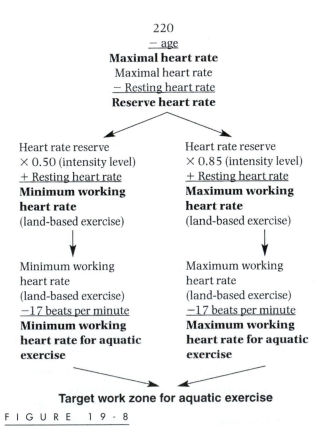

FIGURE 19-8

Karvonen formula for water exercise. (Adapted from Sova R. *Aquatic Activities Handbook*. Boston, Jones & Bartlett, 1993, p. 55.)

DISADVANTAGES OF AQUATIC REHABILITATION

Disadvantages

As with any therapeutic intervention, aquatic therapy has its disadvantages. The cost of building and maintaining a rehabilitation pool, if there is no access to an existing facility, can be very high. Also, qualified pool attendants must be present, and the therapist involved in the treatment must be trained in aquatic safety and therapy procedures.[11,26]

An athlete who requires high levels of stabilization will be more challenging to work with, because stabilization in water is considerably more difficult than on land. Thermoregulation issues exist for the patient who exercises in an aquatic environment. Because the patient cannot always choose the temperature of the pool, the effects of water temperature must be noted for both cool and warm or hot pool temperatures. Water temperatures greater than body temperature cause increase in core body temperature greater than that in a land environment, due to differences in thermoregulation. Water temperatures less than body temperature will decrease core temperature and cause shivering in athletes faster and to a greater degree than the general population, due to their low body fat.[9] Another disadvantage of aquatic exercise utilized for cross-training is that training in water does not allow the athletes to improve or maintain their tolerance to heat while on land.

Contraindications and Precautions

The presence of any open wounds or sores on the patient or patient/client is a contraindication to aquatic therapy, as are contagious skin diseases. This restriction is obvious for health reasons to reduce the chance of infection of the patient/client or others who use the pool.[24,25,31,42] Because of this risk, all surgical wounds must be completely healed or adequately protected using a waterproof barrier before the patient/client enters the pool. An excessive fear of the water would also be a reason to keep a patient/client out of an aquatic exercise program. Fever, urinary tract infections, allergies to the pool chemicals, cardiac problems, and uncontrolled seizures are also contraindications (Tables 19-3 and 19-4). Use caution (or waterproof barrier) with medical equipment access sites such as an insulin pump, osteomies, suprapubic appliances, and G tubes. Patients/clients with a tracheotomy need special consideration; they need to remain in waist to chest depth of water to exercise safely in an aquatic environment.

FACILITIES AND EQUIPMENT

When considering an existing facility or when planning to build one, certain characteristics of the pool should be taken into consideration. The pool should not be smaller than 10 × 12 ft. It can be inground or aboveground as long as access for the pa-

tient/client is well planned. Both a shallow area (2.5 ft) and a deep area (5+ ft) should be present to allow standing exercise and swimming or nonstanding exercise.[7] The pool bottom should be flat and the depth gradations clearly marked. Water temperature will vary depending on the patient/clientele that is served. For the athlete, recommended pool temperature should be 26°–28°C (79°–82°F) but may depend on the available facility.[45] The water temperature suggested by the Arthritis Foundation for their programs is 29°–31°C (85°–89°F).

TABLE 19-3

Contraindications for Aquatic Therapy

Untreated infectious disease (patient has a fever/temperature)
Open wounds or unhealed surgical incisions
Contagious skin diseases
Serous cardiac conditions
Seizure disorders (uncontrolled)
Excessive fear of water
Allergy to pool chemicals
Vital capacity of 1 L
Uncontrolled high or low blood pressure
Uncontrolled bowel or bladder incontinence
Menstruation without internal protection

Reproduced from Irion JM. Aquatic therapy. In: Bandy WD, Sanders B, eds. *Therapeutic Exercise Techniques for Intervention.* Baltimore, Lippincott, Williams & Wilkins, 2001; Sova R. *Aquatic Activities Handbook.* Boston, Jones & Bartlett, 1993; Giesecke C. In: Ruoti RG, Morris DM, Cole AJ, eds. *Aquatic Rehabilitation.* Philadelphia, Lippincott-Raven, 1997; and Thein JM, Thein Brody L. Aquatic-based rehabilitation and training for the elite athlete. *J Orthop Sports Phys Ther* 27(1):32–41, 1998.

TABLE 19-4

Precautions for the Use of Aquatic Therapy

Recently healed wound or incision, incisions covered by moisture-proof barrier
Altered peripheral sensation
Respiratory dysfunction (asthma)
Seizure disorders controlled with medications
Fear of water

Reproduced from Irion JM. Aquatic therapy. *In:* Bandy WD, Sanders B, eds. *Therapeutic Exercise Techniques for Intervention.* Baltimore, Lippincott, Williams & Wilkins, 2001; Sova R. *Aquatic Activities Handbook.* Boston, Jones & Bartlett, 1993: and Thein JM, Thein Brody L. Aquatic-based rehabilitation and training for the elite athlete. *J Orthop Sports Phys Ther* 27(1):32–41, 1998.

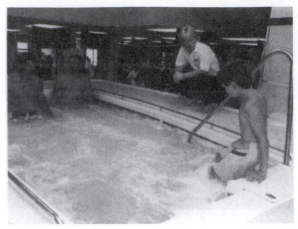

FIGURE 19-9

The SwimEx pool. This pool's even, controllable water flow allows for the application of individualized prescriptive exercise and therapeutic programs. As many as three patients can be treated simultaneously.

Depending on the type of condition, the patient or patient/client's perception of the water temperature may differ.

Some prefabricated pools come with an in-water treadmill or current-producing device (Figs. 19-9 to 19-11). These devices can be beneficial but are not essential to treatment. An aquatic program will benefit from variety of types of equipment to allow increasing levels of resistance and assistance, and also to motivate the patient/client. Catalog companies and sporting goods stores are good resources for obtaining equipment. There are many styles and variations available in regard to equipment: the therapist will need to select equipment depending on the needs of the program. Creative use of actual sport equipment (baseball bats, tennis racquets, golf clubs, etc.) (see Figs. 19-1, 19-12, and 19-19) is helpful to incorporate sport-specific activities that challenge the athlete. Use of mask and snorkel will allow

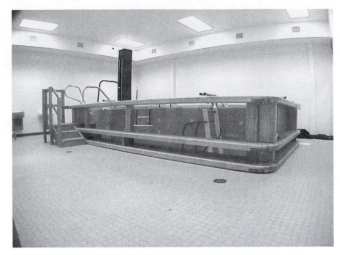

FIGURE 19-11

Custom pool environment.

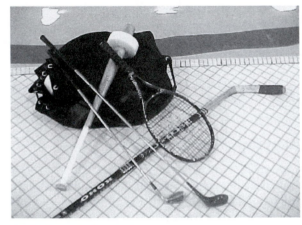

FIGURE 19-12

Sports equipment for use in aquatic environment.

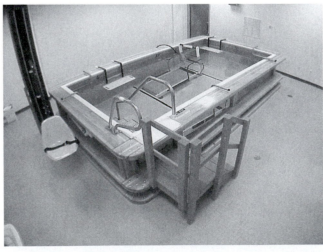

FIGURE 19-10

Custom pool with treadmill.

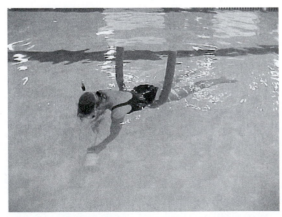

FIGURE 19-13

Prone kayak movement using mask and orkel. Challenges the upper extremities and promotes abilization of the trunk.

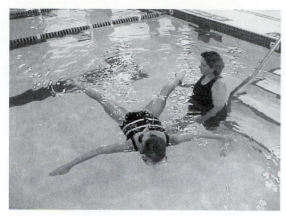

FIGURE 19-14

Prone hip abduction/adduction with manual resistance by athletic trainer. Note use of mask and snorkel, allowing athlete to maintain proper trunk and head/neck position.

options for prone activities/swimming (see Figs. 19-13 and 19-14). Instruction in the proper use of the mask and snorkel is essential for the patient/client's comfort and safety. Equipment aids for aquatic therapy or so-called pool toys are limited in their utilization only by the imagination of the therapist. What is important is to stimulate the patient/client's interest in therapy and to keep in mind what goals are to be accomplished.

The clothing of the therapist is an important consideration. Secondary to the close proximity of the therapist to the patient/client with some treatments, wearing swimwear that covers portions of the lower extremities and upper trunk/upper extremities is an important aspect of professionalism in the aquatic environment. Footwear is another important consideration for the therapist as well as the patient/client. Proper aquatic footwear provides stability, traction, prevents injuries, and maintains good foot position.

WATER SAFETY

There are a number of patients or patients/clients referred for aquatic therapy that are uncomfortable in the water due to minimal experience in aquatic environment. Swimming ability is not necessary to participate in an aquatic exercise program, but instruction of water safety skills will allow for a satisfying experience for the patient/client. Patients and patients/clients may need an exercise bar or floatation noodle to assist with balance during ambulation in water, initially. When adding supine or prone activities into the patient's or patient/client's program, it is important to instruct the individual how to assume that position and return to upright position. This initial act will decrease fear and stress for the patient/client and also decrease stress to injured area.

AQUATIC TECHNIQUES

Aquatic techniques and activities can be designed to begin as active assistive movements and progress to strengthening and eccentric control. Activities are selected based on several factors:

Type of injury/surgery/condition
Treatment protocols, if appropriate
Results/muscle imbalances found in evaluation
Goals/expected return to activities as stated by the patient/client

Aquatic programs are designed similar to land-based programs, with the following components:

Warm-up
Mobility activities
Strengthening activities
Balance or neuromuscular response type of activities
Endurance/cardiovascular activities
Cool down/stretching

With these general considerations in mind, the following sections provide examples of aquatic exercises for the upper extremity, trunk, and lower extremity in a three-phase rehabilitation progression. What has been omitted, in the current discussion from the four-phase rehabilitation scheme used throughout this textbook, is the initial pain control phase. It is assumed that by the time the patient arrives for aquatic therapy, he/she has undergone previous treatment to manage acute injuries and painful conditions. Subsequently, the patient is ready to begin phases two through four of the four-phase approach.

Upper Extremity

The goal of rehabilitation is to restore function by restoring motion and rhythm of movement of all joints of the upper extremity. Aquatic therapy may be used for treatment of the shoulder complex, elbow, wrist, and hand as one of the interventions to accomplish goals along with a land-based program. The following sections describe a rehabilitation progression for shoulder complex dysfunction.

INITIAL LEVEL

The client can be started at chest-deep water to allow for support of the scapular/thoracic area. Walking forward, backward, and sideways will allow for warm-up, working on natural arm swing, and restoration of normal scapulothoracic motions, rotation, and rhythm. Initiation of activities to work on glenohumeral motions can be started at the wall (patient/client with back against the wall); having the patient/client in neck- or shoulder-deep water gives the client physical cues as to posture and quality of movement. The primary goal during the early phase is for the therapist and patient/client to be aware of the amount of movement available without compensatory shoulder elevation. The other options for positions during early treatment are supine and prone. The client will need flotation

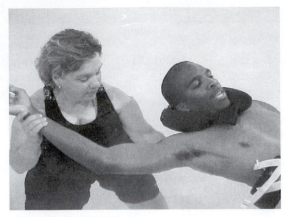

FIGURE 19-15

Range of motion with scapular stabilization.

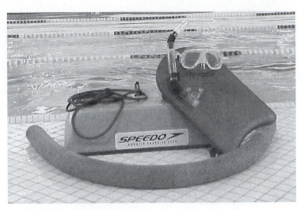

FIGURE 19-17

Other pool equipment: underwater step, mask and snorkel, kickboard, and tubing.

equipment for cervical, lumbar, and lower-extremity support in order to have good positioning when supine (Fig. 19-12).

Supine activities include stretching, mobilization, and range of motion. Stabilizing the scapula with one hand, the therapist can work on glenohumeral motion with the client (Figs. 19-15 and 19-16). The client can initiate active movement in shoulder abduction and extension.

Prone activity can be done depending on the client's comfort in water and use of mask and snorkel. Flotation support around the pelvis allows the client to concentrate on movement. The client is able to perform pendulum type movements, proprioceptive neuromuscular facilitation (PNF) diagonals, and straight-plane movement patterns (flexion/extension and horizontal abduction/adduction) in pain-free range. For the client not comfortable with the prone position, an alternative position is the pendulum position in the standing position.

Deep-water activity can also be integrated for conditioning/endurance building in early stages of rehabilitation. It is important for the client to perform pain-free range when performing endurance type activities.

INTERMEDIATE LEVEL

The program can be progressed to challenge strength by using equipment to resist motion through pain-free range. Increasing the surface area of the extremity or increasing the length of the lever arm will increase the difficulty of the activity. As the client progresses into this phase, the limitations of the standing position become apparent. The athlete can work to the 90° angle but not overhead without exiting the water. It is important for the client to maintain a neutral position of the spine and pelvic area to avoid injury and substitution patterns when performing strengthening activities while standing.

The client will be able to progress with scapular stabilization from standing to supine and prone positions. Supine and prone positioning can allow for more functional movement patterns and core stabilization of the scapular muscles. Flotation assistance from equipment (Fig. 19-18) as well as use of mask and snorkel will allow for proper cervical and spine positioning during prone activities (Figs. 19-13 and 19-14). Activities such as PNF diagonal patterns can be performed with resistance in the pain-free range. Alternate shoulder flexion,

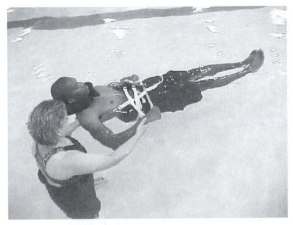

FIGURE 19-16

Internal and external rotation in supine. Note appropriate floatation support for the athlete.

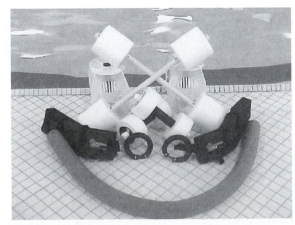

FIGURE 19-18

Equipment used for resistance or floatation.

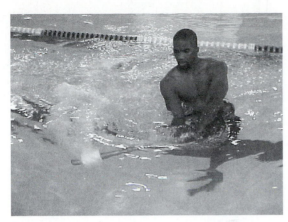

FIGURE 19-19

Sport-specific training using buoyancy cuffs around a bat for resistance.

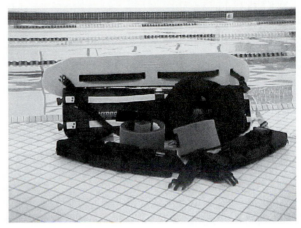

FIGURE 19-20

Flotation equipment.

"kayaking" type motion (Fig. 19-13), and horizontal shoulder abduction/adduction can all be performed using various types of equipment or manual resistance provided by the therapist. Supine positioning allows for work on shoulder extension as well as activities to work on internal and external rotation, at varying degrees of abduction (Fig. 19-16). The land-based program and aquatic program should be coordinated to ensure continued improvement of strength, endurance, and function. The goal of treatment in the intermediate-level activities is development of strength and eccentric control throughout increasing ranges of motion.

FINAL LEVEL

The goal of this level of treatment is high-level functional strengthening and training. Equally important is the transition from the aquatic environment to the land environment. Utilizing sport equipment in treatment, if applicable, will keep an athlete motivated and working toward the goal of returning back to sport (Fig. 19-19). Increasing the resistance by using elastic or flotation attachments will keep it challenging (Figs. 19-18 and 19-20). As in the intermediate level, the client needs to be involved in a strengthening and training program on land.

Spine Dysfunction

The unloading capability of water allows the patient or client ease of movement and some potential relief of symptoms. The patients/clients will need to be shown how to obtain and maintain the neutral spine position in the water even if they have been instructed on land. The neutral spine position is the basis of treatment in land and water and will be progressed in level of difficulty. Activities of the trunk, upper extremities, and lower extremities all challenge trunk stability, strength, total body balance, and neuromuscular control. Directional movement preferences for relief of symptoms, such as extension- or flexion-biased exercises, can be integrated into program. Pregnant patients and clients that experience back pain would benefit from exercising in an aquatic environment.

INITIAL LEVEL

The patient/client in neutral spine position is instructed to take a partial squat position with back against the wall. Use of the pool wall provides the patients/clients with a mechanism to monitor their ability to maintain the neutral position during activities. Upper- and lower-extremity activities can be progressed to incorporate the client's ability to stabilize without increasing symptoms.

Use of deep-water activities can be initiated early in rehabilitation. Client should maintain a vertical position while performing small controlled movements of the upper and lower extremities. The Burdenko approach to aquatic activities utilizes deep-water activities before activities in shallow water. If dealing with radicular (sciatica) type symptoms, a trial of deep-water traction can be done. Flotation support of the upper body and trunk and placement of light weights on the ankles allows for gentle distraction of the lumbar spine (Fig. 19-3). The patient/client can hang while performing small pedaling motions as if bicycling/walking.[29]

Working on normalizing the gait pattern and developing the ability to weight bear equally on the lower extremities in any depth of water comfortable to the client is important early in the therapeutic progression. Incorporation of activities to help centralize the symptoms are important, as well as encouraging the patient to perform only activities that maintain or diminish symptoms during the session. Gentle stretching and rotation movements can be performed in the pain-free motion to increase pelvic and lumbar spine mobility.

INTERMEDIATE LEVEL

At this level the patient/client is progressed away from the wall, and equipment is used to challenge the patient/client's ability to stabilize. Kickboards can be used to mimic pushing, pulling, and lifting motions (Figs. 19-21 and 19-22). Equipment that resists upper-extremity or lower-extremity movements in a single-leg stance or lunge positions challenges the patient/client's balance and stabilization of abdominal and pelvic muscles (Fig. 19-23).

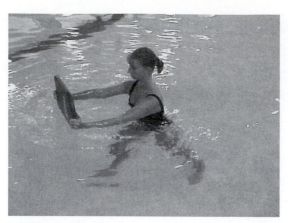

FIGURE 19-21

Trunk stabilization against anterior/posterior forces.

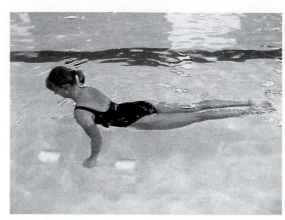

FIGURE 19-24

Tuck-and-roll exercise, extended position.

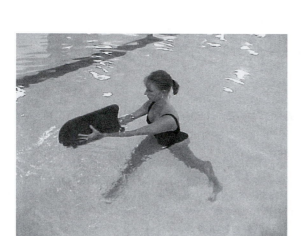

FIGURE 19-22

Trunk stabilization against oblique/diagonal forces.

The client's ability to stabilize can be further challenged using deep-water activities that require maintaining a vertical position while bringing knees to chest and progressing to tucking and rolling type movement (Figs. 19-24 to 19-26). Activities can be created to work on diagonal and rotational motions of the spine and trunk, while maintaining the neutral position.

Activities in a supine position are effective for increasing trunk mobility and then progressing to work on trunk stability using Bad Ragaz techniques (Fig. 19-27).[17] Activities in prone position allow for challenges to the neutral spine position, and the patient/client may need flotation equipment to accomplish that goal. The use of the mask and snorkel will allow for proper positioning of the spine while performing the activities (Fig. 19-18). It is important to monitor and teach the client the neutral spine position with each new position that is introduced in the treatment program. Activities can be simplified or progressed in difficulty according to patients/clients' level of function or their ability to maintain the neutral spine position.

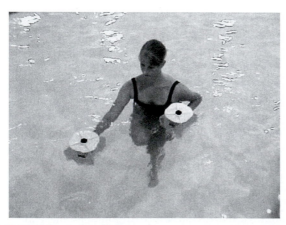

FIGURE 19-23

Challenging lower-extremity neuromuscular control and balance as well as trunk control in single-limb stance, utilizing upper-extremity resistance.

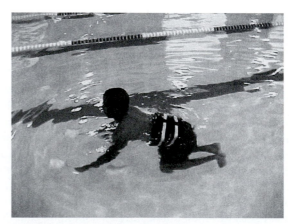

FIGURE 19-25

Tuck-and-roll exercise, tuck position.

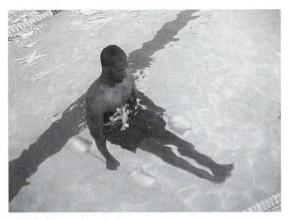

FIGURE   19-26

Tuck-and-roll exercise, pike position.

FINAL LEVEL

Depending on the patient/client's needs and functional goals related to return to a desired level of activity, the program can be modified and progressed. For the patient/client returning to a demanding occupation, development of a program of lifting/pushing/pulling or other needs described by the client can complement a work-conditioning program. For the patient or client returning to a sport, the therapist and athlete can work together to develop specific challenging activities. The therapist needs to be creative with the use of aquatic equipment and should use equipment specific to the athlete's sport to challenge him/her to a higher level of trunk stabilization. It is important to integrate movement patterns that are opposite of the ones the athlete normally performs in his/her sport. (For example, if a gymnast or ice skater predominantly turns or rotates in one direction, have them practice turns in the opposite direction.) The aquatic environment provides the athlete an alternate environment in which to train, which should be encouraged for the serious athlete to avoid overuse type of conditions that can occur. Especially important in this phase is the reintegration of the patient/client back into treatment and training on land, as

the water environment does not allow for normal speeds and forces experienced on land.

Lower-Extremity Injuries

Aquatic therapy is a common modality for rehabilitation of many injuries of the lower extremity because of the properties of unloading and hydrostatic pressure. At an early phase of healing, the client may need to use a flotation belt, vest, exercise bars, noodles, and various other buoyancy devices to provide support (Fig. 19-20), depending on pain and how long they have been non-weightbearing. The aquatic environment allows for limited weight bearing and restoration of gait by calculating the percentage of weight bearing allowed and weight of patient/client and then placing the patient/client in an appropriate depth of water.

INITIAL LEVEL

The expected goals at this phase of rehabilitation are the return of normal motion and early strengthening of affected and unaffected muscles. The restoration of normal and functional gait pattern is also desired. Performing backward and sideways walking adds a functional dimension to the program in addition to traditional forward walking. Range-of-motion activities may involve active motions of the hip, knee, and ankle. Utilizing cuffs, noodles, or kickboards under the foot will assist with increasing motion. Exercises for strengthening noninvolved joints such as hips or ankles can be done with the client who has had a knee injury. However, it is important to remember that resistance may need to be placed above the injured knee to decrease torque forces on the knee. It is important to integrate conditioning and balance activities within this initial level. Standing activities are to be performed with attention to maintaining the spine in a neutral position as well as to challenging balance and neuromuscular control in the lower extremity (Fig. 19-23).

Deep-water activities will allow for conditioning and cross-training opportunities (Figs. 19-3 and 19-28). The patient/client may need more assistance initially with flotation devices, but can progress to decreasing the amount of flotation when able. For the client who must be non-weightbearing secondary to an injury or surgery, the deep water allows for a

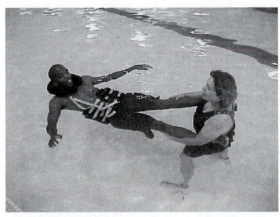

FIGURE   19-27

Bad Ragaz technique for oblique trunk stabilization.

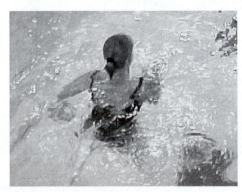

FIGURE   19-28

Deep water running against tether.

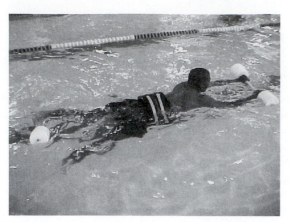

F I G U R E   1 9 - 2 9

Supported single-lower-extremity running movement. Note the appropriate support of the patient/client with buoyancy belts and upper-extremity bell and lower-extremity bell under the stationary lower extremity. Also challenges trunk stabilization.

workout along with maintaining strength in uninvolved joints. Activities can involve running, bicycling, cross-country skiing, and incorporating sport-specific activities (Fig. 19-29).

The therapist can also incorporate activities performed in the supine position. The patients/clients will need to be supported with flotation equipment that will allow them to float evenly. The therapist can stabilize at the feet and have the patient/client work on active hip and knee flexion and extension to work on increasing range of motion at the affected joint (Fig. 19-30). Resistance of hip abduction and adduction can also be performed in a supine position. Again, attention must be paid to the location of applied force. Resistance of the uninvolved leg movement will also allow for strengthening of the injured extremity.

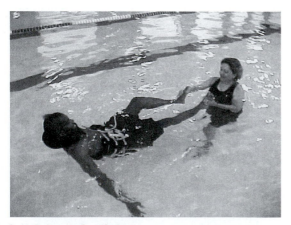

F I G U R E   1 9 - 3 0

Supine alternating hip and knee flexion and extension, using Bad Ragaz technique. Hand contact by therapist gives the patient/client cues for movement.

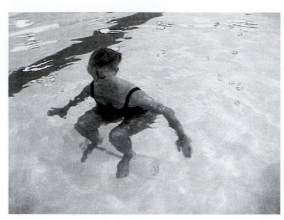

F I G U R E   1 9 - 3 1

Reverse squat, bilateral.

INTERMEDIATE LEVEL

Depending on the injury, surgery, or condition, the client can be progressed to the intermediate level when appropriate. The activities can be progressed by use of weights or flotation cuffs to increase difficulty. As in the initial level, resistance may need to be placed more proximally with anterior crucial ligament injuries/surgeries and other ligament injuries. Performing circuits of straight-plane and diagonal patterns with both lower extremities can be progressed by performing with upper-extremity support on the wall and progressing to no support. The patient/client can stand on an uneven surface, such as a noodle or cuff, to challenge balance and stabilization. Eccentric, closed-chain activities can be performed in the shallow water with the client standing on a noodle or kickboard for single-leg reverse squats, and utilizing a noodle, kickboard, or bar for bilateral reverse-squat motions in deep water (Fig. 19-31) and progressing to a single-leg reverse squat.

Performing deep-water tether running or sprinting forward and backward for increasing periods of time will allow for overall conditioning. The client can progress to running in shallower water depending upon the condition of injury or surgery (Fig. 19-28).

Supine activities can be continued with emphasis on strengthening and stabilization of the trunk, pelvis, and lower extremities. Placement of the therapist's resistance will depend on the client's strength, ability to stabilize, and how much time has elapsed since surgery or injury. Increasing the number of repetitions and/or speed of movement will provide more resistance and work on fatiguing muscle groups of the lower extremity. The prone position provides increased challenges to the client to perform hip abduction and adduction along with hip and knee flexion and extension. The client can use mask and snorkel or flotation equipment to help with positioning while in the prone position (Fig. 19-14).

Sport-specific activities can be integrated into the program for the athlete. While practicing movement patterns needed for sport, the patient/client can start at chest depth and progress to shallow water. As with spine rehabilitation, there is benefit from practicing opposite movement patterns such as turns and jumps. The aquatic environment will allow for early initiation of a structured jumping and landing program. Some adaptations and proper instruction to the patient/client will provide similar positive effects as those seen in land-based programs.[33] Progression to the land-based jump/land program is recommended when appropriate.

FINAL LEVEL

In the final level, the patient/client is involved with a high-level strengthening and training program. The aquatic program can and should be used to complement the land program. The athlete can continue to practice sport-specific activities in varying levels of water. Decreasing the use of flotation equipment can increase the difficulty with deep-water activities. Using buoyancy cuffs on the ankles without using a flotation belt will challenge the athlete's ability to stabilize and perform running in deep water. Endurance training in an aquatic environment is a good alternative for the healthy athlete's conditioning programs and may help prevent further injuries. As with the upper extremity, this phase also requires integration of aquatic- and land-based exercises to successfully transition the athlete to full participation in sport on land.

SPECIAL TECHNIQUES

Bad Ragaz Ring Method

Bad Ragaz technique originated in the thermal pools of Bad Ragaz, Switzerland, in the 1930s but continues to evolve through the years. As a method, it focuses on muscle reeducation, strengthening, spinal traction/elongation, relaxation, and tone inhibition.[17] The properties of water—including buoyancy, turbulence, hydrostatic pressure, and surface tension—provide dynamic environmental forces during activities. The PNF patterns (see Chapter 14) add a three-dimensional aspect to this method. Movement of the client's body through the water provides the resistance.[10] The turbulent drag produced from movement is in direct relation to the client's speed of movement. The therapist provides the movement when the client works on isometric (stabilization) patterns, but the therapist is in the stable/fixed position when the client is performing isokinetic or isotonic activities (Figs. 19-27 and 19-30).[17] Stretching and lengthening responses can be obtained with passive or relaxed response from client; the therapist needs to support and stabilize body segments to obtain desired response.

Awareness of body mechanics and prevention of injury are important to the therapist when performing resistive Bad Ragaz type activities. The therapist should stand in waist-deep water, not deeper than T8-10[17] and wear aqua shoes for traction and stability. The therapist should stand with one foot in front of the other, with knees slightly bent and legs shoulder-width apart, to compensate for the long lever arm force of the client.

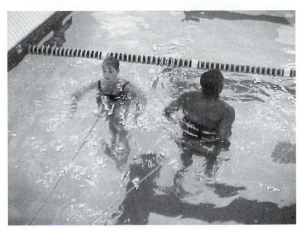

Patients/clients running forward and backward against tubing resistance.

Burdenko Method

The Burdenko method utilizes motion as the principle healing intervention. According to Burdenko,[5] the components of dynamic healing include patterns of movement, injury assessment, and rehabilitation exercises that occur with the client in a standing position; the psychology of the injured client benefiting from pain-free movement, and blood flow and neural stimulation being enhanced by activity.[5] Six essential qualities are necessary for perfecting and maintaining the art of movement: balance, coordination, flexibility, endurance, speed, and strength. Burdenko advocates the presentation of these qualities in exercise activities in the previously stated order. The activities are designed to challenge the center of buoyancy and center of gravity. Treatments/activities are initiated in deep water and incorporate shallow-water activities as client succeeds by demonstrating control of movement while maintaining neutral vertical position. Integration of land exercise along with the aquatic activity addresses functional movement patterns. For further information on this technique, see the section "Suggested Readings" at the end of the chapter.

Halliwick Method

The Halliwick method is commonly used to teach individuals with physical disabilities to swim and to learn balance control in water. Developed by James McMillan, the Halliwick method or concept is based on a "Ten Point Programme."[8] This method is frequently utilized with the pediatric population but portions of the technique can be utilized to improve and restore a patient/client's balance. Use of turbulence forces can assist in developing strategies for maintaining balance or challenge the patient/client to maintain a stable posture during a change in the direction of force. For example, the patient/client maintains a single-leg stance while the therapist or another person

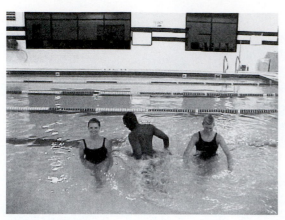

FIGURE   19-33

Balance and neuromuscular control restoration technique for trunk and single lower extremity. This exercise demonstrates the use of the principle of turbulence, generated in the Halliwick technique to challenge the stability of the patient/client.

runs around the patient/client (Fig. 19-33). More information on the Halliwick technique is also available in the "Suggested Readings" section at the end of the chapter.

SPECIAL POPULATIONS

There are many conditions and diagnoses that may benefit from treatment in the aquatic environment. Aquatic therapy interventions can increase a patient/client's level of function. The therapist can be the catalyst for providing an introduction to an environment that can be a temporary rehabilitation tool or lifestyle tool of fitness. The following discussion of the treatment of the pediatric and neurological patient/client is but a brief synopsis and the interested therapist should seek specialized training.

Pediatric Patients and Clients

The aquatic environment provides a fun treatment area for the pediatric patient/client. Examples of congenital pediatric diagnoses that are effectively treated in the aquatic environment include cerebral palsy, spina bifida, and muscular dystrophy. A wide range of additional medical diagnoses may also be appropriate for treatment in this environment. The team of therapists, physicians, and parents can decide on whether it is appropriate to initiate aquatic therapy as a part of the treatment plan. A combination of land and aquatic therapy assists with assessing effectiveness of therapeutic interventions and obtaining functional goals. The major challenge for the therapist is evaluating the pediatric client for water safety. Assessment of the child's ability to accept water to the face, tolerance to being submerged, and breath control are important factors for the aquatic evaluation. The mental adjustment of the child to the water is a

necessary component for successful use of water as a treatment modality. Parents and caregivers may need to find a swim instructor to assist with decreasing fear and increasing comfort of water, with variety of movements.

A variety of approaches such as Halliwick, Bad Ragaz Ring Method, Watsu can be integrated and adapted into treatment program for the pediatric patient/client. Watsu is a passive treatment technique described as Zen Shiatsu in water. It was originally created as a wellness technique and has expanded for utilization with patients and clients. Patients treated with this technique experience relaxation and tone-inhibiting vestibular stimulation.

A treatment program consists of warm up and cool down period, which allows for active stretching and adjustment to the water. Functional motor skills are practiced and integrated into play activities. Water provides constant postural challenges to the child.[37] As with the adult patient or client, the treatment program should progress toward the goals set by the therapist and be readjusted according to patient responses and assessment of progress. It is important to work in collaboration with the multidisciplinary team of personnel who participate in the care of the pediatric client in order to provide synergistic treatment which includes aquatic therapy.

Neurologic Patients and Clients

Benefits of the aquatic environment for the patient/client with neurological involvement include a supportive and safe environment, ease of movement, and an excellent medium in which to practice functional activities. The water allows for the therapist's ease of handling the patient/client with significant neurological involvement. Support offered by the water provides stability and assistance for the therapist who is performing handling techniques to facilitate movement and inhibit tone.

There are a variety of treatment approaches that are effective in accomplishing functional goals. Utilizing the standing and sitting positions encourage and promote postural stability. The first priority is determining the safest and most stable position for the client to begin to work in the water. Practicing functional activities as a whole allows for the patient/client to master the activity while exercising control during the activity and stabilizing multiple body segments. As patient/client progresses, less assistance and support is provided, allowing for increased independence.[35] Like the pediatric population, specialized training is recommended for those therapists who desire to use aquatic rehabilitation as an intervention strategy for their patients and clients with neuromuscular diagnoses.

SUMMARY

Aquatic rehabilitation is usually not the exclusive intervention option for most clients. The aquatic environment offers many positive psychological and physiological effects during the early rehabilitation phase of injury.[30,45] However, in subsequent phases of rehabilitation, it is typical to use combinations of land- and water-based interventions to achieve rehabilitation goals. Because humans function in a "gravity environment," the transition from water to land is necessary for full rehabilitation for most clients. Some clients utilize the aquatic environment for continued strengthening and conditioning programs secondary to a painful response to land-based activities. Examples of this include those patients with pain that occurs with compressive forces at joints (such as cases of disc dysfunction, spinal stenosis, and osteoarthritis), as well as chronic neuromuscular dysfunction such as multiple sclerosis.

This chapter provides information regarding indications and benefits as well as contraindications and precautions of the aquatic environment for rehabilitation. Suggestions and exercises are offered to help the therapist to incorporate aquatic exercise into a rehabilitation program. Utilizing the principles provided and the examples of activities, the therapists can use their judgment, skill, and especially their creativity to develop an exercise program to meet their patient/client's goals. The old English proverb says "We never know the worth of water 'till the well is dry." The worth and value of aquatic therapy as an intervention cannot be fully understood and appreciated until experienced and additional research is completed.

- The buoyant force counteracts the force of gravity as it assists motion toward the water's surface and resists motion away from the surface.
- Because of differences in the specific gravity of the body, the head and chest tend to float higher in the water than the heavier, denser extremities, making compensation with floatation devices necessary.
- The three forces that oppose movement in the water are the cohesive force, the bow force, and the drag force.
- Aquatic therapy allows for fine gradations of exercise, increased control over the percentage of weight bearing, increased range of motion and strength in weak patients/clients, and decreased pain and increased confidence in functional movements.
- Pool size and depth, water temperature, and specific pool equipment will vary depending on clientele being treated and resources available to the therapist.
- Application of the principle of buoyancy allows for progression of exercises.
- Upper- and lower-extremity activities both require and provide a challenge to trunk and core stability.
- The special techniques exclusive to the aquatic environment can be used to complement traditional land-based therapeutic interventions.
- Aquatic therapy can help stimulate interest, motivation, and exercise compliance in pediatric, geriatric, neurological, and athletic patients/clients.
- The aquatic environment is an excellent medium to facilitate speedy functional return to work, activities of daily living, and sport.

- It is typical to use a combination of land- and water-based therapeutic exercise protocols to achieve rehabilitation goals.

REFERENCES

1. Arrigo C, ed. Aquatic rehabilitation. *Sports Med Update* 7(2), 1992.
2. Arrigo C, Fuller CS, Wilk KE. Aquatic rehabilitation following ACL-PTG reconstruction. *Sports Med Update* 7(2):22–27, 1992.
3. Bolton F, Goodwin D. *Pool Exercises.* Edinburgh, Churchill-Livingstone, 1974.
4. Broach E, Groff D, Yaffe R, Dattilo J, Gast D. Effects of aquatics therapy on physical behavior of adult with multiple sclerosis. Paper presented at the 1995 Leisure Research Symposium, San Antonio, TX, 1995. Available at www.indiana.edu/~Irs/Irs95/ebroach95.html. Accessed on October 5, 2005.
5. Burdenko IN. Sport-specific exercises after injuries—the Burdenko method. Paper presented at the Aquatic Therapy Symposium 2002, August 22–25, Orlando, FL, 2002.
6. Butts NK, Tucker M, Greening C. Physiologic responses to maximal treadmill and deep water running in men and women. *Am J Sports Med* 19(6):612–614, 1991.
7. Campion MR. *Adult Hydrotherapy: A Practical Approach.* Oxford, Heinemann Medical, 1990.
8. Cunningham J. Halliwick method. In: Ruoti RG, Morris DM, Cole AJ, eds. *Aquatic Rehabilitation.* Philadelphia, Lippincott-Raven, 1997.
9. Cureton KJ. Physiologic responses to water exercise. In: Ruoti RG, Morris DM, and Cole AJ, eds. *Aquatic Rehabilitation.* Philadelphia, Lippincott-Raven, 1997.
10. Davis BC. A technique of re-education in the treatment pool. *Physiotherapy* 53(2):37–59, 1967.
11. Dioffenbach L. Aquatic therapy services. *Clin Manage* 11(1):14–19, 1991.
12. Dougherty NJ. Risk management in aquatics. *J Health Phys Educ Recreation Dance* (May/June):46–48, 1990.
13. Duffield NH. *Exercise in Water.* London, Bailliere Tindall, 1976.
14. Edlich RF, Towler MA, Goitz RJ, et al. Bioengineering principles of hydrotherapy. *J Burn Care Rehabil* 8(6):580–584, 1987.
15. Eyestone ED, Fellingham G, George J, Fisher G. Effect of water running and cycling on maximum oxygen consumption and 2 mile run performance. *Am J Sports Med* 21(1):41–44, 1993.
16. Fawcett CW. Principles of aquatic rehab: A new look at hydrotherapy. *Sports Med Update* 7(2):6–9, 1992.
17. Garrett G. Bad Ragaz ring method. In: Ruoti RG, Morris DM, Cole AJ, eds. *Aquatic Rehabilitation.* Philadelphia, Lippincott-Raven, 1997.

18. Geigle P, Daddona K, Finken K, et al. The effects of a supplemental aquatic physical therapy program on balance and girth for NCAA division III athletes with a grade I or II lateral ankle sprain. *J Aquatic Phys Ther* 9(1):13–20, 2001.

19. Genuario SE, Vegso JJ. The use of a swimming pool in the rehabilitation and reconditioning of athletic injuries. *Contemp Orthop* 20(4):381–387, 1990.

20. Golland A. Basic hydrotherapy. *Physiotherapy* 67(9):258–262, 1961.

21. Haralson KM. Therapeutic pool programs. *Clin Manage* 5(2):10–13, 1985.

22. Harrison R, Bulstrode S. Percentage weight bearing during partial immersion in the hydrotherapy pool. *Physiother Pract* 3:60–63, 1987.

23. Hertler L, Provost-Craig M, Sestili D, Hove A, Fees M. Water running and the maintenance of maximal oxygen consumption and leg strength in runners. *Med Sci Sports Exerc* 24(5):S23, 1992.

24. Hurley R, Turner C. Neurology and aquatic therapy. *Clin Manage* 11(1):26–27, 1991.

25. Irion JM. Aquatic therapy. In: Bandy WD, Sanders B, eds. *Therapeutic Exercise: Techniques for Intervention.* Baltimore, Lippincott, Williams & Wilkins, 2001.

26. Kolb ME. Principles of underwater exercise. *Phys Ther Rev* 27(6):361–364, 1957.

27. Koszuta LE. From sweats to swimsuits: Is water exercise the wave of the future? *Physician Sports Med* 17(4):203–206, 1989.

28. Levin S. Aquatic therapy. *Physician Sports Med* 19(10):119–126, 1991.

29. McNamara C, Thein L. Aquatic rehabilitation of musculoskeletal conditions of the spine. In: Ruoti RG, Morris DM, Cole AJ, eds. *Aquatic Rehabilitation.* Philadelphia, Lippincott-Raven, 1997.

30. McWaters JG. For faster recovery just add water. *Sports Med Update* 7(2):4–5, 1992.

31. Meyer RI. Practice settings for kinesiotherapy-aquatics. *Clin Kinesiol* 44(1):12–13, 1990.

32. Michaud TL, Brennean DK, Wilder RP, Sherman NW. Aquarun training and changes in treadmill running maximal oxygen consumption. *Med Sci Sports Exerc* 24(5):S23, 1992.

33. Miller MG. Berry DC, Gilders R, Bullard S. Recommendations for implementing an aquatic plyometric program. *Strength Cond J* 23(6):28–35, 2001.

34. Moor FB, Peterson SC, Manueall EM, et al. *Manual of Hydrotherapy and Massage.* Mountain View, CA, Pacific Press, 1964.

35. Morris DM. Aquatic rehabilitation for the treatment of neurologic disorders. In: Cole AJ, Becker BE, eds. *Comprehensive Aquatic Therapy.* Philadelphia, Butterworth-Heinemann, 2004.

36. Nolte-Heuritsch I. *Aqua Rhythmics: Exercises for the Swimming Pool.* New York, Sterling, 1979.

37. Petersen TM. Pediatric aquatic therapy. In: Cole AJ, Becker BE, eds. *Comprehensive Aquatic Therapy.* Philadelphia, Butterworth-Heinemann, 2004.

38. Pöyhönen T, Kyröläinen H, Keskinen KL, Hautala A, Savolainen J, Mälkiä, E. Electromyographic and kinematic analysis of therapeutic knee exercises under water. *Clin Biomech* 16:496–504, 2001.

39. Pöyhönen TK, Keskinen L, Hautala A, Mälkiä E. Determination of hydrodynamic drag forces and drag coefficients on human leg/foot model during knee exercise. *Clin Biomech* 15:256–260, 2000.

40. Robertson JM, Brewster EA, Factora KI. Comparison of heart rates during water running in deep and shallow water at the same rating of perceived exertion. *J Aquatic Phys Ther* 9(1):21–26, 2001.

41. Simmons V, Hansen PD. Effectiveness of water exercise on postural mobility in the well elderly: An experimental study on balance enhancement. *J Gerontol* 51A(5):M233–M238, 1996.

42. Sova R. *Aquatic Activities Handbook.* Boston, Jones & Bartlett, 1993.

43. Speer K, Cavanaugh JT, Warren RF, Day L, Wickiewicz TL. A role for hydrotherapy in shoulder rehabilitation. *Am J Sports Med* 21(6):850–853, 1993.

44. Svendenhag J, Seger J. Running on land and in water: Comparative exercise physiology. *Med Sci Sports Exerc* 24(10):1155–1160, 1992.

45. Thein JM, Thein Brody L. Aquatic-based rehabilitation and training for the elite athlete. *J Orthop Sports Phys Ther* 27(1):32–41, 1998.

46. Town GP, Bradley SS. Maximal metabolic responses of deep and shallow water running in trained runners. *Med Sci Sports Exerc* 23(2):238–241, 1991.

47. Triggs M. Orthopedic aquatic therapy. *Clin Manage* 11(1):30–31, 1991.

48. Wilder RP, Brennan D, Schotte D. A standard measure for exercise prescription and aqua running. *Am J Sports Med* 21(1):45–48, 1993.

SUGGESTED READINGS

Berger MA, deGroot G, Hollander AP. Hydrodynamic drag and lift forces on human hand/arm models. *J Biomech* 28(2):125–133, 1995.

Burdenko J, Connors E. *Ultimate Power of Resistance.* Igor Publishing, 1999 [available only through mail order].

Burdenko J, Miller J. *Defying Gravity.* Igor Publishing, 2001 [available only through mail order].

Campion MR. *Adult Hydrotherapy: A Practical Approach.* Oxford, Heinemann Medical, 1990.

Cassady SL, Nielsen OH. Cardiorespiratory responses of healthy subjects to calisthenics performed on land versus in water. *Phys Ther* 72(7):532–538, 1992.

Christie JL, Sheldahl LM, Tristani FE. Cardiovascular regulation during head-out water immersion exercise. *J Appl Physiol* 69(2):657–664, 1990.

Frangolias DD, Rhodes EC. Maximal and ventilatory threshold responses to treadmill and water immersion running. *Med Sci Sports Exerc* 27(7):1007–1013, 1995.

Green JH, Cable NT, Elms N. Heart rate and oxygen consumption during walking on land and in deep water. *J Sports Med Phys Fitness* 30(1):49–52, 1990.

Martin J. The Halliwick method. *Physiotherapy* 67:288–291, 1981.

Sova R. *Aquatic Activities Handbook.* Boston, Jones & Bartlett, 1993.

CHAPTER 20

Functional Movement Screening

Gray Cook and Lee Burton

OBJECTIVES

After completing this chapter, the therapist should be able to do the following:

- Understand the importance of defining and establishing normal functional movement patterns.
- Develop a knowledge of functional movement screening in normal populations.
- Develop an appreciation of utilizing a performance pyramid to assist and categorize individual weaknesses.
- Understand the philosophy for which the functional movement patterns were established.
- Utilize objective measurements to assess functional movement patterns.
- Utilize the information gained from functional movement screening to assist in developing a holistic approach to therapeutic treatment.

The founders of the physical therapy profession did not have the luxury of documented history or professional texts to use as a guide for practice. They had to gain working knowledge of normal, efficient, functional, and productive human movement and from that perspective, and had to evaluate, rate, and treat dysfunction and disability. Throughout the history of physical therapy, clinicians have drawn upon the data provided to us by normal populations.

The earliest research in growth and development chronicled the sequence of motor development in infants. This information on developmental milestones was gathered by studying large groups of infants as they learned to move within their environment.[11] These milestones served as a basis by which to judge progress and prognosis of patients with movement-related disorders.

In developing theory related to the testing of muscle, Kendall and McCreary did not look at pathological muscle contraction and develop protocols for strengthening.[14] Rather, they first looked at normal contractile qualities and muscular actions and mapped out as many individual muscles as possible for testing, treatment, and exercise purposes. Their observations of normal human physiology and movement provided a baseline for establishment of sound, functional goals. This also allowed for assessment and grading of dysfunction, noted in a particular muscle group.

The information currently employed regarding by therapists balance, proprioception, and equilibrium was derived from testing and observing normal subjects. Isolated joint range of motion values have also been derived from goniometric studies of asymptomatic subjects.[18] Despite our reliance on data derived from normal populations, there is a lack of information related to normal functional movement patterns. Over the last 20 years, this profession has undergone a trend away from traditional isolated strengthening toward an integrated functional approach to therapeutic exercise and assessment incorporating the principles of proprioceptive neuromuscular facilitation, muscle synergy, and motor learning.[13]

In order to properly develop these functional therapeutic exercise protocols, functional movement in normal individuals must be described. It is difficult to develop and refer to protocols as "functional" when a functional evaluation standard does not exist. It seems that most protocols are established based upon isolated, objective, evaluation techniques such as muscle testing, special joint testing, and range of motion measurements. However, adults should be able to utilize this range of motion, joint function and strength into a pain-free deep squat, demonstrating synergistic use of all, as an example.

Substantial efforts have been made to develop functional exercise models which improve squatting, lunging, and single leg stance movements, without understanding what normal movement should be. By documenting the functional movement patterns of individuals who are injury free, a greater understanding of ideal functional movement can be achieved. If data on normal functional movement were available, more efficient intervention strategies to restore functional movement patterns could be developed. Often rehabilitation professionals in industrial and sports medicine settings are far too anxious to perform specific testing for sports and job tasks without first looking at functional movement. It is important to examine and understand fundamental aspects and common denominators of human movement and realize that they are common throughout many activities in varying applications.

In the traditional sports medicine model, preparticipation physicals are followed by performance assessments. This systematic approach does not seem to provide enough baseline information when assessing an individual's preparedness for activity. Commonly, the medical preparticipation or rehabilitation examination only includes information that will exclude an individual from participating in certain activities. The perception of many past researchers was that there were no set standards in determining who was physically prepared to participate in activities.[10,15,20,21] Recently, numerous medical societies have collaborated and attempted to establish more uniformity in this area; however, only baseline medical information is provided.[28] There should also be collaboration in determining what the baseline for fundamental movement should be and if individuals should be allowed to participate when they are unable to perform movements at a basic level.

Once the preparticipation physical is performed, the active individual is then asked to perform performance tests. Commonly recommended performance tests include sit-ups, push-ups, endurance runs, sprints, and agility activities.[1] In many athletic and occupational settings, these performance activities become more specific to the tasks in defined areas of performance.

Performance tests function to gather baseline quantitative information and then attempt to make recommendations and establish goals. The recommendations are based on standardized normative information, which may not be relative to the individual's specific needs. Likewise, in many cases, performance tests provide objective information that fails to evaluate the efficiency by which individuals perform certain movements. Little consideration is given to functional movement deficits, which may limit performance and/or predispose the individual to microtraumatic injury. Prescribed strength and conditioning programs often work to improve agility, speed, and strength, without consideration for perfection or efficiency of underlying functional movement. An example of this would be a person who has an above average score on the sit-up test but is performing very inefficiently, compensating by initiating the movement with the upper body and cervical spine compared to properly using the trunk. Compare this person to an individual who scores above average and is performing very efficiently, who does not utilize compensatory movements to achieve the sit-up. These two individuals would each be deemed "above average" without noting their individual movement inefficiencies. The question arises: if major deficiencies are noted in their functional movement patterns, then should their performance be judged as equal? These two individuals would likely have significant differences in functional mobility and stability; however, without carefully assessing their functional mobility and stability it may be difficult to describe these differences.

Many rehabilitation professionals are guilty of performing job-specific functional capacity examinations without ever looking at functional movement patterns. We may comment that a worker uses very poor lifting mechanics with respect to neutral spine and lower extremity contribution during lifting while failing to observe a significant lack of closed-chain dorsiflexion. This factor alone can cause an individual to have diminished lumbar static and dynamic stability due to compensation. This may be the only way that the individual can perform a lift movement, no matter how much you educate the individual on proper lifting mechanics. Without the proper movement pattern to serve as the foundation for proper lifting mechanics, movement compensations will continue during function.

The main goal in performing preparticipation or performance screenings is to decrease injuries, enhance job performance, and ultimately improve quality of life.[19,20,28] Currently, the research is inconsistent on whether the preparticipation or performance screenings and standardized fitness measures have the ability to do this.[20,21] A reason for this is the standardized screenings' inability to provide individualized, fundamental analysis of an individual's movements. This may be a reason why this type of analysis should be incorporated into the pre-screenings in order to appreciate who has the ability to perform certain essential movements.

In order to better understand an individual's ability to perform during certain activities or tasks, an individualized movement-based assessment could be introduced. To this end, functional movement screening in the normal population will be presented. This type of assessment will serve both as a screening tool for highly active individuals and as an object lesson to help physical therapists learn how to restore, regain, and improve functional movement patterns in individuals who are without symptomatic complaints.

The opportunity to observe the responses of an individual, who is without symptoms but has difficulty in performing functional movement patterns, is an important lesson for today's physical therapist. By performing movement screening on active populations such as laborers, firefighters, safety professionals, athletes of all skill levels, and other highly fit individuals participating in fitness and recreational athletics, a wealth of opportunity exists for the physical therapist to gain much needed knowledge on functional movement patterns.

Hopefully, in time, the techniques developed to restore functional movement patterns in an asymptomatic population will benefit the therapeutic protocols developed to restore functional movement patterns in a symptomatic population. The Functional movement screen (FMS™) is currently being implemented with fit individuals at all levels, athletes of all levels, as well as within military personnel and firefighters.[7] The feedback regarding such screening has been overwhelmingly positive and valuable since the FMS™ examines a missing piece of the puzzle.

Functional Movement   Functional Performance   Functional Skill   Buffer Zone

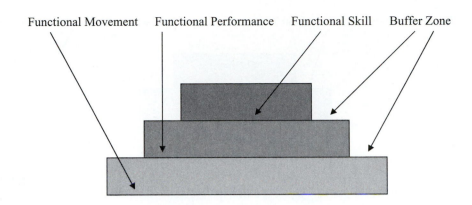

FIGURE 20-1

The optimum performance pyramid.

PERFORMANCE PYRAMID

The performance pyramid is a simple diagram constructed to offer a mental image and understanding of human movement and movement patterns (Fig. 20-1).[6] It is constructed of three rectangles of diminishing size, with one rectangle building upon another.[3] Each of these rectangles represents a certain type of movement. The pyramid must always be constructed from the bottom up and must always have a tapered appearance (a broad base and a narrow top).

The first rectangular pillar is the base platform or foundation. It represents the functional movement patterns or ability to move through fundamental patterns such as squatting, lunging, and stepping. The second rectangular pillar depicts functional performance. Once the ability to move has been established, the efficiency of movement must also be examined. Movement efficiency is defined as power in this movement screen. In active occupational groups, this type of power is measured through activities such as push-ups, sit-ups, or even vertical leap, which is common in athletics. These tests attempt to assess the individual's performance level compared to norms previously established.[1]

It is very important from a training standpoint to be able to compare individuals of different performance areas in a general format. The first two rectangular pillars allow us to make this comparison of functional movement ability and power so that active individuals can learn from each other concerning different training regimes. Moreover, it is important not to get task specific with testing at this level of the performance pyramid. Task specificity at this point of testing reduces the ability to compare individuals to one another as well as the ability to learn from these comparisons. It is also important not to perform too many tests at this level. The more tests you do the more you can overanalyze the person's performance; the purpose is to get an overall assessment of the individual's abilities. A few simple movements illustrate an individual's efficiency at generating power.

The last pillar of the pyramid is functional skill. This pillar constitutes a battery of tests to assess an individual's ability to perform certain functional skills. For example, it may be how job-specific tasks or sports position-specific skills are performed. The idea is to utilize normative data that are related to the specific skill tests and compare them.

The performance pyramid is only a map; it is designed only to give you a direction with which to categorize and identify areas of weakness. Consider four basic appearances of the pyramid (Fig. 1-4).[4] These are simple generalizations, but each represents how the pyramid can help guide the entire evaluation and eventually the conditioning program.

The first pyramid we will discuss is the optimal pyramid, which represents a type of individual whose functional movement patterns (demonstrated by the FMS[TM]), functional performance (demonstrated by performance testing), and functional skill (demonstrated by functional skill testing, sports-specific testing, and statistics) are balanced and adequate (Fig. 20-1). This does not mean that the individual cannot improve; however, any improvement should not upset the balance and appearance of the performance pyramid.

The optimum performance pyramid has a broad base with a slightly smaller rectangular pillar in the middle section and an even smaller rectangular pillar on the top. This broad-base representation demonstrates an individual who has appropriate or optimal functional movement, possessing the ability to explore a full range of movement, and demonstrating body control and movement awareness throughout numerous positions.

In next level, in such an optimal pyramid the individual demonstrates a requisite amount of power. When compared to normative data, this individual also has demonstrated average or above-average general power production. This means the individual utilizes well-coordinated linking movements or kinetic linking. This implies that during a test such as the vertical leap the individual loads the body in a crouched position, throws the arms, slightly extends the trunk, and finally explodes through legs in a well-timed, well-coordinated effort so that optimal efficiency is present. This individual has the potential to learn other kinetic linking movements and power production movements with appropriate time, practice, and analysis.

Finally, the third rectangular pillar, functional skill, demonstrates an average or optimal amount of task-specific or

Functional Movement   Functional Performance   Functional Skill

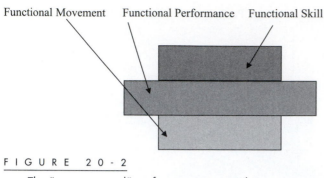

FIGURE 20-2

The "over powered" performance pyramid.

Functional Movement   Functional Performance   Functional Skill

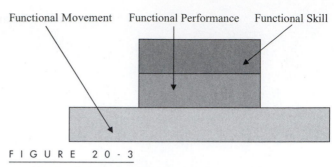

FIGURE 20-3

The "under powered" performance pyramid.

activity-specific skill. Note how the broad base creates a "buffer zone" for the second pillar and the second pillar creates a buffer zone for the top pillar. This buffer zone is extremely important; it implies that the individual exceeds the necessary mobility and stability needed to perform the specific tasks. Without the buffer zone, there may be potential for injury or that power and efficiency are being compromised. This buffer zone simply demonstrates the fact that the individual's functional movements are more than adequate to handle the amount of power that they can generate. Referring to the top of the pyramid, the generated power can more than control the skill that they possess.

The second pyramid is a graphic demonstration of individuals who are "overpowered" (Fig. 20-2). This does not mean that they are too strong—it only means that their ability to generate power exceeds their ability to move freely. The way to rectify this problem is to improve their movement patterns while maintaining their current level of power. This pyramid provides a visual representation of an individual who scores very poorly on mobility and stability tests, but very high on power production (the second pillar) and adequately in skill (the third pillar).

An individual who has these characteristics lacks the ability to move freely in simple and basic positions due to limited flexibility or stability in some of the movement patterns. This causes them to have a less than optimal functional movement score that would appear as a smaller rectangular pillar at the base. This individual's performance does not really have the appearance of a pyramid. The base (functional movement) and the power (functional performance) seem to be inverted in size. This individual is generating a significant amount of power with many restrictions and limitations in functional movement.

Many highly skilled and well-trained individuals will appear this way when their performance is evaluated in the form of a performance pyramid. An example of this type of athlete would be an individual who displays tremendous strength and power when performing traditional weight-training movements such as the bench press and squat. However, this athlete is unable to perform functional movements such as lunging, squatting, or a push-up without compensations. This individual may have never experienced an injury and may be per-

forming at a high level, but if this individual chooses to train, the best focus for training would be on functional movement patterns.

The focus for this type of individual is to remove the limitations to functional movement, which would provide a broader base to the pyramid and create a greater buffer zone. There may not be an immediate tangible improvement in performance; in fact, task-specific performance and power production may remain the same or even go down slightly as mobility and stability improve. However, it is unlikely that this individual would improve in general power production or task-specific skill to any large degree without first improving general fundamental basic movement patterns. Therefore, whether this individual targets functional movement patterns for injury prevention or as a way to realize untapped performance, they will eventually see improvements.

The third pyramid represents a graphic representation of underpowered individuals who have excellent freedom of movement but whose efficiency is poor and could stand improvement (Fig. 20-3). This individual should be involved in training and conditioning that would improve efficiency or power without negatively affecting the movement patterns.

This pyramid is a graphic representation of an individual who demonstrates a broad-base and optimal movement patterns with very poor power production at the second level while demonstrating optimal or above-average skill in a specific movement. This individual has the requisite movement patterns to perform multiple tasks, activities, and skills but lacks the ability to produce power in simple movement patterns. This person would benefit greatly from power, plyometric, or weight training.

It is very important that such an individual maintains functional movement patterns as they gain strength, power, endurance, and speed. This reserve of power will create the buffer zone for task-specific skill while improving their efficiency. Consider the example of a firefighter who has extremely good mobility and stability and honed his skills through practice and expert instruction. This individual must use a very high level of energy expenditure in order to perform at high levels for a short period of time. This individual does not need to be on a mobility or stability program and probably does not need

Functional Movement   Functional Performance   Functional Skill

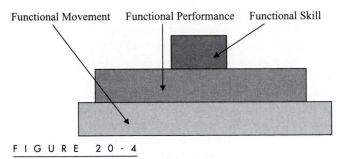

FIGURE 20-4

The "under skilled" performance pyramid.

to work on improving certain tasks specific to firefighting. This individual should create better strength, power, and endurance reserves within the body therefore improving overall strength and wellness.

Such interventions would create a buffer zone between the second and third pillar of the pyramid. This buffer zone would allow the individual to perform at the same level of effectiveness with a higher level of efficiency or a lower level of energy expenditure. This should allow greater effectiveness during job-specific performance.

The last pyramid is a graphic demonstration of individuals who are under-skilled (Fig. 20-4). This is a situation where the movement pattern and efficiency, or power generation, the first two blocks of the pyramid, are adequate. However, analysis of skill demonstrates an overall inability to produce the desired outcome or mastery of skills needed to perform their tasks. Individuals in this category appear to be appropriately conditioned but not appropriately skilled. A training program specifically designed around skill fundamentals and techniques would be the best investment of time for these individuals. This would allow them to develop a greater awareness of the movements needed to perform the skill at a more efficient level. The whole purpose for the testing proposed in this book is to provide a method to acquire information in order to construct a simple performance pyramid. Such a graphic representation will consistently assist in identification of weak areas where training can then be focused. Through training, the performance pyramid will continually change for some individuals, while for others it will remain the same.

Some individuals will have the natural ability to generate power but must consistently work on functional movement patterns to maintain optimal freedom of movement. Other individuals will have excellent natural freedom of movement and movement patterns but need to use supplementary training to maintain a level of power production. Finally, some individuals need to consistently work on fundamentals and task-specific skills, while others are naturally gifted with certain skills and should invest their time in other types of conditioning.

The performance pyramid explains why simply replicating the program of one individual will not consistently yield the level of results it does for another individuals. Many physical therapists, athletic trainers, coaches, and athletes over the years have intuitively used this type of approach to identify the performance area with the greatest weakness and then work on improving that area. The performance pyramid is a simple and effective graphic way to evaluate and illustrate body balance or lack thereof. It also aids in communicating with the athlete regarding his/her deficits.

Functional Movement Screen[5,8,9]

The FMS™ is only an attempt to pinpoint areas of mobility and stability deficits that are being overlooked in our asymptomatic active population. The ability to predict injuries is equally as important as the ability to evaluate and treat injuries. The information gained by functional movement screening of numerous individuals from diverse population groups will provide much needed data toward what is acceptable and what is not with respect to a decline in functional movement patterns across the age spectrum. The development of norms can also alert us to individuals who have developed compensations and are moving inefficiently, which may lead us to focus on their weakness before a microtraumatic injury presents itself. For example, instead of simply looking at balance problems in the elderly, the correlation between balance problems, functional movement patterns, proprioception, posture, strength, and endurance can be examined and correlated. When orthopedic injuries such as anterior cruciate ligament (ACL) tears are sustained by female athletes who participate in soccer and basketball, retrospective correlations can be made between deficiencies and functional movement patterns and incidence and occurrence of ACL trauma.

The FMS™ is an attempt to capture movement pattern quality with a primitive grading system that at least begins the process of functional movement pattern assessment in normal individuals. It is not intended to diagnose but rather to demonstrate limitations or asymmetries with respect to human movement patterns and eventually correlate them with outcomes.

The FMS™ is an evaluation tool that attempts to assess an individual's fundamental movement patterns. This assessment tool fills the void between the preparticipation/preplacement screenings and performance tests by evaluating the individual in a more dynamic and functional capacity. A screening tool such as this offers a different approach to injury prevention and performance predictability. It will lead to individualized and functional recommendations for physical fitness protocols in active population groups.

The test comprises seven fundamental movement patterns that require a balance of mobility and stability. These fundamental movement patterns are designed to provide observable performance of basic locomotor, manipulative, and stabilizing movements. The tests place the individual in extreme positions where weaknesses and imbalances become noticeable if appropriate stability and mobility is not utilized. It has been observed that many individuals who perform at very high levels during activities are unable to perform these simple movements.[7,9] These individuals should be considered to be utilizing compensatory movement patterns during their activities, sacrificing efficient movements for inefficient ones in order to perform at high levels. If these compensations continue, then poor movement patterns will be reinforced leading to poor biomechanics.

The FMS[TM] tests were based upon skills, fundamental proprioceptive, kinesthetic awareness. Each test is a specific movement, which requires appropriate function of the body's kinetic linking system. The kinetic link model is used to analyze movement; it depicts the body as a linked system of interdependent segments, often working in a proximal-to-distal sequence, to impart a desired action at the distal segment.[22] An important aspect of this system is the body's proprioceptive abilities. Proprioception can be defined as a specialized variation of the sensory modality of touch that encompasses the sensation of joint movement and joint position sense.[17] Proprioceptors in each segment of the kinetic chain must be functioning properly in order for efficient movement patterns to occur.

During the growth and development, an individual's proprioceptors are developed through reflexive movements in order to perform basic motor tasks. This development occurs from proximal to distal, the learning to first stabilize the joints in the spine and individual torso and eventually the extremities. This progression occurs due to maturation and learning. An infant learns the fundamental movements by responding to a variety of stimuli through motor control. As the growth and development progresses, the proximodistal process becomes operational and has a tendency to reverse itself. The process of movement regression slowly evolves in a tail-to-head direction.[11] This occurs as individuals gravitate toward specific skills and movements through habit, lifestyles, and/or training.

This can be illustrated within the fire service by the firefighter constantly training certain duties for improved performance. They initially train through voluntary movements, and then as they are repeated, the movement becomes stored as central commands leading to subconscious performance of the task. This subconscious performance involves the highest levels of central nervous system function, which refers to cognitive programming.[17] However, problems arise when the movements and training being "learned" are performed inefficiently or asymmetrically.

An example of this would be a firefighter entering training who does not have the requisite balance of mobility or stability to perform tasks such as the hose drag, stair climb, or the fireman carry. The individual will perform these tasks utilizing compensatory movement patterns in order to overcome the stability or mobility inefficiencies. The compensatory movement pattern will then be developed throughout the training. If this happens, the individual creates a poor movement pattern that will be utilized subconsciously whenever the task is performed. This has the potential to lead to mobility and stability imbalances, which have previously been identified as risk factors for injury.[3,16,23]

An alternative view of what may lead to these poor movement patterns could be previous injuries. Individuals who have suffered from an injury will have a decrease in proprioceptive input if left untreated or treated inappropriately.[17,24] A disruption in proprioceptive performance will have a negative effect on the kinetic linking system. The result will be altered mobility, stability, and asymmetric influences, eventually leading to compensatory movement patterns. This may be a reason why prior injuries have been determined to be one of the more significant risk factors in predisposing individuals to injuries.[24,25]

It is difficult to determine which risk factor has a larger influence on injury, previous injuries, or strength/flexibility imbalances. In either case, both lead to deficiencies in functional mobility and stability. It has been determined that these functional deficits lead to pain, injury, and decreased performance. Cholewicki, Panjabi, and Khachatryn found that limitations in stability in the spine led to muscular compensations, fatigue, and pain.[4] It has been previously determined that spinal instabilities result in degenerative changes due to the muscle activation strategies, which may be disrupted due to previous injury, stiffness, or fatigue.[12] It has been further demonstrated that individuals with previous low-back pain performed timed shuttle runs at a significantly lower pace than individuals who did not have previous low-back pain.[22]

Therefore, an important factor in preventing injuries and improving performance is to quickly identify deficits in mobility and stability because of their influences on creating altered motor programs throughout the kinetic chain. The complexity of the kinetic linking system makes it difficult to evaluate weaknesses using conventional, static methods. Therefore, it has been recommended that functional tests that incorporate the entire kinetic chain need to be utilized to isolate deficiencies in the system.[2,19,24]

The FMS[TM] is designed to identify individuals who have developed compensatory movement patterns in the kinetic chain. This is accomplished by observing right and left side imbalances and mobility and stability weaknesses. The seven movements in the FMS[TM] attempt to challenge the body's ability to facilitate movement through the proximal-to-distal sequence. This course of movement in the kinetic chain allows the body to produce movement patterns more efficiently. The correct movement patterns were initially formed during growth and development. However, due to a weakness in the kinetic linking system, a poor movement pattern may have resulted. Once an inefficient movement pattern has been isolated by the FMS, functional prevention strategies can be instituted to avoid problems such as imbalance, microtraumatic breakdown, and injury.

SCORING

The scoring for the FMS[TM] consists of four possibilities. The scores range from 0 to 3, 3 being the best possible score. The four basic scores are quite simple in philosophy. An individual is given a score of zero if at any time during the testing he/she has pain anywhere in the body. If there is pain, a score of zero is given and the painful area is noted. A score of 1 is given if the person is unable to complete the movement pattern or unable to assume the position to perform the movement. A score of 2 is given if the person is able to complete the movement but must compensate in some way to perform the fundamental movement. A score of 3 is given if the person performs the movement correctly without any compensation. The score sheet contains an area used for comments; this area should be utilized when scoring to make notes about the individual's specific movement problems.

A majority of the tests in the FMS™ test right and left sides respectively, and it is important that both sides are scored. The lower score of the two sides is recorded and counted toward the total; however it is important to note the imbalance between right and left sides on the score sheet.

Three tests that have additional clearing screens are performed, which are graded as positive or negative. These clearing movements only consider pain: if a person has pain then that portion of the test is positive and if there is no pain then it is negative. This does affect the total score for that particular test. If a person has a positive clearing screen test then the score will be zero. It is important to record the scores for each test on the score sheet for future reference, even if the final score is a zero.

The scores for the right and left sides and the scores for the tests, which are associated with the clearing screens, should all be recorded. By documenting all the scores, even if zeros are evident, the sports medicine professional will have a better understanding of the impairment when performing an evaluation. However, it is important to note that only the lowest score is recorded and considered when tallying the total score. The best score that can be attained on the FMS™ is 21.

DEEP SQUAT

Purpose. The squat is a movement common to most athletic events. It is the ready position and required for most power movements involving the lower extremities. The deep squat is a test that challenges total body mechanics when performed properly. The deep squat is used to assess bilateral, symmetrical, functional mobility of the hips, knees, and ankles. The dowel held overhead assesses bilateral, symmetrical mobility of the shoulders as well as the thoracic spine.

Description. The individual assumes the starting position by placing his/her feet approximately shoulder width apart and the feet aligned in the sagittal plane. The individual then adjusts his/her hands on the dowel to assume a 90° angle of the elbows with the dowel overhead. Next, the dowel is pressed overhead with the shoulders flexed and abducted, and the elbows extended. The individual is then instructed to descend slowly into a squat position. The squat position should be assumed with the heels on the floor, head and chest facing forward, and the dowel maximally pressed overhead. As many as three repetitions may be performed. If the criteria for a score of 3 is not achieved, the athlete is then asked to perform the test with a 2 × 6 under the heels.

Tips for testing are

- when in doubt, score it low,
- try not to interpret the score while testing, and
- make sure if you have a question to view individual from the side.

Scores for Deep Squat

SCORE 3 (FIGS. 20-5 AND 20-6)	**SCORE 2 (FIGS. 20-7 AND 20-8)**	**SCORE 1 (FIGS. 20-9 AND 20-10)**
• Upper torso is parallel with tibia or toward vertical • Femur below horizontal • Knees are aligned over feet • Dowel aligned over feet	• Upper torso is parallel with tibia or toward vertical • Femur is below horizontal • Knees are aligned over feet • Dowel is aligned over feet	• Tibia and upper torso are not parallel • Femur is not below horizontal • Knees are not aligned over feet • Lumbar flexion is noted

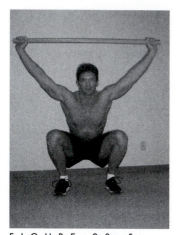

FIGURE 20-5

Deep squat 3: anterior view.

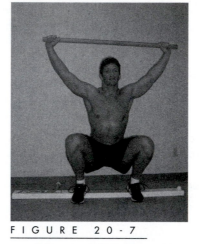

FIGURE 20-7

Deep squat 2: anterior view.

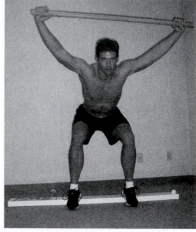

FIGURE 20-9

Deep squat 1: anterior view.

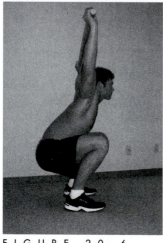

FIGURE 20-6

Deep squat 3: lateral view.

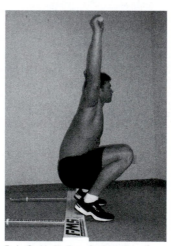

FIGURE 20-8

Deep squat 2: lateral view.

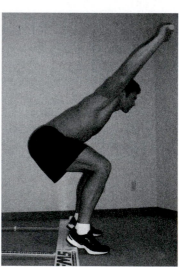

FIGURE 20-10

Deep squat 1: lateral view.

0—The athlete will receive a score of zero if pain is associated with any portion of this test. A medical professional should perform a thorough evaluation of the painful area.

CLINICAL IMPLICATIONS FOR DEEP SQUAT

The ability to perform the deep squat requires closed-kinetic chain dorsiflexion of the ankles, flexion of the knees and hips, and extension of the thoracic spine, as well as flexion and abduction of the shoulders.

Poor performance of this test can be the result of several factors. Limited mobility in the upper torso can be attributed to poor glenohumeral and/or thoracic spine mobility. Limited mobility in the lower extremity including by poor closed-kinetic chain dorsiflexion of the ankles or poor flexion of the hips may also cause poor test performance.

When an athlete achieves a score less than 3, the limiting factor must be identified. Clinical documentation of these limitations can be obtained by using standard goniometric measurements. Previous testing has identified that when an athlete achieves a score of 2, minor limitations most often exist either with closed-kinetic chain dorsiflexion of the ankle or extension of the thoracic spine. When an athlete achieves a score of 1 or less, gross limitations may exist with the motions previously mentioned as well as flexion of the hip.

HURDLE STEP

Purpose. The hurdle step is designed to challenge the body's proper stride mechanics during a stepping motion. The move- ment requires proper coordination and stability between the hips and torso during the stepping motion as well as single leg stance stability. The hurdle step assesses bilateral functional mobility and stability of the hips, knees, and ankles.

Description. The individual assumes the starting position by first placing the feet together and aligning the toes touching the base of the hurdle. The hurdle is then adjusted to the height of the athlete's tibial tuberosity. The dowel is positioned across the shoulders below the neck. The individual is then asked to step over the hurdle and touch their heel to the floor while maintaining the stance leg in an extended position. The moving leg is then returned to the starting position. The hurdle step should be performed slowly and as many as three times bilaterally. If one repetition is completed bilaterally meeting the criteria given next, a 3 is given.

Tips for testing are

- score the leg that is stepping over the hurdle,
- make sure the individual maintains a stable torso,
- make sure the toes keep in contact with the hurdle during and after each repetition,
- tell individual not to lock knees during test,
- maintain proper alignment with the string and the tibial tuberosity,
- when in doubt score low, and
- do not try to interpret the score when testing.

Scores for Hurdle Step

SCORE 3 (FIGS. 20-11 AND 20-12)	SCORE 2 (FIGS. 20-13 AND 20-14)	SCORE 1 (FIGS. 20-15 AND 20-16)
• Hips, knees, and ankles remain aligned in the sagittal plane • Minimal to no movement is noted in lumbar spine • Dowel and hurdle remain parallel	• Alignment is lost between hips, knees, and ankles • Movement is noted in lumbar spine • Dowel and hurdle do not remain parallel	• Contact between foot and hurdle occurs • Loss of balance is noted

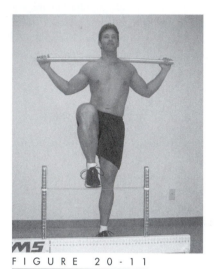

FIGURE   20-11

Hurdle step 3: anterior view.

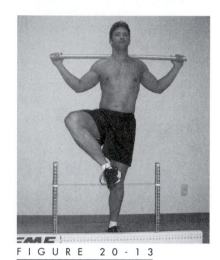

FIGURE   20-13

Hurdle step 2: anterior view.

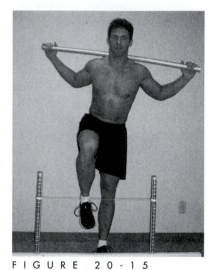

FIGURE   20-15

Hurdle step 1: anterior view

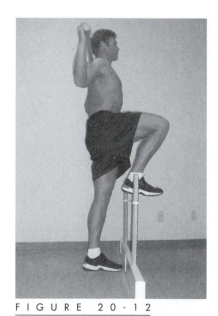

FIGURE   20-12

Hurdle step 3: anterior view.

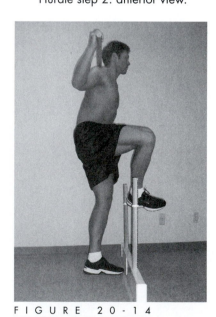

FIGURE   20-14

Hurdle step 2: lateral view.

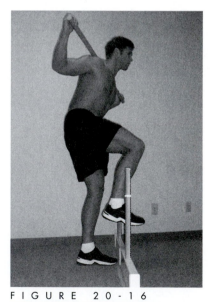

FIGURE   20-16

Hurdle step 1: lateral view.

0—The athlete will receive a score of zero if pain is associated with any portion of this test. A medical professional should perform a thorough evaluation of the painful area.

CLINICAL IMPLICATIONS FOR HURDLE STEP

Performing the hurdle step test requires stance-leg stability of the ankle, knee, and hip as well as maximal closed-kinetic chain extension of the hip. The hurdle step also requires step-leg open-kinetic chain dorsiflexion of the ankle and flexion of the knee and hip. In addition, the athlete must also display adequate balance because the test imposes a need for dynamic stability.

Poor performance during this test can be the result of several factors. It may simply be due to poor stability of the stance leg or poor mobility of the step leg. Imposing maximal hip flexion of one leg while maintaining apparent hip extension of the opposite leg requires the athlete to demonstrate relative bilateral, asymmetric hip mobility.

When an athlete achieves a score less than 3, the limiting factor must be identified. Clinical documentation of these limitations can be obtained by using standard goniometric measurements of the joints as well as muscular flexibility tests such as Thomas test or Kendall's test for hip flexor tightness.[14] Previous testing has identified that when an athlete achieves a score of 2, minor limitations most often exist with ankle dorsiflexion and/or hip flexion with the step leg. When an athlete scores 1 or less, relative asymmetric hip immobility may exist, secondary to an anterior tilted pelvis and poor trunk stability.

IN-LINE LUNGE

Purpose. This test attempts to place the body in a position that will focus on the stresses as simulated during rotational, de-celerating, and lateral type movements. The in-line lunge is a test that places the lower extremities in a scissor style position challenging the body's trunk and extremities to resist rotation and maintain proper alignment. This test assesses hip and ankle mobility and stability, quadriceps flexibility, and knee stability.

Description. The tester attains the individual's tibia length, by either measuring it from the floor to the tibial tuberosity or acquiring it from the height of the string during the hurdle-step test. The individual is then asked to place the end of their heel on the end of the board. The previous tibia measurement is then applied from the end of the toes of the foot on the board and a mark is made. The dowel is placed behind the back touching the head, thoracic spine, and sacrum. The hand opposite to the front foot should be the hand grasping the dowel at the cervical spine. The other hand grasps the dowel at the lumbar spine. The individual then steps out on the board placing the heel of the opposite foot at the indicated mark on the board. The individual then lowers the back knee enough to touch the board behind the heel of the front foot and then returns to starting position. The lunge is performed up to three times bilaterally in a slow controlled fashion. If one repetition is completed successfully then a 3 is given.

Tips for testing are

- the front leg identifies the side being scored,
- dowel remains in contact with the head, thoracic spine, and sacrum during the lunge,
- the front heel remains in contact with the board and back heel touches board when returning to starting position,
- when in doubt score low,
- watch for loss of balance, and
- remain close to individual in case he/she has a loss of balance.

Scores for In-line Lunge

SCORE 3 (FIGS. 20-17 AND 20-18)	SCORE 2 (FIGS. 20-19 AND 20-20)	SCORE 1 (FIGS. 20-21 AND 20-22)

- Dowel contacts remain with L-spine extension
- No torso movement is noted
- Dowel and feet remain in sagittal plane

- Knee touches board behind heel of front foot

- Dowel contacts do not remain with L-spine extension
- Movement is noted in torso
- Dowel and feet do not remain in sagittal plane
- Knee does not touch behind heel of front foot

- Loss of balance is noted

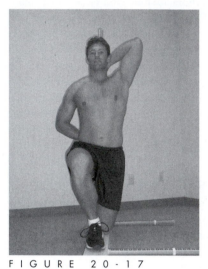

F I G U R E   2 0 - 1 7

In-line lunge 3: anterior view.

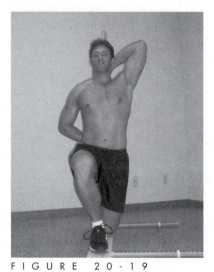

F I G U R E   2 0 - 1 9

In-line lunge 2: anterior view.

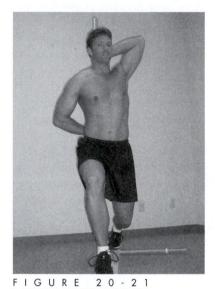

F I G U R E   2 0 - 2 1

In-line lunge 1: anterior view.

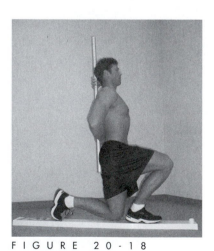

F I G U R E   2 0 - 1 8

In-line lunge 3: lateral view.

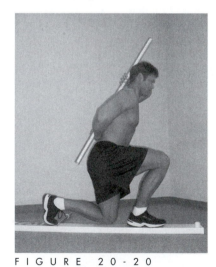

F I G U R E   2 0 - 2 0

In-line lunge 2: lateral view.

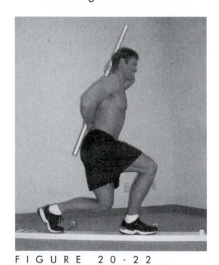

F I G U R E   2 0 - 2 2

In-line lunge 1: lateral view.

0—The athlete will receive a score of zero if pain is associated with any portion of this test. A medical professional should perform a thorough evaluation of the painful area.

CLINICAL IMPLICATIONS FOR IN-LINE LUNGE

The ability to perform the in-line lunge test requires stance-leg stability of the ankle, knee, and hip as well as apparent closed kinetic-chain hip abduction. The in-line lunge also requires step-leg mobility of hip abduction, ankle dorsiflexion, and rectus femoris flexibility. The athlete must also display adequate balance due to the lateral stress imposed.

Poor performance during this test can be the result of several factors. First, hip mobility may be inadequate in either the stance leg or the step leg. Second, the stance-leg knee or ankle may not have the required stability as the athlete performs the lunge. Finally, an imbalance between relative adductor weakness and abductor tightness in one or both hips may cause poor test performance. There may also be limitations in the thoracic spine region, which may inhibit the athlete from performing the test properly.

When an athlete achieves a score less than 3, the limiting factor must be identified. Clinical documentation of these limitations can be obtained by using standard goniometric measurements of the joints as well as muscular flexibility tests such as Thomas test or Kendall's test for hip flexor tightness.[14]

Previous testing has identified that when an athlete achieves a score of 2, minor limitations often exist with mobility of one or both hips. When an athlete scores 1 or less, a relative asymmetry between stability and mobility may occur around one or both hips.

SHOULDER MOBILITY

Purpose. The shoulder mobility screen assesses bilateral shoulder range of motion, combining internal rotation with adduction and external rotation with abduction. It also requires normal scapular mobility and thoracic spine extension.

Description. The tester first determines the hand length by measuring the distance from the distal wrist crease to the tip of the third digit. The individual is instructed to make a fist with each hand, placing the thumb inside the fist. They are then asked to assume a maximally adducted, extended, and internally rotated position with one shoulder, and a maximally abducted, flexed, and externally rotated position with the other. During the test, the hands should remain in a fist and should be placed on the back in one smooth motion. The tester then measures the distance between the two closest bony prominences. Perform the shoulder mobility test as many as three times bilaterally.

Clearing exam. There is a clearing exam at the end of the shoulder mobility test. This movement is not scored; it is simply performed to observe a pain response. If pain is produced, a positive is recorded and a score of zero is given to the entire shoulder mobility test. This clearing exam is necessary because shoulder impingement can sometimes go undetected by shoulder mobility testing alone.

Tips for testing are

- the flexed shoulder identifies the side being scored,
- if the hand measurement is exactly the same as the distance between the two points then score low,
- the clearing test overrides the score on the rest of the test, and
- make sure individual does not try to "walk" the hands toward each other.

Scores for Shoulder Mobility

SCORE 3 (FIG. 20-23)	**SCORE 2 (FIG. 20-24)**	**SCORE 1 (FIG. 20-25)**
• Fists are within one hand length	• Fists are within one and a half hand lengths	• Fists are not within one and half hand lengths

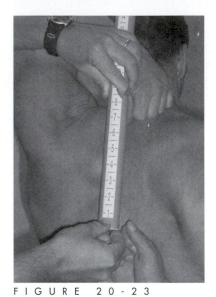 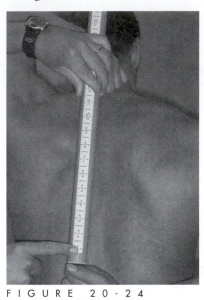 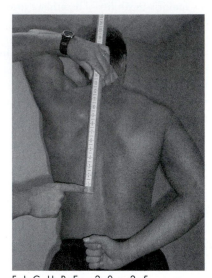

F I G U R E 2 0 - 2 3
Shoulder mobility 3.

F I G U R E 2 0 - 2 4
Shoulder mobility 2.

F I G U R E 2 0 - 2 5
Shoulder mobility 1.

0—The athlete will receive a score of zero if pain is associated with any portion of this test. A medical professional should perform a thorough evaluation of the painful area.

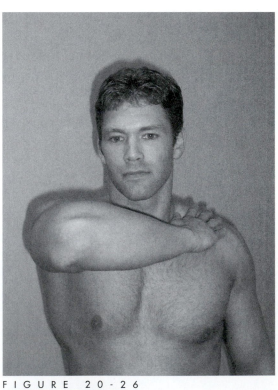

F I G U R E 2 0 - 2 6
Shoulder clearing test.

The individual places his/her hand on the opposite shoulder and then attempts to point the elbow upward (Fig. 20-26). If there is pain associated with this movement, a score of zero is given. It is recommended that a thorough evaluation of the shoulder be done. This screen should be performed bilaterally. If the individual does receive a positive score both scores should be documented for future reference.

CLINICAL IMPLICATIONS FOR SHOULDER MOBILITY

The ability to perform the shoulder mobility test requires shoulder mobility in a combination of motions including abduction/external rotation, flexion/extension, and adduction/internal rotation. It also requires scapular and thoracic spine mobility.

Poor performance during this test can be the result of several causes, one of which is the widely accepted explanation that increased external rotation is gained at the expense of internal rotation in overhead throwing athletes. Excessive development and shortening of the pectoralis minor or latissimus dorsi muscles can cause postural alterations of forward or rounded shoulders. Finally, a scapulothoracic dysfunction may be present, resulting in decreased glenohumeral mobility secondary to poor scapulothoracic mobility or stability.

When an athlete achieves a score less than 3, the limiting factor must be identified. Clinical documentation of these limitations can be obtained by using standard goniometric measurements of the joints as well as muscular flexibility tests such as Kendall's test for pectoralis minor and latissimus dorsi tightness or Sahrmann's tests for shoulder rotator tightness.[14,27]

Previous testing has identified that when an athlete achieves a score of 2, minor postural changes or shortening of isolated axiohumeral or scapulohumeral muscles exist. When an athlete scores 1 or less, a scapulothoracic dysfunction may exist.

ACTIVE STRAIGHT LEG RAISE

Purpose. The active straight leg raise tests the ability to disassociate the lower extremity while maintaining stability in the torso. The active straight leg raise test assesses active hamstring and gastroc-soleus flexibility while maintaining a stable pelvis and active extension of the opposite leg.

Description. The individual first assumes the starting position by lying supine with the arms in an anatomical position and head flat on the floor. The board is placed under the knees. The tester then identifies midpoint between the anterior superior iliac spine (ASIS) and midpoint of the patella. The dowel is then placed at this position perpendicular to the ground. Next, the individual is instructed to lift the test leg with a dorsiflexed ankle and an extended knee. During the test, the opposite knee should remain in contact with the board, the toes should remain pointed upward, and the head remain flat on the floor. Once the end-range position is achieved and the malleolus is located past the dowel, then the score is recorded per the criteria as given next. If the malleolus does not pass the dowel, then the dowel is aligned along the medial malleolus of the test leg, perpendicular to the floor and scored per the criteria given next. The active straight leg raise test should be performed as many as three times bilaterally.

Tips for testing are

- the flexed hip identifies the side being scored,
- make sure leg on floor does not externally rotate at the hip,
- both knees remain extended and the knee on the extended hip remains touching the board, and
- if the dowel resides at exactly the midpoint, score low.

Scores for Active Straight Leg Raise

SCORE 3 (FIG. 20-27)	**SCORE 2 (FIG. 20-28)**	**SCORE 1 (FIG. 20-29)**
• Ankle/dowel resides between mid-thigh and ASIS	• Ankle/dowel resides between mid-thigh and mid-patella/joint line	• Ankle/dowel resides below mid-patella/joint line

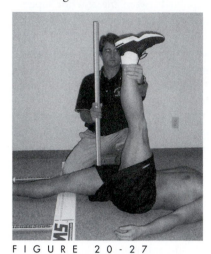

FIGURE 20-27
Active straight leg raise 3.

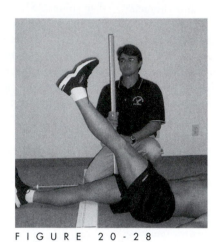

FIGURE 20-28
Active straight leg raise 2.

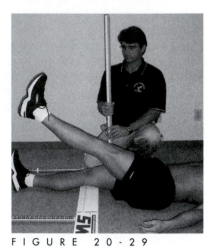

FIGURE 20-29
Active straight leg raise 1.

0—The athlete will receive a score of zero if pain is associated with any portion of this test. A medical professional should perform a thorough evaluation of the painful area.

CLINICAL IMPLICATIONS FOR ACTIVE STRAIGHT LEG RAISE

The ability to perform the active straight leg raise test requires functional hamstring flexibility, which is the flexibility available during training and competition. This is different from passive flexibility, which is more commonly assessed. The athlete is also required to demonstrate adequate hip mobility of the opposite leg as well as lower abdominal stability.

Poor performance during this test can be the result of several factors. First, the athlete may have poor functional hamstring flexibility. Second, the athlete may have inadequate mobility of the opposite hip, stemming from iliopsoas inflexibility associated with an anteriorly tilted pelvis. If this limitation is gross, true active hamstring flexibility will not be realized. A combination of these factors will demonstrate an athlete's relative bilateral, asymmetric hip mobility. Like the hurdle-step test, the active straight leg raise test reveals relative hip mobility; however, this test is more specific to the limitations imposed by the muscles of the hamstrings and the iliopsoas.

When an athlete achieves a score less than 3, the limiting factor must be identified. Clinical documentation of these limitations can be obtained by Kendall's sit-and-reach test as well as the 90–90 straight leg raise test for hamstring flexibility. The Thomas test can be used to identify iliopsoas flexibility.[14]

Previous testing has identified that when an athlete achieves a score of 2, minor asymmetric hip mobility limitations or moderate isolated, unilateral muscle tightness may exist. When an athlete scores 1 or less, relative hip mobility limitations are gross.

TRUNK STABILITY PUSH-UP

Purpose. The trunk stability push-up tests the ability to stabilize the spine in an anterior and posterior plane during a closed-chain upper body movement. It assesses trunk stability in the sagittal plane while a symmetrical upper-extremity motion is performed.
Description. The individual assumes a prone position with the feet together. The hands are then placed shoulder width apart at the appropriate position per the criteria given next. The knees are then fully extended and the ankles are dorsiflexed. The individual is asked to perform one push-up in this position. The body should be lifted as a unit; there should be no "lag" in the lumbar spine when performing this push-up. If the individual cannot perform a push-up in this position, the hands are lowered to the appropriate position per the criteria given next.
Clearing exam. A clearing exam is performed at the end of the trunk stability push-up test. This movement is not scored; it is simply performed to observe a pain response. If pain is

produced, a positive is recorded and a score of zero is given to the entire push-up test. This clearing exam is necessary because back pain can sometimes go undetected by in movement screening.

Tips for testing are

- tell them to lift the body as a unit,

- make sure that original hand position is maintained and the hands do not slide down when they prepare to lift,
- make sure their chest and stomach come off the floor at the same instance,
- when in doubt score it low, and
- the clearing test overrides the test score.

Scores for Trunk Stability Push-Up

SCORE 3 (FIG. 20-30)	SCORE 2 (FIG. 20-31)	SCORE 1 (FIG. 20-32)
• Males perform 1 repetition with thumbs aligned with the top of the forehead • Females perform 1 repetition with thumbs aligned with chin	• Males perform 1 repetition with thumbs aligned with chin • Females perform 1 repetition with thumbs aligned with clavicle	• Males are unable to perform one repetition with hands aligned with chin • Females are unable to perform one repetition with thumbs aligned with clavicle

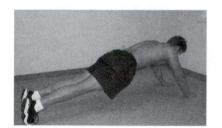

FIGURE 20-30

Trunk stability push-up 3.

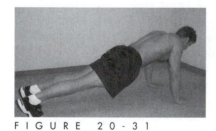

FIGURE 20-31

Trunk stability push-up 2.

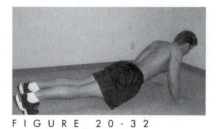

FIGURE 20-32

Trunk stability push-up 1.

0—The athlete will receive a score of zero if pain is associated with any portion of this test. A medical professional should perform a thorough evaluation of the painful area.

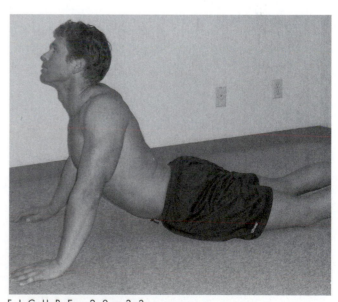

FIGURE 20-33

Spinal extension clearing test.

Spinal extension can be cleared by performing a press-up in the push-up position (Fig. 20-33). If there is pain associated with this motion, a zero is given and a more thorough evaluation should be performed. If the individual does receive a positive score, both scores should be documented for future reference.

CLINICAL IMPLICATIONS FOR TRUNK STABILITY PUSH-UP

The ability to perform the trunk stability push-up requires symmetric trunk stability in the sagittal plane during a symmetric upper-extremity movement. Many functional activities in sports require the trunk stabilizers to transfer force symmetrically from the upper extremities to the lower extremities and vice versa. Movements such as rebounding in basketball, overhead blocking in volleyball, or pass blocking in football are common examples of this type of energy transfer. If the trunk does not have adequate stability during these activities, kinetic energy will be dispersed, leading to poor functional performance as well as increased potential for microtraumatic injury.

Poor performance during this test can be attributed simply to poor stability of the trunk stabilizers. When an athlete achieves a score less than 3, the limiting factor must be identified. Clinical documentation of these limitations can be obtained by using Kendall's or Richardson, Jull, and Hodges tests for upper and lower abdominal and trunk strength.[14,26]

However Kendall's test requires a concentric contraction while a push-up requires an isometric stabilizing reaction to avoid spinal hyperextension. A stabilizing contraction of the core musculature is more fundamental and appropriate than a simple strength test, which may isolate one or two key muscles. It is not necessary to diagnose the muscular deficit at this point. It is only necessary in screening to imply poor trunk stability in the presence of a trunk extension force.

ROTARY STABILITY

Purpose. This test is a complex movement requiring proper neuromuscular coordination and energy transfer from one segment of the body to another through the torso. The rotary stability test assesses multiplane trunk stability during a combined upper- and lower-extremity motion.

Description. The individual assumes the starting position in quadruped with their shoulders and hips at 90° relative to the torso. The knees are positioned at 90° and the ankles should remain dorsiflexed. The board is then placed between the knees and hands so that they are in contact with the board. The individual then flexes the shoulder and extends the same side hip and knee. The leg and hand are only raised enough to clear the floor by approximately 6 in. The elbow, hand, and knee that are lifted should all remain in line with the board. The torso should also remain in the same plane as the board. The same shoulder is then extended and the knee flexed enough for the elbow and knee to touch. This is performed bilaterally for up to three repetitions. If a 3 is not attained, then the individual performs a diagonal pattern using the opposite shoulder and hip in the same manner as described earlier.

Clearing exam. A clearing exam is performed at the end of the rotary stability test. This movement is not scored; it is simply performed to observe a pain response. If pain is produced, a positive is recorded and a score of zero is given to the entire rotary stability test. This clearing exam is necessary because back pain can sometimes go undetected by movement screening.

Tips for testing are

- scoring is identified by the upper-extremity movement on the score sheet, but even if someone gets a 3, both diagonal patterns must be performed and scored. The information should be noted on the score sheet;
- make sure the knee and elbow remain over the board and the back remains flat;
- make sure the elbow and knee touch during the flexion part of the movement;
- provide cueing to let the individual know that he/she does not need to raise the hip and arm above 6 in off of the floor; and
- when in doubt, score low.

Scores for Rotary Stability

SCORE 3 (FIGS. 20-34 AND 20-35)	SCORE 2 (FIGS. 20-36 AND 20-37)	SCORE 1 (FIGS. 20-38 AND 20-39)

- Performs one correct unilateral repetition while keeping spine parallel to board
- Knee and elbow touch in line over the board

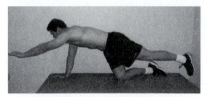

F I G U R E   2 0 - 3 4
Rotary stability 3: extension.

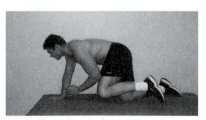

F I G U R E   2 0 - 3 5
Rotary stability 3: flexion.

- Performs one correct diagonal repetition while keeping spine parallel to board
- Knee and elbow touch in line over the board

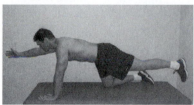

F I G U R E   2 0 - 3 6
Rotary stability 2: extension.

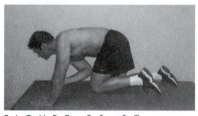

F I G U R E   2 0 - 3 7
Rotary stability 2: flexion.

- Inability to perform diagonal repetitions

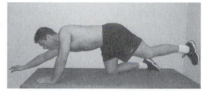

F I G U R E   2 0 - 3 8
Rotary stability 1: extension.

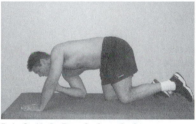

F I G U R E   2 0 - 3 9
Rotary stability 1: flexion.

0—The athlete will receive a score of zero if pain is associated with any portion of this test. A medical professional should perform a thorough evaluation of the painful area.

Spinal flexion can be cleared by first assuming a quadruped position and then rocking back and touching the buttocks to the heels and the chest to the thighs (Fig. 20-40). The hands should remain in front of the body reaching out as far as possible. If there is pain associated with this motion, a zero is given. If the individual does receive a positive score, both scores should be documented for future reference.

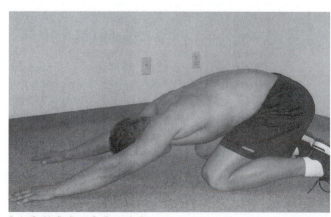

F I G U R E   2 0 - 4 0
Spinal flexion clearing test.

CLINICAL IMPLICATIONS FOR ROTARY STABILITY

The ability to perform the rotary stability test requires asymmetric trunk stability in both sagittal and transverse planes during asymmetric upper- and lower-extremity movement. Many functional activities in sports require the trunk stabilizers to transfer force asymmetrically from the lower extremities to the upper extremities and vice versa. Running and exploding out of a down stance in football and track are common examples of this type of energy transfer. If the trunk does not have adequate stability during these activities, kinetic energy will be dispersed, leading to poor performance as well as increased potential for injury.

Poor performance during this test can be attributed simply to poor asymmetric stability of the trunk stabilizers. When an athlete achieves a score less than 3, the limiting factor must be identified. Clinical documentation of these limitations can be obtained by using Kendall's test for upper and lower abdominal strength.

CONCLUSIONS

The FMS™ can be used as an evaluation tool or for exercise prescription. The physical therapist can use the FMS™ as a tool to interact with highly fit, normal populations to help refine training and develop a more holistic approach to conditioning with the appreciation of movement patterns. The FMS™ can be used as a therapeutic exercise to assist the physical therapist when developing exercise progressions. This will help the physical therapist develop a command of movement pattern restoration. This knowledge can help the physical therapist work with normal populations who want to improve efficiency and performance while increasing their resistance to injury.

The central theme with this type of approach is that a physical therapist, when armed with a wide array of treatment strategies including mobilization, myofascial/soft tissue techniques, stretching, trigger point therapies, modalities, therapeutic exercise, and muscle energy will enjoy a successful practice if these treatment options are considered a means to restoration of function. Total restoration of function is directly dependent on functional movement patterns. Treatment which restores functional movement patterns, without creating secondary symptoms, is the most efficient, effective, and logical path to competent functional performance of all skills.

It is the contention of the authors that it is important during the initial stages of movement screening to watch the distribution of scores and performance by a normal population throughout the structured, simple movements. The therapist must resist the temptation to create multiple screens for each population which caters to their sport, hobby, activity level, age or level of conditioning, or deconditioning. It is of greater therapeutic merit to have a common test battery that presents

the researcher with biomarkers that are predictors of function. A biomarker can define any physical measure that can be utilized as a representative predictor or standard of what may be expected. Medicine has relied on biomarkers with blood chemistry, electromyogram, electrocardiogram, and numerous representations of which is considered normal and abnormal. The FMS™ may provide the first step toward movement-related biomarkers in the early detection of movement impairment and dysfunction. Ideally, subsequent researchers will understand this practical and clinical need in physical therapy and focus upon these biomarkers and develop more powerful clinical assessment tools. The means to this end starts with a focus on capturing functional movement patterns across a normal group of individuals, and studying the distribution of movement pattern behavior across larger populations of active and inactive individuals. This can produce information and create outcomes that hold us to a higher standard in the light of the information gained.

SUMMARY

- In order to fully appreciate functional movement, normal functional movement should be established by assessing assymptomatic population groups.
- A performance pyramid provides a visual representation of how an individual performs during movement, performance, and skill.
- The performance pyramid assist the clinician by placing an individual in a category based on the weakest area.
- The FMS was developed based on fundamental growth and development strategies.
- The FMS consists of seven tests, which offer an analysis of an individual's fundamental movements.
- The results from the FMS can be utilized as an assessment or therapeutic exercise, which will allow the clinician to develop a more holistic approach to therapeutic treatment.

REFERENCES

1. American College of Sports Medicine. *ACSM's Guidelines for Exercise Testing and Prescription*, 6th ed. Philadelphia, PA, Lippincott Williams and Wilkins, 2000.
2. Battie MC, Bigos SJ, Fisher LD, Hansson TH, Jones ME, Wortley MD. Isometric lifting strength as a predictor of industrial back pain reports. *Spine* 14(8):851–856, 1989.
3. Baumhauer JF, Alosa DM, Renstrom PA, Trevino S, Beynnon B. A prospective study of ankle injury risk factors. *Am J Sport Med* 23(5):564–570, 1995.
4. Cholewicki J, Panjabi MM, Khachatryn A. Stabilizing function of trunk flexor-extensor muscles around a neutral spine posture. *Spine* 22(19):2207–2212, 1997.
5. Cook G. Baseline sports-fitness testing. In: Foran B, ed. *High Performance Sports Conditioning*, 1st ed. Champaign, IL, Human Kinetics, 2001.

6. Cook G. Essentials of functional exercise: A four-step clinical model for therapeutic exercise prescription. In: Prentice W, Voight ML, eds. *Techniques in Musculoskeletal Rehabilitation*, 1st ed. New York, McGraw-Hill, 2001, pp. 387—410.

7. Cook, G. *Advance Concepts in Core Training*. Presented at the Functional Training Summit, Providence, RI, 2004.

8. Cook G, Burton L, Fields K, Kiesel K. *The Functional Movement Screen*. Danville, VA, Athletic Testing Services, Inc., 1998.

9. Cook G, Burton L, Fields K, Kiesel K, Van Allen J. *Functional Movement Screening: Upper and Lower Quarter Applications*. Presented at the Mid-America Athletic Trainer's Annual Symposium, Sioux Falls, South Dakota, 1999.

10. Fields KB, Delaney M. Focusing on the pre-participation sports examination. *J Fam Pract* 30(3):304–312, 1989.

11. Gallahue DL, Ozmun JC. *Understanding Motor Development*, 3rd ed. Madison, WI, Brown and Benchmark, 1995.

12. Gardner-Morse M, Stokes I, Laible JP. Role of muscles in lumbar spine stability in maximum extension efforts. *J Orthop Res* 13:802–808, 1995.

13. Gray G. *Lower Extremity Functional Profile*. Adrian, MI, Wynn Marketing, Inc., 1995.

14. Kendall FP, McCreary EK. *Muscles Testing and Function*, 3rd ed. Baltimore, MD, Lippincott Williams and Wilkins, 1983.

15. Kibler WB, Chandler TJ, Uhl T, Maddux RE. A musculoskeletal approach to the preparticipation physical examination: preventing injury and improving performance. *Am J Sport Med* 17(4):525–527, 1989.

16. Knapik JJ, Bauman CL, Jones BH, Harris JM, Vaughn L. Preseason strength and flexibility imbalances associated with athletic injuries in female collegiate athletes. *Am J Sport Med* 19:76–81, 1991.

17. Lephart SM, Pincivero DM, Giraldo JL, Fu FH. The role of proprioception in the management and rehabilitation of athletic injuries. *Am J Sport Med* 25(1):130–138, 1997.

18. Magee DJ. *Orthopedic Physical Assessment*, 4th ed. Philadelphia, PA, Saunders, 2002.

19. Meeuwisse WH. Predictability of sports injuries: What is the epidemiological evidence? *Sports Med* 12(1):8–15, 1991.

20. Meeuwisse WH, Fowler PJ. Frequency and predictability of sports injuries in intercollegiate athletes. *Can J Sport Sci* 13(1):35–42, 1988.

21. Metzl JD. The adolescent preparticpation physical examination: Is it helpful? *Clin Sport Med* 19(4):577–592, 2000.

22. McMullen J, Uhl T. A kinetic chain approach for shoulder rehabilitation. *J Athlet Train* 35(3):329–337, 2000.

23. Nadler SF, Malanga GA, Feinberg JH, Prybicien M, Stitik TP, Deprince M. Relationship between hip muscle imbalance and occurence of low back pain in collegiate athletes: A prospective study. *Am J Phys Med Rehabil* 80(8):572–577, 2001.

24. Nadler SF, Moley P, Malanga GA, Rubbani M, Prybicien M, Fienberg JH. Functional deficits in athletes with a history of low back pain: A pilot study. *Arch Phys Med Rehabil* 88:1753–1758, 2002.

25. Neely FG. Intrinsic risk factors for exercise-related lower limb injuries. *Sports Med* 26(4):253–263, 1998.

26. Richardson C, Hodges P, Hides J. Therapeutic exercise for lumbopelvic stabilization. *A Motor Control Approach for the Treatment and Prevention of Low Back Pain*. Edinburgh, Churchill Livingstone, 2004.

27. Sahrmann SA. *Diagnosis and Treatment of Movement Impairment Syndromes*. St. Louis, MO, Mosby, 2002.

28. The Physician and Sportsmedicine. *The Preparticipation Physical Evaluation*, 3rd ed. New York, McGraw-Hill, 2005.

Functional Exercise Progression and Functional Testing in Rehabilitation

Turner A. Blackburn, Jr and John A. Guido, Jr

O B J E C T I V E S

After completing this chapter, the therapist should be able to do the following:

- Define functional exercise progression.
- Define the SAID principle.
- Outline the need for functional progression and testing.
- Describe the continuum of functional progression for low- and high-level patients.
- Outline a functional progression program for the lower extremity.
- Outline a functional progression program for the upper extremity.
- Outline a functional progression program for the spine.
- Discuss major functional testing research.

The physical therapist plays an important role in helping individuals return to their preinjury level of function. While working to achieve clinically based goals, functional testing is employed to gauge readiness to move through the rehabilitation program and to return to activity. A functional exercise progression can be initiated prior to functional testing or following the results of functional tests. In either case, functional testing or progression should not exceed the healing constraints of the injured tissue. By breaking down functional activities into basic tasks, a safe and effective rehabilitation program can be designed. This chapter examines functional exercise testing and functional exercise progression and provides examples for some common upper- and lower-extremity disorders as well as a sample spine program.

WHAT IS FUNCTIONAL TESTING AND FUNCTIONAL EXERCISE PROGRESSION?

The ultimate goal of any rehabilitation program is to return an individual to the preinjury level of function as quickly and safely as possible. Decreasing pain and swelling—and restoring normal range of motion (ROM), strength, proprioception, and balance—are only part of the plan. Functional testing and a functional exercise progression will complete the rehabilitation program. Functional testing encompasses measuring various activities to provide a baseline for determining progress or to provide normative data with which to compare performance. A functional exercise progression can be defined as a series of activities that have been ordered from basic to complex, simple to difficult, that allows for the reacquisition of a specific task. Many of the exercises in the functional progression may be used for functional testing. Functional testing and functional exercise progression allow the clinician to bridge the gap between basic rehabilitation and a full return to activity.

HOW IS FUNCTIONAL TESTING PERFORMED?

Functional testing and functional exercise progression are used in a variety of physical therapy settings but in very different capacities. Physical therapists practicing in outpatient orthopedic settings use these techniques to help their patients return to activities of daily living (ADLs), work, and sports. In neurologic and geriatric rehabilitation settings, functional testing and functional exercise progression take on a different meaning, being geared more toward ADLs, transfers, and ambulating on level and unlevel surfaces.

Despite these differences, the principles that guide functional testing and exercise progression are the same regardless of the practice setting and level of the patient. Some patients will move further through the program than others, based on their specific rehabilitation goals. There is little basic science and research to guide the physical therapist in designing a functional exercise progression. Rather, common sense prevails and is employed along with the information available regarding healing constraints of various musculoskeletal disorders or the precautions that must be heeded for various medical conditions.

A complete discussion of collagen healing is beyond the scope of this chapter, but in general, many of the injuries encountered in the outpatient setting will heal in 3–6 weeks.[15] In the early phases of the rehabilitation program, appropriate stress must be placed on the healing tissues to ensure proper healing. Our bodies heal according to the specific adaptations to imposed demands (SAID) principle.[9] The imposed demand is therapeutic exercise in the form of a functional progression that will stress the injured tissue to allow it to heal at an adequate length and strength. This enables the individual to handle the demands of return to full function without reinjuring the area. If the functional progression is employed incorrectly, the stress imparted will cause reinjury and impede the patient's progress. Healing constraints may be exceeded or new injuries created during functional testing or exercise progression, and the therapist should be acutely aware of the individual's response to activity. The presence or absence of the cardinal signs of inflammation as well as muscle weakness, loss of motion, and instability of the injured joint should alert the clinician to reassess the activity being performed. The culprit may be one activity that is above the abilities of the patient at that time, or that the overall volume exceeds the ability of the healing structures to accommodate to the stress.

Early in the rehabilitation program, therapeutic techniques should be employed to meet the various clinical goals such as eliminating pain and swelling and restoring full ROM, strength, proprioception, balance, and normal ambulation without deviations or assistive devices. Normal ROM can be assessed with a goniometer by comparing established norms or the range of the uninvolved opposite extremity. Swelling can be assessed via tape measure for circumferential measurements, or with volumetric measures of water displacement. Pain levels can be determined with a visual analog scale.

Strength testing poses a challenge to the clinician. A 5/5 manual muscle test grade may not show true deficits in strength and endurance of the musculature. Isokinetic testing, if available, may be a better alternative and has been shown to correlate with function despite being performed in an open-chain fashion.[20] The authors recommend less than a 30 percent isokinetic deficit in the strength and endurance of the involved versus the uninvolved extremity prior to initiating functional testing activities for athletic endeavors. This form of testing will not be available to all clinicians, and not all patients will need to undergo an isokinetic evaluation. Basic manual muscle testing or the use of a handheld dynamometer to increase objectivity will suffice in many cases. Proprioception at a given joint can be assessed through basic joint repositioning tasks, or can be

measured using the electrogoniometer on the Biodex Multi-Joint System. Balance testing can be performed with or without high-technology equipment. At a minimum, performing a single-leg stance activity for total duration, or counting the number of touchdowns with the opposite lower extremity, can be assessed with a second hand on a watch. There are several excellent balance screens such as the Berg balance scale, the clinical test of sensory interaction for balance, and the functional reach test. There are also several excellent testing devices on the market that will give the clinician information regarding the postural sway envelope and directions of movement such as the Biodex Stability System® and the NeuroCom Balance System (NeuroCom, Inc., Clackamas, OR). Monitored Rehabilitation Systems devices can be used for functional motor control testing and training activities.

When an individual has no pain or swelling, and has reached sufficient ROM, strength, balance, and ambulation without deviations, the clinician can determine if functional testing is appropriate. In some cases, functional testing may be used prior to meeting the clinical goals, provided the individual is not placed at risk for reinjury based on the healing constraints of the injured tissue. The information gained will be valuable to the clinician and the individual in planning further treatment.

SPECIFICS

How is function measured? Functional testing is a onetime, maximal effort that is performed to assess performance.[19] The key is that the test must re-create the activity that the individual will be performing, and must be completed in a controlled environment. The purpose of functional testing is to determine an individual's readiness to return to the preinjury level of function. The information gained will allow the clinician to point out deficits that must be overcome, and to progress the rehabilitation program. Functional testing, like the functional exercise progression, must begin with simple tasks and progress to highly coordinated tasks. At the lowest level, for an individual to perform a sit-to-stand transfer, the leg press or bilateral minisquats can be performed for repetitions for a length of time. This will re-create an individual's daily activities, in this case rising from a chair, commode, or car seat. Testing can be performed through various ranges of motion to re-create the seat heights the individual will encounter. The clinician can also use ambulation itself as a functional test. Ambulation for distance is an important determinant to see if the patient can function in the community. Ambulation measured for time will determine if the patient can cross a street safely or exit an elevator before the door closes.

As another example, the clinician should examine a patient's ability to climb stairs. What functional test can be used to assess this skill? Front or lateral step-ups or step-downs can be used to determine an individual's readiness to complete this task. This test is also easily standardized. Step-ups can be performed with only the heel of the opposite limb touching the ground. A step height can be chosen that equals heights that will be encountered at home, the office, or in the community. Repetitions are counted, or the number of repetitions in a set time can be measured. The results are compared with the uninvolved limb or established norms. Rosenthal et al.[17] reported an intraclass correlation coefficient of 0.99 for the lateral step-up test. Functional testing can be as simple as performing minisquats, ambulation, or lateral step-ups for repetitions, distance, or time.

At the highest level of functional testing in the lower extremity, an athlete may have to complete complex movements such as jump or hop tests, shuttle runs, and agility drills. This part of the rehabilitation process is an integral part of the rehabilitation professional's daily routine in the sports setting and can be easily incorporated to meet patients' needs in the clinic. The results of functional testing will determine when they can return to play. Daniel et al.[4] described the one-leg hop for distance test. One-leg hopping is an example of an activity that places higher demands on the lower extremity than do walking or jogging.[18] Subsequently, many clinicians and researchers have used this test for examining function in varied populations, especially in patients who have undergone anterior crucial ligament (ACL) reconstructions.[18] It is easy to see how important this activity is in terms of a return to athletic competition. This is an ideal test to determine the individual's willingness to accept weight on the involved leg after injury.[19] The one-leg hop for distance and the one-leg timed hop, predominantly used with athletes, have also shown good reliability.[4] A single-leg hop does have its limitations, in that it only describes one movement, whereas most sports require a series of complex maneuvers. Therefore, many authors have attempted to create even higher-level tests to determine readiness to play. Lephart et al.[10] examined three functional testing procedures for the anterior cruciate-deficient athlete. These included the cocontraction maneuver (a shuffling maneuver around a semicircle while tethered to surgical tubing), a carioca (crossover stepping), and a shuttle run (an acceleration and deceleration test). Several investigators have attempted to correlate the results of isokinetic testing and functional activities. Wilk et al.[18] found a positive correlation between isokinetic knee extension peak torque and three functional hop tests (hop for distance, timed hop, and crossover triple hop). The results of this study were further strengthened by Jarvela et al.[7] who assessed muscle performance 5–9 years after ACL reconstruction. They also correlated the strength of the knee extensors and flexors at 60°/second isokinetically with one-legged hop for distance. Both studies suggest that expensive isokinetic devices may not be required for determing the functional status of an athlete.[7,20] Many physical therapy clinics utilize a Total Gym (Engineering Fitness International, Inc., San Diego, CA) for lower-extremity rehabilitation. Munich et al.[13] have created a testing protocol for use on this device. They examined 35 healthy subjects who performed a 20-second test for unilateral squat repetitions and a 50-second squat repetition test for time. Their findings indicate acceptable test–retest reliability for the purpose of evaluating functional ability during the early stages of rehabilitation for lower-extremity conditions. One other consideration during functional testing is determin-

ing an athlete's eccentric control, which is extremely important in changing directions and landing from a jump. Juris et al.[8] had asymptomatic and symptomatic individuals with knee pain perform a maximal controlled leap. This test was performed by having the individual perform a single-leg hop by taking off on the uninjured limb and landing on the injured limb, termed force absorption versus force production. The results of this study demonstrated that individuals with knee pain had difficulty managing force absorption as opposed creating force (force production). If a traditional single-leg hop is examined, the individual does perform force absorption, but if they have lower-extremity weakness, they may not create a large take off force (force production) and therefore not stress the limb in landing. If the forces are lower during the test than those experienced during sports, the athletes may be returned to activity before they are truly ready.

Mattacola et al.[11] studied a group of patients who had undergone ACL reconstruction to determine their performance during two functional tests conducted on the Smart Balance Master (NeuroCom, Inc. Clackamas, OR) as compared to a control group. All of the ACL reconstruction patients were at least 6 months postoperative. Both groups performed the step-up-and-over test (Fig. 21-1) and the forward lunge (Fig. 21-2) on a long force plate. The control group produced significantly more force during the initial step of the step-up-and-over task than the ACL reconstructed group. In the same test, the ACL reconstruction patients were significantly slower when they led with the involved limb. During the forward lunge test, there were no differences between groups in the lunge distance or the contact time. However, the impact index (percentage body weight, indicates eccentric ability of nonstepping leg) and the force impulse (percentage body weight × the time the force is exerted) measurements were significantly greater for the uninvolved leg than the involved leg in the ACL patients. Higher impact and force indices represent better functional ability. Such

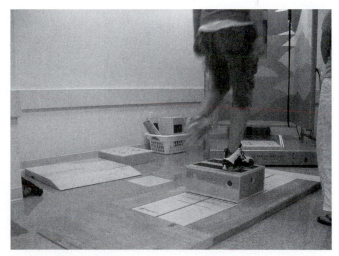

FIGURE 21-1

The step-up-and-over test performed on the Smart Balance Master (NeuroCom, Inc., Clackamas, OR).

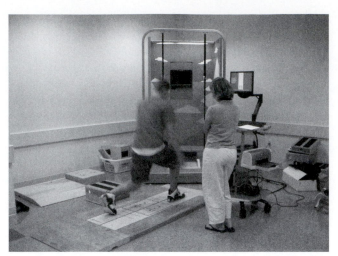

FIGURE   21-2

The forward lunge test performed on the Smart Balance Master (NeuroCom, Inc., Clackamas, OR).

tests, performed on the Smart Balance Master may be useful for screening for functional disability that might persist after ACL reconstruction and not be recognized with more general, clinical functional tests.

In lieu of these tests or sophisticated testing equipment, the physical therapist can have the patient run through a series of progressively difficult tasks such as running straight ahead and backpedaling, performing figure-8 runs, cutting maneuvers, and finally sports-specific tasks.

In the upper extremity, the clinician needs to be more creative to re-create the functional demands an individual may encounter during ADLs or sports. Functional testing can include push-ups for an athlete or overhead activities performed in a specially designed apparatus for an electrician or carpenter. Again, at the lowest level, simple reaching tests can re-create ADLs such as removing items from overhead cabinets. To standardize this, a goniometer can be used to measure ROM at the glenohumeral joint, or a finger ladder to document reach height. A tape measure can be used to measure reach distance. At the highest levels, activities that re-create job tasks, as alluded to, can be performed in the clinic. Measures of specific skills, duration of overhead activity, or speed of activity provide objective evidence of functional ability. For the athlete, both open-chain (throwing activities and racquet sports) and closed-chain (football, wrestling, gymnastics) activities can be reproduced in the clinic. The clinician is only limited by his or her imagination.

Whether testing the upper or lower extremity, begin with bilateral support drills and progress to more demanding unilateral support drills. Always observe for substitution and poor technique, which may signify that the activity is too difficult for the patient at that time, or that the stress is too great on the healing structures. Through functional testing, the therapist can assess speed, strength, agility, and power which when combined equal function.[19] Functional testing can be adapted to meet the needs of every patient with whom we come into contact. Phys-

ical therapists have always performed functional testing with their patients, although they may not have described these activities as such. In the acute care or rehabilitation hospital, as well as in the nursing home, most activities have a functional component and can be used to document functional status. Everything from bed mobility and transfers to ambulation on level and unlevel surfaces can be measured fairly objectively. Two examples of functional testing for the geriatric population include the multiple-sit-to-stand (MSTS) field test and the 6-minute walk test. The MSTS claims to measure leg strength. Netz et al.[14] correlated knee extensor isokinetic strength and endurance with the results of the MSTS. They concluded that the MSTS is not able to predict strength of the knee extensors, but may predict overall endurance of the lower extremities. The results of this study are not surprising since it is well accepted that to measure strength and power, the patient must perform an explosive maneuver. This is obviously not appropriate in an older patient population. In another test of endurance, Bean et al.[1] performed a 6-minute walk test to determine aerobic capacity and function. They found a poor correlation between indirect measures of aerobic capacity but a strong association with functional measures. The results of these two studies provide the clinician with a variety of options for functional testing in the geriatric population.

In the outpatient setting, the activities required for functional testing may be more dynamic, but the principles and goals of treatment are the same. It is easy to take for granted the ease with which ADLs are performed. A functional test can be used to document limitations in ADL tasks, and a functional exercise progression can be implemented to meet the specific needs of the patient. It is imperative to enable individuals to return to their maximum level of function or their preinjury status.

WHAT NOW?

Now that the functional testing procedure has been completed at the appropriate time in the rehabilitation process, what is the next step? Upon completion of functional testing, the clinician must be able to use this information to determine the next step in the rehabilitation process. In one scenario, if the individual completes the tasks adequately, return to work or ADLs without restrictions may be recommended. In another scenario, if the individual is not able to complete the tasks, the clinician must determine where the breakdown occurred. Return to full function is restricted until these tasks can be completed and it is safe for the individual to return to the preinjury activity level. This is where the functional exercise progression should dominate the rehabilitation program. Up until that point, the patient may have been working on and achieved the majority of the clinical goals, but from the results of the functional testing, the patient may not be ready to return to all necessary functional activities.

If the goal activity is kept in mind, whether it is a return to sports or ADLs, the activity can be broken down into small segments that can be performed in the clinic. Once the specific activity has been broken down into required fundamental movements, the individual's injured body part is stressed progressively until function is adequate for a return to work, ADLs, or sports-specific demands.[19] Removing the "conscious mind" from the activity will make the movement pattern more automatic and natural. Some suggestions include throwing a ball for the patient to catch during the activity or having the patient count the fingers held up on your hand. Functional exercises that meet the specific needs of the patient can truly be termed "functional."

The concept of open- versus closed-chain exercise becomes a moot point when discussing functional exercise progression because everything we do is a combination of these two types of activity. Walking requires a combination of movements (the swing phase is open chain, the stance phase is closed chain), as does picking an object up off the floor (the individual braces the body with the uninvolved extremity on a table, which is closed chain, and reaches for the object, which is open chain). The hallmark of closed-chain activities, however, is that they are more closely related to function, incorporating movements that mimic daily activities. Both open- and closed-chain exercise can create concentric, isometric, and eccentric muscular contractions, which are all used for functional tasks. These exercises can also include acceleration and deceleration, which are extremely important principles when discussing functional tasks. Attempting to cross a busy intersection requires acceleration to get across safely. Descending an inclined walkway requires decel-

eration to prevent falls. An advantage that closed-chain exercises have is the addition of appropriate proprioceptive feedback from the muscle and joint mechanoreceptors. Discontinuing the rehabilitation program when the clinic-based rehabilitation goals alone are achieved may be appropriate for some individuals, but this will surely be a disservice to those patients returning to higher levels of function. These patients will have an increased risk for reinjury when they attempt to return to their preinjury level of function without completing a functional exercise progression.[21]

EXAMPLES

This point can be illustrated by discussing some examples of specific patients frequently encountered in the outpatient setting. Assume you are treating a police officer who has suffered a sprain of the medial compartment of his right knee. After valgus stress testing at 30° of flexion and an anterior drawer test with the tibia in external rotation, you determine that there is a slight opening of the joint space—in other words, a grade III ligament sprain with 1+ instability. Functional testing may be appropriate initially in the form of lateral step-ups or minisquats, provided these activities do not cause too great a stress on the healing medial compartment. This will tell you if the individual can perform sit-to-stand transfers from various heights and climb stairs, important aspects of ADL. Table 21-1 describes

TABLE 21-1

Knee Functional Progression

| | CRITERIA FOR RETURN | | |
FUNCTIONAL ACTIVITY	STRENGTH	ROM	OTHER
Sit to stand	3/5 MMT quad 3/5 MMT ham	90° one knee	Sitting balance
	3/5 MMT gastroc	120° hip flexion	Stand balance
Assistive free gait	5/5 MMT quad	Full extension	No pain
	4/5 MMT ham	100° flexion	No swelling
	Lift body weight one leg with heel lift	10° dorsifexion	Nonantalgic gait
	Motor control of knee		Adequate balance
Ascend/descend			10 side-step-downs
Stairs (step over step)			10 side-step-downs
Running	70% quad/ham	Full flexion	30 mins bike
		15° dorsiflexion	50 side-step-downs
			2 miles walking
Sprinting	90% quad/ham		2 miles running
Agility			Successful sprinting
Sports activity			Functional progression of activity

MMT, manual muscle test; gastroc, gastronemius.

lower-extremity criteria needed for return to various functional activities. This particular patient will need to return to high-level functional activities such as chasing and apprehending suspects.

Initially, starting the patient on a regimen of knee isometrics, modalities as needed to control pain and swelling, and flexibility training is an appropriate course. In an earlier discussion, it was stated that adequate collagen healing occurs in 3–6 weeks. The second phase of the rehabilitation program must employ a functional exercise progression to progressively load the injured body part. In relation to Davis' law,[6] the medial compartment will heal along the lines of stress. So, to enable it to heal with appropriate tensile strength and adequate length, activities that involve a valgus stress must be included. To strengthen the surrounding musculature, open-chain exercises are incorporated. However, it is difficult to apply a controlled valgus stress to the knee in the open chain. Therefore, closed-chain exercises are a must. These may include the testing activities themselves, minisquats and lateral step-ups with a valgus stress, the BAPS® board (Biomechanical Ankle Platform System), profitter, and the balance-testing devices. Table 21-2 describes sample lower-extremity functional exercise progression and testing activities.

Once the clinic-based goals have been achieved and the patient is able to ambulate on level and unlevel surfaces without deviation or an assistive device, functional testing is again performed to determine where the patient stands in relation to return to work. Due to the high-level demands this patient will encounter upon his return to full duty as a police officer, we need to perform higher-level functional testing, beginning with jump or hop tests. The jump test is performed with the individual standing on both limbs. He is asked to jump as far as possible in a horizontal fashion (a standing broad jump) and to stick to the landing. The individual should be able to jump a distance equal to his height (or 1.5 times his height).[19] If this task is completed, a single-leg hop can be performed as described by Daniel. Noyes et al.[9] suggest that two types of one-leg hopping tests—for distance and for time—be used to rule out the instability caused by ACL rupture. Table 21-3 describes current functional testing research and conclusions related to functional activity.

If this task is completed and there is less than a 10 percent deficit between limbs, higher-level functional testing can be performed. This will include jogging and backpedaling in a straight line at 25, 50, 75, and 100 percent effort. Then, figure-8 drills

T A B L E   2 1 - 2

Lower-Quarter Functional Progression and Testing Template

LEVELS	SUPPORT	STABILITY	PLANE	RESPONSE	DIRECTION	EXAMPLES
1	Bilateral	Stable	Single	Single	Vertical	Leg press Shuttle Minisquat
2	Bilateral	Unstable	Single	Single	Vertical	DynaDisc Foam roller Biodex stability
3	Unilateral	Stable	Single	Single	Vertical	Leg press Shuttle Minisquat Step-up
4	Unilateral	Unstable	Single	Single	Vertical	Leg press Shuttle Minisquat Step-up
5	Bilateral nonsupport	Stable	Single, multiple	Single, multiple	Vertical, horizontal	Jumping "5 dot drill" Spin hops
6	Unilateral nonsupport	Stable	Single, multiple	Single, multiple	Vertical, horizontal	Jumping "5 dot drill" Spin hops
7	Acceleration, deceleration	Stable				"Suicide" "T-drill" Cocontraction Lateral power hop

Functional Test Research

FUNCTIONAL TEST	RESEARCH
Lateral step-up	ICC.99 (Rosenthal, 1994)
One-leg hop for distance	ICC.99 (Worrell, 1994)
	ICC.96 (Bolga, 1997)
One-leg hop timed	ICC.77 (Worrell, 1994)
	ICC.66 (Bolga, 1997)
One-leg hop triple	ICC.95 (Bolga, 1997)
One-leg hop crossover	ICC.96 (Bolga, 1997)
Four-point run	ICC.98 (Bolga, 1997)
Lateral power hop	ICC.91–92 (Tippett, 1996)
Decreased one-leg timed hop without ACL	Positive correlation (Mangine, 1989)
Decreased one-leg hop distance without ACL	Positive correlation (Barber, 1990)
Decreased one-leg hop distance in post ACL reconstruction	Positive correlation (Sekiya, 1998)
One-leg hop distance and time postlateral ankle sprain	No correlation (Worrell, 1994)
Objective scoring system with postlateral ankle reconstruction	Positive correlation (Kaikkonen, 1994)
One-leg hop distance with decreased quad strength without ACL	Positive correlation (Friden, 1990)
One-leg hop distance with decreased quad strength without ACL	No correlation (Gauffin, 1990)
One-leg hop distance without ACL with a strengthening and coordination program	Positive correlation (Friden, 1991)
One-leg hop distance in reconstructed ACL and laxity	No correlation (Jonsson, 1992)
Cocontraction test and isokinetic strength and power	No correlation (Lephart, 1992)
Cocontraction test and ACL laxity	No correlation (Lephart, 1992)

are employed. Finally, cutting activities are performed, and in this case, emphasizing an open cut (sidestep cut or a "Z" cut) to stress the medial compartment.[21] In the late stages of knee rehabilitation, low-level plyometric activities could be incorporated, such as hopping drills in place, in diagonal patterns, and lateral hops to stress the medial compartment.[21] If these tasks are completed without signs and symptoms of inflammation or hesitancy on the patient's part, a recommendation to return to tactical training and full duty will follow. Clinical outcomes can measure the effectiveness of the clinician's functional exercise progression. Table 21-4 describes various scoring systems that can be employed with knee injuries to document clinical outcomes.

In the upper extremity, we may have a patient who has suffered an anterior glenohumeral shoulder dislocation. Table 21-5 describes a sample progression of activities with criteria for advancement. Assume that this individual is an artist and painting is her medium. Special testing may include an anterior apprehension sign, in this case positive, along with the standard measures of ROM, strength, pain level, and proprioception in the form of joint repositioning. Angular repositioning has been advocated at the glenohumeral joint to determine the input from the mechanoreceptors about the shoulder joint.[3,5]

Functional testing at this early stage may include reaching to a certain height for a specific number of repetitions, or hold-ing the upper extremity at a certain angle for a specific length of time. Both of these activities will re-create the functional demands of painting. In the first stage of the rehabilitation process, just as for the lower-extremity problem, the focus is on decreasing pain and swelling through modalities, increasing ROM as tolerated, and increasing strength through the use of shoulder isometrics. Functional exercise in this phase may take the form of rhythmic stabilization at 90° of flexion and at 45° of abduction. This technique will increase the stability of the shoulder joint by firing the dynamic stabilizers.

Also in this phase, total shoulder girdle strengthening, as tolerated, may begin with emphasis on the scapular stabilizers and rotator cuff musculature. There have been several electromyography studies documenting various exercises for these muscle groups. The authors use a combination of exercises recommended by Mosely et al.[12] for the scapula and those by Blackburn et al.[2] for the rotator cuff. The core exercises for the scapula consist of rows, seated press-ups, scaption, and push-ups with a plus (scapula protraction).[12] The core exercises for the rotator cuff include prone extension with external rotation, prone horizontal abduction with external rotation, and prone external rotation at 90° of abduction.[2] It is up to the clinician to determine the appropriate application of these core strengthening exercises.

In the second phase of the functional exercise progression, increased emphasis is placed on raising the upper extremity in

Knee Scoring Systems

KNEE SCORING SYSTEM	
Lysholm Scale	Developed in 1986 by Lysholm 100-point scale Assesses support with ambulation, limp, stairs, squatting, pain, swelling, atrophy, and instability with walking, running, and jumping Very specific to ADLs
Cincinnati Scale	Developed in 1984 by Noyes Preinjury/surgery to postinjury/surgery comparison Assesses walking, stairs, running, jumping, twisting, sports/work activity level More specific to sports
Methodist Hospital Scale	Developed in 1986 by Shelbourne Assesses 1-mile walk, stairs, jogging, heavy work, ADLs, repetitive jumping, recreational and competitive sports More specific to sports
International Knee Society Scale	Developed in 1986 by the IKDC Assigns an A–D group grading based upon patient subjective assessment, pain, swelling, giving way, ROM, laxity, crepitus, and one-leg hop More specific to ADLs
Combined Rating System	Developed in 1995 by Karlson Cincinnati, HSS, Lysholm, IKDC Assesses pain, swelling, giving way, walk, stairs, squat, run, jump, twist, decelerate, sports, ADLs, locking, function, limp, activity, brace, crutches
Knee Outcome Survey	Scale for disability during ADLs Scale for disability during sports

Shoulder Functional Progression

FUNCTIONAL ACTIVITY	CRITERIA FOR ADVANCEMENT		
	STRENGTH	ROM	OTHER
Active/passive ROM after surgery			Depends on healing restraints
Isometric strengthening	As tolerated	As tolerated	Depends on healing restraints
Elevation of arm after surgery	Successful gravity eliminated	As tolerated	Depends on healing restraints
Elevation of arm with weights	Successful elevation with no weights over three sets of 10 repetitions	As tolerated	Protect healing tissue as necessary
Motor control: blade, tubing, plyoballs	Successful elevation with no weights over three sets of 10 repetitions	As tolerated	Protect healing tissue as necessary
Weight machines/full-body weight	Successful elevation with 3 lb, three sets of 10 repetitions 5/5 MMT	As tolerated	Isokinetics as tolerated
Free weights	Successful weight machine program	As tolerated	
Sports activities	5/5 MMT Isokinetic test WNL	Enough for sport activity	Sufficient healing time No pain, swelling with progressive activity

WNL, within normal limits.

TABLE 21-6

Lumbar Stabilization Progression

FUNCTIONAL ACTIVITY	CRITERIA FOR ADVANCEMENT: LUMBAR STABILIZATION ACTIVITIES
Supine	Abdominal bracing Latissimus dorsi sets Gluteal sets Hip extensions sets "Marching" (hip flexions) "Dying bug" (unilateral hip and arm movement) Pelvic ant/post tilt
Prone	Quadruped with arm flexion Quadruped with hip extension Quadruped with contralateral limb elevation Prone extensions
Seated	Gym ball "Marching" "Dying bug"
Standing	Trunk rotation stabilization with surgical tubing Horizontal adduction and abduction Flexion and extension
Lifting	Table to table Carrying objects Floor to table Table to overhead shelf

the plane of the scapula initially to raising the arm in the sagittal plane. The patient is questioned regarding the duration of time that she spends painting, and estimation can be made as to how many times she must lift her arm in each session. For other individuals, the application of closed-chain exercises for the glenohumeral joint may be appropriate. Closed-chain exercises can be employed to increase the proprioceptive input of the joint mechanoreceptors, which will enhance motor control. Moving a ball on a wall and weight shifting on a table may be low-level activities that are easily implemented. A functional exercise progression may include quadruped activities, the use of the Profitter, and even the Stairmaster for higher-level tasks. The use of the Bodyblade at this stage may also help increase the endurance of the shoulder girdle musculature while enhancing dynamic stability in the sagittal plane. In the final stage of the rehabilitation process for this individual, large muscle group strengthening and endurance exercises are added for the deltoid, pectoralis major, and latissimus dorsi. Final functional testing can be performed to determine whether the patient has the endurance and strength to hold the upper extremity at approximately 90° for repetitions or time.

For the majority of patients seen in the outpatient setting with low back dysfunction, functional testing and a functional exercise progression can return them to their preinjury level of function (Table 21-6). For example, a patient with a bulging disk may present with pain, decreased ROM, and decreased functional status. Functional testing may include lifting tasks or sitting or walking for duration, depending on the individual's occupation. A functional exercise progression in this case would include lumbar stabilization exercises in the supine, sitting, and, ultimately, standing positions. Please refer to Chapter 18 for an in-depth discussion of stabilization of the core.

To provide one more example, suppose you have a new mother who has suffered a sprain/strain of the lumbar region while picking up her child. The immediate postinjury care is dedicated to relieving the pain, inflammation, and muscle spasm, and to restoring ROM. Proper instruction in posture and body mechanics can also begin. The second phase of the program can be initiated quickly, usually within the first 2 weeks, and activities are designed around lifting tasks. A functional exercise program may progress to minisquats to increase lower-extremity strength and endurance, to lifting tasks from various heights, to carrying objects around the clinic. Functional testing, when appropriate, is geared toward lifting an object of equal or greater weight than the infant, from the floor to the table and vice versa. Carrying for distances and holding for time will mimic feeding and nurturing tasks.

SUMMARY

- Functional exercise progression and functional testing are important components of a complete rehabilitation program.
- Taking into account the patient's medical condition, the healing constraints of that condition, and the external environment that must be overcome, tasks can be designed to re-create the functional demands of each individual.
- When the patient is able to perform the goal activity without physical assistance or verbal cueing from the therapist, the entire activity is attempted and practiced.
- The entire formal rehabilitation program does not have to be completed prior to performing functional testing or initiating a functional exercise progression.
- Activities that are compatible with the patient's physical status may be implemented at any time. These techniques are employed by physical therapists regardless of setting and patient diagnosis.
- The use of functional testing and functional exercise progression will enable the patient to return to preinjury level of function as quickly and safely as possible.

REFERENCES

1. Bean JF, Kiely DK, Leveille SG, et al. The 6-minute walk test in mobility-limited elders: What is being measured? *J Geront A Biol Med Sci* 57(11):M751–M756, 2002.

2. Blackburn TA, McLeod WD, White B, et al. EMG analysis of posterior rotator cuff exercises. *Athlet Train* 25:40–45, 1990.

3. Borsa PA, Lephart SM, Kocher MS, et al. Functional assessment and rehabilitation of shoulder proprioception for glenohumeral instability. *J Sport Rehabil* 3:84–104, 1994.

4. Daniel DM, Malcom L, Stone ML, et al. Quantification of knee stability and function. *Contemp Orthop* 5:83–91, 1982.

5. Davies GJ, Dickoff-Hoffman S. Neuromuscular testing and rehabilitation of the shoulder complex. *J Orthop Sports Phys Ther* 18:449–458, 1993.

6. Gould J, Davies G, eds. *Orthopedic and Sports Physical Therapy.* St. Louis, MO, Mosby, 1985.

7. Jarvela T, Kannus P, Latvala K, et al. Simple measurements in assessing muscle performance after an ACL reconstruction. *Int J Sports Med* 23(3):196–201, 2002.

8. Juris PM, Phillips EM, Dalpe C, et al. A dynamic test of lower extremity function following anterior cruciate ligament reconstruction and rehabilitation. *J Orthop Sports Phys Ther* 26(4):184–191, 1997.

9. Kegerreis S. The construction and implementation of functional progression as a component of athletic rehabilitation. *J Orthop Sports Phys Ther* 5:14–19, 1983.

10. Lephart SM, Perrin DN, Fu FH, et al. Functional performance tests for the ACL insufficient athlete. *J Athlet Train* 26:44–50, 1991.

11. Mattacola CH, Jacobs CA, Rund MA, Johnson DL. Functional assessment using the step-up-and-over test and forward lunge following ACL reconstruction. *Orthopedics* 27(6):602–608, 2004.

12. Mosely BJ, Jobe FW, Pink M, et al. EMG analysis of the scapula muscles during a rehabilitation program. *Am J Sports Med* 20:128–134, 1992.

13. Munich H, Cipriani D, Hall L, et al. The test-retest reliability of an inclined squat strength test protocol. *J Orthop Sports Phys Ther* 26(4):209–213, 1997.

14. Netz Y, Ayalon M, Dunsky A, et al. The multiple-sit-to-stand field test for older adults: What does it measure? *Gerontology* 51(4):285, 2005.

15. Noyes FR, Barber SD, Mangine RE. Abnormal lower limb symmetry determined by functional hop tests after anterior cruciate ligament rupture. *Am J Sports Med* 19:513–518, 1992.

16. Reed BV. Wound healing and the use of thermal agents. In: Michovitz S, ed. *Thermal Agents in Rehabilitation.* Philadelphia, FA Davis, 1996, pp. 3–29.

17. Rosenthal MD, Baer LL, Griffith PP, et al. Comparability of work output measures as determined by isokinetic dynamometry and a closed chain kinetic exercise. *J Sport Rehab* 3:218–227, 1994.

18. Rudolph KS, Axe MJ, Snyder-Mackler L. Dynamic stability after ACL injury: Who can hop? *Knee Surg Sports Traumatol Arthrosc* 8:262–269, 2000.

19. Tippett SR, Voight ML. *Functional Progressions for Sports Rehabilitation.* Champaign, IL, Human Kinetics, 1995.

20. Wilk KE, Romaniello WT, Soscia SM, et al. The relationship between subjective knee scores, isokinetic testing and functional testing in the ACL reconstructed knee. *J Orthop Sports Phys Ther* 20:60–73, 1994.

21. Worrell TW, Booher LD, Hench KM. Closed kinetic chain assessment following inversion ankle sprain. *J Sport Rehab* 3:197–203, 1994.

CHAPTER 22

Orthotics in Rehabilitation

Robert Gailey

OBJECTIVES

After completing this chapter, the therapist should be able to do the following:

- Explain the basic mechanical principles that are the foundation for orthotic design.
- Describe the functional considerations for an orthosis based on the client's diagnosis.
- Justify indications, contraindications, advantages, and disadvantages of various orthotic devices.
- Differentiate between materials used in the fabrication of orthotics; this includes the basis for selection of materials for specific purposes.
- Identify various designs of shoewear, lower limb, upper limb, and spinal orthotics and discuss the function of their principal components.

The use of orthotic intervention in rehabilitation spans the history of humans, from the first crude fracture splint made from sticks in the forest to the sophisticated modern day dynamic orthoses fabricated from hybrid materials. Many of the principles have remained the same through time; however, the new materials and structural designs, and breadth of application to a greater number of medical conditions have contributed to the expansive utilization of orthotic intervention. The use of orthotics can be found in almost every aspect of rehabilitation today. With the appreciation and understanding of terminology, principles, materials, generic designs, and the application of orthotics, clinicians can enhance the delivery of health care to their clients.

TERMINOLOGY

The terminology related to medical appliances is fairly straightforward. The prefix "ortho" means to "straighten or correct," with the suffix "tic" referring to the "systematic pursuit of." The term orthosis refers to an exoskeletal appliance applied to a body part, and has replaced the traditional term, "bracing."[24] A brace is considered to be an appliance that allows movement at the joint, whereas a splint does not allow movement at a joint. Through the years, the term "splint" has been used, especially in the area of hand therapy, to mean a short-term orthosis and splints have been described as both static and dynamic. As a result, the terms orthosis, brace, and splint have become inter-changeable across many allied health professions. The orthotist is the person who designs, fabricates, and repairs the orthotic appliance; however, physical and occupational therapists, as well as physicians, may fabricate low-temperature thermoplastic orthotics.

The American Academy of Orthopaedic Surgeons and the American Orthotic and Prosthetic Association developed a standard of nomenclature for orthotic devices.[5,24] The acronyms used for the generic are listed in Table 22-1.

BIOMECHANICAL PRINCIPLES OF ORTHOTIC DESIGN

The biomechanical principles of orthotic design assist in promoting control, correction, stabilization, or dynamic movement. All orthotic designs are based on three relatively simple principles: (1) pressure, (2) equilibrium, and (3) the lever arm principle.[21] However, the complexities of these principles can increase when applied to the human anatomy. These considerations include and are not limited to the forces at the interface between the orthotic materials and the skin, the degrees of freedom of each joint, the number of joint segments, the neuromuscular control of a segment, including strength and tone, the material selected for orthotic fabrication, and the activity level of the client. As a result, the following principles do indeed provide the foundation for all orthotic design and can assist the clinician in visualizing the effects an orthosis will have on a body

TABLE   22-1

Orthotic Acronyms

Lower limb orthoses			
		AFO	Ankle-foot orthosis
FO	Foot orthosis	KAFO	Knee-ankle-foot orthosis
KO	Knee orthosis	HKAFO	Hip-knee-ankle-foot orthosis
HO	Hip orthosis	RGO	Reciprocal gait orthosis
Spinal orthoses			
CO	Cervical orthosis	CTO	Cervical-thoracic orthosis
TO	Thoracic orthosis	CTLSO	Cervicothoraciclumbrosacral orthosis
SO	Sacral orthosis	TLSO	Thoraciclumbrosacral orthosis
SIO	Sacroiliac orthosis	LSO	Lumbrosacral orthosis
Upper extremity orthoses			
HdO	Hand orthosis	WHO	Wrist-hand orthosis
WO	Wrist orthosis	EWHO	Elbow-wrist-hand orthosis
EO	Elbow orthosis	SEO	Shoulder-elbow orthosis
SO	Shoulder orthosis	SEWHO	Shoulder-elbow-wrist-hand orthosis

segment, keeping in mind that the more complicated the orthotic application, the more confounded the various principles become.

1. The *pressure principle* states that pressure is equal to the total force per unit area. Clinically, what this means is that the greater the area of a pad or the plastic shell of an orthosis, the less force will be placed on the skin. Therefore, any material that creates a force against the skin should be of a dimension to minimize the forces on the tissues.

$$P = \frac{\text{Force}}{\text{Area of application}}$$

2. The *equilibrium principle* states that the sum of the forces and the bending moments created must be equal to zero. The practical application is best explained by the most commonly used loading system in orthotics, the three-point pressure system (Fig. 22-1). The three-point pressure or loading system occurs when three forces are applied to a segment in such a way that a single primary force is applied between two additional counterforces with the sum of all three forces equaling zero. The primary force is of a magnitude and located at a point where movement is either inhibited or facilitated, depending on the functional design of the orthosis.

$$\Sigma F = 0$$

3. The *lever arm principle* states that the farther the point of force from the joint, the greater the moment arm and the smaller the magnitude of force required to produce a given torque at the joint. This is why most orthoses are designed with long metal bars or plastic shells that are the length of an adjacent segment. The greater the length of the supporting orthotic structure, the greater the moment or torque that can be placed on the joint or unstable segment.

$$M = F \times d \text{ or } T = F \times d$$

Collectively, these three principles rarely, if ever, act independently of each other. Ideally, when designing or evaluating an orthotic appliance, the clinician should check that (1) there is adequate padding covering the greatest area possible for

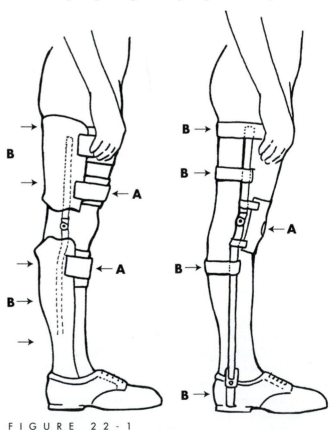

FIGURE   22-1

The three-point pressure system. **A,** primary force. **B,** counterforce application. The sum of all forces will equal zero. Reproduced, with permission from, *Advanced Rehabilitation Therapy,* Inc. Miami, FL.

comfort; (2) the total forces acting on the involved segment should equal zero or that there is equal pressure throughout the orthosis and no areas of irritation to the skin; and (3) the length of the orthosis is suitable to provide an adequate force to create the desired effect and to avoid increased transmission of shear forces against the anatomic tissues.

ORTHOTIC CONSIDERATIONS

The goal of orthotic fitting is to meet the functional requirements of the client with minimal restriction. To meet this goal, the rehabilitation team must evaluate each client individually without preconceived ideas of routine orthotic prescription based purely on the diagnosis. It must be determined whether the appliance will be a temporary device to protect or assist the client until further restorative therapies have been progressed, or in other cases, it might be a permanent or definitive orthosis fabricated for long-term use. The functional considerations for an orthosis typically include one or more of the following.

1. *Alignment:* the correction of a deformity or maintenance of a body segment.
   Clinical examples:
   a) musculoskeletal considerations
      i. Milwaukee brace for scoliosis
      ii. dynamic splint to prevent scar shortening in clients with burns
   b) neurological considerations
      i. tone-reducing AFOs in pediatric clients with cerebral palsy
      ii. CTLSO to prevent motion of the cervical region
2. *Movement:* a joint requires assistance with motion or resistance to excessive motion.
   Clinical examples:
   A. assistance with joint motion
      a) musculoskeletal considerations
         i. AFO with dorsiflexion assist for dorsiflexor weakness
         ii. wheelchair to assist with propulsion
      b) neurological considerations
         i. RGO to assist clients with spinal cord injury with ambulation
         ii. tenodesis splint to assist clients with spinal cord injury
   B. Resistance of joint motion
      a) musculoskeletal considerations
         i. shoe insert for a diabetic patient with foot deformity
         ii. finger splints for arthritic hands
      b) neurological considerations
         i. Swedish knee cage for unstable knee
         ii. arm sling for neurological shoulder
3. *Weight bearing:* to reduce axial loading and reduce the forces placed on a joint.

Clinical examples:
a) musculoskeletal considerations
   i. shoe insert with metatarsal pad for a diabetic with foot deformity
   ii. rocker bottom on the outsole to prevent excessive weight over the metatarsals
b) neurological considerations
   i. patella tendon bearing orthosis for Charcot joints
   ii. heel wedge for the pronated foot of a child with cerebral palsy
4. *Protection:* support or protect a segment against further injury or pain.
   Clinical examples:
   a) musculoskeletal considerations
      i. functional knee brace
      ii. infrapatella strap
   b) neurological considerations
      i. cock-up splints post spinal cord injury
      ii. long leg brace (LLB) for clients with cerebral palsy

There are only a few contraindications for orthotic application: (1) the orthosis cannot provide the required amount of motion, (2) when greater stabilization is required than can be provided, (3) the orthosis actually limits function, therefore, the client is more functional without the appliance, and (4) abnormal pressures from the orthosis would result in injury to the skin and other tissues.

Materials

Over the years several materials have been introduced which offer great strength at reduced weight and, in many cases, are easier to work with during the fabrication process. As a result, the client is fitted with an orthotic appliance that is both functional and, in most cases, cosmetically acceptable. Selecting the appropriate material characteristics for the fabrication of an orthotic device requires careful consideration of a number of factors.[22,24]

1. *Strength:* the maximum external load that can be sustained by a material. The strength of a material is determined by stress, which relates to the magnitude of the applied forces and the amount of material resisting the forces. Depending on the way that a force is applied, stress can be subdivided into several types: tensile, compressive, shear, and flexural (bending) stress. Because the strength of a material can be multidirectional, both the direction and the magnitude of the forces that will be placed on a material must be determined prior to selecting a material.
2. *Stiffness:* the stress–strain or force-to-displacement ratio of a material or simply the amount of bending or compression that occurs under stress. A tension test can be performed on a material to determine the stress–strain curve that reflects the mechanical properties of a material. The stiffness or flexibility of a material is determined by the elasticity and the amount of residual deformation remaining after being placed under tension. Creep is referred to as the

deformation that follows initial loading of a viscoelastic material that occurs over time. Clinically, when greater support is required, a stiffer material is used; when a more dynamic orthosis is desired, a more flexible material is used.

3. *Durability (fatigue resistance):* the ability of a material to withstand repeated cycles of loading and unloading. Fatigue stresses, which are the result of repeated low loads rather than the application of a high load, are the main cause of material breakage. As a result, all materials and many orthotic products are subjected to cyclic testing to determine fatigue strength. Selection of a material for orthotic appliances is frequently based upon the ability of the material to withstand the day-to-day stresses of each individual client.

4. *Density:* the material's weight per unit volume. Generally, the greater the volume or thicker a material, the more rigid and more durable it will be; however, this usually increases the overall weight of the finished orthosis. Some synthetic materials will utilize the arrangement or orientation of the material's properties to increase strength rather than just increasing the volume of material in an effort to minimize the additional weight, yet still increase stiffness.

5. *Corrosion resistance:* the vulnerability of the material to chemical degradation. Most materials will exhibit corrosion over time, metals will rust and plastics will become brittle. Contact with human perspiration and environmental elements such as dirt, temperatures, and water accelerate the wearing effect on materials. Knowing the client's daily environment can assist in material selection.

6. *Ease of fabrication:* the equipment and resources available to work with materials are also very important. Some materials require expensive equipment and familiarity with the properties of the material, such as shrinkage when heated. Others are relatively easy to use with little equipment but may not offer the strength and durability of the more complex materials.

LOWER LIMB ORTHOTICS

Footwear

Shoes are often considered to be the foundation of an orthosis and may also be a corrective device by design. Footwear can be modified to redistribute weight bearing not only throughout the foot and ankle but also can alter the forces transmitted throughout the lower limb. Although consumers often select shoes based on cosmetic or fashion concerns, clinicians should regard a client's footwear as the device that forms the base on which they stand and as a result can have a significant effect on skin, lower limb joints, and posture. Consequently, understanding the components of footwear and the relationship each component may have to the human anatomy is important when evaluating a client.

Often a simple change in footwear style or replacing a worn pair of shoes can benefit a person. If further intervention is necessary, modification to shoes is frequently easily performed and inexpensive. If warranted, custom shoes can be made. Well-designed shoes can frequently promote healing, prevent further injury, and provide an adequate foundation for lower limb orthotics. The basic components of a shoe are illustrated in Figure 22-2. Athletic shoes and custom-designed shoes typically have additional components that are important to athletes and may also prove beneficial to clients in some cases.[20]

Shoe Components

A. Outersole: the hard out layer that protects the plantar surface of the foot and contacts the floor.
B. Innersole: the softer inner layer that interfaces with the plantar surface of the foot.
C. Ball: the widest part of the sole located below the metatarsal heads.

FIGURE 22-2

The anatomy of a shoe. **A,** outer sole. **B,** inner sole. **C,** ball. **D,** uppere. **E,** eyelet. **F,** closure. **G,** heel. **H,** heel counter. **I,** toe box. **J,** shank. Reproduced, with permission from, *Advanced Rehabilitation Therapy,* Inc. Miami, FL.

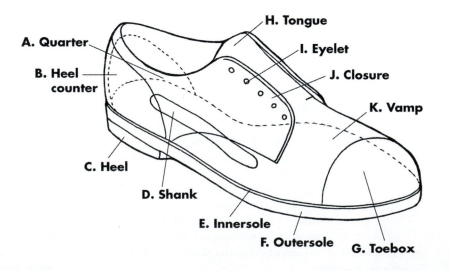

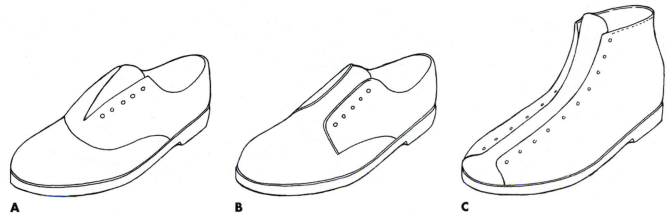

Closure or throat styles of a shoe. **A,** Balmore (Bal). **B,** Blucher. **C,** Lace-to-toe. Reproduced, with permission from, *Advanced Rehabilitation Therapy,* Inc. Miami, FL.

D. Upper: divided into three parts that cover the dorsum of the foot.
    a) Vamp: covers the anterior foot.
    b) Tongue: an extension of the vamp that protects the foot from the eyelet rows and laces.
    c) Quarters: medial and lateral quarters extend posteriorly, under the malleolus in low shoes or cover the malleolus in high shoes, and join at the heel.
E. Eyelet (stays) rows: the laces are contained within the eyelet stays.
F. Closures or throat styles: the portion of the upper that influences the ease of donning and internal adjustability of the shoe (Fig. 22-3).
    a) Balmore (Bal): the tongue is separated from the vamp.
    b) Blucher: the tongue is an extension of the vamp permitting wider opening.
    c) Lace-to-toe: the eyelet stays and tongue extend to the toe permitting the widest opening for donning and may have a high or low quarter.
G. Heel: located posteriorly beneath the outsole under the anatomical heel. A low broad heel provides the greatest stability and assists in evenly distributing the weight between the rear foot and forefoot.
H. Heel counter: a reinforcement cup incorporated into the rear of the upper that helps maintain the anatomical heel in neutral and controls excessive movement.
I. Toe box: a reinforcement material inserted in the vamp to maintain the height of the shoe, protecting the anatomical toes. It may refer to the space provided for the toes within the shoe.
J. Shank: a reinforcement material between the ball and heel of the shoe.
K. Lasts: shoes are constructed over a model of the foot stylized from wood, plaster, plastic, or computer-generated design called a last. The last determines the fit, walking progression, and the outward appearance of the shoe (Fig. 22-4).

a) Medial or inflared last
b) Straight last
c) Lateral or outflared last

Foot Orthoses

Foot orthoses can be classified into three general categories, soft, semirigid, and rigid, depending on the material properties or the degree of flexibility.

1. *Soft:* flexible foam-type materials provide cushioning, improve shock absorption, decrease shear forces and are used to redistribute plantar pressures affording comfort with limited joint control.

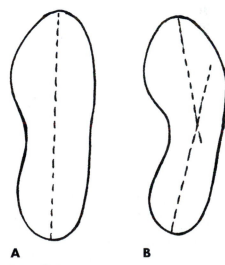

A   **B**

Shoe lasts. **A,** medical or inflared last, **B,** straight last. **C,** lateral or outflared last. Reproduced, with permission from, *Advanced Rehabilitation Therapy,* Inc. Miami, FL.

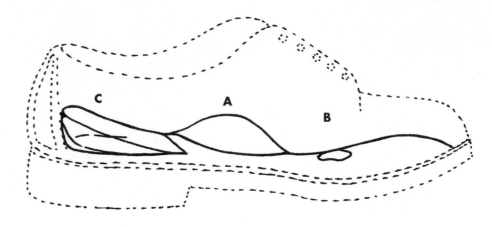

FIGURE 22-5

Internal modifications. **A,** medical longitudinal arch support (cookie/scaphoid pad). **B,** metatarsal pad. **C,** heel cushion. Reproduced, with permission from, *Advanced Rehabilitation Therapy,* Inc. Miami, FL.

2. *Semirigid:* combination of soft and rigid materials, including cork, rubber, or plastics providing some flexibility and shock absorption, however, designed to balance or control the foot.

3. *Rigid:* strong, stiff, and durable materials such as plastics or metals are used to assist with transfer of weight, stabilize flexible deformities, and to control abnormal motion.

Shoe Modifications

Shoe modifications can be either an internal modification where the corrective adaptation is affixed inside the shoe or an external modification, which is attached to the outside of the shoe. Medial supports are incorporated either internally or externally to the shoe with the intention of supporting the anatomical medial longitudinal arch of the foot and shifting the body weight more laterally, decreasing the valgus deformity of the foot, and restraining the depression of the subtalar joint. Conversely, lateral supports are designed to decrease varus deformity of the foot. The lateral aspect of the shoe is reinforced to support the lateral aspect of the foot to shift the body weight more medially.[17]

INTERNAL MODIFICATIONS (FIG. 22-5)

1. *Medical longitudinal arch support (arch cookie/scaphoid pad):* a rubber or leather pad often used in conjunction with a medial longitudinal counter to prevent depression of the subtalar joint by posting the sustentaculum tali and the navicular tuberosity.

2. *Metatarsal pad:* a rubber or semisoft pad that is placed at the apex of the metatarsal shafts, relieves the metatarsal heads from excessive pressure and supports the collapsed transverse metatarsal arch.

3. *Heel cushion:* a viscoelastic material placed in the heel cup of an orthosis or directly into the shoe to accommodate for the inability to achieve a neutral position in the sagittal plane, shock attenuation, and to relieve calcaneal stress fractures or heel pain.

EXTERNAL MODIFICATIONS
Heel Corrections (Fig. 22-6)

1. *Medial heel wedge:* a leather wedged insert incorporated into the heel, used to elevate and maintain the medial margin of shoe to decrease hyperpronation, and designed to shift the weight laterally.

FIGURE 22-6

External modification, heel corrections. **A,** medial heel wedge. **B,** lateral heel wedge. **C,** Thomas heel. **D,** reversed Thomas heel. **E,** heel flares. Reproduced, with permission from, *Advanced Rehabilitation Therapy,* Inc. Miami, FL.

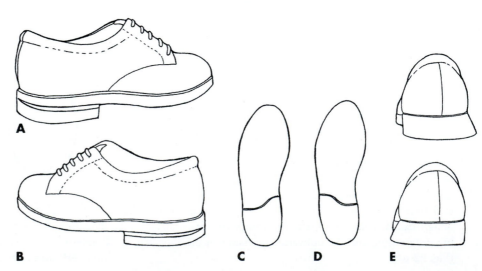

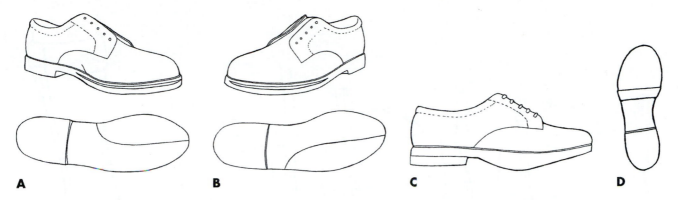

A   **B**   **C**   **D**

FIGURE 22-7

External modifications, outsole corrections. **A,** medial sole wedges. **B,** lateral sole. **C,** rocker bottom wedge. **D,** metatarsal bar. Reproduced, with permission from, *Advanced Rehabilitation Therapy,* Inc. Miami, FL.

2. *Lateral heel wedge:* a leather wedged insert incorporated into the heel, used to elevate and maintain the lateral margin of shoe to decrease supination, and designed to shift the weight medially.

3. *Thomas heel:* the heel of the shoe extends anteriorly 1 in. on the medial aspect to assist with balance, support the longitudinal arch, and assist in maintaining the subtalar joint in a neutral position. The Thomas heel is often coupled with medial heel wedges to assist with stability during ambulation.

4. *Reversed Thomas heel:* opposite to the Thomas heel, the heel is extended 1 in. on the lateral aspect to assist with balance and subtalar joint alignment, and is used in conjunction with lateral heel wedges.

5. *Heel flares:* either medial or lateral extension of the shoe heel that broadens the base of support for greater stability.

Outsole Corrections (Fig. 22-7)

1. *Medial sole wedge:* a crepe or leather wedge used to correct forefoot eversion and promote inversion.

2. *Lateral sole wedge:* a leather wedge used to correct forefoot inversion and promote eversion.

3. *Rocker bottom:* a crepe or leather convex build up under the posterior to the metatarsal heads, intended to redistribute body weight over the entire plantar surface, reduce stress to the forefoot, and assist with rollover during ambulation.

4. *Metatarsal bar:* a flat strip of leather positioned just posterior to the metatarsal heads, designed to transfer the forces from the metatarsophalangeal joints to the metatarsal shafts.

Custom-Molded Inserts

1. *University California Berkeley insert:* a molded plastic design that covers the heel, providing a heel counter for subtalar joint control, that extends to the mid-foot providing support to the medial longitudinal arch (Fig. 22-8).

2. *Custom inserts:* there are a remarkable number of custom or biomechanical inserts available to clinicians today. Some require casting; others use foam impression, and a few use computer imaging. Regardless of how the image of the foot and deformity are obtained, most use semirigid and soft materials to fabricate the insert. Rigid materials are used when maximal control is required. The foot is divided into the rear foot and forefoot. The foot deformity is altered by positioning the rear foot or forefoot with a technique called posting, whereby specific structures of the foot are raised by padding under the soft orthotic shell. Excessive pronation or supination of the foot is corrected by controlling for rear foot and forefoot varus or valgus. The length of the insert varies from posterior to the metatarsal heads to running the full length of the foot.

ANKLE-FOOT ORTHOSES

Ankle-foot orthoses are designed to control the rate and direction of tibial advancement and to maintain an adequate base of support while meeting the specific demands for acceptable gait. There are several designs of AFO constructed from a wide variety of materials with the express purpose of meeting the individual needs of each client. Frequently, standard designs of AFOs are modified for an individual, based on the

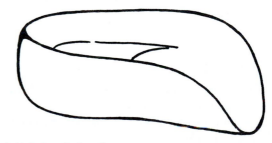

FIGURE 22-8

University California Berkley insert. Reproduced, with permission from, *Advanced Rehabilitation Therapy,* Inc. Miami, FL.

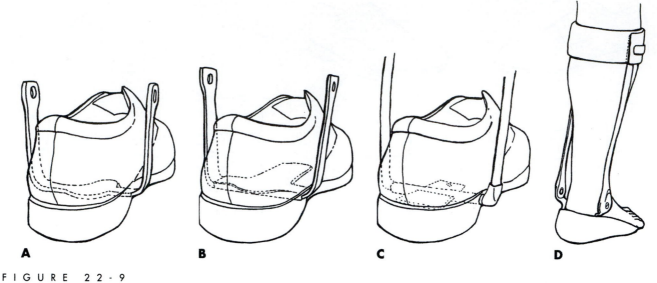

FIGURE   22-9

Shoe and foot attachments. **A,** stirrup (solid). **B,** stirrup (split). **C,** calipere. **D,** molded shoe insert. Reproduced, with permission from, *Advanced Rehabilitation Therapy,* Inc. Miami, FL.

specific requirements of the orthotic prescription. Because of the large variety of AFOs and custom designs, understanding the standard designs and the individual components provides the clinician with a sound foundation for the majority of clients.

Shoe and Foot Attachments (Fig. 22-9)

1. *Stirrup (solid):* a one-piece attachment with a solid metal plate riveted to the sole of the shoe, creating a U-shaped frame that forms the medial and lateral upright.
2. *Stirrup (split):* a two-piece attachment with a metal plate riveted to sole of shoe has two channels to permit donning and doffing of the removable metal uprights. The split stirrup permits use of multiple shoes, providing that the shoes have the receptacle attachment.
3. *Caliper:* very similar to the split stirrup with a metal plate riveted to sole of shoe; however, the uprights are slightly lighter and round.
4. *Molded shoe insert:* a plastic custom-formed footplate attaches directly to the metal uprights with a calf band for proximal support.

Ankle Joints and Controls

STOPS (FIG. 22-10)

1. *Plantarflexion stop:* a posterior stop restricting plantarflexion but allowing full dorsiflexion.
2. *Dorsiflexion stop:* an anterior stop that restricts dorsiflexion but allows full plantarflexion.
3. *Limited motion stop:* an ankle joint that limits motion in all directions.
4. *Free motion joint:* an ankle joint that provides medial lateral stability from the uprights while permitting full

plantarflexion/dorsiflexion. Plastic AFOs use lightweight joints, such as the Gillette or Gaffney joints, that permit free motion, but other mechanisms fabricated into the AFO design, such as posterior stops, have the ability to control motion.

ASSISTS (FIG. 22-11)

1. *Dorsiflexion assist:* a posterior spring assists with dorsiflexion and permits full plantarflexion, which compresses the spring during early stance phase of gait; as the limb moves

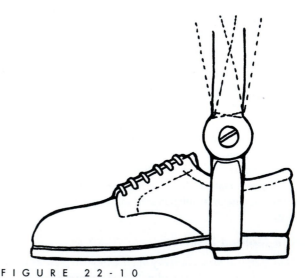

FIGURE   22-10

Ankle joints and controls, Stops. **A,** plantarflexion stop. **B,** dorsiflexion stop. **C,** limited motion stop. **D,** free motion joint. Reproduced, with permission from, *Advanced Rehabilitation Therapy,* Inc. Miami, FL.

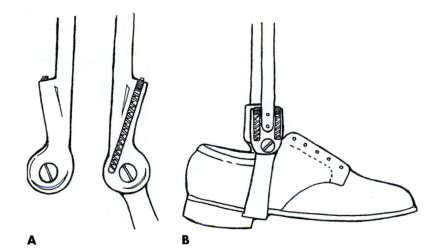

F I G U R E   2 2 - 1 1

Ankle joints and controls, Assists. **A,** dorsiflexion assist. **B,** dorsiflexion/ plantarflexion assist (dual channel). Reproduced, with permission from, *Advanced Rehabilitation Therapy,* Inc. Miami, FL.

A   **B**

into swing phase the spring promotes dorsiflexion. The spring resistance can be adjusted.

2. *Dorsiflexion, plantarflexion assist (dual channel) or Bichannel adjustable ankle locks:* joints with anterior and posterior springs that assist with both plantarflexion and dorsiflexion to varying degrees according to the adjusted settings of the springs. Pins may also be used to replace the spring to limit or control motion in the sagittal plane.

Varus and Valgus Correction (Fig. 22-12)

1. *Medial T-strap:* the leather strap arises from the shoe quarter covering the medial malleolus and buckles to the lateral upright, pushing laterally to correct a valgus (eversion) deformity.

2. *Lateral T-strap:* the leather strap arises from the shoe quarter, covers the lateral malleolus and buckles to the medial upright, pushing medially to correct a varus (inversion) deformity.

3. *Supramalleolar orthoses:* a low-profile supramalleolar orthosis is designed for subtalar joint control to limit varus or valgus. The ankle joint also assists with dorsiflexion during swing. The footplate can be molded for greater rear or forefoot control.

Custom-Molded Thermoplastic Ankle-Foot Orthoses

The vast majority of AFOs today are custom-fitted with high temperature thermoplastic materials such as polyethylene or polypropylene plastic. Plastic AFO designs tend to offer a more intimate fit and can be molded around bony prominence and other anatomical structures, offering greater control of the foot and ankle. The footplates can also be fabricated with arches, postings, counters, and other modifications to support the architecture of the foot and, in the case of central nervous system involvement, potentially reduce tone or spasticity.

The degree of rigidity of the AFO can also be varied by the chemical composition of the plastic or hybrid materials, such as metals or carbon fiber composites, that can be incorporated into the appliance. The thickness of the materials can also determine the stiffness of the AFO. Finally, the shape of the AFO can have an effect. The more anterior the trim lines, the greater the stability. In fact, if an anterior closure is included in the design, a complete cylinder is created, offering maximal control of the tibia over the ankle (Fig. 22-13).[8]

The components of an AFO include the shoe insert, which is often referred to as the footplate. The calf shell runs the length of the posterior leg. If the calf shell is narrow enough to permit bending of the plastic, it is called a posterior leaf spring in that

F I G U R E   2 2 - 1 2

Varus/valgus correction. **A,** medial T-strap. **B,** lateral T-strap. **C,** supramalleolar orthoses. Reproduced, with permission from, *Advanced Rehabilitation Therapy,* Inc. Miami, FL.

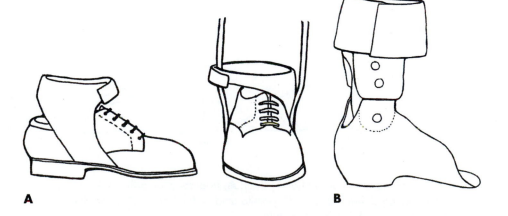

A   **B**

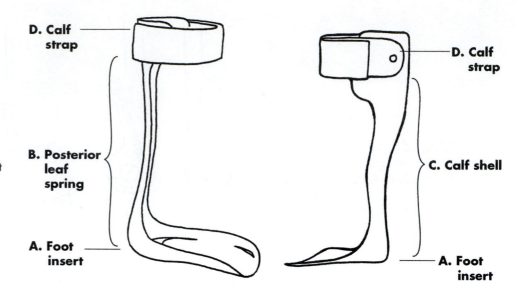

FIGURE 22-13

Ankle-foot orthosis. **A,** foot insert. **B,** calf shell (if flexible, posterior leaf spring). **C,** calf strap. Reproduced, with permission from, *Advanced Rehabilitation Therapy,* Inc. Miami, FL.

D. Calf strap

B. Posterior leaf spring

A. Foot insert

D. Calf strap

C. Calf shell

A. Foot insert

even though movement may take place during weight bearing, the ankle will return to a neutral position when unweighted. The position of the calf shell in relation to the footplate can also have an effect on the knee joint, where the greater the ankle dorsiflexion, the more knee flexion that will occur. Conversely, the greater the plantarflexion at the ankle, the more that knee extension is promoted. The proximal portion of the AFO has

the calf strap, which is typically a Velcro closure, to secure the orthosis and provide some stability (Fig. 22-14).

1. *Floor reaction orthosis AFO:* this design utilizes the joint moments that result from the ground reaction force to create stability at the knee. By placing the ankle in slight plantarflexion, an extension moment is created at the knee.

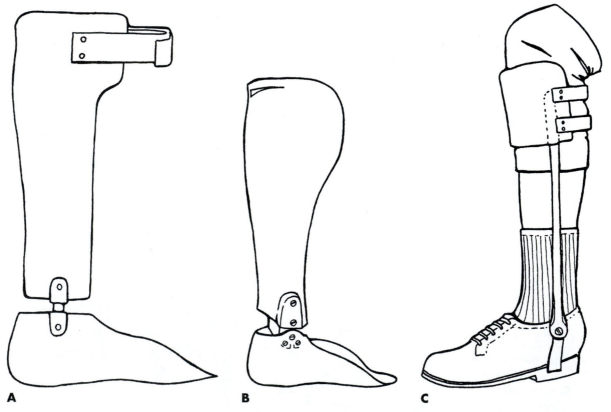

A

B

C

FIGURE 22-14

Custom-molded ankle-foot orthosis (AFO). **A,** floor reaction orthosis AFO. **B,** articulating or hinged AFO. **C,** patella tendom bearing AFO. Reproduced, with permission from, *Advanced Rehabilitation Therapy,* Inc. Miami, FL.

The length and rigidity of the footplate coupled with the plantarflexion angle of ankle, as well as the proximal anterior shell, prevent the tibia from progressing over the foot and promote extension. Typically used with clients who have weak quadriceps in place of using LLBs or KAFOs.

2. *Articulating or hinged AFO:* a variety of mechanical ankle joints as just described are available. The type of joint and design of the foot insert and calf shell control the degree of ankle movement.

3. *Patella tendon bearing AFO:* to reduce the body weight and ground reaction forces transmitted through the ankle, a rigid proximal shell is incorporated which offers a patella tendon bar that rests just inferior to the patella. The ankle is set in slight plantarflexion so that weight is borne through the patella tendon, therefore reducing the weight-bearing forces at the ankle. This design is often prescribed for degenerative joints such as Charcot joint and arthritic ankles.

4. *Tone-reducing AFO:* tone-reducing AFOs have several names depending on the specific design and materials used to construct the orthosis. While some controversy exists over the theoretical neurophysiologic rationale of tone-reducing orthotics, the general principles remain very similar regardless of the specific design. Clients who have spasticity resulting from upper motor neuron lesion dysfunction will present with increased tone, for example, when forces come in contact with particular anatomical structures of the foot such as the metatarsal heads or ball of the foot. Designing an AFO that inhibits tone to increase joint range-of-motion (ROM) to facilitate a more natural gait pattern is the primary consideration. The rationale for tone reducing does vary but tone-reducing AFOs include the following.

   a) *Inhibition of reflexes:* reducing stimulus pressure that increases tone can be accomplished by reducing the pressure over the ball of the foot. This can be accomplished by incorporating into the orthosis spastic inhibitor bars, foam toe separators, and/or metatarsal arch supports to reduce the pressure at the metatarsal heads.

   b) *Pressure over muscle insertions:* increase muscle tone typically plantarflexion, may be reduced when pressure is applied to either side of the insertion of the gastrocnemius–soleus muscle group.

   c) *Inhibitory stretch:* a slow steady stretch may be applied through static mobilization in an attempt to decrease reflexive tone. These AFOs use anterior closures or are bivalved designs that hold the ankle in predetermined stretched position.

KNEE-ANKLE-FOOT ORTHOTICS

The primary purpose of most knee orthotic devices is to provide knee control in one or more planes. Typically, the shoe is the foundation for the KAFO with or without a foot insert and

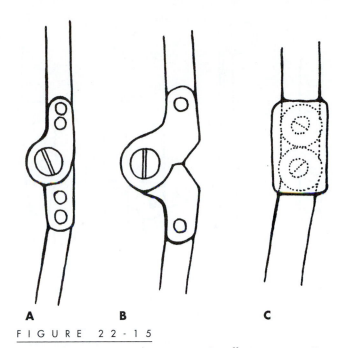

A   **B**   **C**

FIGURE 22-15

Knee joints. **A,** single axis joint. **B,** offset axis joint. **C,** polycentric axis joint. Reproduced, with permission from, *Advanced Rehabilitation Therapy,* Inc. Miami, FL.

ankle joints as described previously. A pair of metal uprights or plastic calf shell connects the foot/ankle components to the mechanical knee joint. The orthosis is suspended by the stabilizing structures, such as the calf bands or shells distally and thigh bands or shells proximally.

Knee Joints (Fig. 22-15)

1. *Single axis joint:* designed to behave like a hinge, preventing movement in the coronal plane, providing medial/lateral stability, while permitting movement in the sagittal plane. Free motion joints allow full knee flexion and extension yet prevent hyperextension. Prescribed for genu varum and valgum.

2. *Offset axis joint:* a single axis joint design with the axis set further posterior from the weight line than the standard single axis joint, promoting maximal knee extension during weight bearing without having to use a mechanical lock. The offset joint is prescribed when greater stability than offered with a single axis joint is warranted.

3. *Polycentric axis joint:* designed to mimic the instantaneous center of rotation present in the anatomical knee, the two-geared mechanical joint is still confined to a uniplanar path. The gliding and rolling motion emulated with the polycentric joint is intended to reduce excessive motion, slippage, and to provide greater comfort than conventional single axis joints afford.

Knee Locking Mechanism (Fig. 22-16)

1. *Drop-ring locks:* the most common locking system. It has small rings that slide down over the proximal portion of

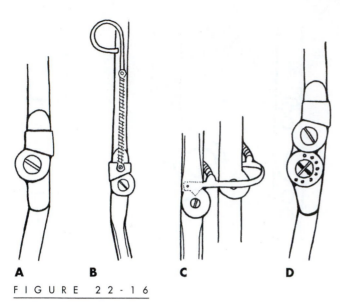

FIGURE 22-16

Knee locking mechanisms. **A,** drop-ring locks. **B,** spring-load pull rod. **C,** pawl or bail locks. **D,** adjustable knee lock. Reproduced, with permission from, *Advanced Rehabilitation Therapy,* Inc. Miami, FL.

a single axis knee joint to maintain full knee extension during standing and may be raised manually to release for sitting or free knee flexion and extension.

2. *Spring-load pull rod:* a spring system with a control rod that can be extended to a height for convenient reach permits easier release of locking mechanism. Often prescribed for clients with poor balance, or dexterity issues that preclude them from using standard locking systems.

3. *Pawl or bail locks:* levers posterior to the knee provide easy release of the locking mechanism for sitting. Clients who have extreme balance disturbances or cannot free their hands in order to operate a locking system during sitting benefit from this type of locking mechanism.

4. *Adjustable knee lock:* a variety of mechanisms are available to preset the knee lock ROM, allowing clinicians to establish the specific knee flexion and extension to prevent reinjury. As greater knee ROM is permitted during the course of rehabilitation, the preset ROM of the knee mechanism can be adjusted to accommodate progress or prevent further injury.

KNEE ORTHOTICS

1. *Rigid knee orthotics (knee cage):* commonly referred to as the "Swedish" knee cage the prefabricated device has a metal frame with canvas or heavy elastic thigh and calf straps and is designed to prevent recurvatum and provide some medial and lateral support. Frequently used with clients having knee instability, preventing further damage or internal derangement to inert structures of the knee while strength is returning.

2. *Knee immobilizer and two-phase/breakdown braces:* fabricated from a variety of fabrics and metal inserts for stability, these orthoses are designed to comfortably restrict all motions of the knee. More sophisticated versions, known as two-phase/breakdown braces, can be either custom-fitted or prefabricated, and are usually used during the immobilization phase of an acute injury and prior to or after surgery. They include knee joints to limit motion as necessary with adjustable hinges and to gradually increase ROM as the person progresses through rehabilitation.

3. *Functional knee braces:* individuals who have returned to activity and require or feel the need for additional stability to protect the knee, wear functional knee braces. Although a topic of controversy with regards as to prophylactic ability of these braces, the major attributes sighted for their use are (1) satisfactory primary and secondary ligament restraint, (2) static compressive joint forces with dynamic forces resulting from muscular contraction, and (3) gproprioceptive and neuromuscular input to integrate cocontraction. The negative aspects of wearing functional knee braces during activity have been identified as (1) brace slippage, (2) bulkiness and weight, (3) heat retention and irritation, (4) excessive medial condylar tightness, (5) calf strap tightness, and (6) brace hinge malalignment with the femoral condyles or knee joint.[20]

4. *Patellofemoral joint:* the primary goals of these braces are to minimize patella compression, assist in guiding patella tracking, and prevent excessive lateral shift. There are a number of brace designs targeted at one or all three of the stated goals for the patellofemoral joint. Generically, there are two types of patellofemoral orthotics (Fig. 22-17).
   * *Elastic sleeves:* running the length of the mid-thigh to mid-calf, this type of brace provides medial dynamic tension and attempts to counterbalance the lateral

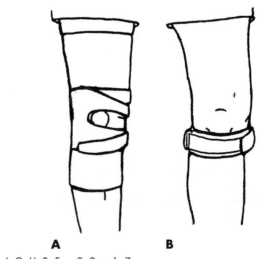

FIGURE 22-17

Knee orthotics. **A,** elastic sleeves. **B,** infrapatella straps. Reproduced, with permission from, *Advanced Rehabilitation Therapy,* Inc. Miami, FL.

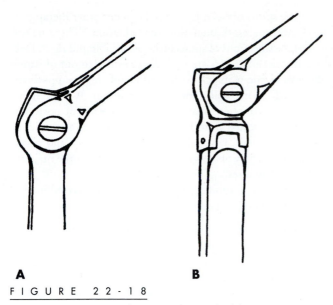

A   **B**

F I G U R E   2 2 - 1 8

Hip joints. **A,** single axis joint. **B,** double axis joint. Reproduced, with permission from, *Advanced Rehabilitation Therapy,* Inc. Miami, FL.

displacement of the patella. The stabilizing component of the brace can be either a series of three adjustable straps, horseshoe-shaped felt or rubber pads, or pneumatic chambers.

- *Infrapatella straps:* a fabric strap with Velcro closure is worn over the patella tendon to support the distal patella, to alter patellofemoral joint mechanics, and facilitate improved tracking to relieve compressive forces between articular forces.
- *Patellar tapping:* one other popular intervention, patellar tapping, is used to assist in correcting patellar orientation and control tracking, and decreases pain and facilitates vastus medialis obliqus.[20]

HIP-KNEE-ANKLE-FOOT ORTHOSES

Hip Joints (Fig. 22-18)

1. *Single axis:* most commonly, hip joints are single axis joints permitting flexion and extension, restricting abduction, adduction, and rotation.
2. *Double axis:* if hip abduction and adduction are desired in addition to flexion and extension, the double axis locks offer two planes of motion with adjustable stops to set limits as needed in each direction.

Hip Locks (Fig. 22-19)

1. *Drop locks:* similar to knee drop lock, a small ring slides down over the axis to lock the joint in extension while in standing.
2. *Two-position hip locks:* designed to lock in full extension and 90° of hip flexion, this locking system proves to be a

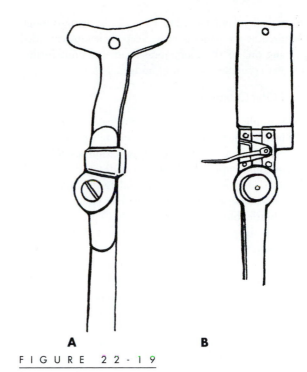

A   **B**

F I G U R E   2 2 - 1 9

Hip locks. **A,** drop locks. **B,** two-position hip locks. Reproduced, with permission from, *Advanced Rehabilitation Therapy,* Inc. Miami, FL.

great asset when poor sitting balance is present, especially in children.

Pelvic Bands

1. *Unilateral band:* when a single limb orthosis requires proximal stability, a rigid band can be incorporated that encircles the pelvis between the iliac crest and greater trochanter, with a flexible belt continues around the waist.
2. *Bilateral band:* most commonly the bilateral pelvic band is used for bilateral HKAFOs where the padded metal band encompasses the pelvis just above the buttock with the posterior band positioned over the sacrum.
3. *Double or pelvic girdle:* when maximal control is required, the entire proximal pelvis is encapsulated from the iliac crest to just proximal to the greater trochanter with varying posteriorly depending or strength and pelvis stability. High-temperature thermoplastics are typically used and custom-molded to each client, ensuring optimal fit.
4. *Silesian belt:* a flexible strap that attaches to proximal portion of the orthosis and encircles the pelvis, assisting to stabilize the orthosis and provide suspension. Although more comfortable than rigid pelvic bands, some stability is sacrificed because of flexible nature of the belt.

Bilateral KAFOs

Often referred to as Craig Scott or LLBs, these orthoses are intended for standing or ambulation in people with spinal cord lesions from the level of L1–T12 to T9–L1–2. A swing-through gait is required as the patients must keep their hips extended as they "hang on" or the iliofemoral ligaments limit further extension, with crutches in front of body.

Reciprocal Gait Orthoses

As the name implies, RGOs are designed to permit a reciprocal gait as opposed to the traditional swing-through gait used with HKAFOs. The patient selection criterion requires stability of the spine, adequate upper limb and shoulder girdle strength and endurance, and a cardiovascular and respiratory system that is free of disease and provides adequate endurance. The types of disabilities often associated with RGO prescription include people with spinal cord injuries levels as high as C8 to T12–L1; however, use of RGOs with the higher levels is rare and most commonly T9 to L1 are candidates. Other diagnoses are myelodyplasia, osteogenesis imperfecta, spinal bifida, paraplegia, muscular dystrophy (not Duchenne type), and cerebral palsy. The three most outstanding contraindications are obesity, hip flexion contractures, and genu varum greater than 15°.

The passive reciprocal motion is facilitated by a variety of mechanisms depending on the individual design. Currently, the three most widely used basic designs are (1) the Louisiana State University RGOs, which have a cable system coupling the passive hip flexion and extension movements that advance the lower limbs in a reciprocal fashion, (2) the Isocentric RGO system, which uses a bar balance system located at the lumbrosacral level of the orthosis, providing the reciprocating hip flexion action; and (3) the advanced reciprocating gait orthosis system, which utilizes a low-profile push–pull cable system that not only provides the reciprocating motion at the hip but also assists with standing through a hip and knee extension assist mechanism. Other RGO systems and variations of the aforementioned orthoses are also used throughout the world.

The suggested advantages of RGOs include increased walking velocity, smoothness of gait, decreased energy expenditure, improved control of lumbar lordosis and hip flexion with a decrease in the risk of flexion contractures, less weight-bearing demand on the shoulder joints from crutch use, improved bowel and bladder function, improved cardiopulmonary mechanics, increased bone density, psychological benefits of standing, and the ability to look eye to eye during personal encounters, as well as increased mobility within narrow confines and on steps.

Disadvantages that have been described include the need for high motivation by the parent and child or the adult patient, excessive perspiration in warm climates, skin irritation, spinal deformity, poor cosmesis, difficult donning/doffing procedures, high metabolic demand, decreased velocity (typically one-fifth of normal walking speed) as compared to using a wheelchair, and multiple orthotist visits and cost.

SPINAL ORTHOTICS

The use of spinal orthotics for back pain, restriction of spinal motion, or postural care has long been a standard of care. Nor-
mally, the spinal orthosis is used to augment other therapies as the clients progress through their rehabilitation.[3] There are two general classifications of spinal orthosis: flexible and rigid. Flexible orthotics or corsets are typically constructed out of strong fabrics or elastic materials with a variety of stiffer supports incorporated, as necessary, for the prescription. A rigid spinal orthotic is used when greater control of motion or posture is required. Fabricated from high-temperature thermoplastics or lightweight metals, with a broad selection of pads and coverings, a wide variety of designs are available to meet the majority of clinical diagnoses.

Flexible corsets and rigid orthoses may offer a combination of the following therapeutic benefits.

1. *Intra-abdominal pressure:* although somewhat controversial,[11,12] the pressure exerted on the abdomen by the corset or rigid orthosis creates a cylinder effect, which in turn, raises the intracavitary pressure,[15,16] and is believed to reduce the intradiscal pressure, especially during forward bending.[18,19]

2. *Muscle relaxation:* the use of a spinal orthosis reduces the need for abdominal contractions as the cylinder effect to support the vertebral column is created passively, therefore, relaxing the abdominal and erector spinae muscles.[14] Performing abdominal muscle contractions can create a flexion moment on the spine that must be restrained by the back extensors, and as a result, increase disk compression.[1,15,16] Decreasing the need for contractile support of the vertebral column may relax the muscles and reduce existing pain.

3. *Restriction of motion:* the primary method employed for motion control is the three-point pressure system. A rigid system is used when cervical, thoracic, and lumbrosacral motions are sought to be limited to the greatest possible degree. The amount of limitation varies between the various designs; however, a reduction in the motion at respective intervertebral segments has been linked to a reduction in pain and spinal instability with the intention of promoting healing.[23] Postoperative spinal orthotics not only limit motion by virtue of the mechanical restraint but, additionally, offer constant proprioceptive feedback, reinforcing positive behaviors.

4. *Postural realignment:* increased intra-abdominal pressure, relaxation of muscle in spasm,[12] and restriction of movement[9] can assist in facilitating improved posture and reduce compensatory postures related to pain. In the case of scoliosis, the use of orthotic intervention may prevent the progression of a spinal curve, stabilize the curvature, and, in many instances, offer some degree of curvature correction, providing the client is compliant.[2]

Flexible Orthoses or Corsets

1. *Sacroiliac corset (binder):* numerous prefabricated designs are available made from a combination of fabric, elastic, laces, and Velcro, offering multiple adjustments. Encircling

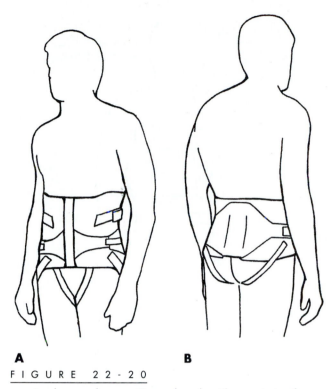

A   **B**

FIGURE 22-20

Lumbosacral corset. Reproduced, with permission from, *Advanced Rehabilitation Therapy,* Inc. Miami, FL.

the waist from the iliac crest to the greater trochanter, and extending anteriorly to the symphysis pubis, they are offered in a variety of widths. Depending on the specific design, intra-abdominal pressure and posture reinforcement promote stability for clients with postpartum or sacroiliac instability. Some versions include a moldable plastic insert for low back pain.

2. *Lumbosacral corset:* constructed from heavy fabrics with laces and hooks for multiple adjustments throughout the garment, the LSO corset is designed to encompass the torso and pelvis. The anterior and lateral trunk containment elevate the intracavitary pressure, while most manufacturers include rigid stays, maintaining a three-point pressure system to restrict motion, or as a reminder to limit motion. The primary use is for back pain clients (Fig. 22-20).

3. *Thoracolumbosacral corset:* relatively the same construction and function as the LSO corset except that the TLSO includes a shoulder strap to restrict spinal motion to the thoracic region as well as to the lumbar spine (Fig. 22-21).

Rigid Orthoses

1. *Lumbrosacral orthoses (Williams) (Extension-lateral control):* fabricated from lightweight metals, such as leather and vinyl, a single three-point pressure system limits trunk extension in the lumbar spine and increases intra-abdominal pressure. Lordosis is decreased to limit lumbar extension, while the pelvic and thoracic bands exert a medial force

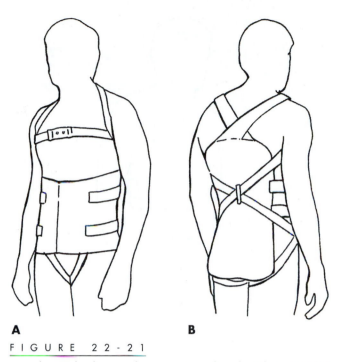

A   **B**

FIGURE 22-21

Thoracolumbosacral corset. Reproduced, with permission from, *Advanced Rehabilitation Therapy,* Inc. Miami, FL.

that tends to limit lateral trunk motions. There is no limitation of trunk flexion, therefore permitting light flexion exercises to increase abdominal strength while wearing the orthosis (Fig. 22-22).

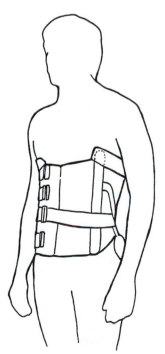

FIGURE 22-22

Lumbrosacral orthoses (Williams) (Extension-lateral control). Reproduced, with permission from, *Advanced Rehabilitation Therapy,* Inc. Miami, FL.

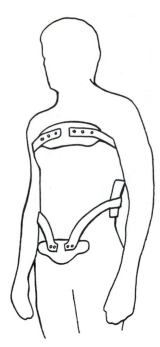

FIGURE 22-23

Jewett (flexion control). Reproduced, with permission from, *Advanced Rehabilitation Therapy,* Inc. Miami, FL.

2.   *Thoraciclumbrosacral orthoses*
   • *Taylor (flexion / extension control):* a pelvic band connects with two posterior uprights terminating at the midscapular level of the thoracic region, with an anterior abdominal closure and axillary straps. Two three-point pressure systems are coupled together to limit both flexion and extension of the lumbar and thoracic spine.
   • *Jewett (flexion control):* a three-point pressure system is created with two pads, one across the sternum and one at the symphysis pubis, providing the counterforce with a single pad posteriorly to promote hyperextension and thus restricting forward flexion (Fig. 22-23).
   • *Plastic body jacket (flexion-extension-lateral-rotary control):* typically fabricated with high-temperature copolymer plastics, a well-fitted body jacket will restrict motion in all planes. Anterior and lateral trunk containment elevate intracavitary pressure, and decrease demands on the vertebral discs. Body jackets are frequently used postsurgically or during an acute trauma. A variety of modifications can be made for comfort such as anterior chest cutouts and altering pelvic trim lines depending on the diagnosis (Fig. 22-24).

CERVICAL ORTHOSES

1.   *Soft collar:* made from soft foam, the collar provides mechanical restraint for cervical flexion and extension and, to a lesser degree, lateral flexion and rotation. Although the soft collar provides minimal restriction to movement, it

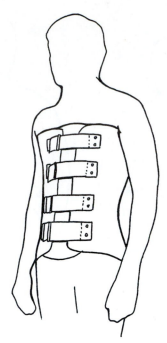

FIGURE 22-24

Plastic body jacket (flexion-extension-lateral-rotary control). Reproduced, with permission from, *Advanced Rehabilitation Therapy,* Inc. Miami, FL.

is a good transitional appliance from more rigid orthoses, and acts as a proprioceptive reminder to the wearer to limit head and neck motions (Fig. 22-25).

2.   *Hard collars (Philadelphia collar):* constructed from semirigid and rigid plastics, depending on the manufacturer. Hard collars provide more rigid stabilization of the cervical spine and typically offer some type of chin and occipital support, with the inferior collar extending to the sternal notch anteriorly and to the T3 spinous process posteriorly. Generally hard collars, like the Philadelphia collar, limit

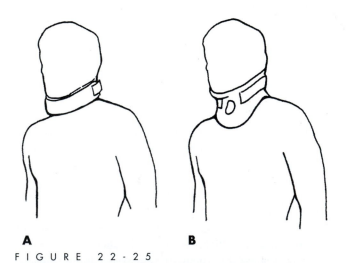

A   **B**

FIGURE 22-25

A, soft collar. **B,** hard collars (Philadelphia collar). Reproduced, with permission from, *Advanced Rehabilitation Therapy,* Inc. Miami, FL.

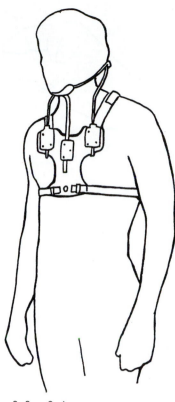

FIGURE 22-26

Cervicothoracic orthoses (sterno-occipital mandibular immobilizer). Reproduced, with permission from, *Advanced Rehabilitation Therapy*, Inc. Miami, FL.

motion much more than soft collars, but on average still permit 40–50 percent of normal cervical ROM, depending on the motion (see Fig. 22-25).[6]

3. *Cervicothoracic orthoses (Sterno-occipital mandibular immobilizer):* sterno-occipital mandibular immobilizer is one of the most common postsurgical appliances. It consists of a rigid metal frame with a chin and occipital rest connected to a chest and back plate, with padded shoulder and trunk straps. The added chest and back plates help to reduce cervical motion by an average of 55–75 percent, depending on the motion (Fig. 22-26).[6]

4. *Halo-cervical orthosis:* the greatest reduction in cervical mobilization occurs with the halo-vest appliance. A cranial ring is secured to the skull using four metal pins. The ring is attached by four metal bars to a plastic vest and is worn continuously. The estimated reduction in all cervical motions is 90–95 percent.[6] It also has the ability to provide distracting forces that aid in the spinal stabilization and in reducing the load of the head on the cervical spine.

Cervicothoraciclumbrosacral Orthosis

The CTLSO is most commonly used for the treatment of scoliosis and kyphosis. Although a number of designs are used for a variety of clients, the Milwaukee brace is without question the most popular. There is extensive literature describing the etiol-

ogy, clinical findings and treatments of scoliosis and kyphosis that extends far beyond the scope of this chapter. Suffice it to say that the Milwaukee brace is designed with a neck ring and occipital pad, connected to four metal upright bars secured to a plastic TLSO, which extends distally, forming a molded pelvic section.

The advantage of the Milwaukee brace is that each component, pelvic, thoracic, and cervical, can be molded or adjusted to slow, or even in some cases, correct scoliotic curve. In the case of idiopathic scoliosis the average 1-year follow-up showed an average 20 percent correction for thoracic curves.[1] The disadvantage to this treatment is that the brace must be worn for 12–18 months, 23 hours a day, with the child being out of the brace only for exercise or athletic activity. The psychological issues and poor acceptance by clients and physicians lead to rejection of scoliotic bracing, even with the more cosmetic, low-profile TLSOs.[4]

Upper Limb Orthotics

Architecture of the Hand

The hand is an extremely complex anatomical structure requiring muscular contractions and joint movement to act in concert with incredible accuracy, coordination, and power. The ability to manipulate the hand to perform the infinite number of functional patterns has, in part, to do with the command of opposition and prehension, two functions that are directly related to the three arches of the hand. The intrinsic muscles and ligaments of the hand and wrist are responsible for maintaining the integrity of the arches of the hand.

Arches of the Hand

1. *Proximal transverse (carpal) arch:* formed by the carpal bones, the capitate bone is considered to be the keystone for this arch, as the annular ligaments secure the bony structures together, providing the stability through the wrist and a mechanical advantage for strength of finger flexors.[7]

2. *Distal transverse (metacarpal) arch:* the intermetacarpal and metaphalangeal volar ligaments along with the metacarpal bones form the distal transverse arch, permitting thumb opposition to the other fingers and rounding of the hand.[7]

3. *Longitudinal (carpometacarpophalangeal) arch:* formed by the intrinsic muscles of the hand and the carpal, metacarpal and phalanges of each digit, the longitudinal arch is the basis for the three-jaw chuck position of the hand. Two other longitudinal arches sometimes described are the oblique arch, where the thumb and fifth digit create an arch during opposition, and when the thumb and index finger form another arch with the web space.[7]

The hand typically functions in four phases: (1) reach, frequently recruiting the motions of the shoulder, the hand is extended as it is about to grasp or manipulate an object, (2) prehension, three patterns of prehension occur—pinch, grasp,

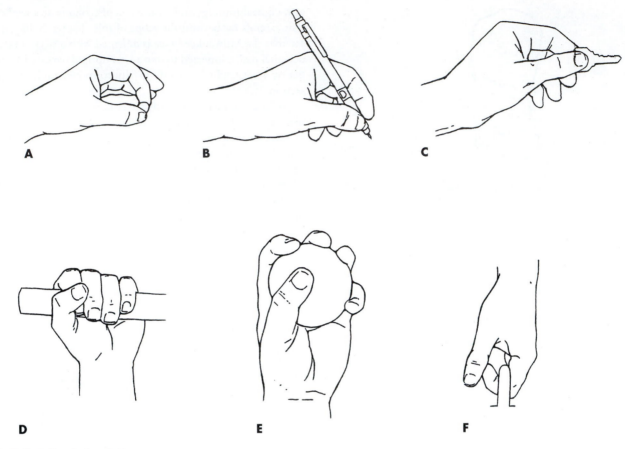

FIGURE 22-27

Prehension. 1. Pinch: **A,** tip. **B,** palmer. **C,** lateral. 2. Grasp: **D,** cylindrical.
E, spherical, 3. Hook: **F,** hook. Reproduced, with permission from, *Advanced Rehabilitation Therapy,* Inc. Miami, FL.

and hook—allowing humans to capture objects in their hands, (3) carry, the ability to move an object from one point to another, and (4) release, the ability to discard or place an object at a specific point or time. The three phases of prehension can be further subdivided into more precise categories (Fig. 22-27).[10]

Pinch

Tip	Index finger to thumb (OK)
Palmar	Index and middle finger to thumb (three-jaw chuck)
Lateral	Thumb to lateral index finger (key grip)

Grasp

Cylindrical	Hand around cylinder
Spherical	Holding a ball

Hook

Hook	PIP joints without thumb (link grip)

UPPER LIMB ORTHOTICS

As stated earlier, when describing upper limb orthotics, it is very common, especially in the case of the hand, to use the term "splint" or "splinting." The use of orthoses and splints are interchangeable in this area.[13] There are two general classifications of splints or orthotics. The first, static orthoses, which do not permit motion and are often referred to as resting or positional splints, are used to position or to hold the wrist and hand. Static splints are commonly fabricated from low-temperature thermoplastics, or, if a permanent orthosis is required, high-temperature copolymer plastics are used. Dynamic orthoses permit movement and are splints that provide a dynamic force, generally using energy-storing materials like rubber bands, spring steel, wound coiled wire, or plastic with memory.

The design variations of upper limb orthoses are quite extensive and require considerable detail and explanation. The orthoses presented are single examples from selected categories of orthoses and are not an attempt to be all-inclusive. Because of the complexity of the hand in terms of anatomy, function, and associated complications with each diagnosis, hand splinting or orthotic fabrication is clearly a specialty that requires careful examination of each client and, in many cases, frequent modifications to the orthosis to meet his/her individual needs.

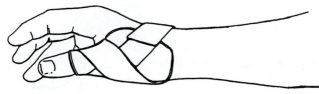

FIGURE 22-28

Hand orthosis (basic or short opponens). Reproduced, with permission from, *Advanced Rehabilitation Therapy,* Inc. Miami, FL.

Hand and Wrist Orthoses

HAND ORTHOSIS (BASIC OR SHORT OPPONENS) (FIG. 22-28)

Fabricated from low-temperature thermoplastics, this orthosis is designed to immobilize the first carpometacarpophalangeal and metacarpophalangeal (MCP) joints, and position the thumb in opposition and abduction to maintain the web space, and the architecture of the hand for future procedures. There is no orthotic wrist control, therefore strong wrist flexor and extensors are required for functional use. Positioning of the hand can be functional for grasp (three-jaw chuck).

Indications include

- inflammation or injury of the thumb
- median nerve lesions
- C6–7 spinal cord lesions
- hemiplegia with loss of thumb opposition

WRIST-HAND ORTHOSIS (LONG OPPONENS SPLINT OR VOLAR FOREARM WRIST ORTHOSIS) (FIG. 22-29)

Constructed from low-temperature thermoplastics, like the short opponens splint, the first carpometacarpophalangeal and MCP joints are immobilized with the thumb in extension and opposition, preserving the web space. The addition of wrist immobilization with a volar wrist control design, maintaining neutral or slight extension, offers less tension to the inflamed tendons, with reduction of movement to the thumb in general. Basically, this splint is a short opponens with wrist control.

Indications include

- DeQuervains's tenosynovitis
- median and ulnar nerve lesions

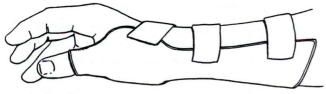

FIGURE 22-29

Wrist-hand orthosis (long opponens splint or volar forearm wrist orthosis). Reproduced, with permission from, *Advanced Rehabilitation Therapy,* Inc. Miami, FL.

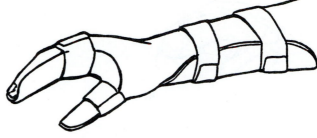

FIGURE 22-30

Volar forearm static wrist-hand orthosis (resting hand sprint). Reproduced, with permission from, *Advanced Rehabilitation Therapy,* Inc. Miami, FL.

- C5–6 spinal cord lesions
- wrist or thumb instability
- degenerative or inflamed wrist thumb joint
- scaphoid or Bennett's fracture-dislocation

VOLAR FOREARM STATIC WRIST HAND ORTHOSIS (RESTING HAND SPLINT (FIG. 22-30)

Commonly referred to as a resting hand splint, the objective of this splint is to place the hand and wrist in a neutral, functional, or lumbrical position, with the MCP joints flexed to 60°–90°, and the proximal interphalangeal and distal interphalangeal joints flexed to 0°–45°. The wrist is in slight extension to neutral. This position maintains the web space, preventing a flat hand or flexion contractures of the hand and is also used to reduce pain and inflammation.

Indications include

- flaccid hand due to paralysis
- burns or healing skin grafts
- Dupuytren's release
- degenerative or inflamed joints
- Volkman's ischemia
- trauma to hand or wrist

WRIST-DRIVEN PREHENSION ORTHOSIS (TENODESIS ORTHOSIS) (FIG. 22-31)

Several designs with a variety of materials from low-temperature thermoplastics to lightweight metals are used to fabricate these orthoses. Designed specifically for clients with spinal cord injury at the C6-7 level and who have the $3^-/5$ to $3^+/5$ extensor carpi radialis muscle strength, necessary to facilitate the passive flexion of the thumb, index, and middle fingers, to create passive three-jaw chuck hand position, or protect the hand for functional tenodesis. The orthotic assist for this motion depends on the design and the required assistance due to weakness. Some clients have the strength, or increase their strength, so that the orthosis is no longer mandatory.

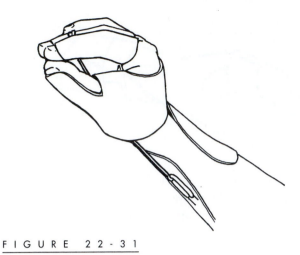

FIGURE 22-31

Wrist-driven prehension orthosis (tenodesis orthosis).
Reproduced, with permission from, *Advanced
Rehabilitation Therapy*, Inc. Miami, FL.

UTENSIL HOLDERS (ADL CUFF, UNIVERSAL SPLINT) (FIG. 22-32)

A custom or prefabricated splint frequently fabricated from
leather and flexible metal. A small sleeve or pouch is located
within the palmer aspect, permitting the placement of eating
utensils, grooming aids, and writing implements. Active shoulder motions and elbow flexion are required to manipulate the
objects placed in the splint.

Indications include

- C5–6 spinal cord lesions
- hemiplegia

EXTERNALLY POWERED PREHENSION ORTHOSIS

Ratchet Orthosis (Pawl Lever) (Fig. 22-33)

Generally indicated for clients with C5 tetraplegia, or when the
extensor muscles of the hand are less than a 3/5 strength grade,
a manually controlled orthosis can be used to provide pinch
in the three-jaw chuck position. Operation of the orthosis is
controlled by a ratchet bar located on the radial side of the
splint. By tapping the knob with the other hand, or on another
stable object, a simple gear system closes the fingers in discrete
increments. A second ratchet button releases the spring-loaded

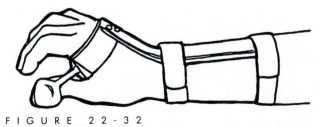

FIGURE 22-32

Utensil holders (ADL Cuff, universal splint). Reproduced,
with permission from, *Advanced Rehabilitation Therapy*,
Inc. Miami, FL.

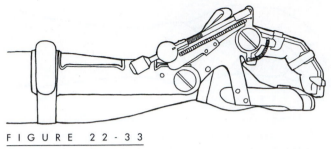

FIGURE 22-33

Ratchet orthosis (Pawl lever) orthsis. Reproduced, with
permission from, *Advanced Rehabilitation Therapy*, Inc.
Miami, FL.

gear system to open the hand. Many feeding, hygiene, and
functional activities, that otherwise would be impossible, can
be performed with this orthosis.

EXTERNALLY POWERED PREHENSION UNIT

The battery-driven externally powered prehension unit is another alternative that allows clients with paralysis or severe
weakness to have hand function with the use of a WHO. The
rechargeable battery power source drives the mechanical closing
and opening of the hand. Gross movements of the upper limb
operate the rocker type electrical switch, producing pronation
to produce prehension and supination to open the hand.

Mobile Arm Support

When shoulder and elbow weakness limits upper limb mobility,
the mobile arm support orthotic system becomes a viable aid.
The appliance clamps to a table or wheelchair, attaches to body
jacket, or can be mounted on the iliac crest with ambulatory
patients. The client must have $2^+/5$ strength of the shoulder or
trunk to depress the elbow, thus elevating the hand by using a
ball-bearing forearm component that permits movement of the
flaccid upper limb and permits horizontal arm adduction and
abduction of the shoulder.

Indications include

- spinal cord lesion
- Guillain-Barré syndrome
- amyotrophic lateral sclerosis
- muscular dystrophy
- poliomyelitis

TONE-REDUCING ORTHOSES (FIG. 22-34)

Tone-reducing or antispasticity splints are prescribed when hypertonicity is present. The primary objective is to reduce flexor
tone, reduce the incidence of contractures, and maintain the
arches by placing the hand and fingers in an extended and abducted position, creating firm pressure to the palmer surface of
the hand. Care must be taken to avoid areas of pressure and
potential skin irritation. The splints are typically worn with a
2-hour on, 2-hour off wearing schedule throughout the day.
A variety of designs include antispasticity ball splint, Snook

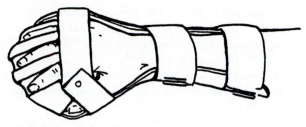

FIGURE 22-34

Tone-reducing orthoses. Reproduced, with permission from, *Advanced Rehabilitation Therapy,* Inc. Miami, FL.

splint, Cone splint (Rood splint), Bobath splint, finger abduction splint, and dynafoam wrist-hand splint.

Elbow Orthosis

STATIC ORTHOSES (SPLINTS)

Frequently custom-fabricated from low-temperature thermoplastics, these splints are formed over the volar surface of the elbow for the purpose of restricting motion, and promote tissue healing. These splints can be removed for topical treatments and hygiene. As ROM returns, the angle of the splint can be adjusted by reforming the plastic shell, a process similar to that of serial casting. Indications for the static splints include burns, fractures, tendon, nerve, vascular repairs and cubital tunnel syndrome.

DYNAMIC ORTHOSES (SPLINTS)

When ROM is lost and there is a need to increase the resting length of the elbow, dynamic splints provide a low-load with prolonged stretch, with the intent of stretching the soft tissues and skin over time. The mechanical or dynamic splints may be utilized in the same fashion as serial casting techniques. This type of splint is used for clients with burns and elbow contractures.

Shoulder Orthoses

ARM SLINGS

Commonly made of fabric construction, an assortment of designs include the figure-eight, universal sling, cuff sling, orthopedic sling, bandana sling, and flail arm sling. They are used to immobilize and promote healing of tissue immediately after injury. For the neurologically involved clients who present with hemiplegia, there are designs such as the hemi arm sling worn to prevent subluxation of the shoulder, while the arm is flaccid.

SHOULDER-ELBOW-WRIST ORTHOSES (AIRPLANE SPLINT)

Shoulder-elbow-wrist orthoses, more commonly referred to as airplane splints, are used to protect the soft tissues of the shoulder and prevent contractures. Most frequently custom fit to the client, although prefabricated kits are available, the shoulder is abducted 70°–90°, with the majority of body weight borne

on the iliac crest and lateral trunk. Custom fabrication permits specific placement of joint angles and can be adjusted as healing progresses throughout rehabilitation.

SUMMARY

- Orthotic appliances are designed based on the biomechanical principles of pressure, equilibrium, and lever arm.
- Functional considerations of orthotics are alignment, movement, weight bearing, and protection.
- Shoes are the foundation of lower limb orthotics and should always be considered in the prescription.
- Foot orthotics maintains or corrects the architecture of foot and can be classified as soft, semirigid, and rigid.
- AFOs are designed to control the rate and direction of tibial advancement to maintain an adequate base of support during walking.
- Knee orthotics are typically designed to control knee movement in more than one plane.
- Hip orthotics are designed to stabilize the pelvis and permit motion for sitting.
- Spinal orthotics can be flexible or rigid and offer a combination of therapeutic benefits including intra-abdominal pressure, muscle relaxation, and restriction of motion.
- Wrist hand orthotics are designed to maintain the architecture of the hand permitting prehension and control of the wrist for upper limb function.

REFERENCES

1. Bartelink DL. The role of abdominal pressure in relieving the pressure on the lumbar intervertebral discs. *J Bone Joint Surg* 39B:718–725, 1957.
2. Blount WP, Moe JH. *The Milwaukee Brace.* Baltimore, MD, Williams & Wilkins, 1973.
3. Cailliet R. Biomechanics of the spine. *Phys Med Rehabil Clin N Am* 3:1–28, 1992.
4. Emans JB, et al. The Boston bracing system for idiopathic scoliosis: Follow-up results in 295 patients. *Spine* 11:172, 1986.
5. Goldberg B, Hsu JD, eds. *Atlas of Orthoses and Assistive Devices/American Academy of Orthopaedic Surgeons*, 3rd ed. St. Louis, MO, Mosby, 1985.
6. Johnson RM, et al. Cervical orthosis: A study comparing their effectiveness in restricting cervical motion in normal subjects. *J Bone Joint Surg* 59A:332–339, 1977.
7. Kapandji IA. *The Physiology of the Joints, Vol. I: Upper Limb*, 2nd ed. Edinburgh, Churchill Livingstone, 1970.
8. Kottke FJ, Lehmann JF, eds. *Krusen's Handbook of Physical Medicine and Rehabilitation*, 4th ed. Philadelphia, WB Saunders, 1990.
9. Lantz SA, Schultz AB. Lumbar spine orthosis wearing: I. Restriction of gross body motion. *Spine* 11:834–837, 1986.

10. Lusardi MM, Nielsen CC. *Orthotics and Prosthetics in Rehabilitation.* Woburn, MA, Butterworth, 2000.

11. McGill SM, Norman RW. Reassessment of the role of intra-abdominal pressure in spinal compression. *Ergonomics* 30:1565–1588, 1987.

12. McGill SM, Norman RW, Sharratt MT. The effect of an abdominal belt on trunk muscle activity and intra-abdominal pressure during squat lifts. *Ergonomics* 33:147–160, 1990.

13. Mckee P, Morgan L. *Orthotics in Rehabilitation: Splinting the Hand and Body.* Philadelphia, FA Davis, 1998.

14. McKenzie AR, Lipscomb PR. Corsets on and off. *J Bone Joint Surg* 61B:384, 1979.

15. Morris JM. Biomechanics of the spine. *Arch Surg* 107:418–423, 1973.

16. Morris JM. Low back bracing. *Clin Orthop* 102:126–132, 1974.

17. Myers RS, ed. *Saunders Manual of Physical Therapy Practice*, 1st ed. Philadelphia, WB Saunders, 1995.

18. Nachemson A, Morris JM. In vivo measurement of intradiscal pressure: Discometry, a method for determining pressure in the lower lumbar discs. *J Bone Joint Surg* A:1077–1092, 1964.

19. Nachemson A, Schultz A, Andersson G. Mechanical effectiveness studies of lumbar spine orthosis. *Scand J Rehabil Med* Suppl 9:139–149, 1983.

20. Nawoczenski DA, Epler ME, eds. *Orthotics in Functional Rehabilitation of the Lower Limb.* Philadelphia, WB Saunders, 1994.

21. New York University Medical Center. *Lower-Limb Orthotics.* New York, NYU Post-Graduate Medical School, Prosthetics and Orthotics, January 1986.

22. Redford JB, Basmajian JV, Trautman P, eds. *Orthotics: Clincal Practice and Rehabilitation Technology.* New York, Churchill Livingstone, 1995.

23. Russek AS. Biomechanical and physiological basis for ambulatory treatment of low back pain. 4:21–26, 1976.

24. Shurr DG, Cook TM. *Prosthetics and Orthotics.* Norwalk, CT, Appleton & Lange, 1990.

CHAPTER 23

Designing Therapeutic Exercise Programs for Home and Clinical Progressions

Andrew Bloch and J. Allen Hardin

O B J E C T I V E S

After completing this chapter, the therapist should be able to do the following:

- Demonstrate an understanding of the historical perspectives and philosophy of home exercise prescription.
- Describe the benefits of home exercise prescription.
- Identify strategies in developing a home exercise program.
- Describe the factors affecting compliance and their relationship to outcomes.
- Identify techniques and guidelines for implementing a home exercise program.
- Describe recent technological advances that enhance the patient education model.
- Design a home exercise program that incorporates the elements described in this chapter.

HISTORICAL PERSPECTIVES

Independent home exercise programs are routinely prescribed by physical therapists as an adjunct to clinical treatment. Research has demonstrated the effectiveness of home exercise programs in the treatment of musculoskeletal conditions with favorable subjective and objective functional outcomes. Adjunct home-based rehabilitation has been shown effective in the treatment of various musculoskeletal conditions including acute ankle sprains, shoulder dysfunction, and chronic low back pain, as well as following total knee arthroplasty, anterior cruciate ligament reconstruction, and arthroscopic partial meniscectomy.[11,12,13,17,18,23,33] In fact, home exercise instruction is a widely accepted practice and considered a critical component in a comprehensive rehabilitation program; *The Guide to Physical Therapy Practice* describes "patient/client-related instruction" as one of three types of interventions that physical therapists provide, in conjunction with the other two interventions, "coordination, communication, and documentation" and "procedural interventions."[2] *The Guide to Physical Therapist Practice* clearly states that home exercise instruction "...should be developed for all patients for whom physical therapy is indicated."[2] Furthermore, the Code of Ethics of the American Physical Therapy Association specifically addresses health promotion and patient education as responsibilities of the physical therapist.[1] Finally, some state practice acts require home exercise prescription be included in a plan of care, specifically stating that physical therapists will provide their patients with a home exercise program.

In the past decade, significant research has been performed examining physical therapy outcomes, which has resulted in the establishment of models aimed at decreasing the number of supervised physical therapy visits. This has created a conflict for physical therapists, a "catch 22" of sorts—organized efforts to utilize home exercise prescription to maximize outcomes have provided insurance companies and other third-party payers the ammunition to support claims that question the medical necessity of many physical therapy services. As physical therapists have attempted to become better at home exercise selection and prescription, it has affected reimbursement. Ultimately, physical therapists should strive to attain recognition as specialists in exercise prescription to create a specialized niche recognized by both medical professionals and the general public alike and described within physical therapists' scope of practice. Until this occurs, the reimbursement-driven uncertainty of managed care will continue to dictate physical therapy plans-of-care, deeming home exercise prescription an inexpensive alternative to supervised physical therapy, rather than a medically necessary adjunct to clinical treatment.

While home exercise prescription is widely utilized and considered an acceptable adjunct to clinical treatment, the reasons behind the use of home exercise programs vary widely. During the 1980s and early 1990s, there was a reimbursement-driven revolution in health care—limitations associated with managed care resulted in drastic reductions in health care benefits. The number of visits patients could attend physical therapy and the reimbursement rates at which providers were paid were significantly limited. As a result, in an attempt to ensure favorable outcomes with fewer supervised therapy sessions, physical therapists were forced to spend a larger portion of their time designing home exercise programs that would supplement clinical treatment.[15] Restricted number of visits and stringent reimbursement remain a part of physical therapy practice today, which continues to affect design and provision of home exercise programs.

PHILOSOPHY OF PATIENT EDUCATION AND EXERCISE PRESCRIPTION

Physical therapists have been, and should continue to be, at the forefront of patient education. Members of various other medical, allied heath, and fitness professions have succeeded in attaining recognition as experts in various specialized areas of care. For example, chiropractors are generally accepted as experts in spinal care, massage therapists as experts in management of soft tissue problems, and personal trainers as experts in fitness. To that end, because of their specialized didactic and clinical training, physical therapists should be recognized as experts in therapeutic exercise prescription and rehabilitation. However, due to the broad-based education provided by most physical therapy curricula encompassing multiple aspects of patient care (cardiopulmonary therapies, integumentary care, musculoskeletal rehabilitation, neuromuscular rehabilitation, etc.), mainstream recognition as experts in therapeutic exercise/rehabilitation has proven to be difficult to attain. Local, state, and national initiatives have focused on educating physicians about the profession of physical therapy rather than concentrating on educating the public, especially prior to physical therapists gaining direct access. In contrast, many of the large prescription drug manufacturers in the United States have demonstrated how patient education initiatives involving direct marketing to the public can be successful; print media and television commercials have aided in increasing brand visibility, name recognition, market share, and ultimately profits.

Physical therapists must shift their efforts from physician-directed education to initiatives directed toward patient education and educating the general public. Many have done so by promoting advanced certifications, specialized training, and/or expertise in physical therapy specialties; however the significance in attaining recognition for expertise in therapeutic exercise prescription is often overlooked. This chapter will serve as a guide and offer insight for practicing clinicians interested in expanding their knowledge of therapeutic exercise prescription and its applications to patient education.

BENEFITS OF HOME EXERCISE PRESCRIPTION

The expected benefits of home exercise prescription include the following[2]:

1. Increased ability to perform a physical task
2. Reduced disability associated with acute or chronic illness/injury
3. Increased functional independence
4. Decreased frequency and intensity of care
5. Decreased level of required supervision for task performance
6. Increased knowledge and awareness of diagnosis, prognosis, interventions, and goals
7. Improved performance levels
8. Improved physical function and health status
9. Reduced risk of recurrence of condition and/or secondary impairments
10. Increased self-management

Many of these expected benefits, when attained, culminate in patient empowerment. The theory of empowerment may perhaps be the most important factor in promoting wellness and ensuring favorable outcomes in rehabilitation from musculoskeletal conditions. Patient empowerment produces a shift in thought, away from therapist dependence to patient participation. The result of such a shift is the establishment of a stronger patient/therapist relationship, which ultimately provides a strengthened foundation to support the physical therapist as a key player in today's ever-changing health care environment. Encouraging patients to become actively involved in treatment and increasing their confidence in performing recommendations may significantly enhance treatment effectiveness.[8] Patients with higher expectations regarding their own outcome tended to be more actively engaged in their own rehabilitation program.[8] In fact, the "Patient Bill of Rights and Responsibilities," a summary of the President's Advisory Commission on Consumer Protection and Quality in the Health Care Industry, encourages patients to be actively involved in their treatment and make informed decisions about their care.[9]

It has been reported that "patients assume two identities" when seeking medical care: "health consumers and active participants in the medical decision making process" (Ref. 26, p. 6). These identities are not mutually exclusive. Because ". . . the right to health must be accompanied by the moral obligation to preserve one's own health . . . ," individual initiatives that promote empowerment should be emphasized, including home exercise programs as an adjunct to clinical rehabilitation.[26] The correlation between patient participation and favorable outcomes is well described. Satisfactory treatment outcomes are dependent on patient consent and cooperation. Because the nature of the profession of physical therapy is one of caring, consent and cooperation should not be difficult to attain. In the case of a patient who has voluntarily sought help and is eager to get better, it is assumed that he/she will have given consent prior to your initial interaction and will be cooperative, enabling the therapist to begin to develop an exercise program.

STRATEGIES FOR DEVELOPING A HOME EXERCISE PROGRAM

Development of a home exercise program is dependent upon two factors: efficiency and efficacy. Efficiency is the production of a desired effect, while efficacy is the capacity to produce a desired effect.

Efficiency relates to the element of time for both the therapist and the patient. *Therapist* efficiency is quantified by the amount of time spent determining the appropriate exercise prescription and instructing the patient in correct performance. *Patient* efficiency is quantified by the amount of time it takes a patient to correctly complete a prescribed program. It has been documented that patients utilizing a videotape method for home exercise instruction, with a therapist available for questions, had self-reported outcomes equal to patients instructed personally by a physical therapist.[27] Favorable outcomes were attained with relatively limited direct patient contact, thereby increasing therapist and patient efficiency.

Efficacy relates to effectiveness. Efficacy is determined by whether or not the desired effects were achieved with the prescribed interventions. The ability of the therapist to be both efficient and effective will result in the creation of an individualized home exercise program in a manner that educates the patient in the least amount of time while still ensuring that a patient performs the prescribed exercises correctly. If so, the result is an empowered, compliant, and satisfied health consumer. A positive correlation exists between information and satisfaction and between satisfaction and compliance. Patients who are encouraged to participate in their own health care are more likely to volunteer information, elicit the best from a practitioner, receive better care, and get better faster with less treatment.[28]

The first step to empowering patients is for the health care provider to become empowered. This paradigm shift is already occurring with the advancements in physical therapy education and postprofessional training as greater numbers of clinicians have been trained in specialized rehabilitation skills and techniques, manual or otherwise, that are routinely utilized in daily clinical practice. As empowered health consumers, patients will undoubtedly perceive value in specialized care administered by a physical therapist during clinical treatment that is unique to that setting; in other words, care that cannot be self-administered or performed in a home exercise program. The authors believe that the employment of specialized skills and techniques during supervised clinical rehabilitation sessions, in conjunction with individualized home exercise prescription, presents the best ap-

proach to rehabilitation of musculoskeletal conditions and represents the true value of physical therapy expertise. Holmes et al. demonstrated that an alternative, graduated treatment model emphasizing a minimal number of office visits and focusing on intensive patient education, home exercise instruction, and specific manual interventions was successful in the management of shoulder dysfunction.[18] The described graduated treatment model included providing a comprehensive program of patient education along with home exercise instruction on the first physical therapy visit. In this report, the patient was empowered to return to his/her prior level of function through compliance to the prescribed treatment regimen. Emphasizing home exercise instruction while ensuring a positive outcome increased both treatment efficiency and efficacy. Although the report described one case, its authors demonstrated that both creating the perception of value in the care a patient received and the specific interventions were effective in eliminating unpleasant symptoms. Both contributed to the result—a satisfied health consumer.

COMPLIANCE AND OUTCOMES

Compliance is traditionally described as how well a patient adheres to a prescribed exercise program or other health-related recommendations.[8] However, the authors of this chapter believe that compliance to a home exercise program must be substantiated by a patient who is not only able to adhere to a prescribed exercise program but also has the ability to demonstrate the exercises with appropriate technique. Empowerment is tantamount in ensuring compliance, while compliance is essential in promoting favorable outcomes. Patients who follow the prescribed treatment program generally have more favorable treatment outcomes.[14] However, noncompliance with physical therapy interventions is common.[7] Compliance was shown to be a limiting factor when Weishaar and colleagues compared the functional outcomes of supervised, clinic-based rehabilitation to unsupervised, home-based rehabilitation in treating male patients with acute ankle sprains.[33] In their study, compliance of the home exercise group was 42 percent, while that of the control supervised group was 56 percent.[33] Although patients are intelligent and well intentioned, it is difficult for anyone to accept a new challenge and stick with it for an extended period of time. To further complicate matters, compliance to a prescribed home exercise program is, at best, difficult to measure. Self-reported compliance is often unreliable. For example, in a patient follow-up, patients asked to rate their actual exercise performance on home programs reported 100 percent compliance.[8] However, when the authors compared what the patients were actually doing to what was there in their records, only 35 percent of patients were determined to be compliant.[8] Likewise, another study demonstrated that subjects' self-perceptions of compliance were far better than actual performance.[16] Genet et al demonstrated that while quantitative compliance with a prescribed home exercise program was considered satisfactory, the effectiveness of the program was limited, explained by a rapid deterioration of qualitative compliance.[11]

FACTORS AFFECTING COMPLIANCE

Health care practitioners must understand reasons for noncompliance if they are to provide supportive care, since compliance is multifactorial. Although physical health variables are considered primary indicators of overall participation in a rehabilitation program, psychological factors have been shown to be the factors that were most important to adherence to a home-based program.[19] Additionally, in a study that in part encouraged patients to describe their experiences and reflect on why they did or did not comply with prescribed physical therapy, Campbell et al. developed a model explaining factors influencing compliance with physical therapy and performance of prescribed home exercises.[7] Results indicated the following[7]:

1. Initial compliance was high because of loyalty to the physical therapist.
2. Reasons for continued compliance involved willingness and ability to accommodate exercises within everyday life, the perceived severity of symptoms, and previous experiences with dysfunction.
3. A necessary precondition for continued compliance was the perception that the physical therapy was effective in reducing unpleasant symptoms.

Prescribing a home exercise program with the expectation that the patient will remain compliant is a challenge faced by many health care practitioners. In essence, the practitioners are attempting to affect behavioral change.[5] Unfortunately, many practitioners believe that simply informing someone of what is good for them will provide the necessary incentive to change their behavior. Realistically however, it is when the perceived benefits outweigh the barriers that the patient will engage in the changed behavior; when the pros associated with performing the exercise program exceed the cons, there is increased likelihood that compliance will be enhanced.[5]

As noted previously, other elements that are related to compliance include environmental factors, physiologic factors, and psychological factors.[22] Environmental factors include sociological and family influences. Physiologic factors include characteristics of the illness or injury. Psychological factors include attitudes toward exercise, levels of confusion, and moods are based on the perceptions of the patient. These behavioral perceptions that impact compliance include perceived susceptibility, severity, benefits, and barriers. It is the combination of many of these factors that manifest in behaviors that range from complete unwillingness to implement an alteration in behavior to total dedication and motivation.

Gaining an understanding of the elements of that factor into behavioral patterns, and therefore affect compliance, is essential when considering home exercise prescription as an adjunct to clinical treatment. Research indicates that reducing or eliminating barriers, clearly conveying personal benefits of compliance, and explaining the relationship between the musculoskeletal condition and the prescribed course of treatment should positively affect compliance.[8,25,29] Ultimately however, the success rate with home exercise programs will be largely dependent upon how the patient perceives his/her condition and the benefits associated with the recommendations provided.[15]

TECHNIQUES FOR IMPLEMENTING A HOME EXERCISE PROGRAM

Therapeutic exercise prescription is both an art and a science. The experienced physical therapist is able to accurately determine the quantity of exercise, including frequency and duration of exercise, as well as the most appropriate method or methods of instruction. Traditionally, clinicians habitually instruct patients in a prescribed "exercise routine" that may include an inappropriate quantity of exercise. For example, it is common practice for patients to be given 10 exercises and instructed to perform 3 sets of 10 repetitions once daily. While this may not seem inappropriate at first, in doing so the therapist has recommended for the patient to perform 450 repetitions per day, an extremely large quantity of exercise. The daunting task for the clinician is to prescribe the exact number of exercises that will enable the patient to reach his/her established short-term goals, promote compliance, and ensure a positive outcome. Prescribing too many exercises will certainly limit compliance, while too few exercises may negatively affect the desired outcome. Results of a recent study indicated that subjects who were prescribed two exercises performed better, as defined by a performance tool score, than subjects who were prescribed eight exercises.[16]

The key to prescribing appropriate home exercise programs lies in proper identification of a patient's functional deficits. Once this has been determined, the goals of home exercise prescription should mirror those of the plan of care. In determining the scope of the home exercise program, the objective functional deficits should be prioritized and home exercises should be prescribed to improve these deficits.

Chapters 6 and 8–11 offer information on identification of and interventions for physiologic impairments that relate to functional deficits. Chapters 7 and 20 offer insights into identification of functional, movement-based deficits. Chapter 21 offers suggestions on functional testing and progressions.

EXERCISE PRESCRIPTION GUIDELINES

There are several guidelines to follow when developing home exercise prescription.

Prescribe One at a Time

As previously described, it is a common mistake for therapists to prescribe a large quantity of exercises on a patient's initial visit and do so very quickly. It is imperative that therapists take the time necessary to instruct in technique and have the patient demonstrate the exercise using the appropriate technique. The significance of this is twofold: it allows the therapist to impart knowledge of the patient's treatment and plan of care as well as provides the opportunity for the patient to begin to take ownership of his/her rehabilitation. Further, taking the necessary time to explain the home exercise program to the patient communicates the importance of the patient's role in his/her own health. There are many ancillary tools that can provide significant support in this process including video and computer-based educational resources.

Keep It Simple

Exercise prescription should emphasize exercises—based on predicted learning styles, comprehension abilities, and fitness level—that can be easily completed with proper technique. Proper technique refers to the patient's ability to demonstrate an exercise without verbal or tactile cueing. If the patient is unsuccessful in properly performing the prescribed exercise, further instruction and/or exercise modification should be utilized to ensure successful performance. Mastery of the prescribed exercise(s) will instill confidence in the patient—confidence both in the patient's ability to perform the exercises and confidence in the therapist's ability to educate and assist the patient in recovery.

Use Professional Materials

Educational materials that are deemed professional, effective, and reliable (or not so) are designated as such quite subjectively. Personal preferences (of the therapist) and availability of resources dictate the methods of instructions and types of materials that are employed in home exercise prescription and other patient education matters. Historically, therapists have given materials that are, by most standards, unprofessional in appearance. The use of stick figures to illustrate exercises, papers that have been photocopied multiple times, often with exercises scratched out and written-over by hand, and illustrations/pictures that demonstrate incorrectly performed exercises are commonplace and should be eliminated completely. In order for patients to understand the significance of home-based exercise, the clinician must use materials that are presentable and easily comprehended. Perception is indeed reality, while the educational materials distributed to patients are a reflection of the therapist's commitment to providing excellent service both inside and outside the clinic.

TECHNOLOGICAL ADVANCES

Although many physical therapists rely primarily on verbal communication with their patients, home exercise prescription instruction is typically accompanied with additional printed materials to assist the patient in exercise performance. This is especially important when a patient has a visual preference for learning; if a visual learner is instructed only using verbal means, success will be limited. Because patients forget a significant amount of what they have been told and to aid in compliance and promote positive outcomes, physical therapists should provide education in as many forms as possible. With technological advances, there are multiple methods to transmit educational materials. Recent technology that utilizes color photos, video demonstration, and Internet transmission is readily available and should be embraced. While the use of technological advances in clinical practice has great appeal, only a tiny fraction of health care providers in the United States utilize an electronic medical record, and relatively few use e-mail and/or the Internet to interact with patients.[6] Although there are a multitude of methods to implement home exercise instruction including videotape, internet-based, and even virtual reality patient instruction, these technological advances are significantly underutilized. It is interesting that this remains the case even though it has been documented that utilizing the latest, cutting-edge technology in patient education and home exercise instruction could provide a way to encourage exercise and treatment compliance and provide safe and motivating therapeutic intervention.[31]

Physical therapists should remain mindful of their patients' comprehension abilities. One problem with a significant amount of written educational materials is that they are frequently written at a level far beyond the average person's comprehension. According to a leading health literacy advocacy group, limited literacy skills are a stronger predictor of an individual's health status than age, income, employment status, education level, or racial/ethnic group.[3] Advances in technology should be utilized to provide home exercise instruction or other educational materials that are appropriate for the patient's comprehension level and promote retention and understanding of the activities being taught.

Physical therapists must keep abreast of ever-changing technology and how to utilize technological advances to improve the delivery of services, including home exercise prescription. Advances in technology have changed the way consumers do business, and the medical professions are no exception. The profession of physical therapy has been impacted significantly. Incorporating technology into daily clinical practice should not be viewed as a burden, rather as a tool to improve the delivery of physical therapy services.

PATIENT EDUCATION MODEL

Utilizing technology as a tool to enhance patient education presents numerous options for clinicians. Factors such as computer availability, Internet accessibility, materials (paper, etc.), and cost have an impact on the methods utilized for exercise prescription and patient education. Factors to consider, with recommendations, are described in the following sections.

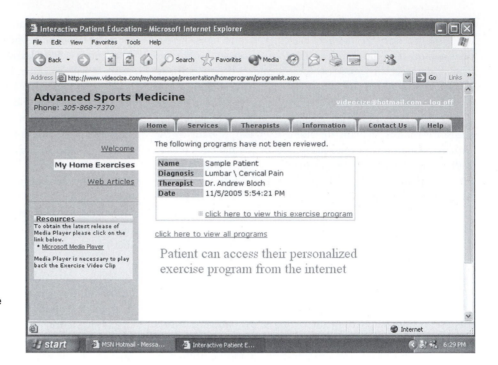

FIGURE 23-1

Example of Internet-based home exercise program. Customized home exercise regimes can include pictures or videos.

Individualized Versus Generic

The proposed model utilizes home exercises to establish and further develop relationships with patients. Most people would prefer to have something that is designed specifically for him/her. Even in instances in which exercise prescriptions are markedly similar, including the patient's name on the material will make an immediate impression and will give the indication that the program was individualized for him/her.

Sketches/Pamphlets Versus Photos

A sketch is widely accepted as an appropriate representation for describing an exercise. However, utilizing photos of individuals

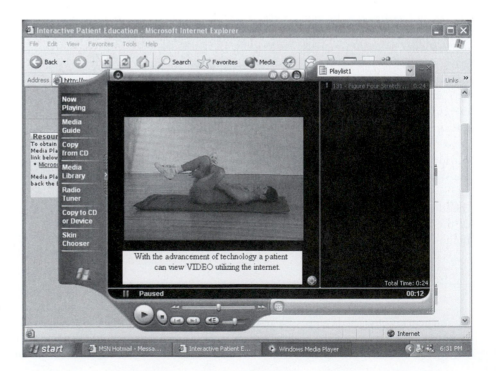

FIGURE 23-2

Example of a computer screen containing what a patient views when watching custom-prescribed exercise videos utilizing the Internet.

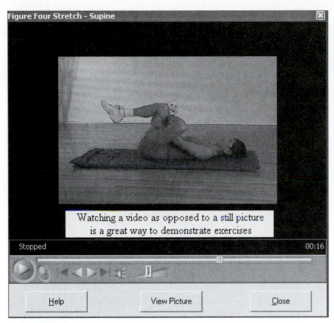

FIGURE 23-3

    Close-up view of still screen image taken from a custom-prescribed video home exercise program.

that are easily recognizable should aid in comprehension and will certainly lend professionalism and credibility to the prescribing clinician.

Color Versus Black and White

While black-and-white depictions are the norm, adding color to any document makes an immediate impact. Although the cost of color documents may certainly be a factor, just as color envelopes have proven successful in direct marketing campaigns, the use of color will create a positive impression that should outweigh the associated costs.

Photos Versus Video

As Internet-based technology and the uses of the Internet continue to evolve, online patient/therapist interaction has evolved. Clinicians now have the ability to e-mail patients their exercise programs, while patients have the ability to view their exercises online and communicate directly with the prescribing clinician. While not all patients have Internet access, this population is certainly the minority. In light of increased Internet accessibility and advances in Internet-based video technology, utilizing state-of-the-art video technology rather than still photos may represent the best choice in home exercise prescription. Figures 23-1 to 23-3 show still-shot video clips.

Standardized Versus Customizable Exercise Programs

Technological advances in software have enabled clinicians to easily edit home exercise programs by taking a photo/video of

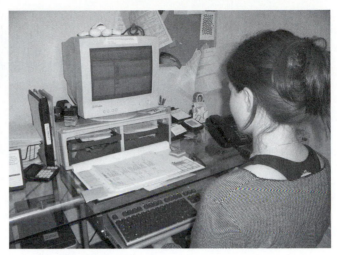

FIGURE 23-4

    Physical therapist creating a custom home exercise program.

a person performing a specific exercise and adding it to the patient's profile. Software manufacturers typically provide this service at no additional cost to customers (Fig. 23-4).

Unmonitored Versus Monitored Compliance

Yet another advantage of technological advances allows patient compliance to be monitored. Clinicians now possess the ability to view whether or not a patient has opened and viewed his/her exercise program. Although compliance is ultimately demonstrated by the patient performing the exercise(s) correctly while supervised, clinicians can better gauge compliance. Additionally, utilization of this feature will demonstrate empathy to the patient, emphasizing the importance of home exercise

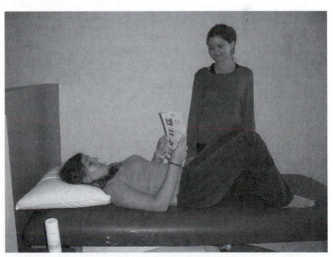

FIGURE 23-5

    Patient referencing color, customized, home exercise program while being instructed in exercises by the physical therapist.

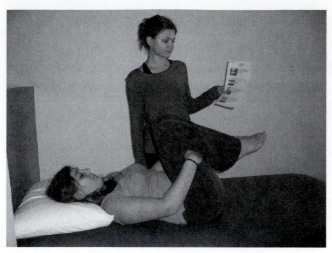

FIGURE 23-6

Physical therapist and patient using custom home exercise program handout for exercise instruction.

performance. This is an important aspect in creating long-term patient/therapist relationships (Figs. 23-5 and 23-6).

SUMMARY

- Therapeutic exercise prescription, particularly in the form of a home exercise program, has become an integral part of any physical therapy plan of care.
- Physical therapists should incorporate state-of-the-art techniques and methods to aid in obtaining recognition as experts in therapeutic exercise prescription and rehabilitation.
- Home exercise prescription will ensure favorable outcomes that will result in enhanced patient compliance and a sense of empowerment.
- Experienced clinicians should utilize the described strategies, techniques, and guidelines for developing and implementing exercise prescription, including the latest technological advances to facilitate patient compliance, demonstrate professionalism, and promote a strong patient/therapist relationship.

REFERENCES

1. American Physical Therapy Association. *Code of Ethics*, HOD 06-00-12-23. Available at www.apta.org. Accessed on September, 2005.
2. American Physical Therapy Association. What types of interventions do physical therapists provide? Guide to physical therapy practice. *Phys Ther* 77(11):1213–1226, 1997.
3. Ask Me 3 Web Site. Available at www.asme3.org. Accessed on September, 2005.
4. Becker MH. Patient adherence to prescribed therapies. *Med Care* 23:539–555, 1985.
5. Blanpied P. Why won't patients do their home exercise programs? *J Orthop Sports Phys Ther* 25:101–102, 1997.
6. Bodenheimer T. Innovations in primary care in the United States. *Br Med J* 326:796–799, 2003.
7. Campbell R, Evans M, Tucker M, et al. Why don't patients do their exercises? Understanding non-compliance with physiotherapy in patients with osteoarthritis of the knee. *J Epidemiol Community Health* 55(2):132–138, 2001.
8. Chen CY, Neufeld PS, Feely CA, Skinner CS. Factors influencing compliance with home exercise programs among patients with upper-extremity impairment. *Am J Occup Ther* 53:171–1780, 1999.
9. Consumer Bill of Rights and Responsibilities. Chapter 4: Participation in Treatment Decisions. President's Advisory Commission on Consumer Protection and Quality in the Health Care Industry. Washington, DC, 1998. Available at www.hcqualitycommission.gov. Accessed on September, 2005.
10. Fischer DA, Tewes DP, Boyd JL, Smith JD, Quick, DC. Home based rehabilitation for anterior cruciate ligament reconstruction. *Clin Orthop Relat Res* 347:194–199, 1998.
11. Genet F, Poiraudeau S, Revel M. Effectiveness and compliance to a center-based short rehabilitation program with a home-based program for chronic low back pain. *Ann Readapt Med Phys* 45(6):265–272, 2002.
12. Goodwin PC, Morrissey MC, Pua Y, et al. Effectiveness of supervised physical therapy in the early period after arthroscopic partial menisectomy. *Phys Ther* 83(6):520–535, 2003.
13. Grant JA, Mohtadi NGH, Maitland ME, Zernicke RF. Comparison of home versus physical therapy-supervised rehabilitation programs after anterior cruciate ligament reconstruction: A randomized clinical trial. *Am J Sports Med* 33(9):1288–1297, 2005.
14. Groth GN, Wilder D, Young VL. The impact of compliance on rehabilitation of mallet finger injuries. *J Hand Ther* 7:21–24, 1994.
15. Halle JS, Thomson BC. Designing home exercise programs. In: Prentice WE, Voight ML, eds. *Techniques in Musculoskeletal Rehabilitation*. New York, McGraw-Hill, 2001, pp. 373–386.
16. Henry KD, Rosemond C, Eckert LB. Effect of number of home exercises on compliance and performance in adults over 65 years of age. *Phys Ther* 79(3):270–277, 1999.
17. Holme E, Magnusson SP, Becher K, et al. The effect of supervised rehabilitation on strength, postural sway, position sense and re-injury risk after acute ankle ligament sprain. *Scand J Med Sci Sports* 9(2):104–109, 1999.
18. Holmes CF, Fletcher JP, Blaschak MJ, Schenck RC. Management of shoulder dysfunction with an alternative model of orthopaedic physical therapy intervention: A case report. *J Orthop Sports Phys Ther* 26(6):347–354, 1997.

19. Jette AM, Rooks D, Lachman M, et al. Home-based resistance training: Predictors of participation and adherence. *Gerontologist* 38(4):412–421, 1998.

20. Kramer JF, Speechley M, Bourne R, Rorabeck C, Vaz M. Comparison of clinic- and home-based rehabilitation programs after total knee arthroplasty. *Clin Orthop* 410:225–234, 2003.

21. Majeed A, Bindman AB. What can primary care in the United States learn from the United Kingdom? Commentary. *Br Med J* 326:799, 2003.

22. Mulder JA. Patient compliance to individualized home exercise programs. *J Fam Pract* 12:991–996, 1981.

23. Oldridge NB. Compliance and exercise in primary and secondary prevention of coronary heart disease: A review. *Prev Med* 11:56–70, 1982.

24. Oldridge NB. Compliance in exercise rehabilitation. *Physianc Sportsmed* 7:95–103, 1979.

25. Prochaska JO, Marcus BH. The transtheroetical model: The applications to exercise. In: Dishman RK, ed. *Advances in Exercise Adherence.* Champaign, IL, Human Kinetics, 1994, pp. 161–180.

26. Rees AM. Communication in the physician-patient relationship. *Bull Med Libr Assoc* 81(1):1–10, 1993.

27. Roddey TS, Olson SL, Gartsman GM, Hanton WP, Cook KF. A randomized controlled trial comparing 2 instructional approaches to home exercise instruction following arthroscopic full-thickness rotator cuff repair surgery. *J Orthop Sports Phys Ther* 32(11):548–559, 2002.

28. Roter DL. Patient participation in the patient-provider interaction: The effect of patient question asking the quality of interaction, satisfaction and compliance. *Health Educ Monogr* 5(4):288, 1977.

29. Samelson TC. Getting information across to patients. *Med Economics* 74:104–108, 1997.

30. Sluijs EM, Kok GJ, van der Zee J. Correlates of exercise: Compliance to physical therapy. *Phys Ther* 73:771–786, 1993.

31. Sveistrup H, McComas J, Thornton M, et al. Experimental studies of virtual reality-delivered compared to conventional exercise programs for rehabilitation. *Cyberpsychol Behav* 6(3):245–29, 2003.

32. Vanderhoff M. Patient education and health literacy. *Phys Ther Magazine* 13(9):42–46, 2005.

33. Weishaar MD, Moore JH. Supervised, clinic-based versus unsupervised, home-based rehabilitation in the treatment of acute grades I and II lateral ankle sprains. Unpublished manuscript, 2005.

34. Wynn KE. Medical College of Ohio: Learning the art of healing through technology. *Phys Ther Magazine* 6:40–44, 1999.

Essentials of Functional Exercise: A Four-Step Clinical Model for Therapeutic Exercise Prescription

Gray Cook and Michael L. Voight

O B J E C T I V E S

After completing this chapter, the therapist should be able to do the following:

- Demonstrate a four-step model designed to promote the practical systematic thinking requisite for the effective therapeutic exercise prescription and progression.

It is widely accepted that therapeutic exercise encompasses a majority of treatment techniques employed in physical medicine. Although many practitioners of physical medicine, such as psychiatrists, chiropractors, and occupational therapists, prescribe or employ physical means to advance and accelerate the rehabilitation process of their patients, the field of physical therapy has always housed a specialized exercise-specific knowledge base. Today's therapist has received instruction and information in general exercise science with emphasis in exercise physiology, kinesiology, and biomechanics. This general knowledge is enhanced by a unique clinical focus on pathologic orthopedic and neurological states and their functional representation. This special focus charges the therapist to consider evaluation of human movement as a complex multisystem interaction and the logical starting point for exercise prescription. Exercise prescription choices must continually represent the specialized training of the therapist through a consistent and centralized focus on human function. Exercise used at the therapeutic level must refine movement, not simply create general exertion with the hope of increased movement tolerance.[4] Moore and Durstine state, "Unfortunately, exercise training to optimize functional capacity has not been well studied in the context of most chronic diseases or disabilities. As a result, many exercise professionals have used clinical experience to develop their own methods for prescribing exercise."[1]

Experience, self-critique, and specialization produce seasoned clinicians with intuitive evaluation abilities and exercise innovations that are sometimes difficult to follow and even harder to ascertain; however, common characteristics do exist.

The clinical expert uses *parallel* (simultaneous) consideration of all factors influencing functional movement. The treatment philosophy is inclusive and adaptable with the ability to address a variety of clinical situations. There is also an understanding that a clinical philosophy is designed to serve, not to be served. The treatment design demonstrates specific attention to the parts (clinical measurements and isolated details) with continual consideration of the whole (restoration of function).[4] Moore and Durstine follow their previous statement by acknowledging that "experience is an acceptable way to guide exercise management, but a systematic approach would be better."[1]

The purpose of this chapter is to demonstrate a four-step model designed to promote the practical systematic thinking requisite for effective therapeutic exercise prescription and progression.[4] The approach will be a *serial* (consecutive) step-by-step method that will, with practice and experience, lead to *parallel* thinking and multilevel problem solving. The intended purpose of this method is to reduce arbitrary trial-and-error exercise attempts and protocol-based thinking. It will give the novice clinician a framework that will guide but not confine clinical exercise prescription. It will provide experienced therapists with a system to observe their particular strengths and weaknesses with respect to exercise dosage and design. Inexperienced and experienced therapists alike will develop practical insight by applying the model and observing the interaction of the systems that produce human movement. The focus is specifically geared to orthopedic physical therapy and the clinical problem-solving strategies used to develop an exercise prescription through an outcome-based, goal-setting process.

All considerations for therapeutic exercise prescription will regard conventional orthopedic exercise standards (biomechanical and physiologic parameters) as well as neurophysiologic strategies (motor learning, proprioceptive feedback, and synergistic recruitment principles) with equal importance. This model will create a mechanism that will necessitate interaction between orthopedic exercise approaches and optimal neurophysiologic techniques. The four-step progression will demonstrate the hierarchy and interaction of the founding principles used in physical therapy (both orthopedic and neurological). For all practical purposes, these four categories help demonstrate efficient and effective continuity necessary in formulation of treatment plan and prompt the therapist to maintain an inclusive open-minded clinical approach.

This chapter is written with the clinic-based practicing therapist in mind. It will help the therapist formulate a clinical exercise philosophy. Some clinicians will discover reasons for success that were intuitive and therefore hard to communicate to other professionals. Others will discover a missing step in the therapeutic exercise-design process. Much of the confusion and frustration encountered by the modern therapist is due to the vast opportunities and treatment options afforded by ever-improving technology and information accessibility. To effectively use the wealth of information the future has yet to bestow, the therapist must adopt an operational framework or personal philosophy regarding therapeutic exercise. If clinical exercise philosophy is based on technology, equipment, or protocols, the scope of problem solving is strictly confined. It will have to continually change, because it has no universal standard or gauge. However, a philosophy based solely on the structure and function of the human body will keep the focus (function) uncorrupted and centralized. Technological developments can only enhance exercise effectiveness as long as the technology, system, or protocol remains true to a holistic functional standard.

The following four principles for exercise prescription are based on human movement and the systems upon which it is constructed. The intention of these four distinct categories is to break down and reconstruct the factors that influence functional movement and to stimulate inductive reasoning, deductive reasoning, and the critical thinking needed to develop a therapeutic exercise progression. Hopefully, these factors will serve the intended purpose of organization and clarity, thereby giving due respect to the many insightful clinicians who have provided the foundation and substance for the construction of this practical framework.[4]

The four principle considerations for therapeutic exercise prescription are the following:

1. Functional evaluation and assessment of conditions of dysfunction (disability) and impairment.
2. Identification and management of motor control.
3. Identification and management of osteokinematic and arthrokinematic limitations.

4. Identification of current movement patterns followed by facilitation and integration of synergistic movement patterns.

FUNCTIONAL EVALUATION, ASSESSMENT, AND DIAGNOSIS

Successful medical intervention is the result of some sort of evaluation or assessment. Physical therapy intervention through exercise prescription is no different. The physical therapy evaluation is the starting point of all exercise recommendations. Saunders states, "Because many different tests, measurements, and sequences for collecting the required data are available, the format chosen largely depends on individual preference. However, a methodical and complete examination is essential."[10] Although each clinician has his/her own individual evaluation style, all must generate the necessary baseline information to proceed with effective treatment choices. Therefore, although one must adhere to a specific evaluation method for personal reliability, that method must provide all the necessary information without a collection or interpretation bias. Clinicians must continually *evaluate* their *evaluations*, because habitual testing and treatment preferences can move the therapist over the line from clinical individuality to personal subjectivity. The functional evaluation is unique in that the primary concern is not signs, symptoms, or structures, as with most medical assessments. In the past, the focus on measuring and altering impairments superceded the more important goals of improving function and reducing disability. A more current emphasis is not on using therapeutic exercise to alter the list of impairments, but rather to use the interventions to improve function and reduce disability that is meaningful to the individual seeking rehabilitation. This type of evaluation process results in a pathomechanical and or pathoanatomic determination of the problem.

The purpose of the functional evaluation is to identify the current level of function. Consider all the possible reasons for that level of function and then decide how function can be positively influenced through intervention. Impairments are isolated movement limitations or abnormalities that can be measured by clinical means. Functional limitations represent a restriction in performance of basic tasks. Instead of considering which exercise can be prescribed to improve an impairment, the rehabilitation provider should consider which impairments are related to reduce function for this patient and which exercises can enhance function by addressing the appropriate impairments. Liebenson states,

> In the majority of soft tissue injuries, functional changes are the only objective findings on which to base treatment and judge progress. Unfortunately, most orthopedic examinations rely on tests that search for structural lesions. Although structural lesions are present in only about 20% of cases, overuse of expensive diagnostic tests is typical in

the search to diagnose such structural pathology. The remaining 80% have no identifiable structural pathologic abnormality and require treatment based on the evaluation of functional deficits.[14]

A brief discussion of the information generated through the evaluation process will negate assimilation errors at this vital stage of the rehabilitation process. As with any treatment, therapeutic exercise prescription must be constructed on a solid and objective evaluation base. The evaluation is not simply the automatic result of collected information but rather careful deliberation upon that information. The information is most effectively managed in definable categories. The categories will give significance and hierarchy to information and help create a uniform direction toward attainment of functional goals through outcome-based exercise treatments. A brief discussion of the categories will demonstrate how clear lines between information groups support organized patient management and objective treatment choices. The goal-setting process is a result of the evaluation, which should encompass both medical and functional information. The primary goal of physical therapy intervention is first to evaluate and then generate a plan of care that restores functional homeostasis. Therefore, we must review and outline the evaluation process before further discussion of exercise. The role of the evaluation in exercise prescription can be better clarified by first defining the roles of the medical evaluation and diagnosis for orthopedic and musculoskeletal conditions compared to the functional diagnosis of the same.[4]

Disablement: The Medical Diagnosis

The medical evaluation and diagnosis is generated by the physician and places the patient in a diagnostic group or category that correlates the anatomic structures, standardized testing procedures, pharmacology, surgery, and so forth. The medical diagnosis along with a medical history usually results in the use of medications or surgery. The medical diagnosis will help the therapist determine *contraindications* affecting therapeutic exercise choices. The "functional diagnosis" is the term that names the primary dysfunction toward which the rehabilitation provider directs treatment. In the rehabilitation model, the therapist examines patients with impairments, functional limitations, and disabilities to determine diagnosis, prognosis, and intervention. If the distinction between the medical and rehabilitation diagnosis is not clear, the process of effective and efficient exercise prescription is not possible. The medical diagnosis does not dictate the type of exercise intervention; it only limits certain types of movement, stress, or physical exertion because of a surgical protocol or anatomic or cellular condition. Because the medical diagnosis is based on physical signs and symptoms and not "functional movement," it cannot provide insight as to specific therapeutic exercise choices. Patients who fall within the same diagnostic categories present a variety of functional movement abilities. This makes it impossible to develop an individualized

therapeutic exercise protocol based solely on a medical diagnosis. Of course, medical diagnostic protocols for exercise do exist, but they are usually generalized and not representative of the full potential of modern rehabilitation.

Two main problems are the following:

1. The medical diagnosis is geared toward a specific biomechanical, physiologic, or anatomic abnormality, not a specific function or movement pattern.
2. Medical "diagnostic" exercise protocols are usually time-based, not function-based. For example, many postsurgical protocols set a time line from the surgical date with recommended exercises based on the days and weeks from the surgical procedure.

This does not challenge the postsurgical exercise protocol. These protocols are based on normative standards designed to help, not hinder. Moreover, it is the sole right of the surgeon to recommend a specific exercise course, but once again it is to limit postsurgical stress and reinforce contraindications. It is the therapist's role to work within the confines of that protocol as long as it does not interfere with efficient and effective treatment. Scientifically based innovation and clinical creativity is usually a welcome addition to most standard protocols whether for consideration of an individual requiring isolated protocol modification or for grounds to challenge the protocol. The therapist and surgeon working together is the only conceivable solution. It is usually a surgeon therapist team that sets postsurgical rehabilitation standards and creates the inventiveness behind continual evolution of most modern postsurgical exercise protocols. Dr. Jerome Ciullo states, "Surgery can correct the original problem but the muscles are still out of balance, so in most cases it is not the surgery that cures you. It is the surgery that allows you to go back to your exercise program."[9] Therefore, a medical diagnosis alone cannot create or determine a therapeutic exercise treatment plan—it can only, at best, limit the available options. From this, the therapist will define impairments or abnormalities at the tissue, organ, or body system level. This will help establish the specific causes of the limitation or dysfunction prior to intervention.[4]

Disablement: The Functional Diagnosis

Functional assessment is obviously required to create a functional diagnosis. It is not simply the reproduction, observation, and appraisal of daily life skills, occupational duties, or sports activities, but a perceptive understanding of the basic movements upon which they are constructed. The word "function" has grown in popularity over the last decade without enjoying the same degree of success with respect to professional clarification or practical understanding. The word implies natural, practical, and purposeful movement, but it has also been used to describe exercise methods at a far greater frequency than evaluation methods. This creates a perplexing question. Most medical treatment is based on and defined by the effect it produces on a particular physical parameter (either chemical or mechanical). The effect can only be measured if an evaluation produces a baseline appraisal of that parameter followed by a reappraisal upon cessation of a treatment cycle. Without a central functional evaluation model, the therapist has no standard or universal functional parameter with which to measure the effectiveness of one particular exercise versus another. The common but sad assumption is that if an exercise replicates a specific task or activity, then that exercise by default is functional.

A better way to define functional exercise is by documenting its positive effects on a functional outcome. This refers to the "functional influence" of an exercise as opposed to its observable similarity to a functional activity. When a functional problem is identified, the therapist does not simply recommend that the activity be repeated by manipulating the parameters of frequency, intensity, and duration. This simple approach may change quantitative measures but will rarely improve qualitative measures "since the body will usually sacrifice movement quality for movement quantity."[5,22] The therapist must break down the functional movement into its fundamental submovements. These submovements, like functional movements, are still multisegmental whole-body movements, but because they are simple and distinguished they are more specific to problem identification. They are distinguished by the particular way each represents a level of motor control as well as the normal developmental parameters needed for acquisition of skill. Skill defined by Sullivan et al., in reference to early motor development, is the "highest level of motor control" that "includes two functions: the manipulation and exploration of the environment."[20]

This broad and general description is then more specifically described as those activities where the distal components (the hands and feet) are mobile as the proximal musculature and joints, as well as the musculature of the spine, remain dynamically stable.[20] For the purposes of this model, the aforementioned definition of skill will be considered *general skill*, because it can be considered a common or basic function of most adult orthopedic patients. The definition becomes more specific when applied to individual adult movement patterns. The many demands of sedentary (static postural demands) and laborious jobs (dynamic physical exertion), as well as the vast array of movement specificity needed for sports and hobbies, should be referred to as *specific skill*. All skillful movement is built on a foundation of *fundamental* movements. This foundation can be simply described by cornerstones called mobility and stability and central pillars called controlled mobility and/or dynamic stability (Fig. 24-1).

The model is constructed to demonstrate the absolute dependence of specific complex movement on its fundamental constituents. Subtle changes in mobility and stability can tilt the entire movement structure.[4] The clinician can assume that functional limitation at a fundamental level is the endowment of the next level. The body and mind, however, are designed to compensate and will absorb the limitation through compensation and substitution. This necessitates the need to return to the most basic level where the limitation remains observable. This may or may not correspond to the level where the limitation first occurred. It also demonstrates that the determinants (mobility, stability, and dynamic stability) of skillful function viewed in isolation sometimes do not appear functional; nevertheless, they are the only unforced paths to restoration of true function. Evaluation and exercise prescription should always consider these as the natural course to skill development and function, as they replicate the normal course of physical development and, more importantly, the primary process of motor learning. "Since normal motor control is acquired during the developmental sequence, when motor control is adversely affected, a recapitulation of the sequence may be the most effective means of reestablishing control."[20]

Functional assessment can be defined as the identification of limitations concerning movement generation or movement control by a deductive process employing both qualitative and quantitative measurements. The ability to test both movement quality and quantity will greatly improve exercise prescription effectiveness. This process involves breaking down the functional movement into the submovements or fundamental movements so the stages of motor control can be viewed and evaluated. This also lends itself nicely to systematic exercise program design. "A functional progression for return to activity can be developed by breaking specific activities down into a hierarchy and then performing them in a sequence that allows for acquisition or reacquisition of skill."[22] Normative data are an essential component to assessment. Developmental specialists have mapped the path to normal motor control, which gives us insight as to the initial sequence of movement abilities and motor learning. "The four major stages of motor control are mobility, stability, controlled mobility and skill."[20] This sequence is helpful and often employed in treatment, but the clinician must also consider available data on normative levels of adult skill or function needed for prognosis and goal setting.

Unfortunately, very little normative data has been gathered on adult populations with specific focus on functional movement *quality*. Quantitative measurements and performance data are helpful, but these data must be balanced and preceded by a quality standard to truly understand and affect (through feedback and treatment) human movement.[11] This is not a new observation. One of the many examples stating a need for more normative quality-based data was by Richter et al. in a 1989 physical therapy journal article.[18] The article dealt with rolling movements in normal adults and attempted to describe normal rolling variance and observe if the rolling represented different developmental steps demonstrated in the use of body segments. The authors stated,

> Physical therapy for patients with neurologic dysfunction often includes the evaluation and teaching of rolling movements. To determine the quality of the rolling pattern, rolling movements must be evaluated against some standard or norm. To date, no reported research exists describing the movement patterns that adults use to roll. Although specific rolling movements have been recommended

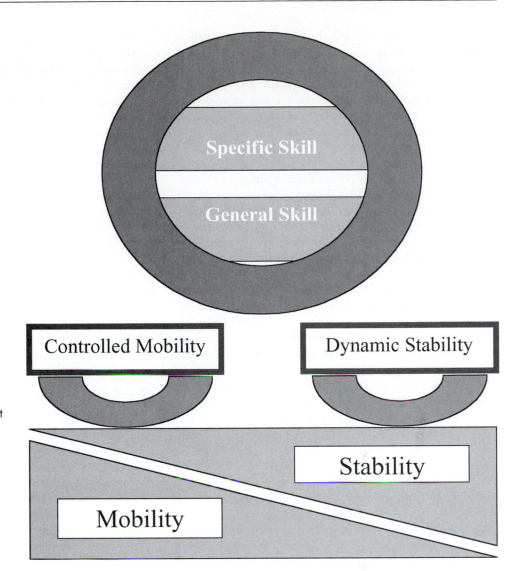

All skillful movement is built on a foundation of *fundamental* movements. This foundation can be simply described by cornerstones called mobility and stability and central pillars called controlled mobility and/or dynamic stability.

for use in treatment, whether these movements are valid representations of healthy individuals' movements is unknown.[18]

Likewise, orthopedic patients are given functional exercises that profess to replicate normal movements, but very few normative quality standards are used. One simple reason for limited qualitative norms, as compared to quantitative norms, may be the problem with data collection. Quantitative norms are easy to obtain once the tester's reliability with a measuring device is achieved. Qualitative norms require much more from the test design and tester. However, with adequate training, high levels of reliability can be achieved.[8,18]

The key to qualitative testing for both clinical and normative research data collection is the practical and employable description of movement. The way a movement is described will determine the amount of quality assigned to that particular movement. The rolling article stated, "If less than 85% of exact agreement was obtained within a body region, we re-

fined the movement pattern description to resolve any possible ambiguities."[18] The functional movement screen (FMS) is an attempt at normative data collection in a healthy physically active population with respect to movement quality. It was designed to set normative standards for specific and general physically active populations in an attempt to monitor movement factors influencing performance and injury factors. It was also specifically designed to detect those movement problems that are not detected in the preparticipation (medical) physical movement by specifically observing functional movement extremes and predictable limitations. Finally, it provides a functional baseline in the event of an injury.[8] The Berg balance measure (BBM) is another excellent example of a qualitative test. Although the FMS and BBM are geared for two different populations, they note the detail of movement description. Distinct lines are drawn between the ability to demonstrate various levels of control.

Whether the physical therapist uses standardized functional testing or creates a new or hybrid test, it is important to understand the need for and contribution of both qualitative and quantitative functional measures. At present, bilateral comparison is a temporary solution for physical therapists who want to employ functional movement patterns for evaluative purposes but are reluctant because of the lack of normative data. Many functional movements and their submovements can be compared in this manner. Consider bilateral qualitative comparison of rolling, single-leg stance, or any fundamental or functional activity that has a right–left component.

The next division of information comes within the physical therapy evaluation itself. This division is between functional evaluation and specific clinical measurements. This will also help to separate and define impairment, functional limitation, and disability. *Impairment* refers to a loss or abnormality at the tissue, organ, or body system level. Functional limitations are restrictions of the ability to perform a physical action, activity, or task in an efficient, typically expected, or competent manner. In contrast, *disability* refers to the inability to perform tasks and activities usually expected in specific social roles that are customary for the individual or expected for one's status or role in the environment. Not all impairments or functional limitations result in disability. It is possible for two individuals with the same disease and similar levels of impairment and functional limitation to have two different levels of disability. One person may remain active in all aspects of life, while the other individual may choose to limit social contact, depend on others for care, and to have a job where it is not possible to use adaptive methods to participate in work tasks.

Through functional assessment, the therapist will recognize and classify impairments, functional limitations, and disability using clinical measurements in an attempt to demonstrate the underlying causes by qualifying and quantifying the impairments. The observation of functional movement should, in most cases, precede clinical measurements, and qualitative testing should precede quantitative measurements. Qualitative assessment can establish a desired level of competence or ability, at which time quantitative assessment will allow comparison bilaterally or with norms and other individuals. Qualitative assessment is particularly useful as a formative evaluation because it helps create instructional experiences and feedback, according to Haywood in her text on *Life Span Motor Development*.[11] This improves the deductive component of movement problem solving, thereby directing the focus on whole movement patterns to consider issues such as synergistic movement, compensatory movement, coordination and balance reactions, and daily activities. Functional movements should usually be described in both qualitative and quantitative terms when possible, whereas clinical measurement is usually reported in the form of quantitative documentation. The observation of mass or whole movements can sometimes redirect and broaden the clinical focus by revealing limitations unrelated to the medical diagnosis but still necessary for improvement or restoration of normal function (Fig. 24-2).[4]

Consider the multiple reasons for the differences in the squatting abilities of these subjects. The knee and ankle range of motion is different to some extent. The sum of their limitation or impairment, however, does not account for gross difference in squat function. It is also possible to have no significant differences in hip, knee, and ankle active range of motion between subjects and still have significantly altered squatting ability. One simple explanation is not lower-quarter mobility but trunk dynamic stability. Secondly, timing, coordination, weight shifting, and balance can determine the ability of multiple joint segments to work together in a functional pattern. A structural or functional asymmetry between limbs can stop a symmetrical pattern altogether instead causing the obvious and predictable weight shift or asymmetrical response, which is expected more often. The squat may not be functional for some lifestyles but it is fundamental to all general and specific skill, because it is a transitional posture and an excellent demonstration of dynamic stability. It is up to the therapists to determine what can be learned from a limitation at this level. Therefore, when possible, a functional or fundamental movement pattern should precede the clinical measurement. Functional and fundamental movement qualitative assessment is the obvious starting point in the deductive reasoning and problem-solving process.

Clinical Measurements

Clinical measurements now use special equipment and/or special test formats to help explain underlying causative factors of dysfunction with greater accuracy than ever before. Balance assessment tools, range-of-motion testing, pain scale testing, and dynamometer-assisted muscle testing may be chosen because of initial qualitative observations by the therapist. The therapist will then use a means of more specific measurement for quantitative testing regarded as reliable and objective. With time, technology will continue to advance the practice of physical therapy. Improvements in clinical measurement and data collection have increased the specificity and convenience of isolated testing. It should not, however, influence the problem-solving process used by the clinician to develop a therapeutic exercise program.

Technological advances will continue to allow the clinician to improve clinical testing and objective data collection. However, the enhanced ability to collect a single piece of data should not change the weight or significance of that data; it should only provide increased sensitivity and objectivity with the same level of importance. This type of mistake is often not intentional but nevertheless a hindrance to problem solving. When one single measurement is favored, the exercise program may be specifically geared toward improving that isolated measure. As the favored measure improves, another equally important parameter may become unmasked, cease to improve, or even decline. A good example of this problem was the introduction of isokinetics. Isokinetics demonstrated a significant advancement in clinical measurement of muscle performance, thereby enabling the therapist to generate data with greater specificity regarding isolated muscle group testing. In addition, this technology also served to improve communication with physicians because the

Subject 1

Clinical measurements of hip flexion do not correlate with hip flexion in functional movement. Unloaded open chain assessment of active and passive range of motion using a goniometer is not representative of the functional movement utilized in squatting.

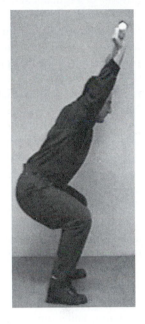

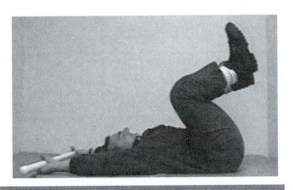

Subject 2

Clinical measurements of hip flexion seem to correlate with hip flexion in functional movement. Unloaded open chain assessment of active and passive hip using a goniometer is representative of the functional movement of squatting.

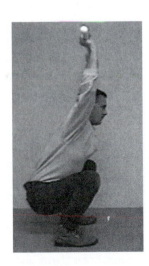

FIGURE 24-2

Unloaded versus loaded lower-extremity active range of motion demonstrated through deep squatting with arms elevated.

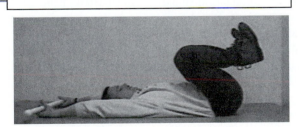

charts and graphs resembled familiar lab results. Objectivity, reliability, and convenience served to confirm the popularity of isokinetics. However, the simple fact remains that it is only one tool for a clinical measurement of a single parameter or impairment. Isolated strength testing does not have the ability to measure function or independently generate a functional diagnosis. This popular clinical measurement tool may have changed the magnitude of muscle testing and given it greater clinical significance than other equally important forms of testing. This is in part due to the fact that manual joint assessment, muscle length testing, postural analysis, trigger point observation, balance and proprioception testing, and other tests lacked the flash and cold reliability of the dynamometer. Because of this, isolated muscle testing may have been weighted with greater significance than other isolated clinical measurements. This error should have been evident long before the research stated, "current literature suggests that a poor correlation exists between the performance of an open kinetic chain strength test and the ability of an individual to perform weight-bearing activities."[16] The lesson is that when greater objectivity is gained on one level (a simple clinical measurement of impairment), it is sometimes lost at a much higher level (functional movement assessment for the purpose of a functional diagnosis).

The last point to be made concerning clinical measurement is the application of two fundamental principles of orthopedic medicine. The first is bilateral comparison, which needs no explanation but should be applied to both structure and function in all cases when possible. Although the information is highly individualized, it is invaluable to the problem-solving process. Nationally published norms and standards are informative, but individualized clinical treatment requires specific attention to a single system. The second principle is just as simple and obvious but often forgotten. It is the complete assessment and clearing of the joints and muscular structures above and below the area in question. Any dysfunction or limitation can greatly influence the rehabilitation process. The clinician may not have control over these limitations but nevertheless needs to be aware of the factors that can potentially limit outcomes. In most cases the proximal and distal joints should also be compared bilaterally as well.

The systematic application of clinical measurements complements the problem-solving process needed for functional evaluation and diagnosis and effective exercise prescription. The previous information may seem oversimplified, but breakdowns of information will improve clinical self-analysis. Most clinicians will agree with this process but may not adhere to it in all clinical situations. Routine case review with these ideas in mind will only improve problem-solving skills.

Pain and Subjective Complaint

Although pain and subjective complaint are significant considerations in exercise prescription, they were intentionally placed after objective functional assessment and clinical measurements (with the exception of the mention of objective pain scale measurement). Subjective complaints are identified while taking the patient's history as well as during functional assessment and clinical measurements. Physical therapists are as close to the subjective complaints of the patient as a health care professional can get. This close proximity can often distort the functional picture. Subjective and objective information must be weighted separately for clarity and precision during the evaluation purposes. The separation will allow comparison and correlation of information and allow the therapist to observe the interaction of pain and function. It is seldom possible to observe a continuous linear relationship between pain and function. The lack of this linear relationship neither automatically indicates magnification or malingering behavior, nor suggests denial of symptoms. Physical therapy is unique in that patients do not just passively discuss their pain and symptoms—they actively confront these problems through movement with supervision and guidance

supported by education. When function is discussed with the patient, the therapist must consider which activities and positions directly affect symptoms and which ones produce some degree of fear or apprehension reported as symptoms. Fear, apprehension, and pain are all strong influences on both temporary and long-term function, and should never be discounted.[3,12] Practical explanations and analogies, along with demonstrations, can usually minimize the effect of this common response.

Liebenson emphasizes, "During functional testing, the effects of movement and position on the behavior of pain, the painful or pain-free range, and the effects of repeated testing should be determined. Sensitivity to various movements and positions, along with any weight-bearing intolerance, should also be determined."[14] However, it is the relationship and interaction of function and symptoms, and not simply the degree of symptomatic response to movement, that should dictate exercise choices. "If the clinician is unable to correlate or match the findings in the various test positions, then the source of the syndrome may be non-mechanical."[17] This could simply implicate acute or subacute chemical irritation or a more involved behavioral or perceptual problem. In chronic cases, if no observable correlation in pain and function can be established, the patient and referral source must be made aware of special circumstances because the scope of physical therapy treatment no longer has a functional or objective goal outside of symptom management.

Finally, therapeutic exercise, like most forms of manual therapy, should not produce pain (unless special circumstances are present and have been discussed with all involved, such as burns). A reproduction of pain, especially during exercise, goes against the natural instincts of human movement as well as the patient's common sense. Those who discuss pain and gain in the same sentence (usually in a fitness setting) are obviously only concerned with exercise quantities, not exercise quality (which is not possible in the presence of pain). Posture, muscle tone, synergistic movements, agonist/antagonist relationships, proprioception, motor learning, and numerous other functional movement determinants are affected when unnecessary and avoidable pain enters the picture. A thorough functional orthopedic physical therapy evaluation will often provoke symptoms (to some degree) to outline both chemical and mechanical irritability of structures. According to Porterfield and DeRosa, "Two of the main goals of the functional assessment are reproducing the pain syndrome with applied stresses, and having the clinician and patient mutually understand the pain pattern".[17] Exercise prescription can then be implemented in such a way as to not provoke symptoms. A review of the principles of chemical and mechanical pain will assist the therapist in the formulation of a ratio of rest/exercise that will best suit the state of the tissue and the attitude of the patient during each stage of recovery. Because of this fact, exercise focus usually takes on one of two general paths, to restore or improve tissue metabolism or to stimulate mechanical efficiency and motor control. It is important to clearly choose one path or the other initially and assess the response and adaptation behavior accordingly.

EVOLUTION OF A CLINICAL EXERCISE PHILOSOPHY

Technological advances will refine objective data, but they will not change the inherent systematic reasoning needed for clinical practice. A comprehensive functional evaluation philosophy will help reduce confusion created by differing physical therapy evaluation and exercise methods. The variety of techniques available to the modern physical therapist in some ways has reduced cohesion and communication in the profession as a whole. Many debates have resulted between therapists because of differing views about exercise treatments. These debates cannot be truly settled until a central evaluation based on functional outcomes is used as a universal standard. A review of the current literature reveals two distinct problems, both relating to functional movement. The following two examples will discuss range of motion and flexibility as a simple example and use cases for debate and consideration.

Examples

EXAMPLE ONE: THE LACK OF NORMATIVE FUNCTIONAL DATA

First, there is a profound lack of normative data regarding functional movement quality. This lack of normal data can possibly allow clinicians to make assumptions about populations based on a small clinical sample or personal experience. The two most common assumptions regarding function concern age and medical diagnosis. Any assumption about a functional limitation without complete qualitative and quantitative evaluation of that limitation will greatly inhibit the ability of the therapist to effectively consider all available exercise options.

First Assumption

"Direct correlation exists between age and function." It is not uncommon to presume that a direct linear correlation is present between age and functional movement. However, research suggests that activity and lifestyle are significant considerations and may play an equal if not greater role than simply considering chronological age.[1,3,11,12] Most geriatric physical therapists do not consider deep squatting (heels flat, thighs below parallel) beneficial or necessary in the treatment of the elderly orthopedic patient. This assumption over time, however, may lead to the notion that deep squatting beyond a certain age is not even possible. Just because deep squatting is not practical does not automatically indicate that it is not possible. The excessive motion of deep squatting may very well be contraindicated for many orthopedic conditions. Nevertheless, it is a fundamental step in the developmental progression and a precursor to ambulation. It is a transitional movement that demonstrates dynamic stability. Dynamic stability precedes ambulation, which is considered a skill. The developmental progression of postures and transitions should be considered on an individual basis and deleted through selective program design and not through age-related functional

assumptions. This will maintain an unprejudiced and flexible exercise philosophy based solely on individual function. An enlightening trip abroad will reveal that deep squatting is often preferred to sitting for both work and recreation by young and old alike. Therefore, lack of deep squatting in all likelihood may be cultural and activity-based and not simply a result of age. Researchers indicate that "the greatest losses (in flexibility) occurred in movements an individual does not habitually perform" and "inactivity is certainly a major factor that may contribute to flexibility decline in old age." Most of these changes are reversible.[11]

Second Assumption

"Diagnosis correlates directly with function." Patients (as well as some medical professionals) usually view the common diagnosis of osteoarthritis as the cause, and not the result, of poor movement patterns. Functional abilities cannot be predicted with any degree of accuracy by only considering structural changes. The clinician cannot assume in cases of nontraumatic arthritis that structural changes preceded functional changes. Consider the words of two physicians on this often oversimplified clinical matter. Janda observes the profound effect of compromised movement relative to an irritant (such as a common sprain or strain) when he states that "joint pain is not a local problem, but affects the entire motor system. Impaired relations within the motor system outlast the elimination of the painful cause."[12] Therefore,

> impairment of central motor control results in defective or uneconomical movement patterns which is one of the main causes of joint dysfunction. Poor movement patterns appear in conjunction with joint dysfunction and alter pressure on joints, therefore leading to further overstrain. Chronic or severe pain may lead to fixation of certain "pain-motor" patterns. Movement patterns can change due to altered CNS function from stress, anxiety, depression or fatigue.[12]

Cailliet makes a similar point when he discusses that "normal use and normal movement place no stress upon soft tissues. Excessive use, abuse, and misuse can cause irritation with resultant pain and disability. Once the neuromuscular pattern is altered, the normal biomechanics of the part is altered and the soft tissue is abused and damaged."[3]

EXAMPLE TWO: QUESTIONABLE VALIDITY OF CURRENT NORMATIVE FUNCTIONAL DATA

The second problem questions the current database available for use. Tests are carried out in the name of function, creating implications that can be prejudiced or incorrect.

Flexibility

Researchers will place individuals in a functional category of either flexible or inflexible based on a single test such as the sit and reach. This test is not representative of an individual's total movement patterns and even less representative of realistic practical movement.[2] When discussing functional categories such as individuals grouped as flexible or inflexible, many factors need to be considered. Significant differences in static and dynamic flexibility, as well as differences in loaded compared to unloaded movements, must be considered.

Stress or Efficiency Testing

Some cardiovascular function tests are conducted without any appropriate *qualitative* biomechanical screen. Posing a question to the validity of the test: Is poor biomechanical efficiency or cardiovascular capacity the major limiting factor of the test? The test does in fact measure physical output, endurance, and work, but if a limitation is detected, it is not qualified because all the parameters affecting efficient movement are not addressed. If a defect or poor score is demonstrated, the tester may automatically assume that the problem is cardiovascular and therefore may prescribe the associated exercise regimen. If, however, the deficit is simply poor biomechanics with a significant loss of movement efficiency, then the major limiting factor of the test has gone unnoticed. A significant improvement in test results could be demonstrated by simply resolving the limiting biomechanical component. This would improve mechanical efficiency and economy, which may change the stress factors on the cardiorespiratory system. Normative data concerning cardiovascular output can possibly be skewed by the unintentional detection of musculoskeletal mechanical dysfunction in the attempt to identify metabolic dysfunction. Brown reminds us that "anatomical changes in the heart (atrophy, lipofuscin accumulation, increased fat and connective tissue) do occur with age but they do not explain the declines in function that have been observed."[1] When testing, one must consider the relationship of cardiac output measured and the work or power produced. This relationship demonstrates efficiency. *Work* is defined as force × distance and, *power* is defined as force × distance/time.[2] Therefore, force and distance are important factors in determining efficiency, necessitating the qualitative and quantitative measurement of those structures producing force (muscles) and allowing distance (joints and connective tissue) prior to the calculation and determination of efficiency problems.

Balance Testing

The popular topic of balance testing in the elderly may need to consider that when range of motion is not optimal, proprioception cannot be optional. Simple restrictions in joint mobility can cause alternative balance strategies and compensations. Often researchers will define functional parameters for the system they are currently studying without full consideration of the functional status of other systems or the comprehensive interaction of multiple systems, which can magnify a small problem in one system.

Four Considerations for Clinical Exercise Philosopy

(1) Some of the greatest advancements in the physical therapy profession have first developed more appropriate evaluations

that eventually led to superior treatment options. A brief historical perspective of orthopedic physical therapy will demonstrate the contributions of James Cyriax and Florence Kendall.[7,13] Both greatly advanced the quality of the physical therapy evaluation process. Their work is so ingrained in the profession that most forms of muscle or joint assessment owe some common trait to their early observations. The Kendalls demonstrated how, through postural assessment and specialized manual muscle testing, a more specific evaluation and exercise prescription could be generated. Cyriax, an orthopedic physician, helped devise a basic methodology for differentiating contractile and noncontractile problems about a joint, which greatly refined the soft-tissue diagnostic process. Both created testing that improved the categorization and communication of functional information with respect to the structure and function relationship.

Since that time, the orthopedic physical therapy evaluation has become highly mechanized and specialized. This has greatly expanded the therapist's ability to evaluate, monitor, communicate, and affect changes in human function. The growth in physical therapy research has produced a wealth of quantitative testing data. This has helped develop many quantitative standards and norms. Much of this data is highly specific. This is the obvious direction for research, because it offers fewer variables and greater specificity. Yet the need for more general functional norms and standards continues to grow. More specifically, the need for qualitative functional norms may be even greater, because qualitative testing lends itself to treatment and education and helps explain the causes for variations in quantitative measurements of performance. Quantitative testing is good for general ranking purposes but offers little insight on the underlying factors influencing the raw score.

(2) It is interesting to observe how normal human movement is appreciated and evaluated throughout the life span. From birth until 2 years of age, the development of movement is considered to proceed along a predictable course.[19] Most agree that a continuum, sequence, or stage model is observable and this progression is clearly defined for clinical purposes. "The developmental sequence has provided the most consistent base for almost all treatment approaches used by physical therapists."[19] Because most of the stages or steps toward the development of posture and movement are defined by clear descriptions, the evaluation of these stages is qualitative in nature. These stages are defined as representations of mobility and stability and the transitional activities that demonstrate the interaction of the two. Various non-weightbearing, weight-shifting, and weightbearing movements display milestones of achievement. As we age, we rank ourselves through more and more quantitative observations. There is a significant quality component to special populations like dance, martial arts, and the skill positions in sports. However, general populations are rarely ranked according to functional movement quality. This has a profound influence on the physical therapy profession, because restoration of qualitative and quantitative function is a primary concern.

A brief contrast between orthopedic and neurological physical therapy will demonstrate the differences in the initial approach of the evaluation process. More specifically, the neurological therapist working with infants and toddlers has an obvious advantage from a qualitative evaluation standpoint, because the developmental sequence and progression is a qualitative standard. Of course, the comparison is unfair, considering the greater variability of the general orthopedic caseload. However, the contrast in theory still serves as a good analogy of qualitative and quantitative evaluation methods. Orthopedic physical therapy does not currently have a centralized or universal, quality-based functional assessment. This may be the central cause of minor divisions in orthopedic physical therapy as a profession. Highly specialized orthopedic physical therapists have honed their skills and improved their training on technique-based philosophies that hold themselves to extremely high standards. However, there is not a functional standard of measurement (qualitative and quantitative combination) that would allow objective comparison of all techniques. In contrast, the neurological physical therapist uses a quality-based functional assessment to monitor and evaluate growth and motor development. The infant, toddler, and child must achieve developmental milestones with respect to mobility, stability, controlled mobility, and skill. A goniometer is not used, and strength tests are not needed to demonstrate success or failure. The patient either achieves a functional milestone or does not. Reasons for pass and fail can be evaluated separately with more specific clinical measurements, but the patient is now in a functional category. The functional category is the logical starting point for functional diagnosis and treatment.

Orthopedic medicine measures the parts with accuracy and reliability and must strive to observe the whole both quantitatively and qualitatively. Observations in science and nature demonstrate that the whole often is not represented by the sum of its parts. Measuring the parts is very scientific and can be tracked with quantitative values. Developmental milestones seem to be pass/fail with ranges of normalcy and require a trained eye to discuss the quality of movement. It is this quality-based assessment tool that sets physical therapists apart from other individuals prescribing exercise. Most individuals with rudimentary exercise training can quantify values such as range of motion, strength, and endurance. The discerning clinician can demonstrate how three different individuals achieving the same quantitative value of a particular performance parameter can do so with varying degrees of quality. The ability to create an equal balance and appreciation for these two forms of movement assessment is, and will continue to be, the defining factor of physical therapy exercise prescription. An analogy for human movement can be observed in today's modern computer. Historically, orthopedics was concerned with hardware (musculoskeletal system), while neurological physical therapy observed and attempted to modify software (motor control). Today the therapist understands that the human hardware can be changed or improved, but if the human software remains the same, movement efficiency is rarely changed or maintained.

(3) Orthopedic manual therapy has contributed greatly to advances in exercise. McKenzie, Kaltenborn, Maitland, Paris, and many others have increased our awareness of joint assessment considering the established osteokinematic model and providing practical treatment options involving arthrokinematic movement. Modern physical therapists have bridged the gap between passive mobilization and active movement, using a combination of mobilization and exercise techniques to achieve accelerated restoration of functional movement. Mulligan has created mobilization techniques that involve a manual mobilizing (sometimes stabilizing) force in the presence of active movement followed by passive stretch.[15] This creative new work demonstrates the disappearing line between mobilization and exercise.[15] Likewise, the new techniques for taping the spine and extremities have moved the science of taping from protective and restrictive to facilitatory and dynamic. The focus is now placed on proprioception, and it complements exercise by not simply reducing symptoms but also by providing continuous tactile feedback.[4] Taping has now moved out of sport-specific applications and is now commonplace for the innovative and aggressive therapist. Taping should be considered an extension of manual therapy by providing mechanical feedback and facilitation as the patient progresses. Taping is complementary to exercise as well. It should follow arthrokinematic rules and replicate anatomy whenever possible.[4]

(4) Kabat and Knott demonstrated in their early work, called proprioceptive neuromuscular facilitation (PNF), how the brain has an affinity for synergistic movements encompassing both spiral and diagonal patterns without consideration of isolated muscle activity or single-plane joint motion. It is unfortunate that many exercise protocols do not employ the inspired theme of PNF at any point in the entire protocol. They go from open-chain, fixed-axis, fitness-styled exercise equipment and recycled home exercises to functional movement patterns without ever first using PNF techniques to refine and stimulate the natural synergistic patterns of movement. PNF has often been considered a hands-on treatment approach, but the idea that a proprioceptive reaction can be improved with movement input rather than visual and auditory input is gaining popularity with hands-off exercise as well (see Chapter 8).[6,22] When clinicians become familiar and comfortable with the techniques of PNF, their exercise skills will improve and their understanding of practical motor learning will be greatly advanced.

INCORPORATION OF FOUR PRINCIPLES

- *Functional evaluation and assessment.* The evaluation must identify a functional problem or limitation resulting in a functional diagnosis. The observation of whole movement patterns, tempered with practical knowledge of key stress points and common compensatory patterns, will improve evaluation efficiency.
- *Identification of motor control.* Orthopedic and sports physical therapy could be greatly advanced by understanding functional milestones and fundamental movements such as those demonstrated during the positions and postures paramount to growth and development. These milestones serve as key representations of functional mobility and

control. They also play a role in the initial setup and design of the exercise program.

- *Identification of osteokinematic and arthrokinematic limitations.* The skills and techniques of orthopedic manual therapy are beneficial in identification of specific arthrokinematic restrictions that would limit movement or impede the motor learning process. Management of myofascial structures will improve osteokinematic movement as well as balance muscle tone between the agonist and antagonist. This will also help the therapist understand the dynamics of the impairment.

- *Integration of synergistic movement patterns.* Once those restrictions and limitations are managed and gross motion is restored, the application of PNF-type patterning will further improve neuromuscular function and control. Considering synergistic movement is the final step in the restoration of function by focusing on coordination, timing, and motor learning.

The application of all four principles in the appropriate sequence will allow the clinician to understand a starting point, consistent progression, and end point for each exercise prescription. This sequence is achieved by using functional activities and fundamental movement patterns as goals. By proceeding in this fashion, the physical therapist will have the ability to evaluate the whole above the parts and then discuss the parts as they apply. The true art of physical therapy is to understand the whole of synergistic functional movement and those therapeutic techniques that will have the greatest positive effect on that movement in the least amount of time. The system is designed to produce musculoskeletal and neuromuscular changes while creating a more favorable motor learning environment.

THE FOUR Ps

The four Ps are actually four simple words starting with the letter "P" that represents the four principles previously mentioned. They serve as quick reminders of the hierarchy, interaction, and application of each principle. The questions of what, when, where, and how with respect to functional movement assessment and exercise prescription are answered in the appropriate order.

1. *Purpose.* Functional evaluation and assessment.
2. *Posture.* Identification of motor control.
3. *Position.* Identification of osteokinematic and arthrokinematic limitations.
4. *Pattern.* Integration of synergistic movement patterns.

Purpose

PRIMARY QUESTIONS

1. *What* functional activity is limited?
2. *What* does the limitation appear to be—a mobility problem or a stability problem?

3. *What* is the dysfunction or disability?
4. *What* fundamental movement is limited?
5. *What* is the impairment?

The word *purpose* is simply a cue to be used both during the evaluation process and the exercise prescription process to keep the clinician intently focused on the greatest single limiting factor of function. It is not uncommon for the therapist to attempt to resolve multiple problems with the initial exercise prescription. However, the practice of identifying the single greatest limiting factor will reduce frustration and also not overwhelm the patient. There may be other factors that have also been identified in the evaluation; however, a major limiting factor or a single weak link should stand out and be the focus of initial therapeutic intervention regarding exercise. Alterations in the limiting factor may produce positive changes elsewhere that can be identified and considered prior to the next exercise progression.

The functional evaluation process should take on three distinct layers or levels. Each of the three levels should involve qualitative observations followed by quantitative documentation when possible. The levels are functional activity assessment, functional or fundamental movement assessment, and specific clinical measurement. Normative data is helpful but bilateral comparison is also effective and serves to demonstrate the functional problem to the patient at each level. Until the physical therapy evaluation, many patients think the problem is simply symptomatic and structural in nature and have no example of dysfunction outside of pain with movement. Moffroid and Zimny suggest, "Muscle strength of the right and left sides is more similar in the proximal muscles whereas we accept a 10% to 15% difference in strength of the distal muscles. . . . With joint flexibility, we accept a 5% difference between goniometric measurements of the right and left sides."[19]

FUNCTIONAL ACTIVITY ASSESSMENT

This is a reproduction of combined movements common to the patient's lifestyle and occupation. They usually fit the definition of general or specific skill. The therapist must have the patient demonstrate a variety of positions and not just those positions that correspond to symptom reproduction. This includes static postural assessment as well as dynamic activity. The quality of control and movement are assessed. Specific measurement of bilateral differences is difficult, but demonstration and observation is helpful for the patient. The therapist should note the positions and activities that provoke symptoms as well as the activities that illustrate poor body mechanics, poor alignment, right–left asymmetries, and inappropriate weight shifting. When the therapist has observed gross movement quality, it may be necessary to also quantify movement performance. Repetition of the activity for endurance comparison, symptom reproduction, or rapidly declining quality will create a functional baseline for bilateral comparison and documentation.

FUNCTIONAL OR FUNDAMENTAL MOVEMENT ASSESSMENT

The therapist must take what is learned through the observation of functional activity and break those movements down to the static and transitional postures seen in the normal developmental sequence. This will reduce activities to the many underlying mobilizing and stabilizing actions and reactions that constitute the functional activity. More simply stated, the activity is broken down into a sequence of primary movements that can be observed independently. It must be noted that these movements still involve multiple joints and muscles. Individual joint and muscle group assessment will be performed during clinical measurements. Martin notes, "The developmental sequence has provided the most consistent base for almost all approaches used by physical therapists."[19] This is a powerful statement and, because true qualitative measurements of normal movement in adult populations are limited, the therapist must look for universal movement similarities. Changes in fundamental movements can affect significant and prompt changes in function and therefore must be considered functional as well. Because the movement patterns of most adults are habitual and specific and therefore not representative of a full or optimal movement spectrum, the clinician must first consider the nonspecific basic movement patterns common to all individuals during growth and development. The developmental sequence is predictable and universal in the first 2 years of life. There are individual differences in rate and quality of the progression. The differences are minimal compared to the variations seen in the adult population with their many habits, occupations, and lifestyles. In addition to diverse movement patterns, the adult population has the consequential complicating factor of a previous medical and injury history. Each medical problem and injury has had some degree of influence on activity and movement. So evaluation of functional activities alone may hide many uneconomical movement patterns, compensations, and asymmetries that when integrated into functional activities are not readily obvious to the clinician. By using the fundamental movements of the developmental progression, the clinician can view mobility and static and dynamic stability problems in a more isolated setting.

Although enormous variations of functional movement quality and quantity exist between specific adult patient populations, most individuals have the developmental sequence in common. The movements used in normal motor development are the building blocks of skill and function. Many of these building blocks can be lost while the skill is maintained or retained at some level (although rarely optimal). We will refer to these movement building blocks as fundamental movements and consider them as precursors to a higher function. Bilateral comparison is helpful when identifying qualitative differences between right and left sides. These movements (like functional activities) can be compared quantitatively as well. Repetition of movement for endurance comparison, symptom reproduction, or rapidly declining quality will create a functional baseline for comparison and documentation.

CLINICAL MEASUREMENTS TO IDENTIFY SPECIFIC PROBLEMS

Clinical measurements should be used to identify specific problems that contribute to limitation of motion or control. Clinical measurements will first classify a patient through qualitative assessment. The parameters that define that classification must then be quantified to reveal impairment. These classifications are called hypermobility and hypomobility and help to create treatment guides considering the functional status, anatomic structures, and severity of symptoms. The therapist should not proceed into exercise prescription without proper identification of one of these general categories. The success or failure of a particular exercise treatment regime is probably more dependent on this classification than the choice of exercise technique or protocol (Fig. 24-3). Janda then provides greater depth of insight to the classification process by identifying muscle groups with common traits and placing them into a functional division. Janda proposes that muscular imbalance progresses in a predictable fashion. "Postural muscles tend to tightness while phasic muscles tend to weakness" (Fig. 24-4).[21]

Once the appropriate clinical classification is produced, specific quantitative measurements will define the level of involvement within the classification and set a baseline for exercise treatment. Periodic reassessments may identify a different major limiting factor or weak link that may require reclassification followed by specific measurement. The new problem or limitation would then be inserted as the purpose for a new exercise intervention. A simple diagram (Fig. 24-5) will help the clinician separate the different levels of function so that intervention and purpose will always be at the appropriate level and assist with clinical decision making relative to exercise prescription.[8]

Functional performance deals with specific parameters that are more extrinsic and achievement-based. It is concerned with repetition of and recovery from a given movement. These are quantitative measures that represent interaction with the environment and a demonstration of work, speed, power, coordination, agility, balance, strength, energy expenditure, and efficiency. The tests employ basic movements previously defined as fundamental (dynamic stability), but basic locomotion (lower extremities) and manipulation (upper extremities), seen as skill by motor development specialists, can also be used. However, the movements should be common so general comparisons of volume and intensity can be observed.

The last category for consideration is specific skill function. For the athlete, this would mean sport-specific analysis as well as position-specific demands. For the industrial patient, it would consider job site ergonomics, job description and responsibilities, as well as norms and averages of production. Other considerations for general populations demonstrate activities of daily living function and specific training for the use of assistive devices and equipment as well as movement for special circumstances. Before entering into specific exercise recommendations, the therapist should demonstrate the specific purpose of exercise intervention. The patient's responses and questions will help the therapist understand the level with which the patient can

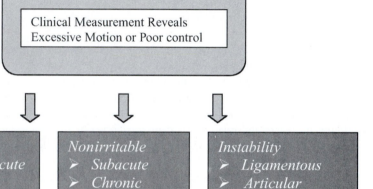

Clinical Measurement
Reveals Reduced Motion

Myofascial hypomobility
➤ Acute *
➤ Chronic

Articular hypomobility
➤ Pericapsular
➤ Subluxation

Clinical Measurement Reveals
Excessive Motion or Poor control

Irritable
➤ Inflamed / Acute
➤ Overused

Nonirritable
➤ Subacute
➤ Chronic

Instability
➤ Ligamentous
➤ Articular

FIGURE 24-3

Biomechancial assessment
and treatment. (SOURCE:
Cook G. *Meadows Manual
Therapy: Biomechanical
Assessment and Treatment.*
NAIOMT Course Notes,
1987.)

Muscles Prone to Tightness	**Muscles Prone to Weakness**
• Gastroc/soleus • Tibialis posterior • Short hip adductors • Hamstrings • Rectus femoris • Iliopsoas • Tensor fasciae latae • Piriformis • Erector spinae (especially lumbar, thoracolumbar, and cervical portions) • Quadratus lumborum • Pectoralis major • Upper portion of trapezius • Levator scapulae • Scalenes • Flexors of the upper limb	• Peronei • Tibialis anterior • Vastus medialis and lateralis • Gluteus maximus, medius, and minimus • Rectus abdominis • Serratus anterior • Rhomboids • Lower portion of the trapezius • Short cervical flexors • Extensors of the upper limb

FIGURE 24-4

Janda's functional division
of muscle groups.

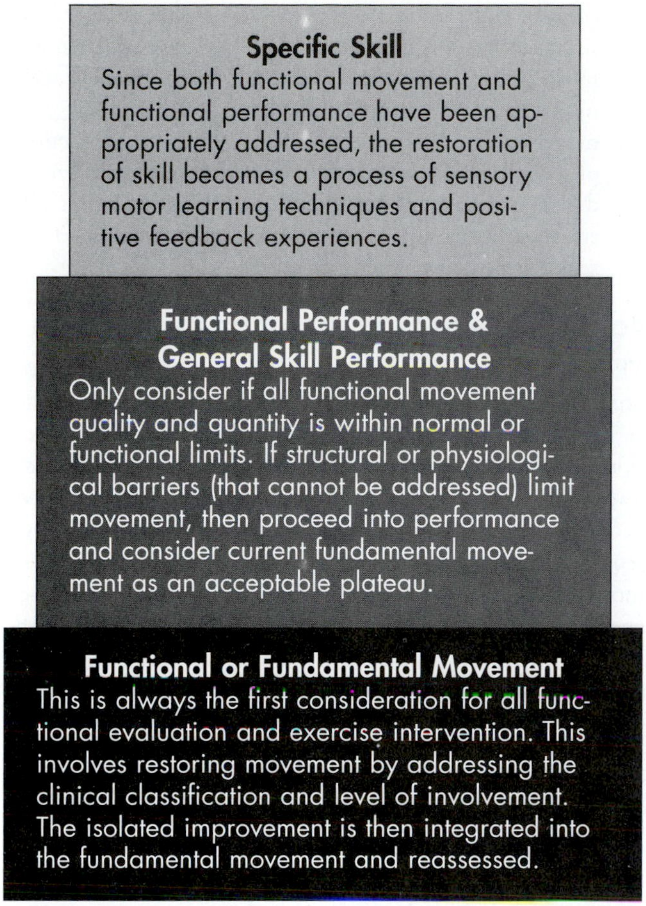

Specific Skill

Since both functional movement and functional performance have been appropriately addressed, the restoration of skill becomes a process of sensory motor learning techniques and positive feedback experiences.

Functional Performance & General Skill Performance

Only consider if all functional movement quality and quantity is within normal or functional limits. If structural or physiological barriers (that cannot be addressed) limit movement, then proceed into performance and consider current fundamental movement as an acceptable plateau.

Functional or Fundamental Movement

This is always the first consideration for all functional evaluation and exercise intervention. This involves restoring movement by addressing the clinical classification and level of involvement. The isolated improvement is then integrated into the fundamental movement and reassessed.

FIGURE 24-5

Levels of function.

appreciate the problem. It is helpful to verbally describe the problem, visually demonstrate the problem, and then let the patient experience dysfunction by performing a movement that illustrates the problem. This will provide an educational experience that involves visual auditory and kinesthetic feedback. Motor learning usually occurs in the presence of three conditions: need or necessity, repetition, and reinforcement. By demonstrating the functional problem through three different sensory examples, the patient might better understand the purpose and necessity of the exercise prescription. Appropriate exercise dosage will enable the patient to perform the volume of exercise needed for repetition with unnecessary stress. The appropriate progression and sequence of exercise will create reinforcement through positive feedback and success. The exercise program should be designed around a predetermined success model with steps designed for the individual's motivation and ability.

Posture

PRIMARY QUESTIONS

1. *When* in the development sequence is the impairment obvious?

2. *When* do the substitutions and compensations occur?
3. *When* in the developmental sequence does the patient demonstrate success?
4. *When* in the developmental sequence does the patient experience difficulty?
5. *When* is the best possible starting point for exercise with respect to posture?

"Posture" is a word to help the therapist consider a much more holistic approach to exercise prescription. Janda creates an interesting point when discussing posture and the muscles responsible for its maintenance. Most discussions regarding posture and postural musculature generally refer to erect standing. However, "erect standing position is so well balanced that little or no activity is necessary to maintain it."[21] Therefore, "basic human posture should be derived from the principle movement pattern, namely gait. Since we stand on one leg for the most of the time during walking, the stance on one leg should be considered to be the typical posture in man; the postural muscles are those which maintain this posture." Janda reports the ratio of single/double-leg stance in gait at 85-to-15 percent. "The muscles which maintain erect posture in standing on one leg are exactly those which show a striking tendency to get tight" (see Fig. 24-4).[21] Infants and toddlers use tonic holding before normal motor development, and maturation produces abilities for the use of cocontraction as a means of effective support. "Tonic holding is the ability of tonic postural muscle to maintain a contraction in their shortened range against gravitational or manual resistance."[20] The adult orthopedic patient may revert to some level of tonic holding following injury or in the presence of pain and altered proprioception. Likewise, those adults who have habitual postures and limited activity may adopt tonic holding for some postures.

Just as Janda uses single-leg stance to observe postural function with greater specificity in contrast to a more conventional double-leg erect standing, the developmental progression can give even greater understanding by looking at the precursors of single-leg stance.[4] As stated previously, fundamental movements are basic representations of mobility, stability, and dynamic stability and include the transitional postures used in growth and development. This approach will help the therapist consider how the mobility or stability problem, which was isolated in the evaluation, has been (temporarily) integrated by substitution and compensation of other body parts. The therapist must remember that motor learning is a survival mechanism. The principles that the therapist will use in rehabilitation to produce motor learning have already been activated by the functional response to the impairment. Necessity or affinity, repetition, and reinforcement have been used to avoid pain or produce alternative movements since the onset of symptoms. Therefore, a new motor program has been activated to manage the impairment and produce some level of function that is usually viewed as dysfunction. It should be considered a natural and appropriate response of the body reacting to limitation or symptoms. The body will sacrifice movement quality to maintain a degree of movement quantity. Considering this, two distinct needs are presented.

POSTURE FOR PROTECTION AND INHIBITION

The therapist must restrict or inhibit the inappropriate motor program. In the case of a control or stability problem, the patient must have some form of support, protection, or facilitation. Otherwise, the inappropriate program will take over in an attempt to protect and respond to the postural demand. Although nearly all adult patients function at the skill level upon evaluation, many qualitative problems are noted. Inappropriate joint loading and locking, poor tonic responses, or even tonic holding can be observed with simple activities. Some joint movements are used excessively, while other joint movements are unconsciously avoided. Many primary stability problems exist in the presence of underlying secondary mobility problems. Moreover, in some cases the mobility problem preceded the stability problem. This is a common explanation for microtraumatic and overuse injuries. It is also why bilateral comparison and assessment of proximal and distal structures is mandatory in the evaluative process. In the case of a mobility problem, a joint is not used appropriately due to weakness or restriction. The primary mobility problem may be the result of compromised stability elsewhere. Motor programs have been created to allow the patient to push on in the presence of the mobility or stability problem. The problems can be managed by mechanical consideration of the mobility and stability status of the patient in the fundamental postures.

- Primary stability problems must be mechanically supported or assisted in some way. This can be done simply by a reduction of partial or complete stress through postural variations. This may include non-weightbearing or partial weight bearing of the spine and extremities or temporary bracing. If the stability problem is only in a particular range of movement, then that movement must be managed. If there is an underlying mobility problem, then it must be managed and temporarily taken out of the initial exercise movement. The alteration of posture can effectively limit complete or partial motion with little need for active control by the patient. The stability problem must be trained independently of the mobility problem or at a great mechanical advantage to avoid compensation. The secondary mobility problem, once managed, should be reintroduced in a nonstressful manner so the previous compensatory pattern is not activated.
- The primary mobility problem must be assisted and managed by manual articular and soft-tissue techniques, when appropriate, and followed by movement to integrate any improved range and benefit from more appropriate tone. If the mobility limitation seems to be the result of weakness, then make sure that the proximal structures can demonstrate the requisite amount of stability prior to strengthening. Then proceed with strengthening or endurance activities with a focus on recruitment, relaxation, timing,

coordination, and reproducibility. Note that the word "resistance" was not used initially. Resistance is not synonymous with strengthening and is only one of many techniques used to improve functional movement in early movement reeducation. However, the subsequent sections on position and pattern will address resistance in greater detail. Use posture to mechanically block or restrict substitution of stronger segments and improve quality at the segment being exercised.

POSTURE FOR RECRUITMENT AND FACILITATION

The therapist must facilitate or stimulate the correct motor program, coordination, and sequence of movement. Although verbal and visual feedback are helpful through demonstration and cueing, kinesthetic feedback is paramount to motor learning.[22] Correct body position or posture will improve feedback. Posture and movement that are early in the developmental sequence will require a less complex motor task and activate a more basic motor program. This will create positive feedback and reinforcement and mark the point (posture) where appropriate and inappropriate actions and reactions meet. From this point, the therapist can manipulate frequency, intensity, and duration or advance to a more difficult posture in the appropriate sequence.

The therapist must also consider developmental biomechanics that divide the movement ability into two categories: internal forces and external forces. "Internal forces include the center of gravity, base of support, and line of gravity." "External forces include gravity, inertia of the body segment, and ground reaction."[6] Considering this, the therapist should evaluate the patient's abilities in the same manner by first observing management of the mass of the body over the particular base provided by the posture. Then progress the patient toward more external stresses like inertia, gravity, and ground reaction forces. This interaction will require various degrees of acceleration production, deceleration control, anticipatory weight shifting, and increased proprioception. Resistance and movement can stress static and dynamic postures, but the therapist should also understand that resistance and movement could be used to refine movement and stimulate appropriate reactions.[22] Postures must be chosen to reduce compensation and allow the patient to exercise below the level where the impairment hinders movement or control. This is easily accomplished by creating "self-limiting" exercises.[4] These exercises require passive or active "locking" by limiting movement of the area the patient will most likely use to substitute or "cheat" with during exercise.

To review, posture identifies the fundamental movements used in growth and development. These movements serve as steps toward skill, which are also helpful in the presence of skill when quality is questionable. A few examples are

- supine-bridging movements,
- rolling to side-lying, rolling to prone, rolling to supine,
- prone on elbows to rolling or reaching, prone press-up,
- quadruped positions, static, dynamic,

- transitions to and from sitting, sitting and reaching,
- kneeling, tall kneeling, half kneeling, add reaching movements,
- squatting movement variations,
- lunging movement variations, and
- single-leg stance, static, dynamic.

By following this natural sequence of movement, the therapist can observe where a mobility or stability problem will first limit the quality of a whole movement pattern. A patient with a mild knee sprain or even a total knee replacement may demonstrate segmental rolling to one side but "log roll" to the other simply to avoid using a flexion adduction medial rotation movement pattern with the involved lower extremity. The therapist has now identified where success and failure meet in the developmental sequence. The knee problem creates a dynamic stability problem in the developmental sequence long before partial or full weight bearing is an issue. It, therefore, must be addressed at that level. The patient is provided with an example of how limited knee mobility can greatly affect movement patterns (like rolling) that seem to require little of the knee. The clinician must define postural levels of success and failure to identify the postural level where therapeutic exercise intervention should start. Otherwise, the therapist could potentially prescribe exercise at a postural level where the patient is creating significant amounts of compensation, substitution, and frustration during exercise. The example of the knee patient is actually a common occurrence and often goes unnoticed. However, by restoring bilateral segmental rolling function, many gait problems will be affected with measurable qualitative and quantitative observations. By using a postural progression, the earliest level of functional limitation can be easily identified and incorporated into the exercise program. Limitations can also be placed on the posture and movement (the self-limiting concept) to limit postural compensation and focus.

Position

PRIMARY QUESTIONS

1. *Where* is the impairment located?
2. *Where* among the structures (myofascial or articular) does the impairment have its greatest effect?
3. *Where* in the range of motion does the impairment have the greatest effect?
4. *Where* is the most beneficial position for the exercise?

The word "position" describes not only the location of the anatomic structure (joint, muscle group, ligament) where impairment has been identified but also the positions (with respect to movement and load) that the greatest and least limitations occur. The limitations can be either reduced strength and control or restricted movement. Orthopedic manual assessment of joints and muscles in various functional positions will demonstrate the influence of the impairment and symptoms throughout the range of movement. The clinician will identify various deficits. Each will be qualified or quantified through

assessment and objective testing and then addressed through the appropriate dosage and positioning for exercise.

To better understand the role of position, consider the single-leg bridge exercise progression. Purpose and posture are clearly defined. Purpose is the obvious reason for exercise intervention, while posture describes the orientation of the body in space. Position refers to the specific mobilizing or stabilizing segment. In the case of the single-leg bridge, the hip is moving toward extension. If range of motion was broken down into thirds, it would only involve the extension third of movement. The flexion third and middle third of movement are not needed, because no impairment was identified in those respective ranges. Not only was the hip in extension, but also the knee was in flexion. This is important, because the hamstring muscle will try to assist hip extension in the end range of movement when gluteal strength is not optimal. However, the hamstrings cannot assist hip extension to any significant degree because of "active insufficiency." Likewise, the lumbar extensors cannot assist the extension pattern due to the passive stretch placed upon them via maximal passive hip flexion on the opposite side. The hip extension proprioception is now void of any inappropriate patterning or compensation from the hamstrings or spinal erectors through the positional use of active and passive insufficiency.[4,13]

Qualitative measures will provide specific information regarding exercise start position, finish position, movement speed and direction, open- and closed-chain considerations, and the need for cueing and feedback. Close observation of osteokinematic and arthrokinematic relationships respecting movement and bilateral comparison is the obvious starting point. Specific identification of the structure and position represent mobility observed by selective tension (active, passive, and resisted movements), and "end feel" of the joint structures would provide specific information about the mechanical nature of limitations and symptoms.[7] Assessment of positional static and dynamic control will describe stability limitations and provide a more specific starting point for exercise. The therapist should map the specific limitations of a segment (muscle/joint complex). The terms "hypermobility" and "hypomobility" create clear *structure* and *function*-based categories (see Fig. 24–3). Quantitative measures will reveal a degree of defect, which can be recorded in the form of a percentage through bilateral comparison and compared to normative data when possible. Range of motion, strength, endurance, and recovery time should be considered along with many other (quantitative) clinical parameters to describe isolated or positional function. This will provide clear communication and specific documentation for goals as well as a tracking device for treatment effectiveness. This information will help define the baseline for initial exercise considerations.

As previously stated, any limitation in mobility or stability will require a bilateral comparison as well as clearing of the joints above and below. The proximal and distal structures must also be compared to their contralateral counterparts. This central point of physical examination is often overlooked. Cyriax noted, "Positive signs must always be balanced by corroborative

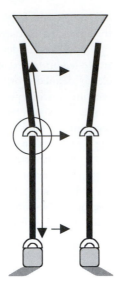

1. Assess right knee
2. Compare to left knee
3. Assess right hip
4. Compare to left hip
5. Assess right ankle
6. Compare to left ankle

F I G U R E   2 4 - 6

Right knee positional comparison.

negative signs." If a lesion appears to lie at or near one joint, this region must be examined for signs identifying its site. It is equally essential for the adjacent joints and the structures about them to be examined so that, by contrast, their normality can be established. These negative findings then reinforce the positive findings emanating elsewhere; only then can the diagnosis be regarded and established" (Fig. 24-6).[7]

Once position and movement options have been established, a trial exercise session should be used to observe and quantify performance prior to prescription. Variables including intensity and duration can be used to establish strength or endurance baselines. Bilateral comparison should be used to document a performance deficit, which is also recorded as percentage. A maximum repetition test (with or without resistance) to fatigue, onset of symptoms, or loss of exercise quality are common examples. This will allow close tracking of home exercise compliance and help establish a rate of improvement. All other factors being addressed, the rate of improvement should be quite large. This is the benefit of correct dosage with regard to prescription of exercise position and appropriate workload. Most of the significant improvement is not due to training volume, tissue metabolism, or muscle hypertrophy. It is the efficient adaptive response of "neural factors."[2] These factors can include motor recruitment efficiency, improved timing, increased proprioceptive awareness, improved agonist/antagonist coordination, appropriate phasic and tonic response to activity, task familiarity, and motor learning as well as psychological factors. Usually, the greater the deficit, the more drastic the improvement. Treatments should be geared to stimulate these changes whenever possible.[5]

Pattern

PRIMARY QUESTIONS

1. *How* is the movement pattern different upon bilateral comparison?

2. *How* can synergistic movement, coordination, recruitment, and timing be facilitated?
3. *How* will this affect the movement limitation?
4. *How* will this affect function?

The word "pattern" will serve as a cue to the clinician to continually consider the functional movements of the human body that occur in unified patterns that occupy three-dimensional space and cross three planes (frontal, sagittal, and transverse).[6] Sometimes this is not easily ascertained by observing the design and usage of fixed axis exercise equipment and the movement patterns suggested in some rehabilitation protocols. The basic patterns of PNF, for both the extremities and the spine, are excellent examples of the brain groups movement. Muscles of the trunk and extremities are recruited in the most advantageous sequence (proprioception) to create movement (mobility) or control (stability) movement. Not only does this provide efficient and economical function, but also it effectively protects the respective joints and muscles from undue stress and strain. Voss et al. clearly and eloquently state,

> The mass movements patterns of facilitation are spiral and diagonal in character and closely resemble the movements used in sports and work activities. The spiral and diagonal character is in keeping with the spiral rotatory characteristics of the skeletal system of bones and joints and the ligamentous structures. This type of motion is also in harmony with the topographical alignment of the muscles from origin to insertion and with the structural characteristics of the individual muscles.[23]

When a structure within the sequence is limited by impairment, the entire pattern is limited in some way. The therapist should document the limited pattern as well as the isolated segment causing the pattern to be limited. The isolated segment is usually identified in the evaluation process and outlined in the "position" considerations. The resultant effect on one or more movement patterns must also be investigated. A review of the basic PNF patterns can be beneficial to the orthopedic therapist. Once a structure is evaluated, look at the basic PNF patterns involving that structure. Multiple patterns can be limited in some way, but usually one pattern in particular will demonstrate significantly reduced function. Obviously, poor function in a muscle group or joint can limit the strength, endurance, and range of motion of an entire PNF pattern to some degree. However, the clinician must not simply view reduced PNF pattern function as an output problem. It should be equally viewed as an input problem. When muscle and joint function are not optimal, mechanoreceptor and muscle spindle are not optimal. This can create an input or proprioceptive problem and greatly distort joint position and muscle tension information. This distorts initial information (before movement is initiated) as well as feedback (once movement is in progress). Therefore, the therapist cannot only consider functional output.

Altered proprioception, if not properly identified and outlined, can unintentionally become part of the recommended

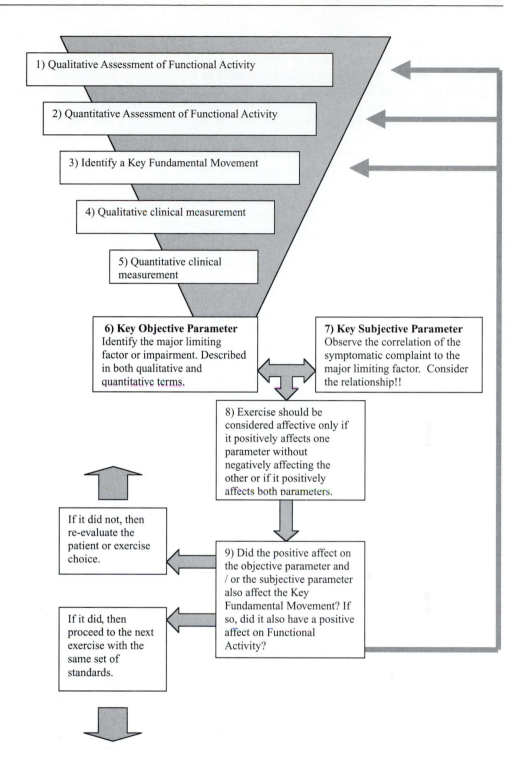

FIGURE 24-7

The deductive process of exercise prescription.

exercises and therefore be reinforced. The therapist must focus on synergistic and integrated function at all levels of rehabilitation. The orthopedic outpatient cannot afford to have a problem simply isolated three times a week for 30 minutes only to reintegrate the same problem at a subconscious level during necessary daily activities throughout the remaining week. PNF-style movement pattern exercise can often be taught as easily as an isolated movement at a significantly greater benefit. Therapeutic exercise is no longer limited by sets as repetitions of the same activity. Successive intervals of increasing difficulty (although not physically stressful) building on the accomplishment of an earlier task will reinforce one level of function and continually challenge the next. A simple movement set focused on isolation of a problem can be quickly followed by a pattern that will improve integration. The integration can be followed by a familiar fundamental movement or functional activity, which may reduce the amount of conscious and deliberate movement and give the therapist a chance to observe subcortical control of mobility and stability as well as appropriate use of phasic and tonic responses (see Chapter 8). By continuously considering the pattern options as well as pattern limitations, the therapist will be able to refine the exercise prescription and reduce unnecessary supplemental movements that could easily be incorporated into pattern-based exercise.

Direction, speed, and amount of resistance (or assistance) will be used to produce more refined patterns. Manual resistance, weighted cable or elastic resistance, weight-shifting activities, and even proprioceptive taping can improve recruitment and facilitate coordination. The therapist should refrain from initially discussing specific structural control like "pelvic tilting" or "scapular retraction." Instead, the therapist should use posture and position to set the initial movement and design proprioceptive feedback to produce a more normal pattern whenever possible (Chapter 8).

SUMMARY

- Hopefully the mastery of functional evaluation and exercise prescription will remain in the rehabilitative domain (Fig. 24-7). This chapter was designed to both describe and define some of the most effective and efficient considerations for functional exercise prescription and progression. Although exercise prescription falls within the scope of many modern health care and fitness professionals, the physical therapist is unique. The four principles in particular serve to describe this distinction.

- In review, the four Ps are actually four simple words starting with the letter "P" that represent each of the four principles. They serve as quick reminders of the hierarchy, interaction, and application of each principle. The questions of what, when, where, and how with respect to functional movement assessment and exercise prescription are answered in the appropriate order
    - ➤ functional evaluation and assessment—*purpose*
    - ➤ identification of motor control—*posture*
    - ➤ identification of osteokinematic and arthrokinematic limitations—*position*
    - ➤ integration of synergistic movement patterns—*pattern*
- Current information has been synchronized to produce a new perspective. This new perspective was specifically designed to improve treatment efficiency and effectiveness. These four principles attempt to assist problem solving by providing a framework that categorizes clinical information in a hierarchy. The information groups are then linked together to demonstrate a natural flow from problem to solution to outcome.
- It is best to first apply the four principles and their primary questions to a case review. This will demonstrate assimilation or sequencing errors related to initial exercise prescription or progression. Likewise, it may also demonstrate individual clinical affinity resulting in efficient use of resources and treatment consistency.
- Once the four principles have been applied to previous cases, the clinician can incorporate all four principles or one principle at a time into his/her current caseload or clinical re-

search. With experience, self-critique, and continued education, the therapist may see the four principles vanish. The clinician will eventually assimilate and implement the four principles in parallel, which refer to simultaneous consideration of the major factors influencing function. The need for a serial step-by-step deduction process is no longer necessary. The steps are still used, but the human mind now has an operative framework and the practical experiences that produce higher and higher levels of intercommunication. This will allow the clinician to move smoothly from evaluation to exercise prescription, progression, and re-evaluation, demonstrating objective improvement in both clinical measurements and functional movement.

- Clinical wisdom is the result of experience and applied knowledge. Intense familiarity and practical observation improve application. To be of benefit, available knowledge must be organized and tempered by an objective and inclusive framework. Hopefully, this framework will provide a starting point and to better organize and apply each clinician's knowledge and experience of functional exercise prescription. In the words of Eden Phillpotts (1862–1960), "The universe is full of magical things patiently waiting for our wits to grow sharper."

REFERENCES

1. American College of Sports Medicine. *Exercise Management for Persons with Chronic Diseases and Disabilities.* Champaign, IL, Human Kinetics, 1997.
2. Baechle TR. *Essentials of Strength Training and Conditioning.* Champaign, IL, Human Kinetics, 1994.
3. Cailliet R. *Soft Tissue Pain and Disability.* Philadelphia, PA, Davis, 1977.
4. Cook G. *The Four Ps (Exercise Prescription). Functional Exercise Training Course Manual.* North American Sports Medicine Institute, ACE, 1997–present.
5. Cook G, Burton L, Fields K. Reactive neuromuscular training for the anterior cruciate ligament-deficient knee: A case report. *J Athl Train* 34:194–201, 1999.
6. Cook G, Fields K. Functional Training for the Torso, National Strength & Conditioning Association, April 1997, 14–19.
7. Cyriax J. Vol I: Diagnosis of soft tissue lesions. *Textbook of Orthopaedic Medicine,* 8th ed. London, Bailliere Tindall, 1982.
8. *FMS Manual.* Danville, VA, ATS, 1998.
9. Glassman S. Advances in treating shoulder injuries. *Adv Phys Ther* 8:11, 1984.
10. Gould JA, III. *Orthopaedic and Sports Physical Therapy,* 2nd ed. St. Louis, MO, Mosby, 1990, p. 169.
11. Haywood KM. *Life Span Motor Development,* 2nd ed. Champaign, IL, Human Kinetics, 1993.
12. Janda V. Pain in the locomotor system. Paper presented at second annual interdisciplinary symposium on rehabilitation in chronic low back disorders, Los Angeles, 1988.

13. Kendall FP, McCreaary KE, Provance PG. *Muscle Testing and Function*, 4th ed. Baltimore, MD, Lippincott Williams & Wilkins, 1993.

14. Liebenson C. *Rehabilitation of the Spine: A Practitioner's Manual.* Media, PA, Lippincott Williams & Wilkins, 1996.

15. Mulligan B. *Manual Therapy, "NAGS", "SNAGS", "MWM."* Wellington, NZ, Plane View Services, 2000.

16. Munich H, Cipriani D, Hall C, Nelson D, Falkel J. The test–retest reliability of an inclined squat strength test protocol. *J Orthop Sports Phys Ther* 26:209–213, 1997.

17. Porterfield JA, DeRosa C. *Mechanical Low Back Pain: Perspectives in Functional Anatomy*, 2nd ed. Chapter 5. Philadelphia, PA, Saunders, 1998.

18. Richter R, VanSant A, Newton R. Description of adult rolling movements and hypothesis of developmental sequences. *Phys Ther* 69:63–76, 1989.

19. Scully R, Barnes M. *Physical Therapy.* Philadelphia, PA, Lippincott Williams & Wilkins, 1989.

20. Sullivan PE, Markos PD, Minor MD. *An Integrated Approach to Therapeutic Exercise: Theory and Clinical Application.* Reston, VA, Reston Publishing Company, 1982.

21. Twomey L. Physical therapy of the low back. In: Janda V, ed. *Muscles and Motor Control in Low Back Pain: Assessment and Management.* New York, Churchill Livingstone, 1987, pp. 253–278.

22. Voight M, Cook G. Clinical application of closed kinetic chain exercise. *J Sport Rehabil* 5:25–44, 1996.

23. Voss DE, Ionta MK, Myers BJ. *Proprioceptive Neuromuscular Facilitation: Patterns and Techniques*, 3rd ed. Philadelphia, PA, Harper Row, 1985.

P A R T 4

Intervention Strategies for Specific Injuries

CHAPTER 25

Rehabilitation of Shoulder Injuries

Rob Schneider, William E. Prentice, and Turner A. Blackburn, Jr

OBJECTIVES

After completing this chapter, the therapist should be able to do the following:

- Review the functional anatomy and biomechanics associated with normal function of the shoulder joint complex.
- Differentiate the various rehabilitative strengthening techniques for the shoulder, including both open- and closed-kinetic-chain isotonic, plyometric, isokinetic, and proprioceptive neuromuscular facilitation (PNF) exercises.
- Compare the various techniques for regaining range of motion (ROM) including stretching exercises and joint mobilizations.
- Administer exercises that may be used to reestablish neuromuscular control.
- Relate biomechanical principles to the rehabilitation of various shoulder injuries/pathologies.
- Discuss criteria for progression of the rehabilitation program for different shoulder injuries/pathologies.
- Describe and explain the rationale for various treatment techniques in the management of shoulder injuries.

FUNCTIONAL ANATOMY AND BIOMECHANICS

The anatomy of the shoulder joint complex allows for tremendous ROM. This wide ROM of the shoulder complex proximal permits precise positioning of the hand distally, to allow both gross and skilled movements. However, the high degree of mobility requires some compromise in stability, which in turn increases the vulnerability of the shoulder joint to injury, particularly in dynamic overhead activities.

The shoulder girdle complex is composed of three bones—the scapula, the clavicle, and the humerus—which are connected either to one another or to the axial skeleton or trunk via the glenohumeral joint, the acromioclavicular (AC) joint, the sternoclavicular (SC) joint, and the scapulothoracic joint (Fig. 25-1). Dynamic movement and stabilization of the shoulder complex require integrated function of all four articulations if normal motion is to occur.

Sternoclavicular Joint

The clavicle articulates with the manubrium of the sternum to form the SC joint, the only direct skeletal connection between the upper extremity and the trunk. The sternal articulating surface is larger than the sternum, causing the clavicle to rise much higher than the sternum. A fibrocartilaginous disk is interposed between the two articulating surfaces. It functions as a shock absorber against the medial forces and also helps to prevent any displacement upward. The articular disk is placed so that the clavicle moves on the disk, and the disk, in turn, moves separately on the sternum. The clavicle is permitted to move up and down, forward and backward, in combination, and in rotation.

The SC joint is extremely weak because of its bony arrangement, but it is held securely by strong ligaments that tend to pull the sternal end of the clavicle downward and toward the sternum, in effect anchoring it. The main ligaments are the anterior SC, which prevents upward displacement of the clavicle; the posterior SC, which also prevents upward displacement of the clavicle; the interclavicular, which prevents lateral displacement of the clavicle; and the costoclavicular, which prevents lateral and upward displacement of the clavicle.[3]

It should also be noted that for the scapula to abduct and upward rotate throughout 180° of humeral abduction, clavicular movement must occur at both the SC and AC joints.

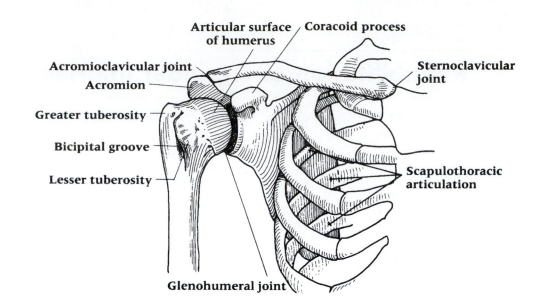

F I G U R E 2 5 - 1

Skeletal anatomy of the shoulder complex.

The clavicle must elevate approximately 40° to allow upward scapular rotation.[56]

Acromioclavicular Joint

The AC joint is a gliding articulation of the lateral end of the clavicle with the acromion process. This is a rather weak joint. A fibrocartilaginous disk separates the two articulating surfaces. A thin, fibrous capsule surrounds the joint.

The AC ligament consists of anterior, posterior, superior, and inferior portions. In addition to the AC ligament, the coracoclavicular ligament joints the coracoid process and the clavicle relative to the acromion. The coracoclavicular ligament is further divided into the trapezoid ligament, which prevents overriding of the clavicle on the acromion, and the conoid ligament, which limits upward movement of the clavicle on the acromion. As the arm moves into an elevated position, there is a posterior rotation of the clavicle on its long axis, which permits the scapula to continue rotating, thus allowing full elevation. The clavicle must rotate approximately 50° for full elevation to occur; otherwise elevation would be limited to approximately 110°.[56]

CORACOACROMIAL ARCH

The coracoacromial ligament connects the coracoid to the acromion. This ligament, along with the acromion and the coracoid, forms the coracoacromial arch over the glenohumeral joint. In the subacromial space between the coracoacromial arch superiorly and the humeral head inferiorly, lies the supraspinatus tendon, the long head of the biceps tendon, and the subacromial bursa. Each of these structures is subject to irritation and inflammation resulting either from excessive humeral head translation or from impingement during repeated overhead activities. In asymptomatic individuals the optimal subacromial space appears to be about 9–10 mm.[57]

Glenohumeral Joint

The glenohumeral joint is an enarthrodial, or ball-and-socket, synovial joint in which the round head of the humerus articulates with the shallow glenoid cavity of the scapula. The cavity is deepened slightly by a fibrocartilaginous rim called the glenoid labrum. The humeral head is larger than the glenoid, and at any point during elevation only 25–30 percent of the humeral head is in contact with the glenoid.[28] The glenohumeral joint is maintained by both static and dynamic restraints. Position is maintained statically by the glenoid labrum and the capsular ligaments, and dynamically by the deltoid and rotator cuff muscles.

Surrounding the articulation is a loose, articular capsule that is attached to the labrum. This capsule is strongly reinforced by the superior, middle, and inferior glenohumeral ligaments and by the tough coracohumeral ligament, which attaches to the coracoid process and to the greater tuberosity of the humerus.[52]

The long tendon of the biceps muscle passes superiorly across the head of the humerus and then through the bicipital groove. In the anatomical position the long head of the biceps moves in close relationship with the humerus. The transverse humeral ligament maintains the long head of the biceps tendon within the bicipital groove by passing over it from the lesser and the greater tuberosities, converting the bicipital groove into a canal.

Scapulothoracic Joint

The scapulothoracic joint is not a true joint; but the movement of the scapula on the wall of the thoracic cage is critical to shoulder joint motion. Contraction of the scapular muscles that attach the scapula to the axial skeleton is essential in stabilizing the scapula, thus providing a base on which a highly mobile joint can function.[38]

Stability in the Shoulder Joint

Maintaining stability, while the four articulations of the shoulder complex collectively allow for a high degree of mobility, is critical for normal function of the shoulder joint. Instability is very often the cause of many of the specific injuries to the shoulder that will be discussed later in this chapter. In the glenohumeral joint, the rounded humeral head articulates with a relatively flat glenoid on the scapula. During movement of the shoulder joint, it is essential to maintain the positioning of the humeral head relative to the glenoid. Likewise it is also critical for the glenoid to adjust its position relative to the moving humeral head while simultaneously maintaining a stable base. The glenohumeral joint is inherently unstable, and stability depends on the coordinated and synchronous function of both dynamic and static stabilizers.[46]

THE DYNAMIC STABILIZERS OF THE GLENOHUMERAL JOINT

The muscles that cross the glenohumeral joint produce motion and function to establish dynamic stability to compensate for a bony and ligamentous arrangement that allows for a great deal of mobility. Movements at the glenohumeral joint include flexion, extension, abduction, adduction, circumduction, and rotation.

The muscles acting on the glenohumeral joint may be classified into two groups. The first group consists of muscles that originate on the axial skeleton and attach to the humerus; these include the latissimus dorsi and the pectoralis major. The second group originates on the scapula and attaches to the humerus; these include the deltoid, teres major, coracobrachialis, subscapularis, supraspinatus, infraspinatus, and teres minor. These muscles constitute the short rotator muscles whose tendons insert into the articular capsule and serve as reinforcing structures. The biceps and triceps muscles attach on the glenoid and affect elbow motion.

The muscles of the rotator cuff, subscapularis, infraspinatus, supraspinatus, and teres minor along with the long head of the biceps function to provide dynamic stability to control the position and prevent excessive displacement or translation of the humeral head relative to the position of the glenoid.[8,43,74]

Stabilization of the humeral head occurs through cocontraction of the rotator cuff muscles. This creates a series of force couples that act to compress the humeral head into the glenoid, minimizing humeral head translation. A force couple involves the action of two opposing forces acting in opposite directions to impose rotation about an axis. These force couples can establish dynamic equilibrium of the glenohumeral joint regardless of the position of the humerus. If an imbalance exists between the muscular components that create these force couples, abnormal glenohumeral mechanics occur.

In the transverse plane a force couple exists between the subscapularis anteriorly and the infraspinatus and teres minor posteriorly (Fig. 25-2). Cocontraction of the infraspina-

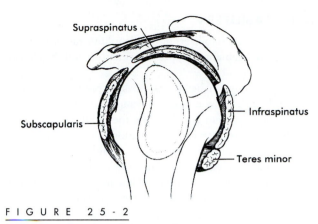

FIGURE 25-2

Transverse plane force couples.

tus, teres minor, and subscapularis muscles both depresses and compresses the humeral head during overhead movements.

In the coronal plane, there is a critical force couple between the deltoid and the inferior rotator cuff muscles (Fig. 25-3). With the arm fully adducted, contraction of the deltoid produces a vertical force in a superior direction, causing an upward translation of the humeral head relative to the glenoid. Cocontraction of the inferior rotator cuff muscles produces both a compressive force and a downward translation of the humerus that counterbalances the force of the deltoid, stabilizing the humeral head. The supraspinatus compresses the humeral head into the glenoid and along with the deltoid initiates abduction on this stable base. Dynamic stability is created by an increase in joint compression forces from contraction of the supraspinatus and by humeral head depression from contraction of the inferior rotator cuff muscles.[8,16,43,74]

The long head of the biceps tendon also contributes to dynamic stability by limiting superior translation of the humerus during elbow flexion and supination.

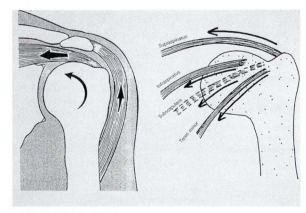

FIGURE 25-3

Coronal plane force couples.

STATIC STABILIZERS

The primary static stabilizers of the glenohumeral joint are the glenohumeral ligaments, the posterior capsule, and the glenoid labrum.

The glenohumeral ligaments appear to produce a major restraint in shoulder flexion, extension, and rotation. The anterior glenohumeral ligament is tight when the shoulder is in extension, abduction, and/or external rotation (ER). The posterior glenohumeral ligament is tight in flexion and ER. The inferior glenohumeral ligament is tight when the shoulder is abducted, extended, and/or externally rotated. The middle glenohumeral ligament is tight when in flexion and ER. Additionally, the middle glenohumeral ligament and the subscapularis tendon limit lateral rotation from 45° to 75° of abduction and are important anterior stabilizers of the glenohumeral joint.[3] The inferior glenohumeral ligament is a primary check against both anterior and posterior dislocation of the humeral head and is the most important stabilizing structure of the shoulder in the overhead athlete.[3]

The tendons of the rotator cuff muscles blend into the glenohumeral joint capsule at their insertions about the humeral head (Fig. 25-4). As these muscles contract, tension is produced, dynamically tightening the capsule and helping to center the humeral head in the glenoid fossa. This creates both static and dynamic control of humeral head movement.

The posterior capsule is tight when the shoulder is in flexion, abduction, internal rotation (IR), or in any combination of these. The superior and middle segment of the posterior capsule has the greatest tension while the shoulder is internally rotated.

The bones and articular surfaces within the shoulder are positioned to contribute to static stability. The glenoid labrum, which is tightly attached to the bottom half of the glenoid and loosely attached at the top, increases the glenoid depth approximately two times, enhancing glenohumeral stability.[41] The scapula faces 30° anteriorly to the chest wall and is tilted upward 3° to enable easier movement on the anterior frontal plane and movements above the shoulder.[28] The glenoid is tilted upward 5° to help control inferior instability.[44]

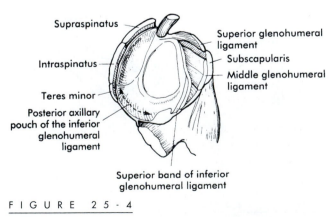

Supraspinatus

Intraspinatus

Teres minor

Posterior axillary
pouch of the inferior
glenohumeral
ligament

Superior glenohumeral
ligament

Subscapularis

Middle glenohumeral
ligament

Superior band of inferior
glenohumeral ligament

FIGURE 25-4

Rotator cuff tendons blend into the joint capsule.

SCAPULAR STABILITY AND MOBILITY

Like the glenohumeral muscles, the scapular muscles play a critical role in normal function of the shoulder. The scapular muscles produce movement of the scapula on the thorax and help to dynamically position the glenoid relative to the moving humerus. They include the levator scapula and upper trapezius, which elevate the scapula; the middle trapezius and rhomboids, which adduct the scapula; the lower trapezius, which adducts and depresses the scapula; the pectoralis minor, which depresses the scapula; and the serratus anterior, which abducts and upward rotates the scapula. Collectively they function to maintain a consistent length–tension relationship with the glenohumeral muscles.[37,38,48]

The only attachment of the scapula to the thorax is through these muscles. The muscle stabilizers must fix the position of the scapula on the thorax, providing a stable base for the rotator cuff to perform its intended function on the humerus. It has been suggested that the serratus anterior moves the scapula while the other scapular muscles function to provide scapular stability.[37,38] The scapular muscles act isometrically, concentrically, or eccentrically, depending on the movement desired and whether the movement is speeding up or slowing down.[44]

Scapulohumeral Rhythm

Scapulohumeral rhythm is the movement of the scapula relative to the movement of the humerus throughout a full range of abduction. As the humerus elevates to 30°, there is no movement of the scapula. This is referred to as the setting phase during which a stable base is being established on the thoracic wall. From 30° to 90°, the scapula abducts and upward rotates 1° for every 2° of humeral elevation. From 90° to full abduction, the scapula abducts and upward rotates 1° for each 1° of humeral elevation. If normal scapulohumeral rhythm is compromised, normal shoulder joint function in moving to a fully elevated position cannot occur, and adaptive compensatory motions can predispose the athlete to injury.[55]

Plane of the Scapula

The concept of the plane of the scapula refers to the angle of the scapula in its resting position, usually 35°–45° anterior to the frontal plane toward the sagittal plane. When the limb is positioned in the plane of the scapula, the mechanical axis of the glenohumeral joint is in line with the mechanical axis of the scapula. The glenohumeral joint capsule is lax, and the deltoid and supraspinatus muscles are optimally positioned to elevate the humerus. Movement of the humerus in this plane is less restricted than in the frontal or sagittal planes, because the glenohumeral capsule is not twisted.[22] Because the rotator cuff muscles originate on the scapula and attach to the humerus, repositioning the humerus into the plane of the scapula increases the length of those muscles, improving the length–tension relationship. This is likely to increase muscle force.[22] It has been recommended that many strengthening exercises for the shoulder joint complex be done in the scapular plane.[22,79,80]

REHABILITATION TECHNIQUES FOR SPECIFIC INJURIES

Sternoclavicular Joint Sprains

PATHOMECHANICS

SC joint sprains are not commonly seen. Although they are rare, the joint's complexity and integral interaction with the other joints of the shoulder complex warrant its discussion. The SC joint has multiple axis of rotation and articulates with the manubrium with an interposed fibrocartilaginous disc. Pathology of this joint can include injury to the fibrocartilage and sprains of the SC ligaments and/or the costoclavicular ligaments.[30]

As stated earlier in this chapter, the SC joint is extremely weak because of its bony arrangement. It is held in place by its strong ligaments, which tend to pull the sternal end of the clavicle downward and toward the sternum. A sprain of these ligaments often results in either a subluxing SC joint or a dislocated SC joint. This can be significant because the joint plays an integral role in scapular motion through the clavicle's articulation with the scapula. Combined movements at the AC and SC joints have been reported to account for up to 60° of upward scapular rotation inherent in glenohumeral abduction.[3]

When this joint incurs an injury, a resultant inflammatory process occurs. The inflammatory process can cause an increase in the joint capsule pressure as well as a stiffening of the joint due to the collagen tissue being produced for the healing tissues. The pathogenesis of this inflammatory process can cause an altering of the joint mechanics as well as an increase in pain felt at the joint. This often results adversely on the shoulder complex.[65]

INJURY MECHANISM

Motor vehicle accidents are the most common source of injuries to the SC joint.[53] The SC joint can be injured by direct or indirect forces, resulting in sprains, dislocations, or physical injuries.[30] Direct force injuries are usually the result of a blow of the anteromedial aspect of the clavicle and produce a posterior dislocation.[30] Indirect force injuries can occur usually when the athlete falls and lands with an outstretched arm in either a flexed and adducted position or extended and adducted position of the upper extremity. The flexed position causes an anterior lateral compression force to the adducted arm, producing a posterior dislocation. The extended position causes a posterior lateral compression force to the adducted arm, leading to an anterior dislocation. Lesser forces can also lead to varying degrees of sprains to the SC joint. There have also been reports of repetitive microtrauma to this joint.[58,65]

REHABILITATION CONCERNS

In addressing the rehabilitation of a patient with a SC joint injury, it is important to address the function of the joint on shoulder complex movement. The SC joint acts as the sole passive attachment of the shoulder complex to the axial skeleton.

As noted earlier in the chapter, the clavicle must elevate approximately 40° to allow upward scapular rotation.[56]

In most cases, the primary problem reported by the injured patient is discomfort associated with end-range movement of the shoulder complex. It is important to identify the cause of the pain (i.e., ligamentous instability, disc degeneration, or ligamentous trauma).

In cases where there is ligamentous instability as well as disc degeneration, the rehabilitation should focus on strengthening the muscles attached to the clavicle in a range that does not put further stress on the joint. Muscles such as the pectoralis minor, sternal fibers of the pectoralis major, and upper trapezius are strengthened to help control the motion of the clavicle during motion of the shoulder complex. Exercises include incline bench, shoulder shrugs, and the seated push-up, in a limited ROM (Figs. 25-22, 25-35, and 25-42). In addition to addressing the dynamic supports of the SC joint, the therapist should employ the appropriate modalities necessary to control pain and the inflammatory process. It is also noteworthy, in case where dislocation or subluxation has occurred, to consider the structures in close proximity to the SC joint. In the case of a posterior dislocation, signs of circulatory vessel compromise nerve tissue impingement, and difficulty in swallowing may be seen. It is important to avoid these symptoms and communicate with the patient's physician regarding any lasting symptoms.[65]

When dealing with ligamentous trauma that lacks instability, the therapist should also address the associated pain with the appropriate modalities and utilize exercises that strengthen muscle with clavicular attachments. In all of the above scenarios, it is important to address the role of the SC joint on shoulder complex movement. A full evaluation of the shoulder complex should be performed to address issues related to scapular elevation. Exercises such as Superman, bent-over row, rhomboids, and push-ups with a plus should be included to help control upward rotation of the scapula (Figs. 25-36 to 25-39). Appropriate progression should be followed while addressing the healing stages for the appropriate tissues.

REHABILITATION PROGRESSION

In the initial stages of rehabilitation, the primary goal is to minimize pain and inflammation associated with shoulder complex motion. The therapist should limit activities to midrange exercises and incorporate the use of therapeutic modalities along with the use of NSAID (nonsteroidal anti-inflammatory drug) intervention from the physician. Ultrasound is often useful for increasing blood flow and facilitating the process of healing. Occasionally a shoulder sling or figure-8 strap can help minimize stress at the joint. During this phase of the rehabilitation progression, the therapist should identify the activity-specific needs of the patient in order to tailor the later phases of rehabilitation to the patient's demands. The patient should also continue to work on exercises that maintain cardiorespiratory fitness.

When the pain and inflammation have been controlled, the patient should gradually engage in a controlled increase of stress to the tissues of the joint. This is a good time to begin low-grade joint mobilizations resisted exercises for the muscles attaching to the clavicle. Exercises in this phase are best done in the midrange to minimize pain. As the patient's tolerance increases, the resistance and ROM can be increased. During this phase it is also important to address any limitations there might be in the athlete's ROM. Emphasis should be placed on restoring the normal mechanics of the shoulder complex during shoulder movements.

As the patient begins to enter the pain-free stages of the progression, the athletic trainer should gradually incorporate activity-specific demands into the exercise program. Examples of this are PNF with rubber tubing (Figs. 25-55 and 25-56), Stair Climber with feet on chair (Fig. 25-44), and rowing machine.

CRITERIA FOR RETURN TO NORMAL ACTIVITY

The patient may return to normal activity when (1) the rehabilitation program has been progressed to the appropriate time and stress for the specific demands of the patient's activity, (2) the patient shows improved strength in the muscles used to protect the SC joint when compared to the uninjured side, and (3) the patient no longer has associated pain with movements of the shoulder complex that will inevitably occur with the demands of his/her activity.

Acromioclavicular Joint Sprains

PATHOMECHANICS

The AC joint is composed of a bony articulation between the clavicle and the scapula. The soft tissues included in the joint are the hyaline cartilage coating the ends of the bony articulations, a fibrocartilaginous disc between the two bones, the AC ligaments, and the costoclavicular ligaments. There have been two conflicting papers regarding the motion available at the joint. Codman reported little movement at the joint, whereas Inman reported exactly the opposite.[13,29] Multiple authors have reported degenerative changes at the AC joint by age 40 in the average healthy adult.[18,62]

The AC joint provides the bridge between the clavicle and the scapula. When an injury occurs to the joint, all soft tissue should be considered in the rehabilitation process. An elaborate grading system has been reported to categorize injuries based on the soft tissue that is involved in the injury (Table 25-1).[60] Through evaluation by X-ray, the patient's injury should be categorized in order to provide the therapist with a guideline for rehabilitation.

INJURY MECHANISM

Type I or type II AC joint sprains are most commonly seen due to a direct fall on the point of the shoulder with the arm at the side in an adducted position or falling on an outstretched arm. The injury mechanism for type III and type IV sprains usually involves a direct impact that forces the acromion process downward, backward, and inward while the clavicle is pushed down against the rib cage. The impact can produce a number of

injuries: (1) fracture of the clavicle, (2) AC joint sprain, (3) AC and coracoclavicular joint sprain, or (4) a combination of the previous injury with concomitant muscle tearing of the deltoid and trapezius at their clavicular attachments.[3] Another possible mechanism for injury to the AC joint is repetitive compression of the joint.[65]

REHABILITATION CONCERNS

Management of AC injuries is dependent on the type of injury.[23] Age, level of activity, and the demand on the patient can also factor into the management of this injury. Most physicians prefer to handle type I and type II injuries conservatively, but some authors have suggested that type I and type II injuries can cause further problems to the patient later in life.[5,15] These injuries might require surgical excision of the distal 2 cm of the clavicle. The therapist should consider when developing a treatment plan (1) the stability of the AC joint, (2) the amount of patient was immobilized, (3) pain, as a guide for the type of exercises being used, and (4) the soft tissue that was involved in the injury. Rehabilitation of these injuries should focus on strengthening the deltoid and trapezius muscles. Additional strengthening of the clavicular fibers of the pectoralis major and that of other muscles that help restore the proper mechanics of the shoulder complex should also be done.

Type I

Treatment for the type I injury consists of ice to relieve pain and a sling to support the extremity for several days. The amount of time in the sling usually depends on the patient's ability to tolerate pain and begin carrying the involved extremity with the appropriate posture. The therapist can have the patient begin active assisted ROM immediately and then incorporate isometric exercises to the muscles with clavicular attachments. This will help restore the appropriate carrying posture for the involved upper extremity. When the patient is able to remove the sling, the therapist should increase the exercise program to incorporate progressive resistive exercises (PREs) for the muscles with clavicular attachments and add exercises to encourage appropriate scapular motion. This will help prevent related shoulder discomfort due to poor glenohumeral mechanics after return to activity.

Type II

The treatment for type II injuries is also nonsurgical. Because this type of injury to the AC joint involves complete disruption of the AC ligaments, immobilization plays a greater role in the treatment of these athletes. There is no consensus as to the duration of immobilization. Some authors have recommended 7–14 days, others have suggested using a sling that not only supports the upper extremity but also depresses the clavicle.[1,65] This debate is fueled by disagreements regarding the time it takes the body to produce collagen and bridge the gap left from the injury. It has been reported that tissue mobilized too early shows a greater amount of type III collagen than the stronger type I collagen.[34] The time needed to heal the soft tissues involved in

TABLE 25-1

Acromioclavicular Sprain Classification

TYPE I
- Sprain of the AC ligaments
- AC ligament intact
- Coracoclavicular ligament, deltoid and trapezius muscles intact

TYPE II
- AC joint disrupted with tearing of the AC ligament
- Coracoclavicular ligament sprained
- Deltoid and trapezius muscles intact

TYPE III
- AC ligament disrupted
- AC joint displaced and the shoulder complex displaced inferiorly
- Coracoclavicular ligament disrupted with a coracoclavicular interspace 25–100% greater than the normal shoulder
- Deltoid and trapezius muscles usually detached from distal end of the clavicle

TYPE IV
- AC ligaments disrupted with the acromioclaricular joint displaced and the clavicle anatomically displaced posteriorly through the trapezius muscle
- Coracoclavicular ligaments disrupted with wider interspace
- Deltoid and trapezius muscles detached

TYPE V
- AC and coracoclavicular ligaments disrupted
- AC joint dislocated and gross displacement between the clavicle and the scapula
- Deltoid and trapezius muscles detached from distal end of the clavicle

TYPE VI
- AC and coracoclavicular ligaments disrupted
- Distal clavicle inferior to the acromion or the coracoid process
- Deltoid and trapezius muscles detached from distal end of the clavicle

this injury must be considered prior to beginning exercises that stress the injury.

Type III

Many authors have recommended a nonoperative approach for this type of injury, most agreeing that a sling is adequate for allowing the patient to rest comfortably.[3] Use of this nonoperative technique has been reported to have limited success. Cox reported improved results without support of the arm in 62 percent of his patients, whereas only 25 percent had relief after 3–6 weeks of immobilization and a sling.[15]

Operative management of this type of injury can be summarized with the following options:

1. Stabilization of clavicle to coracoid with a screw
2. Resection of distal clavicle
3. Transarticular AC fixation with pins
4. Use of coracoclavicular ligament as a substitute AC ligament.

Taft et al. found superior results with coracoclavicular fixation. They found that patients with AC fixation had a higher rate of posttraumatic arthritis than those managed with a coracoclavicular screw.[68]

Type IV, V, and VI

Types IV, V, and VI injuries require open reduction and internal fixation. Operative procedures are designed to attempt realignment of the clavicle to the scapula. The immobilization for this type of injury is longer and therefore the rehabilitation time is longer. After immobilization, the concerns are similar to those previously discussed.

REHABILITATION PROGRESSION

Early in the rehabilitation progression, the therapist should be concerned with application of cold therapy and pressure for the first 24–48 hours to control local hemorrhage. Fitting the patient for a sling is also important to control the patient's pain. Time in the sling depends on the severity of the injury. After the patient has been seen by a physician for differential diagnosis, the rehabilitation progression should be tailored to the type of sprain according to the diagnosis.

Type I, II, and III sprains should be handled similarly at first, with the time of progression accelerated with less severe sprains. Exercises should begin with encouraging the patient to use the involved extremity for activities of daily living and gentle ROM exercises. Return of normal ROM in the patient's shoulder is the first objective goal. The patient can also begin isometric exercises to maintain or restore muscle function in the shoulder. These exercises can be started while the patient is in the sling. Once the sling is removed, pendulum exercises can be started to encourage movement. In type III sprains the therapist should hold off doing passive ROM exercises in the end ranges of shoulder elevation for the first 7 days. The patient should have full passive ROM by 2–3 weeks. Once the patient has full active ROM, a program of PREs should begin. Strengthening of the deltoid and upper trapezius muscles should be emphasized. The therapist should evaluate the patient's shoulder mechanics to identify problems with neuromuscular control and address specific deficiencies as noted. As the patient regains strength in the involved extremity, activity-specific exercises should be incorporated into the rehabilitation program. Gradual return to activity should be supervised by the therapist.

In the case of type IV, V, and VI AC sprains, a postsurgical progression should be followed. The therapist should design a program that is broken down into four phases of rehabilitation with the goal of returning the patient to activity as quickly as possible.[3] Contact with the physician is important to determine the time frame in which each phase may begin. Common surgeries for this injury include open reduction with pin or screw fixation and/or acromioplasty.

The early stage of rehabilitation should be designed with the goal of reestablishing pain-free ROM, preventing muscle atrophy, and decreasing pain and inflammation. ROM exercises may include Codman's exercises (Fig. 25-6), rope and pulley exercises (Fig. 25-9), L-bar exercises (Figs. 25-11 to 25-16), and self-capsular stretches (Figs. 25-18 and 25-19). Strengthening exercises in this phase may include isometrics in all of the cardinal planes and isometrics for medial and lateral rotation of the glenohumeral joint at 0° of elevation (Fig. 25-20).

As rehabilitation progresses, the therapist has the goal of regaining and improving muscle strength, normalizing arthrokinematics, and improving neuromuscular control of the shoulder complex. Prior to advancing to this phase, the patient should have full ROM, minimal pain and tenderness, and a 4/5 manual muscle test for IR, ER, and flexion. Initiation of isotonic PREs should begin. Shoulder medial and lateral rotation (Figs. 25-31 and 25-32), shoulder flexion and abduction to 90° (Figs. 25-26 and 25-28), scaption (Fig. 25-33), bicep curls, and tricep extensions should be included. Additionally, a program of scapular stabilizing exercises should begin. Exercises should include Superman exercises (Fig. 25-36), rhomboids ex-

ercises (Fig. 25-38), shoulder shrugs (Fig. 25-35), and seated push-ups (Fig. 25-42). To help normalize arthrokinematics of the shoulder, complex joint mobilization techniques should be used for the glenohumeral, AC, SC, and scapulothoracic joints (see Figs. 16-10 to 16-20). To complete this phase the patient should begin neuromuscular control exercises (Figs. 25-59 to 25-68), trunk exercises, and a low-impact aerobic exercise program.

During the advanced strengthening phase of rehabilitation, the goals should be to improve strength, power, and endurance of muscles as well as to improve neuromuscular control of the shoulder complex, and preparing the patient to return to specific activities. Prior to advancing to this phase, the therapist should use the criteria of full pain-free ROM, no pain or tenderness, and strength of 70 percent compared to the uninvolved shoulder. The emphasis in this phase is on high-speed strengthening, eccentric exercises, and multiplanar motions. The patient should advance to surgical tubing exercises (Fig. 25-45), plyometric exercises (Figs. 25-46 to 25-51), PNF diagonal strengthening (Figs. 25-53 to 25-58), and isokinetic strengthening exercises (Fig. 25-52).

When the patient is ready to return to activity, the therapist should progressively increase activities that prepare the patient for full functional return. An interval program of activities should be started. Exercises from stage III should be continued. The patient should progressively increase the time of participation in specific activities as tolerated.

CRITERIA FOR RETURN TO NORMAL ACTIVITY

Prior to returning to normal activity the patient should have full ROM and no pain or tenderness. Isokinetic strength testing should meet the demands of the patient's level of activity and the patient should have successfully completed the final phase of the rehabilitation progression.

Clavicle Fractures

PATHOMECHANICS

Clavicle fractures are among the most common fractures. The clavicle acts as a strut connecting the upper extremity to the trunk of the body.[19] Forces acting on the clavicle are most likely to cause a fracture of the bone medial to the attachment of the coracoclavicular ligaments.[4] Intact AC and coracoclavicular ligaments help keep fractures nondisplaced and stabilized.

INJURY MECHANISM

The mechanism can be direct or indirect. Fractures can result from a fall on an outstretched arm, a fall or blow to the point of the shoulder, or less commonly a direct blow.

REHABILITATION CONCERNS

Early identification of the fracture is an important factor in rehabilitation. If stabilization occurs early, with minimal damage and irritation to the surrounding structures, the likelihood of an uncomplicated return to activity increases. Other factors influencing the likelihood of complications are injuries to the AC, coracoclavicular, and SC ligaments. Treatment for clavicle fractures includes approximation of the fracture and immobilization for 6–8 weeks. Most commonly a figure-8 wrap is used, with the involved arm in a sling.

When designing a rehabilitation program for a patient who has sustained a clavicle fracture, the therapist should consider the function of the clavicle. The clavicle acts as a strut offering shoulder girdle stability and allowing the upper extremity to move more freely about the thorax by positioning the extremity away from the body axis.[25] Mobility of the clavicle is therefore very important to normal shoulder mechanics. Joint mobilization techniques are started immediately after the immobilization period in order to restore normal arthrokinematics. The clavicle also serves as an insertion point for the deltoid, upper trapezius, and pectoralis major muscles, providing stability and aiding in neuromuscular control of the shoulder complex. It is important to address these muscles with the appropriate exercises in order to restore normal shoulder mechanics.

REHABILITATION PROGRESSION

For the first 6–8 weeks, the patient is immobilized in the figure-8 brace and sling. If good approximation and healing of the fracture is occurring at 6 weeks, the patient may begin gentle isometric exercises for the upper extremity. Utilization of the involved extremity below 90° of elevation should be encouraged to prevent muscle atrophy and excessive loss of glenohumeral ROM. After the immobilization period, the patient should begin a program to regain full active and passive ROM. Joint mobilization techniques are used to restore normal arthrokinematics (see Figs. 16-10 to 16-12). The patient may continue to wear the sling for the next 3–4 weeks while regaining the ability to carry the arm in an appropriate posture without the figure-8 brace. The patient should begin a strengthening program utilizing progressive resistance as ROM improves. Once full ROM is achieved, the patient should begin resisted diagonal PNF exercises and continue to increase the strength of the shoulder complex muscle, including the periscapular muscles, to enable normal neuromuscular control of the shoulder.

CRITERIA FOR NORMAL RETURN

The patients may return to activity when the fracture is clinically united, full active and passive range of motion (PROM) is achieved, and they have the strength and neuromuscular control to meet the demands of their activity.

Glenohumeral Dislocations/Instabilities (Surgical versus Nonsurgical Rehabilitation)

PATHOMECHANICS

Dislocations of the glenohumeral joint involve the temporary displacement of the humeral head from its normal position in the glenoid labral fossa. From a biomechanical perspective, the resultant force vector is directed outside the arc of contact in the glenoid fossa, creating a dislocating moment of the humeral head by pivoting about the labral rim.[20]

Shoulder dislocations account for up to 50 percent of all dislocations. The inherent instability of the shoulder joint necessary for the extreme mobility of this joint makes the glenohumeral joint susceptible to dislocation. The most common kind of dislocation is that occurring anteriorly. Posterior dislocations account for only 1–4.3 percent of all shoulder dislocations. Inferior dislocations are extremely rare. Of dislocations caused by direct trauma, 85–90 percent are recurring.[63]

In an anterior glenohumeral dislocation, the head of the humerus is forced out of its anterior capsule in an anterior direction past the glenoid labrum and then downward to rest under the coracoid process. The pathology that ensues is extensive, with torn capsular and ligamentous tissue, possibly tendinous avulsion of the rotator cuff muscles, and profuse hemorrhage. A tear or detachment of the glenoid labrum might also be present. Healing is usually slow, and the detached labrum and capsule can produce a permanent anterior defect on the glenoid labrum called a Bankart lesion. Another defect that can occur with anterior dislocation can be found on the posterior lateral aspect of the humeral head called a Hill-Sachs lesion. This is caused by compressive forces between the humeral head and the glenoid rim, while the humeral head rests in the dislocated position. Additional complications can arise if the head of the humerus comes into contact with and injures the brachial nerves and vessels. Rotator cuff tears can also arise as a result of the dislocation. The bicipital tendon might also sublux from its canal as the result of a rupture of the transverse ligament.[63]

Posterior dislocations can also result in significant soft-tissue damage. Tears of the posterior glenoid labrum are common in posterior dislocation. A fracture of the lesser tubercle can occur if the subscapularis tendon avulses its attachment.

Glenohumeral dislocation is usually very disabling. The athlete assumes an obvious disabled posture and the deformity itself is obvious. A positive sulcus sign is usually present at the time of the dislocation, and the deformity can be easily recognized on X-ray. As detailed above, the damage can be extensive to the soft tissue.

INJURY MECHANISM

When discussing the mechanism of injury for dislocations of the glenohumeral joint, it is necessary to categorize the injury as traumatic or atraumatic, and anterior or posterior. An anterior dislocation of the glenohumeral joint can result from direct impact to the posterior or posterolateral aspect of the shoulder. The most common mechanism is forced abduction, ER, and extension that forces the humeral head out of the glenoid cavity.[45] The injury mechanism for a posterior glenohumeral dislocation is usually forced adduction and IR of the shoulder or a fall on an extended and internally rotated arm.

The two mechanisms described for anterior dislocation can be categorized as traumatic or atraumatic. The following acronyms have been described to summarize the two mechanisms.[36]

Traumatic
Unidirectional
Bankart lesion
Surgery required

Atraumatic
Multidirectional
Bilateral involvement
Rehabilitation effective
Inferior capsular shift recommended

The AMBRI group can be characterized by subluxation or dislocation episodes without trauma, resulting in a stretched capsuloligamentous complex that lacks end-range stabilizing ability. Several authors report a high rate of recurrence for dislocations, especially those in the TUBS category.[61]

REHABILITATION CONCERNS

Management of shoulder dislocation depends on a number of factors that need to be identified. Mechanism, chronology, and direction of instability all need to be considered in the development of a conservatively managed rehabilitation program. No single rehabilitation program is an absolute solution for success in the treatment of a shoulder dislocation. The therapist should thoroughly evaluate the injury and discuss those objective findings with the team physician. The initial concern in rehabilitation focuses on maintaining appropriate reduction of the glenohumeral joint. The patient is immobilized in a reduced position for a period of time, depending on the type of management used in the reduction (surgical versus nonsurgical). For the purpose of this section, the discussion will continue with conservative management in mind. The principles of rehabilitation, however, remain constant regardless of whether the physician's management is surgical or nonsurgical. Surgical rehabilitation should be based on the healing time of tissue affected by the surgery. The limitations of motion in the early stages of rehabilitation should also be based on surgical fixation. It is extremely important, because of this, that the therapist and physician communicate prior to the start of rehabilitation. After the immobilization period, the rehabilitation program should be focused on restoring the appropriate axis of rotation for the glenohumeral joint, optimizing the stabilizing muscle's length–tension relationship, and restoring proper neuromuscular control to the shoulder complex. In the uninjured shoulder complex with intact capsuloligamentous structures, the glenohumeral joint maintains a tight axis of rotation within the glenoid fossa.

This is accomplished dynamically with complex neuromuscular control of the periscapular muscles, rotator cuff muscles, and intact passive structures of the joint. Because the extent of damage in this type of injury is variable, the exercises employed to restore these normal mechanics should also vary.[60]

As the therapist helps the patient regain full ROM, a safe zone of positioning should be followed. Starting in the plane of the scapula is safe, because the axis of rotation for forces acting on the joint fall in the center of this plane. The least provocative position is somewhere between 20° and 55° of scapular plane abduction. Keeping the humerus below 55° prevents subacromial impingement, while avoiding full adduction minimizes excessive tension across the supraspinatus/coracohumeral and/or capsuloligamentous complex. As ROM improves, the therapist should progress the exercise program into positions outside the safe zone, accommodating the demands that the patient will need to meet. Specific strengthening should be given to address the muscles of the shoulder complex responsible for maintaining the axis of rotation, such as the supraspinatus and rotator cuff muscles. The periscapular muscles should also be addressed in order to provide the rotator cuff muscles with their optimal length–tension relationship for more efficient usage. In the later stages of rehabilitation, neuromuscular control exercises are incorporated with activity-specific exercises to prepare the patient for return to normal activity.[36]

REHABILITATION PROGRESSION

The first essential to a successful rehabilitation program is to protect the patient from activities that risk reinjury to the glenohumeral joint. A reasonable time frame for return to normal activity is approximately 12 weeks, with unrestricted activity coming closer to 20 weeks. This is variable, depending on the extent of soft-tissue damage and the type of intervention chosen by the patient and physician. Some exercises previously used by the patient might produce undesired forces on noncontractile tissues and need to be modified to be performed safely. Push-ups, pull-downs, and the bench press are performed with the hands in close and avoiding the last 10°–20° of shoulder extension. Pull-downs and military press performed with wide bars and machines are kept in front rather than behind the head. Supine fly exercises are limited to −30° in the coronal plane while maintaining glenohumeral IR. See Table 25-2 for further modifications dependent on directional instability.[3]

TABLE 25-2

Exercise Modification Per Direction of Instability

DIRECTION OF INSTABILITY	POSITION TO AVOID	EXERCISES TO BE MODIFIED OR AVOIDED
Anterior	Combined position of ER and abduction	Fly, pull-down, push-up, bench press, military press
Posterior	Combined position of IR, horizontal adduction, and flexion	Fly, push-up bench press, weight-bearing exercises
Inferior	Full elevation, dependent arm	Shrugs, elbow curls, military press

During phase 1 the patient is immobilized in a sling. This lasts for up to 3 weeks with first-time dislocations. The goal of this phase is to limit the inflammatory process, decrease pain, and retard muscle atrophy. PROM exercises can be initiated along with low-grade joint mobilization techniques to encourage relaxation of the shoulder musculature. Isometric exercises are also started. The athlete begins with submaximal contractions and increases to maximal contractions for as long as 8 seconds. The protective phase is a good time to initiate a scapulothoracic exercise program, avoiding elevated positions of the upper extremity that put stability at risk. Patients should begin an aerobic training regime with the lower extremity, such as stationary biking.

Phase 2 begins after the patient has been removed from the sling. This phase lasts from 3 to 8 weeks postinjury and focuses on full return of active ROM. The program begins with the use of an L-bar performing active assistive ROM (Figs. 25-11 to 25-16). Manual therapy techniques can also begin using PNF techniques to help reestablish neuromuscular control (see Figs. 15-6 to 15-13). Exercises with the hands on the ground can help begin strengthening the scapular stabilizers more aggressively. These exercises should begin on a stable surface like a table, progressing the amount of weight bearing by advancing from the table to the ground (Fig. 25-59). Advancing to a less stable surface like a Biomechanical Ankle Platform System (BAPS board) (Fig. 25-63) or Swiss ball (Fig. 25-64) will also help reestablish neuromuscular control.

At 6–12 weeks the therapist should gradually enter phase 3 of the rehabilitation progression. The goal of this phase is to restore normal strength and neuromuscular control. Prophylactic stretching is done, as full ROM should already be present. Scapular and rotator cuff exercises should focus on strength and endurance. Weight-bearing exercises should be made more challenging by adding motion to the demands of the stabilization. Scapular exercises should be performed with guidance from the therapist. Weight shifting on a Fitter (Fig. 25-61) and closed-kinetic-chain strengthening on a stair climber (Fig. 25-44) for endurance are started. Strengthening exercises progress from PRE to plyometric. Rotator cuff exercises using surgical tubing with emphasis on eccentrics are added.[2] Progression to multiangle exercises is started. A Body Blade is a good rehabilitation tool for this phase (Fig. 25-68), progressing from static to dynamic stabilization and single-position to multiangular dynamic exercises.

Phase 4 is the functional progression. Patients are gradually returned to activity with progressive activity increasing the demands on endurance and stability. This can last as long as 20 weeks, depending on the patient's shoulder strength, lack of pain, and ability to protect the involved shoulder. The physician should be consulted prior to normal return to activity.

CRITERIA FOR RETURN TO NORMAL ACTIVITY

At 20–26 weeks, the patient should be ready for return to normal activity. This decision should be based on (1) full pain-free ROM, (2) normal shoulder strength, (3) pain-free specific ac-

tivities, and (4) ability to protect the patient's shoulder from reinjury.

Multidirectional Instabilities of the Glenohumeral Joint

PATHOMECHANICS

Multidirectional instabilities are an inherent risk of the glenohumeral joint. The shoulder has the greatest ROM of all the joints in the human body. The bony restraints are minimal, and the forces that can be generated in overhead activities far exceed the strength of the static restraints of the joint. Attenuation of force is multifactorial, with time, distance, and speed-determining forces applied to the joint. Thus stability of the joint must be evaluated based on the patient's ability to dynamically control all of these factors in order to have a stable joint. In cases of multidirectional instability, there are two categories for pathology: atraumatic and traumatic. The atraumatic category includes patients who have congenitally loose joints or who have increased the demands on their shoulder prior to having developed the muscular maturity to meet these demands. When forces are generated at the glenohumeral joint that the stabilizing muscles are unable to handle (this occurs most commonly during the deceleration phase of throwing), the humeral head tends to translate anteriorly and inferiorly into the capsuloligamentous structures. Over time, repetitive microtrauma causes these structures to stretch. Lephart et al. document the essential importance of tension in the anterior capsule of the glenohumeral joint as a protective mechanism against excessive strain in these capsuloligamentous structures.[40] They theorized that the loss of this protective reflex joint stabilization can increase the potential for continuing shoulder injury. Increased translation of the humeral head also increases the demand on the posterior structures of the glenohumeral joint, leading to repetitive microtrauma and breakdown of those soft tissues. In this type of instability there will usually be some inferior laxity, leading to a positive sulcus sign. Although the anterior glenoid labrum is usually intact during the early stages of this instability, splitting and partial detachment can develop.[3] The patient usually has some pain and clicking when the arm is held by the side. Any symptoms and signs associated with anterior or posterior recurrent instability may be present.

INJURY MECHANISM

It is generally believed that the cause of multidirectional instability is excessive joint volume with laxity of the capsuloligamentous complex. This laxity might be an inherent condition that becomes more pronounced with the superimposed trauma of activity. This type of instability might also occur due to extensive capsulolabral trauma in patients who do not appear to have laxity of other joints.[58]

REHABILITATION CONCERNS

The rehabilitation concerns for multidirectional instability are similar to those already discussed in relation to shoulder instabilities. The complexity of this program is increased due to the addition of inferior instability. The success of the program is often determined by the patient's tissue status and compliance.[67] Additionally, this program emphasizes the anterior and posterior musculature. These muscles working together are referred to as force couples and are believed to be essential stabilizers of the joint. The rehabilitation program should also address the neuromuscular control of these muscles to promote dynamic stability.[26] Compliance is often an extremely important factor in maintaining good results with this type of instability. The patient must continue to do the exercise program even after symptoms have subsided. If the patient does not, subluxation usually recurs. For cases where conservative treatment is not successful, Neer recommended an inferior capsular shift surgical procedure that has proven successful in restoring joint stability when used in conjunction with a rehabilitation program.[50]

Recently, there has been some controversy regarding surgical management of multidirectional instability. Many orthopedists are choosing to use thermal-assisted capsular shrinkage. Wilk et al.[81] suggest a postoperative rehabilitation program that is based on six factors: (1) type of instability, (2) patient's inflammatory response to surgery, (3) concomitant surgical procedures, (4) precautions following surgery, (5) gradual rate of progression, and (6) team approach to treatment. These factors determine the type and aggressiveness of the program. First, it must be determined whether the instability is congenital or acquired. Congenital instabilities should be treated more conservatively. Second, some patients respond to surgery with excessive scarring and proliferation of collagen ground tissue. Progression should be adjusted weekly, based on assessing capsular end feel. The third factor takes into account any other procedures performed at the time of surgery. Precautions should be followed based on the tissue-healing time of the other procedures. Surgical precautions also should be communicated to the therapist based on the tissues involved; PROM after surgery should be cautious. The authors suggest conservative PROM progression for the first 8-weeks postsurgery. The gradual progression (factor 5) contrasts to one that moves faster and then slows down. The speed of progression should be based on a weekly scheduled assessment of capsular end feel and progress. Factor 6 ensures a successful rehabilitation outcome by open and continuous communication between the patient, surgeon, and therapist.[81]

REHABILITATION PROGRESSION

The rehabilitation program should begin with reestablishing muscle tone and proper scapulothoracic posture. This helps provide a steady base with appropriate length–tension relationships for the anterior and posterior muscles of the shoulder complex acting as force couples. Strengthening of the rotator cuff muscles in the plane of the scapula should progress to higher resistance, starting at 0° of shoulder elevation. As the patient becomes asymptomatic, the therapist should incorporate an emphasis on neuromuscular control exercises like PNF, rhythmic stabilization, and weight-bearing activity to establish cocontraction

at the glenohumeral joint. For successful results, the patients might have to continue a program of maintenance for neuromuscular control for as long as they wish to be asymptomatic.

Postsurgical Management

For a patient who has undergone thermal-assisted capsular shrinkage surgery, a four-phase rehabilitation may be performed.[81] The program also uses a rule of six paradigm.

The first 6 weeks is a protective phase; the goals are prevention of muscle atrophy, initiation of protected motion, soft-tissue healing, and diminished pain and inflammation. During this phase a sling is used for the first 7–10 days and the patient continues to sleep with a sling through day 14. Elbow and wrist exercises are initiated. ROM is done actively or actively assisted starting in the scapular plane (Fig. 25-33), progressing to 160° of elevation, ER at 90° (75°–80°), IR at 90° abduction (60°–65°) by week 6. Extension and cardinal-plane abduction are avoided.

Phase 2 is an intermediate phase from week 6 to 12. The goals of this phase are to restore full ROM, normalize arthrokinematics, improve dynamic stability, and restore basic muscular strength. Full functional ROM should be achieved by week 8 with 180° of flexion, 90°–100° of ER at the 90/90 position, and 60°–65° of IR at the 90/90 position of the upper extremity. Aggressive stretching may be used if the ROM goals are not achieved by week 8. From week 9 to 12, ROM is progressed out of the safe zone to achieve full functional ROM. During this phase, posterior cuff mobility should be monitored and restored to normal. Isotonic strengthening exercises are begun in all planes, scapular stabilizing exercises are started with weights (Figs. 25-34 to 25-38), and dynamic stabilization exercises for the glenohumeral joint (Figs. 25-53 to 25-56), PNF exercises (Figs. 25-59 to 25-68), and closed-kinetic-chain activities are progressed to tolerance. Two-handed plyometric exercises on the Plyoback are also used for strengthening in the later part of this phase (Fig. 25-46).

Phase 3 is the advanced activity and strengthening phase, from week 12 to 20. The goals of this phase include improvement of strength, power, and endurance, enhancement of neuromuscular control, and performance of functional activities. The criteria to enter this phase should include full ROM, no pain, and muscular strength at least 80 percent of the contralateral side.[80] Capsular stretching and flexibility are continued. Strengthening exercises are progressed with PREs. Plyometric exercises are advanced to single-arm activities (Fig. 25-46). Neuromuscular control and dynamic stabilization exercises are advanced (Figs. 25-53 to 25-57).

The final phase is initiated from week 26 to 29. The criteria to enter phase 4 are full ROM, no pain, satisfactory strength as measured by isokinetic testing (Fig. 25-52), and a normal clinical evaluation. Full return is usually achieved in 7–10 months.

CRITERIA FOR RETURN TO FULL ACTIVITY

The criteria for this instability are the same as described for other shoulder instabilities. Burkhead and Rockwood reported an 80 percent success rate using a conservative approach with patients who had atraumatic multidirectional instability.[10,60]

Glenoid Labral Injuries

PATHOMECHANICS

As mentioned above, glenoid labrum injuries can occur during traumatic anterior dislocations. The Bankart lesion occurs in the anterior inferior quadrant of the glenoid. The other labral pathologies occur in the superior labrum. The SLAP or superior labrum anterior–posterior lesion, first described by Andrews in 1985 and defined later by Synder in 1990 involves labral tears that occur in the anterior superior quadrant to the posterior superior quandrant.[2,64]

Injuries to the glenoid labrum can be from trauma such as falls on outstretched arms, lifting heavy weights that stress the long head of the biceps, or from overhead activities such as throwing.[2,62] Synder (Figs. 25-69A–D) described the four most common SLAP injuries as Type I which involves fraying and degeneration of the superior labrum but demonstrates a firm attachment of the labrum and biceps tendon to the glenoid. Type II injury involves a detachment of the superior labrum and biceps from the glenoid rim. Type III injury demonstrates a bucket-handle tear of the labrum with an intact biceps anchor. Type IV injury is a bucket handle tear of the labrum that extends into the biceps tendon.[64]

INJURY MECHANISM

Falls on an outstretched arm can cause damage to the glenoid labrum. Heavy lifting stressing the bicep may also damage the superior labrum. Overhead activities such as throwing are implicated for some types of SLAP tears. These injuries result from repetitive activity with a tight posterior capsule, over rotation of the glenohumeral joint into ER, or capsular laxity.[64]

REHABILITATION CONCERNS

There is not much research to support labral injuries healing on their own especially with SLAP lesions. Appropriate ROM, strengthening, and proprioception activities may reduce symptoms produced by these lesions. Many SLAP lesions do not cause the patient a lot of discomfort except during overhead activities.

In general, postoperative routines for Bankart lesions follow postoperative routines for surgeries for shoulder instability and vary as to the surgeon and surgery type. Basically the repaired tissue must have stress-free time to allow basic healing. There should then be a gradual increase of stress to the healing tissue.

SLAP lesions have varied healing rates depending on injury and type of repair. Type I and III lesions may be arthroscopically debrided. Symptomatic progress of the rehabilitation program is indicated. Type II and IV lesions often utilize fixation devices that serve to reattach the damaged portion of the labrum to the glenoid. Repairs of Type II and IV SLAP lesions require protected healing times best described by the surgeon.

REHABILITATION PROGRESSION

Rehabilitation progression for the glenoid labral injury often follows the shoulder instability routine outlined previously. It is important to follow the surgeon's guidelines for ROM and strength progressions postoperatively. Wilk et al. have outlined postoperative protocols for Type II and IV lesions that are specific to the surgeon's guidelines for motion progression. Overall, ROM, strength, and proprioception programs are added gradually. Return to function and play activities must be carefully monitored and progressed as per the surgeon's guidelines.[81]

Shoulder Impingement

PATHOMECHANICS

Shoulder impingement syndrome was first identified by Dr. Charles Neer,[50] who observed that impingement involves a mechanical compression of the supraspinatus tendon, the subacromial bursa, and the long head of the biceps tendon, all of which are located under the coracoacromial arch. This syndrome has been described as a continuum during which repetitive compression eventually leads to irritation and inflammation that progresses to fibrosis and eventually to rupture of the rotator cuff. Neer has identified three stages of shoulder impingement:

Stage I

- Seen in patients younger than 25 years with report of repetitive overhead activity
- Localized hemorrhage and edema with tenderness at supraspinatus insertion and anterior acromion
- Painful arc between 60° and 119°, increased with resistance at 90°
- Muscle tests revealing weakness secondary to pain
- Positive Neer or Hawkins–Kennedy impingement signs (Figs. 25-70 and 25-71)
- Normal radiographs, typically
- Reversible; usually resolving with rest, activity modification, and rehabilitation program

Stage II

- Seen in patients 25–40 years of age with report of repetitive overhead activity
- Many of the same clinical findings as in Stage I
- Severity of symptoms worse than Stage I, progressing to pain with activity and night pain
- More soft-tissue crepitus or catching at 100°
- Restriction in passive ROM due to fibrosis
- Possibly radiographs showing osteophytes under acromion, degenerative AC joint changes
- No longer reversible with rest; possibly helped by a long-term rehabilitation program

Stage III

- Seen in patients older than 40 years with history of chronic tendinitis and prolonged pain
- Many of the same clinical findings as Stage II
- Tear in rotator cuff usually less than 1 cm

- More limitation in active and passive ROM
- Possibly a prominent capsular laxity with multidirectional instability seen on radiograph
- Atrophy of infraspinatus and supraspinatus due to disuse
- Treatment typically surgical following a failed conservative approach

Neer's impingement theory was based primarily on the treatment of older, nonathletic patients. The older population will likely exhibit what has been referred to as "outside" or "outlet" impingement.[7,50] In outside impingement there is contact of the rotator cuff with the coracoacromial ligament or the acromion with fraying, abrasion, inflammation, fibrosis, and degeneration of the superior surface of the cuff within the subacromial space. There might also be evidence of degenerative processes, including spurring, decreased joint space due to fibrotic changes, and decreased vascularity.

"Inside" or "nonoutlet" impingement is more likely to occur in the younger patient. With inside impingement the subacromial space appears relatively normal. With forced humeral elevation and IR, the rotator cuff can be impinged on the posterior superior glenoid labrum and the humeral head, potentially producing inflammation on the undersurface of the rotator cuff tendon, posterior superior tears in the glenoid labrum, and lesions in the posterior humeral head (Bankart lesion).

The mechanical impingement syndrome as originally proposed by Neer has been referred to as primary impingement. Jobe and Kvnite have proposed that an unstable shoulder permits excessive translation of the humeral head in an anterior and superior direction, resulting in what has been termed secondary impingement.[31] Based on the relationship of shoulder instability to shoulder impingement, Jobe and Kvnite have proposed an alternative system of classification[31]:

Group IA
- Found in recreational patients older than 35 years with pure mechanical impingement and no instability
- Positive impingement signs
- Lesions on the superior surface of the rotator cuff, possibly with subacromial spurring
- Possibly some arthritic changes in the glenohumeral joint

Group IB
- Found in patients over 35 years old who demonstrate instability with impingement secondary to mechanical trauma
- Positive impingement signs
- Lesions found on the undersurface of the rotator cuff, superior glenoid, and humeral head

Group II
- Found in young patients (less than 35 years old) who demonstrate instability and impingement secondary to repetitive microtrauma
- Positive impingement signs with excessive anterior translation of humeral head

- Lesions on the posterior superior glenoid rim, posterior humeral head, or anterior inferior capsule
- Lesions on the undersurface of the rotator cuff

Group III
- Found in young patients (less than 35 years old)
- Positive impingement signs with atraumatic multidirectional, usually bilateral, humeral instabilities
- Demonstrated generalized laxity in all joints
- Humeral head lesions as in Group II but less severe

Group IV
- Found in young patients (less than 35 years old) with anterior instability resulting from a traumatic event but without impingement
- Posterior defect in the humeral head
- Damage in the posterior glenoid labrum

It has also been proposed that wear of the rotator cuff is due to intrinsic tendon pathology, including tendonopathy and partial or small complete tears with age-related thinning, degeneration, and weakening. This permits superior migration of the humeral head, leading to secondary impingement, thus creating a cycle that can ultimately lead to full-thickness tears.[73]

A "critical zone" of vascular insufficiency has been proposed to exist in the tendon of the supraspinatus, which is found at about 1 cm proximal to its distal insertion on the humerus. It has been hypothesized that when the humerus is adducted and internally rotated, a "wringing out" of the blood supply occurs in this tendon. Should this occur repetitively, such as in the recovery phase on a swimming stroke, ultimately irritation and inflammation may lead to partial or complete rotator cuff tears.[59]

It is likely that some as yet unidentified combination of mechanical, traumatic, degenerative, and vascular processes collectively lead to pathology in the rotator cuff.

INJURY MECHANISM

Shoulder impingement syndrome occurs when there is compromise of the subacromial space under the coracoacromial arch. When the dynamic and static stabilizers of the shoulder complex for one reason or another fail to maintain this subacromial space, the soft-tissue structures are compressed, leading to irritation and inflammation. Impingement often occurs in repetitive overhead athletic activities such as throwing, swimming, serving a tennis ball, or spiking a volleyball, or during handstands in gymnastics. There is ongoing disagreement regarding the specific mechanisms that cause shoulder impingement syndrome. It has been proposed that mechanical impingement can result from either structural or functional causes. Structural causes can be attributed to existing congenital abnormalities or to degenerative changes under the coracoacromial arch and might include the following:

- An abnormally shaped acromion (Fig. 25-72). Patients with a type III or hook-shaped acromion are approximately

70 percent more likely to exhibit signs of impingement than those with a flat or slightly curved acromion.[6]

- Inherent capsular laxity compromises the ability of the glenohumeral joint capsule to act as both a static and a dynamic stabilizer.[31]
- Ongoing or recurring tendinitis or subacromial bursitis causes a loss of space under the coracoacromial arch, which can potentially lead to irritation of other uninflamed structures, setting up a vicious degenerative cycle.[65]
- Laxity in the anterior capsule due to recurrent subluxation or dislocation can allow an anterior migration of the humeral head, which can cause impingement under the coracoid process.[77]
- Postural malalignments such as a forward head, round shoulders, and an increased kyphotic curve, which cause the scapular glenoid to be positioned such that the space under the coracoacromial arch is decreased, can also contribute to impingement.

Functional causes include adaptive changes that occur with repetitive overhead activities, altering the normal biomechanical function of the shoulder complex. These include the following:

- Failure of the rotator cuff to dynamically stabilize the humeral head relative to the glenoid, producing excessive translation and instability. The inferior rotator cuff muscles (infraspinatus, teres minor, subscapularis) should act collectively to both depress and compress the humeral head. In the overhead or throwing athlete, the internal rotators must be capable of producing humeral rotation on the order of 7000°/second.[71] The subcapularis tends to be stronger than the infraspinatus and teres minor, creating a strength imbalance in the existing force couple in the transverse plane. This imbalance produces excessive anterior translation of the humeral head. Furthermore, weakness in the inferior rotator cuff muscles creates an imbalance in the existing force couple with the deltoid in the coronal plane. The deltoid produces excessive superior translation of the humeral head, decreasing subacromial space. Weakness in the supraspinatus, which normally functions to compress the humeral head into the glenoid, allows for excessive superior translation of the humeral head.[75]
- Because the tendons of the rotator cuff blend into the joint capsule, we rely on tension created in the capsule by contraction of the rotator cuff to both statically and dynamically center the humeral head relative to the glenoid. Tightness in the posterior and inferior portions of the glenohumeral joint capsule causes an anterosuperior migration of the humeral head, again decreasing the subacromial space. In the overhead athlete, ROM in IR is usually limited by tightness of both the muscles that externally rotate and the posterior capsule. There tends to be excessive ER, primarily due to laxity in the anterior joint capsule.[9]
- The scapular muscles function to dynamically position the glenoid relative to the humeral head, maintaining a normal length–tension relationship with the rotator cuff. As

the humerus moves into elevation, the scapula should also move so that the glenoid is able to adjust regardless of the position of the elevating humerus. Weakness in the serratus anterior, which elevates, upward rotates, and abducts (protracts) the scapula, or weakness in the levator scapula or upper trapezius, which elevate the scapula, will compromise positioning of the glenoid during humeral elevation, interfering with normal scapulohumeral rhythm. Of great importance to scapulohumeral rhythm is the lower trapezius. Along with the serratus anterior, the lower trapezius completes the force couple critical to normal scapular upward rotation and glenoid positioning. Additionally, it is very common for the upper trapezius to overpower the lower and middle trapezius and cause excessive upward displacement of the scapula, which can contribute to subacromial impingement.

- It is critical for the scapula to maintain a stable base on which the highly mobile humerus can move. Weakness in the rhomboids and/or middle and low trapezius, which function eccentrically to decelerate the scapula in high-velocity throwing motions, can contribute to scapular hypermobility. Likewise, weakness in the lower trapezius creates an imbalance in the force couple with the upper trapezius and serratus anterior, contributing to scapular hypermobility.
- An injury that affects normal arthrokinematic motion at either the SC or AC joint can also contribute to shoulder impingement. Any limitation in posterior superior clavicular rotation and/or clavicular elevation will prevent normal upward rotation of the scapula during humeral elevation, compromising the subacromial space.

REHABILITATION CONCERNS

Management of shoulder impingement involves gradually restoring normal biomechanics to the shoulder joint in an effort to maintain space under the coracoacromial arch during overhead activities.[70] The therapist should address the pathomechanics and the adaptive changes that most often occur with overhead activities.

Overhead activities that involve humeral elevation (full abduction or forward flexion) or a position of humeral flexion, horizontal adduction, and IR are likely to increase the pain.[42] The patient complains of diffuse pain around the acromion or glenohumeral joint. Palpation of the subacromial space increases the pain.

Exercises should concentrate on strengthening the dynamic stabilizers, the rotator cuff muscles that act to both compress and depress the humeral head relative to the glenoid[32,49,70] (Figs. 25-31 and 25-32). The inferior rotator cuff muscles in particular should be strengthened to recreate a balance in the force couple with the deltoid in the coronal plane. The supraspinatus should be strengthened to assist in compression of the humeral head into the glenoid (Figs. 25-33 and 25-34). The external rotators, the infraspinatus and teres minor, are generally weaker concentrically but stronger eccentrically than the internal rotators and should be strengthened to recreate a balance in the force couple with the subscapularis in the transverse plane.

The external rotators and the posterior portion of the joint capsule are tight and tend to limit IR and should be stretched (Figs. 25-15, 25-17, and 25-19). There is excessive ER due to laxity in the anterior portion of the joint capsule, and stretching should be avoided. There might be some tightness in both the inferior and the posterior portions of the joint capsule; this can be decreased by using posterior and inferior glenohumeral joint mobilizations (Figs. 25-13, 25-14, 25-16, and 25-17).

Strengthening of the muscles that abduct, elevate, and upward rotate the scapula (these include the serratus anterior, upper trapezius, lower trapezius, and levator scapula) should also be incorporated (Figs. 25-35, 25-39, and 25-40). The lower and middle trapezius and rhomboids should be strengthened eccentrically to help decelerate the scapula during throwing activities (Figs. 25-37 and 25-38). The lower trapezius should also be strengthened to recreate a balance in the force couple with the upper trapezius, facilitating scapular stability (Fig. 25-36).

Anterior, posterior, inferior, and superior joint mobilizations at both the SC and AC joints should be done to assure normal arthrokinematic motion at these joints (see Figs. 16-10 to 16-12).

Strengthening of the lower-extremity and trunk muscles to provide core stability is essential for reducing the stresses and strains placed on the shoulder and arm, and this is also important for the overhead athlete (Fig. 25-40).

REHABILITATION PROGRESSION

In the early stages of a rehabilitation program, the primary goal of the therapist is to minimize the pain associated with the impingement syndrome. This can be accomplished by utilizing some combination of activity modification, therapeutic modalities, and appropriate use of NSAIDs.

The therapist must make some decision about limiting the activity that caused the problem in the first place. Activity limitation, however, does not mean immobilization. Instead, a baseline of tolerable activity should be established. The key is to initially control the frequency and the level of the load on the rotator cuff and then to gradually and systematically increase the level and the frequency of that activity. It might be necessary to initially restrict activity, avoiding any exercise that places the shoulder in the impingement position, to give the inflammation a chance to subside. During this period of restricted activity, the patient should continue to engage in exercises to maintain cardiorespiratory fitness. Working on an upper-extremity ergometer will help to improve both cardiorespiratory fitness and muscular endurance in the shoulder complex.

Therapeutic modalities such as electrical stimulating currents and/or heat and cold therapy may be used to modulate pain. Ultrasound and the diathermies are most useful for elevating tissue temperatures, increasing blood flow, and facilitating the process of healing. NSAIDs prescribed by the team physician are useful not only as analgesics, but also for their long-lasting anti-inflammatory capabilities.

Once pain and inflammation have been controlled, exercises should concentrate on strengthening the dynamic stabilizers of the glenohumeral joint, stretching the inferior and posterior portions of the joint capsule, strengthening the scapular muscles that collectively produce normal scapulohumeral rhythm, and maintaining normal arthrokinematic motions of the AC and SC joints.

Strengthening exercises are done to establish neuromuscular control of the humerus and the scapula (Figs. 25-59 to 25-65). Strengthening exercises should progress from isometric pain-free contractions to isotonic full-range pain-free contractions. Humeral control exercises should be used to strengthen the rotator cuff to restrict migration of the humeral head and to regain voluntary control of the humeral head positioning through rotator cuff stabilization. Seventy-eight scapular control exercises should be used to maintain a normal relationship between the glenohumeral and scapulothoracic joints.[37,38,42]

Closed-kinetic-chain exercises for the shoulder should be primarily eccentric. They tend to compress the joint, providing stability, and are perhaps best used for establishing scapular stability and control.[43]

Gradually, the duration and intensity of the exercise may be progressed within individual patient tolerance limitations, using increased pain or stiffness as a guide for progression, eventually progressing to full-range overhead activities.

CRITERIA FOR RETURN TO NORMAL ACTIVITY

The patient may return to normal activity when (1) the gradual program used to increase the duration and intensity of the workout has allowed him/her to complete a normal exercise regimen without pain; (2) the patient exhibits improved strength in the appropriate rotator cuff and the scapular muscles; (3) there is no longer a positive impingement sign, drop arm test, or empty can test; and (4) the patient can discontinue use of anti-inflammatory medications without a return of pain.

Rotator Cuff Tendinitis and Tears

PATHOMECHANICS

Rotator cuff injury has often been described as a continuum starting with impingement of the tendon that, through repetitive compression, eventually leads to irritation and inflammation and eventually fibrosis of the rotator cuff tendon. This idea began with the work of Codman in 1934 when he identified a critical zone near the insertion of the supraspinatus tendon.[47] Since then many researchers have studied this area and have expanded the information base, leading to the identification of other causative factors.[32,54] Neer is also credited with developing a system of classification for rotator cuff disease. This system seemed to be appropriate until sports therapists began dealing with overhead athletes as a separate entity due to the acceleration of repetitive stresses applied to the shoulder. Disease in the overhead athlete usually results from failure due to one or both of these chronic stresses: repetitive tension or compression of the tissue. We now regard rotator cuff injury in athletics as an accumulation of microtrauma to both the static and the dynamic stabilizers of the shoulder complex. In 1993, Meister and Andrews classified these causative traumas based on the pathophysiology of events leading to rotator cuff failure. Their five categories of classification for modes of failure are primary compressive, secondary compressive, primary tensile overload, secondary tensile overload, and macrotraumatic.[47]

INJURY MECHANISM

Rotator cuff tendonopathy is a gradation of tendon failure, so it is important to identify the causative factors. The following classification system helps group injury mechanisms to better aid the therapist in developing a rehabilitation plan.

Primary compressive disease results from direct compression of the cuff tissue. This occurs when something interferes with the gliding of the cuff tendon in the already tight subacromial space. A predisposing factor in this category is a type III hooked acromion process, a common factor seen in younger patients with rotator cuff disease. Other factors in younger patients include a congenitally thick coracoacromial ligament and the presence of an os acromiale. In younger patients a primary impingement without one of these associated factors is rare. In middle-aged patients, degenerative spurring on the undersurface of the acromion process can cause irritation of the tendon and eventually lead to complete tearing of the tendon. These individuals are often seen because they experience pain during such activities as tennis and golf.

Secondary compressive disease is a primary result of glenohumeral instability. The high forces generated by the overhead activities can cause chronic repetitive trauma to the glenoid labrum and capsuloligamentous structures, leading to subtle instability. Patients with inherent multidirectional instability are also at risk. The additional volume created in the glenohumeral capsule allows for extraneous movement of the humeral head, leading to compressive forces in the subacromial space.

Primary tensile overload can also cause tendon irritation and failure. The rotator cuff resists horizontal adduction, IR, anterior translation of the humeral head, and distraction forces in the deceleration phase of throwing and overhead sports. The repetitive high forces generated by eccentric activity in the rotator cuff while attempting to maintain a central axis of rotation can cause microtrauma to the tendon and eventually lead to tendon failure. This type of mechanism is not associated with previous instability of the joint. Causes for this mechanism often are found when taking a complete history during the evaluation. The therapist might find that the patient had a history of injury to another area of the body where the muscles are used in the deceleration phase of overhead motion.

Secondary tensile disease is often a result of primary tensile overload. In this case the repetitive irritation and weakening of the rotator cuff allows for subtle instability. In contrast to secondary compressive disease of the tendon, the rotator cuff tendon experiences greater distractive and tensile forces because

the humeral head is allowed to translate anteriorly. Over time, the increased tensile force causes failure of the tendon.

Macrotraumatic failure occurs as a direct result of one distinct traumatic event. The mechanism for this is often a fall on an outstretched arm. This is rarely seen in patients with normal, healthy rotator cuff tendons. For this to occur, forces generated by the fall must be greater than the tensile strength of bone that is less than that of young healthy tendon. Such a condition, where the tensile strength of bone is less than tendon, is rarely seen in young patients. It is more common to see a longitudinal tear in the tendon with an avulsion of the greater tubercle.

REHABILITATION CONCERNS

When designing a rehabilitation program for rotator cuff tendonopathy, the basic concerns remain the same regardless of the extent to which the tendon is damaged. Instead, rehabilitation should be based on why and how the tendon has been damaged. Once the cause of the tendonopathy is identified and secondary factors are known, a comprehensive program can be designed. If a comprehensive rehabilitation program does not relieve the painful shoulder, surgical repair of the tendon and alteration of the glenohumeral joint are performed. Surgical rehabilitation is similar to the nonsurgical plan, with the time of progression altered based on tissue healing and tendon histology.

CONSERVATIVE MANAGEMENT

Stage I of the rehabilitation process is focused on reducing inflammation and restricting the activity that caused pain. Pain should not be a part of the rehabilitation process. The therapist may employ therapeutic modalities to aid in patient comfort. A course of NSAIDs is usually followed during this stage of rehabilitation. ROM exercises begin, avoiding further irritation of the tendon. Attention is paid to restoring appropriate arthrokinematics to the shoulder complex. If the injury is a result of a compressive disease to the tendon, capsular stretching may be done (Figs. 25-18 and 25-19). Active strengthening of the glenohumeral joint should begin, concentrating on the force couples acting around the joint; beginning with isometric exercises for the medial and lateral rotators of the joint (Fig. 25-20) and progressing to isotonic exercises if the patient does not experience pain (Figs. 25-31 and 25-32). A towel roll under the patient's arm can help initiate cocontraction of the shoulder muscles, increasing joint stability. Exercises might need to be altered to limit translational forces of the humeral head. Strengthening of the supraspinatus may begin if 90° of elevation in the scapular plane is available (Figs. 25-33 and 25-34). Aggressive pain-free strengthening of the periscapular muscles should also start, as the restoration of normal scapular control will be essential to removal of abnormal stresses of the rotator cuff tendon in later stages. The therapist might want to begin with manual resistance, progressing to free-weight exercises (Figs. 25-35 to 25-39).

In stage II, the healing process progresses and ROM will need to be restored. The therapist might need to be more aggressive in stretching techniques, addressing capsular tightness as it develops. The prone-on-elbows position is a good technique for self-mobilization. This position should be avoided if compressive disease is part of the irritation. If pain continuous to be absent, strengthening gets increasingly aggressive. Isokinetic exercises at speeds greater than 200°/second for shoulder medial and lateral rotation may begin (Fig. 25-52).

Aggressive neuromuscular control exercises are started in this stage: quick reversals during PNF diagonal patterns, starting with manual resistance from the therapist and advancing to resistance applied by surgical tubing (Figs. 25-55 and 25-56). The Body Blade may also be used for rhythmic stabilization (Fig. 25-57).

The exercise program should now progress to free weights, and eccentric exercises of the rotator cuff should be emphasized to meet the demands of the shoulder in overhead activities. Strengthening of the deltoid and upper trapezius muscles can begin above 90° of elevation. Exercises include the military press (Fig. 25-24), shoulder flexion (Fig. 25-26), and reverse flys (Fig. 25-30). Push-ups can also be added. It might be necessary to restrict ROM so the body does not go below the elbow, to prevent excessive translation of the glenohumeral joint. This author prefers combining this exercise with serratus anterior strengthening in a modified push-up with a plus (Fig. 25-39).

In the later part of this stage, exercises should progress to plyometric strengthening. Surgical tubing is used to allow the patient to exercise in 90° of elevation with the elbow bent to 90° (Fig. 25-45). Plyoball exercises are initiated (Figs. 25-46 and 25-47). The weight and distance of the exercises can be altered to increase demands. The Shuttle 2000-1 is an excellent exercise to increase eccentric strength in a plyometric fashion (Fig. 25-50).

Stage III of the rehabilitation focuses on specific activities. The patient should remain pain-free as specific activities are advanced and a gradual return to normal activity achieved.

Postsurgical Management

If conservative management is insufficient, surgical repair is often indicated. The type of repair done depends on the classification of the injury. Subacromial decompression has been described by Neer as a method to stimulate tissue healing and increase the subacromial space.[50] Additional procedures may be done as open repairs of the tendon with appropriate reattachment to bone along with a capsular tightening procedure.

Stage I is often begun with some form of immobilization. This does not mean complete lack of movement. Instead it refers to restricting positions based on the surgical repair. In open repairs, flexion and abduction might be restricted for as long as 4 weeks. When the repair addresses the capsulolabral complex or has been performed under tension due to cuff tissue retraction and subsequent remobilization to achieve repair, the patient might spend up to 2 weeks in an airplane or ablation splint (Fig. 25-73).

Pain control and prevention of muscle atrophy are addressed in this stage. Shoulder shrugs, isometrics, and joint mobilization for pain control can be done. Later in this stage, active assistive exercises with the L-bar and multiangle isometrics are done in the pain-free ROM.

Stage II collagen and elastin components have begun to stabilize. Healing tissue should have a decreased level of elastin and an increased level of collagen by now.[65,81] Regaining full ROM and increasing the stress to healing tissue for better collagen alignment is important in this stage. Having the patient hang from an overhead bar (Fig. 25-5) or using a rope and pulley system (Fig. 25-9) can help achieve desired ROM.

Active ROM exercises are added, progressing from no resistance to resistance with surgical tubing. If a primary repair has been done to the tendon, resisted supraspinatus exercises should be avoided until 10 weeks.

The restoration of normal arthrokinematics and scapulothoracic rhythm is addressed with exercises emphasizing neuromuscular control. The patient can use a mirror to judge progress.

Stage III remains similar to conservative management. However, the time frame might lag getting to this stage.

REHABILITATION PROGRESSION

The rehabilitation progression for conservatively managed rotator cuff injury should follow along with the progression outlined in the section on impingement syndrome. The following progression is the authors' preference for postsurgical progression. The principles followed for rehabilitation progression are based on the dynamics of healing tissue. Depending on the surgical procedure, the time frame for this progression may be altered. A simple way to stage the rehabilitation of the postsurgical patient is by following the rule of six. During the first 6 weeks after the surgery, the goal is to decrease pain, address inflammation, and prevent muscle atrophy. Therapeutic modalities and gentle ROM are initiated.

The second 6-week period (weeks 6–12) begins the stage of rehabilitation where full active and passive ROM need to be achieved prior to maturation of the healing tissue. Other emphasis is placed on regaining normal static and dynamic joint mechanics. Proprioceptive and neuromuscular exercises are used to achieve this goal.

In the last 6 weeks (weeks 12–18), the repair should be mature enough to tolerate progression to activities that prepare the patient for return to normal activity. Speed and control of resisted exercises are increased. Plyometric training and interval progression to specific activities are used.

CRITERIA FOR RETURN TO NORMAL ACTIVITY

Return to normal activity should be based on these criteria: (1) The patient has full active ROM. (2) Normal mechanics have been restored in the shoulder complex. (3) The patient has at least 90 percent strength in the involved shoulder as compared to the uninvolved side. (4) There is no pain present during overhead activity.

Adhesive Capsulitis (Frozen Shoulder)

PATHOMECHANICS

Adhesive capsulitis is characterized by the loss of motion at the glenohumeral joint. The cause of this arthrofibrosis is not well defined. One set of criteria used for diagnosis of a frozen shoulder was described by Jobe et al. in 1996 and included (1) decreased glenohumeral motion and loss of synchronous shoulder girdle motion, (2) restricted elevation (less than 135° or 90°, depending on the therapist), (3) ER 50–60 percent of normal, and (4) arthrogram findings of 5–10 cc volume with obliteration of the normal axillary fold.[33] Other authors have identified histological changes in different areas surrounding the glenohumeral joint.[65] Travell and Simons explained that a reflex autonomic reaction could be the underlying cause, due to the presence of subscapularis trigger points (TPs).[71] The result is a chronic inflammation with fibrosis and rotator cuff muscles that are tight and inelastic.

INJURY MECHANISM

For the purposes of this chapter, we will separate this diagnosis into two categories: primary versus secondary frozen shoulder. Adhesive capsulitis may be considered primary when it develops spontaneously; it is considered secondary when a known underlying condition (e.g., a fractured humeral head) or surgical procedure is present.

Primary frozen shoulder usually has an insidious onset. The patient often describes a sequence of painful restrictions in the shoulder, followed by a gradual stiffness with less pain. Factors that have been found to predispose a patient to idiopathic capsulitis include diabetes, hypothyroidism, and underlying cardiopulmonary involvement.[76] These factors were identified through epidemiological studies and might have more to do with characteristic personalities of these patients. It is rare to see this type of frozen shoulder in the physically active population.

Secondary frozen shoulder is more commonly seen. It has been associated with many different underlying diagnoses. Rockwood and Matsen listed eight categories of conditions that should be considered in the differential diagnosis of frozen shoulder: trauma, other soft-tissue disorders about the shoulder, joint disorders, bone disorders, cervical spine disorders, intrathoracic disorders, abdominal disorders, and psychogenic disorders (Table 25-3).[60]

REHABILITATION CONCERNS

The primary concern for rehabilitation is proper differential diagnosis. Attempting to progress the patient into the strength or functional activities portion of a rehabilitation program can lead to exacerbation of the motion restriction. The single best treatment for adhesive capsulitis is prevention.

Depending on the stage of pathology when intervention is started, the rehabilitation program time frame can be shortened. In all cases, the goals of rehabilitation are the same: first relieving the pain in the acute stages of the disorder, gradually

---

TABLE 25-3

Differential Diagnosis of Frozen Shoulder

TRAUMA
Fractures of the shoulder region
Fractures anywhere in the upper extremity
Misdiagnosed posterior shoulder dislocation
Hemarthrosis of shoulder secondary to trauma

OTHER SOFT-TISSUE DISORDERS ABOUT THE SHOULDER
Tendinitis of the rotator cuff
Tendinitis of the long head of biceps
Subacromial bursitis
Impingement
Suprascapular nerve impingement
Thoracic outlet syndrome

JOINT DISORDERS
Degenerative arthritis of the AC joint
Degenerative arthritis of the glenohumeral joint
Septic arthritis
Other painful forms of arthritis

BONE DISORDERS
Avascular necrosis of the humeral head
Metastatic cancer
Paget's disease
Primary bone tumor
Hyperparathyroidism

CERVICAL SPINE DISORDERS
Cervical spondylosis
Cervical disc herniation
Infection

INTRATHORACIC DISORDER
Diaphragmatic irritation
Pancoast tumor
Myocardinal infarction

ABDOMINAL DISORDER
Gastric ulcer
Cholecystitis
Subphrenic abscess

PSYCHOGENIC

Adapted from Rockwood CA, Matsen FA. *The Shoulder*. Philadelphia, WB Saunders, 1990.

restoring proper arthrokinematics, gradually restoring ROM, and strengthening the muscles of the shoulder complex.

REHABILITATION PROGRESSION

In the acute phase, Codman's exercises and low-grade joint mobilization techniques can be used to relieve pain. This may be accompanied by therapeutic modalities and passive stretching of the upper trapezius and levator scapulae muscles. The therapist may also want to suggest that the patient sleep with a pillow under the involved arm to prevent IR during sleep.

In the subacute phase, ROM is more aggressively addressed. Incorporating PNF techniques such as hold–relax can be helpful. Progressive demands should be placed on the patient with rhythmic stabilization techniques. Wall climbing (Fig. 25-8) and wall/corner stretches (Fig. 25-10) are also good additions to the rehabilitation program. As ROM returns, the program should start to address strengthening. Isometric exercises for the shoulder are often the best way to begin. Progressive strengthening will continue in the next phase.

The final phase of rehabilitation is a progressive strengthening of the shoulder complex. Exercises for maintenance of ROM continue, and a series of strengthening exercises should be added. The rehabilitation program should be tailored to meet the needs of the patient based on the differential diagnosis.

CRITERIA FOR RETURN TO NORMAL ACTIVITY

The patient may return to the previous level of activity once the proper physiological and arthrokinematic motion has been restored to the glenohumeral joint. How long the patient went untreated and undiagnosed will affect how long it takes to reach this point.

Thoracic Outlet Syndrome

PATHOMECHANICS

Thoracic outlet syndrome is the compression of neurovascular structures within the thoracic outlet. The thoracic outlet is a cone-shaped passage, with the greater circumferential opening proximal to the spine and the narrow end passing into the distal extremity. On the proximal end, the cone is bordered anteriorly by the anterior scalene muscles, and posteriorly by the middle and posterior scalene muscles. Structures traveling through the thoracic outlet are the brachial plexus, subclavian artery and vein, and axillary vessels. The neurovascular structures pass distally under the clavicle and subclavius muscle. Beneath the neurovascular bundle is the first rib. At the narrow end of the cone, the bundle passes under the coracoid process of the scapula and into the upper extremity through the axilla. The distal end is bordered anteriorly by the pectoralis minor and posteriorly by the scapula.

Based on the anatomy of the thoracic outlet, there are several areas where neurovascular compression can occur. Therefore, pathology of the thoracic outlet syndrome is dependent on the structures being compressed.

INJURY MECHANISM

In 60 percent of the population affected by thoracic outlet syndrome, there is no report from the patient of an inciting episode.[39] Some of the theories presented by authors regarding the etiology of thoracic outlet syndrome include trauma, postural components, shortening of the pectoralis minor, shortening of the scalenes, and muscle hypertrophy.

There are four areas of vulnerability to compressive forces: the superior thoracic outlet, where the brachial plexus passes over the first rib; the scalene triangle, at the proximal end of the thoracic outlet, where there might be overlapping insertions of the anterior and middle scalenes onto the first rib; the costoclavicular interval, which is the space between the first rib and clavicle where the neurovascular bundle passes (the space can be narrowed by poor posture, inferior laxity of the glenohumeral joint, or an exostosis from a fracture of the clavicle); and under the coracoid process where the brachial plexus passes and is bordered anteriorly by the pectoralis minor.[65]

REHABILITATION CONCERNS

As described, thoracic outlet syndrome is an anatomy-based problem involving compressive forces applied to the neurovascular bundle. Conservative management of thoracic outlet syndrome is moderately successful, resulting in decreased symptoms 50–90 percent of the time. As the first course of treatment, rehabilitation should be based on encouraging the least provocative posture. Leffert advocated a detailed history and evaluation of the patient's activities and lifestyle to help identify where and when postural deficiency is occurring.[39]

Through a detailed history and evaluation of a patient's activity, the therapist can identify the cause of compression in the thoracic outlet. The rehabilitation program should be tailored to encourage good posture throughout the athlete's day. Therapeutic exercises should be used to strengthen postural muscles, such as the rhomboids (Fig. 25-38), middle trapezius (Fig. 25-37), and lower trapezius. Flexibility exercises are also used to increase the space in the thoracic outlet. Scalene stretches and wall/corner stretches (Fig. 25-10) are used to decrease the incidence of muscle impinging on the neurovascular bundle. Proper breathing technique should also be reviewed with the patient. The scalene muscles act as accessory breathing muscles, and improper breathing technique can lead to tightening of these muscles.

REHABILITATION PROGRESSION

The rehabilitation process begins by detailed evaluation of the patient's activities and symptoms. First, the patient is restricted from activities exacerbating the neurovascular symptoms until the patient can maintain a symptom-free posture. During this time an erect posture is encouraged using stretching and strengthening exercises. Gradually, encourage the patient to return to his/her normal activities, for short periods of time, while maintaining a pain-free posture. The time of participation is increased at regular intervals if the patient remains pain-free. This helps build endurance of the postural muscles. Exercising on an upper-body ergometer, by pedaling backward, can help build endurance.

CRITERIA FOR RETURN TO NORMAL ACTIVITY

If the patient responds to the rehabilitation program and can maintain a pain-free posture during a specific activity, participation can be resumed. The patient should have no muscular weakness, neurovascular symptoms, or pain. If the patient fails to respond to therapy, and functionally significant pain and weakness persist, surgical intervention might be indicated. Surgical procedure depends on the anatomical basis for the patient's symptoms.

Brachial Plexus Injuries (Stinger or Burner)

PATHOMECHANICS

The brachial plexus begins at cervical roots c5 to c8 and thoracic root t1. The ventral rami of these roots are formed from a dorsal (sensory) and ventral (motor) root. The ventral rami join to form the brachial plexus. The ventral rami lie between the anterior and middle scalene muscles, where they run adjacent to the subclavian artery. The plexus continues distally passing over the first rib. It is deep to the sternocleidomastoid muscle in the neck.[51] Just caudal to the clavicle and subclavius muscle, the five ventral rami unite to form the three trunks of the plexus: superior, middle, and inferior. The superior trunk is composed of the c5 and c6 ventral roots. The middle trunk is formed by the c7 root, and the inferior trunk is formed by c8 and t1 ventral roots. After passing under the clavicle, the three trunks divide into three divisions that eventually contribute to the three cords of the brachial plexus.

The typical picture of a brachial plexus injury is that of a traction injury. This syndrome is commonly referred to as burner or stinger syndrome. These injuries usually involve the c5 to c6 nerve roots. The patient will complain of a sharp, burning pain in the shoulder that radiates down the arm into the hand. Weakness in the muscles supplied by c5 and c6 (deltoid, biceps, supraspinatus, and infraspinatus) accompany the pain. Burning and pain are often transient, but weakness might last a few minutes or indefinitely.

Clancy et al. have classified brachial plexus injuries into three categories.[12] A grade I injury results in a transient loss of motor and sensory function, which usually resolves completely within minutes. A grade II injury results in significant motor weakness and sensory loss that might last from 6 weeks to 4 months. EMG (electromyogram) evaluation after 2 weeks will demonstrate abnormalities. Grade III lesions are characterized by motor and sensory loss for at least 1 year in duration.

INJURY MECHANISM

The structure of the brachial plexus is such that it winds its way through the musculoskeletal anatomy of the upper extremity as described. Clancy et al. identified neck rotation, neck lateral flexion, shoulder abduction, shoulder ER, and simultaneous scapular and clavicular depression as potential mechanisms of injury.[12]

During neck rotation and lateral flexion to one side, the brachial plexus and the subclavius muscle on the opposite side are put on stretch and the clavicle is slightly elevated about its anterior–posterior axis. If the arm is not elevated, the superior trunk of the plexus will assume the greatest amount of tension. If the shoulder is abducted and externally rotated, the brachial plexus migrates superiorly toward the coracoid process and the scapula retracts, putting the pectoralis minor on stretch. As the shoulder is moved into full abduction, a condition similar to a movable pulley is formed, where the coracoid process of the scapula acts as the pulley. In full abduction, most stress falls on the lower cords of the brachial plexus.[65] The addition of clavicular and scapula depression to the above scenarios would produce a downward force on the pulley system, bringing the brachial plexus into contact with the clavicle and the coracoid process. The portion of the plexus that receives the greatest amount of tensile stress depends on the position of the upper extremity during a collision.

REHABILITATION CONCERNS

Management of brachial plexus injuries begins with the gradual restoration of the patient's cervical ROM. Muscle tightness caused by the direct trauma, and by reflexive guarding that occurs because of pain, needs to be addressed. Gentle PROM exercises and stretching for the upper trapezius, levator scapulae, and scalene muscles should be done. The therapist trainer should be careful not to cause sensory symptoms.

Butler[11] advocates using an early intervention with gentle mobilization of the neural tissues. The goal of early mobilization is to prevent scarring between the nerve and the bed or within the connective tissue of the nerve itself as the nerve heals. He advocates low tensile loads to avoid the possibility of irritating a nerve lesion such as axonotmesis or neurotmesis. More chronic, repetitive injuries may use the neural tension test positions to do mobilizations with higher grades.

Strengthening of the involved muscles is also addressed in the rehabilitation program. Supraspinatus strengthening exercises like scaption (Fig. 25-33) and alternative supraspinatus exercises (Fig. 25-34) should be done. Other exercises for involved musculature are shoulder lateral rotation (Fig. 25-32) for the infraspinatus, forward flexion and abduction to 90° (Figs. 25-26 and 25-28) to strengthen the deltoid, and bicep curls for elbow flexion.

REHABILITATION PROGRESSION

The patient is restricted from activity immediately after the injury. The rehabilitation progression should begin with the restoration of both active and passive ROM at the neck and shoulder. Neural tissue mobilizations utilizing the upper limb tension testing positions should begin with the athlete in the testing positions (see Fig. 10-4).[11] For the median nerve, the testing position consists of shoulder depression, abduction, ER, and wrist and finger extension. For the radial nerve, the elbow is extended, the forearm pronated, the glenohumeral joint internally rotated, and the wrist, finger, and thumb flexed. The position for stretching the ulnar nerve consists of shoulder depression, wrist and finger extension, supination or pronation of the forearm, and elbow flexion. Mobilizations of distal joints, like the elbow and wrist, in large-grade movements should initiate the treatment phase. Progression should include grade 4 and grade 5 mobilizations in later phases of recovery.

As the patient gets return of ROM, strengthening of the neck and shoulder are incorporated into the rehabilitation program. Strengthening should progress from PRE-type strengthening with free weights to exercises that emphasize power and endurance. Functional progression begins with teaching proper technique for activity-specific demands that mimic the position of injury. The progressive return and proper technique are important to the rehabilitation program, as they address the psychological component of preparing the athlete for return to activity.

CRITERIA FOR RETURN TO NORMAL ACTIVITY

Patients are allowed to return to normal activity when they have full, pain-free ROM and full strength.

Myofascial Trigger Points

PATHOLOGY

Clinically, a trigger point is defined as a hyperirritable focus in muscle or fascia that is tender to palpation and may, upon compression, result in referred pain or tenderness in a characteristic "zone." This zone is distinct from myotomes, dermatomes, schlerotomes, or peripheral nerve distribution. TPs are identified via palpation of taut bands of muscle or discrete nodules or adhesions. Snapping of a taut band will usually initiate a local twitch response.[64]

Physiologically, the definition of a TP is not as clear. Muscles with myofascial TPs reveal no diagnostic abnormalities upon EMG examination. Routine laboratory tests show no abnormalities or significant changes attributable to TPs. Normal serum enzyme concentrations have been reported with a shift in the distribution of LDH (lactate dehydrogenase) isoenzymes. Skin temperature over active TPs might be higher in a 5–10-cm diameter.[72]

Travell and Simons classify TPs as follows[72]:

1. *Active Tps*—Symptomatic at rest with referral pain and tenderness upon direct compression. Associated weakness and contracture are often present.
2. *Latent Tps*—Pain is not present unless direct compression is applied. These might show up on clinical exam as stiffness and/or weakness in the region of tenderness.
3. *Primary Tps*—Located in specific muscles.
4. *Associated Tps*—Located within the referral zone of a primary TP's muscle or in a muscle that is functionally overloaded in compensation for a primary TP.

Pathology of a myofascial TP is identified with (1) a history of sudden onset during or shortly after an acute overload stress or chronic overload of the affected muscle; (2) characteristic patterns of pain in a muscle's referral zone; (3) weakness and restriction in the end ROM of the affected muscle; (4) a taut, palpable band in the affected muscle; (5) focal tenderness to direct compression, in the band of taut muscle fibers; (6) a local twitch response elicited by snapping of the tender spot; and (7) reproduction of the patient's pain through pressure on the tender spot.

INJURY MECHANISM

The most common mechanism for myofascial TPs in the shoulder region is acute muscle strain (Table 25-4). The damaged muscle tissue causes tearing of the sarcoplasmic reticulum and release of its stored calcium, with loss of the ability of that portion of the muscle to remove calcium ions. The chronic stress of sustained muscle contraction can cause continued muscle damage, repeating the above cycle of damage. The combined presence of the normal muscle ATP supplies and excessive calcium initiate and maintain a sustained muscle band contracture. This produces a region of the muscle with an uncontrolled metabolism, to which the body responds with local vasoconstriction. This region of increased metabolism and decreased local circulation, with muscle fibers passing through that area,

---

T A B L E   2 5 - 4

Trigger Points of the Shoulder

POSTERIOR SHOULDER PAIN
Deltoid
Levator scapulae
Supraspinatus
Subscapularis
Teres minor
Teres major
Serratus posterior superior
Triceps
Trapezius

ANTERIOR SHOULDER PAIN
Infraspinatus
Deltoid
Scalene
Supraspinatus
Pectoralis major
Pectoralis minor
Biceps
Coracobrachialis

Adapted from Travell JG, Simons DG. Myofascial pain and dysfunction. *The Trigger Point Manual.* Baltimore, Williams & Wilkins, 1983.

causes muscle shortening independent of local motor unit action potentials. This taut band can be palpated in the muscle.

REHABILITATION CONCERNS

The principal mechanism of myofascial TPs is related to muscular overload and fatigue, so the primary concern is identification of the incriminating activity. The therapist should take a detailed history of the patient's daily activity demands.

The cyclic nature of TPs requires interruption of the cycle for successful treatment. Interrupting the shortening of the muscle fibers and prevention of further breakdown of the muscle tissue components should be attempted using modified hold–relax techniques and postisometric stretching. Travell and Simons advocate a spray-and-stretch method, where vapocoolant spray is applied and passive stretching follows. Theoretically, when the muscle is placed in a stretched position and the skin receptors are cooled, a reflexive inhibition of the contracted muscle is facilitated, allowing for increased passive stretching.[72]

After a treatment session where PROM has been achieved, the muscle must be activated to stimulate normal actin and myosin cross-bridging. Gentle active ROM exercises or active assistive exercises with the L-bar might be a good activity to use as posttreatment activity. Normal muscle activity and endurance must be encouraged after ROM is restored. A gradual progression of shoulder exercises with an endurance emphasis should be used.

REHABILITATION PROGRESSION

Treatment progression for TPs should begin with temporary removal from activities that overload the contracted tissue. The patient is then treated with myofascial stretching techniques to increase the length of the contracted tissue. Immediate use of the extended ROM should be emphasized. Strengthening exercises are added once the patient can maintain the normal muscle length without initiating the return of the contracted myofascial band. As strength and function of the involved muscles return, the patient may gradually return to normal activity.

CRITERIA FOR RETURN TO ACTIVITY

The patient may return to activity in a relatively short period of time if he/she can demonstrate the ability to function without reinitiating the myofascial TPs and associated taut bands. Early return without meeting this criterion can lead to greater regionalization of the symptoms.

REHABILITATION TECHNIQUES FOR THE SHOULDER

Stretching Exercises

See Figs. 25-5 to 25-40.

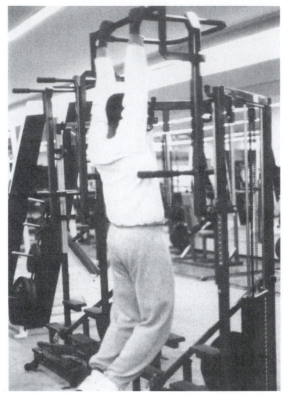

F I G U R E   2 5 - 5

Static hanging. Hanging from a chinning bar is a good general stretch for the musculature in the shoulder complex.

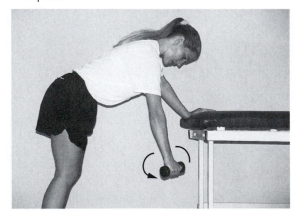

F I G U R E   2 5 - 6

Codman's circumduction exercise. The patient holds a dumbbell in the hand and moves it in a circular pattern, reversing direction periodically. This technique is useful as a general stretch in the early stages of rehabilitation when motion above 90° is restricted.

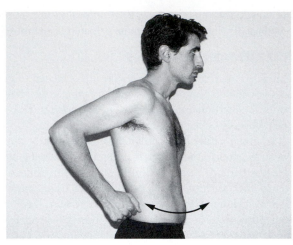

F I G U R E   2 5 - 7

Sawing. The patient moves the arm forward and backward as if performing a sawing motion. This technique is useful as a general stretch in the early stages of rehabilitation when motion above 90° is restricted.

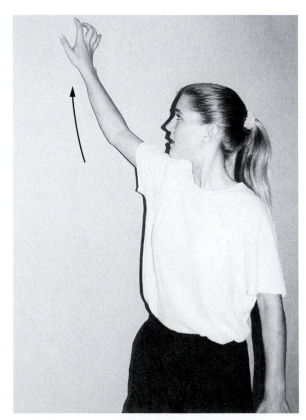

F I G U R E   2 5 - 8

Wall climbing. The patient uses the fingers to "walk" the hand up a wall. This technique is useful when attempting to regain full-range elevation. ROM should be restricted to a pain-free arc.

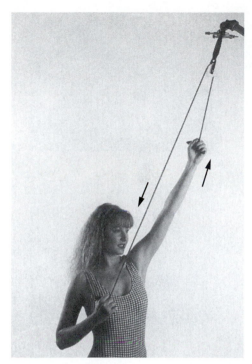

FIGURE   25-9

Rope and pulley exercise. This exercise may be used as an active-assistive exercise when trying to regain full overhead motion. ROM should be restricted to a pain-free arc.

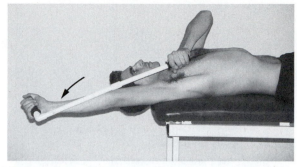

FIGURE   25-11

Shoulder extensor stretch using an L-bar. Used to stretch the latissimus dorsi, teres major and minor, posterior deltoid, and triceps muscles, and the inferior joint capsule.

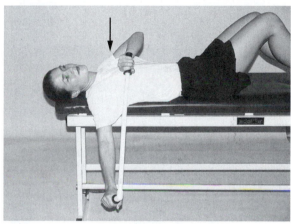

FIGURE   25-12

Shoulder flexors stretch using an L-bar. Used to stretch the anterior deltoid, coracobrachialis, pectoralis major, and biceps muscles and the anterior joint capsule.

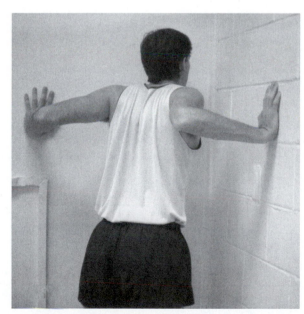

FIGURE   25-10

Wall/corner stretch. Used to stretch the pectoralis major and minor, anterior deltoid, and coracobrachialis, and the anterior joint capsule.

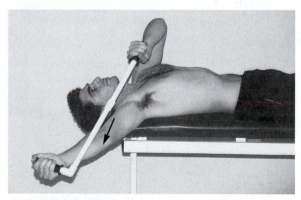

FIGURE   25-13

Shoulder adductors stretch using an L-bar. Used to stretch the latissimus dorsi, teres major and minor, pectoralis major and minor, posterior deltoid, and triceps muscles, and the inferior joint capsule.

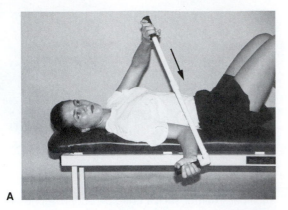

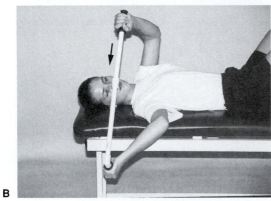

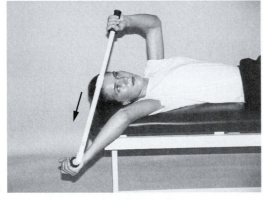

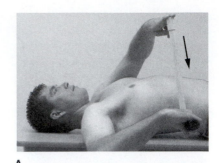

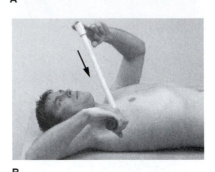

FIGURE   25-15

Shoulder lateral rotators stretch using an L-bar. Used to stretch the infraspinatus, teres minor, and posterior deltoid muscles, and the posterior joint capsule. This stretch should be done at **A,** 90°, **B,** 135°.

FIGURE   25-14

Shoulder medial rotators stretch using an L-bar. Used to stretch the subscapularis pectoralis major, latissimus dorsi, teres major, and anterior deltoid muscles, and the anterior joint capsule. This stretch should be done at **A,** 0°, **B,** 90°, and **C,** 135°.

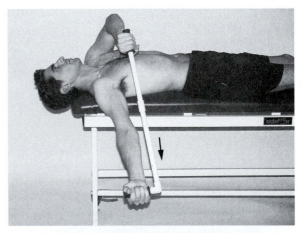

FIGURE   25-16

Horizontal adductors stretch using an L-bar. Used to stretch the pectoralis major, anterior deltoid, and long head of the biceps muscles, and the anterior joint capsule.

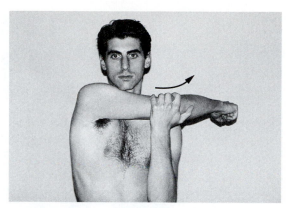

Horizontal abductors stretch. Used to stretch the posterior deltoid, infraspinatus, teres minor, rhomboids, and middle trapezius muscles, and the posterior capsule. This position might be uncomfortable for patients with shoulder impingement syndrome.

Strengthening Techniques

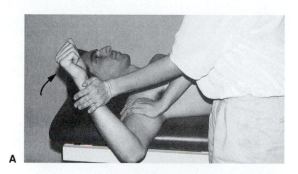

A

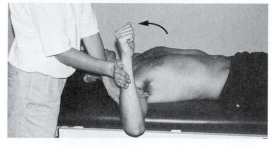

B

F I G U R E   2 5 - 2 0

A, Isometric medial rotation and **B,** isometric lateral rotation are useful in the early stages of a shoulder rehabilitation program when full ROM isotonic exercise is likely to exacerbate a problem. The towel under the arm is used to help establish neuromuscular control and help facilitate scapular stability.

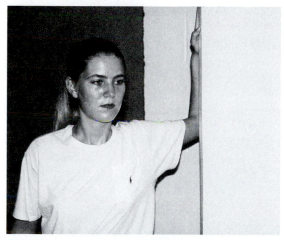

F I G U R E   2 5 - 1 8

Anterior capsule stretch. Self-stretch using the wall.

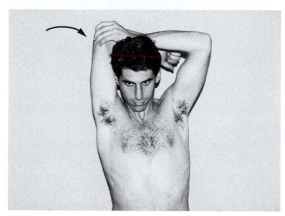

F I G U R E   2 5 - 1 9

Inferior capsule stretch. Self-stretch done with the arm in the fully elevated overhead position. This position might be uncomfortable for patient with shoulder impingement syndrome.

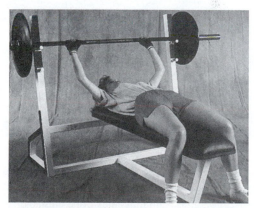

F I G U R E   2 5 - 2 1

Bench press. Used to strengthen the pectoralis major, anterior deltoid, and triceps, and secondarily the coracobrachialis muscles. Performing this exercise with the feet on the bench serves to flatten the low back and helps to isolate these muscles.

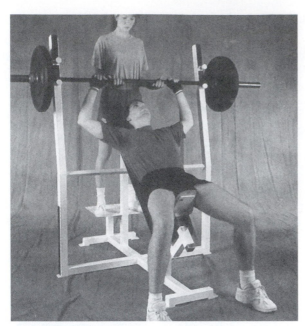

F I G U R E   2 5 - 2 2

Incline bench press. Used to strengthen the pectoralis major (upper fibers), triceps, middle and anterior deltoid, and secondarily the coracobrachialis, upper trapezius, and levator scapula muscles.

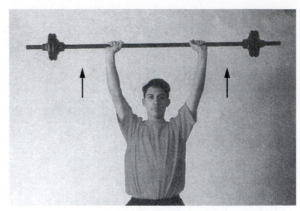

F I G U R E   2 5 - 2 4

Military press. Used to strengthen the middle deltoid, upper trapezius, levator scapula, and triceps.

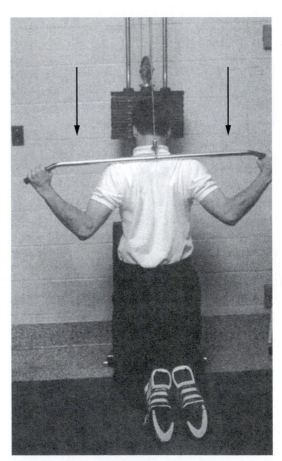

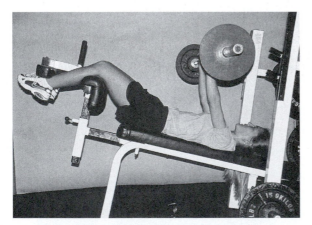

F I G U R E   2 5 - 2 3

Decline bench press. Used to strengthen the pectoralis major (lower fibers), triceps, anterior deltoid, coracobrachialis, and latissimus dorsi muscles.

F I G U R E   2 5 - 2 5

Lat pull-downs. Used to strengthen primarily the latissimus dorsi, teres major, and pectoralis minor and secondarily the biceps muscles. This exercise may be done by pulling the bar down in front of the head or behind the neck. Pulling the bar down behind the neck requires contraction of the rhomboids and middle trapezius. Pull-ups done on a chinning bar can also be used as an alternative strengthening technique.

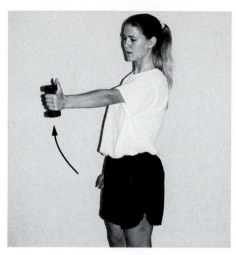

FIGURE 25-26

Shoulder flexion. Used to strengthen primarily the anterior deltoid and coracobrachialis and secondarily the middle deltoid, pectoralis major, and biceps brachii muscles. Note that the thumb should point upward.

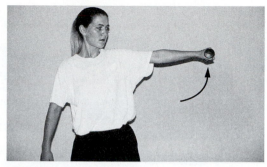

FIGURE 25-28

Shoulder abduction to 90°. Used to strengthen primarily the middle deltoid and supraspinatus and secondarily the anterior and posterior deltoid and serratus anterior muscles. Note that the thumb is in a neutral position.

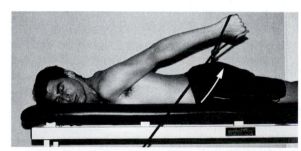

FIGURE 25-27

Shoulder extension. Used to strengthen primarily the latissimus dorsi, teres major, and posterior deltoid and secondarily the teres minor and the long head of the triceps muscles. Note that the thumb should point downward. May be done standing using a dumbbell or lying prone using surgical tubing.

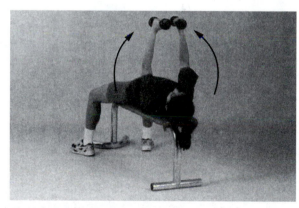

FIGURE 25-29

Flys (shoulder horizontal adduction). Used to strengthen primarily the pectoralis major and secondarily the anterior deltoid. Note that the elbow may be slightly flexed. May be done in a supine position or standing with surgical tubing or wall pulleys behind.

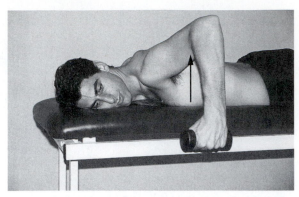

F I G U R E   2 5 - 3 0

Reverse flys (shoulder horizontal abduction). Used to strengthen primarily the posterior deltoid and secondarily the infraspinatus, teres minor, rhomboids, and middle trapezius muscles. May be done lying prone using either dumbbells or tubing. Note that with the thumb pointed upward, the middle trapezius is more active, and with the thumb pointed downward, the rhomboids are more active.

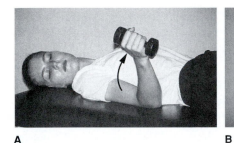
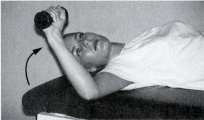
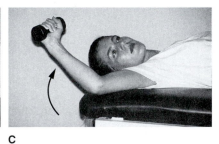

A   **B**   **C**

F I G U R E   2 5 - 3 1

Shoulder medial rotation. Used to strengthen primarily the subscapularis, pectoralis major, latissimus dorsi, and teres major and secondarily the anterior deltoid. This exercise may be done isometrically or isotonically, either lying supine using a dumbbell or standing using tubing. Strengthening should be done with the arm fully adducted at 0°, and also in 90° and 135° of abduction.

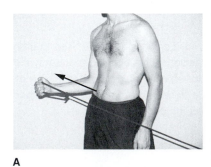
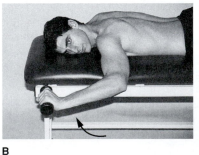
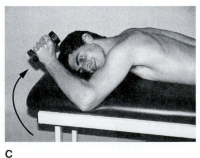

A   **B**   **C**

F I G U R E   2 5 - 3 2

Shoulder lateral rotation. Used to strengthen primarily the infraspinatus and teres minor and secondarily the posterior deltoid muscles. This exercise may be done isometrically or isotonically, either lying prone using a dumbbell or standing using tubing. Strengthening should be done with the arm fully adducted at 0°, and also in 90° and 135° of abduction.

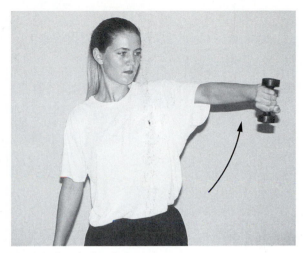

FIGURE 25-33

Scaption. Used to strengthen primarily the supraspinatus in the plane of the scapula and secondarily the anterior and middle deltoid muscles. This exercise should be done standing with the arm horizontally adducted to 45° and the thumb pointing downward.

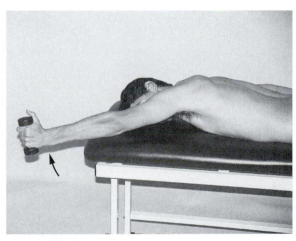

FIGURE 25-34

Alternative supraspinatus exercise. Used to strengthen primarily the supraspinatus and secondarily the posterior deltoid. In the prone position with the arm abducted to 100°, the arm is horizontally abducted in extreme lateral rotation. Note that the thumb should point upward.

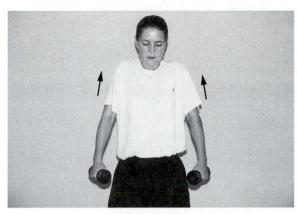

FIGURE 25-35

Shoulder shrugs. Used to strengthen primarily the upper trapezius and the levator scapula and secondarily the rhomboids.

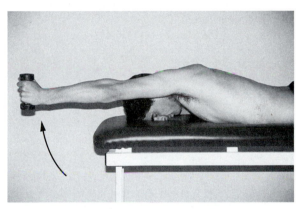

FIGURE 25-36

Superman. Used to strengthen primarily the inferior trapezius and secondarily the middle trapezius. May be done lying prone using either dumbbells or tubing. Note that the thumb is in a neutral position.

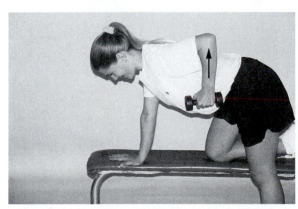

FIGURE 25-37

Bent-over rows. Used to strengthen primarily the middle trapezius and rhomboids. Done standing in a bent-over position with one knee supported on a bench.

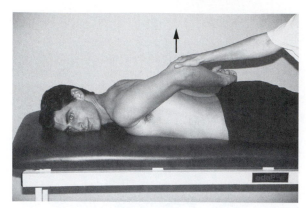

FIGURE 25-38

Rhomboids exercise. Used to strengthen primarily the rhomboids and secondarily the inferior trapezius. Should be done lying prone with manual resistance applied at the elbow.

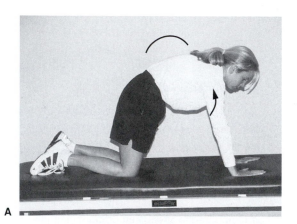

A

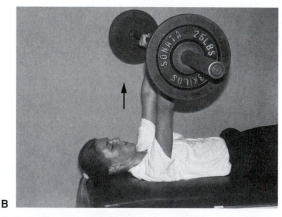

B

FIGURE 25-39

Push-ups with a plus. Used to strengthen the serratus anterior. There are several variations to this exercise, including **A,** regular push-ups and **B,** weight-loaded push-ups with a plus.

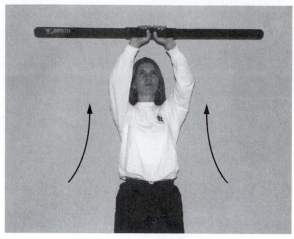

FIGURE 25-40

Scapular strengthening using a Body Blade. Holding an oscillating Body Blade with both hands, the patient moves from a fully adducted position in front of the body to a fully elevated overhead position.

Closed-Kinetic-Chain Exercises

See Figs. 25-41 to 25-44.

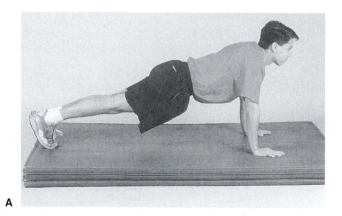

A

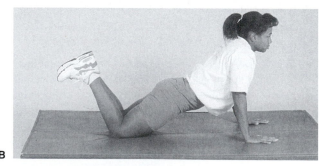

B

FIGURE 25-41

Push-ups. May be done with **A,** weight supported on feet or **B,** modified to support weight on the knees.

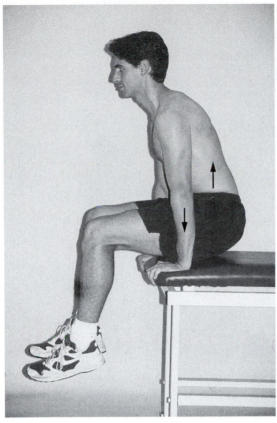

F I G U R E   2 5 - 4 2

Seated push-up. Done sitting on the end of a table. Place hands on the table and lift weight upward off of the table isotonically.

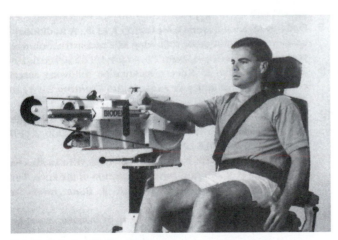

F I G U R E   2 5 - 4 3

Biodex upper-extremity closed-chain device. One of the only isokinetic closed-kinetic-chain exercise devices currently available.

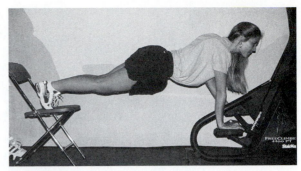

F I G U R E   2 5 - 4 4

Stair Climber with feet on chair. An advanced closed-kinetic-chain strengthening exercise that places the hands on the footplates of a Stair Climber with the feet supported on a chair. Requires substantial upper-body strength.

Plyometric Exercises

See Figs. 25-45 to 25-52.

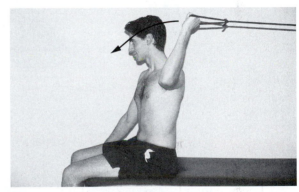

F I G U R E   2 5 - 4 5

Surgical tubing. For example, to strengthen the medial rotators, use a quick eccentric stretch of the medial rotators to facilitate a concentric contraction of those muscles.

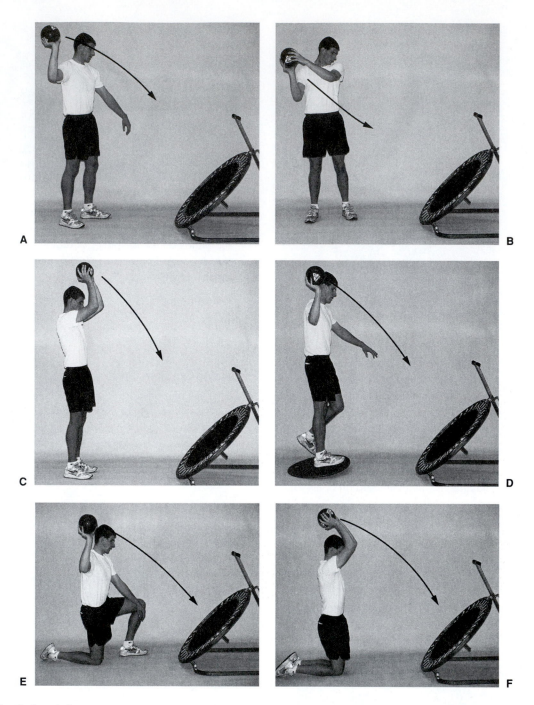

FIGURE 25-46

Plyoback. The patient should catch the ball, decelerate it, and then immediately accelerate in the opposite direction. **A,** Single-arm toss. **B,** Two-arm toss with trunk rotation. **C,** Two-arm overhead toss. **D,** Single-arm toss on unstable surface. **E,** Kneeling single-arm toss. **F,** Kneeling two-arm toss. The weight of the Plyoball should be increased as rapidly as can be tolerated.[73]

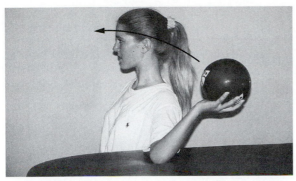

FIGURE 25-47

Seated single-arm weighted-ball throw. The patient should be seated with the arm abducted to 90° and the elbow supported on a table. The sports therapist tosses the ball to the hand, creating an overload in lateral rotation that forces the patient to dynamically stabilize in that position.

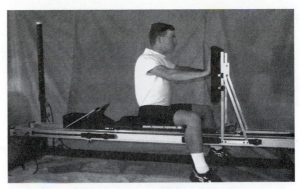

FIGURE 25-50

Shuttle 2000-1. The exercise machine can be used for plyometric exercises in either the upper or the lower extremity.

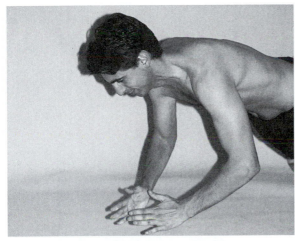

FIGURE 25-48

Push-ups with a clap. The patient pushes off the ground, claps his hands, and catches his weight as he decelerates.

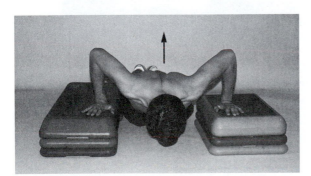

FIGURE 25-49

Push-ups on boxes. When performing a plyometric push-up on boxes, the patient can stretch the anterior muscles, which facilities a concentric contraction.

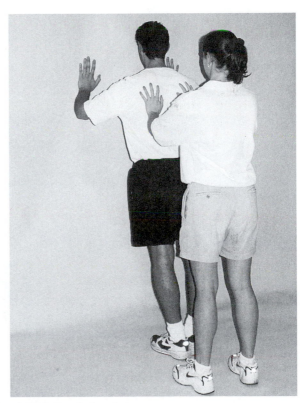

FIGURE 25-51

Push into wall. The therapist stands behind the patient and pushes him toward the wall. The patient decelerates the forces and then pushes off the wall immediately.

Isokinetic Exercises

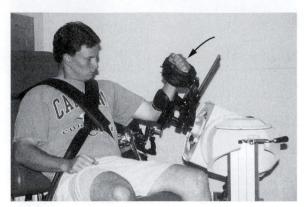

FIGURE 25-52

Isokinetic medial/lateral rotation. When using an isokinetic device for strengthening the shoulder, the patient should be set up such that strengthening can be done in a scapular plane.[21]

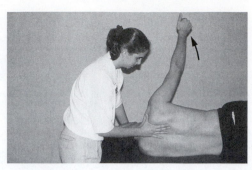

FIGURE 25-54

PNF technique for scapula. As the patient moves through either a D1 or a D2 pattern, the therapist applies resistance at the appropriate scapular border.

PNF Strengthening Techniques

See Figs. 25-53–25-73.

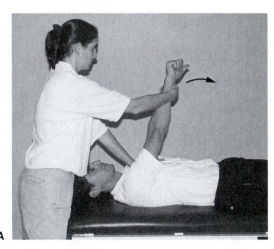

A

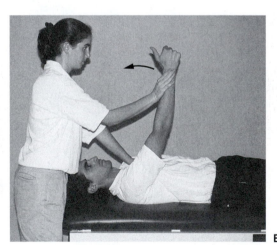

B

FIGURE 25-53

Rhythmic contraction. Using either a D1 or D2 pattern. **A,** The patient uses an isometric cocontraction to maintain a specific position within the ROM. **B,** The therapist repeatedly changes the direction of passive pressure.

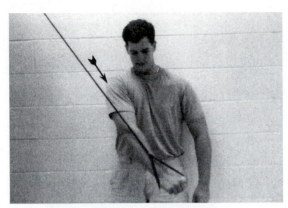

FIGURE   25-55

The patient can use resistance from tubing through a PNF movement pattern.

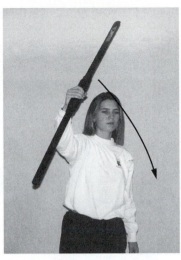

FIGURE   25-57

PNF using a Body Blade. In a standing position, the patient moves an oscillating Body Blade through a D2 pattern.

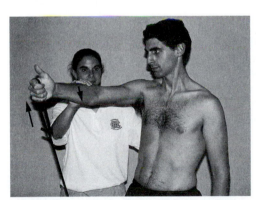

FIGURE   25-56

PNF using both manual resistance and surgical tubing Rhythmic stabilization can be performed as the patient isometrically holds a specific position in the ROM with surgical tubing and force applied by the therapist.

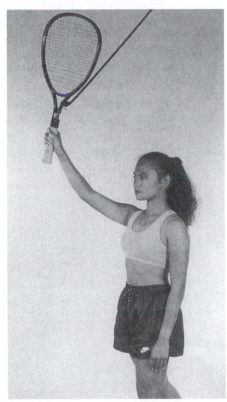

FIGURE   25-58

Surgical tubing may be attached to a tennis racket as the patient practices an overhead serve technique. This is useful as a functional progression technique.

Exercises to Reestablish Neuromuscular Control

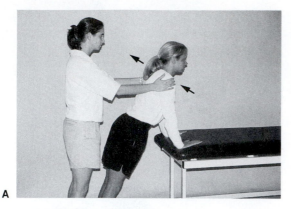
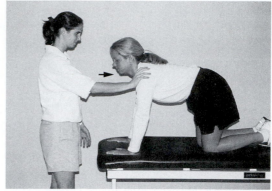
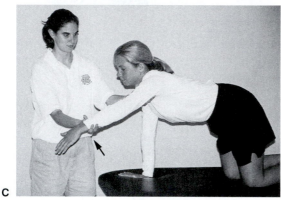
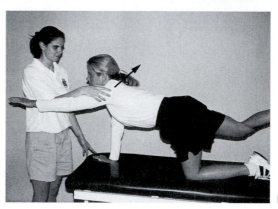

FIGURE   25-59

Weight shifting on a stable surface may be done. **A,** Standing with hands supporting weight on table, **B,** kneeling in a four-point position, **C,** kneeling in a three-point position, and **D,** kneeling in a two-point position. The therapist can apply random directional pressure to which the patient must respond to maintain a static position. In the two- and three-point positions, the arm that is supported in a closed-kinetic-chain is using shoulder force couples to maintain neuromuscular control.

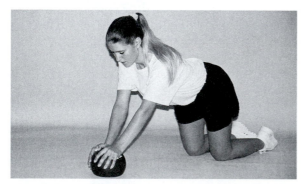

FIGURE   25-60

Weight shifting on a ball. In a push-up position with weight supported on a ball, the patient shifts weight from side to side and/or forward and backward. Weight shifting on an unstable surface facilitates cocontraction of the muscles involved in the force couples that collectively maintain dynamic stability.

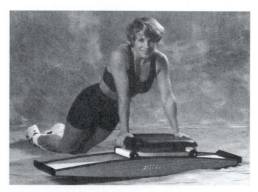

FIGURE   25-61

Weight shifting on a Fitter. In a kneeling position the patient shifts weight from side to side using a Fitter. Weight shifting on an unstable surface facilitates cocontraction of the muscles involved in the force couples that collectively maintain dynamic stability.

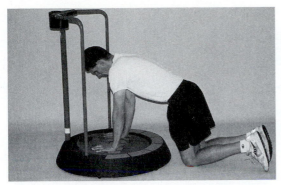

FIGURE 25-62

Weight shifting on a KAT (Kinesthetic Ability Trainer) system. In a kneeling position the patient shifts weight from side to side and/or backward and forward using a KAT. Weight shifting on an unstable surface facilitates cocontraction of the muscles involved in the force couples that collectively maintain dynamic stability.

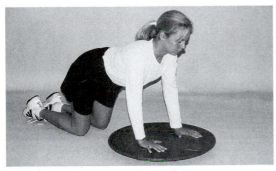

FIGURE 25-63

Weight shifting on a BAPS board. In a kneeling position the patient shifts weight from side to side and/or backward and forward using a BAPS board. Weight shifting on an unstable surface facilitates cocontraction of the muscles involved in the force couples that collectively maintain dynamic stability.

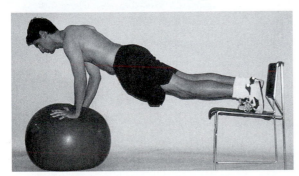

FIGURE 25-64

Weight shifting on a Swiss ball. With the feet supported on a chair, the patient shifts weight from side to side and/or backward and forward using a Swiss ball. Weight shifting on an unstable surface facilitates cocontraction of the muscles involved in the force couples that collectively maintain dynamic stability.

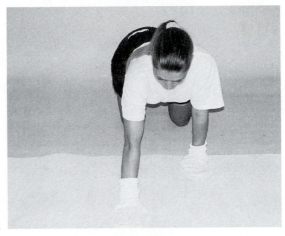

A

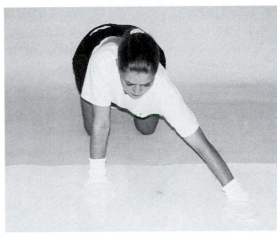

B

FIGURE 25-65

Slide board exercises. **A,** Forward and backward motion. **B,** Wax-on/wax-off motion. **C,** Hands lateral motion. The patient shifts weight from side to side and/or backward and forward using a BAPS board. Weight shifting on an unstable surface facilitates cocontraction of the muscles involved in the force couples that collectively maintain dynamic stability.

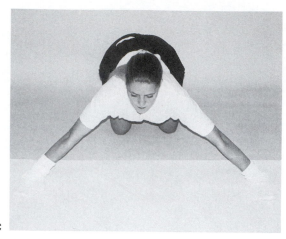

C

FIGURE 25-65

(Continued)

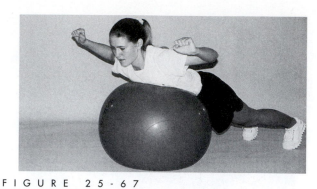

FIGURE 25-67

Swiss ball exercises. The patient lies in a prone position on the Swiss ball and maintains a stable position while lifting the arms in a "W," "T," or "Y" position.

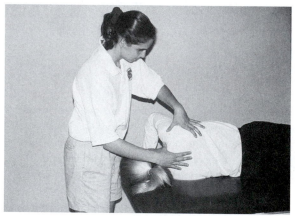

FIGURE 25-66

Scapular neuromuscular control exercises. The patient's hand is placed on the table, creating a closed-kinetic chain, and the therapist applies pressure to the scapula in a random direction. The patient moves the scapula isotonically into the direction of resistance.

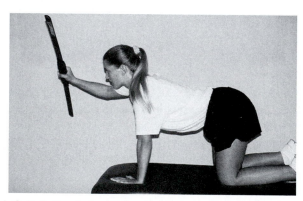

FIGURE 25-68

Body Blade exercises. The patient is in a three-point kneeling position holding an oscillating Body Blade in one hand while working on neuromuscular control in the weight-bearing shoulder.

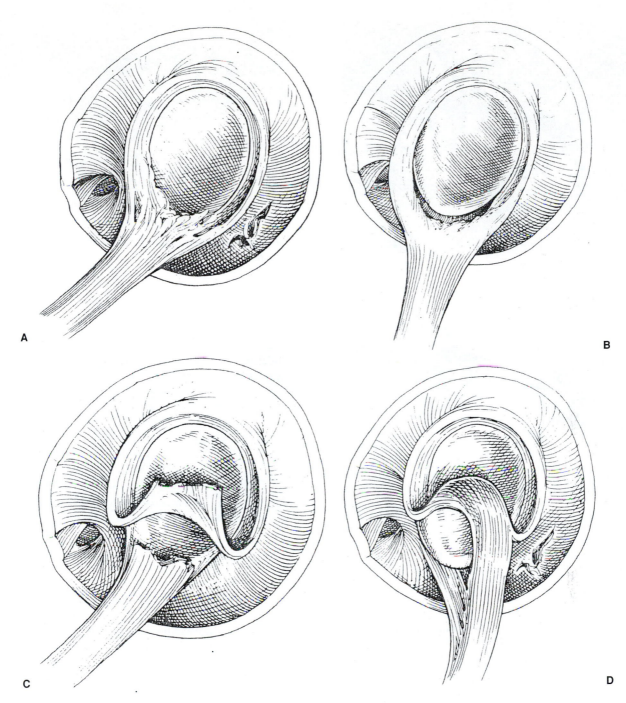

FIGURE 25-69

Graphic representations of the four common types of SLAP lesions of the shoulder.
A, Type I SLAP lesion: fraying of the superior labrum with intact biceps tendon anchor.
B, Type II SLAP lesion: Detachment of the biceps anchor. **C,** Type III SLAP lesion:
Bucket-handle tear of the superior labrum, biceps tendon anchor intact. **D,** Type IV SLAP
lesion: Bucket-handle tear of the superior labrum, extending into biceps tendon anchor.
(Reproduced, with permission from the Arthroscopy Association of North America,
from: Snyder SJ, Karzel RP, Del Pizzo W, Ferkel RD, Friedman MJ. SLAP lesions of the
shoulder. *Arthroscopy* 6(4):274–279, 1990.)

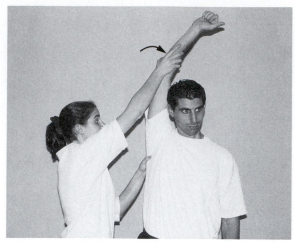

FIGURE   25-70

Neer impingement test.

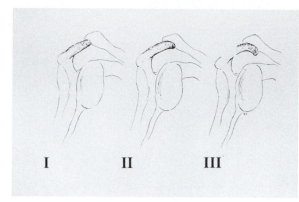

FIGURE   25-72

Acromion shapes. Type I, flat; type II, curved; and type III, hooked.

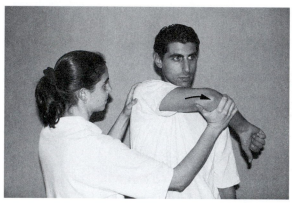

FIGURE   25-71

Hawkins–Kennedy impingement test.

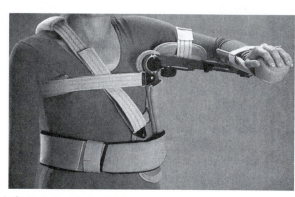

FIGURE   25-73

Airplane splint.

SUMMARY

- The high degree of mobility in the shoulder complex requires some compromise in stability, which in turn increases the vulnerability of the shoulder joint to injury, particularly in dynamic overhead athletic activities.

- In rehabilitation of the SC joint, effort should be directed toward regaining normal clavicular motion that will allow the scapula to abduct and upward rotate throughout 180° of humeral abduction. The clavicle must elevate approximately 40° to allow upward scapular rotation.

- AC joint sprains are most commonly seen in patients due to a direct fall on the point of the shoulder with the arm at the side in an adducted position or falling on an outstretched arm.

- Management of AC injuries depends on the type of injury. Type I and II injuries are usually handled conservatively, focusing on strengthening of the deltoid, trapezius, and the clavicular fibers of the pectoralis major. Occasionally AC

injuries require surgical excision of the distal portion of the clavicle.

- Treatment for clavicle fractures includes approximation of the fracture and immobilization for 6–8 weeks, using a figure-8 wrap with the involved arm in a sling. Because mobility of the clavicle is important for normal shoulder mechanics, rehabilitation should focus on joint mobilization and strengthening of the deltoid, upper trapezius, and pectoralis major muscles.

- Following a short immobilization period, rehabilitation for a dislocated shoulder should focus on restoring the appropriate axis of rotation for the glenohumeral joint, optimizing the stabilizing muscle's length–tension relationship, and restoring proper neuromuscular control of the shoulder complex. Similar rehabilitation strategies are applied in case of multidirectional instabilities, which can occur as a result of recurrent dislocation.

- Management of shoulder impingement involves gradually restoring normal biomechanics to the shoulder joint in an effort to maintain space under the coracoacromial arch during overhead activities. Techniques include strengthening of the rotator cuff muscles, strengthening of the muscles that abduct, elevate, and upward rotate the scapula, and stretching both the inferior and the posterior portions of the joint capsule.

- The basic concerns of a rehabilitation program for rotator cuff tendonopathy are based on why and how the tendon has been damaged. If a comprehensive rehabilitation program does not relieve the painful shoulder, surgical repair of the tendon and alteration of the glenohumeral joint are performed. Surgical rehabilitation is similar to the nonsurgical plan, with the time of progression altered, based on tissue healing and tendon histology.

- In cases of adhesive capsulitis, the goals of rehabilitation are relieving the pain in the acute stages of the disorder, gradually restoring proper arthrokinematics, gradual restoration of ROM, and strengthening the muscles of the shoulder complex.

- Rehabilitation for thoracic outlet syndrome should be directed toward encouraging the least provocative posture combined with exercises to strengthen postural muscles (rhomboids, middle trapezius, upper trapezius) and stretching exercises for the scalenes to increase the space in the thoracic outlet in order to reduce muscle impingement on the neurovascular bundle.

- Management of brachial plexus injuries includes the gradual restoration of cervical ROM and stretching for the upper trapezius, levator scapulae, and scalene muscles.

- After identifying the cause of myofascial TPs, rehabilitation may include a spray-and-stretch method with passive stretching, gentle active ROM exercises or active assistive exercises, encouraging normal muscle activity and endurance, and gradual improvement of muscle endurance.

REFERENCES

1. Allman FL. Fractures and ligamentous injuries of the clavicle and its articulations. *J Bone Joint Surg* 49A:774, 1967.
2. Anderson L, Rush R, Shearer L. The effects of a TheraBand exercise program on shoulder internal rotation strength. *Physl Ther* 72(Suppl 6):540, 1992.
3. Andrews JR, Wilk KE, eds. *The Athlete's Shoulder*. New York, Churchill Livingstone, 1994.
4. Bateman JE. *The Shoulder and Neck*. Philadelphia, WB Saunders, 1971.
5. Bergfeld JA, Andrish JT, Clancy WG. Evaluation of the acromioclavicular joint following first and second degree sprains. *Am J Sports Med* 6:153, 1978.
6. Bigliani L, Kimmel J, McCann P. Repair of rotator cuff tears in tennis players. *Am J Sports Med* 20(2):112–117, 1992.
7. Bigliani L, Morrison D, April E. The morphology of the acromion and its relation to rotator cuff tears. *Orthop Trans* 10:216, 1986.
8. Blackburn T, McCloud W, White B. EMG analysis of posterior rotator cuff exercises. *Athlet Train* 25(1):40–45, 1990.
9. Brewster C, Moynes D. Rehabilitation of the shoulder following rotator cuff injury or surgery. *J Orthop Sports Phys Ther* 18(2):422–426, 1993.
10. Burkhead W, Rockwood C. Treatment of instability of rotator cuff injuries in the overhead athlete. *J Bone Joint Surg* 74A:890, 1992.
11. Butler D. *The Sensitive Nervous System*. Adelaide, Australia, Noigroup, 2000.
12. Clancy WG, Brand RI, Bergfeld JA. Upper trunk brachial plexus injuries in contact sports. *Am J Sports Med* 5:209, 1977.
13. Codman EA. Ruptures of the supraspinatus tendon and other lesions in or about the subacromial bursa. In: Codman EA, ed. *The Shoulder*. Boston, Thomas Todd, 1934.
14. Cools AM, Witvrouw EE, DeClercq GA, Voight ML. Scapular muscle recruitment pattern: EMG response of the trapezius muscle to the sudden shoulder movement before and after a fatiguing exercise. *J Orthop Sports Phys Ther* 32(5):221–229, 2002.
15. Cox JS. The fate of the acromioclavicular joint in athletic injuries. *Am J Sports Med* 9:50, 1981.
16. Culham E, Malcolm P. Functional anatomy of the shoulder complex. *J Orthop Sports Phys Ther* 18(1):342–350, 1993.
17. Davies G, Dickoff-Hoffman S. Neuromuscular testing and rehabilitation of the shoulder complex. *J Orthop Sports Phys Ther* 18(2):449–458, 1993.
18. Depalma AF. *Surgery of the Shoulder*, 2nd ed. Philadelphia, Lippincott Williams & Wilkins, 1973.
19. Dvir Z, Berme N. The shoulder complex in elevation of the arm: A mechanism approach. *J Biomech* 11:219–225, 1978.
20. Duncan A. Personal communication, August 1997.
21. Favorito P, Langenderfer M, Colosimo A, Heidt R, Jr, Carlonas R. Arthroscopic laser-assisted capsular shift in the treatment of patients with multidirectional shoulder instability. *Am J Sports Med* 30:322–328, 2002.
22. Greenfield B. Special considerations in shoulder exercises: Plane of the scapula. In: Andrews J, Wilk K, eds. *The Athlete's Shoulder*. New York, Churchill Livingstone, 1993.
23. Gryzlo SM. Bony disorders: Clinical assessment and treatment. In: Jobe FW, ed. *Operative Techniques in Upper Extremity Sports Injuries*. St. Louis, MO, Mosby, 1996.
24. Hageman P, Mason D, Rydlund K. Effects of position and speed on concentric isokinetic testing of the shoulder rotators. *J Orthop Sports Phys Ther* 11:64–69, 1989.
25. Hart DL, Carmichael SW. Biomechanics of the shoulder. *J Orthop Sports Phys Ther* 6(4):229–234, 1985.
26. Hawkins R, Bell R. Dynamic EMG analysis of the shoulder muscles during rotational and scapular strengthening exercises. In: Post M, Morey B, Hawkins R, eds. *Surgery of the Shoulder*. St. Louis, MO, Mosby, 1990.

27. Hawkins R, Kennedy J. Impingement syndrome in athletes. *Am J Sports Med* 8:151, 1980.

28. Howell S, Kraft T. The role of the supraspinatus and infraspinatus muscles in glenohumeral kinematics of anterior shoulder instability. *Clin Orthop* 263:128–134, 1991.

29. Inman VT, Saunders JB, Abbott LC. Observations on the function of the shoulder joint. *J Bone Joint Surg* 26:1, 1944.

30. Jobe FW, ed. *Operative Techniques in Upper Extremity Sports Injuries*. St. Louis, MO, Mosby, 1996.

31. Jobe F, Kvnite R. Shoulder pain in the overhand and throwing athlete: The relationship of anterior instability and rotator cuff impingement. *Orthop Rev* 18:963, 1989.

32. Jobe F, Moynes D. Delineation of diagnostic criteria and a rehabilitation program for rotator cuff injuries. *Am J Sports Med* 10(6):336–339, 1982.

33. Jobe FW, Schwab DM, Wilk KE, Andrews JE. Rehabilitation of the shoulder. In: Brotzman SB, ed. *Clinical Orthopedics Rehabilitation*. St. Louis, MO, Mosby, 1996.

34. Kannus P, Josza L, Renstrom P, et al. The effects of training, immobilization and remobilization on musculoskeletal tissue: 2. Remobilization and prevention of immobilization atrophy. *Scand J Sports Sci* 2:164–176, 1992.

35. Keirns M. Conservative management of shoulder impingement. In: Andrews J, Wilk K, eds. *The Athlete's Shoulder*. New York, Churchill Livingstone, 1993.

36. Kelley MJ. Anatomic and biomechanical rationale for rehabilitation of the athlete's shoulder. *J Sport Rehabil* 4:122–154, 1995.

37. Kibbler WB. Role of the scapula in the overhead throwing motion. *Contemp Orthop* 22:525–532, 1998.

38. Kibler WB. The role of the scapula in athletic shoulder function. *Am J Sports Med* 26(2):325–337, 1998.

39. Leffert RD. Neurological problems. In: Rockwood CA, Matsen FA, eds. *The Shoulder*. Philadelphia, WB Saunders, 1990.

40. Lephart SM, Warner JP, Borsa PA, Fu FH. Proprioception of the shoulder joint in healthy, unstable, and surgically repaired shoulders. *J Shoulder Elbow Surg* 3(6):371–380, 1994.

41. Lew W, Lewis J, Craig E. Stabilization by capsule ligaments and labrum: Stability at the extremes of motion. In: Masten F, Fu F, Hawkins R, Rosemont IL, eds. *The Shoulder: A Balance of Mobility and Stability*. American Academy of Orthopedic Surgery, 1993.

42. Litchfield R, Hawkins R, Dillman C. Rehabilitation for the overhead athlete. *J Orthop Sports Phys Ther* 18(2):433–441, 1993.

43. Ludewig PM, Cook TM. Translations of the humerus in persons with shoulder impingement syndromes. *J Orthop Sports Phys Ther* 32(6):248–259, 2002.

44. Magee D, Reid D. Shoulder injuries. In: Zachazewski J, Magee D, Quillen W, eds. *Athletic Injuries and Rehabilitation*. Philadelphia, WB Saunders, 1995.

45. Matsen FA, Thomas SC, Rockwood CA. Glenohumeral instability. In: Rockwood CA, Matsen FA, eds. *The Shoulder*. Philadelphia, WB Saunders, 1990.

46. McCarroll J. Golf. In: Pettrone FA, ed. *Athletic Injuries of the Shoulder*. New York, McGraw-Hill, 1995.

47. Meister K, Andrews JR. Classification and treatment of rotator cuff injuries in the overhead athlete. *J Orthop Sports Phys Ther* 18(2):413–421, 1993.

48. Moseley J, Jobe F, Pink M. EMG analysis of the scapular muscles during a shoulder rehabilitation program. *Am J Sports Med* 20:128–134, 1992.

49. Mulligan E. Conservative management of shoulder impingement syndrome. *Athlet Train* 23(4):348–353, 1988.

50. Neer C. Anterior acromioplasty for the chronic impingement syndrome in the shoulder: A preliminary report. *J Bone Joint Surg* 54A:41, 1972.

51. Nicholas JA, Hershmann EB, eds. *The Upper Extremity in Sports Medicine*. St. Louis, MO, Mosby, 1990.

52. O'Brien S, Neeves M, Arnoczky A. The anatomy and histology of the inferior glenohumeral ligament complex of the shoulder. *Am J Sports Educ* 18:451, 1990.

53. Omer GE. Osteotomy of the clavicle in surgical reduction of anterior sternoclavicular dislocations. *J Trauma* 7(4):584–590, 1967.

54. Ozaki J, Fujimoto S, Nakagawa Y. Tears of the rotator cuff of the shoulder associated with pathological changes in the acromion: A study of cadavers. *J Bone Joint Surg* 70A:1224, 1988.

55. Paine R, Voight M. The role of the scapula. *J Orthop Sports Phys Ther* 18(1):386–391, 1993.

56. Peat M, Culham E. Functional anatomy of the shoulder complex. In: Andrews J, Wilk K, eds. *The Athlete's Shoulder*. New York, Churchill Livingstone, 1993.

57. Petersson C, Redlund-Johnell I. The subacromial space in normal shoulder radiographs. *Acta Orthop Scand* 55:57, 1984.

58. Pettrone FA, ed. *Athletic Injuries of the Shoulder*. New York, McGraw-Hill, 1995.

59. Rathburn J, McNab I. The microvascular pattern of the rotator cuff. *J Bone Joint Surg* 52B:540, 1970.

60. Rockwood C, Matsen F. *The Shoulder, Vols. 1 and 2*. Philadelphia, WB Saunders, 1990.

61. Rowe CR. Prognosis in dislocation of the shoulder. *J Bone Joint Surg* 38A:957, 1956.

62. Salter EG, Shelley BS, Nasca R. A morphological study of the acromioclavicular joint in humans [abstract]. *Anat Rec* 211:353, 1985.

63. Skyhar M, Warren R, Altcheck D. Instability of the shoulder. In: Nicholas A, Hershmann EB, eds. *The Upper Extremity in Sports Medicine*. St. Louis, MO, Mosby, 1990.

64. Snyder SJ, Katzel KP, Del Pizzo W, Feckel RD, Friedman MJ. SLAP lesions of the shoulder. *Arthroscopy* 6(4):274–279, 1990.

65. Souza TA. *Sports Injuries of the Shoulder: Conservative Management*. New York, Churchill Livingstone, 1994.

66. Stevens JH. The classic brachial plexus paralysis. In: Codman EA, ed. *The Shoulder*. Boston, Thomas Todd, 1934, pp. 344–350.

67. Sutter JS. Conservative treatment of shoulder instability. In: Andrews J, Wilk KE, eds. *The Athlete's Shoulder*. New York, Churchill Livingstone, 1994.

68. Taft TN, Wilson FC, Ogelsby JW. Dislocation of the AC joint, an end result study. *J Bone Joint Surg* 69A:1045, 1987.

69. Takeda Y, Kashiwguchi S, Endo K, Matsuura T, Sasa T. The most effective exercise for strengthening the supraspinatus muscle. *Am J Sports Med* 30:374–381, 2002.

70. Thein L. Impingement syndrome and its conservative management. *J Orthop Sports Phys Ther* 11(5):183–191, 1989.

71. Townsend H, Jobe F, Pink M. EMG analysis of the glenohumeral muscles during a baseball rehabilitation program. *Am J Sports Med* 19(3):264–272, 1991.

72. Travell JG, Simons DG. Myofascial pain and dysfunction. *The Trigger Point Manual*. Baltimore, Williams & Wilkins, 1983.

73. Uthoff H, Loeher J, Sarkar K. The pathogenesis of rotator cuff tears. In: Takagishi N, ed. *The Shoulder*. Philadelphia, Professional Post Graduate Services, 1987.

74. von Eisenhart-Rothe R, Jager A, Englmeier K, Vogl TJ, Graichen H. Relevance of arm position and muscle activity in three-dimensional glenohumeral translation in patients with traumatic and atraumatic shoulder instability. *Am J Sports Med* 30:514–522, 2002.

75. Warner J, Michili L, Arslanin L. Patterns of flexibility, laxity, and strength in normal shoulders and shoulders with instability and impingement. *Am J Sports Med* 18(4):366–375, 1990.

76. Warren RF. Neurological injuries in football. In: Jordan BD, Tsiaris P, Warren RF, eds. *Sports Neurology*. Rockville, MD, Aspen, 1989.

77. Wilk K, Andrews J. Rehabilitation following subacromial decompression. *Orthopaedics* 16(3):349–358, 1993.

78. Wilk K, Arrigo C. An integrated approach to upper extremity exercises. *Orthop Phys Ther Clin N Am* 9(2):337–360, 1992.

79. Wilk K, Arrigo C. Current concepts in the rehabilitation of the athletic shoulder. *J Orthop Sports Phys Ther* 18(1):365–378, 1993.

80. Wilk K, Arrigo C. Current concepts in rehabilitation of the shoulder. In: Andrews J, Wilk K, eds. *The Athlete's Shoulder*. New York, Churchill Livingstone, 1993.

81. Wilk K, Reinhold M, Dugas JR, Andrews JR. Rehabilitation following thermal-assisted capsular shrinkage of the glenohumeral joint: Current concepts. *J Orthop Sports Phys Ther* 32(6):268–287, 2002.

82. Wilk K, Voight M, Kearns M. Stretch shortening drills for the upper extremity. Theory and application. *J Orthop Sports Phys Ther* 17(5):225–239, 1993.

TREATMENT PROTOCOL FOR THERMAL ASSISTED CAPSULAR SHRINKAGE OF THE GLENOHUMERAL JOINT

Injury Situation: A 34-year old male assembly line worker, who performs a repetitive overhead motion in his job, complains of posterior shoulder pain. After 3 months of using ice and NSAID therapy he goes to see his physician. On initial visit he complains of posterior cuff pain whenever he externally rotates. He has 165° of ER and 35° of IR. Horizontal adduction of the humerus is only 15°. Tenderness is present along the posterior glenohumeral joint line. He also has a positive apprehension sign and relocation test. The patient is diagnosed by an orthopedist with posterior impingement secondary to multidirectional instability of the glenohumeral joint.

Phase One—Acute Phase

GOALS: Allow soft-tissue healing, diminish pain and inflammation, initiate protected motion, retard muscle atrophy.

Estimated length of time (ELT): day 1 to week 6

For the first 2 weeks the patient uses a sling full time for 7–10 days, sleeping with it for the full 2 weeks. Exercises include hand and wrist ROM and active cervical spine ROM. During this phase, cryotherapy is used before and after treatments. Passive and active assisted ROM for the glenohumeral joint is cautiously performed in a restricted ROM. Shoulder rotation is done in the scapular plane; ER is to neutral and IR is allowed to 25° or 30° for the first week. Moist heat can be used prior to therapy after 10 days. At 2 weeks, ROM is progressed cautiously; flexion is allowed to 90°, ER to 25°, IR to 45° in the scapular plane. Passive ROM is performed by the therapist and active assisted ROM by the patient.

During this phase, ROM is progressed based on the end feel the therapist gets when evaluating the patient. With a hard end feel, the therapist may choose to be more aggressive; a soft end feel dictates slower progression. ROM is not the main focus of this phase. By weeks 5 and 6 the therapist should be able to progress to 160° of elevation, 75°–80° of ER, and 60°–65° of IR. Rotation should be progressed out of the safe zone to 90° of elevation.

Shoulder strengthening begins early in this phase with rhythmic stabilization, scapular stabilizing exercises, isometric exercises for the rotator cuff muscles, and PNF control exercises in a restricted ROM. By the end of this phase, exercise for the external rotators and scapular stabilizers should move to unweighted isotonic exercises.

Phase Two—Intermediate Phase

GOALS: Restore full ROM, restore functional ROM, normalize arthrokinematics, improve dynamic stability, improve muscular strength.

ELT: weeks 7–12

During this phase the patient's ROM is progressed to fully functional by 8 weeks: flexion to 180°, 90°–100° of ER at 90° of abduction, and 60°–65° of IR. Aggressive stretching may be used during this phase if the goal is not met by 8 weeks. This may include joint mobilization and capsular stretching techniques. From week 9 to 12, the therapist begins to gradually progress ROM exercises to a position functional for this assembly line worker.

In this phase, strengthening exercises include PRE in all planes of shoulder motion and IR and ER resisted exercises at the 90/90 positions. Resistance progresses from isotonic to plyometric. Plyometric exercises are initiated with two-handed drills progressing to single-handed plyometric throwing activities. Rhythmic stabilization drills continue to be progressed with increasing difficulty. Aggressive strengthening may be initiated if ROM goals are achieved. Weight activities, including push-ups, bench press (without allowing the arm to drop below the body), and latissimus pull-downs in front of body, may begin. Exercises should be performed asymptomatically. If symptoms of pain or instability occur, a thorough evaluation of the patient should be performed and the program adjusted accordingly.

Phase Three—Advanced Phase

GOALS: Improve strength, power, and endurance; enhance neuromuscular control; functional activities.

ELT: weeks 12–20

The criteria used to allow the patient to progress to this phase are full ROM, no pain or tenderness, and muscular strength at least 80 percent of the contralateral side. All strengthening exercises are progressed. The patient should maintain established ROM and should continue stretching exercises.

Criteria for Return to Function

GOALS: Complete elimination of pain and full return to function.

ELT: weeks 20

1. Full function ROM
2. No pain or tenderness
3. Satisfactory muscular strength
4. Satisfactory clinical exam

TREATMENT PROTOCOL FOR ANTERIOR GLENOHUMERAL DISLOCATION

Injury Situation: A 42-year old female slipped on a patch of ice and attempted to prevent herself from falling. She demonstrated a position of abduction and ER. She immediately felt her shoulder give way and felt a pop and a tearing sensation with intense pain. There was a flattened deltoid contour. Palpation of the axilla revealed prominence of the humeral head. The patient was unable to touch the opposite shoulder with the hand of the affected arm. The shoulder was immediately immobilized by paramedics without attempting reduction. The patient was then referred to a physician for reduction after X-rays ruled out fracture. After the dislocation was reduced and immobilized, physical therapy was initiated the following day.

Phase One—Acute Phase

GOALS: To control pain and swelling and to begin to regain ROM.

ELT: 1–5 days.

RICE (rest, ice, compression, elevation) should be applied immediately and should continue to be used for the next several days. Initial management of an interior shoulder dislocation requires immediate immobilization in a position of comfort using a sling with a folded towel or small pillow placed under the arm. Protective sling immobilization should continue for approximately one week after reduction. In anterior dislocations, the arm should be maintained in a relaxed position of adduction and IR. While the shoulder is immobilized, the patient is instructed to perform isometric exercises for strengthening the internal and external rotator muscles. Codman's pendulum exercises and sawing exercises can help the athlete regain ROM as pain allows.

Phase Two—Intermediate Phase

GOALS: To achieve full ROM and increase strength.

ELT: 5–12 days.

Ice and electrical stimulation should be used to modulate pain. Low-intensity ultrasound may also be used to facilitate healing. The patient may continue to wear the sling but should be progressively weaned from it as pain allows. ROM exercises using a T-bar can be instituted as early as tolerated. Wall climbing and rope and pulley exercises can also be used to regain motion. The strengthening program should progress from isometrics to resistive rubber tubing and then to dumbbells and other resistance devices as quickly as can be tolerated. Exercises should concentrate on strengthening the rotator cuff. Weight shifting with the hands on the ground can help the patient to begin strengthening the scapular stabilizers and reestablishing neuromuscular control.

Phase Three—Advanced Phase

GOALS: To regain normal strength and return to full activity.

ELT: 12 days to 3 weeks.

Electrical stimulation can be used for muscle reeducation. Ultrasound can be used for deep heating to increase blood flow to clean up the injured area. Ice should be used after exercise.

Strengthening exercises should progress from resisted isotonics to isokinetics at greater speeds. Functional D1 and D2 PNF strengthening patterns should be used, adjusting resistance to the patient's capabilities. Plyometric activities using weighted balls can be used to work on more dynamic control. Closed-kinetic-chain exercises using weight shifting on a ball or balance device improve neuromuscular control.

Criteria for Return to Function

1. The shoulder should have full ROM and be pain-free
2. Shoulder strength should be near normal
3. Normal functional activities should not produce pain
4. Protective shoulder braces may be used to help limit shoulder motion

C H A P T E R   2 6

Rehabilitation of the Elbow

Todd S. Ellenbecker, Tad Pieczynski, and Anna Thatcher

O B J E C T I V E S

After completing this chapter, the therapist should be able to do the following:

- Discuss the functional anatomy and biomechanics associated with normal function of the elbow.
- Identify the various techniques for regaining range of motion including stretching exercises and joint mobilizations.
- Perform specific clinical tests to identify ligamentous laxity and tendon pathology in the injured elbow.
- Discuss criteria for progression of the rehabilitation program for different elbow injuries.
- Demonstrate the various rehabilitative strengthening techniques for the elbow, including open- and closed-kinetic chain isometric, isotonic, plyometric, isokinetic, and functional exercises.

INTRODUCTION

Treatment of elbow injuries in active individuals requires an understanding of the mechanism of injury, the anatomy and biomechanics of the human elbow and upper-extremity kinetic chain, as well as a structured and detailed clinical examination to identify the structure or structures involved. Treatment of the injured elbow of both a younger adolescent patient and an older active patient requires this same approach. This approach consists of understanding the specific anatomical vulnerabilities present in the young athletes' elbow as well as the effects of years of repetitive stress and the clinical ramifications these stresses produce in the aging elbow joint. An overview of the most common elbow injuries as well as a review of the musculoskeletal adaptations of the elbow will provide a platform for the discussion of examination and most specifically treatment concepts for patients with elbow injury. The important interplay between the elbow and shoulder joints in the upper-extremity kinetic chain will be reviewed throughout this chapter to support the comprehensive examination and treatment strategies of the total arm strength treatment concept.

FUNCTIONAL ANATOMY AND BIOMECHANICS

Anatomically, the elbow joint comprises three joints. The humeroulnar joint, humeroradial joint, and the proximal ra-

dioulnar joint are the articulations that make up the elbow complex (Fig. 26-1). The elbow allows for flexion, extension, pronation, and supination movement patterns about the joint complex. The bony limitations, ligamentous support, and muscular stability will help to protect it from vulnerability of overuse and resultant injury.

The elbow complex comprises three bones: the distal humerus, proximal ulna, and proximal radius. The articulations among these three bones dictate elbow movement patterns.[109] It is also important to mention that the appropriate strength and function of the upper quarter (cervical spine to the hand, including the scapulothoracic joint) needs to be addressed when evaluating the elbow specifically. The elbow complex has an intricate mechanical articulation between the three separate joints of the upper quarter to allow for function to occur.

In the elbow, the joint capsule plays an important role. The capsule is continuous (Fig. 26-2A) among the three articulations and highly innervated.[78,82] This is important not only for support of the elbow joint complex but also for proprioception of the joint. The capsule of the elbow functions as a neurological link between the shoulder and the hand within the upper-extremity kinetic chain. Therefore, function of the capsule has an effect on upper-quarter activity and is an obvious portion of the rehabilitation process if injury does occur.

Humeroulnar Joint

The humeroulnar joint is the articulation between the distal humerus medially and the proximal ulna. The humerus has

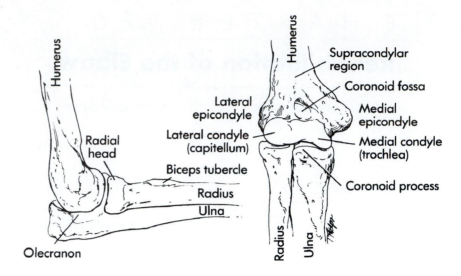

FIGURE 26-1

Articulations of the elbow joint complex.

distinct features distally. The medial aspect has the medial epicondyle and an hourglass-shaped trochlea, located anteromedial on the distal humerus.[2,45] The trochlea extends more distal than the lateral aspect of the humerus. The trochlea articulates with the trochlear notch of the proximal ulna.

Because of the more distal projection of the humerus medially, the elbow complex demonstrates a carrying angle that is essentially an abducted position of the elbow in the anatomic position. The normal carrying angle (Fig. 26-3) is 10°–15° in females and 5° in males.[7]

Radiocapitellar Joint (Humeroradial Joint)

The radiocapitellar or humeroradial joint is the articulation of the distal lateral humerus and the proximal radius. The lateral aspect of the humerus has the lateral epicondyle and the

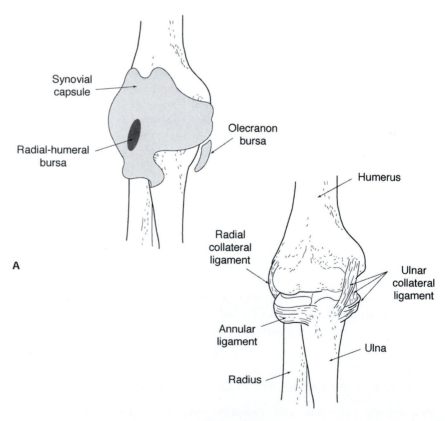

FIGURE 26-2

A, Elbow joint capsule. **B,** Medial ulnar collateral ligament complex.

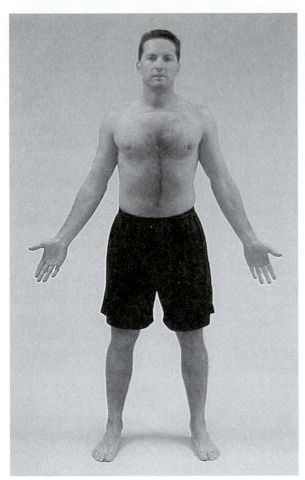

FIGURE 26-3

Carrying angle of the human elbow.

capitellum, which is located anteriolateral on the distal humerus. With flexion, the radius is in contact with the radial fossa of the distal humerus, whereas in extension, the radius and the humerus are not in contact.

Proximal Radioulnar Joint

The proximal radioulnar joint is the articulation between the radial notch of the proximal lateral aspect of the ulna, the radial head, and the capitellum of the distal humerus. The proximal and distal radioulnar joints are important for supination and pronation. Proximally, the radius articulates with the ulna by the support of the annular ligament, which attaches to the ulnar notch anteriorly and posteriorly. This ligament circles the radial head and adds support. The interosseous membrane is the connective tissue that functions to complete the interval between the two bones. When there is a fall on the outstretched arm, the interosseous membrane can shift forces off the radius—the main weight-bearing bone of the forearm—to the ulna. This prevents the radial head from having forceful contact with the capitellum. Distally, the concave radius articulates with the con-

vex ulna. With supination and pronation, the radius moves on the more stationary ulna.

Ligamentous Structures

The stability of the elbow starts with the joint capsule and excellent bony congruity inherent to the three articulations of the human elbow. The capsule is loose anteriorly and posteriorly to allow for movement in flexion and extension.[113] The joint capsule is taut medially and laterally due to the added support of the collateral ligaments.

The medial (ulnar) collateral ligament (MUCL) is fan shaped in nature and has three bands (Fig. 26-2B). The anterior band of the MUCL is the primary stabilizer of the elbow against valgus loads when the elbow is near extension.[113] The posterior band of the MUCL becomes taut after 60° of elbow flexion and assists in stabilizing against valgus stress when the elbow is in a flexed position. The oblique band of the MUCL does not technically cross the elbow joint and this does not provide extensive stabilization to the medial elbow like the anterior and posterior bands.

The lateral elbow complex consists of four structures. The radial collateral ligament attachments are from the lateral epicondyle to the annular ligament. The lateral ulnar collateral ligament is the primary lateral stabilizer and passes over the annular ligament into the supinator tubercle. It reinforces the elbow laterally, as well as re-enforcing the humeroradial joint.[92,113] The accessory lateral collateral ligament passes from the tubercle of the supinator into the annular ligament. The annular ligament, as previously stated, is the main support of the radial head in the radial notch of the ulna. The interosseous membrane is a syndesmotic tissue that connects the ulna and the radius in the forearm. As previously mentioned, this structure prevents the proximal displacement of the radius on the ulna and transmits force between the radius and ulna.

Dynamic Stabilizers of the Elbow Complex

The elbow flexors are the biceps brachii, brachialis, and brachioradialis muscles (Fig. 26-4). The biceps brachii originates via two heads proximally at the shoulder: the long head from the supraglenoid tuberosity of the scapula and the short head from the coracoid process of the scapula. The insertion is achieved by a common tendon at the radial tuberosity and lacertus fibrosis to origins of the forearm flexors. The functions of the biceps brachii are flexion of the elbow and supination the forearm.[117] The brachialis originates from the lower two-thirds of the anterior humerus and inserts on the coronoid process and tuberosity of the ulna. It functions to flex the elbow. The brachioradialis, which originates from the lower two-thirds of the lateral humerus and attaches to the lateral styloid process of the distal radius, functions as an elbow flexor as well as a weak pronator and supinator of the forearm.

The elbow extensors are the triceps brachii and the anconeus muscles. The triceps brachii has long, medial, and lateral

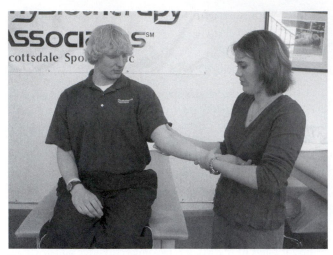

F I G U R E   2 6 - 4

Valgus stress test to evaluate the medial ulnar collateral ligament complex.

heads. The long head originates at the infraglenoid tuberosity of the scapula, the lateral and medial heads to the posterior aspect of the humerus. The insertion is via the common tendon posteriorly at the olecranon. Through this insertion along with the anconeus muscle that assists the triceps, extension of the elbow complex is accomplished.

CLINICAL EXAMINATION OF THE ELBOW

While it is beyond the scope of this chapter to describe a complete elbow examination, several important components necessary in the comprehensive examination of the athletes elbow will be discussed. Structural inspection of the athletes elbow must include a complete and thorough inspection of the entire upper extremity and trunk, due to the reliance of the entire upper-extremity kinetic chain on the core for power generation and force attenuation during functional activities.[31] Adaptive changes are commonly encountered during clinical examination of the athletic elbow, particularly in the unilaterally dominant upper extremity athlete. In these athletes, use of the contralateral extremity as a baseline is particularly important to determine the degree of actual adaptation that may be a contributing factor in the patient's injury presentation.

Anatomical adaptation of the athlete's elbow can be categorized into four main categories for the purpose of this chapter. These include range of motion (ROM), osseous, ligamentous, and muscular. Each will be presented in the context of the clinical examination of the patient with elbow dysfunction.

Range of Motion Adaptations

King et al.[68] initially reported on elbow ROM in professional baseball pitchers. Fifty percent of the pitchers they examined were found to have a flexion contracture of the dominant elbow with 30 percent of subjects demonstrating a cubitus valgus de-

formity. Chinn et al.[20] measured world-class professional adult tennis players and reported significant elbow flexion contractures on the dominant arm, but no presence of a cubitus valgus deformity.

More recently, Ellenbecker et al.[32] measured elbow extension in a population of 40 healthy professional baseball pitchers and found flexion contractures averaging 5°. Directly related to elbow function was wrist flexibility, which Ellenbecker et al.[32] reported as significantly less in extension on the dominant arm due to tightness of the wrist flexor musculature, with no difference in wrist flexion ROM between extremities. Ellenbecker and Roetert[35] measured senior tennis players aged 55 years and older and found flexion contractures averaging 10° in the dominant elbow, as well as significantly less wrist flexion ROM. The higher utilization of the wrist extensor musculature is likely the cause of limited wrist flexor ROM among the senior tennis players, as opposed to the reduced wrist extension ROM from excessive overuse of the wrist flexor muscles inherent in baseball pitching.[40,98]

More proximally, measurement of ROM of humeral rotation in the older overhead athlete is also recommended. Several studies have shown consistent alterations of shoulder rotational ROM in the overhead athlete.[36,66,100] Ellenbecker et al.[36] have shown statistically greater dominant-shoulder external rotation and less internal rotation in a sample of professional baseball pitchers. Despite these differences in internal and external rotation ROM, the total rotation (internal rotation + external rotation) between extremities remained equal, such that any increases in external rotation ROM were matched by decreases in internal rotation ROM in this uninjured population. Elite level tennis players had significantly less internal rotation and no significant difference in external rotation on the dominant arm, and an overall decrease in total rotation ROM on the dominant arm of approximately 10°. Careful monitoring of proximal glenohumeral joint ROM is recommended for the athlete with an elbow injury.

Based on the findings of these descriptive profiles, the finding of an elbow flexion contracture and limited wrist flexion or extension ROM, as well as reduced glenohumeral joint internal rotation, can be expected during the examination of the older athlete from a unilaterally dominant upper-extremity sport. Careful measurement during the clinical examination is recommended to determine baseline levels of ROM loss in the distal upper extremity. This careful measurement serves to determine if rehabilitative interventions are needed as well as to assess progress during rehabilitation.

Osseous Adaptation

In a study by Priest et al.,[94] 84 world-ranked tennis players were studied using radiography, and an average of 6.5 bony changes were found on the dominant elbow of each player. Additionally, they reported two times as many bony adaptations, such as spurs, on the medial aspect of the elbow as compared to the lateral aspect. The coronoid process of the ulna was the number one site of osseous adaptation or spurring. An average of 44 percent increase in thickness of the anterior humeral cortex was found on the dominant arm of these players, with an 11 percent increase in cortical thickness reported in the radius of the dominant tennis playing extremity.

Additionally, in an MRI study, Waslewski et al.[118] found osteophytes at the proximal or distal insertion of the ulnar collateral ligament in 5 out of 20 asymptomatic professional baseball pitchers, as well as posterior osteophytes in 2 out of 20 pitchers.

Ligamentous Laxity

Manual clinical examination of the human elbow to assess medial and lateral laxity can be challenging, given the presence of humeral rotation and small increases in joint opening that often present with ulnar collateral ligament injury. Ellenbecker et al.[32] measured medial elbow joint laxity in 40 asymptomatic professional baseball pitchers to determine if bilateral differences in medial elbow laxity exist in healthy pitchers with a long history of repetitive overuse to the medial aspect of the elbow. A Telos stress radiography device was used to assess medial elbow joint opening, using a standardized valgus stress of 15 daN (kPa) with the elbow placed in 25° of elbow flexion and the forearm in a supinated position. The joint space between the medial epicondyle and coronoid process of the ulna was measured using anterior-posterior radiographs by a musculoskeletal radiologist and compared bilaterally, with and without the application of the valgus stress. Results showed significant differences between extremities with stress application, with the dominant elbow opening 1.20 mm, and the nondominant elbow opening 0.88 mm. This difference, while statistically significant, averaged 0.32 mm between the dominant and nondominant elbow and would be virtually unidentifiable with manual assessment. Previous research by Rijke et al.[99] using stress radiography had identified a critical level of 0.5 mm increase in medial elbow joint opening in elbows with ulnar collateral ligament injury. Thus, the results of the study by Ellenbecker et al.[32] do support this 0.5-mm critical level, as asymptomatic professional pitchers in their study exhibited less than this 0.5 mm of medial elbow joint laxity.

Muscular Adaptations

Several methods can be used to measure upper-extremity strength in athletic populations. These can range from measuring grip strength with a hand grip dynamometer to the use of isokinetic dynamometers to measure specific joint motions and muscular parameters. Increased forearm circumference was measured on the dominant forearm in world-class tennis players,[20] as well as in the dominant forearm of senior tennis players.[71]

Isometric grip strength measured using a hand grip dynamometer has revealed unilateral increases in strength in elite adult and senior tennis players as well. Increases ranging from 10 to 30 percent have been reported using standardized measurement methods.[20,28,31,71]

Isokinetic dynamometers have been used to measure specific muscular performance parameters in elite level tennis players and baseball pitchers.[28,31,33,34] Specific patterns of unilateral muscular development have been identified by reviewing the isokinetic literature from different populations of overhead athletes. Ellenbecker[28] measured isokinetic wrist and forearm strength in mature adult tennis players who were highly skilled, and found 10–25 percent greater wrist flexion and extension as well as forearm pronation strength on the dominant extremity as compared to the nondominant extremity. Additionally, no significant difference between extremities in forearm supination strength was measured. No significant difference between extremities was found in elbow flexion strength in elite tennis players, but dominant arm elbow extension strength was significantly stronger than the nontennis-playing extremity.[33]

Research on professional throwing athletes has identified significantly greater wrist flexion and forearm pronation strength on the dominant arm by as much as 15–35 percent when compared to the nondominant extremity,[31] with no difference in wrist extension strength or forearm supination strength between extremities. Wilk, Arrigo, and Andrews[120] reported 10–20 percent greater elbow flexion strength in professional baseball pitchers on the dominant arm, as well as 5–15 percent greater elbow extension strength as compared to the nondominant extremity.

These data help to portray the chronic muscular adaptations that can be present in the senior athlete who may present with elbow injury, as well as help to determine realistic and accurate discharge strength levels following rehabilitation. Failure to return the dominant extremity-stabilizing musculature to its preinjury status (10 percent to as much as 35 percent greater than the nondominant) in these athletes may represent an incomplete rehabilitation and prohibit the return to full activity.

CLINICAL EXAMINATION METHODS

In addition to the examination methods outlined in the previous section, including accurate measurement of both distal and proximal joint ROM, radiographic screening, and muscular strength assessment, several other tests should be included in the comprehensive examination of the elbow of the older active patient. While it is beyond the scope of this chapter to completely review all of the necessary tests, several will be highlighted based on their overall importance. The reader is referred to Morrey[82] and Ellenbecker and Mattalino[31] for more complete chapters solely on examination of the elbow.

Clinical testing of the joints proximal and distal to the elbow allows the examiner to rule out referred symptoms and ensure that elbow pain is from a local musculoskeletal origin. Overpressure of the cervical spine in the motions of flexion/extension and lateral flexion/rotation, as well as quadrant or Spurling's test combining extension with ipsilateral lateral flexion and rotation, are commonly used to clear the cervical spine and rule out radicular symptoms.[42]

Additionally, clearing the glenohumeral joint, and determining whether concomitant impingement or instability is present, is also highly recommended.[31] Use of the Sulcus sign[79] to determine the presence of multidirectional instability of the glenohumeral joint, along with the subluxation/relocation sign[58] and load and shift test, can provide valuable insight into the status of the glenohumeral joint. The impingement signs of Neer[84] and Hawkins and Kennedy[49] are also helpful to rule out proximal tendon pathology.

In addition to the clearing tests for the glenohumeral joint, full inspection of the scapulothoracic joint is recommended. Removal of the patient's shirt or examination of the patient in a gown with full exposure of the upper back is highly recommended. Kibler et al.[67] has recently presented a classification system for scapular pathology. Careful observation of the patient at rest and with the hands placed upon the hips, as well as during active overhead movements, is recommended to identify prominence of particular borders of the scapula, as well as a lack of close association with the thoracic wall during movement.[64,65] Bilateral comparison provides the primary basis for identifying scapular pathology; however in many athletes, bilateral scapular pathology can be observed.

The presence of overuse injuries in the elbow occurring with proximal injury to the shoulder complex or with scapulothoracic dysfunction is widely reported,[27,31,82,85,86] and thus a thorough inspection of the proximal joint is extremely important in the comprehensive management of elbow pathology.

Elbow Joint: Special Tests

Several tests specific for the elbow should be performed to assist in the diagnosis of elbow dysfunction. These include Tinel's test, varus and vaglus stress tests, Milking test, valgus extension overpressure test, bounce home test, and provocation tests. The Tinel's test involves tapping of the ulnar nerve in the medial region of the elbow over the cubital tunnel retinaculum. Reproduction of paresthesia or tingling along the distal course of the ulnar nerve indicates irritability of the ulnar nerve.[82]

The valgus stress test (Fig. 26-4) is used to evaluate the integrity of the ulnar collateral ligament. The position used for testing the anterior band of the ulnar collateral ligament is characterized by 15°–25° of elbow flexion and forearm supination. The elbow flexion position is used to unlock the olecranon from the olecranon fossa and decreases the stability provided by the osseous congruity of the joint. This places a greater relative stress on the medial ulnar collateral ligament.[83] Reproduction of medial elbow pain, in addition to unilateral increases in ulnohumeral joint laxity, indicates a positive test. Grading the test is typically performed using the American Academy of Orthopedic Surgeons guidelines of 0–5 mm grade I, 5–10 mm grade II, and greater than 10 mm grade III.[32] Performing the test using a position of greater than 25° of elbow flexion will increase the

amount of humeral rotation during performance of the valgus stress test and lead to misleading information to the clinician's hands. The test is typically performed with the shoulder in the scapular plane, but can be performed with the shoulder in the coronal plane, to minimize compensatory movements at the shoulder during testing. The milking sign is a test the patient performs on himself, with approximately 90° of elbow flexion. By reaching under the involved elbow with the contralateral extremity, the patient grasps the thumb of their injured extremity and pulls in a lateral direction, thus imposing a valgus stress to the flexed elbow. Some patients may not have enough flexibility to perform this maneuver, and a valgus stress can be imparted by the examiner to mimic this movement, which stresses the posterior band of the ulnar collateral ligament.[83]

The varus stress test is performed using similar degrees of elbow flexion and shoulder and forearm positioning. This test assesses the integrity of the lateral ulnar collateral ligament, and should be performed along with the valgus stress test, to completely evaluate the medial/lateral stability of the ulnohumeral joint.

The valgus extension overpressure test has been reported by Andrews et al.[7] to determine whether posterior elbow pain is caused by a posteromedial osteophyte abutting the medial margin of the trochlea and the olecranon fossa. This test is performed by passively extending the elbow while maintaining a valgus stress to it. This test is meant to simulate the stresses imparted to the posterior medial part of the elbow during the acceleration phase of the throwing or serving motion. Reproduction of pain in the posteromedial aspect of the elbow indicates a positive test.

The use of provocation tests can be applied when screening the muscle tendon units of the elbow. Provocation tests consist of manual muscle tests to determine pain reproduction. The specific tests, used to screen the elbow joint of a patient with suspected elbow pathology, include wrist and finger flexion and extension as well as forearm pronation and supination.[27] These tests can be used to provoke the muscle tendon unit at the lateral or medial epicondyle. Testing of the elbow at or near full extension can often recreate localized lateral or medial elbow pain secondary to tendon degeneration.[70] Reproduction of lateral or medial elbow pain with resistive muscle testing (provocation testing) may indicate concomitant tendon injury at the elbow and would direct the clinician to perform a more complete elbow examination.

REHABILITATION TECHNIQUES FOR SPECIFIC INJURIES

Overuse injuries constitute most of the elbow injuries in the athletic elbow patient, with one of the most common being humeral epicondylitis.[31,88] Repetitive overuse is one of the primary etiological factors evident in the history of most patients with elbow dysfunction. Epidemiological research on adult tennis players reports incidences of humeral epicondylitis ranging from 35–50 percent.[19,47,62,69,95] The incidence reported in elite junior players is significantly less (11–12 percent).[123]

PATHOMECHANICS

Etiology of Humeral Epicondylitis

Reported in the literature as early as 1873 by Runge,[103] humeral epicondylitis or "tennis elbow", as it is more popularly known, has been studied extensively by many authors. Cyriax in 1936 listed 26 causes of tennis elbow,[22] while an extensive study of this overuse disorder by Goldie in 1964 reported hypervascularization of the extensor aponeurosis and an increased quantity of free nerve endings in the subtendinous space.[41] More recently, Leadbetter[75] described humeral epicondylitis as a degenerative condition consisting of a time dependent process including vascular, chemical, and cellular events that lead to a failure of the cell-matrix healing response in human tendon. This description of tendon injury differs from earlier theories where an inflammatory response was considered as a primary factor; hence the term "tendonitis" was used as opposed to the term recommended by Leadbetter[75] and Nirschl.[86]

Nirschl[85,86] has defined humeral epicondylitis as an extraarticular tendinous injury characterized by excessive vascular granulation and an impaired healing response in the tendon, which he has termed "angiofibroblastic hyperplasia." In the most recent and thorough histopathological analysis, Nirschl and colleagues[70] studied specimens of injured tendon obtained from areas of chronic overuse and reported that these specimens did not contain large numbers of lymphocytes, macrophages, and neutrophils. Instead, tendonosis appears to be a degenerative process characterized by large populations of fibroblasts, disorganized collagen, and vascular hyperplasia.[70] It is not clear why tendonosis is painful, given the lack of inflammatory cells, and it is also unknown why the collagen does not mature or heal typically.

Structures Involved in Humeral Epicondylitis

Nirschl[86] has described the primary structure involved in lateral humeral epicondylitis as the tendon of the extensor carpi radialis brevis. Approximately one-third of cases involve the tendon of the extensor digitorum communis.[70] Additionally, the extensor carpi radialis longus and extensor carpi ulnaris can be involved as well. The primary site of medial humeral epicondylitis is the flexor carpi radialis, pronator teres, and flexor carpi ulnaris tendons.[85,86]

Recent research has described in detail the anatomy of the lateral epicondylar region.[17,43] The specific location of the extensor carpi radialis brevis tendon lies inferior to the tendinous origin of the extensor carpi radialis longus, which can be palpated along the anterior surface of the supracondylar ridge just proximal or cephalid to the extensor carpi radialis brevis tendon on the lateral epicondyle.[17] Greenbaum et al.[43] describe the pyramidal slope or shape of the lateral epicondyle and explain how both the extensor carpi radialis brevis and the extensor communis originate from the entire anterior surface of the lateral epicondyle. These specific relationships are important for the clinician to bear in mind when palpating for the region of maximal tenderness during the clinical examination process. While detailed recent reports are not present in the literature regarding the medial epicondyle, careful palpation can be used to discriminate between the muscle tendon junctions of the pronator teres and flexor carpi radialis. Additionally, palpation of the medial ulnar collateral ligament, which originates from nearly the entire inferior surface of the medial epicondyle and inserts into the anterior medial aspect of the coronoid process of the ulna, should be performed. Understanding the involved structures, as well as a detailed knowledge of the exact locations where these structures can be palpated, can assist the clinician in better localizing the painful tendon or tendons involved.

Dijs et al.[25] reported with lateral epicondylitis on 70 patients. They reported the area of maximal involvement in these cases: the extensor carpi radialis longus in only 1 percent and the extensor carpi radialis brevis in 90 percent. The body of the extensor carpi radialis tendon was implicated in 1 percent of cases, and 8 percent were over the muscle tendon junction over the most proximal part of the muscle of the extensor carpi radialis brevis.

Epidemiology of Humeral Epicondylitis

Nirschl[85,86] reports that the incidence of lateral humeral epicondylitis is far greater than that of medial epicondylitis in recreational tennis players and in the leading arm of golfers (left arm in a right handed golfer). Medial humeral epicondylitis is far more common in elite tennis players and throwing athletes, due to the powerful loading of the flexor and pronator muscle tendon units during the valgus extension overload inherent in the acceleration phase of those overhead movement patterns. Additionally, the trailing arm of the golfer (right arm in a right handed golfer) is more likely to have medial symptoms than lateral.

REHABILITATION PROGRESSION: HUMERAL EPICONDYLITIS

Following the detailed examination, a detailed rehabilitation program can commence. Three main stages of rehabilitation can conceptually be applied for the patient, which include protected function, total arm strength, and the return to activity phase. Each will be discussed in greater detail in this section of the chapter with specific highlights on the therapeutic exercises utilized during each stage of the rehabilitation process.

PROTECTED FUNCTION PHASE

During this first phase in the rehabilitation process, care is taken to protect the injured muscle tendon unit from stress, but not function. Nirschl[85,86] cautions against the use of an immobilizer or sling due to the further atrophy of the musculature and negative effects on the upper-extremity kinetic chain. Protection of the patient from offending activities is recommended, with cessation of throwing and serving suggested for medial-based humeral symptoms. Allowing the patient to bat or hit 200 backhands allows for continued activity while minimizing stress to the injured area. Very often however, sport activity must cease entirely to allow the muscle tendon unit time to heal and to most importantly allow formal rehabilitation to progress. Continued work or sport performance can severely slow the progression of resistive exercise and other long-term treatments in physical therapy.

Use of modalities is very helpful during this time period; however agreement on a clearly superior modality or sequence of modalities has not been substantiated in the literature.[17,73] A meta-analysis of 185 studies on treatment of humeral epicondylitis showed glaring deficits in the scientific quality of the investigations, with no significantly superior treatment approach identified. While many modalities or sequences of modalities have anecdotally produced superior results, there is a tremendous need for prospective, randomized, controlled clinical trials to better identify optimal methods for intervention. Modalities such as ultrasound,[12,88] electrical stimulation and ice, cortisone injection,[62,88] nonsteroidal anti-inflammatory drugs,[101] acupuncture,[18] transverse friction massage,[53] and dimethyl sulfoxide application[93] have all been reported to provide varying levels of effectiveness in the literature. Boyer and Hastings,[17] in a comprehensive review of the treatment of humeral epicondylitis, reported no significant difference with the use of low-energy laser, acupuncture, extracorporeal shockwave therapy, or steroid injection.

The use of cortisone injection has been widely reported in the literature during the pain reduction phase of treatment of this often-recalcitrant condition. Dijs et al.[25] compared the effects of traditional physical therapy and cortisone injection in 70 patients diagnosed with humeral epicondylitis. In their research, 91 percent of patients who received the cortisone injection received initial relief, as compared with 47 percent who reported relief from undergoing physical therapy. The recurrence rate in their study however, after only 3 months, showed 51 percent in the cortisone injection group, and only 5 percent in the physical therapy group had a return of primary symptoms. Similar findings were reported in a study by Verhaar et al.[116] comparing physical therapy consisting of Mills Manipulation and cross friction massage with corticosteroid injection in a prospective, randomized, controlled clinical trial in 106 patients with humeral epicondylitis. At 6 weeks, 22 of 53 subjects reported a complete relief from the cortisone injection, while only 3 subjects had complete relief from this type of physical therapy treatment. At 1 year, there were no differences between treatment groups regarding the course of treatment. This study shows the short-term benefit from the corticosteroid injection, as well as the ineffectiveness of physical therapy using manipulation and cross friction massage.

Several additional recent studies deserve further discussion as they also can be used to direct clinicians in the development of appropriate interventions. Nirschl et al.[87] studied the effects of iontophoresis with Dexamethasone in 199 patients with humeral epicondylitis. Results showed that 52 percent of the subjects in the treatment group reported overall improvement on the investigators' improvement index, with only 33 percent of the placebo group reporting improvement 2 days after the series of treatments with iontophoresis. One month following the treatment, there was no statistical difference in the overall improvement in the patients in the treatment group versus the control group. One additional finding from this study that has clinical relevance was the presence of greater pain relief in the group that underwent six treatments in a 10-day period, as opposed to subjects in the treatment group who underwent treatment over a longer period of time. While this study does support the use of iontophoresis with Dexamethasone, it does not report substantial benefits during follow-up.

Haake et al.[46] studied the effects of extracorporeal shock wave therapy in 272 patients with humeral epicondylitis in a multicenter prospective randomized control study. They reported that extracorporeal shock wave therapy was ineffective in the treatment of humeral epicondylitis. Similarly, Basford et al.[9] used low-intensity Nd:YAG laser irradiation at 7 points along the forearm three times a week for 4 weeks and also reported it to be ineffective in the treatment of lateral humeral epicondylitis.

Based on this review of the literature, it appears that no standardized modality or modality sequence has been identified in the literature that is clearly statistically more effective than any other at the present time. Clinical reviews by Nirschl[85,86] and Ellenbecker and Mattalino[31] advocate the use of multiple modalities, such as electrical stimulation and ultrasound, as well as iontophoresis with Dexamethesone, to assist in pain reduction and encourage local increases in blood flow. The copious use of ice or cryotherapy following increases in daily activity is also recommended. The use of therapeutic modalities and also cortisone injection, if needed, can only be seen as one part of the treatment sequence, with increasing evidence being generated favoring progressive resistive exercise.

Exercise is one of the most powerful modalities used in rehabilitative medicine. Research has shown increases in local blood flow following isometric contraction of the musculature at levels as submaximal as 5–50 percent of maximum voluntary contraction both during the contraction and for periods of up to 1 minute postcontraction.[56] Two studies have shown superior results in the treatment of humeral epicondylitis using progressive resistive exercise compared with ultrasound.[39] In a study by Svernl and Adolffson,[111] 38 patients with lateral humeral epicondylitis were randomly assigned to a contract relax stretching or eccentric exercise treatment group. Result of their study showed a 71 percent report of full recovery in the eccentric exercise group, as compared to the group that performed contract-relax stretching, which only found 39 percent of the subjects rating themselves as fully recovered. These studies support the heavy reliance on the successful application of progressive, resistive exercise in the treatment of humeral epicondylitis.

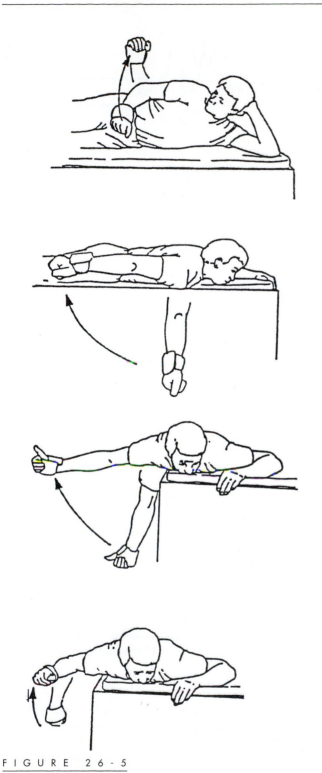

FIGURE 26-5

Rotator cuff exercises used during rehabilitation of elbow injuries.

TOTAL ARM STRENGTH REHABILITATION

Early application of resistive exercise for the treatment of humeral epicondylitis mainly focuses on the important princi-

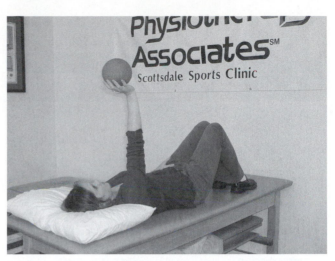

FIGURE 26-6

Serratus press exercise used to recruit and strengthen the serratus anterior.

ple that states that "proximal stability is needed to promote distal mobility."[110] The initial application of resistive exercise actually consists of specific exercises to strengthen the upper-extremity proximal force couples.[54] The rotator cuff (deltoid and rotator cuff musculature) and lower trapezius force couples are targeted to enhance proximal stabilization using a low–resistance, high-repetition exercise format (i.e., three sets of 15 RM loading [RM = repetition maximum]). Specific exercises such as side-lying external rotation, prone horizontal abduction, and prone extension, both with externally rotated humeral positions and prone external rotation, all have been shown to elicit high levels of posterior rotator cuff activation during electromyogram research(Fig. 26-5).[8,14,112] Additionally, exercises such as the serratus press (Fig. 26-6) and manual scapular protraction and retraction resistance (Fig. 26-7A and B) can be safely applied without stress to the distal aspect of the upper extremity during this important phase of rehabilitation. The use of cuff weights allows some of the rotator cuff and scapular exercises to be performed with the weight attached proximal to the elbow, to further minimize overload to the elbow and forearm during the earliest phases of rehabilitation if needed for some patients.

The initial application of exercise to the distal aspect of the extremity follows a pattern that stresses the injured muscle-tendon unit last. For example, the initial distal exercise sequence for the patient with lateral humeral epicondylitis would include wrist flexion and forearm pronation, which provides most of the tensile stress to the medially inserting tendons which are not directly involved in lateral humeral epicondylitis (Fig. 26-8). Gradual addition of wrist extension and forearm supination, as well as radial and ulnar deviation exercises, are added as signs and symptoms allow. Additional progression is based on the elbow position utilized during distal exercises. Initially, most patients tolerate the exercises in a more pain-free fashion with the elbow placed in slight flexion, with a progression to more extended and functional elbow positions, as signs and

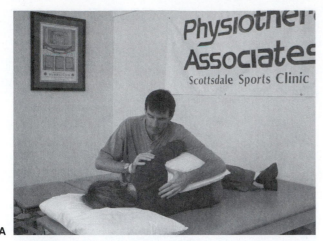

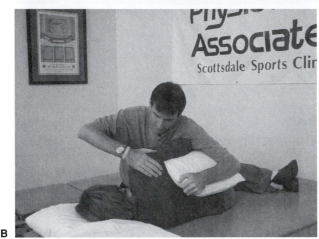

FIGURE 26-7

A, Manual scapular protraction exercise. **B,** Manual scapular retraction exercise.

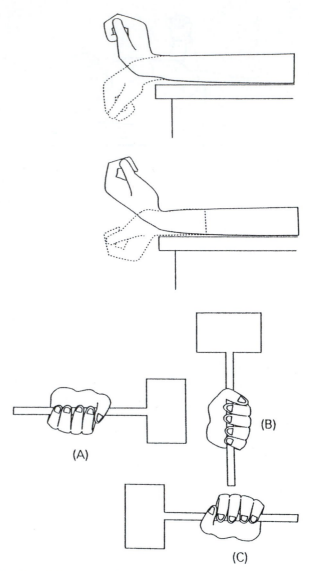

FIGURE 26-8

Distal upper extremity isotonic exercise patterns including wrist flexion and extension, radial and ulnar deviation as well as forearm pronation and supination.

symptoms allow. These exercises are performed with light weights, often as little as 1 lb or 1 kg, as well as tan or yellow Theraband emphasizing both the concentric and eccentric portions of the exercise movement. According to the research by Svernl and Adolffson,[111] the eccentric portion of the exercise may actually have a greater benefit than the concentric portion; however, more research is needed before a greater and clearer understanding of the role isolated eccentric exercise plays in the rehabilitation of degenerative tendon conditions is fully understood. Multiple sets of 15–20 repetitions are recommended to promote muscular endurance.

Once the patient can tolerate the most basic series of distal exercises (wrist flexion/extension, forearm pronation/supination, and wrist radial/ulnar deviation), exercises are progressed to include activities that involve simultaneous contraction of the wrist and forearm musculature with elbow flexion/extension ROM. These include exercises such as exercise ball dribbling (Fig. 26-9), Body Blade (Hymanson, TX), Boing (OPTP, Minneapolis, MN) (Figs. 26-10 and 26-11), Theraband (Hygenic Corp, Akron, OH), resistance bar external

oscillations (Fig. 26-12) (which combine wrist and forearm stabilization with posterior rotator cuff and scapular exercise), and seated rowing (Fig. 26-13). Additionally, the use of closed kinetic-chain exercise for the upper extremity is added to promote cocontraction and mimic functional positions with joint approximation (Figs. 26-14 to 26-16).[29]

In addition to the resistive exercise, the use of gentle passive stretching to optimize the muscle tendon unit length is indicated. Combined stretches with the patient in the supine position are indicated to elongate the biarticular muscle tendon units of the elbow, forearm and wrist using a combination of elbow, and wrist and forearm positions (Fig. 26-17A and B). Additionally, stretching the distal aspect of the extremity in varying positions of glenohumeral joint elevation is also

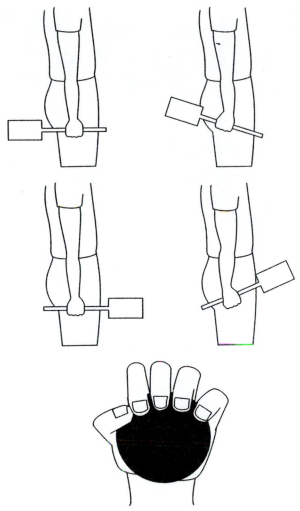

FIGURE 26-8

(*continued*)

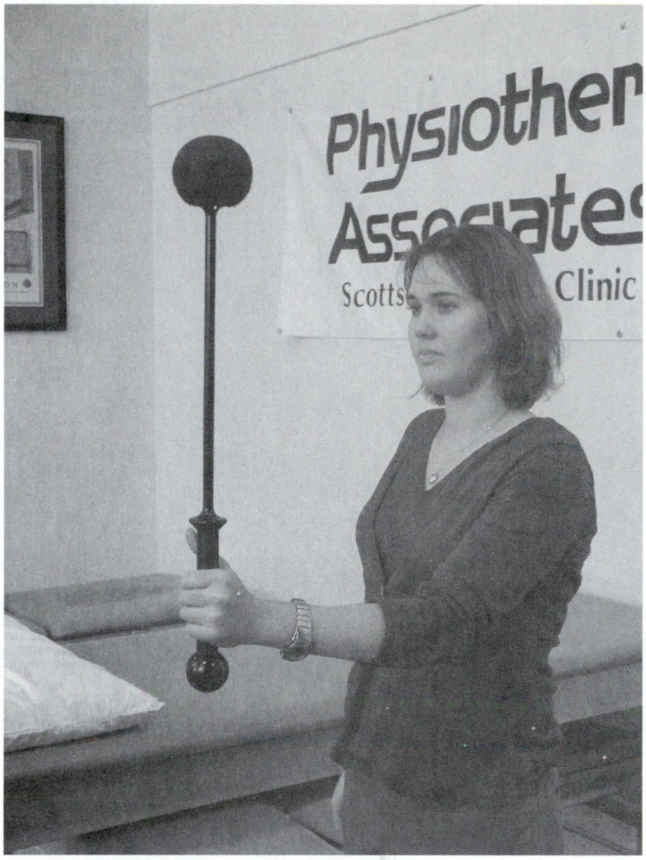

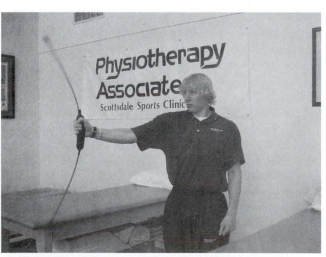

FIGURE 26-10

Oscillatory exercise using the boing device.

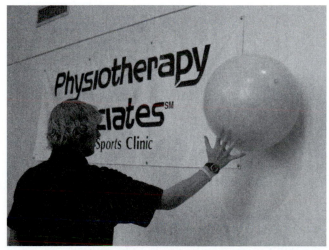

FIGURE 26-9

Ball dribbling using an exercise ball to promote rapid contraction of the musculature in an endurance-oriented fashion.

FIGURE 26-11

Oscillatory exercise using the body blade device.

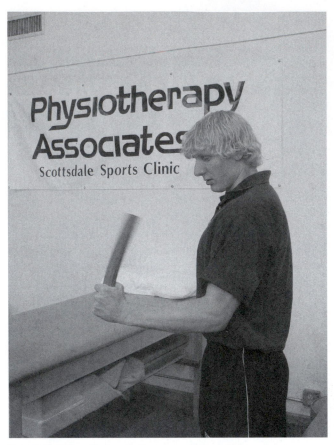

FIGURE 26-12

Oscillatory exercise using the Theraband flex bar. Oscillations can be performed in a sagittal and frontal plane direction to target specific muscle group activation.

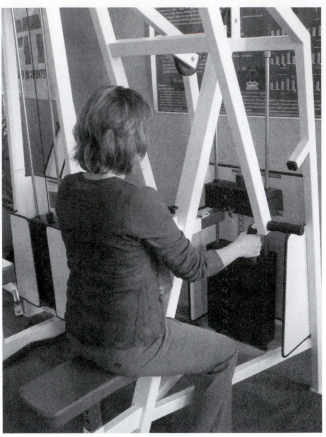

FIGURE 26-13

Seated rowing exercise used for proximal stabilization and total arm strength.

Return to Activity Phase

Of the three phases in the rehabilitation process for humeral epicondylitis, return to activity is the one that is most frequently ignored or cut short, resulting in serious consequences for

indicated.[31] Mobilization of the ulnohumeral joint can also be effective in cases where significant flexion contractures exist. Use of ulnohumeral distraction with the elbow near full extension will selectively tension the anterior joint capsule (Fig. 26-18).[16]

As the patients tolerate the distal isotonic exercise progression pain-free at a level of 3–5 lbs or medium level elastic tubing or bands, as well as demonstrate a tolerance to the oscillatory type exercises in this phase of rehabilitation, they are progressed to the isokinetic form of exercise. Advantages of isokinetic exercise are the inherent accommodative resistance and utilization of faster, more functional contractile velocities, in addition to providing isolated patterns to elicit high levels of muscular activation. The initial pattern of exercise used anecdotally has been wrist flexion/extension (Fig. 26-19), with forearm pronation/supination (Fig. 26-20) added after successful tolerance of a trial treatment of wrist flexion/extension. Contractile velocities ranging between 180° and 300° per second, with six to eight sets of 15–20 repetitions, are used to foster local muscular endurance.[38] In addition to isokinetic exercise, plyometric wrist snaps (Fig. 26-21) and wrist flips (Fig. 26-22) are utilized to begin to train the active elbow for functional and sport specific demands.

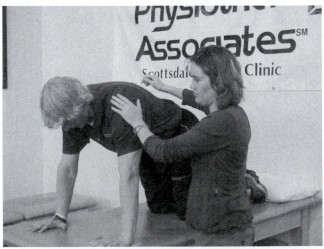

FIGURE 26-14

Quadruped rhythmic stabilization exercise.

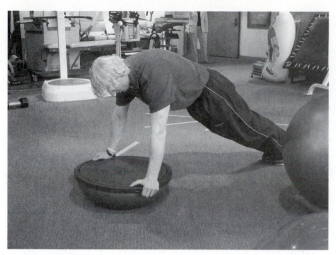

FIGURE 26-15

Closed chain upper extremity exercise using the BOSU platform.

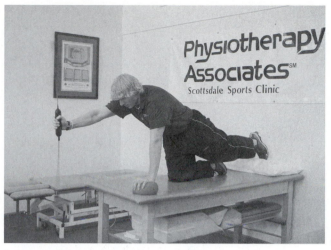

FIGURE 26-16

Pointer closed-chain upper extremity exercise using the body blade to promote instability in the open-chain limb and a medicine ball under the closed-chain limb.

reinjury and the development of a "chronic" status for this injury. Objective criterion for entry into this stage are tolerance of the previously stated resistive exercise series, objectively documented strength equal to the contralateral extremity with either manual muscle testing, or preferably isokinetic testing distal grip strength measured with a dynamometer, and functional ROM. It is important to note that often in the elite athlete, chronic musculoskeletal adaptations exist which prevent attainment

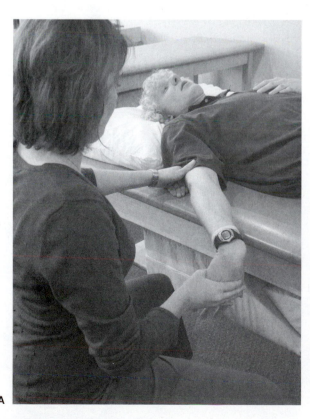

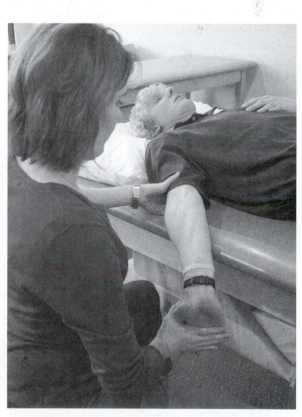

A   B

FIGURE 26-17

Passive stretching of the wrist and forearm musculature (**A**) wrist flexion and pronation to stretch the wrist extensors, and (**B**) wrist extension and supination to stretch the flexors and pronators of the distal upper extremity.

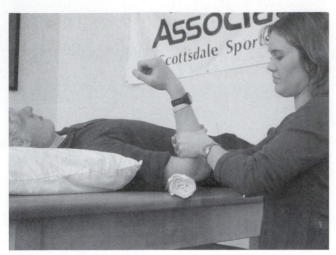

FIGURE 26-18

Ulnohumeral joint distraction mobilization. Altering the position of elbow flexion and extension selectively stresses portions of the anterior and posterior capsule.

of full elbow ROM. Recall that this is often secondary to the osseous and capsular adaptations discussed earlier in this chapter.

Characteristics of interval sport return programs include alternate day performance, as well as gradual progressions of intensity and repetitions of sport activities. For example, utilizing low-compression tennis balls such as the Pro-Penn Star Ball (Penn Racquet Sports, Phoenix, AZ) or Wilson Gator Ball (Wilson Sporting Goods, Chicago, IL) during the initial contact phase of the return to tennis decreases impact stress and increases tolerance to the activity. Performing the interval program under supervision, either during therapy or with a knowledgeable teaching professional or coach, allows for the biomechanical evaluation of technique and guards against overzealous intensity levels, which can be a common mistake in well-intentioned,

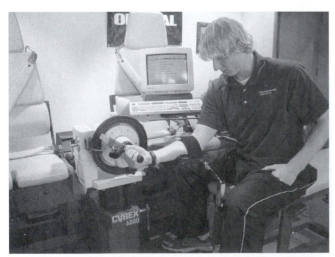

FIGURE 26-19

Isokinetic wrist flexion/extension exercise on the Cybex 6000 isokinetic dynamometer.

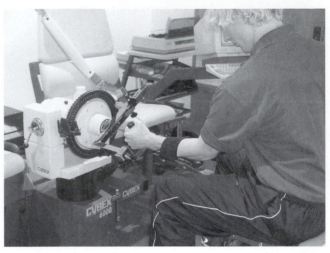

FIGURE 26-20

Isokinetic forearm pronation/supination exercise on the Cybex 6000 isokinetic dynamometer.

motivated patients. Using the return program on alternate days, with rest between sessions, allows for recovery and decreases reinjury.

Two other important aspects of the return to sport activity are the continued application of resistive exercise and the

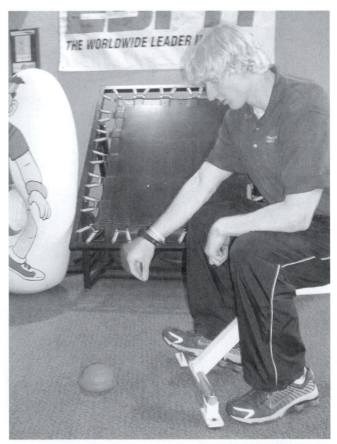

FIGURE 26-21

Plyometric wrist snap used for explosive training of the wrist and finger flexor muscle groups.

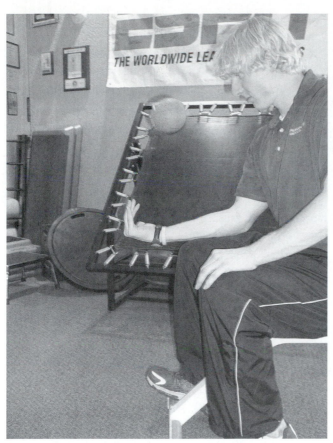

FIGURE 26-22

Plyometric wrist flip used for explosive training of the wrist and finger flexor muscle groups.

modification or evaluation of the patient's equipment. Continuation of the total arm strength rehabilitation exercises using elastic resistance, medicine balls, and isotonic or isokinetic resistance is important to continue to enhance not only strength but also muscular endurance. Inspection and modification of the patient's tennis racquet or golf clubs is also important. For example, lowering the string tension several pounds and ensuring that the player use a more resilient or softer string, such as a coreless multifilament synthetic string or gut, is widely recommended for tennis players with upper-extremity injury histories.[85,86,88] Grip size is also very important with research showing changes in muscular activity with alteration of handle or grip size.[1] Measurement of proper grip size has been described by Nirschl as corresponding to the distance between the distal tip of the ring finger along the radial border of the finger to the proximal palmar crease.[85] Nirschl has also recommended the use of a counterforce brace (Fig. 26-23) to decrease stress on the insertion of the flexor and extensor tendons during work or sport activity.[44]

POSTOPERATIVE REHABILITATION PROGRESSION

In a study of over 3000 cases of humeral epicondylitis, Nirschl[86] has reported that 92 percent respond to nonoperative treatment.

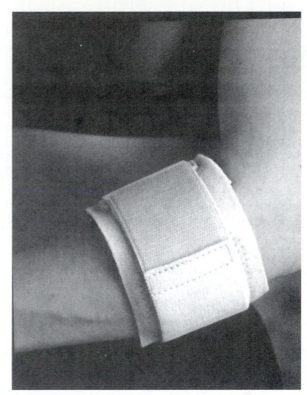

FIGURE 26-23

Counterforce brace applied the elbow for a patient with lateral humeral epicondylitis.

Characteristics of patients who often require surgical correction for this condition are failure of nonoperative rehabilitation programs, minimal relief with corticosteroid injection, and intense pain in the injured elbow even at rest. Surgical treatment for lateral humeral epicondylitis, as reported by Nirschl,[86] involves a small incision from the radial head to 1 inch proximal to the lateral epicondyle. Through this incision, Nirschl removes the pathological tissue he termed *angiofibroblastic hyperplasia*, without disturbing the attachment of the extensor aponeurosis to preserve stability of the elbow.[86] Vascular enhancement is afforded by drilling holes into the cortical bone in the anterior lateral epicondyle to cancellous bone level. Postoperative immobilization is brief (48 hours), with early motion of the wrist and fingers on postoperative day 1, progressing to elbow active assistive ROM during the first 2–3 weeks. Resistive exercise is gradually applied after the third postoperative week, with a return to normal daily activities expected at 8 weeks postoperatively and a return to sport activity several months thereafter.[85,86]

Rehabilitation Following Elbow Arthroscopy

Repetitive stresses to the athletic elbow often result in loose body formation and osteochondral injury, in addition to the more commonly reported tendon injury resulting in humeral epicondylitis. Andrews and Soffer[4] report that the most common indications for elbow arthroscopy are loose body removal and removal of osteophytes. Posteromedial decompression includes the excision of osteophytes, with or without resection of additional posteromedial bone from the proximal olecranon.[3] Early emphasis on regaining full-extension ROM is possible due to the minimally invasive arthroscopic procedure. The senior author's postoperative protocol following arthroscopic procedures of the elbow is presented in Appendix 1. Progressive application of resistive exercise to increase both strength and local muscle endurance forms the bulk of the rehabilitation protocol. Use of early shoulder and scapular stabilization is also recommended in these patients in preparation to the return to overhead activities and aggressive functional activity following discharge.

Outcomes following elbow arthroscopy for posteromedial osteophyte and loose body removal were reported by Oglive-Harris et al.,[91] where 21 patients were followed on an average of 35 months postoperatively, rendering good and excellent results in 7 and 14 patients, respectively. O'Driscoll and Morrey[90] reported that arthroscopic removal of loose bodies was of benefit in 75 percent of all patients; however when loose bodies were not secondary to some other intra-articular condition, 100 percent of patients rated the procedure as beneficial. Andrews and Timmerman[5] reviewed the results of 73 cases of arthroscopic elbow surgery in professional baseball pitchers. Eighty percent of players were able to return to full activity, pitching at their preinjury level for at least one season. Further review of these patients found that 25 percent returned for additional surgery, often requiring stabilization and reconstruction of the ulnar collateral ligament due to valgus instability. This important study shows the close association between medial elbow laxity and posterior medial osteochondral injury and highlights the importance of identifying subtle instability in the athletic elbow.

Reddy et al.[96] retrospectively reviewed a sample of 172 patients who underwent elbow arthroscopy and had a mean follow-up of 42 months. Fifty-six percent of patients had an excellent result, which allowed them a full return to activity, with 36 percent having a good result. A 1.6 percent complication rate was reported, with an overall conclusion that this procedure is both safe and efficacious for the treatment of osteochondral injury of the elbow.

Ellenbecker and Mattalino[31] measured muscular strength at a mean of 8 weeks postoperatively in eight professional baseball pitchers following arthroscopic removal of loose bodies and posteromedial olecranon spur resection. Results showed a complete return of wrist flexion/extension strength and forearm pronation/supination strength at 8 weeks following arthroscopy. This allows for a gradual progression to interval sport return programs between 8 and 12 weeks postoperatively.

VALGUS EXTENSION OVERLOAD INJURIES

Repeated activities such as overhead throwing, tennis serving, or throwing the javelin can lead to characteristic patterns of osseous and osteochondral injury in both the older active patient, as well as the adolescent elbow. These injuries are commonly referred to as valgus extension overload injuries.[122]

Pathomechanics

As a result of the valgus stress incurred during throwing or the serving motion, traction placed via the medial aspect of the elbow can create bony spurs or osteophytes at the medial epicondyle or coronoid process of the elbow.[10,52,107] Additionally, the valgus stress during elbow extension creates impingement, which leads to the development of osteophyte formation at the posterior and posteriormedial aspects of the olecranon tip, causing chondromalacia and loose body formation.[122] The combined motion of valgus pressure with the powerful extension of the elbow leads to posterior osteophyte formation, due to impingement of the posterior medial aspect of the ulna against the trochlea and olecranon fossa. Joyce[61] has reported the presence of chondromalacia in the medial groove of the trochlea, which often precedes osteophyte formation. Erosion to subchondral bone is often witnessed when olecranon osteophytes are initially developing. Injury to the ulnar collateral ligament and medial muscle-tendon units of the flexor-pronator group can also occur with this type of repetitive loading.[52,124]

During the valgus stress that occurs to the human elbow during the acceleration phase of both the throwing and serving motions, lateral compressive forces occur in the lateral aspect of the elbow, specifically at the radio-capitellar joint. Of great concern in the immature pediatric throwing athlete is osteochondritis dissecans and Panner's Disease.[31,61] Both of these injuries are covered in Chapter 34. In the older adult elbow, the radiocapitellar joint can be the site of joint degeneration and osteochondral injury from the compressive loading.[52] This lateral compressive loading is increased in the elbow with medial ulnar collateral ligament laxity or ligament injury.[31]

ULNAR COLLATERAL LIGAMENT INJURY

Pathomechanics/Mechanism of Injury

Attenuation of the ulnar collateral ligament can produce valgus instability of the elbow, which can lead to medial joint pain, ulnar nerve compromise, and lateral radiocapitellar and posterolateral osseous dysfunction, which is a severely restricting injury to the throwing or racquet sport athlete. The repetitive valgus loading that occurs in the elbow during the acceleration phase of the throwing or serving motion can attenuate this structure. Sprains and partial thickness tears of the medial ulnar collateral ligament can occur and progress to complete tears and avulsions of the ligament from its bony attachments.[31]

Rehabilitation Concerns

Nonoperative rehabilitation of the athlete with an ulnar collateral ligament sprain also involves the primary stages outlined in the rehabilitation of humeral epicondylitis. During the initial stage of rehabilitation, immobilization of the elbow is often a characteristic part of the process to decrease pain and enhance healing. Either an immobilizer or hinged brace is used to limit end ranges of elbow extension and flexion. Modalities are again used to assist in the healing process, as are gentle ROM, submaximal isometrics, and manual resistance of both wrist and forearm midrange movements.

Rehabilitation Progression

Use of a total arm strength rehabilitation protocol is indicated to facilitate both muscular strength and endurance to the elbow, forearm, and wrist. In addition to previously mentioned exercises, particular attention is given to eccentric muscle work of the wrist flexors and forearm supinators to attempt to dynamically support the attenuated ulnar collateral ligament. Due to the intimate association between the flexor carpi ulnaris and the unlar collateral ligament, early strengthening in the pattern of wrist flexion and ulnar deviation may provoke symptoms; however, later in rehabilitation, the repeated use of exercises to strengthen the muscles directly overlying the injured ligament to provide dynamic stabilization is highly recommended.[23]

Progression to plyometric exercises, which impart a submaximal, controlled valgus stress to the medial aspect of the elbow such as a 90/90 shoulder and elbow medicine ball toss in later stages of rehabilitation, attempts to simulate loads placed on the medial elbow (Fig. 26-24). Use of the isokinetic dynamometer for distal strengthening is also recommended, with additional training focused on the shoulder for internal/external rotation with the arm abducted 90° and elbow flexed 90° (Fig. 26-25). Use of this position imparts a controlled valgus stress to the elbow in addition to strengthening the rotator cuff.[30]

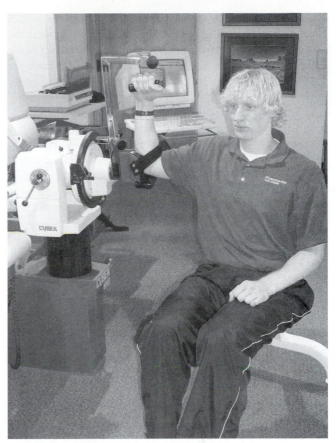

FIGURE 26-25

Isokinetic 90/90 internal/external rotation training position on the Cybex isokinetic dynamometer.

A complete return of ROM and isokinetically documented appropriate elbow, forearm, and wrist strength are required before an interval program is initiated. Reoccurrence of pain, feelings of instability, or neural irritation with throwing or functional activity identify the patient as a potential candidate for an ulnar collateral ligament repair or reconstruction.

Postoperative Rehabilitation Following Ulnar Collateral Ligament Reconsruction

Operative procedures for the athlete with valgus instability of the elbow have focused on direct primary repair of the ligament[72] as well as utilization of an autogenous graft for reconstruction of the medial elbow. Conway et al.,[21] Jobe et al.,[59] and Regan et al.[97] reported that the palmaris tendon used as the autogenous graft, harvested from the ipsilateral forearm, fails at higher loads (357 N) and is four times as strong as the anterior band of the ulnar collateral ligament, which fails at 260 N.

In a retrospective study by Conway et al.,[21] out of 71 throwing athletes who underwent either surgical repair or reconstruction of the ulnar collateral ligament, 87 percent were found to have a mid-substance tear of the ulnar collateral ligament, 10 percent had a distal ulnar avulsion, and only 3 percent

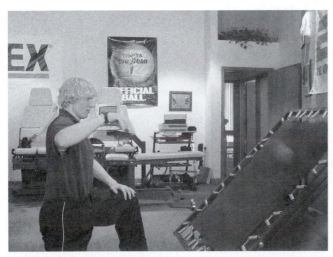

FIGURE 26-24

Plyometric 90/90 medicine ball toss to simulate loads placed to the medial elbow in the later stages of rehabilitation only to prepare the overhead athlete for a return to throwing.

avulsed from the medial epicondyle. Thirty-nine percent of these athletic elbows had calcification and scar formation in the ulnar collateral ligament with 16 percent demonstrating an osteophyte to the posteromedial olecranon most likely from the increased valgus extension overload secondary to ulnar collateral ligament attenuation.

The clinical evaluation of these patients preoperatively resulted in a positive valgus stress test in 8 of the 14 patients who underwent an ulnar collateral ligament repair, and 33 of 56 patients who underwent autogenous reconstruction. Valgus stress radiographs were also used in the preoperative evaluation with greater emphasis placed upon the subjective and clinical evaluation.[21] Fifty percent of these athletes demonstrated a flexion contracture that limited full elbow extension.

SURGICAL TECHNIQUE FOR ULNAR COLLATERAL LIGAMENT RECONSTRUCTION

The surgical technique used to reconstruct the ulnar collateral ligament is described extensively by Conway et al.,[21] Jobe et al.,[59] and Jobe and ElAttrache.[57] A 10-cm medial incision over the medial epicondyle is used to provide exposure with careful dissection and protection of the ulnar nerve carried out before the ulnar collateral ligament is addressed. If a primary repair is performed, adequate normal-appearing ligamentous tissue is required to allow for direct repair. If inadequate ligamentous tissue is present, a reconstruction is performed. Additional exposure is required to perform the reconstruction, which is obtained by transection of the flexor/pronator tendinous origin.

This has important ramifications with respect to rehabilitation. The removal of this tendinous origin results in a greater amount of time required for healing, and a longer time period before resistive exercise of the flexor/pronator muscles and forearm supination and wrist extension ROM can be performed.

Calcification within the ligament and surrounding soft tissues is also removed with relocation of the ulnar nerve performed by removing it from the cubital tunnel. The ulnar nerve is mobilized from the level of the arcade of Struthers to the interval between the two heads of the flexor carpi ulnaris. The attachment sites of the anterior band of the ulnar collateral ligament are identified and tunnels are drilled in the medial epicondyle and proximal ulna to approximate the anatomical location of the original ligament. The graft taken from the ipsilateral palmaris longus (if available) is then placed in a figure of eight fashion through the tunnels. The ulnar nerve is carefully transposed so that no impingement or tethering occurs. Reattachment of the flexor pronator origin is then performed. The elbow is immobilized in a position of 90° of flexion, neutral forearm rotation, with the wrist left free to move.

Rehabilitation Concerns

The elbow remains immobilized for the first 10 days postoperatively with gentle gripping exercises allowed in order to prevent further disuse atrophy. Active and passive ROM of the elbow, wrist, and shoulder are performed at 10 days postoperatively.

Close monitoring of the ulnar nerve distribution in the distal upper extremity is recommended due to the transposition of the nerve that frequently accompanies surgical reconstruction of the MUCL. As discussed in the surgical summary previously, care is taken to protect the graft by gradually progressing elbow extension ROM to 30° by week 2 and finally to terminal ranges by 4–6 weeks postoperatively. Protection of the graft from large stresses is recommended, even though loss of extension ROM is an undesirable postoperative result. Therefore, progressive increases in elbow extension ROM and the use of gentle joint mobilization and contract-relax stretching techniques are warranted to achieve timely, optimal elbow extension. Due to the reattachment of the flexor-pronator tendinous insertion, limited ROM into wrist extension and forearm supination is performed for the first 6 weeks until healing of the flexor-pronator insertion takes place.

Rehabilitation of the postoperative elbow should also include activities to restore proprioceptive function to the injured joint. Kinesthesia is the perceived sensation of the position and movement of joints and muscles and an important part in the coordination of movement patterns in the peripheral joints. Simple use of exercises such as angular replication and end-range reproduction can be used early in rehabilitation, without visual assistance, to stimulate mechanoreceptors in the postoperative joint. These procedures are utilized early in the rehabilitation process concomitant with ROM and joint mobilization. Loss of kinesthetic awareness in the upper extremity following injury has been objectively identified by Smith and Brunolli.[108]

Rehabilitation Progression

The progression of resistive exercise follows previously discussed exercises beginning with multiple angle isometrics at week 2 and submaximal isotonics during the fourth postoperative week. Utilization of the total arm strength concept is followed, with proximal weight attachment for glenohumeral exercises to prevent stresses placed across the elbow. No glenohumeral joint, internal or external rotation strengthening for at least 6 weeks to as many as 16 weeks postoperatively, is allowed due to the valgus stress placed upon the elbow with this movement pattern. During 8–12 weeks following surgery, both concentric and eccentric exercises are performed in the elbow extensors and flexors, as well as a continued total arm strengthening emphasis, with all distal movement patterns described in nonoperative rehabilitation of humeral epicondylitis being applied (pages 523–524). Plyometric exercises, ball dribbling, and closed-chain exercises are also used during this time frame.

Isokinetic training is introduced at 4 months postoperatively, with isokinetic testing applied to identify areas needing specific emphasis.[120,121] Progression of isokinetic training patterns by these authors again follows from wrist extension/flexion to forearm pronation/supination, and finally elbow extension/flexion. The isokinetic dynamometer is also used at 4–6 months postoperatively for shoulder internal/external rotation strengthening with 90° of abduction and 90° of elbow flexion to impart a gentle, controlled valgus stress to the elbow. At 4 months postoperatively, throwing athletes begin an interval-throwing program to prepare the elbow for the stresses of functional activity.

The duration of rehabilitation postoperatively is often 6 months to a year. A slow revascularization of the graft through a sheath of granulation tissue that grows from the tissue adjacent to the site of implantation encircles the graft is the rationale provided by Jobe et al.[59] for their time-based rehabilitation program. They are convinced that at least 1 year is required for the tendon graft and its surrounding tissues to develop sufficient strength and endurance to function as a ligament in the medial elbow.

Outcomes Following Ulnar Collateral Ligament Reconstruction

In their series of 56 reconstructed elbows, Conway et al.[21] reported baseball players return to throwing 15 ft by 4.5 months, with competition at 12.5 months postoperatively. The athlete with a repaired ulnar collateral ligament performed throwing activities of 15 ft at 3 months and competed at 9 months. Overall, an excellent result was achieved in 64 percent of the operative elbows of elite athletes. An excellent result was defined as achieving a level of activity equal to or greater than preinjury level. Bennett et al.[11] reported improved stability in 13 of 14 cases of ulnar collateral ligament reconstruction in an active adult and working population, with improved stability reported in all cases of direct repair by Kuroda and Sakamaki.[72] A flexion contracture was reported in as many as 50 percent of the athletes at a mean of 6 years following an autogenous ulnar collateral ligament reconstruction.[21] Conway et al.[21] did not feel that this finding limits performance, since elbow ROM during throwing ranges from 120° to 20°, although conscious effort during rehabilitation is given to regain as much extension as possible during the time-based rehabilitation program.

ELBOW DISLOCATIONS

Failure of the normally stable osseous, ligamentous, capsular, and muscular constraints at the elbow ultimately can lead to dislocation in response to a macrotrauma.

Pathomechanics

The elbow is the second most commonly dislocated large joint behind the shoulder in the adult population and the most commonly dislocated joint in children under the age of 10.[77] It is reported that 7 out of every 100,000 people suffer an elbow dislocation.[60] Inherent in any elbow dislocation is a degree of instability present at the joint. Rehabilitation and treatment is predicated upon regaining full functional mobility while maintaining elbow joint stability.

Mechanism of Injury

Elbow dislocations are typically the result of trauma as the person falls onto an outstretched arm. Two specific mechanisms of injury have been reported. Hyperextension along with an axially directed force causes the olecranon to act as a fulcrum, levering the trochlea over the coronoid process.[77] A posterolateral rotary-directed force can produce a rotational displacement of the ulna on the humerus leading to dislocation.[89] A combination of axial compression, elbow flexion, valgus stress, and forearm supination produces this type of displacement. Concomitant injuries associated with elbow dislocations include fractures, soft tissue tear or rupture of ligaments, muscles, and joint capsule, vascular and neural compromise, as well as articular cartilage defects. Following the dislocation event, the elbow typically presents with significant swelling, severe pain, and structural deformity with the forearm appearing shortened upon observation.

Classification

Traditionally, elbow dislocations are classified according to the direction of ulnar displacement relative to the humerus. The overwhelming majority of cases involve a posterior dislocation versus the rare incidence of both anterior and lateral dislocation. Posterior dislocations are further subdivided into posterior, posteromedial, and posterolateral groups. Approximately 90 percent of all elbow dislocations are posterior and posterolateral.[6] Other classifications include simple versus complete dislocations. Simple dislocations involve minimal disruption of the congruity of bony and soft-tissue restraints, which usually allow for early initiated motion and rehabilitation. Complete dislocations involve the destruction of the bony restraints and soft tissue, particularly the ulnar collateral ligament. The ulnar collateral ligament and bony articulation provide the majority of stability at the elbow absorbing 54 percent and 33 percent of the valgus forces at 90° of elbow flexion and 31 percent each at 0° of elbow flexion.[83] Complete dislocations generally require a longer immobilization and recovery period to allow for healing of the primary restraints. Further classification is used to describe posterolateral instability as it progresses to dislocation. This classification is divided into three stages and based upon a circular disruption of bone and soft tissue that starts laterally and progresses toward the medial side of the elbow.[89] Stage 1 involves a partial or complete rupture of the lateral collateral ligament resulting in subluxation. In stage 2, the entire lateral collateral ligament is ruptured along with part of the anterior and posterior capsule leading to a *perched* dislocation. *Perched* refers to the position of the coronoid process as it sits "perched" on the posterior aspect of the trochlea. Stage 3 posterolateral dislocations are considered complete dislocations. Stage 3A involves all soft tissues around the elbow including the posterior band of the ulnar collateral ligament with the exception of the anterior band. In stage 3B, complete disruption of both lateral and ulnar collateral ligament complexes results in gross multidirectional instability.

Rehabilitation Concerns

Immediate care of elbow dislocations initially involves reduction, evaluation of the neurovascular triad for compromise, and further assessment of ligamentous stability. Radiographs and MRI are obtained to determine the extent of bony and soft-tissue damage. The elbow is typically placed in a posterior splint at 90° flexion and immobilized until cleared to begin ROM activities. Severe damage to bony and soft-tissue restraints may require surgical intervention.

Rehabilitation Progression

Elbow rehabilitation guidelines following dislocation comprise three distinct phases as proposed by Harrelson and Leaver-Dunn.[48] Phase 1 is the *immediate motion phase* and generally starts anywhere from 1–10 days postinjury. Early active ROM (all planes) within a protected and pain-free range is initiated to prevent adhesion formation and flexion contracture, which causes subsequent loss of motion and pain. For simple dislocations, immediate motion protocols have been shown to produce favorable results including return of full motion, early return to athletic and competitive activities, and low incidence of recurrent instability.[102,114,115] Passive ROM is not indicated early due to the possibility of heterotopic ossification. Management of pain and inflammation is conducted with ice, compression, and use of modalities. Strengthening activities can include gripping, shoulder and wrist isotonics, and gentle multiangle submax-to-max isometrics for both elbow flexion and extension. All exercises should be completed in a pain-free ROM. Care should be taken to avoid valgus stresses at the elbow. The posterior splint is usually discharged, however a hinged elbow brace may be utilized to protect ROM within the limits of stability.

Phase 2 consists of the *intermediate phase* from days 10–14. During this period chief concern is achieving full elbow ROM particularly extension. Strength, endurance, and power exercise are progressed to include elbow isotonics in all planes. Progressive resistive exercises are to be incorporated for the shoulder, wrist, and elbow. Inclusion of proprioceptive activities, rhythmic stabilization, plyometrics, and eccentric isotonics during the latter parts of this phase helps retrain the dynamic elbow stabilizers. Phase 3 is the *advanced strengthening phase* beginning from week 2 to 6. During this phase preparation is made for a gradual return to sport or activity. Exercise progression is to include sport specific activities and drills along with continued progressive resistive exercise. At this time, an interval-throwing program may be initiated for those returning to overhand throwing activities. Wilk and Arrigo,[119] have also included a *return to activity phase* as part of a general rehabilitation protocol. Sport-specific exercise and tests are conducted to determine appropriate stability requirements on the elbow. Upon clinical examination by the physician, ROM should be full and no pain present. Medical doctor clearance is ultimately required for return to activity. Bracing or taping may continue to be used to ensure stability and joint protection.

ELBOW FRACTURES

Pathomechanics/Mechanism of Injury

Fractures that will affect function at the elbow joint may occur at the distal humerus, capitellum, coronoid, olecranon, radial head and neck, supracondylar region, lateral condyle, and medial epicondyle. These fractures occur in both children and adults as the result of an acute traumatic injury, such as a direct collision or a fall on an outstretched hand. A thorough clinical examination and radiographs are important in obtaining a correct diagnosis so that appropriate treatment can be given. Clinical signs and symptoms of a fracture include history of traumatic onset, pain, swelling, tenderness, and ecchymosis. Elbow stability and neurovascular status should also be assessed immediately following injury. The presence of the posterior fat pad sign on radiographs has been suggested as a sign of an intracapsular elbow fracture in pediatric patients even if no fracture is seen on the radiograph. Effusion within the elbow joint elevates the posterior fat pad, making it visible on radiographs. In a prospective study, the presence of a posterior fat pad on radiographs was indicative of a fracture in 76 percent of the children evaluated. These results suggest that the children with an elevated posterior fat pad sign should be treated as though a nondisplaced elbow fracture is present, even if the fracture is not evident on radiographs.[106]

Types of Elbow Fractures

SUPRACONDYLAR FRACTURES

Supracondylar fractures are the most common elbow fractures that occur in children and account for 60 percent of all elbow fractures.[26,80] They often occur in children around 7 years old.[24] The mechanism of injury is a fall on a hyperextended arm with pronation.[24,26] Since the supracondylar ridge is only 2–3 mm thick in children,[26] it has a high risk for injury with a hyperextension mechanism. The Gartland classification system is used to divide supracondylar fractures into three types.[26,80] Type I fractures are nondisplaced and usually treated with 3 weeks of immobilization. Type II fractures are moderately displaced, but there is contact between the fragments as the posterior periosteal hinge is intact. A complete displacement is classified as type III. Posteromedial displacement is associated with radial nerve injuries, and posterolateral displacement is associated with brachial artery or median nerve injury. Reduction and surgical stabilization is required for type III, and possibly for type II fractures.[26,80] Three to four weeks of immobilization is recommended following surgery.[24] Complications following supracondylar injury may include cubitus varus, transient nerve injury, and compartment syndrome.[26]

Full elbow ROM can be difficult to regain after supracondylar fractures and rehabilitation may last several months.[24] Loss of ROM will vary based on patient age, injury severity, and concomitant injuries. Keppler et al.[63] investigated the effectiveness of physiotherapy in regaining elbow ROM after uncomplicated, operative treatment supracondylar humeral fractures without neurovascular injury in children between the ages of 5 and 12 years. At 12 and 18 weeks following surgery, results showed a significant improvement in elbow ROM in those children receiving physiotherapy compared to those not receiving treatment. However, at a 1-year follow-up, there was no significant difference between the children who had received physiotherapy and those who did not.

LATERAL CONDYLE FRACTURES

Lateral condyle fractures account for 12–20 percent of elbow fractures in children[13,26,74,80] and are the second most common elbow fracture.[74] These fractures result from a fall on an outstretched hand with forearm supination.[80,81] A varus force may cause the extensor muscles and collateral ligament to avulse the lateral condyle.[26,81] Lateral condyle fractures are classified by the Milch system into two types based on the location of the fracture line.[26,80,81] Milch type I fractures occur when the fracture line is lateral to the trochlear groove or in the trochlear groove. Milch type II fractures extend medial to the trochlea, allowing lateral subluxation of the ulna and elbow instability. Proper classification in children may be difficult to assess because the trochlea is not ossified until the child is approximately 10 years old.[81]

Lateral condyle fractures with less than 2-mm displacement may be treated nonoperatively with immobilization if fracture healing is monitored.[26,74] For fractures displaced more than 2 mm, surgery is recommended.[74,80] Surgical treatment may involve open reduction and internal fixation[13,80] or intraoperative arthrography followed by closed reduction and percutaneous pinning, with no consensus for the optimal technique in the literature.[13] Complications following lateral condyle fractures may include delayed union, nonunion, avascular necrosis of the lateral condyle, and stiffness.[26,80]

MEDIAL EPICONDYLE FRACTURES

Medial epicondyle fractures account for 8–10 percent of pediatric elbow fractures[80] and are most common in children between the ages of 9 and 15 years.[26] They are caused by a fall on an outstretched hand with forced wrist hyperextension and valgus stress at the elbow.[80] Associated elbow dislocation occurs in 50 percent of cases.[80] Possible complications to be aware of after medial epicondyle fractures include ulnar nerve irritation, elbow instability, nonunion, and stiffness.

Fractures with displacement up to 2 mm can be treated with immobilization. Surgery is a consideration for fractures displaced greater than 2 mm.[26] Farsetti et al.[37] performed a long-term follow-up comparison of medial epicondyle fractures displaced greater than 5 mm treated surgically versus nonsurgically. Subjects were divided into three treatment groups: (1) nonsurgical treatment consisting of immobilization, (2) open reduction and internal fixation of the fragment, and (3) excision of the osteocartilaginous fragment.

Outcome measures included ROM, forearm muscle atrophy, elbow stability, grip strength, radiographs to assess epicondylar nonunion and posttraumatic arthritis, and electromyography if symptoms of nerve impairment were present. At an average follow-up of 34 years (range 18–48), results showed patients treated with cast immobilization and patients treated with open reduction and internal fixation had similar functional outcomes, despite a high incidence of nonunion of the medial epicondyle in patients treated with cast immobilization only. A good functional outcome was defined as full or minimally restricted pain-free elbow motion, stable manual valgus stress testing, normal ipsilateral grip strength, minimal-to-no forearm muscle atrophy, and no radiographic signs of osteoarthritis. Good results were found in 16 out of 19 patients in the immobilization group and 15 out of 17 patients following open reduction internal fixation. No good results were found in patients treated with excision of the epicondylar fragment. Due to poor long-term outcomes, surgical excision of the medial epicondyle should be avoided. Nonunion did not have negative effects on function. A study by Lee et al.[76] also showed good to excellent results in subjects aged 7–17 years who had sustained medial epicondyle fractures (with greater than 5 mm displacement) that were treated operatively.

RADIAL HEAD AND NECK FRACTURES

Radial head and neck fractures occur secondary to a fall on an outstretched hand with valgus stress.[26,80] Treatment is determined by the amount of displacement and angulation between the radial head and shaft. Nondisplaced fractures usually have no residual deficits despite minimal treatment. It has also been shown that displaced Mason type I radial head or neck fractures have good long-term outcomes with conservative treatment.[50] Sanchez-Sotelo[105] recommends nonoperative treatment for radial head fractures in adults with less than 2 mm displacement, less than 30 percent involvement of the articular surface, angulation of less than 30°, and no instability. An angulation of 30° or greater may be an indication for surgical consideration.[80] When treating displaced or comminuted radial head fractures, the clinician should be aware of possible associated injuries, including osteochondral and ligamentous injury.[55] Following radial fractures, complications may include malunion, radial head overgrowth, avascular necrosis, and nonunion.[80]

Rehabilitation Concerns

STRATEGIES TO REGAIN ELBOW ROM FOLLOWING IMMOBILIZATION

The amount and rate of progression of rehabilitation following an elbow fracture will be determined by several factors including severity of injury, length of immobilization, concomitant injuries, age of patient, and level of sport activities. The primary focus of rehabilitation is on optimizing the return of elbow ROM and strength, with progression to functional daily and sport activities as needed.

Elbow ROM may not be completely regained following traumatic injury. Decreased ROM may be due to osseous structures, but is usually due to the joint capsule or soft-tissue structures (muscles, tendons, ligaments). The viscoelastic properties of soft tissue must be considered during treatment to regain elbow ROM. These properties include strain rate dependency, creep, stress relaxation, elastic deformation, and plastic deformation. Strain rate is the dependence of material properties on the rate or speed in which a load is applied. Rapidly applied forces will cause stiffness and elastic deformation whereas gradually applied forces will result in plastic deformation.

Creep is defined as the continued deformation of soft tissue with the application of a fixed load (e.g., traction and dynamic splinting). Stress relaxation is the reduction of forces, over time, in a material that is stretched and held at a constant length (e.g., serial casting and static splinting). Elastic deformation is the elongation produced by loading that is recovered after the load is removed. There is no long-term effect on tissues. Plastic deformation is the elongation produced under loading that will remain after the removal of a load, resulting in a permanent increase in length.[15]

A study by Bonutti et al.[15] evaluated the effectiveness of a patient-directed static progressive stretching program in the treatment of elbow contractures. Subjects had elbow contractures for 1 month to 42 years that did not respond to previous treatment consisting of physical therapy, dynamic splinting, serial casting, surgery, or a combination of these treatments. The orthosis providing a static progressive stretch was worn for 30 minutes with the patient increasing the amount of stretch every 5 minutes as tolerated. Separate 30-minute sessions were used in patients requiring flexion and extension improvement. Results showed an average improvement of 17° extension and 14° flexion. Improved results were seen in 4–6 weeks, with continued improvement in patients using the orthotic 3 months or more. There was no change in ROM in subjects 1 year after

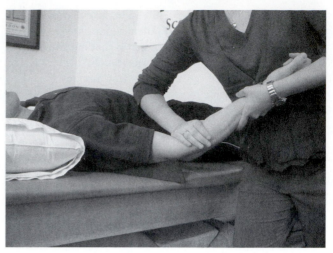

FIGURE 26-26

Posterior glide of the ulnohumeral joint.

discontinuation of the orthosis, suggesting that the plastic deformation of soft tissue occurred and the elongation of tissue was maintained over time.

Manual rehabilitation techniques for improving elbow ROM include passive ROM and joint mobilizations. Passive range is performed in elbow flexion, extension, supination, and pronation. Care should be taken with passive ROM into extension, as end range stretching of the flexors can potentially contribute to heterotrophic ossification, as discussed previously. Elbow joint mobilizations may be used to restore joint arthrokinematics. Joint distraction (Fig. 26-18 already listed), posterior glides of the ulna (Fig. 26-26), medial and lateral ulna glides (Fig. 26-27A and B), radial distraction (Fig. 26-28), and dorsal and ventral glides of the proximal radioulnar (Fig. 26-29) joint are used to increase elbow ROM.[31] Shoulder passive ROM should also be performed early in the rehabilitation process to

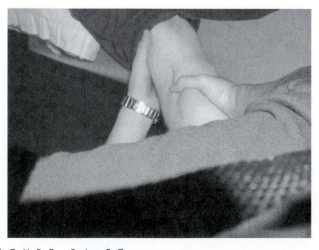
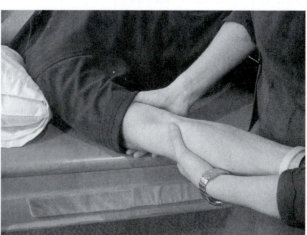

FIGURE 26-27

Lateral and medial glides of the ulnohumeral joint. **A,** Lateral glide. **B,** Medial glide.

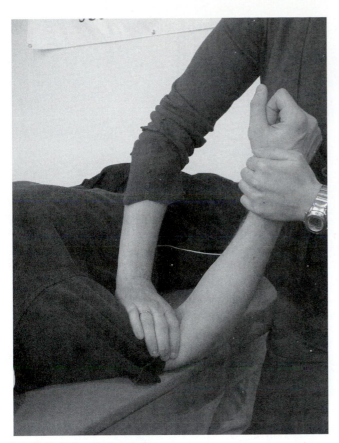

FIGURE 26-28

Radial distraction mobilization.

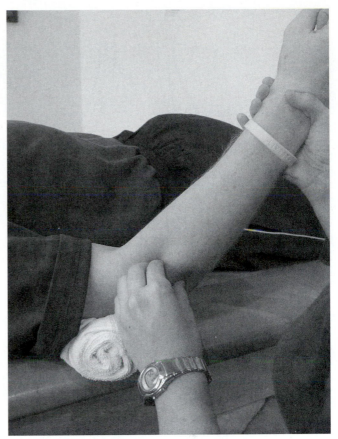

FIGURE 26-29

Dorsal and ventral glides of the proximal radioulnar joint.

prevent glenohumeral capsular hypomobility, especially if the injury required prolonged immobilization.

PEDIATRIC CONSIDERATIONS

When diagnosing and treating pediatric elbow injuries, consideration must be given to bone maturation and growth. In young children, the elbow joint is cartilaginous with the appearance of apophyseal ossification centers between the ages of 2 and 10 years. It is important to be aware of the apophyseal ossification centers at the elbow so that they are not misinterpreted as fractures on a radiograph. The ossification centers with the date of appearance in parentheses include the capitellum (2 years), radial head (4 years), medial epicondyle (5 years), trochlea (7 years), olecranon (9 years), and lateral epicondyle (10 years).[26] Since the soft tissues surrounding the apophyses are stronger than the cartilage present at the apophyses, injurious forces causing a sprain or strain in an adult may cause an avulsion fracture in children. The most common site for an avulsion fracture is the medial epicondyle. Medial epicondyle avulsion fractures occur in young throwing athletes due to an acute valgus stress and flexor-pronator muscle contraction.[51] There is an acute onset of medial elbow pain after forceful contraction such as during a baseball pitch. The avulsion commonly occurs during late cocking or early acceleration phase of throwing. A "pop" may be heard at time of injury. If a medial epicondyle

avulsion fracture is suspected, it is important to assess the ulnar nerve, point tenderness of the medial epicondyle, swelling, ecchymosis, and valgus instability.

The Salter-Harris classification system[104] is commonly used to describe acute physeal injuries (Fig. 26-30). There are five types of fractures in this classification, with type II fractures being the most common. Type I fractures occur when the epiphysis separates completely from the metaphysis. The mechanism of injury involves shear, torsion, and avulsion forces. Treatment consists of casting with excellent prognosis unless vascular damage is present. In a type II fracture, the fracture line extends along the growth plate and into the metaphysis. The triangular-shaped metaphyseal fragment is referred to as the Thurston-Holland sign. Type III fractures are intra-articular and extend from the joint surface to the weak zone of the growth plate and reaches the periphery of the plate. There is good prognosis with proper reduction and intact vascular supply. Surgery may be needed for type III fractures. Type IV fractures are characterized by the fracture extending from the joint surface through the epiphysis, across the full thickness of the growth plate, and through a portion of the metaphysis. Surgery is required for this type of fracture, and there is usually a poor prognosis unless the growth

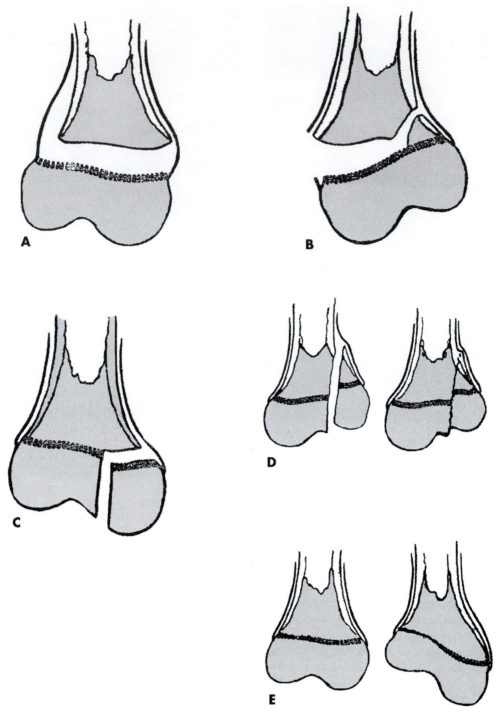

F I G U R E   2 6 - 3 0

Salter-Harris fracture classification. (**A**) Type I. (**B**) Type II. (**C**) Type III. (**D**) Type IV. (**E**) Type V.

plate is completely and accurately aligned. A type V fracture is rare and involves crushing of the growth plate, which inhibits further growth.

Similar to elbow fractures in adults, treatment of pediatric elbow fractures will vary based on location and type of fracture. Protection of the open growth plates is an important consid-eration to optimize long-term outcomes. Prolonged immobi-lization following injury can be more conservative in children than adults, as children will not develop the amount of stiffness and soft-tissue contractures as adults. Pediatric injuries may re-quire less rehabilitation due to decreased ROM restriction when compared to adults.

APPENDIX 1: POSTOPERATIVE PROTOCOL FOR ELBOW ARTHROSCOPY AND REMOVAL OF LOOSE BODIES

Acute Phase

Primary goals

1. Reduce pain and postoperative edema
2. Regain joint ROM and muscle length
3. Initiate submaximal resistive exercise as tolerated

POSTOPERATIVE DAYS 1 AND 2

A. Removal of bulky postoperative dressing and replacement with Ace wrap.
B. Electric stimulation and ice to decrease pain/inflammation.
C. Initiation of ROM exercise for the glenohumeral joint, elbow, forearm, and wrist.
D. Initiation of submaximal strengthening exercises including:
   1. putty
   2. isometric elbow and wrist flexion/extension
   3. isometric forearm pronation/supination

POSTOPERATIVE DAYS 2–7

A. ROM and joint mobilization to terminal ranges for the elbow, forearm, and wrist (avoid overaggressive elbow extension passive range of motion)
B. Begin progressive resistance exercise program with 0–1 lb weight and three sets of 15 repetitions
   1. wrist flexion curls
   2. wrist extension curls
   3. radial deviation
   4. ulnar deviation
   5. forearm pronation
   6. forearm supination
C. Upper body ergometer

Intermediate Phase

Primary goals

1. Begin total arm strength training program
2. Emphasize full elbow ROM

POSTOPERATIVE 1–3 WEEKS

A. Continue progressive resistance exercise program adding:
   1. elbow extension
   2. elbow flexion
   3. isolated rotator cuff program (Jobe exercises)
   4. seated row
   5. manual and isotonic scapular program
   6. closed-chain, upper-extremity program

Advanced/Return to Activity Phase

Primary goals

1. Advance strengthening progression of distal upper extremity
2. Prepare patient for return to functional activity with simulation of joint angles and muscular demands inherent in intended sport activity

POSTOPERATIVE 4–8 WEEKS

A. Isokinetic exercise introduction using wrist flexion/extension and forearm pronation/supination movement patterns
B. Upper-extremity plyometrics with medicine balls
C. Isokinetic test to formally assess distal strength
D. Interval sport return program
   1. criterion for advancement:
      a. full, pain-free ROM
      b. 85–100 percent return of muscle strength
      c. no provocation of pain on clinical exam
E. Upper-extremity strength and flexibility maintenance program

APPENDIX 2: POSTOPERATIVE REHABILITATION FOLLOWING ULNAR COLLATERAL LIGAMENT RECONSTRUCTION USING AUTOGENOUS GRAFT

Postoperative Week 1

Brace. Posterior splint applied immediately postoperatively with elbow placed in 90° of flexion. Progression to hinged ROM brace dependent on patient tolerance. ROM brace to remain locked at 90° for week 1.

Rehab.

–Modalities to decrease elbow swelling and control pain
–ROM forearm pronation/supination and wrist flexion/extension
–ROM glenohumeral joint and scapulothoracic joint mobilization
–Shoulder isometrics (No internal rotation or external rotation due to valgus stress on elbow)
–Gripping exercises with balls or putty

Postoperative Week 2

Brace. ROM set in hinged elbow brace from 30–100°

Rehab.

–Continue with above exercises and ROM
–Initiate isometric muscular work of wrist flexion/extension, radial/ulnar deviation, and elbow flexion/extension within ROM available at ulnohumeral joint

–Initiate closed-chain exercise over Swiss balls (wax-on/off) with limited weight bearing over extremity

–Begin scapular protraction/retraction manual resistance in side lying with the elbow in 90° of elbow flexion

Postoperative Week 3

Brace. Hinged elbow brace is opened to 15–110°. (ROM in brace is gradually increased 5° in extension and 10° in flexion each week unless otherwise specified by physician.)

Rehab. No changes in exercises during this time period.

Postoperative Week 4–5

Brace. Hinged elbow brace set at 10°–120°.

Rehab.

–Begin submaximal isotonic exercise for wrist flexion/extension, radial/ulnar deviation and forearm pronation/supination with light 1 pound weight or theratubing (yellow or red).

–Begin shoulder isotonic exercise program with prone extension, prone horizontal abduction and standing scaption to 80° elevation as tolerated. Continue to avoid rotational strengthening patterns, due to valgus stress at ulnohumeral joint. Weight attachment proximal to elbow with cuff weights recommended for introduction.

–Initiate seated rowing using Theratube or machine/cables.

Postoperative Week 6

Brace. * Hinged elbow brace set at 0°–130°.

Rehab.

–Begin elbow flexion/extension isotonics using available ranges and avoiding a "bounce home" type movement at end range extension.

–Initiate shoulder internal rotation and external rotation patterns using both isotonic machine or cables (submax), Theratube (yellow or red to start), and initiation of side lying external rotation pattern.

–Begin ball dribbling off ground using Swiss balls, body blade, Theraband resistance bar oscillation, and BOING using patterns of radial/ulnar deviation and pronation/supination with varied shoulder positions less than 90° of elevation.

Postoperative Weeks 10–12

Rehab.

–Plyometric program initiated using Swiss ball, progressing to medicine ball. Patterns consisting of initially a 2-hand chest pass and progressing to side throws, wood chops, and eventually eccentric arm deceleration with contralateral arm throwing.

*Discontinuation of hinged elbow brace occurs between 6 and 10 weeks postoperative, as designated by referring physician.

–Continuation of shoulder, elbow, forearm and wrist isotonics.

–Rhythmic stabilization techniques using both open and closed chain environments.

–Closed-chain step-up progression.

Postoperative Week 12

Rehabilitation.

–Initiation of isokinetic training using the pattern of wrist flexion/extension at speeds ranging from 180°–300° per second. ROM stops used at 0°–35° wrist extension and 0°–55° wrist flexion. Upon successful completion of wrist flexion/extension during several trial treatments, isokinetic forearm pronation and supination is initiated using ROM stops of 0°–50° of pronation and supination.

–Shoulder isokinetic internal rotation/external rotation is initiated submaximally using speeds between 210° and 300° per second in the modified base position.

Postoperative Week 14 (Return to Activity Phase)

Rehab.

–Initiation of elbow extension/flexion isokinetics using speeds between 180° and 300° per second and ROM stops at 10° extension and 125° flexion.

–Initiation of interval sport return programs.

–Continuation of upper-extremity strengthening programs and maintenance of particularly elbow extension ROM.

–A return to competitive levels of throwing or racquet sports is not expected until at least 6 months following surgery.

SUMMARY

- The elbow joint is composed of the humeroulnar joint, humeroradial joint, and the proximal radioulnar joint. Motions in the elbow complex include flexion, extension, pronation, and supination.

- Fractures in the elbow may occur from a direct blow or falling on an outstretched hand. They may be treated by casting or in some cases by surgical reduction and fixation. Following surgical fixation, the patient may require 12 weeks for rehabilitation.

- Valgus extension overload injuries occur during the acceleration phase of the throwing motion and can result in the development of posterior medical osteophytes and loose bodies in the athletic elbow. Treatment via arthroscopy is followed by early immediate ROM and a progression of strength and functional training to restore full function to the elbow.

- The ulnar collateral ligament is injured as a result of a repetitive valgus force. Reconstruction is vital to competitive throwing patients.

- Elbow dislocations result from elbow hyperextension from a fall on an extended arm, with the radius and ulna dislocating posteriorly. The degree of stability present will determine the course of rehabilitation. If the elbow is stable, a brief period of immobilization is followed by rehabilitation. An unstable dislocation requires surgical repair and thus a longer period of immobilization.

- Medial epicondylitis results from repetitive microtrauma to the common flexor and pronator tendons during pronation and flexion of the forearm and wrist.

- Lateral epicondylitis (*tennis elbow*) occurs with concentric or eccentric overload of the wrist extensors and supinators, most commonly the extensor carpi radialis brevis tendon.

REFERENCES

1. Adelsberg S. An EMG analysis of selected muscles with rackets of increasing grip size. *Am J Sports Med* 14:139–142, 1986.

2. An KN, Morrey BF. Biomechanics of the elbow. In: Morrey BF, ed. *The Elbow and Its Disorders*. Philadelphia, PA, Saunders, 1993.

3. Andrews JR, Heggland EJH, Fleisig GS, Zheng N. Relationship of ulnar collateral ligament strain to amount of medial olecranon osteotomy. *Am J Sports Med* 29(6):716–721, 2001.

4. Andrews JR, Soffer SR. *Elbow Arthroscopy*. St. Louis, MO, Mosby-Yearbook Inc., 1994.

5. Andrews JR, Timmerman LA. Outcome of elbow surgery in professional baseball players. *Am J Sports Med* 23:407–4134, 1995.

6. Andrews JR, Wilk KE, Groh G. Elbow rehabilitation. In: Brotzman SB, ed. *Clinical Orthopaedic Rehabilitation*. Philadelphia, PA, Mosby-Yearbook Inc., 67–71, 1996.

7. Andrews JR, Wilk KE, Satterwhite YE, Tedder JL. Physical examination of the thrower's elbow. *J Orthop Sports Phys Ther* 6: 296–304, 1993.

8. Ballentyne BT, O'Hare SJ, Paschall JL, et al. Electromyographic activity of selected shoulder muscles in commonly used therapeutic exercises. *Phys Ther* 73:668–682, 1993.

9. Basford JR, Sheffield CG, Cieslak KR. Laser therapy: A randomized, controlled trial of the effects of low intensity Nd: YAG laser irradiation on lateral epicondylitis. *Arch Phys Med Rehabil* 81:1504–1510, 2000.

10. Bennett GE. Elbow and shoulder lesions of baseball players. *Am J Surgery* 98:484–492, 1959.

11. Bennett JB, Green MS, Tullos HS. Surgical management of chronic medial elbow instability. *Clin Othop Rel Research* 278:62–68, 1992.

12. Bernhang AM, Dehner W, Fogarty C. Tennis elbow: A biomechanical approach. *Am J Sports Med* 2:235–260, 1974.

13. Bhandari M, Tornetta P, Swiontkowski MF. Displaced lateral condyle fractures of the distal humerus. *J Orthop Trauma* 17:306–308, 2003.

14. Blackburn TA, McLeod WD, White B, et al. EMG analysis of posterior rotator cuff exercises. *Athlet Train* 25:40–45, 1990.

15. Bonutti PM, Windau JE, Ables BA, Miller BG. Static progressive stretch to reestablish elbow range of motion. *Clin Orthop Relat Res* 303:128–134, 1994.

16. Bowling RW, Rockar PA. The elbow complex. In: Davies GJ, Gould JA, eds. *Orthopaedic and Sports Physical Therapy*. St. Louis, MO, Mosby, 1985, pp. 476–496.

17. Boyer MI, Hastings H. Lateral tennis elbow: Is there any science out there? *J Shoulder Elbow Surg* 8:481–491, 1999.

18. Brattberg G. Acupuncture therapy for tennis elbow. *Pain* 16:285–288, 1983.

19. Carroll R. Tennis elbow: Incidence in local league players. *Br J Sports Med* 15:250–255, 1981.

20. Chinn CJ, Priest JD, Kent BE. Upper extremity range of motion, grip strength, and girth in highly skilled tennis players. *Phys Ther* 54:474–482, 1974.

21. Conway JE, Jobe FW, Glousman RE, Pink M. Medial instability of the elbow in throwing athletes. *J Bone Joint Surg* 74A(1):67–83, 1992.

22. Cyriax JH, Cyriax PJ. *Illustrated Manual of Orthopaedic Medicine*. London, Butterworths, 1983.

23. Davidson PA, Pink M, Perry J, Jobe FW. Functional anatomy of the flexor pronator muscle group in relation to the medial collateral ligament of the elbow. *Am J Sports Med* 23(2):245–250, 1995.

24. de las Heras J, Duran D, de la Cerdo J, Romanillos O, Martinez-Miranda J, Rodriguez-Merchain EC. Supracondylar fractures of the humerus in children. *Clin Orthop Relat Res* 432:57–64, 2005.

25. Dijs H, Mortier G, Driessens M, DeRidder A, Willems J, Devroey TA. Retrospective study of the conservative treatment of tennis elbow. *Medica Physica* 13:73–77, 1990.

26. Do T, Herrara-Soto J. Elbow injuries in children. *Curr Opin Pediatr* 15:68–73, 2003.

27. Ellenbecker TS. Rehabilitation of shoulder and elbow injuries in tennis players. *Clin Sports Med* 14:87–110, 1995.

28. Ellenbecker TS. A total arm strength isokinetic profile of highly skilled tennis players. *Isokinetics Exerc Sci* 1:9–21, 1991.

29. Ellenbecker TS, Davies GJ. *Closed Kinetic Chain Exercise*. Champaign, IL, Human Kinetics, 2001.

30. Ellenbecker TS, Davies GJ, Rowinski MJ. Concentric versus eccentric isokinetic strengthening of the rotator cuff: Objective testing versus functional test. *Am J Sports Med* 16(1):64–69, 1988.

31. Ellenbecker TS, Mattalino AJ. *The Elbow in Sport*. Champaign, IL, Human Kinetics, 1997.

32. Ellenbecker TS, Mattalino AJ, Elam EA, Caplinger RA. Medial elbow laxity in professional baseball pitchers: A bilateral comparison using stress radiography. *Am J Sports Med* 26(3):420–424, 1998.

33. Ellenbecker TS, Roetert EP. Isokinetic profile of elbow flexion and extension strength in elite junior tennis players. *J Orthop Sports Phys Ther* 33(2):79–84, 2003.

34. Ellenbecker TS, Roetert EP. Isokinetic profile of wrist and forearm strength in female elite junior tennis players. Platform presentation presented at the APTA Annual Conference and Exposition, Washington DC, June 2003.

35. Ellenbecker TS, Roetert EP. Unpublished data from the USTA on Range of Motion of the Elbow and Wrist in Senior Tennis Players, 1994.

36. Ellenbecker TS, Roetert EP, Bailie DS, Davies GJ, Brown SW. Glenohumeral joint total rotation range of motion in elite tennis players and baseball pitchers. *Med Sci Sports Exerc* 34(12):2052–2056, 2002.

37. Farsetti P, Potenza V, Caterini R, Ippolito E. Long-term results of treatment of fractures of the medial humeral epicondyle in children. *J Bone Joint Surg* 83(9):1299–1305, 2001.

38. Fleck SJ, Kraemer WJ. Designing resistance training programs. Champaign, IL, Human Kinetics, 1987.

39. Gam AN, Warming S, Larsen LH, et al. Treatment of myofascial trigger points with ultrasound combined with massage and exercise. A randomized controlled trial. *Pain* 77(1):73–79, 1998.

40. Glousman RE, Barron J, Jobe FW, et al. An electromyographic analysis of the elbow in normal and injured pitchers with medial collateral ligament insufficiency. *Am J Sports Med* 20:311–317, 1992.

41. Goldie I. Epicondylitis lateralis humeri. *Acta Chir Scand Suppl* 339:1–114, 1964.

42. Gould JA, Davies GJ. Orthopaedic and sports rehabilitation concepts. In: Gould JA, Davies GJ, eds. *Orthopaedic and Sports Physical Therapy.* St. Louis, MO, Mosby, 1985, pp. 181–198.

43. Greenbaum B, Itamura J, Vangsness CT, Tibone J, Atkinson R. Extensor carpi radialis brevis. *J Bone Joint Surg BR* 81(5):926–929, 1999.

44. Groppel JL, Nirschl RP. A biomechanical and electromyographical analysis of the effects of counter force braces on the tennis player. *Am J Sports Med* 14:195–200, 1986.

45. Guerra JJ, Timmerman LA. Clinical anatomy, histology, & pathomechanics of the elbow in sports. *Oper Tech Sports Med* 4:69–76, 1996.

46. Haake M, Konig IR, Decker T, et al. Extracorporeal shock wave therapy in the treatment of lateral epicondylitis: A randomized multicenter trial. *J Bone Joint Surgery* 84:1982–1991, 2002.

47. Hang YS, Peng SM. An epidemiological study of upper extremity injury in tennis players with particular reference to tennis elbow. *J Formos Med Assoc* 83:307–316, 1984.

48. Harrelson GL, Leaver-Dunn D. Elbow rehabilitation. In: Andrews JR, Harrelson GL, Wilk KE, eds. *Physical Rehabilitation of the Injured Athlete,* 2nd ed. Philadelphia, PA, Saunders, 1998, pp. 554–588.

49. Hawkins RJ, Kennedy JC. Impingement syndrome in athletes. *Am J Sports Med* 8:151–158, 1980.

50. Herbertson P, Josefsson PO, Hasserius R, Karlsson C, Besjakov J, Karlsson MK. Displaced mason type I fractures of the radial head and neck in adults: A fifteen-to thirty-three-year follow-up study. *J Shoulder Elbow Surg* 14:73–77, 2005.

51. Hughes PE, Paletta GA. Little leaguer's elbow, medial epicondyle injury, and osteochondritis dissecans. *Sports Med Arthroscopy Rev* 11:30–39, 2003.

52. Indelicato PA, Jobe FW, Kerlan RK, Carter VS, Shields CL, Lombardo SJ. Correctable elbow lesions in professional baseball players: a review of 25 cases. *Am J Sports Med* 7:72–75, 1979.

53. Ingham K. Transverse cross friction massage. *Phys Sports Med* 9(10):116, 1981.

54. Inman VT, Saunders JB de CM, Abbot LC. Observations on the function of the shoulder joint. *J Bone Joint Surg AM* 26:1–30, 1944.

55. Itamura J, Roidis N, Mirzayan R, Vaishnzv S, Learch T, Shean C. Radial head fractures: MRI evaluation of associated injuries. *J Shoulder Elbow Surg* 14:421–424, 2005.

56. Jensen BR, Sjogaard G, Bornmyr S, Arborelius M, Jorgensen K. Intramuscular laser-Dopler flowmetry in the supraspinatus muscle during isometric contractions. *Eur J Appl Physiol Occup Physiol* 71(4):373–378, 1995.

57. Jobe FW, Elattrache NS. Diagnosis and treatment of ulnar collateral ligament injuries in athletes. In: Morrey BF, ed. *The Elbow and its Disorders,* 2nd ed. Philadelphia, PA, Saunders, 1993, pp. 566–572.

58. Jobe FW, Kvitne RS. Shoulder pain in the overhand or throwing athlete: The relationship of anterior instability and rotator cuff impingement. *Orthop Rev* 28(9):963–975, 1989.

59. Jobe FW, Stark H, Lombardo SJ. Reconstruction of the ulnar collateral ligament in athletes. *J Bone Joint Surg* 68A:1158–1163, 1986.

60. Josefsson PO, Nilsson BE. Incidence of elbow dislocations. *Acta Orthop Scand* 57:537–538, 1986.

61. Joyce ME, Jelsma RD, Andrews JR. Throwing injuries to the elbow. *Sports Med Arthrosc Rev* 3:224–236, 1995.

62. Kamien M. A rational management of tennis elbow. *Sports Med* 9:173–191, 1990.

63. Keppler P, Salem K, Schwarting B, Kintzl L. The effectiveness of physiotherapy after operative treatment of supracondylar humeral fractures in children. *J Pediatr Orthop* 25: 314–316, 2005.

64. Kibler WB. The role of the scapula in athletic shoulder function. *Am J Sports Med* 26(2):325–337, 1998.

65. Kibler WB. Role of the scapula in the overhead throwing motion. *Contemp Orthop* 22(5):525–532, 1991.

66. Kibler WB, Chandler TJ, Livingston BP, Roetert EP. Shoulder range of motion in elite tennis players. *Am J Sports Med* 24(3):279–285, 1996.

67. Kibler WB, Uhl TL, Maddux JWQ, Brooks PV, Zeller B, McMullen J. Qualitative clinical evaluation of scapular dysfunction: A reliability study. *J Shoulder Elbow Surg* 11:550–556, 2002.

68. King JW, Brelsford HJ, Tullos HS. Analysis of the pitching arm of the professional baseball pitcher. *Clin Orthop* 67:116–123, 1969.

69. Kitai E, Itay S, Ruder A, et al. Ann epidemiological study of lateral epicondylitis in amateur male players. *Ann Chir Main* 5:113–121, 1986.

70. Kraushaar BS, Nirschl RP. Tendinosis of the elbow (tennis elbow). Clinical features and findings of histopathological, immunohistochemical and electron microscopy studies. *J Bone Joint Surgery AM* 81:259–278, 1999.

71. Kulund DN, Rockwell DA, Brubaker CE. The long term effects of playing tennis. *Physician Sports Med* 7:87–92, 1979.

72. Kuroda S, Sakamaki K. Ulnar collateral ligament tears of the elbow joint. *Clin Orthop Rel Research* 208:266–271, 1986.

73. Labelle H, Guibert R, Joncas J, Newman N, Fallaha M, Rivard CH. Lack of scientific evidence for the treatment of lateral epicondylitis of the elbow. *J Bone Joint Surg* 74-B:646–651, 1992.

74. Launay F, Leet A, Jacopin S, Jouve J, Bollini G, Sponseller PD. Lateral humeral condyle fractures in children: A comparison to two approaches in treatment. *J Orthop Ped* 24:385–391, 2004.

75. Leadbetter WB. Cell matrix response in tendon injury. *Clin Sports Med* 11:533–579, 1992.

76. Lee H, Shen H, Chang J, Lee C, Wu S. Operative treatment of displaced medial epicondyle fractures in children and adolescents. *J Shoulder Elbow Surg* 14:178–185, 2005.

77. Linscheid RL, O'Driscoll SW. Elbow dislocation. In: Morrey BF, ed. *The Elbow and Its Disorders*, 2nd ed. Philadelphia, PA, Saunders, 1993, pp. 441–452.

78. Magee DJ. Elbow. In: Magee DJ, ed. *Orthopedic Physical Assessment*. Philadelphia, PA, Saunders, 1997.

79. McFarland EG, Torpey BM, Carl LA. Evaluation of shoulder laxity. *Sports Med* 22:264–272, 1996.

80. Milbrandt TA, Copley LA. Common elbow injuries in children: Evaluation, treatment, and clinical outcomes. *Curr Opin Orthop* 15:286–294, 2004.

81. Mirsky EC, Karas EH, Weiner L. Lateral condyle fractures in children: Evaluation of classification and treatment. *J Orthop Trauma* 11(2):117–120, 1997.

82. Morrey BF. *The Elbow and its Disorders*, 2nd ed. Philadelphia, PA, Saunders, 1993.

83. Morrey BF, An KN. Articular and ligamentous contributions to the stability of the elbow joint. *Am J Sports Med* 11:315, 1983.

84. Neer CS. Impingement lesions. *Clin Orthop* 173:70–77, 1973.

85. Nirschl RP. In: Morrey BF, ed. *The Elbow and its Disorders*, 2nd ed. Philadelphia, PA, Saunders, 1993, pp. 537–552.

86. Nirschl RP. Elbow tendinosis/tennis elbow. *Clin Sports Med* 11:851–870, 1992.

87. Nirschl RP, Rodin DM, Ochiai DH, Maartmann-Moe C. Iontophoretic administration of Dexamethasone Sodium Phosphate for acute epicondylitis: A randomized, double blinede, placebo controlled study. *Am J Sports Med* 31(2):189–195, 2003.

88. Nirschl R, Sobel J. Conservative treatment of tennis elbow. *Physician Sports Med* 9:43–54, 1981.

89. O'Driscoll SW. Elbow instability. *Hand Clin* 10:405–415, 1994.

90. O'Driscoll SW, Morrey BF. Arthroscopy of the elbow. *J Bone Joint Surg* 74-A:84–94, 1992.

91. Oglive-Harris DJ, Gordon R, MacKay M. Arthroscopic treatment for posterior impingement in degenerative arthritis of the elbow. *Arthroscopy* 11(4):437–443, 1995.

92. Olsen BS, Sojbjerg JO, Dalstra M, Sneppen O. Kinematics of the lateral ligamentous constraints of the elbow joint. *J Shoulder Elbow Surg* 5:333–341, 1996.

93. Percy EC, Carson JD. The use of DMSO in tennis elbow and rotator cuff tendinitis. A double blind study. *Med Sci Sports Exerc* 13:215–219, 1981.

94. Priest JD, Jones HH, Nagel DA. Elbow injuries in highly skilled tennis players. *J Sports Med* 2(3):137–149, 1974.

95. Priest JD, Jones HH, Tichenor CJC, et al. Arm and elbow changes in expert tennis players. *Minnesota Med* 60:399–404, 1977.

96. Reddy AS, Kvitne RS, Yocum LA, ElAtrache NS, Glousman RE, Jobe FW. Arthroscopy of the elbow: A long term clinical review. *Arthrosc* 16(6):588–594, 2000.

97. Regan WD, Korinek SL, Morrey BF, An KN. Biomechanical study of ligaments around the elbow joint. *Clin Orthop* 271:170–179, 1991.

98. Rhu KN, McCormick J, Jobe FW, et al. An electromyographic analysis of shoulder function in tennis players. *Am J Sports Med* 16:481–485, 1988.

99. Rijke AM, Goitz HT, McCue FC. Stress radiography of the medial elbow ligaments. *Radiology* 191:213–216, 1994.

100. Roetert EP, Ellenbecker TS, Brown SW. Shoulder internal and external rotation range of motion in nationally ranked junior tennis players: A longitudinal analysis. *J Strength Cond Res* 14(2):140–143, 2000.

101. Rosenthal M. The efficacy of flurbiprofen versus piroxicam in the treatment of acute soft tissue rheumatism. *Curr Med Res Opin* 9:304–309, 1984.

102. Ross G, McDevitt ER, Chronister R, et al. Treatment of simple elbow dislocation using an immediate motion protocol. *Am J Sports Med* 27(3):308–311, 1999.

103. Runge F. Zur genese unt behand lung bes schreibekramp fes Berl Kun *Woschenschr* 10:245, 1873.

104. Salter RB, Harris WR. Injuries involving the epiphyseal plate. *J Bone Joint Surg* 45:587–632, 1963.

105. Sanchez-Sotelo J, Barwood SA, Blaine TA. Current concepts in elbow fracture care. *Curr Opin Orthop* 15:300–310, 2004.

106. Skagus DL, Mirzayan R. The posterior fat pad sign in association with occult fracture of the elbow in children. *J Bone Joint Surg* 10:1429–1433, 1999.

107. Slocum DB. Classification of the elbow injuries from baseball pitching. *Am J Sports Med* 6:62, 1978.

108. Smith R, Brunulli J. Shoulder kinesthesia after anterior glenohumeral dislocation. *Phys Ther* 69(2):106–112, 1989.

109. Stroyan M, Wilk KE. The functional anatomy of the elbow complex. *J Orthop Sports Phys Ther* 17:279–288, 1993.

110. Sullivan PE, Markos PD, Minor MD. *An Integrated Approach to Therapeutic Exercise: Theory and Clinical Application.* Reston, VA, Reston Publishing Company, 1982.

111. Svernl AB, Adolfsson L. Non-operative treatment regime including eccentric training for lateral humeral epicondylalgia. *Scand J Med Sci Sports* 11(6):328–334, 2001.

112. Townsend H, Jobe FW, Pink M, et al. Electromyographic analysis of the glenohumeral muscles during a baseball rehabilitation program. *Am J Sports Med* 19:264–272, 1991.

113. Tullos HS, Ryan WJ. Functional anatomy of the elbow. In: Zarins B, Andres JR, Carson WD, eds. *Injuries to the Throwing Arm.* Philadelphia, PA, Saunders, 1985.

114. Uhl TL. Uncomplicated elbow dislocation rehabilitation. *Athlet Ther Today* 5(3):31–35, 2000.

115. Uhl TL, Gould M, Gieck JH. Rehabilitation after posterolateral dislocation of the elbow in a collegiate football player: A case report. *J Athlet Train* 35(1):108–110, 2000.

116. Verhaar JAN, Walenkamp GHIM, Kester ADM, Linden AJVD. Local corticosteroid injection versus Cyriax-type physiotherapy for tennis elbow. *J Bone Joint Surg BR* 77:128–132, 1995.

117. Warfel JH. Muscles of the arm. *The Extremities, Muscles, and Motor Points.* Philadelphia, PA, Lea & Febinger, 1993.

118. Waslewski GL, Lund P, Chilvers M, Taljanovic M, Krupinski E. MRI Evaluation of the Ulnar Collateral Ligament of the Elbow in Asymptomatic, Professional Baseball Players. Presented at the AOSSM Meeting, San Diego, CA, 2002.

119. Wilk KE, Arrigo CA. Rehabilitation of elbow injuries. In: Andrews JR, Harrelson GL, Wilk KE, eds. *Physical Rehabilitation of the Injured Athlete*, 3rd ed. Philadelphia, PA, Saunders, 2004, pp. 590–618.

120. Wilk KE, Arrigo CA, Andrews JR. Rehabilitation of the elbow in the throwing athlete. *J Orthop Sports Phys Ther* 17:305–317, 1993.

121. Wilk KE, Azar FM, Andrews JR. Conservative and operative rehabilitation of the elbow in sports. *Sports Med Arthrosc Rev* 3:237–258, 1995.

122. Wilson FD, Andrews JR, Blackburn TA, McCluskey G. Valgus extension overload in the pitching elbow. *Am J Sports Med* 11(2):83–88, 1983.

123. Winge S, Jorgensen U, Nielsen AL. Epidemiology of injuries in danish championship tennis. *Int J Sports Med* 10:368–371, 1989.

124. Wolf BR, Altchek DW. Elbow problems in elite tennis players. *Tech Shoulder Elbow Surg* 4(2):55–68, 2003.

CHAPTER 27

Rehabilitation of the Wrist, Hand, and Fingers

Jeanine Biese and Anne Marie Schneider

OBJECTIVES

After completing this chapter, the therapist should be able to do the following:

- Discuss key concepts of functional anatomy and biomechanics involved in the normal wrist and hand.
- Relate biomechanical and tissue-healing principles to the rehabilitation of various wrist and hand conditions.
- Discuss criteria for progression of the rehabilitation program for specific hand and wrist injuries.
- Describe the rationale for specific splinting techniques in the management of selected wrist and hand conditions.

FUNCTIONAL ANATOMY AND BIOMECHANICS

The hand is an intricate balance of muscles, tendons, and joints working in unison. This balance combines mobility, stability, and dexterity to allow the hand to perform a multitude of activities. Any disruption of this balance due to various injuries or conditions can greatly alter the appearance and ability of the hand to function. At work, the hand is the most frequently injured body part.[1] Hand conditions can occur as a single injury, over time as in cumulative trauma, or because of a disease process.

Treatment of hand conditions requires a complete history and evaluation. These evaluations can include subjective and objective assessments that assist the physician and therapist in determining the specific hand dysfunction and disease. A diagnosis of "hand pain" or "wrist pain" does the client a disservice and may lend itself to treatment that is not specific to the condition. The reader is referred to the text, "*Rehabilitation of the Hand and Upper Extremity* (5th ed.),"[2] for a complete discussion of evaluations and assessments.

Treatment of the hand is based on the phases of wound healing. The initial phase is the inflammatory phase, and usually lasts 5 days. It is typically a time of vascular dilation and edema.[3,4] This is often a time of immobilization, such as a bulky surgical dressing. This phase can be prolonged in cases of mishandling or aggressive therapy. Diabetes or specific medications can also prolong the phases of wound healing.

The second phase is the fibroplasia phase, which typically lasts from 5 to 21 days.[3,4] During this phase, the fibroblasts lay down collagen in a random network. Depending on the specific diagnosis, special protected motion exercises may be allowed during this time. For example, a newly repaired flexor tendon usually initiates a program of passive range of motion (PROM) in a protective splint during this time to avoid stress or rupture to the repair.[4]

The third phase is the maturation phase and usually begins at 3 weeks. It continues for 6–12 months and beyond. Here the randomly oriented collagen matures and develops strength with intermolecular cross-linking.[3,4] Adhesions can be formed during this time. Treatment protocols (such as some flexor tendon protocols) are often progressed during this time. Care should be taken to balance the application of stress to the newly healing tissues with avoiding damage to the structure.

The Wrist

The wrist is the connecting link between the hand and forearm.[5] The wrist joint comprises eight carpal bones that are arranged in two rows. They normally articulate with radius and the triangular fibrocartilage of the ulna proximally, and the metacarpals distally.

There is an intricate relationship between the carpal bones. Ligaments interconnect the carpal bones, as well as connect the carpal bones to the radius and ulna.[6,7] During range of motion (ROM) the carpal bones demonstrate complex kinematics.

With radial deviation, the distal row is displaced radially, while the scaphoid and the lunate of the proximal row move palmarly.[7] This is reversed in ulnar deviation when the distal row is displaced ulnarly and the scaphoid and lunate of the proximal row move in an ulnar direction. This is referred to as "conjunct rotation."[7] The total arc of motion for radial and ulnar deviation averages approximately 50°, 10°–20° radially and 20°–35° ulnarly.[7]

Flexion and extension occur through synchronous movement of proximal and distal rows. The capitate, radius, and scaphoid move in the same plane during flexion and extension. The total excursion is equally distributed between the midcarpal and radiocarpal joints when measured by means of the capitolunate/radiolunate joint column.[7] Berger points out that when the movement is measured through the radioscaphoid-STT (scaphoid, trapezium, trapezoid) joint, more than two-thirds of the ROM occurs through the radioscpahoid joint.[7] The ROM for both flexion and extension is normally 65°–80° in each direction.[7,8] Functional movement of the wrist, or the amount of wrist movement needed to do most daily living activities is much less, and was found by Ryu et al.[9] to be 40° of flexion, 40° of extension, and a combined arc of 40° of radial and ulnar deviation. It is important that the therapist remembers not to sacrifice joint stability and increase joint pain in an attempt to increase ROM. A pain-free stable joint with adequate functional motion will serve the client's functional activities better than a joint with greater ROM, greater pain, and less stability.

Cross sections through the wrist reveal that tendons of the extensor carpi ulnaris (ECU) at the ulnar aspect of the wrist, and the extensor pollicis brevis (EPB) and abductor pollicis longus (APL) on the radial side are in the "collateral" position.[10] This anatomical arrangement provides medial and lateral stability to the wrist. Electromyography (EMG) studies demonstrate that the ECU, EPB, and APL are active in wrist flexion and extension. These muscles show only small displacement with wrist flexion and extension, and assist in joint stability by means of this isometric contraction.[10] Their function can be described as an adjustable collateral system. The ECU shows activity in ulnar deviation and the APL and EPB in radial deviation.[10]

Stability of the ulnar side of the wrist is provided by the triangular fibrocartilage complex (TFCC).[5] This ligament arises from the radius and inserts into the base of the ulnar styloid, the ulnar carpus, and the base of the fifth metacarpal.[5] This ligament complex is the major stabilizer of the distal radioulnar joint (DRUJ) and is a load-bearing column between the distal ulna and ulnar carpus.[5] Injury to the triangular fibrocartilage can result in pain with pronation and supination of the forearm and pain with ulnar deviation. Diagnostically, this pain may be reduced when the examiner depresses and provides support to the ulna during pronation and supination (Figs. 27-1A and B). Treatment for this condition is discussed later in this chapter.

The flexor carpi ulnaris (FCU) insertion into the pisiform, a sesamoid bone, is unique in that it is the only muscle with a tendon insertion into the wrist. The proximity of this easily pal-pated bone to the ulnar nerve can sometimes be troublesome in cases of blows to the area or a pisiform fracture. In cases of ulnar nerve compression, symptoms should be differentiated to determine if the problem arises from Guyon's canal (located under the pisiform) or at the cubital tunnel of the elbow. Compression of the ulnar nerve at the cubital tunnel is a more common condition.

The dorsal wrist has an extensor retinaculum (fascia) with six extensor compartments that are separated by septa.[11] The purpose of the retinaculum is to prevent bowstringing or subluxation of the tendons during wrist movement. The fibro-osseous tunnels or compartments position and maintain the extensor tendons in their synovial sheaths.[11] The sixth compartment houses the ECU, the fifth is a pulley for the extensor digiti minimi, the fourth contains extensor digitorum communis (EDC) and indices, the third contains extensor pollicis longus (EPL). More radially, the second compartment contains extensor carpi radialis and longus. One of the most common wrist conditions is located in the first compartment. Here, the EPB and APL make up the radial border of the anatomical snuffbox. Stenosing tenosynovitis of the first dorsal compartment is called de Quervain's disease and in two studies made up one-third of all cases of tenovaginitis affecting the hand and wrist.[12,13]

Volarly, the long finger flexors, long thumb flexor, median nerve, and radial artery pass through the carpal tunnel. The carpal tunnel consists of a concave arch of carpal bones. The roof of this arch includes the transverse carpal ligament, forearm fascia, and the distal aponeurosis of the thenar and hypothenar muscles.[14] The carpal tunnel is the site of one of the most common hand pathologies, carpal tunnel syndrome. Any condition that increases pressure in the tunnel can lead to compression of the median nerve. This can result in pain and paresthesia in the median nerve distribution.

The Hand

The metacarpophalangeal (MP) joints allow for several planes of motion including flexion, extension, abduction, adduction, as well as a slight degree of pronation and supination. The metacarpal head has a convex shape, which fits with a shallow concave proximal phalanx. The stability of the MP joint is provided by its capsule, collateral ligaments, accessory collateral ligaments, volar plate, and musculotendinous units. The collateral ligaments are laterally positioned and are dorsal to the axis of rotation. In extension, the collateral ligament is lax; in flexion, it is taut.[15] If the MP joint is immobilized in extension, the lax collateral ligament can tighten, which can make MP flexion difficult once mobilization has begun. MP flexion is considered the "safe position" to prevent this tightening of the collateral ligaments but care should be taken to consider the specific condition when immobilizing the MP joint. For example, an extensor tendon laceration (zones 5 and 6) needs to be placed in 0° of MP extension to protect the repair (Fig. 27-2).

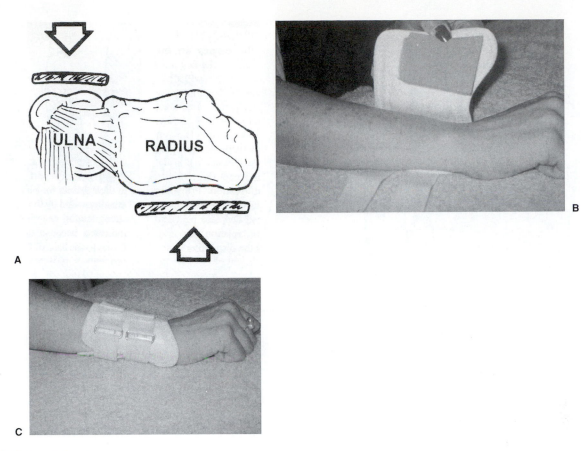

FIGURE 27-1

A, Injury to the triangular fibrocartilage can result in forearm pain with pronation and supination, as well as with wrist ulnar deviation. Instability of the DRUJ can be supported with a soft splint that provides compression of the distal ulna in a volar direction and a counterforce to the distal radius in a dorsal direction. (Reprinted, with permission, from Biese J. In: Mackin EJ, Callahan AD, Skirven TM, Schneider LH, Osterman AL, eds. *Rehabilitation of the Hand and Upper Extremity*, 5th ed. St. Louis, MO, Mosby, 2002, pp. 1846–1857. Concept courtesy of Judy Leonard, OTR, CHT, and redrawn from Melvin JL. *Rheumatic disease: Occupational Therapy and Rehabilitation*, 2nd ed. Philadelphia, FA Davis, 1982.) **B,** A prefabricated wrist wrap splint (Count'R-force) with padding at the dorsal ulna and the volar wrist is very helpful in managing painful pronation and supination due to disruption of the triangular fibrocartilage. **C,** The wrist wrap splint allows partial wrist movement while supporting the distal ulna.

Several tendons cross the MP joints. On the flexor surface, the flexor digitorum superficialis (FDS) and flexor digitorum profundus (FDP) are held closely to the bones by pulleys. These pulleys prevent bowstringing during finger flexion. The A-1 pulley (Fig. 27-3) is the site of tendon drag or locking in the case of a trigger finger. The FDS flexes the proximal interphalangeal (PIP) joint, and the FDP flexes the distal interphalangeal (DIP) joint. Injuries to the flexor tendons are categorized by zones (Fig. 27-4). Zone 1 injuries involve only FDP, whereas zone 2 can involve both FDS and FDP. Tendon nutrition in zone 1 and 2 relies largely on synovial diffusion due to the limited vascularity. This diffusion is increased with digit motion, and supports the concept of protective motion to enhance tendon healing. Zones 3–5 have greater vascularity than zones 1 and 2 and often heal with less complications. The interosseous muscles are lateral to the MP joints and are responsible for abduction and adduction of the MP joints. The lumbrical muscles are volar to the axis of rotation of the MP joint, but then insert into the lateral bands and are dorsal to the PIP and DIP joints. Their function is MP joint flexion and interphalangeal (IP) joint extension. (This is also the reason you can have IP extension with radial nerve palsy.) The extensor mechanism crosses the MP joint dorsally. Sagittal bands hold the EDC tendons centrally. Injuries and treatment to the extensor tendons are also categorized by zones (see Fig. 27-2). An easy way to remember this system is to locate the odd-numbered zones over the joints.

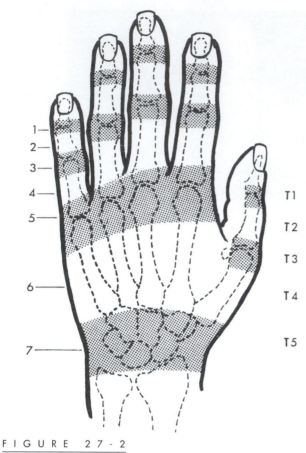

FIGURE   27-2

The extensor tendon zones. (Reprinted, with permission, from Kleinert HE, Schepel S, Gill T. *Surg Clin N Am* 61:267, 1981.)

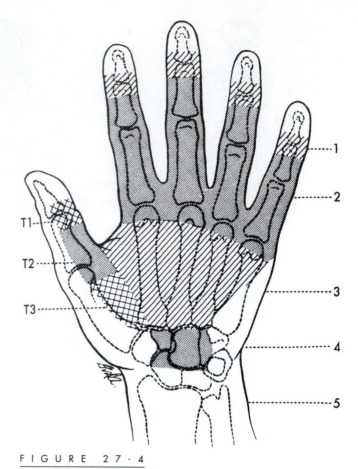

FIGURE   27-4

The flexor tendon zones. (Reprinted, with permission, from Kleinert HE, Schepel S, Gill T. *Surg Clin N Am* 61:267, 1981.)

The Fingers

The IP joints are bicondylar hinge joints allowing flexion and extension. Collateral and accessory collateral ligaments stabilize the joints on the lateral aspect. The collateral ligaments are taut in extension and lax in flexion. This is important when splinting the PIP joint. If it is not a contraindication with the injury (as with PIP fracture dislocation), the joint should be splinted in full extension to help prevent flexion contractures.

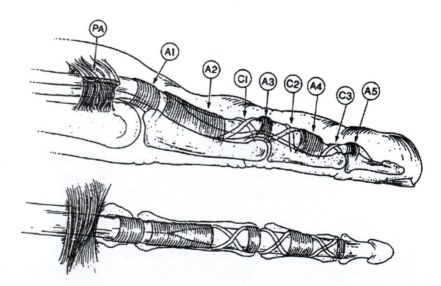

FIGURE   27-3

The pulleys of the flexor tendons. (Reprinted, with permission, from Strickland JW. Development of flexor tendon surgery: Twenty-five years of progress. *J Hand Surg* 25:214–235, 2000.)

On the flexor surface, the FDS bifurcates proximal to the PIP joint, allowing the FDP to become more superficial as it continues to insert on the distal phalanx, providing DIP flexion. The FDS inserts on the middle phalanx for PIP flexion. Five annular pulleys and three cruciate pulleys between the MP and DIP joints prevent bowstringing of the tendons. These pulleys keep the tendon close to the bone and provide the mechanical advantage for composite digit flexion (see Fig. 27-3).

On the extensor surface, the common extensor tendons cross the MP joints and then divide into three slips. The central slip inserts on the dorsal middle phalanx, allowing for PIP extension. The two lateral slips, called the lateral bands, receive attachments from the lumbricals, travel dorsal and lateral to the PIP joint, rejoin after the PIP joint, and insert as the terminal extensor into the DIP joint. This delicately balanced system serves to extend the IP joints. Disruption of this system greatly alters the balance and mechanics of the tendons, and can result in boutonnière (PIP flexion with DIP hyperextension) and swan neck deformities (PIP hypertension with DIP flexion).

The Thumb

The thumb is responsible for 40–50 percent of the function of the hand.[16] The thumb's ability to oppose the digits, grasp, and pinch is due to the thumb's unique ability to balance this mobility with joint stability. The thumb carpal metacarpal joint is a biconcave saddle joint that allows for ROM in a wide variety of planes. This great degree of motion is combined with excellent joint stability, especially during pinching activities, due to the strong joint capsule and supporting ligaments. When a disease process such as osteoarthritis or rheumatoid arthritis compromises this stability, the thumb collapses into deformities.

There are four extrinsic thumb muscles, which include EPL, EPB, APL, and FPL (flexor pollicis longus). The five intrinsic muscles that add to the unique mobility and dexterity of the thumb are abductor pollicis brevis, opponens pollicis, abductor pollicis, adductor pollicis, and flexor pollicis brevis. The thumb, like the other digits, has a series of pulleys for the flexor tendons. The A-1 pulley at the MP joint of the thumb is the site of a common condition called trigger thumb (see Fig. 27-3). This is when the flexor tendon drags or locks due to stenosing tenosynovitis at the A-1 pulley. Due to the tenosynovitis, the tendon becomes too large to glide through the pulley. The tendon then drags or locks as the digit flexes.

REHABILITATION TECHNIQUES FOR SPECIFIC INJURIES

Distal Radius Fractures

PATHOMECHANICS

Fractures of the distal radius can be described in many different ways, by several classification systems. It is important that the therapist has an understanding of the type of fracture and how different types of fractures need to be treated. Some of the questions the therapist may ask include the following. Is the fracture intra-articular or extra-articular? Displaced or nondisplaced? Simple or comminuted? Open or closed? Is the radius shortened? Is the ulna also fractured? Answers to these questions will help the therapist select interventions and determine expected outcomes.

Extra-articular nondisplaced fractures tend to heal without incident with immobilization. When the treating physician allows wrist active range of motion (AROM), the initial joint stiffness is usually brief, and most cases progress to a good outcome. As the fractures become more involved, either intra-articular or comminuted, the chances of full return of motion and hand function are decreased.

The normal anatomic radius is tilted volarly. If in a fracture the volar tilt becomes dorsal, motion will be affected, and can lead to midcarpal instability, decreased strength, increased ulnar loading, and a dysfunctional DRUJ.[17]

The normal anatomic radius is longer than the ulna. If in a comminuted fracture the radius is shortened, there is a high potential for disability.[17,18,20] Radial shortening may lead to DRUJ pain, especially with pronation and supination activities. This can result in reduced grip strength due to pain and limited use of the hand.

In more involved fractures, an external fixator may need to be applied by the surgeon to reduce and align the fracture. The external fixator will attach to the radius and to the second metacarpal shaft. Length may be restored and held with the traction bars of the external fixator. The type of fracture, size of the fragments, and displacement determine initial (cast versus fixator) treatment. Once reduced, the fractures need to be closely monitored to be sure that reduction is being maintained. Periodic adjustments by the surgeon to the external fixator can assure proper tension and positioning of the fracture.

Rehabilitation following a distal radius fracture is similar regardless of the method of fixation (cast, open reduction internal fixation (ORIF), or external fixator). While in the cast or external fixator, ROM and edema control of noninvolved joints is essential, so that when immobilization is discontinued, rehabilitation can be concentrated on the wrist and forearm. Slings are not usually recommended as they can contribute to shoulder stiffness. With an external fixator, some patients and surgeons prefer the addition of a custom fabricated wrist splint that allows additional comfort and support. (Fig. 27-5B). This splint is easily removed by the patient with Velcro straps for skin care. The pins and/or external fixator sites should be cleaned daily. Surgeons recommend various techniques such as sterile water, peroxide, clean water, or a combination. The therapist should confer with surgeon as to their preferred method of pin care, and instruct the patient in this technique. In some cases, low-temperature splinting material can be fit over the external fixator to prevent it from being bumped (especially at night). This guard is also secured with Velcro straps.

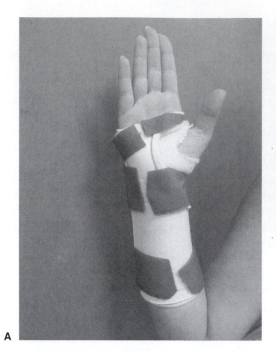

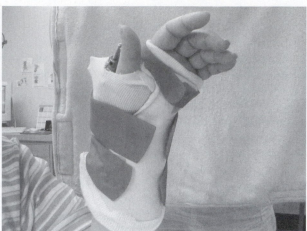

FIGURE   27-5

A, A wrist splint is used for a variety of conditions. With conservative management of carpal tunnel syndrome it can be beneficial to keep the wrist in a neutral position at night. After a healed wrist fracture, wrist extension limitations can be treated effectively with serial night splinting. In the clinic, the splint is molded while the wrist is held in comfortable maximum extension. The night splint gently stretches the wrist into progressively more extension. The splint is remolded at each therapy visit as gains in extension are made. **B,** A wrist splint can be used in combination with an external fixator for additional support and patient comfort.

INJURY MECHANISM

As is true of most wrist injuries, most distal radius fractures occur from a fall on an outstretched hand. It may be a high-impact event, but with a low-impact event, the presence of this condition in the middle-aged population may indicate a need for a bone density test. This test may rule out the possibility of osteoporosis and the need to seek the appropriate treatment.

REHABILITATION CONCERNS

Early and proper reduction and immobilization is of utmost importance. The fracture must be closely watched initially to be sure the reduction is being maintained. Early ROM to noninvolved joints is imperative. This helps prevent muscle atrophy, aids in muscle pumping to decrease edema, and most importantly maintains motion, so treatment can focus on the wrist once fracture is healed and fixation is removed.

Other concerns include complications of carpal tunnel syndrome or complex regional pain syndrome.[19,21] If either is present and first noted in the therapy clinic, referral should be made back to the physician as soon as possible. Both conditions are best managed by early detection and intervention. One other complication, which usually occurs late in a seemingly inconsequential nondisplaced distal radius fracture, is an EPL rupture.[19] It is thought that this occurs from the EPL rubbing through bone around the fracture site near Lister's tubercle. In such a condition, the patient would be unable to actively extend the thumb IP joint, and surgical intervention is required.

REHABILITATION PROGRESSION

Rehabilitation may be initiated while the wrist is immobilized. This should include shoulder ROM in all planes, elbow flexion and extension, and finger flexion and extension. Finger exercises should include isolated MP flexion, composite flexion (full fist), and intrinsic minus fisting (MP extension with IP flexion) (Exercises 27-1A–D). Coban or an Isotoner glove may be used for edema control if necessary.

As previously mentioned, if a fixator or pins are present, pin site care may be performed depending on physician preference. A different applicator should be used on each pin to prevent possible spread of infection. Some physicians allow patients to shower with the fixator in place (not soaking while bathing), while other physicians prefer a plastic bag over the pin site and fixator.

Once immobilization is discontinued (approximately 6 weeks for casting, 6–8 weeks with an external fixator, or 4–6 weeks if ORIF with plate and screws), ROM to the wrist is begun. This includes active wrist flexion, extension, radial and ulnar deviation, and forearm pronation and supination (Exercises 27-2A and B, 27-3A and B, and 27-4A and B). Wrist extension should be taught with digit (especially MP) flexion (Exercise 27-2A). This isolates the wrist extensors rather than using the EDC. Extrinsic tightness of the finger extensors can occur if tightness and/or adhesions are evident due to scarring at the fracture site. This is most commonly seen with plate fixation. AROM to decrease extrinsic extensor tightness requires simultaneous wrist flexion with digit flexion. Forearm rotation (supination and pronation) should be instructed to be done with the elbow held close to the side of the body to avoid compensation from the shoulder (Exercises 27-3A and B).

PROM is dependent upon the stability of the fracture and physician preference. A lightweight hammer or mallet in the hand during pronation and supination exercises is a helpful tool to gently stretch and increase this motion (Exercises 27-5A and B). Gentle joint mobilizations to the radius and ulna are also helpful in increasing motion as well (Exercises 27-14A–F). When stretching forearm rotation passively, gentle pressure should be applied at the distal radius, proximal to the wrist, not at the hand. This will avoid placing unnecessary torque across the carpus (Exercises 27-6A and B). Gentle wrist distraction combined with flexion and extension is very effective in increasing ROM in a pain-free range. Contract and relax techniques are also helpful in obtaining ROM.

Splinting can be an effective tool in increasing ROM in patients who are not progressing. Wrist extension limitations can be treated effectively with serial night splinting (Fig. 27-5A). The splint is molded in while the wrist is held in comfortable maximum extension. The night splint gently stretches the wrist into progressively more extension. The splint is remolded at each therapy visit as gains in extension are made. This technique is not used to obtain normal end ranges due to the possibility of increasing pressure on the median nerve with prolonged wrist extension. It is very effective in cases that are having difficulty obtaining a functional range (40°). Static progressive splinting can be also utilized periodically during the day to increase wrist ROM. Daytime static progressive splinting for wrist flexion and/or extension (Fig. 27-6) is usually worn for 20–30 minutes, two to three times daily. The patient adjusts this splint as gains are made. This type of splint is also available commercially. Static progressive or dynamic pronation and supination splinting is done in cases that are not obtaining a functional range. These splints are usually worn for 20–30 minutes, two to three times a day as to not interfere with functional use of the hand.

Active motion can be progressed to strengthening after adequate ROM is achieved. Strengthening a wrist with limited motion too soon may result in strength with less than ideal ROM. All strengthening exercises should be pain free and can include light weights, Theraband, or tubing and can be graded for wrist and forearm motions. This can be in conjunction with com-

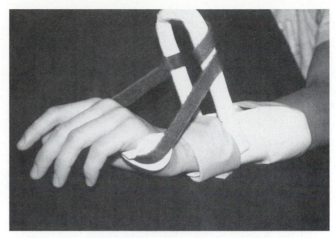

FIGURE 27-6

Static progressive splinting can be utilized periodically during the day to increase wrist ROM. Daytime static progressive splinting for wrist flexion and/or extension is usually worn for 20–30 minutes, two to three times daily. The patient adjusts this splint as gains are made. This splint demonstrates static progressive extension.

fortable progressive weight bearing such as wall push-ups that progress to the countertop, and then to a floor mat (see Exercises 27-9A and B). Weight bearing on a ball and gentle ball rolling can be the next progression (Exercise 27-10). Putty is available in a variety of grades, from soft to hard, to provide different levels of resistance. The type of putty for grip strengthening should be soft enough to provide a pain-free level of resistance (Exercise 27-7). If the patients aggravate pain in an attempt to increase strength, the pain will limit their function during activities of daily living (ADL). Pain will also reduce grip strength measurements. Most patients will continue to gain grip strength when working with submaximal effort and light putty resistance.

Athletes, particularly those in contact sports, can require additional protection as they resume athletic activity. Care must be taken to avoid returning the athlete to the field of play too quickly. Many referees will not allow a rigid splint or cast to be used as a possible weapon on the field of play. A soft cast or various padding materials may be utilized. The best care for both the patient and the other team players should be considered. Families may want their children in high-school sports to return to play too quickly. The patient and family should be cautioned to avoid the possibility of additional injury or chronic conditions that may result from premature return to the field of play.

Scaphoid Fracture

PATHOMECHANICS

Fractures of the scaphoid account for 60 percent of all carpal injuries.[20,22,25] The prognosis is related to the site of the fracture, obliquity, displacement, and promptness of diagnosis and treatment. The blood supply of the scaphoid comes distal to proximal. Fracture through the proximal one-third of the scaphoid may result in delayed union or avascular necrosis

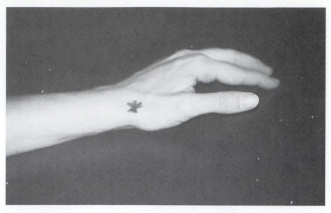

FIGURE 27-7

The * indicates the anatomic snuffbox under which the scaphoid is positioned. This area will be painful to palpation with scaphoid fracture.

secondary to the limited blood supply. It can take 20 weeks or longer for a proximal fracture to heal.[22] Displacement of the fracture usually occurs at the time of injury and can be treated using ORIF.

Surgical treatment is usually necessary if the fracture results in a nonunion. Not treating the fracture can lead to carpal instability and periscaphoid arthritis.[23,24] Diagnosis is often difficult and not easily confirmed with a standard radiograph. A bone scan may be needed for definitive diagnosis. Patients usually have wrist pain with this fracture, especially when palpated in the anatomic snuffbox (Fig. 27-7).

INJURY MECHANISM

Scaphoid fractures result from a fall on an outstretched hand in wrist hyperextension and radial deviation.[25]

REHABILITATION CONCERNS

Of primary concern is proper diagnosis. Scaphoid fractures often do not show upon initial radiographs and many go undiagnosed or misdiagnosed as wrist sprains. The typical patient has a history of a fall on an outstretched hand and has pain in the anatomic snuffbox, but the initial radiograph is negative. Bone scans may be needed to confirm the diagnosis.[26]

Nonunions can result in cases that are misdiagnosed as a wrist sprain, or are undertreated.[26] Greater concern about nonunion exists when the fracture is at the proximal pole due to the limited or absent blood supply in that region. Scaphoid nonunion may lead to carpal instability or periscaphoid arthritis.

REHABILITATION PROGRESSION

Once the diagnosis has been made, the treatment of the nondisplaced scaphoid is casting. The scaphoid can take a long time to heal. Casting usually continues for at least 6 weeks, which is followed by fabrication of a custom thumb spica splint (Fig. 27-8) for continued protection. Fractures to the proximal pole of the scaphoid may require an additional 3–6 months of splinting.[26]

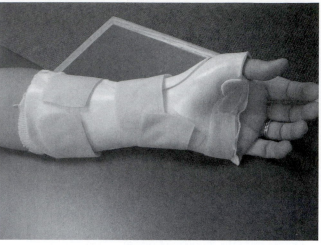

FIGURE 27-8

A forearm-based thumb spica splint includes the thumb and wrist. It may also include the thumb IP joint in some cases. It is most commonly used for a scaphoid fracture, thumb metacarpal fracture, or de Quervain's tendonitis.

The initiation of the wrist AROM program is determined by the surgeon, based on evidence of fracture healing. The thumb spica splint is worn between exercises and at night. AROM exercises of wrist flexion, wrist extension (with finger flexion to isolate wrist extensors), and radial and ulnar deviation are completed in a pain-free range (Exercises 27-2 and 27-4). Thumb flexion and extension, abduction and adduction, and opposition to each finger are also initiated (Exercises 27-8A–C). Due to the long casting and splinting time, there is a tendency for the patients to be aggressive with their exercise programs upon removal of immobilization, in a mistaken attempt to speed functional return. It is typical to have ligament injuries associated with the scaphoid fracture and aggressive PROM can increase pain by possibly compromising the newly healed ligaments. Progressing wrist PROM to the point of pain can compromise long-term function. Grip strength measurements are often diminished in the presence of pain. Strengthening exercises are delayed until healing is complete, adequate ROM has been achieved, and pain is under control. Joint stability should not be sacrificed for an increase in ROM. This fracture is typically very difficult for athletes who are frustrated by the slow healing of this bone and the long amount of time in a splint or cast. Care should be taken not to return this patient back to the sport too quickly.

Rehabilitation after ORIF is the same progression as nonsurgical. The period of immobilization may be less because of the repair of the scaphoid with rigid fixation.

Lunate Dislocations

PATHOMECHANICS

Stability of the carpus is dependent upon the maintenance of bony architecture interlaced with ligaments.[26,27] Most carpal dislocations are the dorsal perilunate type, in fact, many believe that a lunate dislocation is the end of a perilunate dislocation.[26,27] The lunate dislocates palmarly due to the loss of ligamentous stability. It is very common for reduction to be lost over time with this injury, so percutaneous pinning or ORIF is often recommended.[26,27]

Median nerve compression is frequently associated with this injury. The palmarly displaced lunate puts pressure on the nerve. Symptoms may continue for several weeks following reduction of the lunate secondary to swelling and contusion of the nerve.

INJURY MECHANISM

A violent hyperextension of the wrist is the injury mechanism.[6,17] A fall on the outstretched hand produces a translational compressive force when the lunate is caught between the capitate and the dorsal aspect of the distal radius articular surface.[17] If the lunate does not fracture, a periscaphoid or lunate dislocation may occur.

REHABILITATION CONCERNS

The primary concern is early surgical repair. Complications if not surgically corrected include pain, weakness, wrist clicking, and carpal translocation.[27] Carpal tunnel syndrome, if present, is usually addressed at the time of surgery. ROM of noninvolved joints must be maintained during immobilization.

REHABILITATION PROGRESSION

Progression is very similar to the rehabilitation of distal radius fractures and other wrist injuries. Following cast and pin (if applicable) removal, pain-free AROM is begun. Motions that need to be addressed for AROM are flexion, extension, radial deviation, ulnar deviation, supination, and pronation (Exercises 27-2A and B, 27-3A and B, and 27-4A and B). Care should be taken with lunate dislocations to encourage a stable pain-free wrist. As previously mentioned, aggressive stretching and strengthening can compromise newly healed ligaments.

The severity of this injury and need for ORIF (secondary to frequent loss of reduction if not repaired) will require at least 8 weeks for rehabilitation. At 8 weeks, the wrist may be taped for support and protection (Fig. 27-9). A soft splint that allows partial ROM can also be very helpful as the patient gradually returns to pain-free activity. One way to obtain this type of splint is to remove the metal stays from a prefabricated cloth splint. This soft splint then allows gentle support and partial ROM.[29]

Hamate Fractures

PATHOMECHANICS

A hook of the hamate fracture is more common than fractures of the hamate body.[26,27,31,33b] The hook is the attachment for the pisohamate ligament, short flexor, and opponens to the small finger and the transverse carpal ligament.[5] Because of

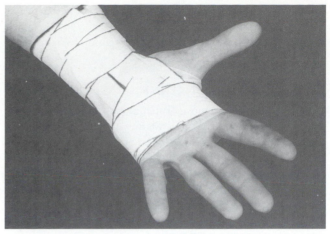

FIGURE 27-9

Wrist taping may be done when extra support is needed for activities as the patient weans from rigid splint.

these attachments, if there is a hamate hook fracture, there are deforming forces on the fragment with intermittent tension. This makes it nearly impossible to align and immobilize the fractures, and as a result, they often do not heal.[5] The hook can be palpated on the volar surface of the hand at the base of the hypothenar eminence deep and radial to the pisiform.

The hamate is in close proximity to the ulnar nerve and artery on the ulnar side, and flexor tendons to the ring and small finger in the carpal canal on the radial side (Fig. 27-10). There is a possibility of an ulnar neuropathy, tendonitis, or tendon rupture with this injury.[30,31]

INJURY MECHANISM

The suspected injury mechanism is a shearing force transmitted from a handle of a club to the hamate. It will often occur when striking an unexpected object, for example a rock or tree root

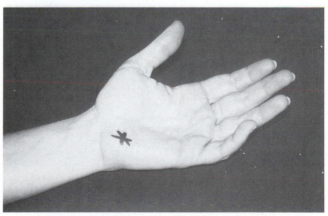

FIGURE 27-10

The * indicates the point that will elicit pain with palpation for a hamate hook fracture. Some pain may also be referred to the ulnar wrist.

by a golfer. It most frequently occurs in golfers but may occur in any stick sport such as baseball or field hockey. There is also a rare possibility of a stress fracture due to tension from ligament and muscle attachments.[9]

REHABILITATION CONCERNS

Of first concern is diagnosis. Patients may have felt a snap or pop. They will have localized tenderness over the hamate hook, ulnar-sided wrist pain, and weakness of grip that increases over time. A carpal tunnel view radiograph will confirm the diagnosis, but some patients have difficulty dorsiflexing the wrist for this view due to pain.[26] The therapist must also watch for signs of ulnar neuritis or neuropathy and flexor tendon rupture.

REHABILITATION PROGRESSION

Treatment of nondisplaced acute hamate hook fractures consists of casting for 6–8 weeks.[26,32,33a] A displaced fracture usually requires excision.[31,34] Treatment following excision is edema control with a compressive dressing and fabrication of a wrist splint.[31] A few days after the stitches are removed, scar management techniques are initiated. This can include scar massage (2–5 minutes, five times per day), and use of silicone or mineral oil products at night to soften the scar. Silicone or mineral oil based products such as Silipos, Cica-Care (Fig. 27-11), or Otoform (Fig. 27-12) is fit to the scar and held in place with Tubigrip (elasticized stockinet) at night. It is important that the scar pad be in direct contact with the skin, without an interface of lotion. Lotion can break down the silicone or mineral oil product. Patients who have persistent pain may benefit from padded bike gloves as they return to their sports. This glove

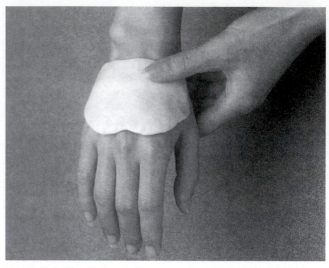

F I G U R E   2 7 - 1 2

Otoform is used as a scar control pad. A catalyst is then added to the "putty." It is then mixed and formed directly to the scar area. It hardens in a few minutes and is then secured with Coban or Tubigrip. It is usually worn at night for scar control. It may also be worn during sports activities for additional protection to a sensitive area.

protects the sensitive area while allowing a gradual return to such sport activities as golf or tennis (Fig. 27-13).

Injuries to the Distal Radioulnar Joint

PATHOMECHANICS

The distal radioulnar joint is a complex system. The design of the structures at the DRUJ allows for forearm pronation and supination while providing the necessary stability to the ulnar side of the wrist. The TFCC at the distal ulna provides support and stability to the DRUJ. Pain in this area can be due to fractures of the ulna, arthritis, synovitis, dislocation, DRUJ instability, tendonitis, and/or tears of the TFCC.[35] A complete evaluation by an experienced hand surgeon is often needed to make an accurate diagnosis. Some of these conditions can be evaluated by a radiograph, but others are difficult to diagnose, largely due to the soft-tissue involvement. The distal ulna is more prominent in pronation and less prominent in supination when palpated. When the DRUJ looses stability due to a disruption of the TFCC, the ulna can displace during ROM, make a popping or clicking noise, and/or have significant pain, limiting ADL. Injuries are often overlooked and patients often become frustrated when there is a delay in diagnosis and treatment.

INJURY MECHANISM

A fracture to the distal radius can commonly include an injury to the DRUJ. This may include a fracture to the ulnar styloid or an injury to the TFCC. Arthritis at the DRUJ can result in pain with pronation and supination. Injuries and tears to the

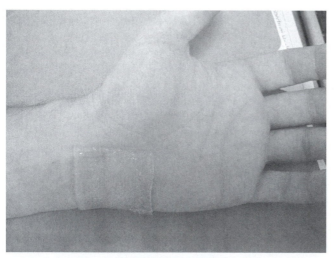

F I G U R E   2 7 - 1 1

Silicone or mineral oil based products such as Silipos or Cica-Care is fit to the scar and held in place with Tubigrip (elasticized stockinet) at night. It is important that the scar pad be in direct contact with the skin, without an interface of lotion. Lotion can break down the silicone or mineral oil product.

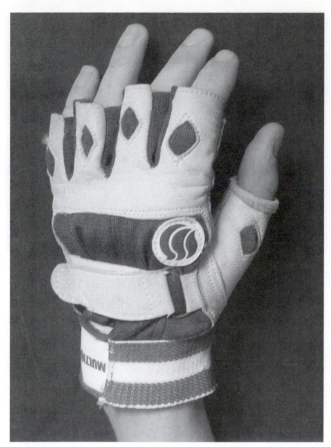

FIGURE 27-13

Patients that have persistent pain may benefit from padded bike gloves as they return to their sports. This glove protects the sensitive area while allowing a gradual return to such activities as golf or tennis.

TFCC can be a result of excessive load in wrist ulnar deviation and forearm rotation activities.

REHABILITATION CONCERNS

Surgical intervention can include arthroscopy, ulnar resection, ulnar shortening, hemiresection interposition arthroplasty, fusion with proximal pseudoarthrodesis, repair to the TFCC, and tethering of the distal ulna.[35–38] Each procedure will have an individualized and specific period of immobilization with specific casting and/or splinting (specified by the surgeon), followed by gentle and gradual return of ROM. The therapist should contact the surgeon to determine when gentle AROM can be initiated. It is important to avoid aggressive ROM that can stretch out ligaments that provide the necessary stability to the DRUJ. All ROM should be kept pain free, as stability was a major area of concern prior to surgery.

Patients with persistent pain at the distal ulna should be tested to determine if depression and support of the ulna during pronation and supination could relieve their symptoms (Fig. 27-1A).[27] Manually depressing the ulna can reduce pain by providing support to weakened ligaments. A simple wristband

that provides padding at the dorsal ulna and volar radius can be very helpful in decreasing pain and providing support to the TFCC (Fig. 27-1B).[27]

REHABILITATION PROGRESSION

The key to successful management of injuries to the DRUJ is gradual progression in a pain-free range. Motions that need to be addressed for AROM are flexion, extension, radial deviation, ulnar deviation, supination, and pronation (Exercises 27-2A and B, 27-3A and B, and 27-4A and B). Strengthening exercises are delayed until healing is complete, adequate ROM has been achieved, and pain is under control. Joint stability should not be sacrificed for an increase in ROM. Care should be taken not to return this patient back to work, sport, or other activities too quickly. The wristband (described in Figs. 27-1B and C) can be helpful in returning a patient to activities by decreasing any persistent pain with forearm rotation.

Carpal Tunnel Syndrome

PATHOMECHANICS

Carpal tunnel syndrome is compression of the median nerve at the level of the wrist. The carpal tunnel is made up of the carpal bones dorsally and transverse carpal ligament volarly. Located in the carpal tunnel are the FDS and FDP to all digits, FPL, median nerve, and median artery.[36] If the space within the carpal tunnel is decreased due to inflammation, cyst, tumor, scar tissue, fracture, edema, or other conditions, the median nerve can be compressed. In two studies, when wrist intratunnel pressures were measured, it was found that even a small change in wrist position could increase intratunnel pressures. Studies by Burke et al.[40] and Weiss et al.[41] found that the lowest intratunnel pressure is with the wrist in a near neutral position. This information should influence the night splinting design. Many prefabricated splints place the wrist in far too much wrist extension, possibly aggravating symptoms. Symptoms of classic carpal tunnel are numbness and tingling in the median nerve distribution, pain or waking at night, and clumsiness or weakness in the hand. Symptoms may increase with static positioning (e.g., driving or reading a newspaper),[39] vibration, activation of the lumbricals,[42] and changes in joint position.[41] Diagnosis is made by history, Phalen's test (Fig. 27-14), Tinel's sign, nerve conduction studies, direct pressure over the carpal tunnel (Fig. 27-15), and EMGs. It is important to note that negative EMG and nerve conduction studies are not always conclusive. One study by Grundberg has shown that 11.3 percent of the patients with negative tests had positive clinical and surgical findings.[48]

INJURY MECHANISM

Conditions and injuries that contribute to median nerve compression due to elevated carpal pressures include tenosynovitis, fracture, carpal dislocation, cysts, tumor, diabetes, alcoholism, pregnancy, menopause, thyroid disorders, obesity, vibration, external forces, tendon load, and changes in joint position.[42,49,50]

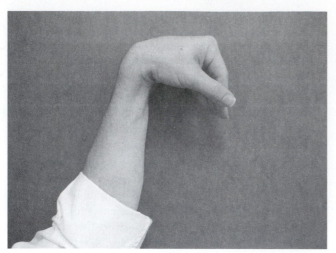

F I G U R E   2 7 - 1 4

Phalen's test for carpal tunnel syndrome is full wrist flexion, which increases the pressure in the carpal canal. The test is positive if there is numbness and tingling in the median nerve distribution within 60 seconds.

REHABILITATION CONCERNS

Conservative treatment is tried first and consists of night splinting with the wrist in a neutral position (Fig. 27-5A) and relative rest from aggravating sources (if known). Occasionally physicians will recommend full-time wrist splinting. Prefabricated splints may need to be adapted as they often place the wrist in extension as opposed to a near neutral position. Custom fabricated splints can be accurately molded to place the wrist in $2 \pm 9°$ of extension,[41] with 3° of ulnar deviation as outlined by Burke et al.[40] and Weiss et al.[41] In some cases, it is also necessary to limit movement of digits 2–5 because of the action of the lumbricals moving into the carpal tunnel, with digit flexion.[42] Including the MP joints in extension within the splint has been reported to be effective in decreasing symptoms (Fig. 27-16).[47]

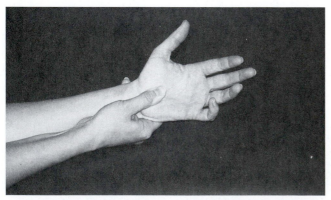

F I G U R E   2 7 - 1 5

Firm pressure over the carpal tunnel may elicit numbness or tingling in the median nerve distribution. It alone is not indicative of carpal tunnel syndrome, but provides additional information regarding symptoms.

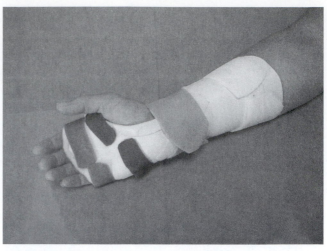

F I G U R E   2 7 - 1 6

In some cases of carpal tunnel syndrome, it is necessary to limit movement of digits 2–5 due to the action of the lumbricals moving into the carpal tunnel with digit flexion.[42] Including the MP joints in extension within the splint has been reported to be effective in decreasing symptoms.[47]

Nerve gliding exercises described by Butler[51] should only be used with extreme caution as not to aggravate symptoms. It is difficult for most patients to keep these nerve gliding techniques symptom free. Forced nerve gliding may result in increased inflammation, fibrosis, and edema[52] to the nerve that will aggravate as opposed to improve symptoms. Activity analysis to determine activities that increase symptoms should be done to see if changes in technique would help to decrease or avoid symptoms. Grip strengthening has been found to be contraindicated by several authors due to the action of the lumbricals increasing pressure in the carpal tunnel.[47]

If conservative treatment fails, a carpal tunnel release may be performed. There are two standard approaches to this release. The open technique exposes and releases the transverse carpal ligament and the endoscopic technique uses portals to view and then release the transverse carpal ligament. Surgeon preference determines the type of procedure selected, with advocates in both camps reporting advantages and disadvantages to each procedure.[46] The lack of visualization of the nerve has been a critique of the endoscopic technique, with the possibility of complications such as an incomplete release[43] or the possibility of injury to the median nerve and other structures.[44] Critics of the open technique report longer return to work time and greater scar tenderness.[45–47] Rehabilitation is dictated by the individual needs of each patient rather than by the surgical technique utilized. Rehabilitation following release consists of wound care, scar massage, and ROM exercises.[46,47] Tendon gliding exercises are done to improve ROM, prevent adhesions, and decrease edema. Start with full finger extension, and then hook fist to maximize FDP pull-through in relation to FDS, and then long fist to maximize FDS pull-through, and then composite fist. Full extension should be performed between each position and should be kept pain free (Exercises 27-1A–D). The FDS is also isolated by holding all but one digit in extension and flexing each digit at the PIP joint individually (Exercise 27-11). Wrist AROM should also be performed in a pain-free range (Exercises 27-2A and B).

REHABILITATION PROGRESSION

The postoperative progression after carpal tunnel release involves a gradual return to normal use. Grip strengthening and repetitive strengthening exercises should be avoided to prevent inflammation and aggravation of preoperative symptoms.[47] Returning to work will require an evaluation of the conditions that may have aggravated the symptoms. Padded work gloves can be helpful in decreasing vibration and protecting sensitive incision sites (Fig. 27-13). Workstation adaptations may be needed to avoid awkward and repetitive movements whenever possible.

Ganglion Cysts

PATHOLOGY

A ganglion cyst is the most common soft-tissue tumor in the hand.[53] It is a synovial cyst arising from the synovial lining of a tendon sheath or joint. The etiology is unclear. They are most common on the dorsal radial wrist, but may also be volar (Fig. 27-17). They originate deep in the joint and may be symptomatic before they appear at the surface.

Treatment by the physician is aspiration or surgical removal of the cyst. Recurrence rates are variable. In adults multiple aspirations are suggested, with success rates of 51–85 percent.[54,55] If multiple aspirations are not successful and cysts recur, the cyst may be surgically excised. The level of pain will often dictate the course of treatment.

INJURY MECHANISM

The cause of a ganglion cyst remains unclear. Pain and/or diminished function are the usual indications for treatment.

REHABILITATION CONCERNS

Cyst aspiration usually decreases pain and many patients gradually return to full ROM. Following a ganglion cyst excision, patients may need to be seen for gentle ROM, edema management, and scar control. ROM emphasis should be on wrist flexion and extension and finger flexion and extension (Exercises 27-1A–D and 27-2A and B). Patients who have undergone a removal of their dorsal ganglions can have difficulty with wrist flexion due to pain and dorsal wrist adhesions. A combination of heat and stretch with the wrist and digits placed in comfortable flexion is very effective in increasing wrist ROM without increasing pain (Fig. 27-18). The digits are gently wrapped into flexion with an ace bandage, and then the wrist is placed on the hot pack with appropriate toweling in comfortable wrist flexion. A second hot pack with appropriate toweling is placed on top with the weight of the hot pack encouraging wrist flexion. Scar management and desensitization may be done with lotion, scar massage, and gentle vibration. Less noxious stimuli should be applied first, with a gradual increase in texture being applied as tolerated by the patient. Scar control pads such as Otoform (Fig. 27-12), Silipos, or Cica-Care (Fig. 27-11) sheeting may

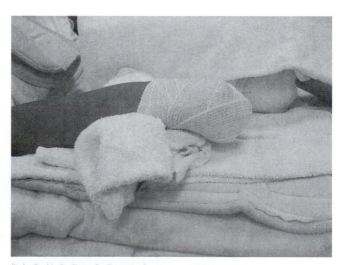

F I G U R E   2 7 - 1 8

A combination of heat and stretch with wrist flexion and digits placed in comfortable flexion (with an ace bandage) is very effective in increasing ROM without increasing pain. The digits are gently wrapped into flexion with an ace bandage, and then the wrist is placed on the hot pack with appropriate toweling in comfortable wrist flexion. A second hot pack with appropriate toweling is placed on top with the weight of the hot pack encouraging wrist flexion. This is usually applied for 20 minutes.

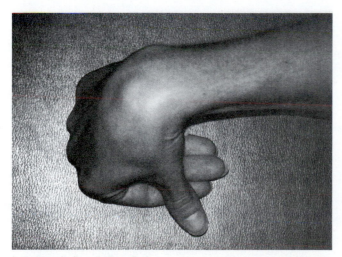

F I G U R E   2 7 - 1 7

This is a dorsal wrist ganglion which varies in size and shape.

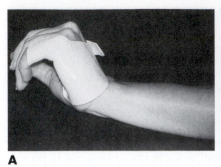
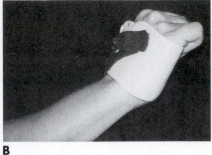
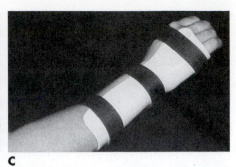

A **B** **C**

FIGURE 27-19

A boxer's fracture splint often protects the ring and small finger proximal phalanxes and metacarpals, including the MP joint. **A,** The splint may be modified for a neck fracture (immobilizing the involved MP joint), **B,** metacarpal shaft fracture (may need only the metacarpal in the splint leaving the wrist and MP joints free), or **C,** metacarpal base fracture (may need to include the wrist, usually leave the MP joints free).

also be used and held in place with Coban or Tubigrip type products.

REHABILITATION PROGRESSION

Pain from a ganglion cyst may limit ROM and some activities. Asymptomatic patients are less likely to seek treatment. If symptomatic, it may be aspirated by the physician with instruction in gentle AROM and gradual return to activity. If the ganglion recurs, it may be aspirated again.

If the ganglion is excised, sutures are removed at approximately 10 days. The above stated exercises assist with return of ROM. Gentle grip strengthening (Exercise 27-7) may be done after adequate ROM and pain reduction are achieved. Most patients with good ROM gradually return to their previous ADL. Scar management techniques may be needed until scar maturation is complete.

Boxer's Fracture

PATHOMECHANICS

A boxer's fracture is a fracture of the fifth metacarpal neck, the most commonly fractured metacarpal.[56] On impact with a solid object, the metacarpal will frequently shorten and angulate. Because of the large degree of mobility of the fifth metacarpal, less than perfect anatomic reduction is acceptable, and can result in adequate hand function.

INJURY MECHANISM

This injury occurs most frequently from contact against an object with a closed fist. It can also be the result of a fall. Many patients who sustain this fracture because of a hostile encounter are often ashamed to admit the true cause of the injury.

REHABILITATION CONCERNS

If the injury is open, the risk of infection is serious due to contact with the opponent's teeth and/or saliva. If the injury is closed, treatment consists of proper immobilization, edema control,

and ROM of noninvolved joints. PIP joint extension can be problematic especially of the fifth digit. In some cases, ORIF is required. Postoperatively, proper splinting, edema control, and AROM of uninvolved joints are important.[35,56]

Treatment is immobilization in a plaster gutter splint, or in a thermoplastic splint fabricated by a hand therapist (Figs. 27-19A–C). The latter is often preferred, as it allows for skin hygiene, wrist ROM, and IP joint ROM. The splint only immobilizes the ring and small finger MP joints and places the MP joints in comfortable flexion. In some cases, a removable second splint is utilized to gently place the PIP joints in extension at night. This can be very helpful in preventing PIP joint flexion contractures (Fig. 27-20). The splint should be remolded as edema decreases. Splinting is continued for approximately 4–6

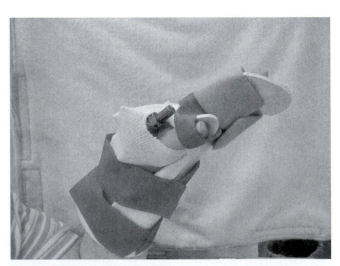

FIGURE 27-20

In some cases, a removable second splint is utilized to gently place the PIP joints in extension at night. This can be very helpful in preventing PIP joint flexion contractures in some cases of wrist or metacarpal fractures.

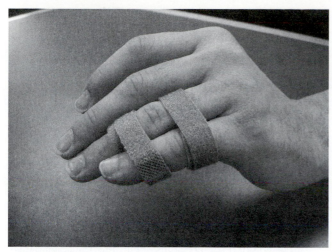

FIGURE 27-21
Buddy taping may be utilized when MP AROM is allowed following a boxers fracture to encourage or maintain proper digit alignment.

weeks. An open wound should be monitored for infection and the physician contacted immediately if evident. The physician often places patients on a course of antibiotics when an open wound is present.

REHABILITATION PROGRESSION

During time of immobilization, ROM to noninvolved joints is maintained by active exercises. The surgeon, based on the stability of the fracture or surgical fixation, should determine the initiation of MP AROM to the involved digit. At approximately 6 weeks, the splint is discontinued but may be used as needed for protection during heavier activities. Buddy taping (Fig. 27-21) may be done when MP AROM is allowed to encourage proper digit alignment. A patient may gradually resume normal activity without the splint when there is evidence of radiographic healing. Gentle grip strengthening exercises with putty (Exercise 27-7) can be initiated with a healed fracture usually at the 6–8 week point.

De Quervain's Tenosynovitis

PATHOMECHANICS

De Quervain's tenosynovitis is an inflammation in the first dorsal compartment affecting APL and EPB.[57,58] Finklestein's test,[59] which involves thumb flexion into the palm with passive wrist ulnar deviation, can assist with the diagnosis (Fig. 27-22). It may be helpful to compare the level of pain elicited to the noninjured side. This test alone cannot confirm the diagnosis, as it can be uncomfortable in the normal population. The results of the Finklestein's test must be considered in conjunction with other clinical findings.

INJURY MECHANISM

Repeated wrist movements may cause de Quervain's tenosynovitis. Less frequent causes include a direct blow to the radial

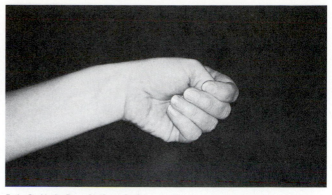

FIGURE 27-22
Finklestein's test will be positive for pain in de Quervain's tenosynovitis. Passive flexion of the thumb with wrist ulnar deviation is the provocative position.[58,59] Always compare to the noninvolved side, as this test can be uncomfortable normally.

styloid, acute strain as in lifting, or a ganglion in the first dorsal compartment.[51,57,58]

REHABILITATION CONCERNS

Initial treatment is rest from aggravating activities. Modalities for edema reduction and pain control such as ultrasound and ice are widely utilized by clinicians for this condition. Ice is used for its ability to manage inflammation and pain. Michlovitz[60,61] reports that ultrasound at lower intensities most likely produces its therapeutic effects by the phenomenon known as microstreaming. This is reported to cause changes in cell permeability and may help to promote healing. Michlovitz[60] discusses that low-dose pulsed ultrasound may be effective in acute and subacute rehabilitation of tendonitis, but stresses that further study is needed.[61] In addition, an analysis of activities should be done to determine aggravating activities and avoid or adapt as necessary.

Splinting for de Quervain's tenosynovitis includes the thumb MP and carpometacarpal (CMC) joints, and the wrist (Figs. 27-8). Some authors advocate including the IP joint of the thumb in the splint as well.[62,64] Splinting is usually full time except for hygiene for the first 4–6 weeks. Many patients need to be reminded not to "fight" their splint but to relax and let it support them. Resisting the splint can aggravate symptoms. Many patients have a combined condition that includes irritation of the superficial branch of the radial nerve. This nerve irritation can be very troubling for the patient. Hypersensitivity may be so severe that the patient may be unable to lightly touch the area. These patients will be unable to tolerate ice to the area. Clinical use of a transcutaneous electrical nerve stimulation (TENS) unit may be very helpful for pain control for these patients until the nerve symptoms subside. As the pain from the tendon is reduced after 4–6 weeks, the patient slowly decreases the splint wearing time. Activity is resumed gradually, while avoiding aggravating activities. If pain is persistent, splinting is continued. Patients who do not respond to conservative management may be candidates for a surgical release of the first dorsal compartment.

Various surgical techniques are utilized to release the first dorsal compartment. Some surgeons hope to prevent the complication of a tendon subluxation with an internal tendon sling to help stabilize the release. This surgery will require a thumb spica splint for 6 weeks postoperatively, with the initiation of gentle thumb and wrist AROM usually at the 4-week point.[63] AROM consists of gentle thumb opposition, thumb flexion and extension (Exercises 27-8A–C), and wrist flexion and extension (Exercises 27-2A and B). If the release to the first dorsal compartment does not include an internal sling, then gentle AROM as described above can begin after the sutures are removed. This is usually 10–14 days after surgery. Some physicians prefer a thumb spica splint for a few weeks after this type (no internal sling) of surgery. The patient gradually resumes normal activity around the 6th week.[64] It is important that the therapist consult with the physician as to the preferred postoperative protocol.

Complications from surgery include hypersensitivity, complex regional pain syndrome, incomplete release, tendon subluxation, and injury to the radial sensory nerve.[64] Radial sensory nerve injury will present itself as a very different type of pain than the patient had before surgery. The patient may complain of numbness, or pain that is burning, shooting, or electrical in nature. Care should be taken to avoid any pressure from splints or straps to the superficial branch of the radial nerve in the preoperative or postoperative splinting programs.

REHABILITATION PROGRESSION

Early strengthening exercises should be avoided or symptoms could be exacerbated. Increased symptoms are likely to limit return to normal activity. Patients should have pain-free ROM in the affected part as the primary goal. Aggravating activities should be addressed and adapted as appropriate. Some patients, who have difficulty returning to activities because of nerve pain, appreciate the support and protection of a soft neoprene splint (Fig. 27-23). This soft splint allows good ROM but provides gentle support and padding to an area that can be hypersensitive. This splint allows more activity, as the patient is not fearful of bumping or hitting the hand accidentally during daily living activities.[29]

Ulnar Collateral Ligament Sprain (Gamekeeper's Thumb or Skier's Thumb)

PATHOMECHANICS

The ulnar collateral ligament (UCL) injury to the MP joint of the thumb is one of the most common ligament injuries.[65–71] The injury can be classified as grade I or II, in which the majority of the ligament remains intact. Grade III is a complete disruption of the UCL and surgical repair is recommended. It is most often the distal attachment of the ligament where the rupture occurs.[68,69]

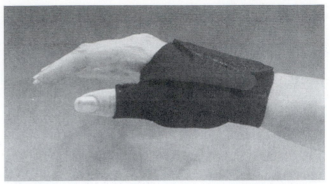

F I G U R E   2 7 - 2 3

Some patients, who have difficulty returning to activities because of nerve pain, appreciate the support and protection of a soft neoprene splint. This soft splint allows good ROM but provides gentle support and padding to an area that can be hypersensitive. This splint will then allow more activity as the patient is not fearful of bumping or hitting the hand accidentally during daily living activities.[29] (Reprinted, with permission, from Biese J. Soft splints: Indications and techniques. In: Mackin EJ, Callahan AD, Skirven TM, Schneider LH, Osterman AL, eds. *Rehabilitation of the Hand and Upper Extremity*, 5th ed. St. Louis, MO, Mosby, 2002, pp. 1846–1857. Photo and splint courtesy of North Coast Medical, Inc., Morgan Hill, CA.)

The patient will complain of pain or tenderness on the ulnar side of the MP joint. If the ligament is completely torn, one must also be concerned about a Stener lesion. This is where the torn UCL protrudes beneath the adductor aponeurosis. This places the aponeurosis between the ligament and its insertion. If this occurs, reattachment will not occur and surgery is needed.[70]

This injury is referred to as skier's thumb as well as gamekeeper's injury. Gamekeeper's injury occurs most frequently from chronic repeated stress on the UCL[71] while skier's thumb occurs most commonly as an acute injury.[68]

INJURY MECHANISM

UCL injuries occur when a torsional load is applied to the thumb.[6] It frequently occurs in pole sports (e.g., skiing) where the thumb is abducted to hold the pole (or stick in other sports) and the patient falls and tries to catch himself/herself on an outstretched hand, landing on an abducted thumb (Fig. 27-24).[66–71] Defensive backs in football may sustain this injury while abducting the thumb before making a tackle.[69]

REHABILITATION CONCERNS

Early diagnosis and treatment are important. An unstable thumb or Stener lesion,[70,71] if not treated, will become chronically and painfully unstable with weak pinch and arthritis as a possible result.[67]

Treatment for incomplete (grade I or II) tears is immobilization in a thumb spica cast or splint (Fig. 27-25) for 4–6

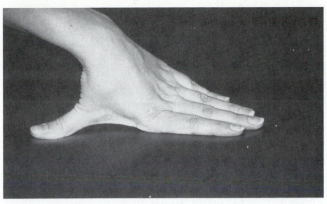

FIGURE 27-24

The UCL provides support for the ulnar MP joint. A fall on an abducted thumb may cause injury or rupture.

weeks, depending on the preferences of the physician. Care should be taken to avoid MP radial deviation during the immobilization phase to prevent stretching out the healing UCL.

Treatment for complete injury (grade III, unstable MP joint) is often a surgical repair. Late reconstruction is not as successful as early surgery, so early operative treatment is usually recommended.[71] Postoperatively, a thumb spica cast is usually worn for 4 weeks, with an additional 2–4 weeks of splinting, depending on the preferences of the physician. This splint is worn full time except for gentle exercise sessions of active thumb flexion and extension.

The initial concerns during the initial 5–6 weeks post injury include protective immobilization, controlling edema, and maintaining motion in all noninvolved joints. Once the physician allows AROM, it is important to avoid radial stress on the thumb. Radial deviation can stretch out the newly healed UCL.

REHABILITATION PROGRESSION

Some patients, as they return to sports or specific activities, prefer to continue to wear a thin hand-based thumb spica splint to (Fig. 27-25) to prevent reinjury during higher intensity activities. This splint should be fabricated by a hand therapist, to provide the necessary protection with light (1/16 in.) splinting materials. Many skiers find that the splint can easily fit under their ski glove and gradually wean from the splint over time. Care should be taken to avoid any stress to the healed UCL during the entire rehabilitation program.

Flexor Digitorum Profundus Avulsion (Jersey Finger)

PATHOMECHANICS

Jersey finger is a rupture of the FDP tendon from its insertion on the distal phalanx. It most frequently occurs at the ring finger. It may be avulsed with or without a bone fragment. If avulsed with bone, depending on size of fragment, the tendon will usually not retract back into the palm, as it is "caught" on the pulley system of the finger. If no bone or only very small fleck of bone is avulsed, the tendon can retract back into the palm. This is the most common.[73] Each time the patient tries to flex the finger, the muscle contracts but the insertion is not attached. This brings the insertion closer to its origin.

To evaluate and isolate FDP function and integrity prior to surgery, hold the MP and PIP joints of affected finger in full extension, and then have the patient attempt to flex the DIP joint. If it flexes, it is intact. If not, it is ruptured (Exercise 27-13A).

INJURY MECHANISM

Forceful hyperextension of the fingers while tightly gripping into flexion is the injury mechanism (Fig. 27-26).[74]

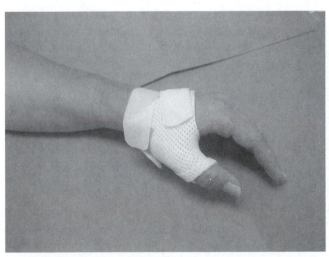

FIGURE 27-25

A hand-based thumb spica splint is utilized for protection of the UCL. This condition is often referred to as gamekeeper's thumb or skier's thumb.

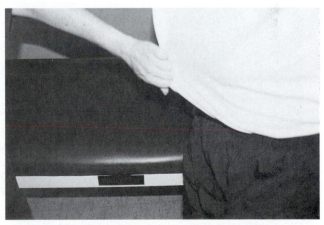

FIGURE 27-26

A jersey finger (FDP avulsion) injury is named for the injury mechanism—forced hyperextension with finger flexion—as in trying to grab a shirt during a tackle in the sport of football. The position of the DIP joint after injury will be extension or hyperextension.

REHABILITATION CONCERNS

This can be a very complex injury to treat following surgical repair. The surgery should be performed by an experienced hand surgeon,[74] with subsequent rehabilitation performed by an experienced hand therapist. Close communication between the hand surgeon and the hand therapist is necessary. All protocols are guidelines and as such may need to be altered if complications such as infection, poor tendon glide, or excellent tendon glide occur. With this injury, unlike most others, the better a person is doing (full active tendon glide), the more he/she is held back and protected. Good tendon glide is indicative of less scarring, which means there is less healing at the repaired tendon, less tensile strength, and increased chance of rupture. If a tendon is reruptured, it must be repaired with less chance of a successful outcome. Proper patient education is necessary. Instruction in what to expect, reasons for specific exercises, and consequences must be conveyed.

REHABILITATION PROGRESSION

The following are guidelines. They are not all-inclusive, nor are they an indication that anyone can treat this injury. For more specific information on this detailed protocol, readers are encouraged to read the article by Evans on zone I flexor tendon rehabilitation.[73,74]

Between 2 and 5 days postoperatively, the bulky dressing should be removed and a dorsal blocking splint fabricated to hold the wrist in 30°–40° of flexion, MP joints in 30° of flexion, and IP joints with full extension (Figs. 27-27A and B). The affected DIP joint is splinted at 45° of flexion with a second dorsal splint that extends from the PIP joint to the fingertip,

and secured with Coban or tape at the middle phalanx only. Exercises for the first three weeks are (1) passive DIP flexion in the splint from 45° to 75° of flexion; (2) full composite passive flexion, then extend MP joints passively to a modified hook position; (3) passive flexion of MP joints with active extension of PIP joints to 0°; and (4) strap or hold noninvolved fingers to the top of the splint and position the involved digit's PIP joint in flexion passively, then actively hold the joint in flexion. This last exercise is referred to as a place and hold for FDS (which is not injured in zone 1). All exercises in the home program should be done with the splint on, at a frequency of 10 repetitions every waking hour. The patients should not use their injured hand for any activity, extend the wrist or fingers without the splint, or actively flex the fingers. All of the preceding could cause tendon rupture. In addition, during the first weeks, Coban and Tubigrip can be used for edema control and scar control. Scar massage may be performed in the splint. The dressing and cleaning of the dorsal blocking splint may be completed at home if the patient is able to understand proper positioning techniques (i.e., avoiding active wrist and MP extension outside of the splint). The DIP splint should remain in place for the first 3 weeks.

During visits to the therapist, the home program is reviewed and the therapist completes wrist tenodesis (digit passive flexion with wrist extension, and wrist flexion with digit relaxed in natural extension) (Exercises 27-12A and B). Place and hold to the distal phalanx is allowed only with the supervision of the therapist and only to approximately 15–20 g of force.[74]

Between 3 and 4 weeks post repair, the digital splint is discontinued but the protective dorsal blocking splint is continued. Between 4 and 6 weeks, tendon gliding exercises are initiated (Exercises 27-1A–D). DIP blocking should initially

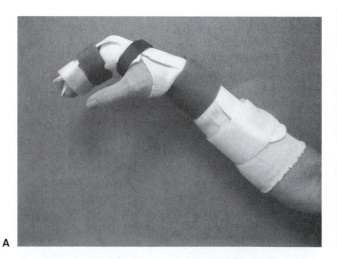
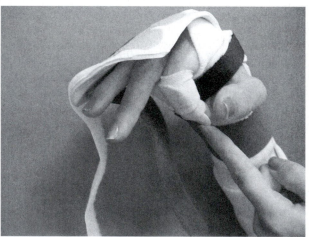

FIGURE 27-27

A, Flexor tendon splint is usually applied between 2 and 5 days postoperatively. The bulky dressing should be removed with a dorsal blocking splint fabricated to hold the wrist in 30°–40° of flexion, MP joints in 30° of flexion, and IP joints with full extension.[73,74] **B,** The affected DIP joint is splinted at 45° of flexion with a second dorsal splint that extends from the PIP joint to the fingertip, and is secured with Coban or tape at the middle phalanx only. This protocol was developed by Evans[73,74] and should be referred to for further information.

be done very gently to avoid pressure at the repair site (Exercise 27-13A).[74] At this time, the splint is remolded to place the wrist in neutral with the MP joints in less flexion.[74]

At 6–7 weeks the splint is discontinued, light ADL may be done with the injured hand, and tendon gliding exercises including DIP blocking are continued. Patients are excited to be out of their splints and may overdo during this phase. It is a prime time for tendon ruptures. By 12 weeks, patients should be back with full tendon gliding and gradual return to activities. Activities and sports in which a sudden force may pull on flexed fingers such as rock climbing, windsurfing, water skiing, or dog walking, should not be done until 14–16 weeks postoperatively.

Mallet Finger

PATHOMECHANICS

A mallet finger is the avulsion of the terminal extensor tendon, which is responsible for extension of the DIP joint.[11] It may occur with or without fracture of bone. If there is a large fracture fragment where the fracture fragment is displaced greater than 2 mm, or the DIP joint has volar subluxation on X-ray, the injury will require ORIF.

There is no alternate mechanism for extending the DIP joint. Presenting complaint is inability to extend the DIP joint (Fig. 27-28).

Treatment is splinting the DIP joint in slight hyperextension (Figs. 27-29A and B) for 6–8 weeks with no flexion of the DIP joint.[75,76] If the DIP joint is flexed even once during the splinting period, the 6 weeks starts again at that time.

INJURY MECHANISM

The injury mechanism is forced flexion of the DIP joint while it is held in full extension.[76] It frequently happens when a ball or some other object strikes the fully extended digit. It also may occur when tucking in bedding.

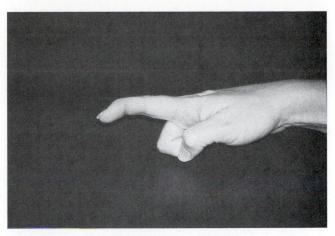

FIGURE 27-28
A mallet finger deformity with DIP flexion.

REHABILITATION CONCERNS

Rehabilitation of the mallet finger requires excellent splinting/casting skills and good patient compliance. There is a tendency to minimize this condition and many patients are noncompliant. A splint/cast should be custom made, be comfortable to the patient, not cause skin breakdown, and if removable, be able to be applied by the patient with the DIP held in hyperextension during the donning procedure. The splint must hold the DIP joint in slight hyperextension. Skin integrity needs to be monitored with the splint being modified or redesigned if irritation occurs. Because of this challenge, we have begun to utilize a waterproof QuickCast material that allows full time wear even while bathing. The QuickCast material must be heated up with a hair dryer (using a heat gun is too hot for this material) and quickly applied to the digit held in slight DIP hyperextension (Figs. 27-30A–E). Patients return weekly for cast changes. If the cast becomes loose between cast

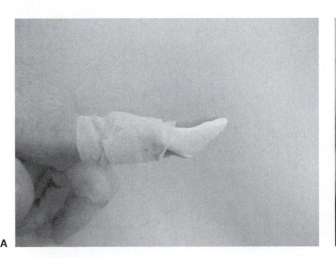
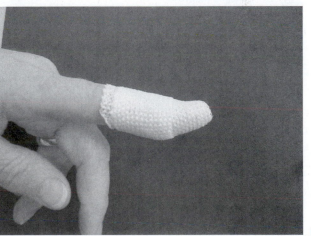

A   B

FIGURE 27-29

A, A mallet finger splint must hold the DIP in slight hyperextension. Skin integrity needs to be monitored with the splint being modified or redesigned if irritation occurs. **B,** A waterproof QuickCast material allows full-time wear even while bathing.

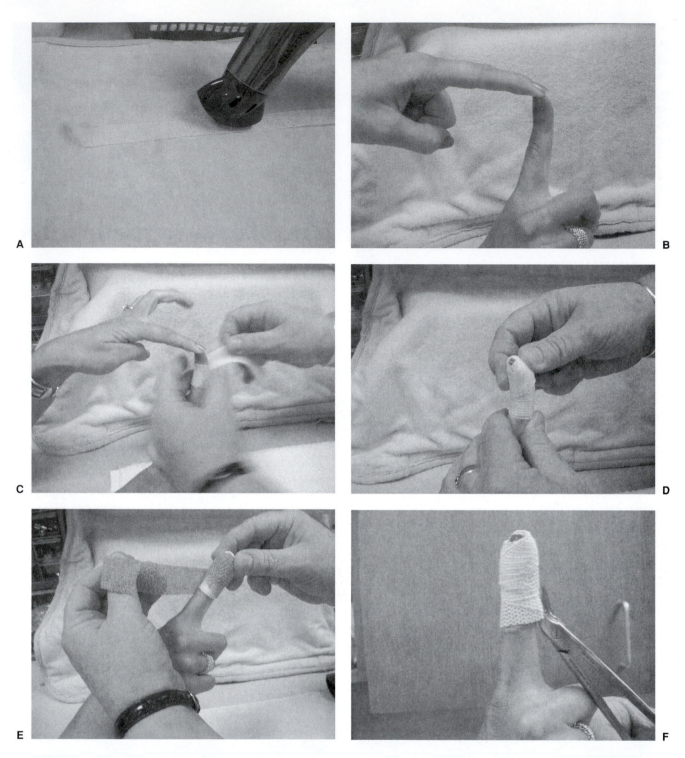

FIGURE 27-30

A, The QuickCast material must be heated up with a hair dryer (using a heat gun is too hot for this material). **B,** The digit held in slight DIP hyperextension at all times. **C** and **D,** The cast is quickly applied and the position of slight hyperextension maintained as the splint cools. Patients return weekly for cast changes. **E,** If the cast becomes loose between cast changes, it can be held snug by an over wrap of Coban. ROM of noninvolved fingers and joints should be maintained. PIP flexion with the DIP cast will not put tension on the injury and should be encouraged. **F,** The cast is removed with a special short scissors.

changes, it can be held snug by an overwrap of Coban. ROM of noninvolved fingers and joints should be maintained. PIP flexion with the DIP cast will not put tension on the injury and should be encouraged.

REHABILITATION PROGRESSION

Once the tendon is healed, often at approximately 6–8 weeks, splint weaning is initiated. If an extensor lag is present, splinting should be continued, or the physician evaluates as to the possibility of surgery. Splint weaning is initiated with a schedule of 2 hours on, 2 hours off, and continued night splinting. If no extension lag develops, then the time out of the splint is gradually increased. Night splinting is often continued for 3–4 weeks after full-time splinting is discontinued. Gentle DIP joint AROM consists of initiating light use of the hand. No attempts to passively flex the DIP joint or to stretch out the tendon with DIP joint blocking should be attempted. Full ROM is usually gained through regular functional hand use. Athletes should wear a DIP joint splint for no less than 8 weeks. Athletes may need cast changes with each game or practice due to perspiration. The therapist can instruct the team's athletic trainer in the QuickCast technique to reduce the number of visits to the clinic.

Boutonnière Deformity

PATHOMECHANICS

The posture of a finger with a boutonnière deformity is PIP joint flexion and DIP joint hyperextension (Fig. 27-31). It is caused by interruption of the central slip. Normally the central

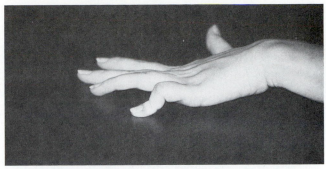

FIGURE   2 7 · 3 1

A boutonnière deformity may start as a PIP contracture. It can in time result in hyperextension of the DIP joint.

slip will initiate extension of flexed PIP joints. When the central slip is disrupted, the extensor muscle displaces proximally and shifts the lateral bands shift volarly. The FDS is then unopposed without an intact central slip and will flex the PIP joint. The lateral bands displace volarly and may become fixed as the deformity progresses. This then makes passive correction very difficult. The DIP joint hyperextends because all the force to extend the PIP is transmitted to the DIP joint.[11]

Once a fixed deformity is present, it is much more difficult to treat. Many patients do not seek immediate medical attention, mistakenly feeling that the finger was jammed and would be fine in several days or weeks.

Treatment for the acute injury is uninterrupted splinting of the PIP joint in full extension for 6–8 weeks (Figs. 27-32A and B). The DIP joint is left free or blocked in slight flexion

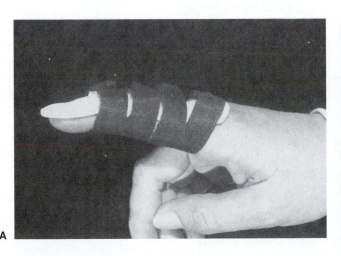

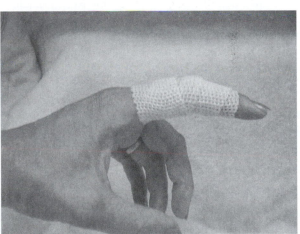

FIGURE   2 7 · 3 2

A, Treatment for the acute boutonnière injury is uninterrupted splinting of the PIP joint in full extension for 6–8 weeks. The DIP joint is left free or blocked in slight flexion without strapping to encourage DIP flexion. This will synergistically relax the extrinsic and intrinsic extensor tendon muscles and exercises the oblique retinacular ligament.[9]

B, Chronic injures usually require serial casting to gradually obtain full PIP extension.

without strapping to encourage DIP flexion. This will synergistically relax the extrinsic and intrinsic extensor tendon muscles and exercises the oblique retinacular ligament.[9] Chronic injures usually require serial casting to gradually obtain full PIPextension.

INJURY MECHANISM

Injury occurs when the extended finger is forcibly flexed, such as when being hit by a ball or because of a fall when striking the finger on another object.[67,77]

REHABILITATION CONCERNS

Of primary concern is early and proper diagnosis and treatment. Radiographs can help to rule out a fracture or a PIP joint dislocation. It is also very important to splint the PIP in full extension. As edema decreases, frequent splint modifications are needed to assure full PIP joint extension. If diagnosis is made late and there is a fixed PIP flexion contracture, serial casting may be the best conservative measure to restore extension. Serial casting lends itself nicely to QuickCast as it is waterproof and more easily accepted by the patient. Following return of full extension, the finger is then placed in a removable splint for the splint-weaning program. Weaning from the splint is gradual, with return to the splint if an extension lag develops at the PIP joint.

REHABILITATION PROGRESSION

Weaning from the splint after 6–8 weeks may be initiated with a 2 hours on and 2 hours off schedule and night splinting continuing for several weeks. Gentle PIP joint AROM begins gradually, observing for the development of PIP joint extension lags. If an extension lag develops, the patient returns to the splint. If the extension lag is persistent, the patient should be referred to the surgeon for evaluation. Splint-weaning programs that progress without an extension lag can gradually return to using the hand for light activities. Night splinting may continue for 12 weeks and beyond.

PROTOCOLS

De Quervain's Tendonitis Conservative Management Protocol

ACUTE PHASE

The initial treatment is rest from aggravating activities. This includes full-time splinting for 4–6 weeks (Figs. 27-8 and 27-33) with splint removal for bathing and skin care. The forearm-based splint includes the wrist, and thumb carpal-metacarpal (CMC) and MP joints. Some authors include the thumb IP joint in the splint. The patient using a 10 cm analog scale usually reports the presplinting pain level. Modalities to decrease inflammation may be utilized by the clinician during this phase as well. Goals for the acute phase include the following:

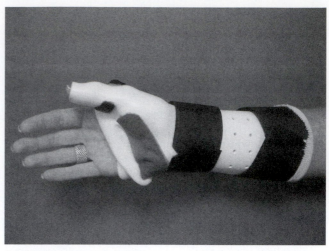

F I G U R E   2 7 - 3 3

Splinting for de Quervain's tenosynovitis includes the thumb MP joints, CMC joints, and the wrist. Some authors advocate including the IP joint of the thumb in the splint as well.[55,64] Splinting is usually full time except for hygiene for the first 4–6 weeks. Many patients need to be reminded not to "fight" their splint but to relax and let it support them. Resisting the splint can aggravate symptoms.

1. The patient's pain level is reduced while wearing the splint.
2. The patient is independent with the home splinting program, and the splint fits comfortably.
3. The patient does not resist the support of the splint during ADL.

INTERMEDIATE PHASE

After 4–6 weeks of splint wear, if the patient reports a decrease in pain (with a pain analog scale), weaning from the splint is initiated. This begins with a schedule of 2 hours on and 2 hours off, during the day, with continued night splinting. Painful activities are avoided, and night splinting continues. The time out of the splint gradually increases, as dictated by reduced pain levels. If the symptoms return during the splint-weaning program, the physician should be contacted to determine if full-time splinting should be resumed, or if surgery is an option. The goal of the intermediate phase is

• the patient will wean from the splint during the day without an increase in pain.

ADVANCED PHASE

The patient gradually weans from the night splint and returns to ADL. Aggravating activities (including work) are evaluated and avoided or adapted as necessary to prevent recurrence of the condition. The goal of the advanced phase is

• the patient returns to ADL and weans from the night splint without an increase in pain.

RETURN TO FUNCTION

Strengthening exercises should be avoided to prevent reirritation to the involved tendons. Once the patient returns to pain-free ADL, formal strengthening programs are usually not needed. Work as well as all activities should be carefully analyzed and adapted as possible to avoid recurrence of painful symptoms. The goal of the return to function phase is

- return to ADL and work activities without a recurrence of symptoms.

Mallet Finger Conservative Management Protocol

ACUTE PHASE

Rehabilitation for a mallet finger requires precise splinting or casting. The splint or QuickCast must be applied in slight DIP hyperextension. The splint or QuickCast will be worn full time for the next 6–8 weeks. The hyperextension position must be maintained at each weekly splint/cast change. When patients are wearing a splint, the patient should do skin care at least once a day. If the patient is wearing a QuickCast, it will need to be changed by the therapist at least once a week. Many patients are unable to obtain the position of slight DIP hyperextension at the initial therapy visit. This will require serial splinting or casting until the position is obtained (Figs. 27-30A–F). The goals of the acute phase are as follows:

1. Obtain a position of passive DIP slight hyperextension.
2. Independence in the home splinting/casting program.
3. The patient will understand the anatomical importance of maintaining the DIP joint in the hyperextension position continuously throughout the 6–8 week program.

INTERMEDIATE PHASE

The cast/splinting program continues for 6–8 weeks until full active DIP extension is achieved. At the 6 week point, the DIP active extension position is carefully tested by having the digit supported in hyperextension by the examiner (Fig. 27-30B), and then very briefly removing this support to observe for full active DIP extension. If full DIP active extension is achieved, the patient moves on to the advanced phase (if allowed by the treating physician). If the DIP flexes slightly, support is immediately reapplied by the examiner and the splint/cast reapplied. The physician should be contacted as to the need to continue

the splinting program or the possibility of surgery. The goal of the intermediate phase is

- the patient achieves full active DIP extension.

ADVANCED PHASE

After full active DIP extension has been achieved by means of the continuous DIP splint/cast program, weaning from the splint/cast is initiated. Weaning proceeds by gradually decreasing the amount of time in the splint/cast and observing for DIP extension lags. The patient will usually begin by removing the splint/cast for 2 hours, three times a day, but continues to wear the splint/cast at night. After 3–4 days, if full DIP extension is maintained, the wearing schedule or time out of the splint/cast is increased to 4 hours, three times a day, and continues at night. This weaning procedure continues until the daytime splint/cast is gradually discontinued, but night splinting remains.

If at any point during the weaning program, the DIP demonstrates an extension lag, the splint/cast is reapplied and the physician is contacted. The patient may be a candidate for surgery if the splint/cast program has been unsuccessful. Some physicians and/or patients may prefer another trial month of the full-time splint/cast program as opposed to surgery. The goal of the advanced phase is

- the patient will successfully wean from the cast/splint while maintaining full DIP active extension of the involved digit.

RETURN TO FUNCTION

The advanced phase ends with successful weaning from the daytime DIP splint/cast program. During the return to function phase the patient gradually weans from the night splint/cast. One option is to wear the night splint/cast every other night and gradually increase the number of nights out of the splint. This continues until night splinting is eliminated and full active DIP extension is maintained. DIP blocking exercises are avoided to avoid stress to the newly healed tendon. The patient gradually returns to using the digit for progressively more involved ADL. Once again (as stated previously), any return of the DIP extension lag is reported to the surgeon.

Anne Marie Schneider wishes to thank Dr. Wallace Andrew of Raleigh Orthopaedic Clinic for his support, knowledge, and willingness to answer her countless questions.

Jeanine Biese wishes to thank the staff at Rehabilitation Professionals in Grand Rapids, Michigan, the Faculty at Grand Valley State University, and Dr. Donald Condit for all of their help and encouragement with this project.

EXERCISES

REHABILITATION TECHNIQUES

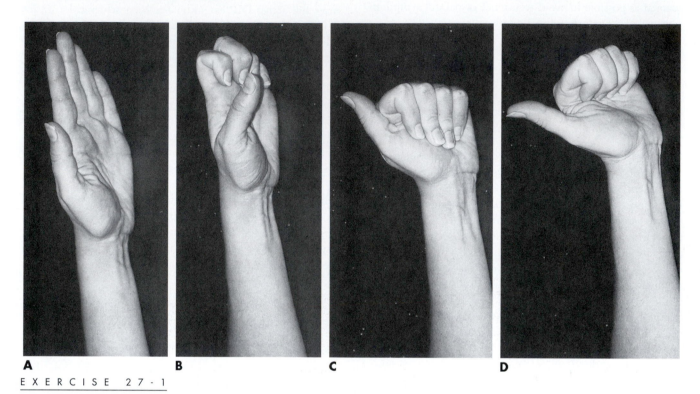

A   **B**   **C**   **D**

E X E R C I S E   2 7 - 1

Tendon gliding exercises allow for maximum gliding of the FDS and FDP. **A,** Start with full composite finger extension. **B,** Move to hook fisting, which gives maximum differential tendon gliding between FDS and FDP. **C,** Return to extension, move to long fisting with MP and PIP flexion and DIP extension for maximum FDS tendon glide. **D,** Return to extension, and then to composite flexion with full fisting, which gives the maximum glide of the FDP tendon.

E X E R C I S E   2 7 - 2

A, Wrist extension encourages exercise of the common wrist extensor tendons (ECRL, ECRB, and ECU). MP flexion should be maintained to eliminate EDC contribution and to isolate the wrist musculature. Active wrist extension is first done without a weight. **B,** Later in the rehabilitation program (depending on the protocol) weights may be added.

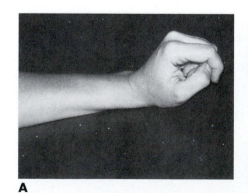

A

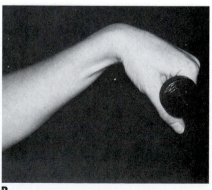

B

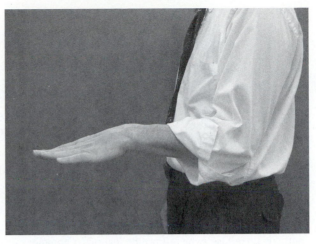

A

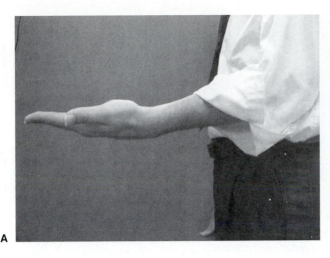

B

EXERCISE 27-3

A, Active supination exercises the supinator and the biceps. It should be done with elbow at 90° of flexion with the humerus by the side. This eliminates shoulder rotation. **B,** Active pronation exercises should also be done in the same position.

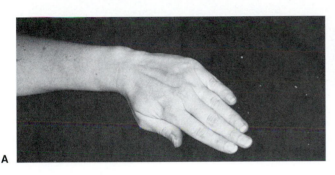

A

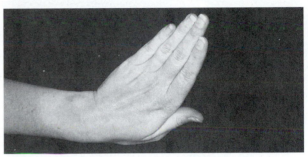

B

EXERCISE 27-4

A, Wrist radial deviation to exercise the FCR and ECRL. **B,** Wrist ulnar deviation to exercise the ECU and FCU.

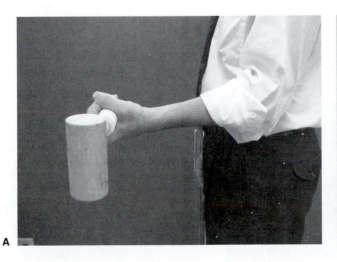

A

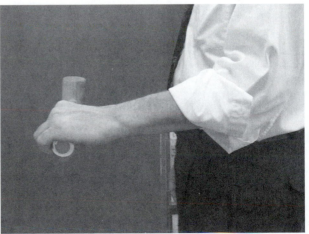

B

EXERCISE 27-5

A, Passive supination can be done with a hammer. The lever action of the hammer assists with the passive motion. **B,** Passive pronation is also done with the hammer.

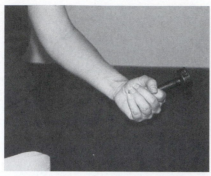
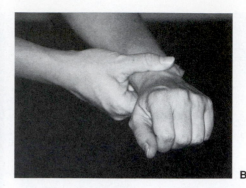

E X E R C I S E   2 7 - 6

A, Supination and pronation can be progressed by using a hammer or weights for strengthening. The hammer provides an additional lever due to being heavier on one end. This exercise, when using the lever of a hammer can also assist with passive motion. **B,** Passive stretching for pronation and supination should be done by applying pressure proximal to the wrist, applying pressure over the radius results in torquing the wrist.

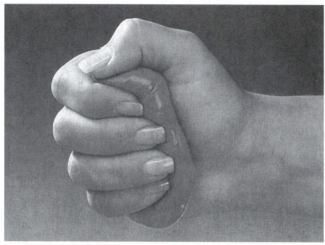

E X E R C I S E   2 7 - 7

This is a putty exercise for grip strengthening. Putty gives resistance throughout the entire ROM. Putty can be used for a variety of exercises for the intrinsic and extrinsic musculature.

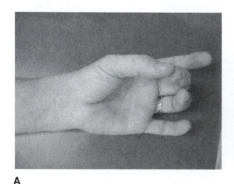
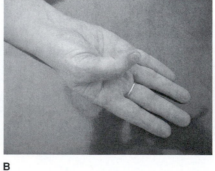
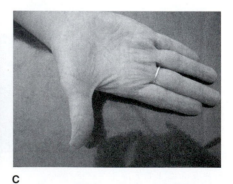

E X E R C I S E   2 7 - 8

Some of the more common AROM exercises to the thumb include **A,** Opposition. **B,** Flexion. **C,** Extension.

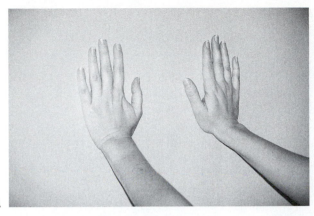
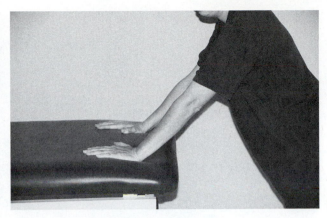

A   B

EXERCISE 27-9

A, Wall push-ups encourage wrist motion and general upper body strengthening. They also encourage weight bearing and closed-chain activities. **B,** Push-ups can be progressed from the wall to a table or countertop. This encourages gradual progression of increased weight bearing to the extremity.

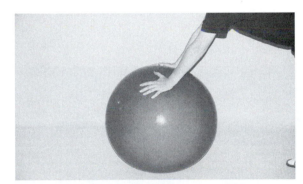

EXERCISE 27-10

Push-ups on a ball encourage upper extremity control.

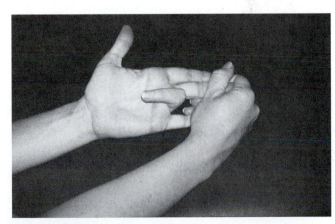

EXERCISE 27-11

To isolate active movement of the FDS, the noninvolved fingers are held in full extension, allowing only the involved finger to flex.

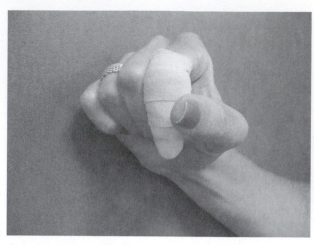
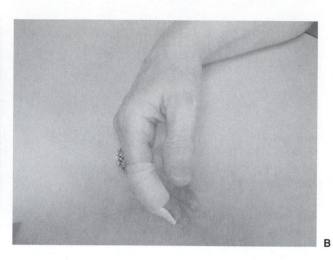

A   **B**

E X E R C I S E   2 7 - 1 2

With a Jersey finger repair (flexor tendon) during therapy the therapist reviews the home program, and helps the patient to complete wrist tenodesis. **A,** digit passive flexion with wrist extension. **B,** wrist flexion with digit in relaxed natural extension) with the distal splint in place. Place and hold to the distal phalanx is allowed only with the supervision of the therapist and only to 15–20 g of force.[74]

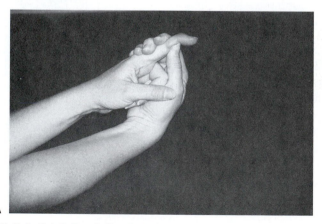
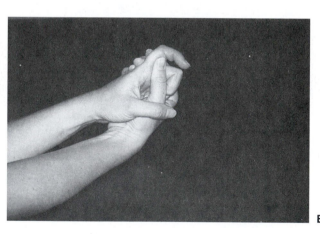

A   **B**

E X E R C I S E   2 7 - 1 3

A, Blocked DIP exercises encourage FDP pull-through. Stabilizing the middle phalanx allows the flexion force to concentrate at the DIP joint. **B,** Blocked PIP exercises encourage FDS pull-through. Stabilizing the proximal phalanx then allows the flexion force to act at the PIP joint.

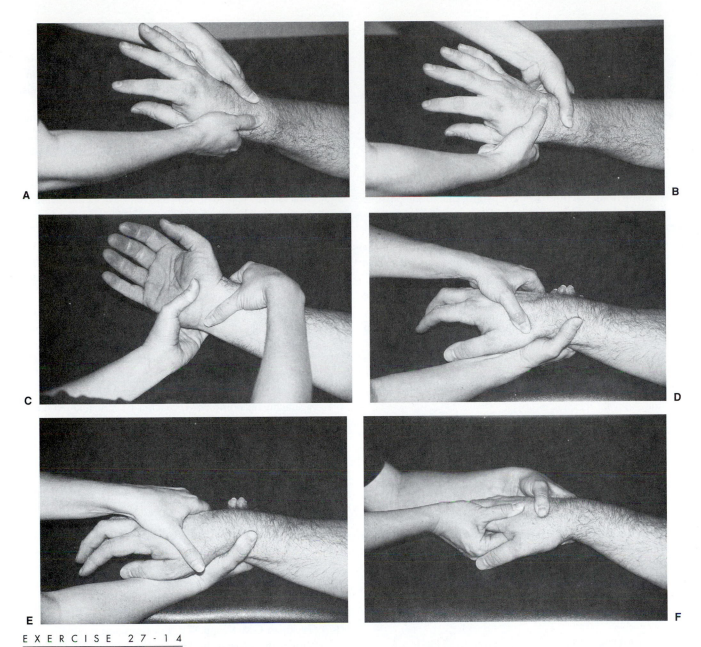

EXERCISE 27-14

A, Distal anterior/posterior radial glides. Distal anterior/posterior radial glides are done with one hand stabilizing the ulna and the other gliding the radius. These glides help to increase pronation. **B,** Radiocarpal joint anterior glides. Radiocarpal joint anterior glides help to increase wrist extension. **C,** Radiocarpal joint posterior glides. Radiocarpal joint posterior glides help to increase wrist flexion. **D,** Carpometacarpal joint anterior/posterior glides can help to increase mobility of the hand. **E,** Radiocarpal joint ulnar glides. Radiocarpal joint ulnar glides help to increase radial deviation. **F,** Radiocarpal joint radial glides. Radiocarpal joint radial glides help to increase ulnar deviation.

SUMMARY

- Distraction of the wrist while performing PROM after a healed wrist fracture may help to increase motion and decrease pain.
- Scaphoid fractures may not be obvious on an initial radiograph. Some scaphoid fractures are misdiagnosed as wrist sprains. Proper immobilization is important in the long-term outcome.
- Lunate dislocations can result in median nerve compressions.
- Hamate hook fractures are very painful due to the possible irritation to the ulnar nerve.
- Carpal tunnel syndrome is usually treated by rest and night splints that place the wrist in a neutral wrist position.
- Postoperatively, patients with dorsal ganglion cysts can have difficulty with wrist flexion due to pain and scarring.
- Boxer's fractures with an open wound have a high incidence of infection.
- De Quervain's tenosynovitis should be immobilized for 4–6 weeks.
- The goal in the treatment of UCL injuries (gamekeeper's thumb and skier's thumb) is stability of the MP joint. Care should be taken to avoid any thumb MP radial deviation.
- Conservative management of a mallet finger requires a cooperative compliant patient. DIP flexion is not allowed at any time during the 6–8 week splinting or casting program.
- Flexor tendon injuries are very labor-intensive and significant injuries. Be sure an experienced hand surgeon and hand therapist are involved in the care, and be sure that the patient is aware of what to expect.
- Early treatment of the boutonnière deformity is essential, as is a proper splint position. The PIP joint should be fully extended with the DIP joint free or in slight flexion. Serial casting can be very effective in increasing extension in chronic boutonnière deformities.

REFERENCES

1. Storock GS, Lomardi DA, Hauser RB, Eisen EA, Herrick RF, Mittleman MA. Acute traumatic occupational hand injuries: Type location and severity. *J Occup Env Med* 44(4):345–351, April 2002.
2. Mackin EJ, Callahan AD, Skirven TM, Schneider LH, Osterman AL, eds. *Rehabilitation of the Hand and Upper Extremity*, 5th ed. St. Louis, MO, Mosby, 2002.
3. Smith KL, Price JL. Care of the hand wound. In: Mackin EJ, Callahan AD, Skirven TM, Schneider LH, Osterman AL, eds. *Rehabilitation of the Hand and Upper Extremity*, 5th ed. St. Louis, MO, Mosby, 2002.
4. Pettengil KM, Van Strien G. Postoperative management of flexor tendon injuries. In: Mackin EJ, Callahan AD, Skirven TM, Schneider LH, Osterman AL, eds. *Rehabilitation of the Hand and Upper Extremity*, 5th ed. St. Louis, MO, Mosby, 2002.
5. Zemel NP. Fractures and ligament injuries of the wrist. In: Jobe FW, Pink MM, Glousman RE, eds. *Operative Techniques in Upper Extremity Sports Injuries*. St. Louis, MO, Mosby, 1996.
6. Cahalan TD, Cooney WP. Biomechanics. In: Jobe FW, Pink MM, Glousman RE, et al., eds. *Operative Techniques in Upper Extremity Sports Injuries*. St. Louis, MO, Mosby, 1996.
7. Berger AB. Anatomy and kinesiology of the wrist. In: Mackin EJ, Callahan AD, Skirven TM, Schneider LH, Osterman AL, eds. *Rehabilitation of the Hand and Upper Extremity*, 5th ed. St. Louis, MO, Mosby, 2002, pp. 77–87.
8. Sarrafian S, Melamed JL, Goshgarian GM. Study of wrist motion in flexion and extension. *Clin Orthop* 126:153, 1977.
9. Ryu JY, Cooney WP, Askew LJ, An KN, Chao EY. Functional ranges of motion of the wrist joint. *J Hand Surg* 16A:409, 1991.
10. Kauer JM. Functional anatomy of the wrist. *Clin Orthop Relat Res* 149:9–20, 1980.
11. Rosenthal EA. The extensor tendons: Anatomy and management. In: Hunter JM, Mackin EJ, Callahan AD, eds. *Rehabilitation of the Hand: Surgery and Therapy*, 4th ed. St. Louis, MO, Mosby, 1995.
12. Lapidus PW, Fenton R. Stenosing tenovaginitis at the wrist and fingers: Report of 423 cases in 369 patients with 354 operations. *Arch Surg* 64:475, 1952.
13. Lipscomb PR. Tenovaginitis at the radial styloid process. *Ann Surg* 134:110, 1951.
14. Cobb TK, Dalley BK, Posteraro RH, Lewis RC. Anatomy of the flexor retinaculum. *Hand Surg* 18A:91, 1993.
15. Kaplan EM. *Joints and Ligaments in Functional and Surgical Anatomy of the Hand*. Philadelphia, Lippincott, 1965.
16. Verdan C. The reconstruction of the thumb. *Surg Clin North Am* 48:1033, 1968.
17. Frykman GK, Kropp WE. Fractures and traumatic conditions of the wrist. In: Hunter JM, Mackin EJ, Callahan AD, eds. *Rehabilitation of the Hand: Surgery and Therapy*, 4th ed. St. Louis, MO, Mosby, 1995.
18. Gartland JJ, Werley CW. Evaluation of healed Colles' fractures. *J Bone Joint Surg Br* 43:245, 1961.
19. Kozin SH, Wood MB. Early soft tissue complications after fractures of the distal part of the radius. *J Bone Joint Surg Am* 75:144, 1993.
20. Bohler L. *The Treatment of Fractures*, 4th ed. Baltimore, William Wood, 1942.
21. Frykman G. Fracture of the distal radius including sequelae—shoulder-hand-finger syndrome, disturbance in the distal radioulnar joint, and impairment of nerve function: A clinical and experimental study. *Acta Orthop Scand Suppl* 108:1, 1967.
22. Mazet R, Hohl M. Fractures of the carpal navicular:

Analysis of 91 cases and review of the literature. *J Bone Joint Surg Am* 45:82, 1967.

23. Palmer AK, Dobyns JH, Linscheid RL. Management of post-traumatic instability of the wrist secondary to ligament rupture. *J Hand Surg* 3:507, 1978.

24. Volz RG, Lieb M, Benjamin J. Biomechanics of the wrist. *Clin Orthop Relat Res* 149:112–117, 1980.

25. Weber ER, Chap EY. An experimental approach to the mechanism of scaphoid waist fractures. *J Hand Surg* 3A:142, 1978.

26. Dell PC, Dell RB. Management of carpal fractures and dislocations. In: Mackin EJ, Callahan AD, Skirven TM, Schneider LH, Osterman AL, eds. *Rehabilitation of the Hand and Upper Extremity*, 5th ed. St. Louis, MO, Mosby, 2002, pp. 1171–1184.

27. Dray GJ, Eaton RG. Dislocations and ligament injuries in the digits. In: Green DP, ed. *Operative Hand Surgery, Vol. 1*, 3rd ed. New York, Churchill Livingstone, 1993.

28. Bryan RS, Dobyns JH. Less commonly fractured carpal bones. *Clin Orthop Relat Res* 149:108–109, 1980.

29. Biese J. Soft splints: Indications and techniques. In: Mackin EJ, Callahan AD, Skirven TM, Schneider LH, Osterman AL, eds. *Rehabilitation of the Hand and Upper Extremity*, 5th ed. St. Louis, MO, Mosby, 2002, pp. 1846–1857.

30. Crosby EB, Linscheid RI. Rupture of the flexor profundus tendon of the ring finger secondary to ancient fracture of the hook of the hamate: Review of the literature and report of two cases. *J Bone Joint Surg Am* 56:1076–1078, 1974.

31. Stark HH, Chow E, Zemel NP, Rickard TA, Ashworth CR. Fracture of the hook of the hamate. *J Bone Joint Surg Am* 71:1202–1207, 1989.

32. McCue FC, Bougher WN, Kulund DN, Gieck JH. Hand and wrist injuries in the patient. *Am J Sports Med* 7:275–286, 1979.

33a. Bishop AT, Beckenbaugh RD. Fracture of the hamate hook. *J Hand Surg Am* 13(1):135–139, 1988.

33b. Bohler L. *The Treatment of Fractures*, 4th ed. Baltimore, William Wood, 1942.

34. Watson HK, Rogers WD. Nonunion of the hook of the hamate, an argument for bone grafting the nonunion. *J Hand Surg Am* 14:486–490, 1989.

35. Meyer FN, Wilson RL. Management of nonarticular fractures of the hand. In: Hunter JM, Mackin EJ, Callahan AD, eds. *Rehabilitation of the Hand: Surgery and Therapy*, 4th ed. St. Louis, MO, Mosby, 1995.

36. Frykman GK, Waiking BE. The distal radioulnar joint. In: Mackin EJ, Callahan AD, Skirven TM, Schneider LH, Osterman AL, eds. *Rehabilitation of the Hand and Upper Extremity*, 5th ed. St. Louis, MO, Mosby, 2002.

37. Cooney WP, Linschied RI, Dobyns JH. Triangular fibrocartilage tears. *J Hand Surg* 19(1):143–154, 1994.

38. Trumble TE, Gilbert M, Vedder N. Ulnar shortening combined with arthroscopic repairs in the delayed management of triangular fibrocartilage complex tears. *J Hand Surg* 22A:807–813, 1997.

39. Hunter JM, Davlin LB, Fedus LM. Major neuropathies of the upper extremity: The median nerve. In: Hunter JM, Mackin EJ, Callahan AD, eds. *Rehabilitation of the Hand: Surgery and Therapy*, 4th ed. St. Louis, MO, Mosby, 1995.

40. Burke DT, Burke MM, Stewart GW, Cambre A. Splinting for carpal tunnel syndrome: In search of the optimal angle. *Arch Phys Med Rehabil* 75:1241, 1994.

41. Weiss ND, Gordon L, Bloom T, So Y, Rempel DM. Position of the wrist associated with the lowest carpal tunnel pressure: Implication for splint design. *J Bone Joint Surg* 77A:1695, 1995.

42. Ham SJ, Kolkman WF, Heeres J, den Boer JA. Changes in the carpal tunnel due to action of the flexor tendons: Visualization with magnetic resonance imaging. *J Hand Surg* 21A:977, 1996.

43. Van Heest A, Waters P, Simmons D, Schwartz JT. A cadaveric study of the single-portal endoscopic carpal tunnel release. *J Hand Surg* 20A:363, 1995.

44. Murphy RX, Jr, Jennings JF, Wukich DK. Major neurovascular complications of endoscopic carpal tunnel release. *J Hand Surg* 19A:114, 1994.

45. Brown RA, Gelberman RH, Seiler JG, et al. Carpal tunnel release: A prospective, randomized assessment of open and endoscopic methods. *J Bone Joint Surg* 75A:1265, 1993.

46. Hayes EP. Carpal tunnel syndrome. In: Mackin EJ, Callahan AD, Skirven TM, Schneider LH, Osterman AL, eds. *Rehabilitation of the Hand and Upper Extremity*, 5th ed. St. Louis, MO, Mosby, 2002.

47. Evans RB. Therapist's management of carpal tunnel syndrome. In: Mackin EJ, Callahan AD, Skirven TM, Schneider LH, Osterman AL, eds. *Rehabilitation of the Hand and Upper Extremity*, 5th ed. St. Louis, MO, Mosby, 2002.

48. Grundberg AB. Carpal tunnel decompression in spite of normal electromyography. *J Hand Surg* 8A:348, 1983.

49. Lam N, Thurston A. Association of obesity, gender, age, and occupation with carpal tunnel syndrome. *Aug N Z J Surg* 68:190,1998.

50. Weinstein SM, Herring SA. Nerve problems and compartment syndromes in the hand, wrist, and forearm. *Clin Sports Med* 11(1):161–188, 1992.

51. Butler DS. *Mobilization of the Nervous System*. Melbourne, Churchill Livingstone, 1991.

52. Totten PA, Hunter JM. Therapeutic techniques to enhance nerve gliding in thoracic outlet syndrome and carpal tunnel syndrome. *Hand Clin* 7:505, 1991.

53. Bush DC. Soft-tissue tumors of the hand. In: Hunter JM, Mackin EJ, Callahan AD, eds. *Rehabilitation of the Hand: Surgery and Therapy*, 4th ed. St. Louis, MO, Mosby, 1995.

54. Zubowicz VN, Ishii CH. Management of ganglion cysts by simple aspiration. *J Hand Surg* 12:618, 1987.

55. Korman J, Pearl R, Hentz VR. Efficacy of immobilization following aspiration of carpal and digital ganglion. *J Hand Surg* 17:1097, 1992.

56. Jupiter JB, Belsky MR. Fractures and dislocations of the hand. In: Browner BD, Jupiter JB, Levine AM, Trafton PG, eds. *Skeletal Trauma*. Philadelphia, WB Saunders, 1992.

57. Baxter-Petralia P, Penney V. Cumulative trauma. In: Stanley BG, Tribuzi SM, eds. *Concepts in Hand Rehabilitation*. Philadelphia, FA Davis, 1992.

58. Kirkpatrick WH, Lisser S. Soft-tissue conditions: Trigger fingers and de Quervain's disease. In: Hunter JM, Mackin EJ, Callahan AD, eds. *Rehabilitation of the Hand: Surgery and Therapy*, 4th ed. St. Louis, MO, Mosby, 1995.

59. Finklestein H. Stenosing tendovaginitis at the radial styloid process. *J Bone Joint Surg* 12:509, 1930.

60. Michlovitz S. Is there a role for ultrasound and electrical stimulation following injury to tendon and nerve? *J Hand Ther* 18:2, 2005.

61. Michlovitz S. Ultrasound and selected physical agent modalities in upper extremity rehabilitation. In: Mackin EJ, Callahan AD, Skirven TM, Schneider LH, Osterman AL, eds. *Rehabilitation of the Hand and Upper Extremity*, 5th ed. St. Louis, MO, Mosby, 2002, pp. 1745–1763.

62. Witt J, Pess G, Gelberman RH. Treatment of de Quervain tenosynovitis: A prospective study of the results of injection of steroid and immobilization in a splint. *J Bone Joint Surg* 73:219, 1991.

63. Condit D. Personal communication, June 2005.

64. Peterson Lee M, Nazzer-Sharif S, Zelouf DS. Surgeon's and therapist's management of tendonopathies in the hand and wrist. In: Mackin EJ, Callahan AD, Skirven TM, Schneider LH, Osterman AL, eds. *Rehabilitation of the Hand and Upper Extremity*, 5th ed. St. Louis, MO, Mosby, 2002, pp. 931–953.

65. Rettig AC. Current concepts in management of football injuries of the hand and wrist. *J Hand Ther* 4(2):42–50, 1991.

66. Smith RJ. Posttraumatic instability of the metacarpophalangeal joint of the thumb. *J Bone Joint Surg* 59:14–21, 1977.

67. Wright HH, Retting AC. Management of common sports injuries. In: Hunter JM, Mackin EJ, Callahan AD, eds. *Rehabilitation of the Hand: Surgery and Therapy*, 4th ed. St. Louis, MO, Mosby, 1995.

68. Husband JB, McPherson SA. Bony skier's thumb injuries. *Clin Orthop Relat Res* 327:79–84, 1996.

69. McCue FC, Nelson WE. Ulnar collateral ligament injuries of the thumb. *Physician Sports Med* 21:67–80, 1993.

70. Stener B. Displacement of the ruptured ulnar collateral ligament of the metacarpophalangeal joint of the thumb. *J Bone Joint Surg Br* 44:869–879, 1962.

71. Campbell CS. Gamekeeper's thumb. *J Bone Joint Surg Br* 37:148–149, 1955.

72. Culp RW, Taras JS. Primary care of flexor tendon injuries. In: Hunter JM, Mackin EJ, Callahan AD, eds. *Rehabilitation of the Hand: Surgery and Therapy*, 4th ed. St. Louis, MO, Mosby, 1995.

73. Evans RA. Study of the zone I flexor tendon injury and implications for treatment. *J Hand Ther* 3:133, 1990.

74. Evans RA. Zone I flexor tendon rehabilitation with limited extension and active flexion. *J Hand Ther* 18:2, 2005.

75. Doyle JR. Extensor tendons—acute injuries. In: Green DP, ed. *Operative Hand Surgery*, 2nd ed. New York, Churchill Livingstone, 1988.

76. Stark HH, Bayer JH, Wilson JN. Mallet finger. *J Bone Joint Surg* 44:1061, 1962.

77. Wilson RL, Hazen J. Management of joint injuries and intraarticular fractures of the hand. In: Hunter JM, Mackin EJ, Callahan AD, eds. *Rehabilitation of the Hand: Surgery and Therapy*, 4th ed. St. Louis, MO, Mosby, 1995.

CHAPTER 28

Rehabilitation of the Groin, Hip, and Thigh

Timothy F. Tyler and Gregory C. Thomas

O B J E C T I V E S

After completing this chapter, the therapist should be able to do the following:

- Discuss the functional anatomy and biomechanics of the groin, hip, and thigh.
- Discuss injuries to the groin, hip, and thigh and describe the biomechanical changes that occur during and after injury.
- Discuss and describe the functional injury evaluation of the groin, thigh, and hip.
- Articulate the role previous injury may play in subsequent injuries in the athlete.
- Describe the at-risk populations and the mechanism of injury for muscle strains, muscle contusions, and acetabular labral injuries.
- Demonstrate application of various intervention strategies for a wide variety of hip pathologies including muscle strains and contusions and acetabular labral injuries.
- Apply principles of prevention and wellness using screening for imbalances and preseason-strengthening programs for susceptible populations.
- Apply principles of stretching, strengthening, open- and closed kinetic-chain exercises, plyometrics, isokinetics, and proprioceptive neuromuscular facilitation exercises to the hip complex as a part of comprehensive rehabilitation.

INTRODUCTION

The occurrence of injuries to the hip, pelvis, and thigh are relatively small when compared to the other lower-extremity regions.[1–5] While statistically less prevalent, a hip pathology can cause immediate gait abnormalities, lead to chronic pain, and give rise to premature degeneration in the hip joint itself. These injuries can vary significantly depending on the specific sporting activity involved.[6] Contact sports will have a high incident of traumatic injuries such as fractures, contusions, and dislocations, whereas endurance sports like running, swimming, and biking can lead to stress and overuse injuries. No matter what the injury, proper diagnosis and intervention is key in returning the athlete back to their sport(s) of choice. The purpose of this chapter is to identify common hip pathologies and direct an appropriate and concise rehabilitation program to optimize a patient's recovery time.

ANATOMY AND BIOMECHANICS

The primary function at the hip joint is to support the weight of the head, arm, and trunk, while also serving as the connection between the lower extremities and pelvic girdle. The anatomical design of the hip is well suited to handle this task as well as the increased loads that can be transmitted during athletic competition.[7] Joint impact forces such as running produces loads of up to three to five times body weight.

The joint itself is the articulation between the acetabulum of the pelvis and the head of the femur. These two segments form a diarthrodial ball and socket joint with three degrees of freedom: flexion/extension in the sagital plane, abduction/adduction in the frontal plane, and medial/lateral rotation in the transverse plane.

The cuplike concavity of the acetabulum is formed by the fusion of three bones: ilium, ischium and pubis. These bones typically unite by the late teenage years.[8] The resulting socket is located on the lateral aspect of the pelvic bone and has an angular orientation of inferior and anterior. The femoral component of the joint has an angular orientation of superior and anterior. These orientations represent the angles of inclination and torsion respectfully. The angle of inclination is measured in the frontal plane between the axis of the head/neck and the axis of the shaft. Normal angles range between 125° and 135°. A pathological increase in inclination is called *coxa valga*, and a decrease is referred to as *coxa vara*. The angle of torsion is measured in the transverse plane between the axis of the head/neck of the femur and the axis through the femoral condyles. It can best be viewed by looking down the length of the femur from top to bottom. Normal angles of torsion are between 10° and 15° with an increase termed anteversion and a decrease called retroversion.[7] Both normal and abnormal angles are properties of the femur and independent of the hip joint.

The femoral and acetabular surfaces correspond well to each other, but given the increased need for stability at this joint, an accessory structure is needed. The entire periphery of the acetabulum is rimmed by a ring of wedge-shaped fibrocartlidge called the acetabular labrum. This labrum not only deepens the socket but also increases the concavity of the socket through its triangular shape. This structural stability is reinforced by the hip joint capsule and its ligaments.

The capsule is attached proximally to the entire periphery of the acetabulum beyond the labrum. The distal end covers the head and neck like a sleeve and attaches to the base of the femoral neck. This capsule is considered to have three reinforcing ligaments: two anteriorly and one posteriorly. The two anterior ligaments are the iliofemoral ligament and pubofemoral ligament. These are often referred to as the Y ligament of Bigelow. The ischiofemoral ligament is the posterior capsular ligament.[7] Femoroacetabular anomalies may occur at the hip joint. These morphological variances include an abnormal femoral head interacting with a normal acetabulum, or conversely, a normal femoral head acting on an abnormally formed acetabulum.[9]

Movements at the hip joint consist of arthrokinematic and osteokinematic actions. The arthrokinematics that occur within the joint can best be visualized as the movement of the convex head of the femur within the concavity of the acetabulum. Thus the convex on concave rule states that arthrokinematic motions are opposite of the osteokinematic movements. Hip flexion created by primary movers such as the iliopsoas, rectus femoris, tensor fascia lata, and sartorius occurs in the anterior direction around the coronal axis. During hip flexion there is a posterior glide of the humeral head. Full range through flexion is approximately 125°.

The hip extensors are made up of the gluteus maximus and hamstrings, which consist of the biceps femoris, semimembranosus, and semitendinosus. Extension occurs posteriorly around the coronal axis causing an anterior glide of the femoral head. Normal range for extension is 10°.

Abduction of the hip is brought about by the primary actions of the gluteus medius and gluteus minimus. This move-

ment occurs away from the midsagittal plane in the lateral direction. Normal range is approximately 45° with inferior movement of the humeral head.

The gracilis, adductor magnus, longus, and brevis produce osteokinematic adduction toward the midsagittal plane. This results in a superior arthrokinematic femoral head glide within the acetabulum. Adduction range on average is 10°.[7,10,11]

The final motion of the hip is hip rotation that occurs in the transverse plane of motion and is often overlooked. More importance has been given to the patients' ability to control hip rotation during function movements. In patients with patellofemoral pain syndrome, it has been suggested that a theoretical mechanism for pathology may be weak femoral external rotators which allow the femur to be in relative internal rotation and influence patellar alignment and kinematics. In fact, the role of the hip rotator muscles is frequently overlooked when addressing prevention and rehabilitation of lumbar spine injuries. Weak and/or shortened hip rotators may contribute to abnormal lumbopelvic posture and cause compensatory motion in the lumbar spine during daily activities. The detrimental effects of inadequately conditioned and prepared hip rotators may predispose the athlete to lumbar spine injuries. The small external rotators of the hip (piriformis, obturator internus, obturator externus, gemellus superior, gemellus inferior, and quadratus femoris) sometimes get fatigued or overpowered by the large internal rotators of the hip (gluteus maximus, gluteus medius, and gluteus minimus) creating muscle imbalance.

Hip Muscular Strains

A muscle strain, also called a pull or tear, is a common injury, particularly among people who participate in sports. The thigh has three sets of strong muscles: the hamstring muscles posteriorly, the quadriceps muscles anteriorly, and the adductor muscles medially. The hamstring and quadriceps muscle groups are particularly at risk for muscle strains because they cross both the hip and knee joints. They are also used for high-speed activities such as track and field events, football, basketball, ice hockey, and soccer.

Most commonly, the mechanism of injury for muscle strains in the hip area is when a stretched muscle is forced to contract suddenly. A fall or direct blow to the muscle, overstretching, and overuse can tear muscle fibers resulting in a strain. The risk of muscle strain increases if the patient had a prior injury in the area, performs inadequate warm-up before exercising or attempts to do too much too quickly. Strains may be mild, moderate, or severe depending on the extent of the injury. Signs and symptoms may include pain over the injured muscle (the most common symptom of a hip strain), increased pain level with muscular contraction, swelling and discoloration (depending on the severity of the strain), and a loss of strength in the muscle.

Evaluation of hip muscle strains can be challenging when overlapping conditions exist. A muscle that is painful on contraction and painful when stretched may be strained. Certain exercises or stretches in specific ways, which stress the involved muscle, can help determine which muscle is injured. A radiograph or other diagnostic test may be used to rule out the possibility of a stress fracture of the hip, which has similar symptoms, including pain in the groin area, with weight bearing. In most cases, no additional tests are needed to confirm the diagnosis.

In general, interventions are chosen and rehabilitation programs designed to relieve pain, restore range of motion (ROM), and restore strength, in that order. Rest, ice, compression, elevation (RICE) is standard protocol for mild-to-moderate muscle strains. Gently massaging the area with ice may also help decrease swelling. Nonsteroidal anti-inflammatary drugs (NSAIDs) can be taken to reduce swelling and ease pain. Compression shorts/sleeve or a compression bandage may also be helpful to decrease swelling and provide support. If walking causes pain, consider limiting weight bearing and using crutches for the first day or two after the injury.

Adductor Muscle Strains

Adductor muscle strains can result in missed playing time for athletes in many sports. Adductor muscle strains are encountered most frequently in ice hockey and soccer.[12–14] These sports require a strong eccentric contraction of the adductor musculature during competition.[15,16] Recently, adductor muscle strength has been linked to the incidence of adductor muscle strains. Specifically, the strength ratio of the adduction-abduction muscles groups has been identified as a risk factor in professional ice hockey players.[17] Intervention programs can lower the incidence of adductor muscle strains but cannot avoid them altogether. Therefore, proper injury treatment and rehabilitation must be implemented to limit the amount of missed playing time and avoid surgical intervention.[18]

Adductor Musculature

The group of muscles along the inner thigh is referred to as the adductor muscle group. This group of six muscles includes the pectineus, adductor longus, adductor brevis, adductor magnus, gracillis, and obturator externus. All of the adductor muscles are innervated by the obturator nerve except for the pectineus, which gets its motor intervention from the femoral nerve. These muscles originate in the inguinal region at various points on the pubis. They travel inferior to insert along the medial femur. The main action of this muscle group is to adduct the thigh in the open kinetic chain and stabilize the lower extremity to perturbations in the closed kinetic chain. Each individual muscle can also provide assistance in femoral flexion and rotation.[8,19] The adductor longus is thought to be the most frequently injured adductor muscle.[20] Its lack of mechanical advantage may make it more susceptible to strain.

Adductor Muscle Injury

A groin strain is defined as pain on palpation of the adductor tendons or the insertion on the pubic bone, or both, and groin pain during adduction against resistance.[18,21,22] Groin strains and muscle strains in general are graded as a first-degree strain if there is pain but minimal loss of strength and minimal restriction of motion. A second-degree strain is defined as tissue damage that compromises the strength of the muscle, but not including complete loss of strength and function. A third-degree strain denotes complete disruption of the muscle tendon unit. It includes complete loss of function of the muscle.[23] A thorough history and a physical examination is needed to differentiate groin strains from athletic pubalgia, osteitis pubis, hernia, hip-joint osteoarthrosis, rectal or testicular referred pain, piriformis syndrome, or presence of a coexisting fracture of the pelvis or the lower extremities.[20–23] Imaging studies can sometimes be useful to rule out other possible causes of inguinal pain.[24]

Adductor Muscle Strain Incidence

The exact incidence of adductor muscle strains in sport is unknown. This is due in part to athletes playing through minor groin pain and the injury going unreported. In addition, overlapping diagnosis can also skew the exact incidence. Groin strains are among the most common injuries seen in ice hockey players.[25–27] It has been documented that groin strains accounted for 10 percent of all injuries in elite Swedish ice hockey players.[28] Furthermore, Molsa[29] reported that groin strains accounted for 43 percent of all muscles strains in elite Finish ice hockey players. Tyler et al.[17] published the incidence of groin strains in a single National Hockey League (NHL) team of 3.2 strains per 1000 player-game exposures. In a larger study of 26 NHL teams, Emery et al.[13] reported, the incidence of adductor strains in the NHL has increased over the last 6 years. The rate of injury was greatest during the preseason compared to regular and postseason play. Prospective soccer studies in Scandinavia have reported a groin strain incidence between 10 and 18 injuries per 100 soccer players.[30] Ekstrand and Gillquist[14] documented 32 groin strains in 180 male soccer players representing 13 percent of all injuries over the course of 1 year. Adductor muscle strains, certainly, are not isolated to these two sports.

RISK FACTORS

Previous studies have shown an association between strength and/or flexibility and musculoskeletal strains in various athletic populations.[14,31,32] Ekstrandt and Gillquist[14] found that preseason hip abduction ROM was decreased in soccer players who subsequently sustained groin strains compared with uninjured players. This is in contrast to the data published on professional ice hockey players that found no relationship between passive or active abduction ROM (adductor flexibility) and adductor muscle strains.[17,33]

Adductor muscle strength has been associated with a subsequent muscle strain. Tyler et al.[17] found that preseason hip adduction strength was 18 percent lower in NHL players who subsequently sustained groin strains as compared to those who remained uninjured. The hip adduction to abduction strength ratio was also significantly different between the two groups.

Adduction strength was 95 percent of abduction strength in the uninjured players but only 78 percent of abduction strength in the injured players. Additionally, in the players who sustained a groin strain, preseason adduction to abduction strength ratio was lower on the side which subsequently sustained a groin strain compared with the uninjured side. Adduction strength was 86 percent of abduction strength on the uninjured side but only 70 percent of abduction strength on the injured side. Conversely, another study on adductor strains on ice hockey players found no relationship between peak isometric adductor torque and the incidence of adductor strains.[33] Unlike the previous study this study had multiple testers using a hand held dynamometer, which would increase the variability and decrease the likelihood of finding strength differences. However, the results of Emery et al.[33] did demonstrate that players who practiced during the off season were less likely to sustain a groin injury as were rookies in the NHL. The final risk factor was the presence of a previous adductor strain. Tyler et al.[17] also linked preexisting injury as a risk factor, as in their study four of the nine groin strains (44 percent) were recurrent injuries. This is consistent with the results of Seward et al.[34] who reported a 32 percent recurrence rate for groin strains in athletes participating in Australian Rules Football.

PREVENTION

Now that researchers have identified players at risk for a future adductor strain, the next step is to design an intervention program to address all risk factors. Tyler et al.[25] were able to demonstrate that a therapeutic intervention of strengthening the adductor muscle group could be an effective method for preventing adductor strains in professional ice hockey players. Prior to 2000 and 2001, season's professional ice hockey players were strength tested. Thirty-three of these 58 players were classified as "at risk" which was defined as having an adduction-abduction strength ratio of less than 80 percent and placed on an intervention program. The intervention program consisted of strengthening and functional exercises aimed at increasing adductor strength (Table 28-1). The injuries were tracked over the course of the two seasons. In the present study there were three adductor strains which all occurred in game situations. This gives an incidence of 0.71 adductor strains per 1000 player-game exposures. Adductor strains accounted for approximately 2 percent of all injuries. In contrast, there were 11 adductor strains and an incidence of 3.2 adductor strains per 1000 player-game exposures in the previous two seasons prior to the intervention. In those prior two seasons, adductor strains accounted for approximately 8 percent of all injuries. This was also significantly lower than the incidence reported by Lorentzon et al.[28] who found adductor strains to be 10 percent of all injuries. Of the three players who sustained adductor strains, none of the players had sustained a previous adductor strain on the same side. One player had bilateral adductor strains at different times during the first season. This study demonstrated that a therapeutic intervention of strengthening the adductor muscle group can be an effective method for preventing adductor strains in professional ice hockey players.

TABLE 28-1

Adductor Strain Injury Prevention Program

Warm-up	Bike
	Adductor stretching
	Sumo squats
	Side lunges
	Kneeling pelvic tilts
Strengthening program	Ball squeezes (legs bent to legs straight)
	Different ball sizes
	Concentric adduction with weight against gravity
	Adduction in standing on cable column or elastic resistance
	Seated adduction machine
	Standing with involved foot on sliding board moving in sagittal plane
	Bilateral adduction on sliding board moving in frontal plane (i.e., bilateral adduction simultaneously)
	Unilateral lunges with reciprocal arm movements
Sports-specific training	On ice kneeling adductor pulls together
	Standing resisted stride lengths on cable column to simulate skating
	Slide skating
	Cable column crossover pulls
Clinical goal	Adduction strength at least 80% of the abduction strength

REHABILITATION

Despite the identification of risk factors and strengthening intervention for ice hockey players, adductor strains continue to occur in all sports.[24] The high incidence of recurrent strains could be due to incomplete rehabilitation or inadequate time for complete tissue repair. Hömlich et al.[18] demonstrated that a passive physical therapy program of massage, stretching, and modalities were ineffective in treating chronic groin strains. By contrast, an 8–12 week active strengthening program consisting of progressive resistive adduction and abduction exercises, balance training, abdominal strengthening, and skating movements on a slide board proved more effective in treating chronic groin strains. An increased emphasis on strengthening exercises may reduce the recurrence rate of groin strains. An adductor muscle strain injury program progressing the athlete through the phases of healing has been developed by Tyler et al.[25] and anecdotally seems to be effective (Table 28-2). This type of treatment regime combines modalities and passive treatment

T A B L E   2 8 - 2

Adductor Strain Postinjury Program

Phase I (acute)	RICE for first ~48 hours after injury
	NSAIDs
	Massage
	Transcutaneous electrical nerve stimulation (TENS)
	Ultrasound
	Submaximal isometric adduction with knees bent→with knees straight progressing to maximal isometric adduction, pain-free hip PROM in pain-free range
	Non-weightbearing hip progressive resistive exercises without weight in antigravity position (all except abduction), pain-free, low-load, high-repetition exercise
	Upper body and trunk strengthening
	Contralateral lower extremity (LE) strengthening
	Flexibility program for noninvolved muscles
	Bilateral balance board
Clinical milestone	Concentric adduction against gravity without pain
Phase II (subacute)	Bicycling/swimming
	Sumo squats
	Single limb stance
	Concentric adduction with weight against gravity
	Standing with involved foot on sliding board moving in frontal plane
	Adduction in standing on cable column or Theraband
	Seated adduction machine
	Bilateral adduction on sliding board moving in frontal plane (i.e., bilateral adduction simultaneously)
	Unilateral lunges (sagittal) with reciprocal arm movements
	Multiplane trunk tilting
	Balance board squats with throwbacks
	General flexibility program
Clinical milestone	Involved lower extremity PROM equal to that of the uninvolved side and involved adductor strength at least 75% that of the ipsilateral abductors.
Phase III (sports-specific training)	Phase II exercises with increase in load, intensity, speed, and volume
	Standing resisted stride lengths on cable column to simulate skating
	Slide board
	On ice kneeling adductor pulls together
	Lunges (in all planes)
	Correct or modify ice-skating technique
Clinical milestone	Adduction strength at least 90–100% of the abduction strength and involved muscle strength equal to that of the contralateral side

PROM, passive range of motion.

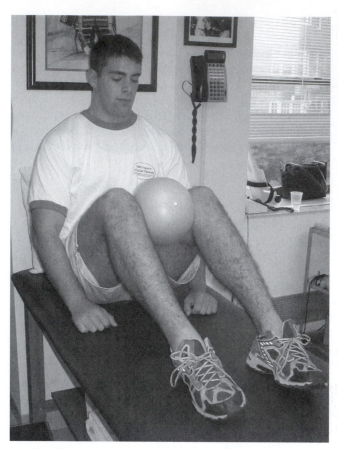

FIGURE 28-1

Ball squeeze.

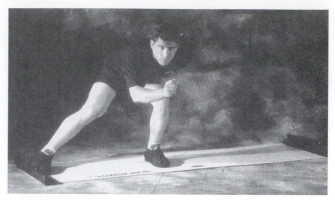

FIGURE 28-3

Slide board.

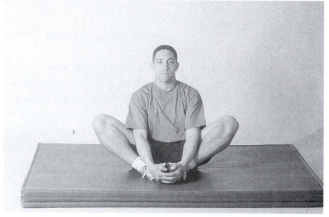

FIGURE 28-4

Hip adductor stretch.

immediately, followed by an active training program emphasizing eccentric resistive exercise. This method of rehabilitation program has been supported throughout the literature.[22,24] Exercises for this injury are shown in Figures 28-1 to 28-3. Stretches are shown in Figures 28-4 to 28-6.

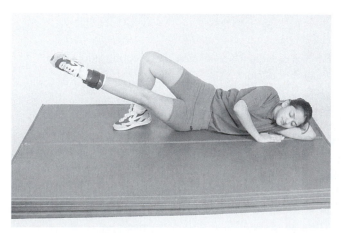

FIGURE 28-2

Hip adduction.

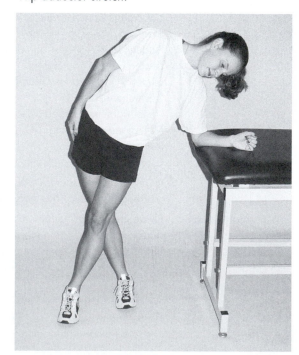

FIGURE 28-5

Standing hip abduction stretch.

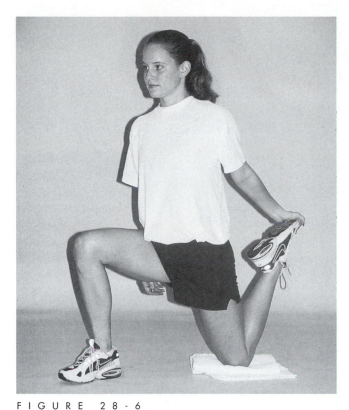

FIGURE 28-6

Hip flexor stretch.

Hamstring Musculature

The Hamstrings actually comprise three separate muscles: the biceps femoris, semitendinosus, and semimembranosus. These muscles originate just underneath the gluteus maximus on the pelvic bone and attach on the tibia and fibula. The hamstrings are primarily fast-twitch muscles, responding to low repetitions and powerful movements. The primary functions of the hamstrings are knee flexion and hip extension.

Hamstring Muscle Injury

Hamstring muscle strains commonly result from a wide variety of sporting activities, particularly those requiring rapid acceleration and deceleration. An eccentric load to the muscle causes the majority of these injuries. Garrett et al.[23,35] demonstrated that, in young athletes, hamstring muscle strains typically involve myotendinous disruption of the proximal biceps femoris muscle. Other authors have also shown experimentally that the weak link of the muscle complex is the myotendinous junction.[23,36] Although apophyseal fractures of the ischial tuberosity have been reported in young athletes, the majority of hamstring muscle strains are first- and second-degree strains.[37]

Hamstring Muscle Strain Incidence

Hamstring muscle strains are among the most common injuries in sports involving high-speed movement and physical contact. Hamstring strains are by far the most commonly seen muscle strains in Australian Rules Football with an incidence of 8.05 injuries per 1000 player-game-hours. Soccer players are also susceptible to hamstring strains with an incidence of 3.0 per 1000 player-game-hours for hamstring strains. Overall, any athlete who sprints as part of their sport may contribute to the incidence of hamstring strains.

RISK FACTORS

Factors causing hamstring muscle injury have been studied for many years. Age and previous injury were identified as the main risk factors for hamstring strains injury among elite football players from Iceland.[38] It has been suggested that muscle weakness, strength imbalance, lack of flexibility, fatigue, inadequate warm-up, and dyssynergic contraction may predispose an athlete to a hamstring strain.[39]

Fatigue has been implicated in the pathogenesis of muscle strain injury. Because muscle strains have been observed to occur either late in training or late in competitive matches, muscle fatigue has been indicated as a risk factor. Another study suggests that the injuries occur either early in games or training or late in games or training with inadequate warm-up and muscle fatigue, respectively, being the hypothesized reasons.[40] However, there is little quantitative data to support these statements. Croisier et al.[41] has suggests that the persistence of muscle weakness and imbalance may give rise to recurrent hamstring muscle injuries and pain. These authors feel that when there is insufficient eccentric braking capacity of the hamstring muscles compared with the concentric motor action of the quadriceps muscles, the muscle may be at risk for injury.

Ekstrand and Gillquist[42] prospectively studied male Swedish soccer players and found hamstrings to be the muscle group most often injured. They noted that minor injuries increased the risk of having a more severe injury within 2 months. Others have noted a recurrence rate of 25 percent for hamstring injuries in intercollegiate football players.[43]

PREVENTION

Most clinicians prescribe warm-up and stretching to help reduce the incidence of muscle strains. The evidence supporting this idea is weak and largely based on retrospective studies.[44] In fact, following hamstring injury, the affected extremity and muscle group are significantly less flexible than the uninjured side, but there are no differences in isokinetic strength.[45] However, Jonhagen et al.[46] found decreased flexibility and lower eccentric hamstring torques in runners who sustained a hamstring strain when compared with uninjured subjects matched for age and speed. The role of stretching and warm-up in injury prevention needs to be better understood so that optimal strategies can be developed.

REHABILITATION

There is no consensus for rehabilitation of the hamstring muscles after strain. However, a rehabilitation program consisting of progressive agility and trunk stabilization exercises has been

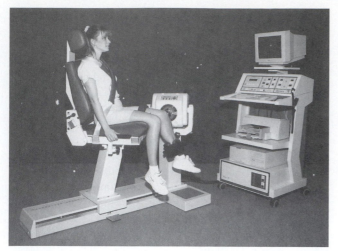

F I G U R E   2 8 - 7

Multiangle isometrics on Biodex.

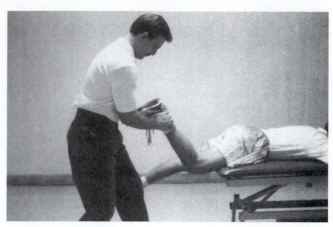

F I G U R E   2 8 - 8

Manual eccentric hamstring strengthening.

shown to be more effective than a program emphasizing isolated hamstring stretching and strengthening in promoting return to sports and preventing injury recurrence in athletes suffering an acute hamstring strain.[47] The aim of the physical therapy is to restore full pain-free ROM and strength throughout the ROM. In addition, as a complement to the usual restoration of function we emphasize restoring eccentric muscle strength and correction of agonist/antagonist imbalances in the rehabilitation process. We recommend the inclusion of eccentric exercises at an elongated position of the hamstring muscles, submaximally, as soon as the patient can tolerate it. Our rationale is based on basic science animal research[48] and imaging studies of human muscle tissue[23] that have indicated incomplete healing following muscle strains. Fibrosis at the injury site is thought to be related to the risk of reinjury. Based on these observations, interventions aimed at remodeling the muscle tissue may be effective in reducing the risk associated with having had a prior muscle strain. Eccentric muscle contractions have been shown to result in muscle-tendon junction remodeling in an animal model[49] and more recently have been shown to cause intramuscular collagen remodeling in humans.[50] Therefore, an eccentrically biased training program for previously injured muscles could theoretically reduce recurrence rates and would be worth studying in future research.

Rehabilitation would start with relative rest and protection of the injured muscle phase lasting from 1 to 3 days. Returning to exercise in this stage can lead to reinjury and disruption of the healing tissue. Multiangle isometrics, as shown in Figure 28-7, should be initiated to properly align the regenerating muscle fibers and limit the extent of connective tissue fibrosis. Rest, ice, compression, and elevation, along with anti-inflammatory medication, are helpful during the immediate stages of treatment. Heat, electrical stimulation, and ultrasound modalities can also be used in conjunction with each other during the rehabilitation program to facilitate a return to competition. Heat is effective at increasing tissue temperature prior to stretching and

exercise. Electric stimulation can be used to control edema and pain. Ultrasound is used as a deep-heating agent during the subacute (intermediate) phase to decrease spasm and prevent soft-tissue shortening.

An effective strengthening program should treat the hamstrings as a two-joint muscle and focus on concentric and eccentric contractions. Exercises for this are shown in Figures 28-8 to 28-10. Although lack of flexibility has been identified as a factor leading to hamstring injuries, the effectiveness of preexercise muscle stretching in reducing injuries has recently been questioned. In fact, recent studies cite decreased strength/power up to 1 hour following passive stretching.[45] In theory, this decrease in force production is thought to result from the relaxation of the muscle tendon unit. Therefore, prior to athletic competition, a general warm-up (jogging, cycling) to increase tissue temperature followed by dynamic stretching that includes sports-specific movements is recommended. Examples of dynamic stretches for the legs include forward or backward lunges, high-knee

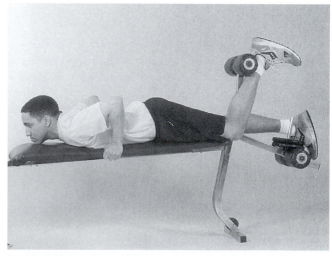

F I G U R E   2 8 - 9

Hamstring prone.

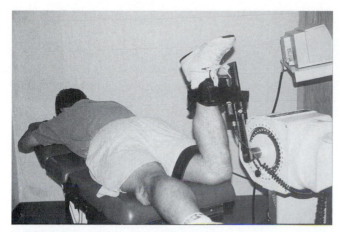

FIGURE 28-10

Isokinetic hamstring strengthening.

marching, and straight-leg kicks. Static stretching should be performed after the athletic activity. Stretches are shown in Figures 28-11 to 28-13.

Quadriceps Strain

The quadriceps is a group of four muscles that sit on the anterior aspect of the thigh. They are the vastus medialis, intermedius, lateralis, and finally the rectus femoris. The quadriceps attach to the front of the tibia via the patella tendon and originate at the top of the femur. The exception is the rectus femoris which actually crosses the hip joint and originates on the pelvis. The function of the quadriceps as a whole is to extend the knee. The rectus femoris not only functions to extend the knee but also acts as a hip flexor because it crosses the hip joint. Any of these muscles can strain (or tear) but probably the most common is the rectus femoris. The grading system is the same as the adductor strains. A grade III tear is felt as an abrupt, sudden, acute pain that occurs during activity (often while sprinting). It may be accompanied by swelling or bruises on the thigh. The rehabilitation of quadriceps strains follows the same principles as the

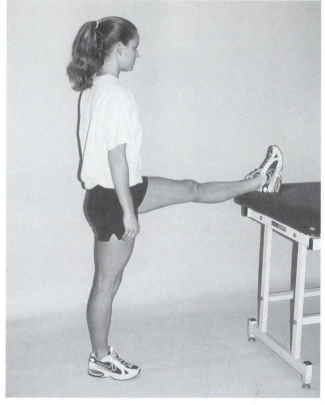

FIGURE 28-12

Standing hamstring band stretch.

rehabilitation process of adductors and hamstring strains. Exercises for this type of injury initially are shown in Figures 28-14 and 28-15. Advanced exercises can be as given in Figures 28-16 through 28-18. Stretches are shown in Figures 28-4 through 28-6.

Avulsion Fractures

Avulsion fractures are the result of a sudden, forceful eccentric or unbalanced contraction of a musculo-tendonous unit at its

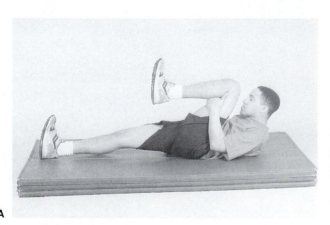

A   **B**

FIGURE 28-11

Supine hamstring stretches. **A,** Flexed knee position. **B,** Active knee extension to stretch hamstring.

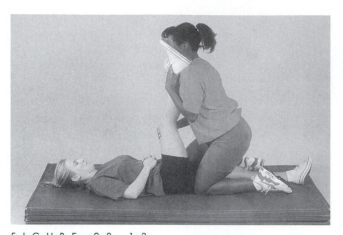

F I G U R E   2 8 - 1 3

Passive hamstring.

attachment at an apophysis. Traction epiphyses, or apophyses, are bony projections of forming bone that do not contribute to longitudinal growth of the bone. These epiphyseal plates are weaker than their associated ligaments; for this reason, injuries that would result in torn ligaments or tendons in adults may produce traumatic separation of the apophyses in adolescents. These injuries account for up to 15 percent of children's fractures.[51]

The ischial apophysis is the site of hamstring and adductor magnus origin and is the last apophysis to unite.[52] An avulsion

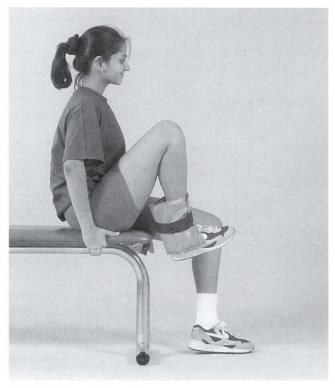

F I G U R E   2 8 - 1 4

Hip flexor stretch.

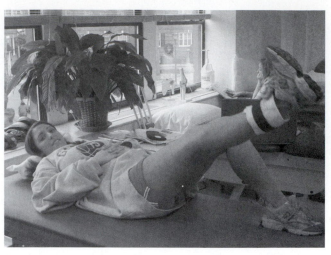

F I G U R E   2 8 - 1 5

Straight leg raises.

here is the result of a violent or forceful hip flexion while the knee is extended. This injury is commonly seen in hurdlers, sprinters, cheerleaders, and dancers.

The athlete will give a history report of a traumatic event that caused an acute onset of pain. They present with tenderness over the ischial tuberosity and pain with a straight leg raise. An antalgic gait may be evident as well as statements of pain with sitting. Definitive diagnosis is performed radiographically. In older adults with no history of traumatic incident a systemic or pathological cause needs to be reviewed.[53]

Treatment for this injury begins with rest along with pain-free active range of motion (AROM) and PROM and protected weight bearing with crutches if needed.[54] With a reduction of

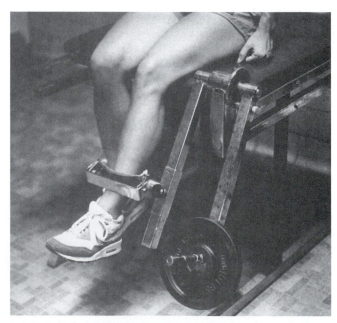

F I G U R E   2 8 - 1 6

Knee extension.

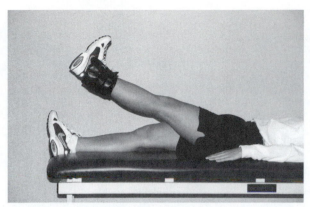

FIGURE 28-17

Leg raises.

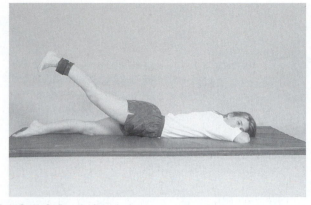

FIGURE 28-19

Hip extension.

pain, initiation of light strengthening and gentle stretching can be prescribed. Exercises shown in Figures 28-2, 28-14, 28-15, and 28-19 illustrate such interventions. Stretching shown in Figure 28-13 may also be helpful. Normalization of gait cycle is progressed throughout healing time. Progressive resistant exercises are introduced with return of ROM and cessation of pain (Figs. 28-9 and 28-20). A steady advancement to sport-specific activities should concentrate on strengthening, proprioceptive

training, and finally plyometrics (exercises shown in Figs. 28-21 to 28-23). Patients should not return to competition until full ROM and strength is restored.[24]

Another avulsion fracture in the pelvis involves the anterior inferior iliac spine (AIIS). This injury cost commonly occurs in kicking sports. The AIIS is the origin of the reflected head of rectus femoris. The tension load occurs in the kicking mechanics with a sudden contraction of the rectus while the hip is extended and the knee is flexed. Examination may reveal an antalgic gait pattern along with local tenderness and pain with resisted hip flexion.

Avulsion of the anterior superior iliac spine (ASIS) involves the same mechanics of hip extension with flexed knee, but involves a forceful contraction of the sartorious muscle. This is found in sprinters during high-speed hip extension. The athlete will present with palpable tenderness over the anatomical landmark.

Both injuries respond well to conservative treatment that involves initial rest and cessation of injuring activity. Rehabilitation is similar to that of the ischial avulsion fracture

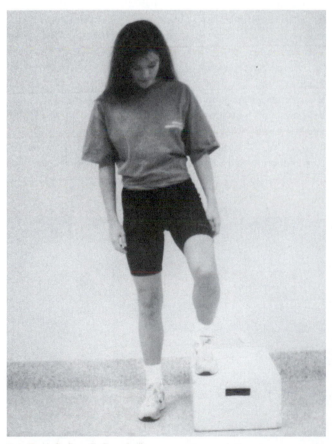

FIGURE 28-18

Step up.

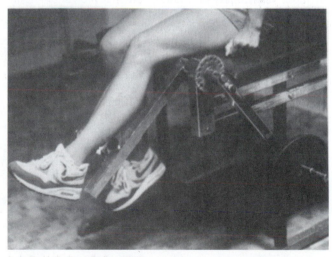

FIGURE 28-20

Progressive resistant exercise.

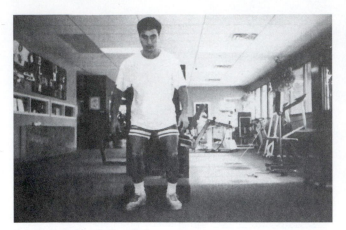

FIGURE 28-21

Plyometric exercise 1.

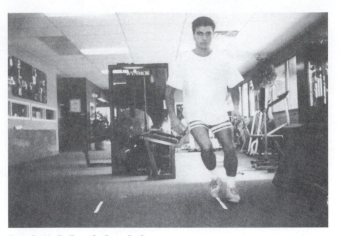

FIGURE 28-23

Plyometric exercise 3.

with emphasis on pain-free progression (exercises shown in Figs. 28-2, 28-14, 28-15, and 28-19).

Hip Pointer

A hip pointer occurs from a traumatic blow or fall to the iliac crest. It is also referred to as a contusion of the iliac crest. The impact causes bleeding from ruptured capillaries and infiltration of blood into muscles, tendons, and other soft tissues, i.e., subperiostal and subcutaneous regions.[8] The iliac crest has a minimal amount of overlying fatty or muscular tissue, which makes it more susceptible to injury than other more protected areas of the body. Hip pointers occur most commonly in contact sports such as football, rugby, hockey, but also occurs in noncontact sports such as volleyball as a result of a fall or dig onto the hip or side.

The signs and symptoms include a sudden onset of pain after a traumatic hit or fall onto that side. Pain is often localized (point tender) and may present with swelling and ecchymosis at the injury site. The athlete may present physically

with guarding, decreased strength, pain with resistance, and gait abnormalities.[55]

Three grades of contusion can be distinguished based on physical findings. A grade I hip pointer presents with a normal gait and posture, but with complaints of pain, palpable tenderness, and minimal swelling. Grade II injuries are more painful with noticeable swelling and abnormal gait patterns. ROM is limited and trunk movement is painful. The posture may be flexed to the injured side. Finally a grade III presents with severe pain, increased swelling, ecchymosis, limited ROM, and a slow and shortened stride length during gait.

Initial rehabilitation should consist of ice, compression, NSAIDs, and rest in a position of comfort (Fig. 28-24). An assistive device may be utilized if gait is too painful. As pain decreases, interventions should focus on return of full ROM and stretching of all adjacent musculature (Figs. 28-6, 28-25, and 28-26). Modalities may be utilized as needed to aid in pain reduction and tissue healing.[56,57] Progression to strength and aerobic training should be implemented with emphasis on

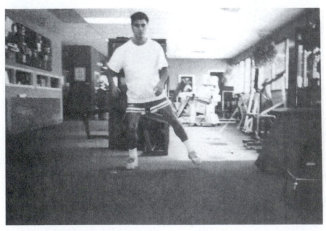

FIGURE 28-22

Plyometric exercise 2.

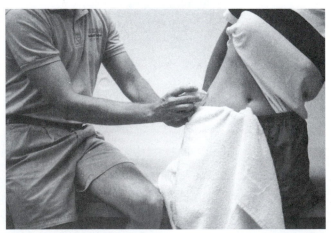

FIGURE 28-24

Hip ice massage.

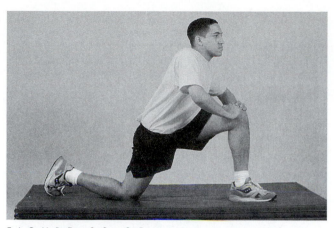

FIGURE 28-25

Hip flexion stretch.

pain-free activity. As pain continues to subside, activities should be increased with a transition to sport-specific training. With a return to sports a protective pad will be worn to prevent reinjury to the area.

Quadriceps Contusion

PATHOMECHANICS

Because the quadriceps muscle is in the front of the thigh, a direct blow to the area that causes the muscle to compress against the femur can be very disabling.[1,31] A direct blow to the anterior portion of the muscle is usually more serious and disabling than a direct blow to the lateral quadriceps area because of the differences in muscle mass present in the two areas. Blood vessels that break cause bleeding in the area where muscle tissue has been damaged.[3] If not treated correctly or if treated too aggressively, a quadriceps contusion can lead to the formation of myositis ossificans (see Section "Myositis Ossificans" later in the chapter). Ice hockey players are especially susceptible to this injury due to the velocity of the puck and players causing high impact.

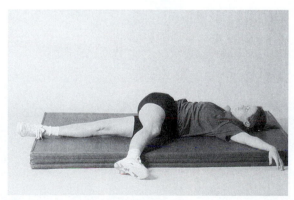

FIGURE 28-26

Hip abduction stretch.

At the time of injury, the patient may develop pain, loss of function to the quadriceps mechanism, and loss of knee flexion ROM. How forceful the blow was at the time of injury will determine the grade of injury.

INJURY MECHANISM

A patient with a grade I contusion may present a normal gait cycle, negative swelling, and only mild discomfort on palpation. The patient's active knee flexion ROM while lying prone should be within normal limits. Resistive knee extension while sitting and lying supine with the knee bent over the end of a table may not cause discomfort.

A patient with a grade II contusion may have a normal gait cycle. Attempting to continue activity will likely cause the injury to become progressively disabling. If the gait cycle is abnormal, the patient will splint the knee in extension and avoid knee flexion while bearing weight because the knee feels like it will give out. This patient may also externally rotate the extremity to use the hip adductors to pull the leg through during the swing-through phase. This move may be accompanied by hiking the hip at push-off, which causes tilting of the pelvis in the frontal plane. Swelling may be moderate to severe, with a noticeable defect and pain on palpation. While the patient is lying prone, AROM in the knee may be limited, with possibly only 90° of motion. Resistive knee extension while sitting and lying supine with the knee bent over the end of a table may be painful, and a noticeable weakness in the quadriceps mechanism may be evident.

A patient with a grade III contusion may herniate the muscle through the fascia to cause a marked defect, severe bleeding, and disability. The patient may not be able to ambulate without crutches. Pain, severe swelling, and a bulge of muscle tissue may be present on palpation. When the patient is lying prone, knee flexion AROM may be severely limited. Active resistive knee extension while the patient is sitting and lying supine with the knee bent over the end of a table may not be tolerated, and severe weakness may be present. If a grade III quadriceps contusion is diagnosed, a possible fracture should be ruled out.[58]

REHABILITATION CONCERNS AND PROGRESSION

A patient with a grade I quadriceps contusion should begin ice and 24-hour compression immediately. Twenty-four hour compression should be continued until all signs and symptoms are absent. Gentle, pain-free quadriceps stretching exercises (see exercises shown in Figs. 28-6 and 28-25) may be performed on the first day. The knee should be braced in full available flexion to avoid the accumulation of blood and prevent myositis ossificans. Progressive resistive strengthening exercises may also be performed as soon as possible, usually on the second day, in the order given and pain-free (see exercises in Figs. 28-15 and 28-16 to 28-27) flexion with knee both extended and flexed (see exercises in Figs. 28-17 to 28-28), and isokinetics (see exercises in Figs. 28-7 and 28-10). This patient's AROM should be carefully monitored. A patient with a grade I quadriceps contusion may try to continue normal activities, but compression and

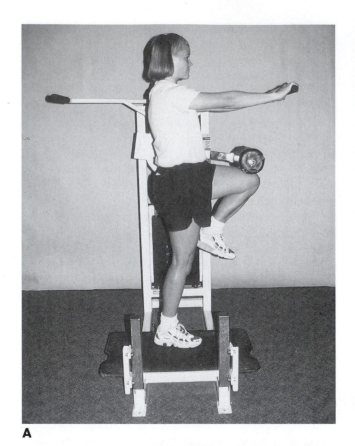

A

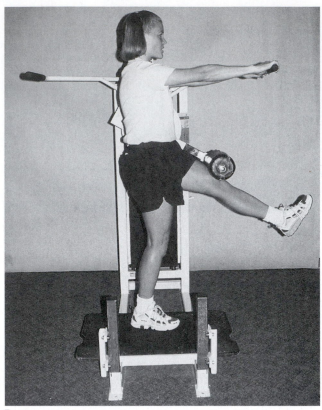

B

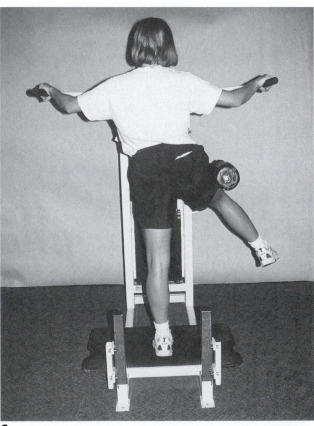

C

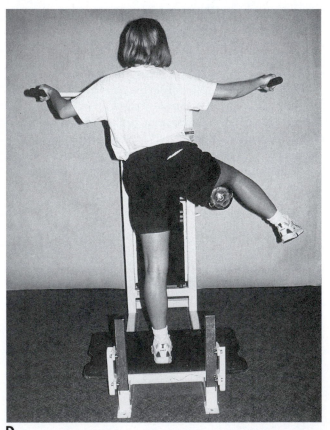

D

F I G U R E   2 8 - 2 7

Multihip strengthening.

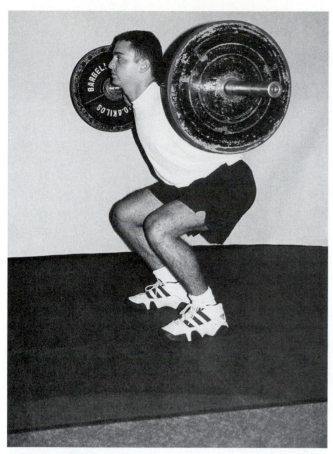

FIGURE   28-28

Squat.

protective padding should be worn until the patient is symptom free.

A patient with a grade II contusion should be treated very conservatively. Crutches should be used until a normal gait can be accomplished free of pain. Ice, 24-hour compression, and electrical muscle stimulation modalities may be started immediately to decrease swelling, inflammation, pain, and to promote ROM.[29] Compression should be applied at all times to minimize bleeding into the area. Pain-free quadriceps isometric exercises may be performed as soon as possible, usually within the first 3 days. Between days 3 and 5, ice is continued with pain-free AROM while the patient is sitting and lying prone. AROM lying supine with the knee bent over the end of a table can be added. Passive stretching is contraindicated at this time and not used until the later phases of rehabilitation. Massage and heat modalities are also contraindicated in the early phases because of the possibility of promoting bleeding and eventually myositis ossificans. At approximately day 5, the patient may perform straight leg raises without weights and then progress to weights, pain free (see exercise in Fig. 28-15). As AROM increases and approaches 95°–100° of knee flexion, swimming, aquatic therapy, and biking may be performed if the seat height is adjusted to the patient's available ROM. Between days 7 and 10, heat in the form of hot packs, ultrasound, or whirlpool may be used, as long as swelling is absent and the patient is ap-

proaching full AROM while lying prone. Pain-free quadriceps progressive resistive strengthening exercises may be performed in the order given (see exercises in Figs. 28-15 to 28-27), flexion with knee both extended and flexed (see exercises in Figs. 28-17 to 28-28), and isokinetics (see exercises in Figs. 28-7 and 28-10) may be added. Ice or heat modalities, with AROM, should be continued before all exercises as a warm-up. Pain-free quadriceps stretching exercises should not be rushed and can be started between 10 and 14 days as needed (see exercises in Figs. 28-6 and 28-25). A patient with a grade II quadriceps contusion may require 3-21 days for rehabilitation, depending upon the severity of the injury. Jogging, slide board (see exercise in Figs. 28-3), plyometrics (see exercises in Figs. 28-21 to 28-23), and functional activities may be used after the 14th day. Compression and protective padding should be worn during physical activity until the patient is symptom free.

A patient with a grade III quadriceps contusion should use crutches, rest, ice, 24-hour compression, and electrical muscle stimulation modalities immediately to decrease pain, bleeding, and swelling and to counteract atrophy.[29] The patient may begin pain-free isometric quadriceps exercises between days 5 and 7. Ice and 24-hour compression should be continued from the very first day through day 7, with pain-free AROM exercises, while the patient is sitting and lying prone, added about day 7. AROM lying supine with the knee bent over the end of a table can also be added. At approximately day 10, the patient may perform straight leg raises without weights and then progress to weights by day 14 (see exercise in Fig. 28-15). Electrical muscle stimulation may be very helpful in this phase to counteract muscle atrophy and reeducate muscle contraction. Again, as AROM increases and approaches 95°–100° of knee flexion, swimming, aquatic therapy, and biking may be performed if the seat height is adjusted to the patient's available ROM. After day 14, the patient may use heat in the form of hot packs or whirlpool, as long as the swelling has decreased and the patient has gained AROM. At approximately the third week of rehabilitation, pain-free quadriceps progressive resistive strengthening exercises may be performed in the order presented (see exercises in Figs. 28-15 to 28-27), flexion with knee both extended and flexed (see exercises in Figs. 28-17 to 28-28), and isokinetics (see exercises in Figs. 28-7 and 28-10). Pain-free quadriceps stretching may also be performed (see exercises in Figs. 28-6 and 28-25) if the patient is careful not to overstretch the quadriceps muscles. A patient with a grade III quadriceps contusion may require 3 weeks to 3 months for rehabilitation. In general, at approximately week 3, the patient may begin jogging, slide board (see exercise in Fig. 28-3), plyometrics (see exercises in Figs. 28-21 to 28-23), and functional activities. Again, compression and protective padding should be worn during all competition until the patient is symptom free.[59]

Myositis Ossificans

PATHOMECHANICS AND INJURY MECHANISM

With a severe direct blow or repetitive direct blows to the quadriceps muscles that cause muscle tissue damage, bleeding, and injury to the periosteum of the femur, ectopic bone production may occur.[1,21] In 3–6 weeks, calcium formation may be seen on X-ray films. If the trauma was to the quadriceps muscles only and not the femur, a smaller bony mass may be seen on radiographs.[1]

If quadriceps contusion and strain are properly treated and rehabilitated, myositis ossificans can be prevented. Myositis ossificans can be caused by trying to "play through" a grade II or III quadriceps contusion or strain and by early use of stretching exercises into pain, ultrasound, and other heat modalities.[60]

REHABILITATION CONCERNS AND PROGRESSION

After 1 year, surgical removal of the bony mass may be helpful. If the bony mass is removed too early, the trauma caused by the surgery may actually enhance the condition.

After radiographic diagnosis, intervention should follow that for a grade II or III quadriceps contusion or quadriceps strain (see treatment and rehabilitation for grade II and III quadriceps contusions and strains).[59] The bony mass usually stabilizes after the sixth month.[18] If the mass does not cause disability, the patient should be closely monitored and follow the treatment and rehabilitation programs outlined in grade II and III quadriceps contusions and strains. It has also been recommended that myositis can be treated using acetic acid with iontophoresis.[39]

HIP DISLOCATION

The capsule and ligaments of the hip joint permit little or no distraction even upon strong traction forces. The joint is also very difficult to traumatically dislocate (unlike the glenohumeral joint). Under circumstances where the joint surfaces are neither maximally congruent nor in a closed-pack position, the hip joint is at risk for traumatic dislocation. This position of particular vulnerability occurs when the hip joint is flexed, internally rotated and adducted.[7] In this position, a strong force up the femoral shaft toward the joint may push the femoral head out of the acetabulum. This is found predominantly in motor vehicle accidents due to the seated position of an individual within the car. Upon a head on collision the dashboard provides the load down the femoral shaft dislocating the hip joint.

While rare in athletics, two general categories of hip dislocation exist: anterior and posterior.[61] Anterior dislocations compose only 10 percent of cases and occur in contact sports as a result of a violent force that send the hip into extension, abduction, and lateral rotation.[24,62] The more prevalent posterior dislocation occurs with excessive loads applied to a flexed, adducted, and internally rotated joint. This mechanism is found also in contact sports where the athlete has a high-speed uncontrolled fall onto a flexed knee such as in a gang tackle.

When a posterior dislocation is sustained, the athlete presents with severe pain in the hip region with inability to walk or move the involved leg. The affected limb will appear shortened, flexed, adducted, and internally rotated. Of great concern with this injury is the compromise of hip vascularity and the close relationship of the sciatic nerve. These two components make hip dislocations a medical emergency. The dislocated hip can occlude the lateral circumflex artery, which is the primary provider of circulation to the femoral head. This reduced flow can lead to avascular necrosis of the femoral head. Adults whose hips are reduced within 8 hours from the time of injury have a low incidence of avascular necrosis. Those whose reduction occurred longer than 8 hours have up to approximately a 40-percent chance of this complication.[51] Stretching or compression of the sciatic nerve as a result of this injury may lead to paralysis of hamstrings and muscularity distal to the knee that is innervated by the nerve.[63]

Medical treatment includes rapid reduction and hospitalization along with possible traction or immobilization in a hip splica cast until the joint is pain free, which is approximately 1–3 weeks. Following this initial time line, rehabilitation will begin with simple assisted ROM to maintain normal flexibility. Pain-free use of isometrics or muscular stimulation can be utilized to prevent excessive atrophy and aid in muscular reeducation acutely (see exercises in Figs. 28-29 and 28-30).[56,57] Crutch ambulation with progressive weight bearing is implemented with advancement to gait normalization. Progressive resistance exercises can begin with return of painless ROM and

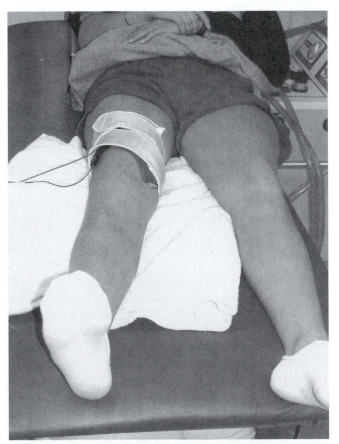

FIGURE 28-29

Quadriceps set with assisted electric stimulation.

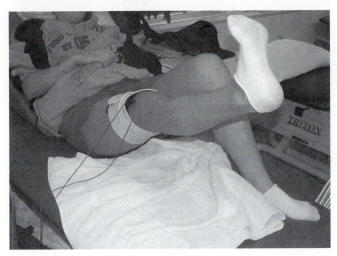

FIGURE 28-30

Straight leg raise with assisted electric stimulation.

concentration focused on proximal hip musculature (see exercises in Figs. 28-2, 28-14, 28-15, 28-19, and 28-31). Advancement of exercise can progress as tolerated and with pain-free motions.

Labral Tears

PATHOMECHANICS AND INJURY MECHANISM

The acetabular labrum is a fibrocartilage ring around the rim of the acetabulum, located in the socket of the hip joint. It has the job of increasing the congruency of the hip joint, acting as a shock absorber during weight bearing.[64] The acetabular labrum can be torn if there is a twisting movement while the hip joint is bearing weight, and it frequently occurs during soccer activity. Golfers and ice hockey players are also susceptible to labral tears that can result in arthritis if not treated, according to a study reported at the annual meeting of the Radiological Society of North America in Chicago.

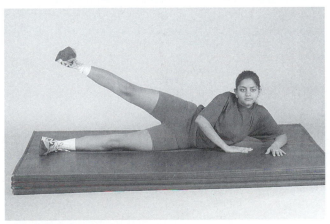

FIGURE 28-31

Hip abduction.

The onset of pain is immediate and usually located at the front of the hip joint. As with all hip problems, the pain may become diffuse and difficult to pinpoint. If the front of the hip joint is affected, there may be a pinching sensation when the patient flexes the hip by bringing the knee up to the chest. A mechanical catching or giving way sensation in the hip may also occur. Symptoms usually occur when the hip is changing position. The pain may be reproduced in sport during activities that require concomitant weight bearing and twisting, i.e., driving a golf ball.[65]

Labrum tears can be the result of an underlying anatomic abnormality of the hip. Since a torn labrum not only causes pain and instability but also disturbs the mechanical function of the hip in its own right and predisposes to arthritis, a symptomatic labral tear is an indication for treatment both to prevent arthritis and improve symptoms. Nonoperative treatment of labral tears can be successful if the tear is small and stable. If nonoperative means are not successful, the results of hip arthroscopy have to be reported to be good.[66] A return to sports is usually possible between 2 and 3 months after the operation.

Although hip arthroscopy usually can allow symptom-relieving trimming of the torn labrum in a minimally invasive way, if the torn labrum occurred because of an underlying anatomic abnormality in the hip, it is usually advisable to correct the underlying anatomic hip abnormality first.[67]

REHABILITATION CONCERNS AND PROGRESSION

An emerging surgical trend hip arthroscopy is becoming more common, especially among athletes. The application of this minimally invasive technique, combined with advances in MRI, is considered a significant advancement in treating many forms of chronic hip injuries. Although the surgery is new and emerging, the rehabilitation progression should take into consideration the basic science principles of soft-tissue healing (Table 28-3).

Following surgery, the patient is instructed to use bilateral crutches with partial weight bearing as tolerated for the first 2 weeks. Then, they are progressed to one crutch for 1 week, until they regain normal gait. Gait training to restore normal gait is paramount at this point in the rehabilitation. Some surgeons utilize a hip brace to restrict hip flexion ROM. During the second week, the patient may also begin some easy pool walking and stationary biking without resistance (exercise in Fig. 28-32).

Independent ambulation is encouraged at the 3-week mark. Aerobic activity is increased to 30 minutes along with the activation of active assistive hip ROM exercises. Any explosive movements or rotational hip torque could potentially damage the hip capsule and labrum and are therefore to be avoided. During the first 4 to 6 weeks, pain-free exercise is recommended to avoid a synovitis, tendonitis, or overstretching.

At 2 weeks postoperatively, light hip isotonics and more weight-bearing exercises such as bridges and single-leg bridges are initiated (see exercises in Figs. 28-2, 28-14, 28-19, 28-31, and 28-33). Strengthening of the hip extensors, abductors, and external rotators are emphasized along with light stretching

T A B L E   2 8 - 3

Arthroscopic Hip Labral Repair Rehabilitation Guidelines

Weight bearing (WB) status	Foot flat with 20 lb of pressure Duration 2–4 weeks
Continuous passive motion (CPM)	Start 30°–70° Increase as tolerated 0°–90° Duration 2 weeks
Sleeping	Ace wrap feet when sleeping for 2 weeks
Brace	Daytime use Set at 0°–90° of hip flexion
Stationary bicycle	Immediate postoperatively 1–2 times/day × 15–20 minutes Avoid pinching in front of hip by setting seat high
Pool exercises	Begin postoperative day 14 or as soon as sutures are removed and wound is healed
Range of motion	Examine stool internal rotation—day 3 (may push early internal rotation within pain limits) Examine stool external rotation—day 7 (limit to 30° enternal rotation) 2–3 sets × 12–15 repetitions Quadriceps rocking—day 7 AROM—within limits of brace or as tolerated if no brace is worn PROM—within available pain-free limits after brace is removed

Strength	Quad sets/ankle pumps—day 1
	Isometrics in neutral day 7 (within painful limits)
	Bridges—day 7–10
	Isotonic weight equipment day 14
	    Except for leg press begin at 6 weeks
	    Shuttle/pilates begin at 3–4 weeks dependent on WB
	Trunk Strength
	    Transverse abdominus
	    Side supports
	    Trunk and low-back stabilization as tolerated

Function	No straight leg raises for 4 weeks May begin pool walking in chest-high water Avoid antalgic gait Be aware of weakness of gluteus medius, side supports, and transverse abdominus strength in sagittal, coronal, and transverse planes
Balance	As soon as WB is permitted begin working on both double and single leg balance with eyes open and eyes closed 10 repetitions × 5 seconds is a good place to start

General considerations
- Typically requires 3 months of supervised therapy
- **Month 1: tissue healing phase (1–2 × per week)**

Goals:	Pain control Decrease tissue inflammation Decrease swelling Maintenance of motion (flexion 0°–90°; internal rotation as tolerated; enternal rotation 0°–30°)

- **Month 2: early functional recovery (2–3 × per week)**

Goals:	Full PROM Progress to full AROM Early strength gains Avoid flexor tendonitis and abductor tendonitis

Continued

TABLE 28-3

(Continued)

• **Month 3: late functional recovery (2–3 × per week)**

Goals: Advance strength gains—focus on abductor and hip flexor strength
                                Balance and proprioception
                                Continue to monitor for development of tendonitis
                                Progress to sport-specific activity in months 3 and 4 depending on strength
                                Do not progress to running until abductor strength is equal to contralateral side
                                Progression to sport-specific activities requires full strength return and muscle coordination

Precautions

                                • Avoid anything which causes either anterior or lateral impingement
                                • Be aware of low-back of sacroiliac joint dysfunction
                                • Pay close attention for the onset of flexor tendonitis and abductor tendonitis
                                • Patients with preoperative weakness in proximal hip musculature are at increased risk
                                  for postoperative tendonitis
                                • Modification of activity with focus on decreasing inflammation takes precedent if
                                  tendonitis occurs

for hamstrings, hip flexors, quadriceps, and the iliotibial band (ITB). The straight leg exercise is avoided until the forth week following surgery, due to potential for high compressive loading (see exercise in Fig. 28-15). ROM is pushed for internal rota-tion but progressed more slowly for external rotation. Trunk strengthening is begun at this time with emphasis on the trans-verse abdominals and the back extensors.

At 6 weeks, the patient begins light internal-external hip-rotation stretching, which marks the first time stretches that are introduced to the postoperative hip beyond the AROM (see stretches in Figs. 28-34 to 28-36). Eight weeks following surgery, lower-extremity strength work, which included squats, Romanian dead lifts, four-way hip exercises, lunges, and lat-eral step work, is initiated (see exercises 28-17, 28-18, 28-37, and 28-38). The lifting program emphasizes lighter weights and higher repetitions and is designed to build endurance and avoid positions that could potentially aggravate the hip. Avoid any-thing that causes either anterior or lateral impingement. The physical therapist should be aware of overlapping condition

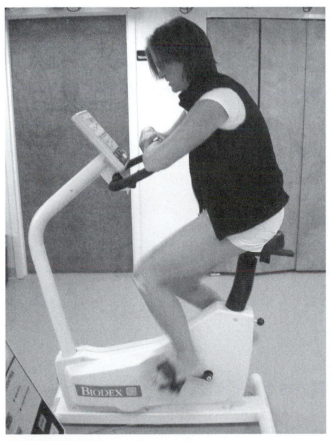

FIGURE 28-32

Stationary bike.

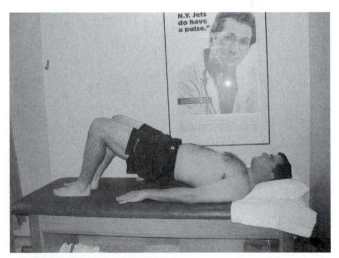

FIGURE 28-33

Bridges.

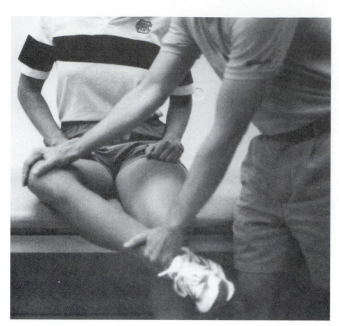

F I G U R E   2 8 - 3 4

Hip IR stretch.

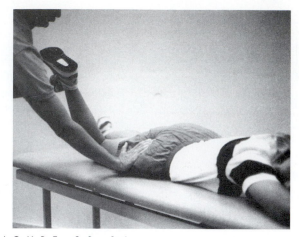

F I G U R E   2 8 - 3 6

Piriformis prone.

such as low-back pain and sacroiliac dysfunction. In addition, monitoring for the onset of flexor tendonitis and abductor tendonitis can help prevent failures. Keep in mind that patients with preoperative weakness in proximal hip musculature are at increased risk for postoperative tendonitis.[67]

Following hip arthroscopy, patients should avoid weight-bearing twists and turns on the hip for up to 3 months after surgery. Although not evidence based, similar to a healing meniscus, this compression with rotation is likely not beneficial to a healing labrum of patients in age groups and of all occupations. It is recommended that patients attempt to keep

their movements within the midline, certainly for a 6-week period. They can then gradually introduce rotational movements to the hip, but such movements must be under their own control. Rotational therapeutic exercises should start with non-weightbearing exercises and progress cautiously to full weight bearing (refer to exercises in Figs. 28-39 and 28-40). At the 3–4

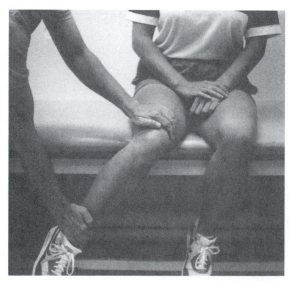

F I G U R E   2 8 - 3 5

Hip ER stretch.

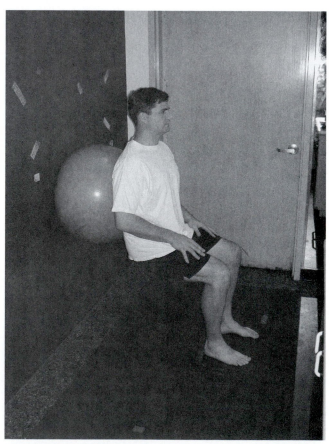

F I G U R E   2 8 - 3 7

Ball squats.

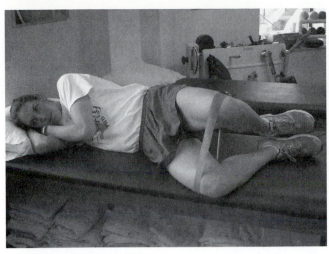

FIGURE   28-38

Clam shells.

month point, assuming no set-backs, patients are allowed to return to unprotected, full activities provided full strength and coordination have returned.

INCIDIOUS INJURIES

Bursitis

Bursae are lined with synovium and are synovial fluid filled sacs that exist normally at sites of friction between tendons and bone as well as between these structures and the overlying skin.[51] It is analogous to filling a balloon with oil and rubbing it between your fingers. The purpose of the bursae is to dissipate friction caused by two or more structures moving against one another.[8] The development of a bursitis is the product of one of two mechanisms. The most common being inflammation secondary to excessive friction or shear forces as a result of overuse. Posttraumatic bursitis is the other mechanism, and

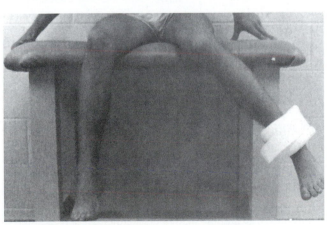

FIGURE   28-39

Straight hip IR.

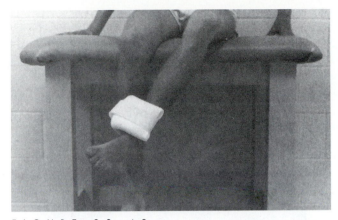

FIGURE   28-40

Straight hip ER.

stems from direct blows and contusions that cause bleeding in the bursae with resultant inflammation. The three major bursae around the hip joint that are susceptible to bursitis are the iliopsoas bursa, ischial bursa, and the greater trochanteric bursa.

TROCANTERIC BURSITIS

The greater trochanteric bursa lies between the gluteus maximus, tensor gascia lata, and the surface of the greater trochanter. Its location on the lateral aspect of the hip exposes it to contact injuries in sports such as football, soccer, and ice hockey. More commonly though it is seen in the clinic as an overuse injury found in runners, bikers, and cross-country skiers. It may also be found in individuals with an increased Q-angle, prominent trochanters, or a leg-length discrepancy. It is the repetitive motion of hip flexion and extension on an excessively compressed bursa that gives rise to irritation and inflammation. This can occur with tightness in tissues around the hip, for example the ITB pulling across the hip, or hip adductors bringing the thigh into a more midline position. Poor running mechanics or continuous running on banked surfaces that brings the lower extremity into an increased adducted position can also cause undo strain at the hip.

Signs and symptoms of trochanteric bursitis include warmth and reported pain at the greater trochanter region of the hip. Pain with hip abduction resistance, palpable tenderness at lateral hip, pain with gait and possible swelling or ecchymosis at the surface of the greater trochanter, as well as pain with lying on affected side may be present.[68,69]

Intervention begins by taking a thorough history from the patient to determine activity level, length of onset, or mechanism of possible traumatic incident. Examination is then performed to check for ROM, tenderness, tightness, and weakness in surrounding soft-tissue structures. It is necessary to analyze gait and stair patterns as well as possibly analyzing running mechanics if subjective complaints warrant.

Initial home rehabilitation for the individual will consist of rest, ice, and non-steroidal anti-inflammatories. Clinical

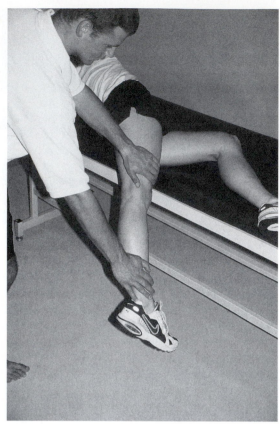

FIGURE 28-41

ITB stretch.

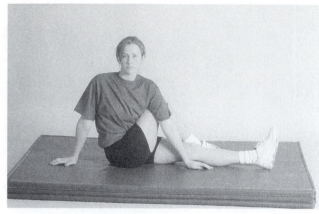

FIGURE 28-42

Self ITB.

ILIOPSOAS (ILIOPECTINEIAL) BURSITIS

Iliopsoas (*iliopectineal*) bursitis is most often due to excessive activity. It is thought to be irritated by the iliopsaos muscle passing over the iliopectineal eminence. This rubbing may also be associated with a snapping hip. Pain is reported in the inguinal area and can radiate into femoral triangle. Associated palpable tenderness can be present by placing the hip in flexion and external rotation. This position can also help relieve symptoms. Treatment includes the rest, NSAIDs, and stretching of the iliopsoas (see stretches in Figs. 28-6 and 28-25). Strengthening of any muscle imbalances can be initiated in pain-free arcs (see exercises in Figs. 28-2, 28-14, 28-15, 28-19, and 28-31).

Snapping Hip Syndrome

Snapping hip syndrome (*coxa saltans*) can arise from two different sources: intra-articular and extra-articular. Intra-articular causes include loose bodies, osteocartilaginous exotosis, labral tears, synovial chondromatosis, and subluxation of the hip. More common though is the extra-articular causes of a "snapping hip." This occurs primarily when, but not exclusively to, the ITB snapping over the greater trochanter during hip flexion and extension. Hip adduction and knee extension will tighten the ITB and accentuate the snapping sensation. This continuous pathomechanical movement can lead directly to trochenteric bursitis. A second extra-articular source comes from the iliopsoas tendon as it passes just in front of the hip joint. This tendon can catch on the pelvic brim (iliopectineal eminence) and cause a snap when the hip is flexed.[71]

This syndrome is common in ballet dancers where 44 percent of reported hip pain involved a snapping or clicking. Most complaints concerned the sensation with only one-third reporting pain.[72] The condition can present itself with specific flexion movements of the thigh such as sit-ups. Both have signs and symptoms of an audible snap or click either laterally or anterior deep in the groin which may or may not be painful. They may also present with an associated bursitis.

treatment will emphasize modalities for inflammation, i.e., ultrasound, stretching of appropriate structures such as the ITB and adductors (see exercises in Figs. 28-4, 28-5, and 28-41), as well as slow integration into progressive resistive exercises for encompassing hip musculature (see exercises in Figs. 28-2, 28-14, 28-15, 28-19, and 28-31).[57,70] If the underlying cause is due to a leg-length discrepancy, it should be corrected with the appropriate device. Upon normalization of ROM and flexibility, a gradual return to sport-specific activities should be implemented. Full return to sports should emphasize prevention with a regular stretching program (see stretching in Fig. 28-42) or appropriate padding for traumatic injuries.

ISHIAL BURSITIS

Ischial bursitis while uncommon may occur as a complication of an injury to the hamstring insertion into the ischial tuberosity or as a direct trauma to a fall or hit. The symptoms include pain while sitting and localized tenderness. It is important to distinguish this bursitis from a hamstring tear at the origin. Initial treatment consists of rest, ice, and NSAIDs. Sitting cushion may be utilized as needed. General stretching of the hamstrings and progressive resistant exercises are implemented as pain subsides (see stretching in Figs. 28-11 to 28-13 as well as exercises in Figs. 28-2, 28-14, 28-15, 28-19, and 28-31).

Treatment for a patient with snapping hip syndrome begins with a thorough examination. During the subjective evaluation, the clinician must question the patient to determine which actions exacerbate symptoms during daily activities and athletics. The objective examination is designed to determine the severity of pathology and to perform a biomechanical assessment. The information gathered in this portion of the examination can be used to guide specific elements of the treatment program. Muscle-tendon length and strength, joint mobility testing, and palpation of the injured area are key to a proper examination. Biomechanical assessment of the patient includes both static (posture) and dynamic (gait/functional movement) elements. Perform static inspection of the entire lower extremity. Particular areas of attention during this portion of the examination include observation of genu recurvatum, knee flexion contracture, biomechanical abnormalities of the foot, hip flexion contracture, and the amount of internal or external rotation present in the lower extremity during static stance. Also take note of leg length. Gait analysis allows the clinician to confirm the findings of static examination and observe if a movement dysfunction is present. Functional movements (e.g., squatting, stair accent/descent) may further demonstrate to the clinician the severity of the movement dysfunction.[72]

Once identification of contributing factors has been completed, treatment can be directed toward those factors. Intervention during the acute phase consists of standard anti-inflammatory care and the elimination of activities that exacerbate symptoms. Physical therapy modalities (e.g., ice, ultrasound, electrical stimulation, iontophoresis) may be used during this time.[56,57] Activity modification depends on the severity of the pathology. Crutches may be used in severe cases, while simply decreasing the time and intensity of the aggravating activity is commonly used in less severe cases. Muscle weakness and/or tightness in the thigh or pelvis is addressed with a strengthening and stretching program (see exercises in Figs. 28-2, 28-14, 28-15, 28-19, and 28-31 and stretches in Figs. 28-42 and 28-43). Biomechanical abnormalities of the foot may require an orthotic to assist with foot stabilization or control (refer to Chapter 31). Leg length deformities commonly require a lift in the shoe to assist with balancing the entire lower extremity. For those patients with a symptomatic snapping hip and trochanteric bursitis unresponsive to conservative therapy, a surgical procedure has been described as an effective method of treatment in this specific population.[73]

OSTEITIS PUBIS

The anterior connection between the two pubic bones of the pelvis creates the pubic symphysis. This along with the sacroiliac joint completes the closure of the pelvic ring. Generally, there is little motion at this joint. Excessive forces, however, may occur to produce injury or dislocation. Osteitis pubis is the result of inflammation at the pubic symphysis. It is most often encountered in postoperative patient who have undergone invasive procedures around the pelvic region. In athletes, this pathology may present as a type of overuse injury or stress frac-

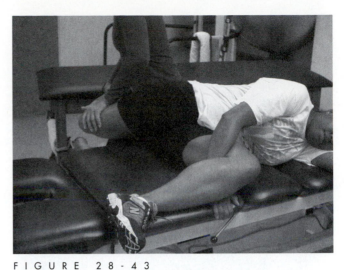

FIGURE 28-43
Passive Ober's stretch.

ture. It is seen mainly in distance runners, soccer players, and in other sports requiring pivoting and kicking. The constant repetitive force at the symphysis can be the cause of inflammation and pain. The stress may also be caused by traction on muscles whose origins arise from the pubis symphysis region.[24]

Patients report pain in the groin region that may radiate down the medial thigh and is exacerbated with sporting activities. There is palpable tenderness over the pubic symphysis and statements of clicking or popping with various movements. Pain may also be present during normal gait, stair climbing, or lying on ones side. The examination should focus on subjective and objective findings as well as the effects that occur on other *activities of daily living* (ADL).[74]

Early treatment involves rest and the use of NSAIDs.[75] As pain subsides, intervention should concentrate on the deficits found and pelvic stabilization. Closed-chain exercises may be started for stabilization prior to moving to open-chain motions (see exercises in Figs. 28-17, 28-33, 28-37, 28-44, and 28-45 to 28-48). Because the inflammation may be due to traction at muscular origins, exercises should be modified based off subjective complaints of discomfort. Corticosteroid injection may be utilized if symptoms do not resolve with noninvasive treatment.[76]

APOPHYSITIS

Apophysitis is an inflammatory response to overuse and chronic traction at an apophysis in athletic children (see discussion of avulsion fractures). The injury is characterized with an insidious onset and palpable tenderness at the bony landmark. There may or may not be accompanying swelling present. Treatment will consist of relative rest from high-intensity activity with management of inflammation and pain. Graded progression of flexibility with open- and closed-chain strengthening activities implemented (see exercises in Figs. 28-2, 28-14, 28-15, 28-17, 28-19, 28-31, 28-33, 28-37, and 28-44). With a cessation of pain, a return to sports program begins. Training is tailored

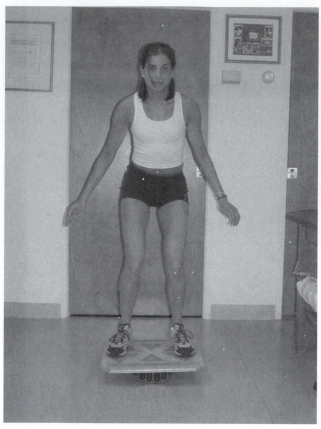

FIGURE 28-44

Balance board stability training.

for specific sports and monitored for the return of pain and irritation. If this is encountered, training is reduced to pain-free levels.

FEMORAL NECK STRESS FRACTURE

Bone is a specialized type of connective tissue that is capable of only a limited number of reactions to a large number of abnormal conditions. The basic nature of these reactions is best considered at a microscopic or cellular level. There are just four basic ways in which bone can react to abnormal conditions: (1) local death, (2) an alteration in bone deposition, (3) alteration in bone reabsorbtion, and (4) mechanical failure (fracture). Wolf's law states that intermittent stresses applied to bone result in architectural remodeling to allow adaptation to the new mechanical environment.[51] Thus bone is in a constant state of change with bone deposition being completed by osteoblasts while at the same time allowing for bone reabsorbtion by osteoclasts. This dynamic remodeling is based on applied stresses that occur in response to weight bearing and muscle contractions. Thus maintenance of healthy bone mass and structure relies on a balance between osteoclastic and osteoblastic activity.[77]

A stress fracture is a metabolic event in which an overuse repetitive injury exceeds the intrinsic ability of the bone to repair itself.[78,79] It is this stage where osteoclastic activity exceeds osteoblastic activity and leads to a stress fracture.[80–82] While femoral neck stress fractures are rare, representing only 5 percent of all stress fractures, they do commonly occur in endurance athletes.[83,84] It is often associated with participation in sports involving running, jumping, or other lower-extremity repetitive stress.

Two types of stress fractures can occur in the femoral neck. They are described as transverse, which presents on the tension side of the neck, or compression fractures, which occur on the medial side of the femoral neck.[85] The tension fractures have a poor prognosis and are treated aggressively with open reduction and internal fixation. The fractures on the compression side heal well and respond favorably to noninvasive treatment.[85]

This section will cover rehabilitation of compression femoral neck stress fractures. An athlete with a possible stress fracture will present with reports of pain in groin and thigh, which is exacerbated with activities. It is important to obtain a detailed history to pinpoint any increased training regimes

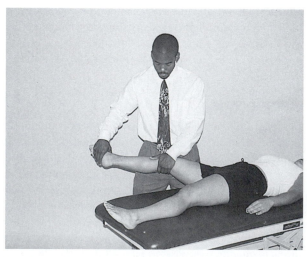
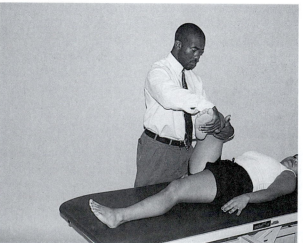

FIGURE 28-45

D1 flexion.

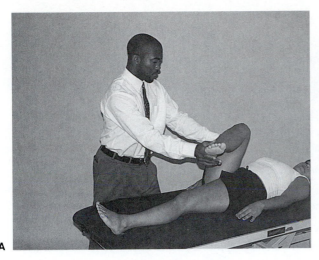
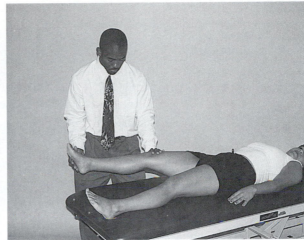

FIGURE 28-46

D1 extension.

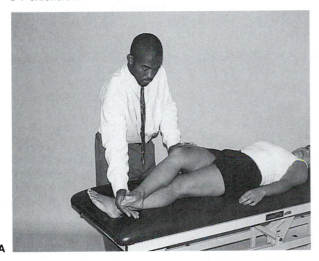
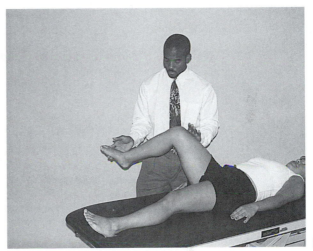

FIGURE 28-47

D2 flexion.

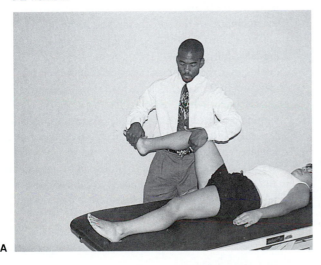
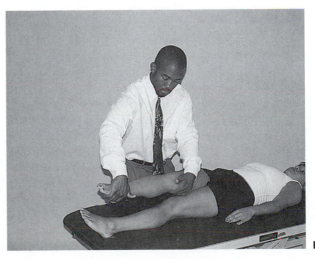

FIGURE 28-48

D2 extension.

TABLE   28-4

Protocol for Return to Running After a Hip or Pelvis Injury

RUNNING TIME MISSED (WEEK)	MODIFICATION OF RUNNING PROGRAM
<1	No modification of preinjury training
1–2	Decrease 25% from preinjury mileage
2–3	Decrease 50% from preinjury mileage first week, 25% second week
≥4	Week 1: Walk 1–2 miles, alternating 1 min fast and 1 min normal pace
	Week 2: Walk 2–3 miles, alternating 1.5 min jog with 1.5 min walk
	Week 3: If no pain occurs, substitute 10 min jog every other day in lieu of walk/jog, incorporate rest days as needed
	Week 4: Same as week 3, but increase jog to 15 min every other day in lieu of walk/jog
	Week 5: Jog 15 min and alternate with 25 min every other day, incorporate rest days as needed
	Week 6: Jog 20 min and alternate with 30 min every other day, incorporate rest days as needed
	Week 7: Jog 20 min and alternate with 35 min every other day, incorporate rest days as needed
	Week 8: Jog 20 min and alternate with 40 min every other day, incorporate rest days as needed
	Week 9: Resume training at preinjury level if training errors have been corrected

Adapted from James SL. Running injuries of the knee. *Instr Course Lect* 47:407–417, 1998.

or changes in gear or equipment used in the training program. The patient may have an antalgic gait pattern or possible lurch and a decrease in available ROM secondary to pain.

Initial treatment of a diagnosed fracture includes rest, ice, NSAIDs, and cessation of painful activity. ROM and progressive resistant exercises are carried out within pain-free limits (see exercises in Figs. 28-2, 28-14, 28-15, 28-19, and 28-31). Crutches with non-weightbearing ambulation can be prescribed until relief of pain in gait cycle. As pain reduces, a gradual increase from non-weightbearing to touchdown weight bearing to partial weight bearing to discontinuation of crutches is implemented. Utilization of cross training, or active rest, can be accomplished by activities such as water running, stationary bike riding, and upper-body ergometer training. Activity resumption requires recovery periods that allow for tissue healing and adaptation (see exercise in Figs. 28-17, 28-32, 28-37, and 28-44). A return to running should be initiated and monitored toward the end of rehabilitation. Training and rest days are key components in returning the athlete based off this injury etiology. See Table 28-4 for a return-to-running protocol. Increasing training volume by no more than 10 percent per week allows adaptation to mechanical stress as speed and intensity are gradually reintroduced.[24]

SUMMARY

- Soft-tissue injuries to the hip, thigh, and groin can be extremely disabling and often require a substantial amount of time for full rehabilitation.
- Early return after soft-tissue injury to the thigh often exacerbates the problem.
- Previous injury to the soft tissues about the hip and thigh predispose athletes to additional injury, especially if not rehabilitated fully.
- Pathologies of the acetabular labrum are more common than once thought and often treated with arthroscopic surgery and subsequent rehabilitation.
- Snapping or clicking hip syndrome occurs most commonly when the ITB snaps over the greater trochanter causing trochanteric bursitis.
- Hip dislocations are rare, but require careful rehabilitation in order to return the patient/client to full function.
- The femur is subject to stress fractures (uncommon) and avulsion fractures.
- Different patterns of injury exist in the skeletally mature (adult) patient than in the skeletally immature patient (children and adolescents).

- Protection after soft tissue injury is important to prevent further injury (padding, wrapping, compression shorts/ sleeves).

REFERENCES

1. Berend KR, Vail TP. Hip arthroscopy in the adolescent and pediatric athlete. *Clin Sports Med* 20(4):763–778, 2001.

2. Byrd JW, Jones KS. Hip arthroscopy in athletes. *Clin Sports Med* 20(4):749–761, 2001.

3. Culpepper MI, Niemann KM. High school football injuries in Birmingham, Alabama. *South Med J* 76(7):873–875, 878, 1983.

4. Gomez E, DeLee JC, Farney WC. Incidence of injury in Texas girls' high school basketball. *Am J Sports Med* 24:684–687, 1996.

5. DeLee JC, Farney WC. Incidence of injury in texas high school football. *Am J Sports Med* 20:575–580, 1992.

6. Anderson K, Strickland SM, Warren R. Hip and groin injuries in athletes. *Am J Sports Med* 29(4):521–533, 2001.

7. Norkin CC, Levangie PK. *Joint Structure and Function*, 2nd ed. Philadelphia, F.A. Davis Company, 1992.

8. Moore KL. *Clinically Oriented Anatomy*, 3rd ed. Baltimore, MD, Lippincott Williams & Wilkins, 1992.

9. Ganz R, Parvizi J, Beck M, Leunig M, Notzli H, Siebenrock K. Femoroacetabular impingement: A cause for osteoarthritis of the hip. *Clin Orthop Relat Res* 417(12):112–120, 2003.

10. Sahrmann, SA. *Diagnosis and Treatment of Movement Impairment Syndromes.* St. Louis, MO, Mosby, 2002.

11. lSmith ZK, Weiss EL, Lehmkuhl DL. *Brunstrom's Clinical Kinesiology*, 5th ed. 1996.

12. Lynch SA, Renstrom PA. Groin injuries in sport: Treatment strategies. *Sports Med* 28(2):137–144, 1999.

13. Emery CA, Meeuwisse WH, Powell JW. 1. Groin and abdominal strain injuries in the National Hockey League. *Clin J Sport Med* 9:151–156, 1999.

14. Ekstrand J, Gillquist J. The avoidability of soccer injuries. *Intl J Sports Med* 4:124–128, 1983.

15. Sim FH, Chao EY. Injury potential in modern ice hockey. *Am J Sports Med* 6(6):378–384, 1978.

16. Tegner Y, Lorentzon R. Ice hockey injuries: Incidence, nature and causes. *Brit J Sports Med* 25(2):87–89, 1991.

17. Tyler TF, Nicholas SJ, Campbell RJ, McHugh MP. The association of hip strength and flexibility on the incidence of groin strains in professional ice hockey players. *Am J Sports Med* 29(2):124–128, 2001.

18. Holmich P, Uhrskou P, Ulnits L, et al. Effectiveness of active physical training as treatment for long-standing adductor-related groin pain in athletes: Randomized trial. *Lancet* 353:339–443, 1999.

19. Kendall FP, McCreary EK. *Muscles: Testing and Function* 3:1983.

20. Renstrom P, Peterson L. Groin injuries in athletes. *Brit J Sports Med* 14:30–36, 1980.

21. Lynch SA, Renstrom PA. Groin injuries in sport: Treatment strategies. *Sports Med* 28(2):137–144, 1999.

22. Meyers WC, Ricciardi R, Busconi BD, et al. *Groin Pain in Athletes.* 1999, pp. 281–289.

23. Speer KP, Lohnes J, Garrett WE. Radiographic imaging of muscle strain injury. *Am J Sports Med* 21(1):89–96, 1993.

24. Anderson K, Strickland SM, Warren R. Hip and groin injuries in athletes. *Am J Sports Med* 29(4):521–533, 2001.

25. Tyler TF, Campbell R, Nicholas SJ, Donellan S, McHugh MP. The effectiveness of a preseason exercise program on the prevention of groin strains in professional ice hockey players. *Am J Sports Med* 30(5):680–683, 2002.

26. Jorgenson U, Schmidt-Olsen S. The epidemiology of ice hockey injuries. *Brit J Sports Med* 20(1):7–9, 1986.

27. Sim FH, Simonet WT, Malton JM, Lehn T. Ice hockey injuries. *Am J Sports Med* 15(1):30–40, 1987.

28. Lorentzon R, Wedren H, Pietila T. Incidences, nature, and causes of ice hockey injuries: A three year prospective study of a Swedish elite ice hockey team. *Am J Sports Med* 16:392–396, 1988.

29. Molsa J, Airaksinen O, Nasman O, Torstila I. Ice hockey injuries in Finland. A prospective epidemiologic study. *Am J Sports Med* 25(4):495–499, 1997.

30. Nielsen A, Yde J. Epidemiology and traumatology of injuries in soccer. *Am J Sports Med* 17:803–807, 1989.

31. Knapik JJ, Bauman CL, Jones BH, Harris JM, Vaughan L. Preseason strength and flexibility imbalances associated with athletic injuries in female athletes collegiate athletes. *Am J Sports Med* 19(1):76–81, 1991.

32. Orchard J, Marsden J, Lord S, Garlick D. Preseason hamstring muscle weakness associated with hamstring muscle injury in Australian footballers. *Am J Sports Med* 25(1):495–499, 1997.

33. Emery CA, Meeuwisse WH. Risk factors for groin injuries in hockey. *Med Sci Sports Exerc* 33(9):1423–1433, 2001.

34. Seward H, Orchard J, Hazard H. Collinson: Football injuries in Australia at the elite level. *Med J Australia* 159:298–301, 1993.

35. Garrett WE, Jr. Muscle strain injuries: Clinical and basic aspects. *Med Sci Sports Exerc* (22):436–443, 1990.

36. De Smet AA, Best TM. MR imaging of the distribution and location of acute hamstring injuries in athletes. *Am J Roentgenol* (174):393–399, 2000.

37. Wootton JR, Cross MJ, Holt KW. Avulsion of the ischial apophysis. The case for open reduction and internal fixation. *J Bone Joint Surg* 72B:625–627, 1990.

38. Arnason A, Sigurdsson SB, Gudmundsson A, Holme I, Engebretsen L, Bahr R. Risk factors for injuries in football. *Am J Sports Med* 32(1):5–16, 2004.

39. Verrall GM, Slavotinek JP, Barnes PG, Fon GT, Spriggins AJ. Clinical risk factors for hamstring muscle strain injury:

A prospective study with correlation of injury by magnetic resonance imaging. *Br J Sports Med* 35(6):435–439, 2001.

40. Baumhauer JF, Alosa DM, Renstrom AF, et al. A prospective study of ankle injury risk factors. *Am J Sports Med* 23:564–570, 1995.

41. Croisier JL. Factors associated with recurrent hamstring injuries. *Sports Med* 34(10):681–695, 2004.

42. Ekstrand J, Gillquist J. Soccer injuries and their mechanisms: A prospective study. *Med Sci Sports Exerc* 15(3): 267–270, 1983.

43. Heiser TM, Weber J, Sullivan G, et al. Prophylaxis and management of hamstring muscle injuries in intercollegiate football players. *Am J Sports Med* 12(5):368–370, 1984.

44. Dadebo B, White J, George KP. A survey of flexibility training protocols and hamstring strains in professional football clubs in England. *Br J Sports Med* 38(4):388–394, 2004.

45. Worrell TW, Smith TL, Winegardner J. Effect of hamstring stretching on hamstring muscle performance. *J Orthop Sports Phys Ther* 20(3):154–159, 1994.

46. Jonhagen S, Nemeth G, Eriksson E. Hamstring injuries in sprinters. The role of concentric and eccentric hamstring muscle strength and flexibility. *Am J Sports Med* 22(3):262–266, 2005.

47. Sherry MA, Best TM. A comparison of 2 rehabilitation programs in the treatment of acute hamstring strains. *J Orthop Sports Phys Ther* 34(3):116–125, 2004.

48. Nikolau P, Macdonald B, Glisson R, Seaber A, Garrett W. Biomechanical and histological evaluation of muscle after controlled strain injury. *Am J Sports Med* 15(1):9–14, 1987.

49. Frenette J, Cote CH. Modulation of structural protein content of the myotendinous junction following eccentric contractions. *Int J Sports Med* 21(5):313–320, 2000.

50. Mackey A, Donnelly A, Turpeenniemi-Hujanen T, Roper H. Skeletal muscle collagen content in humans following high force eccentric contractions. *J Appl Physiol* 97(1):197–203, 2004.

51. Salter RB. *Textbook of Disorders and Injuries of the Musculoskeletal System*, 3rd ed. Baltimore, MD, Williams and Wilkins, 1999.

52. Kujala UM, Orava S, Karpakka J, et al. Ischial tuberosity apophysittis and avulsion among athletes. *Int J Sports Med* 18(2):149–155, 1997.

53. Ly JQ, Bui-Mansfield LT, Taylor, DC. Radiologic demonstration of temporal development of bizarre parosteal osteochondromatous proliferation. *Clin Imaging* 28(3):216–218, 2004.

54. Mc Bryne AM, Jr. Stress fractured in runners. *Clin Sports Med* 4:737–752, 1985.

55. O'Kane JW. Anterior hip pain. *Am Fam Physician* 60(6): 1687–1696, October 15, 1999.

56. Hecox B, Mehreteab TA, Weisberg J. *Physical Agents: A Comprehensive Text for Physical Therapists.* Upper Saddle River, NJ, Prentice Hall, 1994.

57. Cameron MH. *Physical Agents in Rehabilitation: From Research to Practice.* Philadelphia, PA, WB Saunders, 1999.

58. Vanden Bossche L, Vanderstraeten G. Heterotopic ossification: A review. *J Rehabil Med* 37(3):129–136, 2005.

59. Berg E. Deep muscle contusion complicated by myositis ossificans (a.k.a. heterotopic bone). *Orthop Nurs* 19(6): 66–67, 2000.

60. Cetin C, Sekir U, Yildiz Y, Aydin T, Ors F, Kalyon TA. Chronic groin pain in an amateur soccer player. *Br J Sports Med* 38(2):223–224, 2004.

61. Chudick S, Answorth A, Lopez V, et al. Hip dislocations in athletes. *Sports Med Arthroscopic Rev* 10:123–133, 2002.

62. Scudese VA. Traumatic anterior hip redislocation. A Case Report. *Clin Orthop* 88:60–63, 1972.

63. Tennent TD, Chambler AF, Rossouw DJ. Poterior dislocation of the hip while playing basketball. *Brit J Sports Med* 32(4):342–343, 1998.

64. Keene GS, Villar RN. Arthroscopic anatomy of the hip: An in vivo study. *Arthroscopy* 10(4):392–399, 1994.

65. Byrd JW, Jones KS. Diagnostic accuracy of clinical assessment, magnetic resonance imaging, magnetic resonance arthrography, and intra-articular injection in hip arthroscopy patients. *Am J Sports Med* 32(7):1668–1674, 2004.

66. Byrd JW. Hip arthroscopy in athletes. *Instr Course Lect* 52:701–709, 2003.

67. Byrd JW, Jones KS. Prospective analysis of hip arthroscopy with 2-year follow-up. *Arthroscopy* 16(6):578–587, 2000.

68. Shbeeb MI, Matteson EL. Trochanteric bursitis (greater trochanter pain syndrome). *Mayo Clin Proc* 71(6):565–569, 1996.

69. Shbeeb MI, O'Duffy JD, Michet CJ, Jr, O'Fallon WM, Matteson EL. Evaluation of glucocorticosteroid injection for the treatment of trochanteric bursitis. *J Rheumatol* 23(12):2104–2106, 1996.

70. Gerber JM, Herrin SO. Conservative treatment of calcific trochanteric bursitis. *J Manipulative Physiol Ther* 17(4):250–252, 1994.

71. Schaberg JE, Harper MC, Allen WC. The snapping hip syndrome. *Am J Sports Med* 12(5):1984.

72. Reid DC. Prevention of hip and knee injuries in ballet dancers. *Sports Med* 6(5):295–307, 1988.

73. Zoltan DJ, Clancy WG, Jr, Keene JS. A new operative approach to snapping hip and refractory trochanteric bursitis in athletes. *Am J Sports Med* 14(3):201–204, 1986.

74. Fricker PA, Taunton JE, Ammann W. Osteitis pubis in athletes. Infection, inflammation or injury? *Sports Med* 12(4):266–279, 1991.

75. Batt ME, McShane JM, Dillingham MF. Osteitis pubis in collegiate football players. *Med Sci Sports Exerc* 27(5):629–633, 1995.

76. Holt MA, Keene JS, Graf BK, Helwig DC. Treatment of osteitis pubis in athletes. Results of corticosteroid infections. *Am J Sports Med* 23(5):601–606, 1995.

77. Junqueira LC, Carneiro J, Kelly RO. *Basic Histology*, 9th ed. New York, NY, Long, 1998.

78. Monteleone GP, Jr. Stress fractures in the athletes. *Orthop Clin North Am* 26:423–432, 1995.

79. Haverstock BD. Stress fractures of the foot and ankle. *Clin Podiatric Med Surg* 18:273–284, 2001.

80. Maitria RS, Johnson DL. Stress fractures. Clinical history and physical examination. *Clin Sports Med* 16(2):259–274, 1997.

81. Knapp ME. Late treatment of fractures and complications. 2. *Postgrad Med* 40(2):A113–A118, 1966.

82. Shin AY, Gillingham BL. Fatigue fractures of the femoral neck in athletes. *J Am Acad Orthop Surg* 5(6):293–302, 1997.

83. Volpin G, Hoerer D, Groisman G, Zaltsman S, Stein H. Stress fractures of the femoral neck following strendious activity. *J Orthop Trauma* 4:394–398, 1990.

84. Benell KL, Malcolm SA, Thomas SA, et al. Risk factors for stress fractures in track and field athletes. Twelve month prospective study. *Am J Sports Med* 24:810–818, 1996.

85. Fullerton LR, Snoway HA. Femoral neck stress fractures. *Am J Sports Med* 16:365–377, 1998.

CHAPTER 29

Rehabilitation of the Knee

Mark De Carlo and Ryan McDivitt

OBJECTIVES

After completing this chapter, the therapist should be able to do the following:

- Describe the applied anatomy of the lower extremity as it relates to the knee.
- Understand the functional biomechanics associated with normal function of the knee.
- Utilize a general rehabilitation progression when treating knee injuries.
- Integrate a comprehensive understanding of pathomechanics and mechanism of injury into the rehabilitation of ligamentous and meniscal injuries.
- Integrate a comprehensive understanding of pathomechanics and mechanism of injury into the rehabilitation of patellofemoral and extensor mechanism injuries.
- Justify the use of external supports to augment the rehabilitation process.
- Implement a functional progression to ensure safe return to activity.

FUNCTIONAL ANATOMY OF THE KNEE

A thorough understanding of functional anatomy is required to effectively evaluate and treat patients with knee pathologies. A comprehensive body of knowledge obtained from cadaveric studies and surgical observations has led to significant improvements in the management of patients with knee injury. This section will describe knee anatomy in a logical sequence, beginning with skeletal anatomy and progressing to the muscles, menisci, ligaments, and other related structural anatomy.

Skeletal Anatomy

FEMUR

The three bony components that comprise the knee include the femur, tibia, and patella (Fig. 29-1). The medial and lateral condyles form the distal aspect of the femur and articulate with the medial and lateral tibial plateaus. The anterior surface of the femoral condyles articulates with the posterior surface of the patella.

Although both femoral condyles are convex, each possesses distinct structural characteristics. The medial femoral condyle is longer in the sagittal plane and has greater surface area (Fig. 29-2). The increased length of the medial femoral condyle permits rolling and external rotation of the tibia during knee

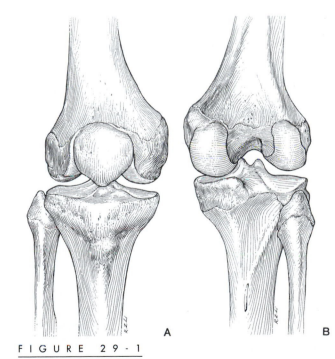

FIGURE 29-1

Bony components of the right knee. (Reproduced from Tria AJ, Jr, Klein KS. *An Illustrated Guide to the Knee.* New York, Churchill Livingstone, 1992, p. 4, with permission from Elsevier.)

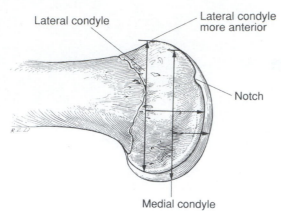

FIGURE 29-2

Increased length of the medial femoral condyle depicted by a lateral view of the right knee. (Reproduced from Tria AJ, Jr, Klein KS. *An Illustrated Guide to the Knee.* New York, Churchill Livingstone, 1992, p. 5, with permission from Elsevier.)

extension and contributes to the stability of the tibiofemoral joint in terminal extension. The medial femoral condyle angles away from the longitudinal axis of the femur at a valgus angulation of approximately 10° (Fig. 29-3). The lateral femoral condyle is wider in the frontal plane and narrower in the sagittal

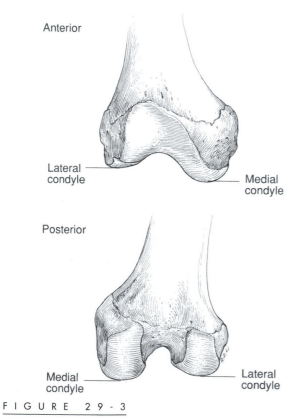

FIGURE 29-3

Angulation of the medial femoral condyle away from the longitudinal axis of the femur. (Reproduced from Tria AJ, Jr, Klein KS. *An Illustrated Guide to the Knee.* New York, Churchill Livingstone, 1992, p. 5, with permission from Elsevier.)

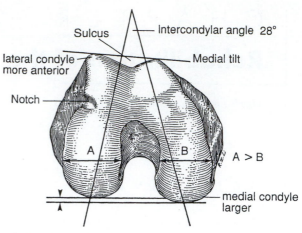

FIGURE 29-4

The lateral femoral condyle projects further anterior to provide a bony block to the patella. Also depicted is the increased frontal plane width of the lateral femoral condyle and length of the medial femoral condyle. (Reproduced from Tria AJ, Jr, Klein KS. *An Illustrated Guide to the Knee.* New York, Churchill Livingstone, 1992, p. 5, with permission from Elsevier.)

plane. In the longitudinal axis of the femur, the lateral femoral condyle projects anteriorly to act as a buttress against excessive lateral displacement of the patella (Fig. 29-4).

The medial and lateral femoral epicondyles protrude superiorly from the femoral condyles. These bony prominences contribute to medial–lateral stability of the knee by serving as attachment sites for the collateral ligaments. Lying anterior and inferior to the adductor tubercle, the medial epicondyle is the attachment site for the medial collateral ligament (MCL) and the medial head of the gastrocnemius (Fig. 29-5). The lateral

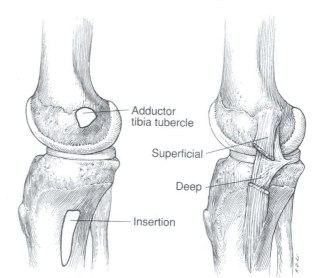

FIGURE 29-5

Attachment sites of the medial collateral ligament. (Reproduced from Tria AJ, Jr, Klein KS. *An Illustrated Guide to the Knee.* New York, Churchill Livingstone, 1992, p. 9, with permission from Elsevier.)

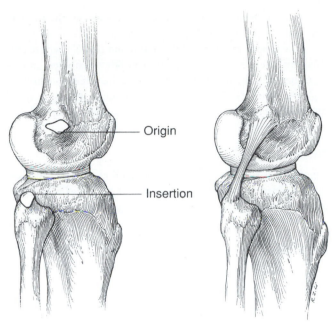

Attachment sites of the lateral collateral ligament. (Reproduced from Tria AJ, Jr, Klein KS. *An Illustrated Guide to the Knee*. New York, Churchill Livingstone, 1992, p. 9, with permission from Elsevier.)

femoral epicondyle provides an attachment site for the lateral collateral ligament (LCL), popliteus, and lateral head of the gastrocnemius (Fig. 29-6).

The anterior surface of the distal femur is characterized by the trochlea or central sulcus (Fig. 29-7). The central sulcus articulates with the posterior aspect of the patella to form the patellofemoral joint. Incongruency of the patellofemoral joint contributes to the inherent risk of patellar subluxation.

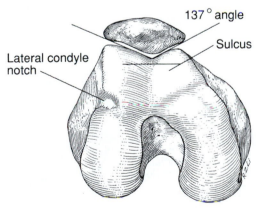

The trochlea of the distal femur articulates with the posterior surface of the patella. (Reproduced from Tria AJ, Jr, Klein KS. *An Illustrated Guide to the Knee*. New York, Churchill Livingstone, 1992, p. 7, with permission from Elsevier.)

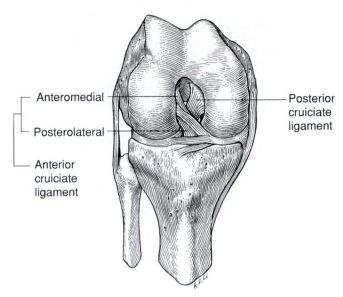

The cruciate ligaments attach to the walls of the intercondylar notch. (Reproduced from Tria AJ, Jr, Klein KS. *An Illustrated Guide to the Knee*. New York, Churchill Livingstone, 1992, p. 10, with permission from Elsevier.)

The intercondylar notch divides the medial and lateral femoral condyles. The cruciate ligaments cross and attach within this space. The anterior cruciate ligament (ACL) attaches to the lateral wall of the intercondylar notch, while the posterior cruciate ligament (PCL) attaches to the medial wall of the intercondylar notch (Fig. 29-8).

TIBIA

The tibial plateau, consisting of asymmetric medial and lateral surfaces, is relatively flat with a 9° posterior slope. The larger medial tibial plateau is oval and concave in both the frontal and sagittal planes. The lateral tibial plateau is concave in the frontal plane and flat to convex in the sagittal plane (Fig. 29-9).

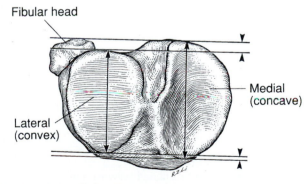

Superior view of the tibial plateau showing increased surface area of the medial tibial plateau. (Reproduced from Tria AJ, Jr, Klein KS. *An Illustrated Guide to the Knee*. New York, Churchill Livingstone, 1992, p. 6, with permission from Elsevier.)

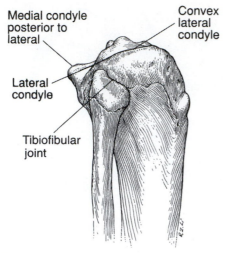

FIGURE 29-10

A posterolateral flare of the lateral tibial condyle articulates with the head of the fibula. (Reproduced from Tria AJ, Jr, Klein KS. *An Illustrated Guide to the Knee.* New York, Churchill Livingstone, 1992, p. 6, with permission from Elsevier.)

A posterolateral flare at the lateral tibial condyle accommodates articulation with the fibula (Fig. 29-10).

The tibial eminence lies between the medial and lateral tibial plateaus (Fig. 29-11). This roughened elevation projects superiorly in a compact linear shape. An anteroposterior depression in the tibial eminence is the attachment site for the ACL. During knee movement, the elevated tibial eminence positions itself in the intercondylar notch of the femur to provide bony stability to the tibiofemoral joint.

The tibial tuberosity lies anterior and inferior to the tibia plateau along the shaft of the tibia. This prominence is the insertion site for the extensor mechanism through the patellar tendon.

The articular surfaces of the femur and tibia are covered by thick hyaline cartilage, permitting smooth, frictionless movement between the femoral condyles and the tibial plateau during knee motion. The properties of articular cartilage help to dissipate the forces of joint compression caused during weight-bearing activity.

FIBULA

The fibula is situated posterior and lateral to the tibia and has limited function in weight bearing at the knee. The fibular head is an attachment site for muscles and ligaments, including the biceps femoris and LCL.

PATELLA

The patella is a triangular-shaped sesamoid bone that lies within the tendon of the extensor mechanism. The patella is the largest sesamoid bone in the body and serves a protective role for the knee joint. The patella's most important function is to increase the distance of the lever arm of the extensor mechanism from the joint axis, thereby enhancing the force production of the quadriceps by 15–30 percent.[46]

The anterior surface of the patella is widely vascularized, giving it a roughened appearance. The large superior pole of the patella accounts for approximately 75 percent of patellar height (Fig. 29-12). It protects the trochlea and femoral condyles from direct impact.

The posterior articular surface of the patella consists of three distinct facets (Fig. 29-13). A vertical ridge divides the posterior surface into medial and lateral patellar facets. The convex shape of the facet accommodates the concave trochlea. Each facet can be further divided into superior, middle, and inferior zones. The lateral facet is wider to accommodate the shape of the lateral femoral condyle. The medial facet is thicker

FIGURE 29-11

The tibial eminence is situated between the medial and lateral tibial plateau. (Reproduced from Tria AJ, Jr, Klein KS. *An Illustrated Guide to the Knee.* New York, Churchill Livingstone, 1992, p. 6, with permission from Elsevier.)

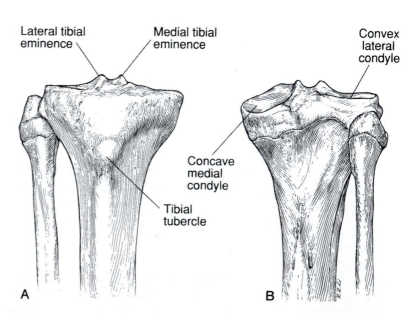

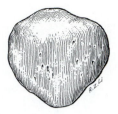

FIGURE   29-12

The superior pole of the patellar constitutes 75 percent of patellar height. (Reproduced from Tria AJ, Jr, Klein KS. *An Illustrated Guide to the Knee*. New York, Churchill Livingstone, 1992, p. 7, with permission from Elsevier.)

than its lateral counterpart. The medial and lateral facets are attachment sites for the joint capsule, patellofemoral ligaments, synovium, retinaculum, and vastus medialis and lateralis muscles, respectively. The third facet, considered the "odd" facet, lies medially and is separated from the inferior and medial zones by a small vertical ridge.

Hyaline cartilage covers the convex patellar surfaces and is approximately 4–5-mm thick; it is the thickest of any area in the body. This articular cartilage is designed to assist in smooth motion of the patella in the trochlea.

Muscular Anatomy

The muscular anatomy is most easily divided into quadrants corresponding to their anterior, posterior, lateral, or medial locations. These muscles create gross movement at the knee and provide dynamic protection to supporting structures of the tibiofemoral joint, including the ligaments and menisci.

ANTERIOR COMPARTMENT

The quadriceps muscle group comprises the largest portion of the anterior compartment of the knee and consists of four muscles: the rectus femoris, vastus medialis, vastus lateralis (VL), and vastus intermedialis. These muscles attach to the tibia through

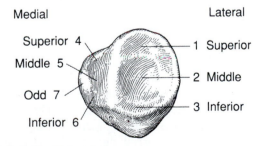

FIGURE   29-13

The posterior surface of the patella consists of a medial, lateral, and odd facet. (Reproduced from Tria AJ, Jr, Klein KS. *An Illustrated Guide to the Knee*. New York, Churchill Livingstone, 1992, p. 7, with permission from Elsevier.)

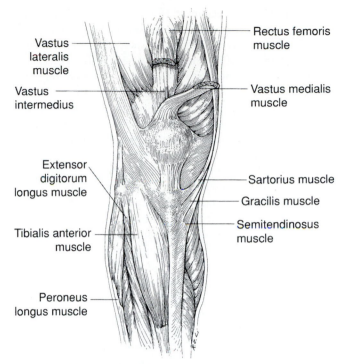

FIGURE   29-14

Anterior knee musculature depicting fiber direction of the vastus lateralis and vastus medialis muscles. (Reproduced from Tria AJ, Jr, Klein KS. *An Illustrated Guide to the Knee*. New York, Churchill Livingstone, 1992, p. 18, with permission from Elsevier.)

a common patella tendon and are innervated by the femoral nerve.

The most anterior of the quadriceps muscles is the rectus femoris, which originates from the anterior inferior iliac spine and the superior rim of the acetabulum. The three other heads border the rectus femoris distally. The rectus femoris, characterized as a two-joint muscle, performs both hip flexion and knee extension.

The VL, the largest head of the quadriceps muscles, originates on the anterior inferior greater trochanter, the intertrochanteric line, the lateral lip of the linea aspera, and the intermuscular septum. The fibers run in a 12°–15° lateral direction to the femur with a portion of the distal attachment terminating into the lateral retinaculum (Fig. 29-14).[54] Dominance of the VL along with tightness in the lateral retinaculum can result in excessive lateral displacement of the patella.

The vastus medialis originates at the lower end of the anterior intertrochanteric line, linea aspera, and intermuscular septum, while a division originates from the medial supracondylar line and adductor longus and adductor magnus tendon. The distal portion of the vastus medialis, the vastus medialis obliquus (VMO), has fibers that run in a 60°–65° medial direction to the femur.[54] The VMO together with the vastus medialis longus, which has a fiber direction of 15°–18° medial to the femur, primarily functions to maintain dynamic patellar alignment.

The vastus intermedialis originates on the anterior medial and lateral surfaces of the femoral diaphysis. Its fibers run almost entirely in a vertical direction and contribute to extension of the knee.

The quadriceps muscles converge into the superior pole of the patella and form the quadriceps tendon. Continuing distally, the patellar tendon extends from the inferior patellar pole to the tibial tuberosity. The tendon is widest at the apex of the patella and tapers slightly as it attaches into the tibial tuberosity.

The quadriceps eccentrically control knee flexion. In this mode of muscular contraction, the quadriceps absorb compressive forces and decelerate the weighted extremity. The fiber direction of the VMO serves to control patellar tracking through varying degrees of knee motion. Maintaining dynamic balance of the quadriceps is critical to limit the dominance of lateral structures.

The sartorius is also part of the anterior compartment and is innervated by the femoral nerve. It is a superficial, narrow muscle that is credited as being the longest muscle in the body. The sartorius originates from the anterior superior iliac spine and obliquely crosses the anterior thigh downward and medially to insert on the anterior medial aspect of the tibia. The sartorius, semitendinosus, and gracilis muscles form a common insertion on the tibia called the pes anserinus. The pes anserine bursa lies directly under these tendons and can be a source of irritation. As a two-joint muscle, the sartorius performs flexion, abduction, and external rotation at the hip and internally rotates the flexed knee.

POSTERIOR COMPARTMENT

The hamstrings comprise the posterior muscles of the knee (Fig. 29-15). These muscles include the semimembranosus, semitendinosus, and biceps femoris. With the exception of the short head of the biceps femoris, the hamstrings originate from the ischial tuberosity and are innervated by the tibial division of the sciatic nerve. The short head of biceps femoris originates from the posterolateral lip of the linea aspera and receives innervation by the peroneal division of the sciatic nerve.

The semimembranosus performs flexion and internal rotation of the knee and extension and internal rotation of the hip. It resists excessive hip abduction and external rotation of the tibia and provides dynamic support to the posterior capsule. The semimembranosus attaches on the anterior medial aspect of the medial tibia and sends a slip to the posterior horn of the medial meniscus. During knee flexion, the semimembranosus assists with retraction of the medial meniscus. The semitendinosus arises furthest posteriorly off the ischial tuberosity and attaches on the proximal medial tibia at the pes anserinus. The semitendinosus provides additional valgus stability to the knee, assists with flexion and internal rotation of the knee, and extends of the hip.

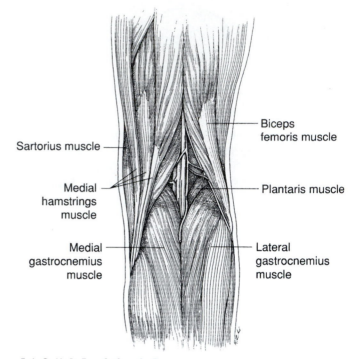

F I G U R E   2 9 - 1 5

Posterior knee musculature. (Reproduced from Tria AJ, Jr, Klein KS. *An Illustrated Guide to the Knee.* New York, Churchill Livingstone, 1992, p. 20, with permission from Elsevier.)

The biceps femoris resides on the lateral side of the posterior compartment, opposite to the semimembranosus and semitendinosus. The tendons of the short and long heads converge to travel distally and anteriorly, splitting around the inferior portion of the LCL and attaching at the fibular head and lateral tibial condyle. The biceps femoris externally rotates the tibia and contributes to knee flexion and hip extension. The biceps femoris also functions to prevent excessive adduction of the tibia and anterior displacement of the lateral tibial condyle, and provides dynamic support to the posterolateral knee.

Other posterior muscles that influence the knee joint are the popliteus and the gastrocnemius. The popliteus, innervated by the tibial nerve, arises from the anterior lateral femoral condyle and oblique popliteal ligament and inserts just proximal to the soleus muscle on the posterior tibia. This triangular-shaped muscle is the deepest muscle of the knee and provides dynamic support to the posterolateral capsule. The primary action of the popliteus muscle during weight bearing is external rotation of the femur and knee flexion, which enables the knee to unlock from terminal extension. During non-weightbearing activities, the popliteus internally rotates the tibia and flexes the knee.

The gastrocnemius consists of medial and lateral heads that originate from the posterior aspect of the medial and lateral

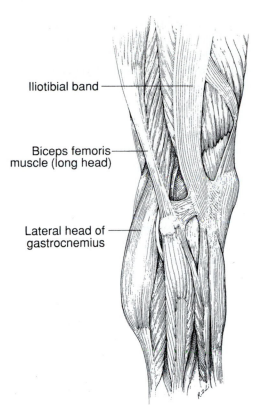

F I G U R E   2 9 - 1 6

Lateral knee musculature. (Reproduced from Tria AJ, Jr, Klein KS. *An Illustrated Guide to the Knee*. New York, Churchill Livingstone, 1992, p. 19, with permission from Elsevier.)

femoral condyles, adjacent femur, and joint capsule. The common tendon anchors into the posterior calcaneus. While the gastrocnemius is viewed primarily as an ankle plantar flexor, it also assists in knee flexion. The gastrocnemius is innervated either by separate branches of the tibial nerve to each head or by a common stem of the nerve.

LATERAL COMPARTMENT

The lateral compartment, consisting of the tensor fascia lata (TFL) and gluteus medius, plays an important role in knee function. The superior gluteal nerve supplies innervation to both muscles. The TFL originates from the external lip of the iliac crest and outer anterior superior iliac spine, while inserting into the iliotibial band (ITB). The ITB inserts on the lateral femoral condyle with fascial attachment to the lateral joint capsule, Gerdy's tubercle on the tibia, and fibula (Fig. 29-16). The TFL influences the biomechanics of the hip and patellofemoral joint mainly because of the relative flexibility of the ITB. A bursa lies between the ITB and lateral femoral condyle and can be a source of irritation secondary to soft tissue imbalances. The TFL flexes, abducts, and internally rotates the hip. The iliotib-

ial tract is an active knee extensor in the last 30° of terminal extension. It also serves as an active knee flexor and decelerator of knee extension beyond 30° of flexion.

The gluteus medius originates from the outer surface of the ilium between the iliac crest and the anterior and posterior gluteal line and inserts on the oblique ridge of the lateral aspect of the greater trochanter. While the primary action of the gluteus medius is hip abduction, function of the gluteus medius varies depending on which fibers are being activated. The anterior fibers internally rotate and flex the hip while the posterior fibers externally rotate and extend the hip. The gluteus medius acts as a primary stabilizer of the pelvis and influences the biomechanical relationship between the hip, knee, ankle, and subtalar joint.

MEDIAL COMPARTMENT

The hip adductor muscles are located in the medial compartment of the thigh and innervated by the obturator nerve. The majority of these muscles do not cross the knee joint or directly influence knee range of motion (ROM). The gracilis is the only hip adductor muscle that crosses the joint line by inserting on the proximal tibial diaphysis (Fig. 29-17). The gracilis is part of the pes anserinus complex and participates in hip

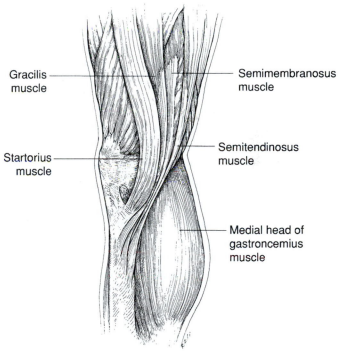

F I G U R E   2 9 - 1 7

Medial knee musculature. (Reproduced from Tria AJ, Jr, Klein KS. *An Illustrated Guide to the Knee*. New York, Churchill Livingstone, 1992, p. 19, with permission from Elsevier.)

adduction and internal rotation, tibial internal rotation, and knee flexion.

Meniscal Anatomy

The menisci are semilunar fibrocartilages that serve to absorb shock and transmit load in the tibiofemoral joint. The menisci increase the articular surface area during joint contact and provide joint lubrication through forced fluid circulation during weight bearing and non-weightbearing activities. In addition, the menisci restrain secondary motion and improve joint stability at the tibiofemoral joint by increasing the concavity of the tibial plateau. Joint geometry as well as meniscal attachment to the semimembranosus allows the menisci to move posteriorly during flexion and anteriorly during extension. Although often considered avascular, the peripheral rim of the menisci is vascularized by capillary extensions from the superior and inferior medial and lateral geniculate arteries (Fig. 29-18). Healing can occur in small, peripheral meniscal tears that receive adequate blood supply. The menisci obtain nutrients through compressive and distractive forces typical of normal knee kinematics during gait.

The medial meniscus is semicircular in shape with a wider posterior horn than anterior horn. It is approximately 3.5 cm in length, and approximately 30 percent of the peripheral rim is vascularized.[2] The anterior horn of the medial meniscus attaches into the intercondylar fossa of the tibia, the coronary ligament, and quadriceps expansion from the patella. The middle one-third of the meniscus attaches to the deep layer of the medial capsule. The posterior horn is attached to the posterior intercondylar fossa and semimembranosus tendon. The extensive capsular attachment to the medial meniscus allows approximately 6 mm of anteroposterior movement of the meniscus, resulting in a higher incidence of tears to the posterior horn.

The circular-shaped lateral meniscus covers more tibial plateau surface area than the medial meniscus (Fig. 29-19). The anterior horn of the lateral meniscus attaches firmly to the intercondylar fossa. Peripherally, it blends with the quadriceps expansion from the patella and coronary ligaments of the tibia. Posteriorly, it attaches to the popliteus tendon by way of the capsule. The posterior horn of the lateral meniscus attaches anteriorly to the intercondylar eminence of the tibia and posteriorly to the femur via the meniscus femoral ligaments. The middle one-third of the lateral meniscus has minimal capsular attachment, which allows approximately 12 mm of anterior–posterior meniscus movement.

Ligamentous Anatomy

Four main ligaments provide static stability to the knee and protect the knee from excessive tensile loads. The collateral ligaments provide passive restraint to the knee in the frontal plane while the cruciate ligaments provide passive restraint in the sagittal plane. To appreciate the structural complexity of the collateral ligaments, the layers of the capsular complex must

be identified. The capsular complex can be divided into three highly unified levels: the superficial aponeurotic level, the middle tendinous level, and the deep capsular level.

The MCL comprises the middle layer of the medial capsular complex, forming distinct vertical and oblique bundles (Fig. 29-20). The vertical fibers arise from the femoral epicondyle and descend to attach on the medial tibial border just posterior to the pes anserinus tendons. The oblique fibers lie posterior to the vertical fibers and have a common insertion on the femoral epicondyle. These fibers, however, insert inferior to the articular surface on the posterior medial aspect of the tibia.

The medial capsular complex protects the knee against excessive valgus forces. The superficial layers of the MCL are the first to sustain injury in a valgus stress. The fibers are taut in extension and relaxed in flexion. With tibial internal rotation, the fibers are positioned in a vertical manner and relaxed, whereas the fibers are oblique and taut in external rotation.

Hughston and Eilers[39] identified the posterior oblique ligament (POL) as a separate and distinct part of the medial capsular ligament complex (Fig. 29-21). These fibers traverse from the tibia in a superior and medial direction to their attachment on the femur. Hughston and Eilers[39] noted that the POL is the "keystone" of medial knee stability, with the semimembranosus offering dynamic medial support. When the knee is fully extended, the POL is taut. The vertical fibers of the MCL lose little tension during knee flexion because of the elliptical area of attachment on the medial epicondyle and its common flexion axis with the cruciate ligaments. In contrast, the POL is lax in flexion. It is reinforced dynamically during flexion by the semimembranosus, which provides support to the posteromedial capsule with valgus and external rotation forces.

The arcuate ligament is a thickening of the posterolateral capsule. The posterior aspect attaches to the fascia of the popliteal muscle and the posterior horn of the lateral meniscus. This arcuate ligament serves to reinforce the posterolateral joint capsule.

The LCL is a shorter bundle of fibers that attaches proximally near the lateral epicondyle of the femur and slopes posteriorly and inferiorly to the fibular head (Fig. 29-22). The LCL is taut from flexion to extension and offers protection against excessive varus stress of the knee during tibial rotation.

The cruciate ligaments cross within the intercondylar notch and are named for their attachment sites on the tibia (Fig. 29-23). The ACL lies in an anterior direction from the femur to tibia, whereas the PCL runs posteriorly from the femur to tibia. The cruciate ligaments, while contained within the joint capsule, are extrasynovial, with the synovial lining passing in front of the ligaments (Fig. 29-24).

The ACL attaches to the lateral femoral condyle and to the anterior medial tibial eminence in an oblique fashion. The tibial insertion is connected to the anterior horn of the medial meniscus. Various portions of this ligament are taut throughout the entire range of knee motion. The anteromedial bundle is taut in flexion while the larger posterolateral bundle is taut with the knee in extension. On average, the ligament is 4 cm in length

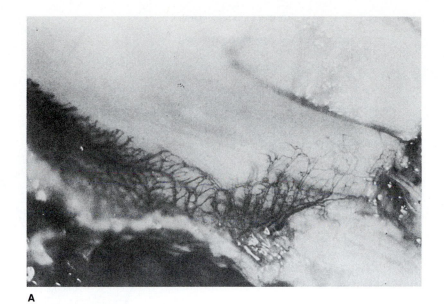

A

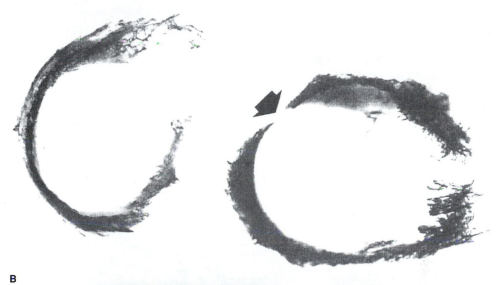

B

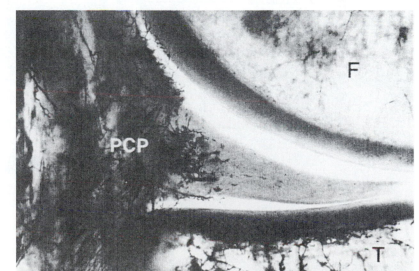

C

FIGURE 29-18

The menisci receive blood supply at the periphery. (Reproduced from Timm K. The knee. In: Richardson JK, Iglarsh ZA, eds. *Clinical Orthopaedic Physical Therapy*, Philadelphia, WB Saunders, 1994, pp. 409–410, with permission from Elsevier.)

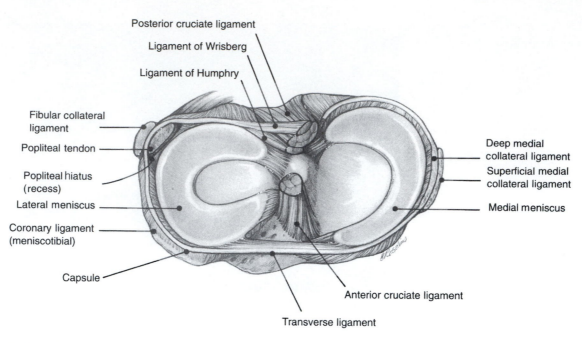

Posterior cruciate ligament

Ligament of Wrisberg

Ligament of Humphry

Fibular collateral ligament

Popliteal tendon

Popliteal hiatus (recess)

Lateral meniscus

Coronary ligament (meniscotibial)

Capsule

Deep medial collateral ligament

Superficial medial collateral ligament

Medial meniscus

Anterior cruciate ligament

Transverse ligament

FIGURE 29-19

Superior view of the circular-shaped menisci. (Reproduced from Scott WN. *The Knee.* St. Louis, MO, Mosby, 1994, p. 20, with permission from Elsevier.)

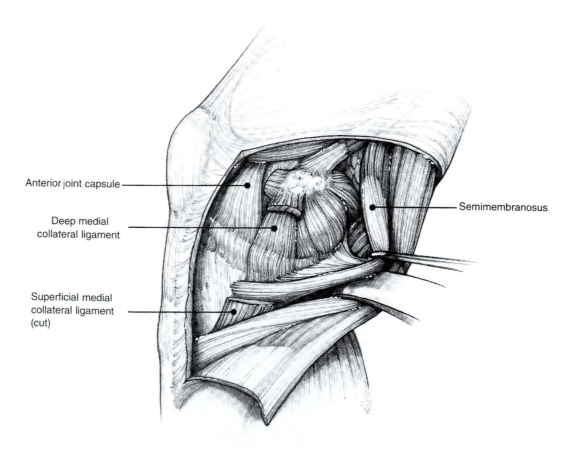

Anterior joint capsule

Deep medial collateral ligament

Superficial medial collateral ligament (cut)

Semimembranosus

FIGURE 29-20

Middle layer of the medial capsular complex. (Reproduced from Scott WN. *The Knee.* St. Louis, MO, Mosby, 1994, p. 37, with permission from Elsevier.)

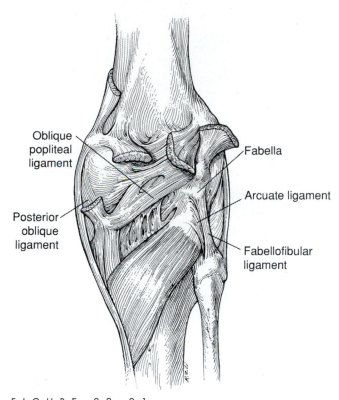

FIGURE 29-21

Posterior ligaments of the knee, including the posterior oblique and arcuate ligaments. (Reproduced from Tria AJ, Jr, Klein KS. *An Illustrated Guide to the Knee*. New York, Churchill Livingstone, 1992, p. 14, with permission from Elsevier.)

and 1 cm in thickness at the midsection.[31] The primary function of the ACL is to minimize anterior tibial translation and internal rotation of the tibia, consistent with the injury mechanism to this ligament. The ACL also serves as a secondary restraint for valgus/varus stress with collateral ligament damage.

The PCL originates from the medial femoral condyle and attaches to the middle to posterior portion of the tibial plateau. In contrast to the fibers of the ACL, the fibers of the PCL are oriented more vertically, primarily because of its high attachment in the intercondylar notch. The anterolateral bundle is taut in flexion while the posteromedial bundle becomes taut in extension. The PCL is designed to limit knee hyperextension and posterior tibial translation. It tends to be slightly thicker than the ACL, which may account for the lower incidence of injury to the PCL.

Related Structural Anatomy

The medial and lateral retinacula are defined sections of the anterior capsule of the knee joint. They originate from the patella of the vastus medialis and lateralis, respectively, and extend to the tibia. The medial and lateral retinacula each send

a slip transversely off the patella to form the medial and lateral patellofemoral ligaments (Fig. 29-25). The patellofemoral ligaments are generally thin, secondary to the stress relief provided by the dynamic support of the quadriceps. The thicker patellotibial ligaments receive no relief dynamically. The medial patellotibial ligament originates at the medial inferior patella and extends inferiorly to the tibia. The lateral patellotibial ligament connects the ITB distally to the patella proximally.[88] The lateral retinaculum, in conjunction with the lateral patellofemoral and patellotibial ligaments, dominates the medial stabilizing structures. The function of the medial retinacular system is to provide static restraint to excessive patellar mobility.

The infrapatellar fat pad lies deep to the patellar tendon. It extends superiorly to the peripatellar fold (middle portion) of the synovial membrane and can extend beyond the midpoint of the articular surface of the patella. The fat pad extends into the ligamentum mucosa posteriorly. The ligamentum mucosa is formed by the convergence of the medial and lateral aspects of the synovial lining. In full knee extension, the infrapatellar fat pad protrudes anteriorly on each side of the patellar tendon (Fig. 29-26) and is relatively mobile with connections to the menisci. It acts as a dynamic shock absorber and helps to distribute synovial fluid over the joint surface during knee flexion and extension.

PLICAE

The plicae (medial patellar, infrapatellar, and suprapatellar) are embryological remnants of synovial structures and serve no function in knee pathomechanics (Fig. 29-27). These structures are usually reabsorbed in early gestation, although sometimes this process is disrupted. Often, the plicae are clinically insignificant, although they can restrict joint flexion. The medial patellar plica can become thickened or inflamed if impingement occurs at the medial femoral condyle. The infrapatellar plica, also referred to as the ligamentum mucosum, is located in the intercondylar area of the knee just anterior to the ACL. It widens as it inserts distally into the fat pad. The inferior plica is the most common remnant and is usually asymptomatic. The suprapatellar plica is located at the posterior aspect of the quadriceps tendon.

FUNCTIONAL BIOMECHANICS OF THE KNEE

The study of biomechanics, along with functional anatomy, is a cornerstone to knee rehabilitation. A complete understanding of joint articulations, arthrokinematics, and the structures responsible for controlling movement is essential for the clinician to make sound decisions in the diagnosis and treatment of musculoskeletal disorders. Despite the relative simplicity of a hinge-type joint, the knee provides an interesting biomechanical study due to the intricacies required to maintain stability without good bony support along with attenuating forces greater

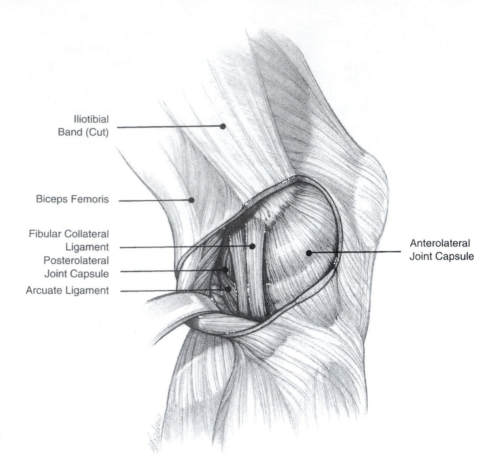

Iliotibial
Band (Cut)

Biceps Femoris

Fibular Collateral
Ligament
Posterolateral
Joint Capsule
Arcuate Ligament

Anterolateral
Joint Capsule

F I G U R E   2 9 - 2 2

Lateral stabilizers of the knee,
including the lateral collateral
ligament. (Reproduced from
Scott WN. *The Knee*. St. Louis,
MO, Mosby, 1994, p. 41, with
permission from Elsevier.)

than four times the weight of the body. The patellofemoral
joint and the pain syndromes often associated with the knee
also present an interesting study. A solid knowledge of the
supporting structures and stress placed on the patellofemoral
joint provide the framework for rehabilitation program
design.

Tibiofemoral Joint

TIBIOFEMORAL ARTICULATION: MENISCI-FEMORAL CONDYLES

The condyles of the distal femur articulate with the shallow,
concave tibial plateau, resulting in significant tibiofemoral joint

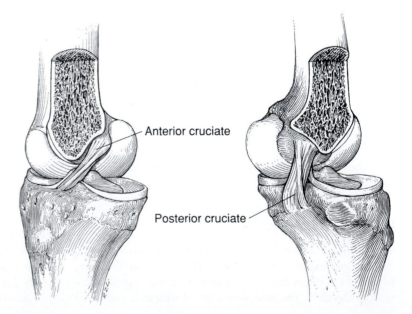

Anterior cruciate

Posterior cruciate

F I G U R E   2 9 - 2 3

Lateral cutaway view of the cruciate
ligaments. (Reproduced from Tria AJ, Jr, Klein
KS. *An Illustrated Guide to the Knee*. New
York, Churchill Livingstone, 1992, p. 11, with
permission from Elsevier.)

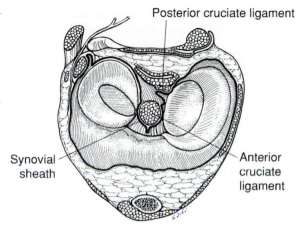

FIGURE 29-24

The synovial lining passes anterior to the extrasynovial cruciate ligaments. (Reproduced from Tria AJ, Jr, Klein KS. *An Illustrated Guide to the Knee.* New York, Churchill Livingstone, 1992, p. 10, with permission from Elsevier.)

incongruence. Tibiofemoral stability would be insufficient if left solely to the skeletal structure. The medial and lateral menisci provide additional congruency to the joint through their semicircular shape and peripheral thickness, thus forming a wedge surrounding the femoral condyles.

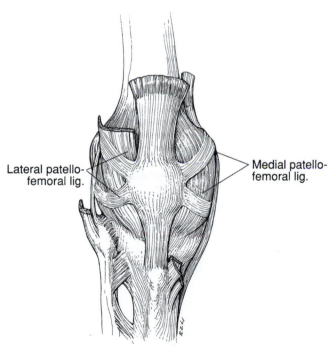

FIGURE 29-25

The medial and lateral patellofemoral ligaments are formed by the retinacula. (Reproduced from Tria AJ, Jr, Klein KS. *An Illustrated Guide to the Knee.* New York, Churchill Livingstone, 1992, p. 13, with permission from Elsevier.)

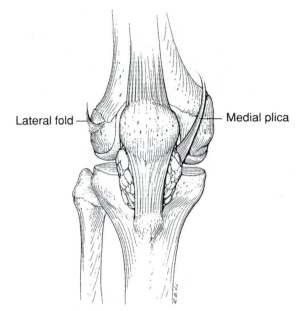

FIGURE 29-26

The fat pad protrudes to each side from under the patellar tendon in full extension. (Reproduced from Tria AJ, Jr, Klein KS. *An Illustrated Guide to the Knee.* New York, Churchill Livingstone, 1992, p. 17, with permission from Elsevier.)

The contact area of the menisci varies significantly during knee ROM. In weight bearing, the total contact area of the menisci decreases with knee flexion. Although mean surface area increases in non-weightbearing conditions, total menisci

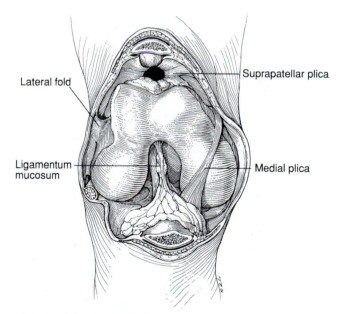

FIGURE 29-27

Synovial plicae viewed with the knee in flexion. (Reproduced from Tria AJ, Jr, Klein KS. *An Illustrated Guide to the Knee.* New York, Churchill Livingstone, 1992, p. 17, with permission from Elsevier.)

contact area also decreases during knee flexion. Following a meniscectomy, surface contact area decreases, resulting in a greater amount of stress upon the contact surface.

AXIAL FORCES

The ability of the tibiofemoral joint to withstand forces imposed by the superincumbent weight of the body combined with the ground reaction force transmitted through the distal extremity requires interaction of multiple structural factors. The longitudinal axis of the femur extends laterally to medially to the tibiofemoral articulation, resulting in an oblique angle formed 5°–10° away from vertical. It would seem that this alignment would produce a greater load on the lateral femoral condyle; however, a close look at the mechanical axis that connects the head of the femur with the superior surface of the talus contradicts this. The mechanical axis, which is the true line of weight bearing and determines the angle of force distribution, produces

approximately equal weight bearing on the lateral and medial compartments of the tibiofemoral joints during bilateral stance.

ARTHROKINEMATICS

Arthrokinematics is a description of the accessory motion that occurs between articulating surfaces. The accessory motions of rolling and gliding of the joint surfaces occur in combination during the osteokinematic motion at the knee. This combination allows the articulating surfaces to stay in contact and permit maximal osteokinematic motion.

Arthrokinematic motion plays a prominent role in sagittal plane movements of the tibiofemoral joint. During knee flexion in the closed kinetic chain (CKC), the convex femur moves on a fixed, concave tibia. When a convex surface is moving on a concave surface, rolling and gliding occur in opposite directions. Because of this relationship, the femur must glide anteriorly to counteract the posteriorly directed roll that is occurring (Fig. 29-28). Without the anterior glide of the femur, tibiofemoral

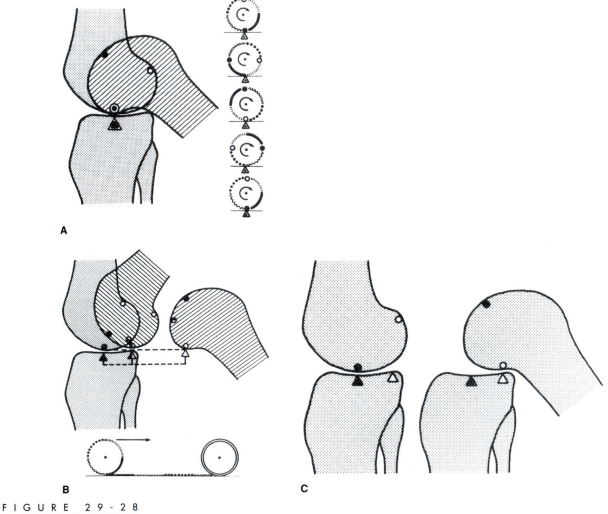

A

B

C

F I G U R E   2 9 - 2 8

Arthrokinematic motion. **A,** Anterior gliding of the femur on the tibia. **B,** Posterior rolling of the femur on the tibia. **C,** Both gliding and rolling. (Reproduced from Scott WN. *The Knee*. St. Louis, MO, Mosby, 1994, p. 77, with permission from Elsevier.)

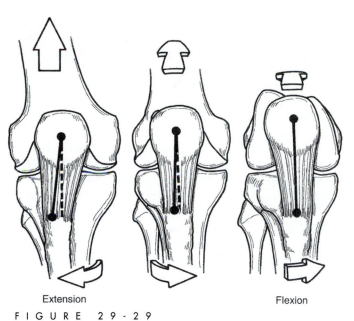

Extension   Flexion

FIGURE 29-29

The tibia externally rotates as the knee moves into terminal extension, creating a "screw-home" mechanism. (Reproduced from Scott WN. *The Knee*. St. Louis, MO, Mosby, 1994, p. 22, with permission from Elsevier.)

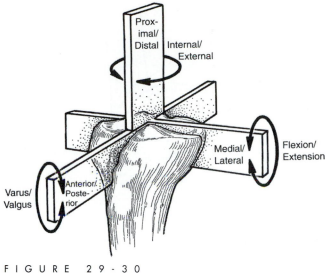

FIGURE 29-30

Knee motion in each plane occurs around an axis. (Reproduced from Scott WN. *The Knee*. St. Louis, MO, Mosby, 1994, p. 17, with permission from Elsevier.)

flexion would be limited, as the femur would roll off the posterior tibia. During CKC knee extension, the femur rolls anteriorly and glides posteriorly. In the open kinetic chain (OKC), the concave tibia moves on the convex femur as rolling and gliding occur anteriorly with extension and posteriorly with flexion.

Although rolling and gliding must both occur to keep the tibia and femur in contact, the rolling and gliding do not happen simultaneously as the knee flexes. At the initiation of flexion, pure rolling occurs between the joint surfaces, with gliding becoming more prominent to terminal flexion. Once the gliding starts in early flexion, the ratio between rolling and gliding is 1:2, progressing to a 1:4 ratio at terminal flexion.

Screw-home mechanism: Near terminal knee extension, arthrokinematic motion occurs in the transverse plane. Because the medial femoral condyle is 1–2 cm longer than the lateral femoral condyle, the lateral femoral condyle completes all of its motion when the knee is at 30° of flexion in a weight-bearing position. As the knee continues to extend and glide on the medial femoral condyle, it pivots on the fixed lateral femoral condyle, thus producing medial femoral rotation on the fixed tibia.

Rotation at terminal extension, called the screw-home mechanism (Fig. 29-29), is an involuntary motion that occurs because of bony geometry. The screw-home mechanism is crucial for knee stability, locking the tibiofemoral joint into a close-packed position. As the femur internally rotates on the fixed tibia, the femoral condyles become closely united and congruent with the menisci, the tibial tubercles becomes lodged in the intercondylar notch, and the ligaments become taut. For the tibiofemoral joint to flex from terminal extension, the joint must first unlock. While this is also an automatic motion caused by the bony structure of the femoral condyles, the popliteus can initiate the lateral rotation of the femur on a fixed tibia to begin the unlocking of the tibiofemoral joint.

KINEMATIC MOTION OF THE TIBIOFEMORAL JOINT

Flexion/extension: Tibiofemoral motion occurs in the three cardinal planes (Fig. 29-30). Flexion/extension, occurring in the sagittal plane, is the largest motion. Sagittal plane ROM varies among patients. De Carlo and Sell[19] reported that females average 6° of recurvatum to 143° of flexion and males average 5° of recurvatum to 140° of flexion. During sagittal plane motion, the instantaneous axis of rotation of the knee also varies. A study of a series of roentgenograms illustrated that the instantaneous axis of rotation forms a semicircle (Fig. 29-31).[49] An abnormal instantaneous axis of rotation can result from internal derangement in the tibiofemoral joint, causing a compensatory attenuation of static supporting structures of the knee. These abnormal stresses on the articulating surfaces can result in early degenerative changes.

Rotation: Motion in the transverse plane is influenced by the position of the knee in the sagittal plane. In the close-packed position (terminal extension), motion in the transverse plane cannot occur. Rotation is greatest at 90° of knee flexion. In this position, lateral rotation averages 45° and medial rotation averages 30°.[49] The axis for tibiofemoral rotation runs longitudinally through the medial tibial intercondylar tubercle.

Abduction/adduction: Only a small amount of tibiofemoral motion occurs in the frontal plane. Similar to rotation, this motion is dictated by the position of the knee in the sagittal plane. Abduction and adduction, primarily limited by ligaments, reach a maximum at 30° of knee flexion. The muscles do not contribute motion to the frontal plane.

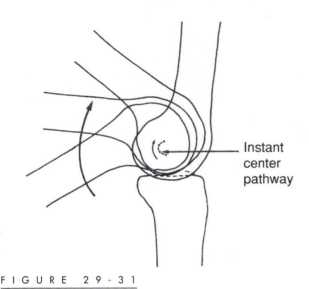

FIGURE   29-31

Normal instantaneous axis of rotation forms a semicircle. (Reproduced from Scott WN. *The Knee*. St. Louis, MO, Mosby, 1994, p. 76, with permission from Elsevier.)

KNEE STABILITY

Stability of the tibiofemoral joint is of primary concern in the orthopedic setting. Although the bony structures of the knee contribute to stability in terminal extension, the knee must rely on soft tissues for stability during most of the degrees of movement. Injury to these structures (the menisci, muscles, and ligaments) often results in debilitating instability.

A review of the literature related to knee stability reveals varied and often contradictory information on the roles of different support structures. The differences in results are because studies often test knee stability in a static scenario and in varied positions. Although describing the stabilizers individually provides a "clean and neat" presentation, one must remember that most of the structures work together to provide knee stability in all motions.

Menisci: The menisci contribute mainly to force distribution and dissipation, although they can provide a degree of stability to the tibiofemoral joint. Johnson et al.[44] have made clinical observations that joint laxity can result after meniscectomy. The belief that the medial and lateral menisci act as anterior and posterior wedges to prevent anteroposterior movement is supported by several studies which found that resection of the medial meniscus resulted in more instability than resection of the lateral meniscus.[52,53,86] The studies often found that resection of the ACL exposed a greater reliance on the menisci for stability, but that the medial supporting structures must be intact for more effective stability.

Muscular contributions: As the tibiofemoral joint becomes loaded, stability can be gained from multiple dynamic structures. The main muscular contributors to anteroposterior stabilization are the quadriceps, hamstring, gastrocnemius, and popliteus muscles. The quadriceps complex resists posteriorly directed forces on the tibia, while the hamstrings, gastrocne-

mius, and popliteus resist anterior displacement of the tibia. The popliteus and the semimembranosus, as a result of their multiple connections, are particularly crucial in the stability of the posterior tibiofemoral joint.

The muscles that contribute to medial stability as the knee flexes are part of the pes anserine complex (Fig. 29-32). The iliotibial tract, popliteus, and biceps femoris provide lateral stability (Fig. 29-33), but the popliteus is the main contributor, particularly in the posterolateral direction. It is uncertain what effect the dynamic structures have on rotational stabilization, but the position and action of the popliteus and hamstring muscles would suggest a minor contribution to rotational stability.

Ligaments and stability: The role of ligaments in knee stability has been widely substantiated in the scientific literature as well as by practical clinical observations of ligament disruption. Ligaments enhance knee stability by their ability to restrict tensile forces along the orientation of their fibers. Knee stability is reliant on multiple ligamentous, meniscal, muscular, or bony structures. This is an important factor to consider when studying the biomechanics of ligaments, because no ligament acts alone in limiting knee motion, nor does one ligament limit one plane of movement.

The MCL is the primary stabilizer against valgus stress. Studies in which the superficial fibers of the MCL were disrupted showed an increase in knee valgus following an externally directed force. The superficial fibers also limited external rotation of the tibia, whereas sectioning the deeper fibers of the MCL did not significantly increase valgus movement or external rotation.[37] Secondary restraints include the ACL, PCL (especially at terminal extension), and the lateral compartment due to the increased compressive forces.[76]

The LCL has been shown to be the primary restraint to varus forces. The restraining effect of the LCL increases as the knee flexes. The LCL's maximal contribution in limiting lateral joint opening is 69 percent at 25° of knee flexion. The ACL and PCL contribute as secondary stabilizers and provide maximal protection against varus forces at 8° of flexion, but then decrease as the knee flexes. The lateral joint capsule, particularly the posterior portion, contributes to stability, but this effect also decreases with increased knee flexion.[32] Other secondary restraints include the medial compartment through compression and the popliteus, ITB, and biceps femoris.

It has been well established that the ACL is the primary restraint to anterior translation of the tibia. The anteromedial and posterolateral bundles allow the ACL to be taut during all ranges of knee motion. At 90° of flexion, the ACL contributes 85 percent of the restraining force and this force increases up to 30° of flexion. Clinically, this property is demonstrated by the classic Lachman test that examines ACL integrity by placing an anteriorly directed force to the tibia with the knee in 20°–30° of flexion.[10] The MCL and LCL provide minimal secondary ligamentous support with other contributions from the posterior capsule, ITB, and hamstrings.

The PCL is responsible for restricting the majority (94 percent) or posterior tibial translation. If the PCL is not present,

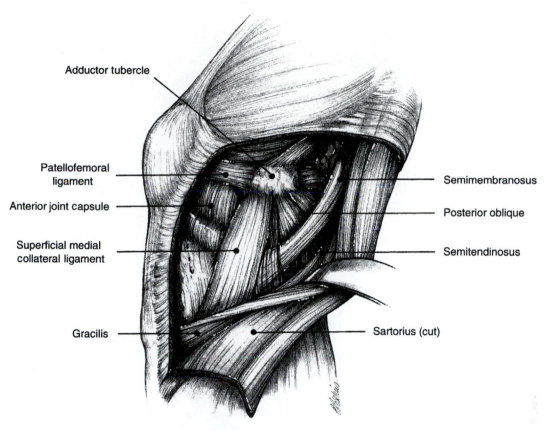

F I G U R E   2 9 - 3 2

Medial dynamic stabilizers of the knee. (Reproduced from Scott WN. *The Knee.* St. Louis, MO, Mosby, 1994, p. 36, with permission from Elsevier.)

the popliteus and posterolateral capsule provide most of the support, with minor contributions of the MCL, LCL, posteromedial capsule, and medial capsule.

As noted previously, ligaments limit movement in the direction of the fibers. Because there is not a ligament aligned in the transverse plane, it is evident that a combination of ligaments and other structures must work to restrict tibiofemoral rotation. The ACL has been shown to be the primary restraint of tibial internal rotation, with secondary restraint provided by the posteromedial capsule and the LCL.[55] The posterolateral capsule and the MCL are the primary restraints for external tibial rotation.

Patellofemoral Joint

FUNCTIONS OF THE PATELLA

The patella possesses very unique characteristics that are required for normal function of the knee. The patella functions to increase the distance (lever arm) from the joint axis, increase leverage of the quadriceps through gliding in the trochlear, provide a smooth articular surface, and provide a bony shield to the trochlea and condyles of the distal femur during knee flexion.

The length of the lever arm changes from knee flexion to extension, modulating the force production that the patella

provides. In full flexion, there is little anterior displacement of the quadriceps tendon. Thus, the patella contributes only 10 percent to the length of the lever arm in this position. As the knee extends, the patella migrates superiorly and anteriorly in the trochlear groove, leading to a greater mechanical advantage. The mechanical advantage reaches its peak at 45° of knee flexion, where the patella contributes 30 percent to the lever arm. As the knee nears terminal extension, the effect of the patella on quadriceps force (Fq) decreases to the point where the quadriceps muscles must generate 60 percent more force to perform the last 15° of knee extension. The inability of weakened quadriceps to perform this motion is demonstrated by a quadriceps lag during a straight-leg raise.

PATELLOFEMORAL CONTACT AREAS

As the knee goes through a ROM, various portions of the patella articulate with the trochlea (Fig. 29-34). Goodfellow et al.[33] described the contact surfaces of the patellofemoral joint at different points of knee flexion during weight-bearing conditions. At terminal extension, the patella lies slightly lateral and proximal to the trochlea without contact. The patella engages with the bony groove between 10°–20° of flexion. The area of contact is initiated at the inferior pole of the patella and moves superiorly on the retropatellar surface until 90° of flexion, where the major

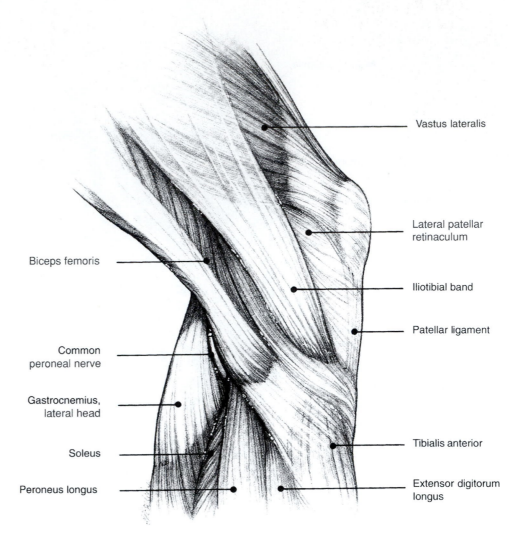

Vastus lateralis

Lateral patellar retinaculum

Iliotibial band

Patellar ligament

Biceps femoris

Tibialis anterior

Common peroneal nerve

Gastrocnemius, lateral head

Soleus

Extensor digitorum longus

Peroneus longus

F I G U R E   2 9 - 3 3

Lateral dynamic stabilizers of the knee. (Reproduced from Scott WN. *The Knee.* St. Louis, MO, Mosby, 1994, p. 40, with permission from Elsevier.)

contact point is on the superior pole. The contact of the patella from lateral to medial also varies with knee motion. During the first 90° of flexion, the contact is exclusively lateral. After 90°, the contact moves medially to the odd facet.

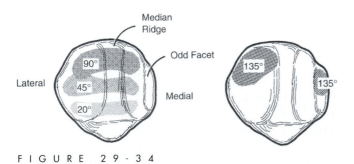

Median Ridge

Odd Facet

Lateral

90°

45°

20°

135°

135°

Medial

F I G U R E   2 9 - 3 4

Patellofemoral contact areas during varying degrees of flexion. (Reproduced from Scott WN. *The Knee.* St. Louis, MO, Mosby, 1994, p. 22, with permission from Elsevier.)

PATELLOFEMORAL JOINT REACTION FORCE AND JOINT STRESS

The amount of force that the posterior surface of the patella encounters with various activities has been well documented. Clinically, understanding the ROM and load optimal for patellofemoral joint contact forces is very useful in treating patellofemoral disorders that result from abnormal force on the posterior surface of the patella. Patellofemoral joint reaction force[85] (Fpf) is determined by the following equation:

$$Fpf = kXFq$$

At a specific point of knee ROM, the amount of Fq multiplied by the angle of knee flexion (X) equals Fpf, or Fpf = kXFq. k is a constant that is predetermined for each angle of knee flexion.

The amount of force that the patella encounters does not fully reveal the amount of stress placed on the patella. *Joint surface stress* is determined by the amount of force placed on a given area of joint surface. This relationship is expressed by the equation force/area = stress. Thus, the less area to which a force is applied, the greater amount of stress is applied to the joint. The amount of stress that is on a given point of the patella has important clinical implications. It is the amount of stress, not simply the joint reaction force, that can inflict abnormal wear or pain on the posterior surface of the patella.[36]

OKC joint reaction force: During OKC function, Fpf increases as the knee extends from 90° of knee flexion. At 90° of flexion, the patellar tendon and quadriceps muscles are perpendicular to each other and Fq tends to result in a low Fpf. As the knee extends from 90° to 60° of knee flexion, Fq must increase, resulting in increased Fpf. After 60° of knee flexion, Fq levels off and Fpf is relatively unchanged to end range.

OKC joint stress: As a result of decreased joint surface area contact during knee extension, joint stress increases from 90° of flexion to approximately 20° of extension. Typically, there is little to no patellar contact area past 20° of flexion to terminal extension, thus joint stress often does not occur during this range. For the patients who do maintain some contact in this ROM, joint stress will be very high due to the small contact area.

CKC joint reaction force: Investigation of joint reaction force in the CKC shows that in contrast to the OKC, Fpf decreases as the knee extends. This decrease in force is greatest between 30° and 90° of flexion. Fpf decreases at a lesser rate past 30° of flexion, particularly because there is relatively no contact between the articulating surfaces of the patellofemoral joint past 20°.[85]

CKC joint stress: As in the OKC, joint surface contact area increases as the knee extends from 90° of flexion. However, the Fq required for knee extension decreases faster than the contact area decreases, resulting in a decrease of joint stress. Realizing when the patellofemoral joint is subjected to stress is crucial for exercise prescription to minimize the amount of injury to patellofemoral articular cartilage.

FUNCTIONAL IMPLICATIONS OF JOINT REACTION FORCE AND STRESS

Understanding the amount of Fpf and joint stress that are encountered with daily tasks can be useful in educating patients who have anterior knee pain. As a result of the elastic pull of the proximal and distal tendon units, there is a substantial amount of force present during sitting.[40] This increased stress accounts for a patient's subjective complaint of anterior knee pain during prolonged sitting. Although sitting can impose a low load with long duration pressure on the patellofemoral joint, dynamic movements frequently cause abnormal stress and injury. During gait, the joint reaction force is typically 50 percent of the body weight as the knee flexes to 10°–15° during initial contact.[40] Stair ambulation, which requires increased Fq and knee flexion, can produce far greater Fpf. As the knee reaches 60° of flexion during stair ambulation, joint reaction force can be as much as 3.3 times the body weight.[17,40] As the knee approaches 130° of flexion in deep-squatting activities, joint reaction force may reach 7.8 times the body weight.[17,40]

FORCE DISSIPATION

The patellofemoral joint is subjected to varying extremes of joint reaction force over small areas. Fortunately, the trochlea and articulating surface of the patella possess multiple properties responsible for dissipating patellofemoral joint stress. When compressed, articular cartilage allows fluid to flow freely within the matrix and permits the cartilage to expand laterally. The patella benefits from thickened articular cartilage that easily expands laterally during compression. As knee flexion increases, the patella will seat more deeply into the trochlea and contact more surface area, which reduces the stress at a given point. This property also contributes to greater patellofemoral joint stability. Because of the large amount of permeability and compressibility of the articular cartilage, there is greater stress on the matrix that composes the cartilage. Unfortunately, chronic wear to the matrix can lead to degeneration and eventual patellar lesions.

PATELLAR STABILITY

Static stabilization: The articulation of the patella with the trochlea represents the greatest contribution to patellar stability. The trochlea acts as a trough for the patella to glide within. There is a greater degree of dynamic muscle pull from the proximal–lateral direction, necessitating increased support to prevent excessive lateral movement. This support is provided in part by the large anterior extension of the lateral femoral condyle. A lack of lateral femoral condyle height can contribute to chronic patella subluxation or dislocation.

The lack of bony contact between the patella and trochlea from 20° of flexion to terminal extension results in a dependence on soft tissue restraints. Investigators have described the medial and lateral extensor retinacula as the primary restraints to excessive patellar movement in the frontal plane.[90] The added support of medial and lateral patellofemoral ligaments present in a portion of the population will reinforce the retinacula.[17,67]

Dynamic stabilization: The dynamic musculotendinous stabilizers are oriented in a longitudinal fashion proximal and distal to the patella. The single distal stabilizer, the patellar tendon, contains the patella inferiorly. Proximally, the quadriceps generate a superior pull through the quadriceps tendon.[17,27] The combination of these longitudinal forces provides stability during knee flexion by seating the patella into the trochlear groove. However, the longitudinal pull may decrease stability by pulling the patella out of the trochlear groove during knee hyperextension.

Based on the pull of the quadriceps muscle, an imbalance of the vastus lateralis and vastus medialis oblique can result in abnormal tracking of the patellofemoral joint and disrupt stability as the knee approaches terminal extension. Recent literature has been controversial regarding the role of this mechanism in aiding the stability of the patellofemoral joint and decreasing anterior knee pain, as well as optimal treatment techniques.[7,56,83]

INFLUENCE OF PROXIMAL AND DISTAL JOINT POSITION ON THE PATELLOFEMORAL JOINT

Hip and femur: Changes in the position of the femur at the hip joint can alter the orientation of the trochlea. The osteokinematics of the femur in the frontal and transverse planes can affect the directional force of the quadriceps on the patella. Clinically, the most common abnormal movement pattern is hip adduction and internal rotation, causing an inward collapse of the knee and medial displacement of the trochlea. The insertion of the quadriceps at the tibial tubercle remains fixed, resulting in a more laterally aligned patella.

Kendall et al.[47] have cited dominance of the hip internal rotators and adductors as possible sources of this faulty movement pattern. In addition, positional weakness or increased length of the hip abductors and external rotators, particularly the posterior fibers of the gluteus medius, contributes to the inward collapse knee.

Tibia and foot: Rotation of the tibia can also influence the alignment of the patellofemoral joint. As the tibia rotates either medially or laterally against a fixed femur, the patella can either glide or rotate in the direction of the tibial tubercle. Whether glide or rotation occurs depends upon the proximal fixation of the patella.

Rotation of the tibia has several influences. The proximal tibia will laterally rotate with a dominance of muscle action of the biceps femoris or TFL–ITB. Medial rotation can be caused by the predominance of the semitendinosus and semimembranosus. Distally, tibial rotation is influenced by the position of the subtalar joint. Pronation will lead to medial rotation of the tibia, thus positioning the patella medially relative to the trochlea.

QUADRICEPS ANGLE

The quadriceps (Q) angle is the angle formed between a line connecting the anterior superior iliac spine to the midpoint of the patella and a line that connects the tibial tubercle with the midpoint of the patella (Fig. 29-35). A 15° angle between these two lines is considered normal.[1,17] A Q angle greater than 20° can contribute to pathology in the patellofemoral joint. A large Q angle can cause displacement of the patella laterally, resulting in a bowstringing effect against the lateral femoral condyle during quadriceps contraction.[42,51]

There are several concerns when using the Q angle as a diagnostic tool. A large Q angle has not been shown to predispose a knee to patellofemoral pain, nor do all patients with patellofemoral pain have a large Q angle. Also, the measure assumes that the patella is centered in the trochlea; however, a laterally subluxed patella can result in a false positive finding.[34]

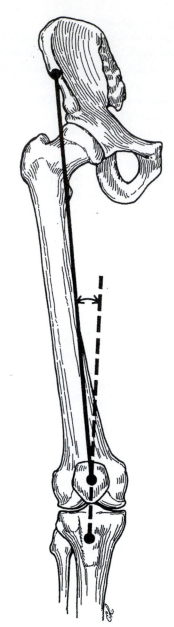

FIGURE 29-35

The quadriceps angle. (Reproduced from Scott WN. *The Knee.* St. Louis, MO, Mosby, 1994, p. 46, with permission from Elsevier.)

GENERAL REHABILITATION PROGRESSION FOLLOWING LIGAMENTOUS AND MENISCAL INJURY

When treating knee injuries, the clinician should utilize a progression that considers the physiologic effects of the rehabil-

itation. Pain and inflammatory control, ROM, gait training, strengthening exercises, agility drills, and sport-specific exercises must all be implemented in a sequence that adheres to a criterion-based rehabilitation protocol. If the rehabilitation deviates from a criterion-based approach, the body will respond with adverse affects such as inflammation, swelling, pain, and further injury.

For purposes of this section, the general treatment plan has been divided into four phases. Many rehabilitation protocols set a time line to determine when it is appropriate to advance to the next phase. However, movement between phases should be criterion-based, requiring the patient to meet the goals outlined in each phase and not on a prespecified period of time. Advancing a patient into a later stage without full ROM or controlled swelling may delay the entire rehabilitation process. A skilled clinician knows when to advance an accelerated patient, delay a patient who has plateaued or regressed, or provide some overlap between phases.

Phase I

In the past, the majority of acute injuries requiring surgery were often repaired within days of the initial insult. As a result, patients were undergoing surgery with swelling and inflammation, ROM deficits, antalgic gait patterns, and muscular weakness. Immediate surgery following an ACL tear often led to a severe arthrofibrosis.[81] With most injuries that require surgery, delaying surgery until the knee has passed the acute inflammatory stage and regained near normal ROM and strength can contribute to an optimal outcome.

Preoperative rehabilitation involves both mental and physical preparation. The patient must be given time to experience the psychological responses to injury as well as become emotionally prepared for the challenges of surgery and postoperative rehabilitation. Patient education about the surgical and rehabilitative procedures is of utmost importance. Using anatomical models or other resources, the clinician should explain the injury as well as the surgical technique. The patient should also have a detailed understanding of the postoperative rehabilitation program and goals. The patient must exhibit a positive attitude and have a sense of control over his/her situation. The clinician should also establish a good rapport with the patient during this time.

From a physical standpoint, the initial focus should be placed on the elimination of swelling and restoration of ROM. In the early stages of rehabilitation, a knee CryoCuff (Aircast Inc., Summit, NJ) is an easy and effective way to control pain and swelling by means of cold and compression (Fig. 29-36). Compression garments and ice bags can also be used. Pain is often the main deterrent to motion and can lead to muscular and neurogenic inhibition, weakness and atrophy, and altered neuromuscular patterns.

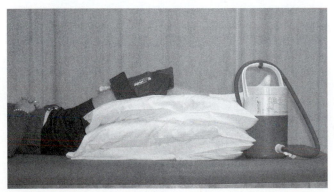

FIGURE 29-36

CryoCuff application provides cold and compression.

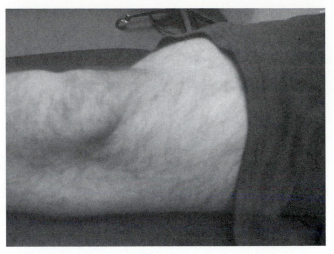

FIGURE 29-37

Quadriceps setting is isometric quadriceps contraction performed in full extension for early strengthening and recruitment.

ROM exercises should begin almost immediately after the injury, with a greater emphasis placed on regaining extension. Among the many exercises to improve passive extension are heel props and prone hangs. Typically, flexion can be improved through exercises such as heel slides. ROM should be the focus of treatment until both legs are symmetrical. It has been shown that returning full ROM prior to surgery decreases postoperative complications.[74,80]

Once full ROM is restored and swelling and pain are minimal, basic level strengthening can begin. A resistive exercise continuum should be utilized, beginning with low-level isometric strengthening. Isometric quadriceps contraction from a long-sitting position, or quad sets, is an exercise often employed after a major knee injury (Fig. 29-37). As strength and weight bearing improve, the patient can begin selective CKC exercises, such as minisquats, step-downs, and calf raises. Gait training can also begin during this period. As weight bearing becomes tolerable, gait should be practiced in a normal heel-to-toe pattern, with emphasis on obtaining full extension at heel strike. Low-impact aerobics, such as stationary bicycle and stair machines, are also appropriate at this time.

The preoperative phase also includes measurement and testing of both extremities. Strength testing is achieved typically through an isokinetic strength assessment. Single-leg hop test is another functional measure that can be utilized. Other measurements that should be taken include ligament arthrometry, ROM, and subjective knee questionnaire.

Phase II

Phase II follows many of the principles of the preoperative phase. This phase also includes those patients whose injuries do not require surgery or who choose a nonoperative course of treatment. Immediate postinjury status is often thought of as the protection phase. Phase II is characterized by pain modulation,

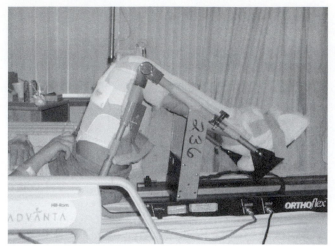

FIGURE 29-38

Continuous passive motion device permits early motion.

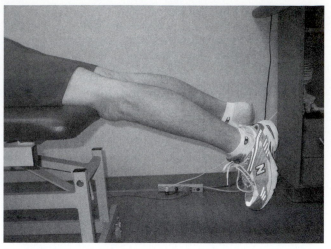

FIGURE 29-40

The prone hang is performed with the patient's distal thighs at the edge of the table.

restoration of normal ROM, basic strengthening, and restoration of normal gait.

Pain modulation can take place through a number of modalities. Ice, compression, and elevation are staples during this period to control pain and swelling. Limiting ROM and weight-bearing status through an immobilizer, brace, or crutches can appropriately protect and rest the joint, depending on the type of injury. The effects of pain and swelling and the effectiveness of a CryoCuff were discussed earlier in the preoperative section.

The importance of early ROM, except when contraindicated, cannot be overstated. Motion is often considered the key to recovery. Often after surgery, a continuous passive motion (CPM) device is applied to the knee to begin early motion through a small arc (Fig. 29-38). When dealing with knee injuries and especially surgical patients, an immediate emphasis is placed on regaining terminal knee extension. Not only does terminal knee extension facilitate a normal gait pattern, it also

helps to prevent scar tissue from forming in the femoral notch and becoming a permanent block to extension.[29] In addition, lack of full extension has been linked to quadriceps weakness, anterior knee pain, and crepitus.[75] This has led to a market of extension boards and devices aimed at achieving the motion (Fig. 29-39). Exercise instruction may include prone hangs and heel props. Prone hangs allow passive knee extension from a prone position with the involved knee and lower leg off the end of the table (Fig. 29-40). In this gravity-assisted position, the weight of the extremity is utilized in gaining extension. An ankle cuff weight can be added for assistance. Heel props are performed with the heel of the extremity propped onto a bolster, lifting the gastrocnemius and distal thigh from the table (Fig. 29-41). This position allows the knee to relax into full extension. A weight or strap can be affixed superior to the patella for assistance.

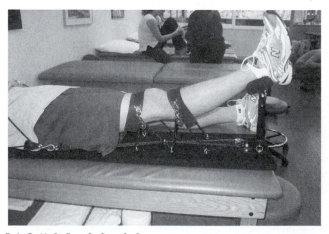

FIGURE 29-39

Extension board utilized to gain full hyperextension.

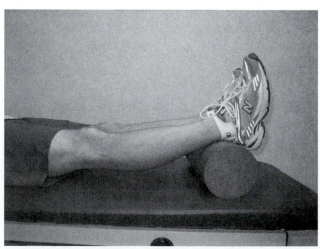

FIGURE 29-41

The heel prop is an early extension exercise.

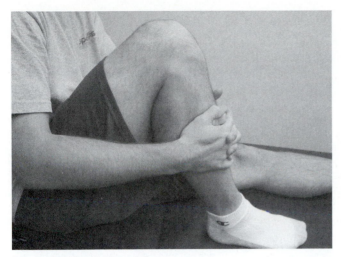

FIGURE 29-42

Heel slides are an effective means of obtaining knee flexion.

Although not as urgent a concern as extension, obtaining flexion is also important. Flexion can be improved through heel slides, wall slides, and active-assistive knee flexion in sitting. Heel slides are performed from a long-sitting position with the knee in flexion. The patient grasps the lower leg and passively pulls it into further flexion (Fig. 29-42). This can also be performed with a towel. Wall slides involve the patient in a supine position with legs extended up a wall. The injured leg slowly slides down the wall with assistance from the uninjured leg (Fig. 29-43). Active-assistive knee flexion is performed in a short-sitting position. From this position, the noninjured leg can pull the injured leg into even more flexion. A stationary bicycle also can be used as a mechanical means of attaining flexion. With both feet strapped into the pedals, the patient can use the contralateral leg to propel the knee into flexion. The clinician should adjust the seat to a position that is challenging to the patient. As this position becomes easy, the seat can be lowered, increasing the amount of flexion required at the knee to complete a revolution. If a full revolution cannot be completed, a rocking strategy can be employed. An alternating forward and backward pedaling motion is used until the knee gets "over the top" of the first revolution.

Along with ROM, a few associated concepts to consider are flexibility and joint mobility. Improving flexibility means increasing the ability of soft tissue structures to elongate through a range of joint motion. A lack of soft tissue elongation may or may not be a result of the injury; however, balancing the available ROM is critical for normal biomechanics to occur at the knee. Mobilization of the patellofemoral and tibiofemoral joints may also be necessary for restoration of accessory motion, especially after a period of immobilization. Grade I–II mobilizations are oscillations applied at less than full joint mobility and can be useful in pain control and preventing restrictions of joint motion during the early phases of rehabilitation. Grade III–IV mobilizations are taken to the end of physiologic joint motion and are used to correct restrictions to joint motion.

Basic strengthening to regain leg control and improve quadriceps tone is also important during the early rehabilitation period. Exercises to improve leg control include quad sets, straight-leg raises, and active knee flexion and extension. Straight-leg raises are performed with the patient in a long-sitting position and the knee in full extension. The patient contracts the quadriceps muscle, much like performing a quad set, and then raises the leg 6–12 in off the table (Fig. 29-44). The straight-leg raise should be performed slowly in a controlled manner. Partial to full knee extension and flexion exercises are to be completed during this time, with ROM depending on the status of the articular cartilage and menisci. Sitting knee

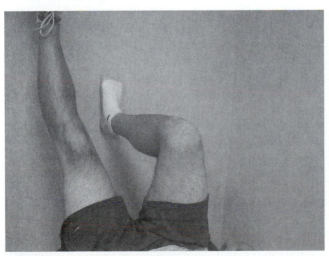

FIGURE 29-43

Wall slides are performed by slowly sliding the foot down the wall.

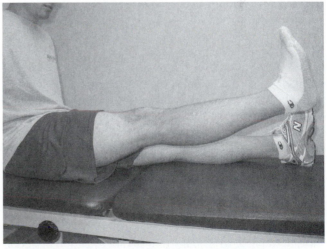

FIGURE 29-44

Straight leg raise performed by initiating a quad set and maintaining knee extension while raising the leg off the table.

extensions are performed in a pain-free ROM off the edge of the table. With both flexion and extension, active assistance can be provided from the contralateral extremity.

Restoration of gait can be critical in positively affecting many aspects of early rehabilitation. During the early postinjury period, the patient should ambulate with crutches until gait can be normalized. The clinician should encourage both full knee extension at heel strike and full-weightbearing as tolerated during the stance phase of gait, which in turn contribute to the facilitation of quadriceps function. If the patient is having difficulty obtaining full extension at heel strike, backward walking can be a means of obtaining active knee extension. Early weight bearing also allows for compression and motion at the knee joint, which are conducive to cartilage nutrition and normal physiologic stresses to osseous and soft tissue structures about the knee.

Toward the end of phase I, the patient should be encouraged to progress to full-weightbearing without crutches. Practicing in front of a mirror may enhance the patient's ability to ambulate normally. Stance phase during normal ambulation is one of the most basic forms of CKC quadriceps strengthening. By achieving this goal, the patient is able to regain good quadriceps tone and leg control, making it possible to implement more challenging strengthening exercises. The benefits of CKC exercise have been widely demonstrated. Bilateral minisquats are performed with the feet shoulder-width apart and toes pointing forward. The patient slowly bends the hip and knees to one-quarter of a typical full squat, maintaining the knees in a position posterior to the toes (Fig. 29-45). This minisquatting activity can be performed near a stable object at arm level for balance. Bilateral leg press is similar to the bilateral one-quarter knee bends in muscular activity. Bilateral calf raises are appropriate for strengthening the triceps surae musculature. The patient can begin this exercise from a flat surface and advance to standing on a stable object with heels hanging off the edge for a greater ROM. The patient should elevate as high as possible, contracting tightly at the top. Unilateral stance of the involved extremity, if tolerable, can be used to begin improving balance and proprioception.

Working toward leg control and normal gait is aimed at improving the patient's function. Depending on the injury, a knee brace or taping of the patella may be appropriate to assist in returning function to the patient. Cross-training activities such as swimming, biking, or stair machine may be appropriate to initiate muscular endurance and aerobic capacity. Swimming is contraindicated in surgical patients with unhealed wounds.

Phase III

Once the goals of phase II are achieved, the patient can move forward to phase III. If full terminal knee extension or flexion are still lacking, the clinician must emphasize the importance of full ROM prior to more strenuous strengthening activities. If this criterion is not followed, the body may respond adversely. The focus of phase III is advanced strengthening.

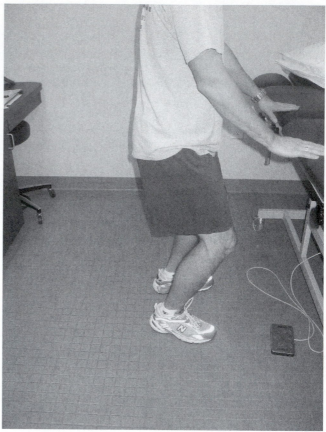

FIGURE 29-45

Bilateral one-quarter squats permit early CKC strengthening of the quadriceps.

Strengthening activities of phase II are continued with increased repetition and resistance. The patient should be encouraged to place more weight on the involved side as tolerated, in a progression toward unilateral strengthening. Once the patient has sufficient leg control to perform a unilateral knee bend without difficulty, weight room activities may commence. The clinician should consider a combination of OKC and CKC activities, as well as concentric and eccentric muscular strengthening. Chapter 14 provides an introductory discussion of OKC and CKC exercises.

OKC exercise facilitates isolated quadriceps muscle strengthening. However, caution must be exercised, as patellofemoral compressive forces are distributed over a small contact area with progressive knee extension.[73] OKC extension exercises also produce an anterior shear force that significantly loads the ACL, particularly in the last 30° of extension. Thus, patients should begin performing leg extension exercises between approximately 45° and 90° of flexion. The patient should perform full terminal extension only if there is sufficient quadriceps strength and proper alignment to complete the exercise without pain.

CKC exercise is preferred for a more functional rehabilitation of the lower extremity. During these types of exercises, patellofemoral compressive forces become larger as flexion increases.[73] CKC exercises have been shown to reduce shear forces across the tibiofemoral joint through cocontraction and axial loading.[6] Thus, patients should begin performing CKC exercise from 0° to approximately 45°. A more advanced patient may go beyond 45°–90° of knee flexion if the exercise can be completed without pain.

Concentric muscular contraction involves shortening of the muscle fibers, resulting in joint approximation. Often, concentric activity is viewed as positive work and functions to accelerate the limb. In contrast, eccentric muscular contraction involves lengthening of the muscle fibers, resulting in an increase in the joint angle. Eccentric activity is often viewed as negative work and functions to decelerate the limb. Since contraction refers to a shortening of muscle fibers, it may be more accurate to describe eccentric activity as a "controlled lengthening" rather than a "lengthening contraction."

Frequently, emphasis in rehabilitation is placed solely on concentric activity. However, eccentric activity is dominant in running, tennis, and throwing. Eccentric control is needed when landing from a jump in activities such as basketball, track and field, volleyball, and gymnastics, and is recognized as important for efficient gait. In fact, many simple activities of daily living require eccentric activity, such as bending over to pick up an object or descending stairs.

Cavagna et al.[12] recognized the potential force of eccentric activity as they described the stretch-shorten cycle. The authors stated that muscle stretch loads potential energy into elastic elements that is transferred into kinetic energy during the concentric phase, thereby raising the peak potential force. This is the premise behind plyometric activity. For example, consider an athlete performing a standing vertical leap. During the knee and hip flexion phase, the athlete is storing potential energy as the muscles lengthen eccentrically. This allows the athlete to jump higher than if the athlete were to jump from a static position of knee and hip flexion.

Using both OKC and CKC exercises, a skilled clinician can effectively incorporate exercises that work the muscles around the knee through an entire ROM, while safely maintaining the integrity of the joints and cartilage. The clinician can also utilize both concentric and eccentric muscular activity, preparing the patient for tasks inherent to both home activities and sports participation. The clinician should integrate each of these aspects into the strengthening component of a rehabilitation program.

Advanced strengthening should emphasize unilateral strengthening exercises, including leg press, step-downs, calf raises, and leg extensions. When performing leg press and leg extensions, the patient may assist the injured leg by using the uninvolved leg through the concentric phase. This is an easy and safe way to emphasize the eccentric portion of the lift. Step-downs are performed by having the patient stand on a step with the affected extremity. The patient slowly lowers the contralateral leg to the floor while maintaining good biomechanical alignment of the lower extremity and then returns to the starting position (Fig. 29-46). Initially, the height of the step should be small (2–4 in) and should increase as the exercise

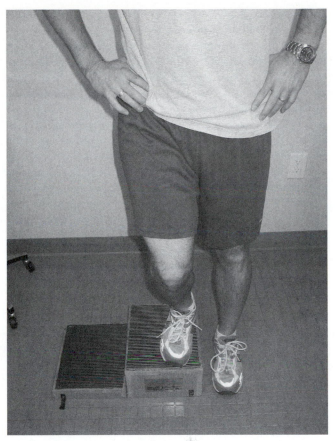

FIGURE 29-46

Step-downs can be made more challenging by increasing the height of the step.

becomes easier. The clinician can also increase the difficulty of the exercise by having the patient perform the step-down to the front or back of the step.

From an aerobic standpoint, exercising on a stair machine or stationary bicycle is either initiated or progressed to greater intensity levels. Aerobic machines with variable resistance can be used as a means of moderate speed strengthening. If wounds have healed, the patient can also begin swimming and performing other hydrotherapy activity.

Toward the end of phase III, the patient can begin some early agility drills. Jumping rope, straight-ahead jogging, or easy position drills for athletes are appropriate at this time. During this period, the patient should maintain full ROM, continue to minimize pain and swelling, and demonstrate a normal gait pattern. As strength and quadriceps tone continue to improve, the patient may progress to light squatting and lunges.

Phase IV

A functional return to prior activity status is the goal of the final phase. The patient can progress, once meeting the goals of phase III and maintaining the objectives, from the previous phase. Phase IV is characterized by a functional progression that includes activity- or sport-specific exercises, agility drills, and balance and proprioceptive training.

The patient continues advanced strengthening throughout the entire final phase. Once the patient has attained 65–70 percent strength in the involved leg through an isokinetic strength assessment (refer to Chapter 12 for additional Isokinetic information), agility activities and sports drills can be advanced safely. Weight room activities and home strengthening exercises should progress from high repetition/low weight to low repetition/high weight. Moderate speed strengthening and cardiovascular conditioning should be continued during this period.

All activities and exercises during this phase should be functional, specific, and progressive. Whether the patient is a mail carrier or a football linebacker, the rehabilitation needs to focus on the tasks required for that individual to return to his/her prior activity status. A mail carrier may be required to lift moderately heavy objects and walk long distances, while a linebacker requires explosive power and high-speed change of direction. Solo sport activities, such as shooting a basketball or hitting a tennis ball, are appropriate during this time.

Advanced agility drills can include lateral shuffles, cariocas, crossover drills, and backward running. By focusing on agility activities rather than on jogging, the patient is more apt to improve areas of confidence, moderate speed strength, quickness, and sport-specific skills. By avoiding the repetition and redundancy of jogging and making the activity purposeful and specific, the patient is often able to better absorb joint compressive forces.

As the patient progresses, agility training becomes more vigorous. Figure of eights and half-to-full-speed running should be included at this time. Typically, a functional progression will follow a scheme that gradually increases speed increments from half to three-quarter, to full-speed activity. Chapter 21 provides additional suggestions for functional progressions. Making certain the patient performs activities with proper technique is paramount during this phase. Jumping movements should be performed straight up and down with no lateral moments at the knee. The patient should maintain the trunk over knees and knees over feet while keeping the hips, knees, and ankles in a straight line. The patient should land on the balls of the feet instead of flat-footed and assume a position of slight flexion in the hips and knees.

During return to activity, the clinician should attempt to challenge the patient's balance. Perturbation activities performed on a wobble board, foam, or trampoline are appropriate. Performing the exercise unilaterally or with eyes closed can increase difficulty of the activity. These types of exercises can improve joint stabilization patterns through cocontractions of the quadriceps and hamstrings. The patient also improves body awareness through an enhancement in proprioceptive information. Chapter 11 provides additional information regarding neuromuscular training.

Before a full return to prior activity level, the patient's involved extremity should be reevaluated. Isokinetic strength assessment, single-leg hop, ligament arthrometry, ROM, and subjective knee questionnaire should all be compared to preoperative or preinjury status. The patient should have full ROM, acceptable ligament stability, and 80 percent strength bilaterally before returning to competitive athletic or recreational activities. The patient should complete a sport- or occupation-specific functional progression prior to full return.

SPECIFIC REHABILITATION TECHNIQUES FOR LIGAMENTOUS AND MENISCAL INJURY

Medial Collateral Ligament Sprain

PATHOMECHANICS

Although current research on knee ligament injuries focuses on ACL injuries, the MCL remains the most commonly injured ligament of the knee.[97] Successful management of MCL injuries often depends on establishing the existence of an isolated lesion, with no associated damage to other knee structures, particularly the ACL. Isolated MCL injuries can heal spontaneously, without the need for surgical correction, even in complete ligament ruptures when the fragmented ends of the damaged tissue are not in close approximation.

The MCL can tear midsubstance or at either the femoral or tibial attachment sites. About 65 percent of MCL sprains occur at the proximal insertion site on the femur. On the basis of location of the injury, rehabilitation can vary substantially. MCL injuries occurring midsubstance or near femoral origin tend to develop more stiffness and readily incur ROM loss. Restoration of full motion should be monitored closely within the first few weeks following injury. In contrast, injuries at the tibial attachment tend to heal with residual laxity and thus have easier return of ROM. As a result, additional protection may be required to allow the MCL to heal.

Diagnosis of MCL sprains can usually always be made by physical evaluation. The grade of ligament injury is determined by the amount of joint laxity. In a grade I sprain the MCL is tender due to microtears; however, there is no increased laxity and there is a firm end point. A grade II sprain involves an incomplete tear with some increased laxity with valgus stress at 30° of flexion and minimal laxity in full extension, yet there is still a firm end point. There is tenderness to palpation, hemorrhage, and pain on valgus stress test. A grade III sprain is a complete tear with significant laxity on valgus stress in full extension. No end point is evident, and pain is generally less than that experienced with grade I or II sprains. Significant laxity with valgus stress testing in full extension indicates injury to the medial joint capsule as well as the cruciate ligaments.

MECHANISM OF INJURY

Injury to the MCL occurs as a result of valgus stress to the knee from either a contact or noncontact force. The most common mechanism of injury is by a direct lateral contact, which is frequent during contact sports such as football. A direct force to the outside of the knee can result in a valgus stress to the medial aspect of the knee that exceeds the strength of the ligament. The patient will usually explain that the knee was hit on the lateral side with the foot planted and that there was immediate pain on the medial side of the knee that felt more like a "pulling" or "tearing" than a "pop."

Less commonly, the MCL is injured through a noncontact mechanism that occurs when the foot is planted and an indirect rotational force is coupled with an increased valgus stress at the knee. This mechanism is common in sports that involve cutting maneuvers such as soccer, basketball, and football.

REHABILITATION CONCERNS

Traditionally, standard of care for MCL injuries was surgical management. Since the early 1990s, the treatment of MCL sprains has changed considerably. The current approach is non-surgical and includes limited immobilization with early ROM and strengthening exercises. Shelbourne and Patel[79] found the best approach for management of a combined MCL/ACL injury is achieved by treating the MCL injury nonsurgically and performing a delayed reconstruction of the ACL.

Patient advancement will vary according to the location of the tear, degree of ligamentous instability, concomitant injuries involved, age, and activity demands. A patient with a grade III tear at the femoral attachment site typically will have more difficulty restoring motion, while patients with tears at the tibial insertion tend to have more instability.

Grade I injuries may be progressed as tolerated with or without the use of a hinged knee brace. Grade II injuries can be progressed as tolerated, depending on the patient's signs and symptoms. These injuries will display increased valgus laxity but retain a firm end point. A hinged knee brace can be used early in the rehabilitation, although an immobilizer may be used for patient comfort. Grade III injuries will be immobilized in 30° of flexion for 1–3 weeks. This protection provides a stable environment for proper healing and tightening of the injured ligamentous complex. The physician and clinician should collaborate on patient progression at each clinical visit, as overlapping of the three phases is very common and has been built in to this progression.

REHABILITATION PROGRESSION

Phase I: 0–3 Weeks

Phase I is characterized by protection, early healing, and restoring ROM. The clinical goals are to minimize pain and swelling and to attain full-weightbearing and normal gait with or without a brace or immobilizer. The clinician will test bilateral ROM during this phase.

A CryoCuff is to be used as much as possible throughout the day for control of pain and swelling. A stockinette can be worn to assist in swelling control. Anti-inflammatory medications can be taken as prescribed by the physician. Immobilization at this time is dependent on the patient's instability and pain. For patients with a grade I MCL injury, bracing is used as needed. Patients with a grade II injury use a brace and possibly an immobilizer. Grade III injuries are managed with a cast or immobilizer. Immobilization times will vary depending on the severity of instability.

The patient may be allowed to bear weight as tolerated with or without protective devices, depending on pain status. ROM exercises are performed three times daily (prone hangs, heel props, wall slides, and heel slides). If an immobilization period is required, ROM exercise is performed afterward.

Phase II: 1–5 Weeks

Phase II rehabilitation focuses on restoring full ROM and beginning a strengthening program that utilizes both OKC and CKC exercises. Clinical goals include no swelling, full ROM, normal gait, pain-free activities of daily living, and initiation of strengthening and proprioception activities. The clinician will again test bilateral ROM throughout this phase.

ROM exercises are continued during this period. The patient should begin to exhibit a normal gait pattern without assistance from a hinged brace, although a brace can be worn as needed for comfort. Strengthening exercises begin bilaterally and are progressed to a unilateral exercise. The regimen consists of minisquats, step-downs, toe raises, leg press, and leg extensions. Proprioceptive activities and nonimpact aerobic training such as stationary bicycle, stair machine, and elliptical trainers are initiated at this time.

By the end of phase II, the patient should possess full ROM, including terminal extension. Stockinette use can be discontinued at the end of this phase if no swelling is present. The patient should continue use of the CryoCuff after exercise and for pain control as needed.

Phase III: 2–8 Weeks

The final phase consists of a progressive return to functional activities. The goals of phase III include pain-free activities of daily living without a brace, weight room strengthening, completing a functional progression with a brace, and return to sport or work with a brace. The clinician will administer the functional progression and isokinetic strength assessment. The patient should be free from pain with daily activity at this time.

Strengthening should be performed unilaterally, continuing the exercises from phase II. Most phase III activities are performed in the weight room and include unilateral leg press to 90°, step-downs from a 2–4-in step height, unilateral leg extensions, squats to 90° performed in a squat rack, lunges, and stair machine.

Easy agility drills are initiated at this time and should be completed with a hinged knee brace. Activities should include jump rope, backward running, lateral slides, cariocas, cutting movements, and a jogging to sprinting progression.

Successful completion of a functional progression constitutes the end of this phase. At this time, the patient can return to full activity. A functional knee brace will be utilized depending on the demands of the individual's activity or sport and degree of injury. The patient will need to continue a regular strengthening program even after full return to activity.

Lateral Collateral Ligament Sprain

PATHOMECHANICS

Fortunately, the lateral aspect of the knee is well supported by secondary stabilizers, and isolated injury to the LCL is rare. When it does occur, the clinician must rule out other ligamentous injuries. Isolated sprain of the LCL is the least common of all knee ligament sprains.[61] LCL sprains result in disruption at the fibular head either with or without an avulsion in approximately 75 percent of the cases, with 20 percent occurring at the femur, and only 5 percent as midsubstance tears.[90] It is not uncommon to see associated injuries of the peroneal nerve because the nerve courses around the head of the fibula. A complete disruption of the LCL often involves injury to the posterolateral joint capsule as well as the PCL and occasionally the ACL.

The amount of laxity evident on a varus stress test determines the severity of injury to the LCL. Grading the extent of LCL laxity follows the same I–III grading scale as the MCL.

MECHANISM OF INJURY

An isolated LCL injury is almost always the result of a varus stress applied to the medial aspect of the knee. Occasionally, a varus stress may occur during weight bearing when weight is shifted away from the side of injury, creating stress on the lateral structures. Patients who sustain an LCL sprain will report that they heard or felt a pop and that there was immediate lateral pain. Swelling will be immediate and extra-articular, with no joint effusion unless there is an associated meniscus or capsular injury.

REHABILITATION CONCERNS

Grade I injuries may be progressed as tolerated with or without the use of a hinged knee brace. Grade II injuries can be progressed as tolerated, depending on the patient's signs and symptoms. These injuries will display increased valgus laxity but retain a firm end point. A hinged knee brace can be used early in the rehabilitation, although an immobilizer may be used for patient comfort. Grade III injuries may be managed nonoperatively with bracing for 4–6 weeks, limited to 0°–90° of motion; however, grade III LCL tears with associated ligamentous injuries that result in rotational instabilities are usually managed by surgical repair or reconstruction. This is certainly the case if the patient has chronic varus laxity and intends to continue participation in athletics or if there is a displaced avulsion.

REHABILITATION PROGRESSION

The rehabilitation progression following LCL sprains should follow the same course as was previously described for MCL sprains. In the case of a grade III LCL sprain that involves multiple ligamentous injury with associated instability that is surgically repaired or reconstructed, the patient should be placed in a postoperative brace, with partial-weightbearing for 4–6 weeks. At 6 weeks, a rehabilitation program involving a carefully monitored gradual sport-specific functional progression should

begin. In general, the patient may return to full activity at about 6 months.

Anterior Cruciate Ligament Sprain

PATHOMECHANICS

The healing potential of a torn ACL is very poor.[26] Healing potential for a partially torn ACL can be favorable when certain conditions exist, but only 15 percent of all ACL injuries are partial tears.[23] In addition, healing requires 2–3 months following injury. Because of the poor healing conditions, the torn ACL often leads to anterior laxity, rotary instability, and meniscal tears when left untreated. Very few athletes can participate at a high level with a nonfunctional ACL.[38] Giving-way episodes are often the result, damaging the meniscus and articular cartilage within the joint.

Convincing evidence suggests that an active individual with a torn ACL is susceptible to meniscal injury.[11] Shelbourne and Gray[77] reported that the results of ACL reconstruction 9 years after surgery strongly correlated with the status of the meniscus and articular cartilage. Patients who underwent ACL reconstruction without meniscal tears requiring removal or articular cartilage damage had significantly better long-term results compared to patients who had surgery with meniscus removal or severe articular cartilage damage. Patients with normal meniscus and articular cartilage at the time of surgery had subjective scores equal to a normal control group without knee injuries.

The temporary stability of a nonoperated ACL tear is often referred to as the "honeymoon period." When treated nonoperatively, an active individual will likely become symptomatic. The present laxity will lead to instability, causing giving-way episodes with ensuing swelling and pain. Damage to the meniscus and articular cartilage is highly probable following such episodes. Meniscal damage is associated with half of acute cases and 90 percent of chronic ACL deficiencies of greater than 10 years duration.[23] Similarly, 30 percent of acute ACL injuries and 70 percent of ACL-deficient knees of 10 years postinjury display articular cartilage lesions.[23] The relationship of long-term joint arthrosis to ACL deficiency is not fully understood. However, the alteration of knee biomechanics can lead to areas of overload, causing articular cartilage breakdown. Depending on the length of follow-up, detectable osteoarthritis in ACL injuries ranges from 15 to 65 percent.[18,25]

As with MCL and LCL sprains, the severity of the injury is indicated by the degree of laxity or instability. Rotational instability will also be present as indicated by a positive pivot shift. The patient will most often report feeling and hearing a pop and a feeling that the knee "gave out." There is also significant pain, and hemarthrosis will occur within 1–2 hours.

MECHANISM OF INJURY

The most common injury mechanism to the ACL involves a noncontact valgus and external rotation stress to the knee as the foot is planted on the ground. The classic example of this mechanism happens in football when a running back plants the foot to make a cut and avoid being tackled. Occasionally, the mechanism of injury involves deceleration, valgus stress, and internal rotation. Knee hyperextension combined with internal rotation can also produce a tear of the ACL.

External contact forces to the tibiofemoral joint can result in a combined knee injury of which an ACL rupture is a component. Typically, this injury is a result of lateral or hyperextension force to the knee, which frequently results in complete rupture of both the ACL and MCL, plus a longitudinal tear of the lateral meniscus, all of which require surgical reconstruction. Another common mechanism occurs when an athlete is unexpectedly bumped right before landing from a jump, causing a premature contraction of the quadriceps and landing upon an anteriorly translated tibia. A discussion of ACL injuries in athletic females is presented in Chapter 36.

REHABILITATION CONCERNS

Although successful treatment options exist following ACL injury, an appropriate plan of care continues to be debated. For the sedentary individual, a more conservative approach may be considered in which the acute phase of the injury is allowed to pass and then the individual undergoes a vigorous rehabilitation program. If normal function does not return and the knee remains unstable, then reconstructive surgery is considered.

Most active and athletic patients prefer a more aggressive approach. The ideal patient is a young, motivated, and skilled athlete who is willing to make the personal sacrifices necessary to successfully complete the rehabilitation process. Thus, successful surgical repair and reconstruction of the ACL-deficient knee is dependent to a large extent upon patient selection.

In the case of a partially torn ligament, the medical community is split on treatment approach. Some feel that a partially damaged ACL is incompetent and that the knee should be viewed as if the ligament were completely gone. Others prefer a prolonged initial period of immobilization and limited motion, hoping that the ligament will heal and remain functional. Decisions to treat a patient nonoperatively should be based on the individual's preinjury status and a willingness of that patient to engage only in activities such as jogging, swimming, or cycling that will not place the knee at high risk. This is clearly a case where the patient may wisely seek several opinions before choosing the treatment course.

Surgical technique is crucial to a successful outcome. The improper placement of the tendon graft by only a few millimeters can prevent the return of normal motion. The type of graft chosen will also affect postoperative rehabilitation in terms of tensile strength, harvest site comorbidity, and revascularization.

Traditional rehabilitation following ACL reconstruction is based on the work of Paulos et al.[66] in which phases of rehabilitation correspond to healing time frames of animal models. The traditional model emphasized limited ROM and weight bearing as well as delayed strengthening and return to activity. Return to sports typically occurred within 6–12 months. In 1990, Shelbourne and Nitz[78] reported positive outcomes with an accelerated rehabilitation program that emphasized immediate ROM and full extension, immediate weight bearing as tolerated, early CKC strengthening, and return to sporting activities by 2 months and full competition within 4–6 months.

The following rehabilitation progression is based the accelerated program used at the authors' clinic.

REHABILITATION PROGRESSION

Phase I: Preoperative

The preoperative phase objectives focus on physically preparing the knee for surgery and mentally preparing the patient to deal with the surgery and postoperative rehabilitation. Restoration of full ROM and normal strength prior to reconstruction are key components of this phase, with emphasis on obtaining full ROM before strengthening. The patient should attempt to control swelling during this time. This phase is also an opportunity for the clinician to educate the patient on the basic principles of rehabilitation, which include full hyperextension and full flexion, early weight bearing, and OKC and CKC strengthening.

Preoperative testing should be undertaken to provide a baseline for objective comparison later in the rehabilitation process. The clinician should measure bilateral ROM, including full terminal knee extension. A KT-1000 can be used to determine ligament laxity in each knee. Isokinetic strength evaluation, isometric leg press, and single-leg hop test on the noninvolved leg are all performed prior to surgery.

Gaining full ROM is the first goal during this period. Extension exercises include heel props, towel stretches, and prone hangs. An extension board or other extension device can be used if gaining full extension is difficult. Exercises aimed at gaining flexion include heel slides, wall slides, and supine flexion hangs. In conjunction with ROM exercises, activities to develop quadriceps control are initiated. Active heel lifts and standing knee lock-outs produce quadriceps strength and develop early extension habits. Once full ROM with minimal swelling is obtained, CKC strengthening can begin. The patient can perform leg press, minisquats, step-downs, stationary bike, and stair machine activities.

Phase II: 1–14 Days

Phase II begins immediately after surgery to 2 weeks postoperatively. At discharge, goals for the patient are to achieve full passive knee extension and 110° of flexion, perform an independent straight-leg raise, and weight bear as tolerated. A CPM machine is utilized the day of surgery and is set from 0° to 30° flexion (Fig. 29-38). A CryoCuff is donned immediately after surgery to control pain and swelling. The patient's leg remains in the CPM and CryoCuff except when motion exercises. The patient remains lying down with the knee elevated in the CPM throughout the 1st week except when getting up to go to the bathroom. During this time, the patient is encouraged to fully weight bear as tolerated with crutches if needed.

Initially, extension exercises are performed six times daily. The knee is allowed to fully extend into terminal extension for

10 minutes during each bout with a heel prop. Towel stretches are also used to help gain extension. Knee flexion exercises begin with the knee rested in the CPM at 110°, completed six times daily. The patient can further increase flexion by pulling the leg toward the buttocks and holding for 3 minutes. Leg control is initiated with exercises that emphasize active quadriceps contractions such as quad sets, straight-leg raises, and active heel height. The patient should report to physical therapy 1 week postoperatively with full terminal extension and flexion to 110°, minimal swelling, soft tissue healing, and normal gait.

Exercise progression for knee extension ROM becomes a critical factor during this time. The patient continues to push toward full hyperextension equal to the opposite leg by means of towel stretches, heel props, and prone hangs. A standing knee lock-out is performed by standing with the weight shifted to the reconstructed leg while fully locking the knee into extension by contracting the quadriceps (Fig. 29-47). Obtaining full extension and normal gait early in the rehabilitation process enables the patient to regain quadriceps tone and leg control that set the pace for the entire rehabilitation program. Once full knee extension and normal ambulation are obtained, more challenging leg control exercises such as minisquats and knee extensions are implemented. Knee flexion continues to progress through heel slides, wall slides, and supine flexion hangs.

Criteria for completion of phase II consist of full terminal extension, flexion to 130°, minimal swelling, soft tissue healing, normalized gait including stairs, and the ability to lock the operated knee into extension. The clinician should also test bilateral knee ROM.

Phase III: 2–4 Weeks

Clinical goals for phase III are full ROM, including terminal knee extension, and continued strengthening. The patient should work toward being able to sit back onto the heels. Again, ROM should be measured and documented at the end of this phase.

If full passive terminal extension or full flexion is not yet attained, other measures should be taken to meet these goals. Because of the importance of attaining full ROM, especially extension, additional clinic visits may need to be scheduled. An extension board or other extension device can be used at home and during clinic visits to restore full extension. Supine flexion hangs are the most common method of regaining terminal flexion. The patient can gauge proximity to full terminal flexion by sitting back onto the heels (Fig. 29-48).

Leg control through quadriceps strength is targeted with the addition of step-down exercises. High frequency and high repetitions are utilized to stimulate the patellar tendon graft harvest site. Progression to unilateral step-downs is determined by maintaining full ROM and minimal swelling.

Phase IV: 4–8 Weeks

Phase IV is characterized by improved strength and the initiation of functional activities. Full ROM including terminal extension should be maintained throughout this phase. Quadriceps tone should continue to improve with visible quadriceps definition returning. Once 70 percent quadriceps strength has been demonstrated, a proprioceptive and agility program can begin. A sport-specific functional progression can be set up toward the end of this phase.

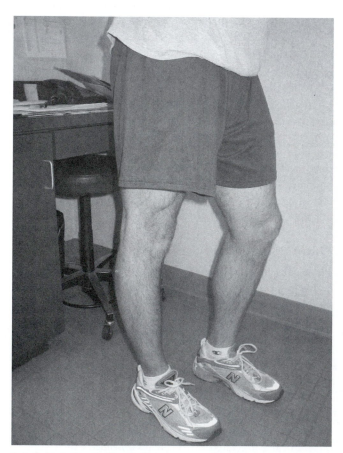

FIGURE 29-47

Standing knee lock-out facilitates extension in weight bearing.

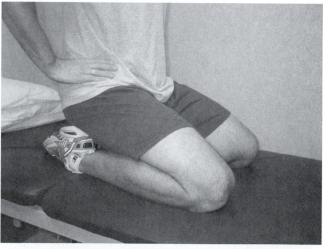

FIGURE 29-48

Sitting back on one's heels to achieve terminal knee flexion and assess flexion ROM.

Postoperative testing at 4 weeks includes a subjective knee questionnaire, bilateral ROM, and KT-1000 arthrometry. The first isokinetic evaluation following surgery occurs during this time frame at speeds of 180°/second and 60°/second. An isometric leg press test is also performed at this time.

During this period, strengthening exercises progress from bilateral to unilateral in an effort to emphasize strength of the quadriceps and patellar tendon graft site. The exercise regimen consists of unilateral leg press, unilateral knee extensions, unilateral step-downs, and lunges. Stair machines, stationary bicycle, and elliptical trainers can be used for aerobic conditioning and moderate speed strengthening.

Controlled agility training activities are initiated based upon the patient's subjective knee rating and strength testing scores. Agility training and limited sports participation not only help the patient to regain quickness and functional movement patterns but also restore confidence in returning to previous functional status. Agility drills may include form running in shortened distances, backward running, lateral slides, crossovers, and single-leg hopping. Individual athletic drills should be sport specific, such as shooting a basketball or dribbling a soccer ball. For specifics on current jump training programs advocated for female athletes, refer to Chapter 36. This component of rehabilitation is not only for athletes, but should also be tailored to meet the demands each patient will face upon return to prior activity level.

Phase V: 8 Weeks and On

Return to full activity is the focus of the final phase. The goals for the patient are to maintain full ROM, continue quadriceps strengthening, and increase activities as appropriate. Testing at this time includes a subjective knee questionnaire, bilateral ROM, KT-1000 arthrometry, isokinetic strength test, and isometric leg press. The single-leg hop test should be initiated 2 months postoperatively for functional comparison between legs. The single-leg hop is performed for distance with takeoff and landing from the same leg.

Exercises to maintain full ROM and continuous strength and conditioning are adjusted according to the patient's needs. A functional progression is integrated to meet the unique needs of each patient. The patient, family, coach, and athletic trainer need to be educated when and how to modify activity based upon subjective and objective knee findings. Return to full, nonrestricted activities is the ultimate goal of the patient and clinician in pursuit of a successful outcome. The patient will periodically follow-up in the clinic for reassessment, strength testing, and research purposes.

Posterior Cruciate Ligament Sprain

PATHOMECHANICS

Isolated tears of the PCL are uncommon and injuries to the PCL are usually the result of a combined ligament injury. The majority of PCL tears occur on the tibia (70 percent), whereas 15 percent occur on the femur and 15 percent are midsubstance

tears.[90] In the PCL-deficient knee, there is an increased likelihood of medial side meniscus lesions and chondral defects.[30]

As with other ligament sprains, the severity of the injury is indicated by the degree of laxity. Grade II and III sprains will demonstrate increased laxity with the posterior drawer, posterior sag, and reverse pivot shift tests when compared to the opposite knee. Increased laxity is typically associated with combined ligament injuries and meniscus tears.

MECHANISM OF INJURY

In athletics, the most common mechanism of injury to the PCL is with the knee in a position of forced hyperflexion with the foot plantar flexed. The PCL may also be injured when the tibia is forced posteriorly on the fixed femur or the femur is forced anteriorly on the fixed tibia. It is also possible to injure the PCL when the knee is hyperflexed and a downward force is applied to the thigh. Forced hyperextension will usually result in injury to both the PCL and ACL. If an anteromedial force is applied to a hyperextended knee, the posterolateral joint capsule may also be injured. If enough valgus or varus force is applied to the fully extended knee to rupture either collateral ligament, it is possible that the PCL may also be torn.

After PCL injury, the patients will likely indicate that they heard a pop. Unlike ACL injuries, patients sustaining injury to the PCL will often feel that the injury was minor and that they can return to activity immediately. There will be mild to moderate swelling occurring within 2–6 hours.

REHABILITATION CONCERNS

Perhaps the greatest concern in rehabilitating a patient with an injured PCL is the fact that the arthrokinematics of the joint are altered, and this change can eventually lead to degeneration of both the medial compartment and the patellofemoral joint.

The treatment of PCL injuries remains unclear because of the uncertainty about the natural history and because of the lack of consistent and reproducible surgical results. Patients sustaining grade I or II PCL injuries should initially undergo nonoperative treatment as most athletes return to functional activity independent of degree of laxity. In addition, nonoperative treatment results are often similar to those for operative treatment. Many patients with an isolated PCL tear do not seem to exhibit any functional performance limitations and can continue to compete athletically, whereas others occasionally are limited in performing normal daily activities.[30] Parolie and Bergfield[65] reported a success rate of over 80 percent with nonoperative treatment and that knee stability was not related to return to sport or patient satisfaction.

Nonoperative treatment of PCL should follow a course of rehabilitation similar to that of the general progression presented earlier in the chapter. In the early phase, hamstring exercises should be avoided and knee extension should be performed in an arc of 0°–60° to prevent increased tibiofemoral shear forces. Bracing may be useful to prevent subtle subluxation in patients who report pain during rehabilitation, but is generally not recommended. For patients with a significant sag sign, it may be necessary to splint the knee in extension in order to promote healing in a shortened position. Often, there is minimal functional limitation and the patient may progress rapidly through the rehabilitative process with minimal pain and swelling.

Operative treatment of acute or chronic grade II or III isolated PCL tears remains controversial. Furthermore, there are typically associated ligamentous injuries with increased posterior laxity. Therefore, PCL reconstructions are most often performed secondary to combined ligamentous instability, making the rate of performing isolated PCL reconstruction minimal. The decision to undergo operative treatment should be based on the functional participation status of the individual and associated risk factors that may produce arthritic changes.

REHABILITATION PROGRESSION

Phase I: Preoperative

Phase I includes preoperative rehabilitation and objective testing. The goals of this phase include restoring full ROM and quadriceps strength, minimizing swelling and pain, and educating the patient in the basic principles of PCL rehabilitation. Unlike patients with ACL injury, most patients with an isolated PCL injury do not have preoperative ROM limitations, quadriceps atrophy and weakness, or significant effusion. A functional PCL brace may be worn to assist in preventing posterior tibiofemoral shear forces. Strengthening exercises can progress as in the general progression with caution against hamstring dominated exercises and active knee flexion beyond 60°. Preoperative testing consists of bilateral ROM, ligament arthrometry, and isokinetic strength evaluation.

Phase II: 1–14 Days

The goals of phase II include controlling swelling and pain through the use of cryotherapy, improving gait quality, improving quadriceps control, and gradually returning flexion ROM.

The patient wears a CryoCuff and compression garment immediately postoperative through the 1st week. Cryotherapy can be weaned to six to eight times per day after the 1st week of surgery. The patient will ambulate with crutches and an immobilizer, progressing from weight bearing as tolerated to full-weightbearing throughout the first 2 weeks. Extension ROM is maintained by lying the leg flat for 10 minutes, three to four times per day. The patient can work on passive flexion from 0° to 60°, three to four times per day. Strengthening exercises to facilitate the early return of quadriceps strength include quad sets, straight-leg raises, and knee extensions from 0° to 60° of knee flexion. The patient is seen in the clinic 1 week postoperative to evaluate and modify the rehabilitation program as needed.

Phase III: 2–4 Weeks

The patient is seen in the clinic again 2 weeks following surgery for the second postoperative visit. The goals of phase III include attaining symmetrical hyperextension, increasing flexion to 90°, improving quadriceps strength, restoring patellar mobility, and restoring normal gait.

Cryotherapy is continued four to six times per day and a compression garment is worn in order to minimize residual swelling and pain. The patient gradually begins to increase knee flexion passively, which can be done in a sitting position by placing a small bolster in the popliteal crease and gently pulling the distal tibia back. This technique will ensure anterior placement of the tibia during flexion. Heel props or prone hangs can begin approximately three times per day in order to obtain symmetrical hyperextension. Patellar mobilization is also initiated in order to restore normal patellar glide and prevent contracture. Restoration of normal hyperextension and patellar glide is essential for proper patellofemoral biomechanics.

The patient may begin CKC strengthening that includes minisquats, calf raises, step-ups/-downs, and leg press in addition to the strengthening exercises of phase II. The goals of strength training in this phase include muscle reeducation and protection of healing tissue. Active knee flexion and hamstring strengthening must be avoided in this phase. Gait quality is assessed and progressed from full-weightbearing with immobilizer to full-weightbearing with a functional PCL brace locked at 70° of flexion.

Phase IV: 4–8 Weeks

The patient will be seen in phase IV for the third and fourth visits at the 4th and 6th postoperative week. Goals of phase IV include gradual return of full flexion and aggressive strengthening. Cryotherapy is continued two to three times per day and after exercise. The flexion block on the PCL brace may be removed at this time. Extension ROM is maintained by performing heel props, while full flexion is obtained by using the popliteal bolster and performing heel slides. The bolster may be removed once 120° of flexion is achieved. The intensity of the current OKC and CKC strengthening exercises may be increased, and isolated hamstring strengthening can be initiated at the end of this phase if needed. Step machine may be initiated using the PCL brace, and swimming may also begin following adequate healing of the incision. ROM is measured during each clinical visit, and knee ligament arthrometry is conducted at the 6th postoperative week.

Phase V: 8 Weeks and On

Phase V consists of weeks 8 through the 1st postoperative year. The goals of phase V include restoration of normal flexibility and a gradual return to sports, emphasizing return of power and endurance. Typically, the patient will experience a gradual return to full activity between 3 and 6 months postoperation.

ROM exercises may be weaned down once full ROM is obtained and a comprehensive flexibility program is begun on a daily basis. The functional PCL brace may be removed and the aforementioned CKC strengthening exercises are performed with increased intensity, three times per week. Isotonic hamstring strengthening may be begun if rendered appropriated by the clinician. Stationary bike and a jogging progression are initiated to improve cardiorespiratory endurance. Running may begin in the pool progressing to the treadmill and land as tolerated. The principle of specificity is very important in order to prepare the athlete for high-speed movements, jumping, and rapid change in direction required by the individual sport. Proprioceptive training needs to be addressed to improve static and dynamic balance deficiencies. Functional strength deficits need to be addressed if they are encountered in this phase. The patient must safely pass a functional progression before return to sports.

The patient is seen in this phase at 2, 3, and 6 months postoperative, and 1 year after surgery for objective measurement and follow-up. A subjective knee questionnaire, ROM, ligament arthrometry, isometric strength evaluation, and single-leg hop test are performed at each of these visits. These tests are useful to make an informed decision regarding the safe return of the athletes to physical activity.

Meniscal Injury

PATHOMECHANICS

The medial meniscus has a much higher incidence of injury than the lateral meniscus, which may be attributed to the coronary ligaments that attach the meniscus peripherally to the tibia and also to the capsular ligament. The lateral meniscus does not attach to the capsular ligament and is more mobile during knee movement. Because of the attachment to the medial structures, the medial meniscus is prone to disruption from valgus and torsional forces.

A meniscus tear often results in immediate joint-line pain with an effusion developing gradually over 48–72 hours. Initially, pain is described as a "giving-way" feeling. The torn meniscus may become displaced and wedge itself between the articulating surfaces of the tibia and femur, thus imposing a chronic locking or "catching" of the joint. A knee that is locked at 10°–30° of flexion may indicate a tear of the medial meniscus, whereas a knee that is locked at 70° or more may indicate a tear of the posterior portion of the lateral meniscus. A positive McMurray's test usually indicates a tear in the posterior horn of the meniscus.

Chronic meniscal lesions may also display recurrent swelling and obvious muscle atrophy around the knee. The patient may complain of an inability to perform a full squat or to change direction quickly when running without pain, a sense of the knee collapsing, or a "popping" sensation. Displaced meniscal tears can eventually lead to serious articular degeneration with major impairment and disability. Such symptoms and signs usually warrant surgical intervention.

MECHANISM OF INJURY

Acute meniscus injuries are most often caused by coupled compression and rotation. As a result of these forces, the meniscus becomes pinched within the tibiofemoral joint and tears. Noncontact mechanisms include a plant and cut maneuver or jumping, common in sporting activities. A contact mechanism is usually the result of a direct blow or force to the knee that causes a valgus, varus, or hyperextension force combined with rotation while the knee is in a weight-bearing position.

Meniscal lesions can be longitudinal, oblique, or transverse. Stretching of the anterior and posterior horns of the meniscus can produce a vertical–longitudinal or "bucket-handle" tear. A longitudinal tear may also occur by forcefully extending the knee from a flexed position, while the femur is internally rotated. During extension, the medial meniscus is suddenly pulled back, causing the tear. In contrast, the lateral meniscus can sustain an oblique tear by a forceful knee extension with the femur externally rotated.

REHABILITATION CONCERNS

Three surgical treatment choices are possible for the patient with a damaged meniscus: partial meniscectomy, meniscal repair, and meniscal transplantation. It was not too long ago that the accepted surgical treatment for a torn meniscus involved total removal of the damaged meniscus. However, total meniscectomy has been shown to cause premature degenerative arthritis. With the advent of arthroscopic surgery, the need for total meniscectomy has been virtually eliminated. Surgical management of meniscal tears should include every effort to minimize loss of any portion of the meniscus.

The location of the meniscal tear often dictates whether surgical treatment will involve a partial meniscectomy or a meniscal repair. Tears that occur within the inner one-third of the meniscus will have to be resected because they are unlikely to heal, even with surgical repair, because of avascularity. Tears in the middle one-third of the meniscus, and particularly in the outer one-third, may heal well following surgical repair because they have a good vascular supply. Partial meniscectomy of a torn meniscus is much more common than meniscal repair.

Rehabilitation following meniscal repair commands restricted joint motion through 6 weeks to allow for healing. An upper body ergometer can be used to maintain cardiorespiratory endurance during this period. During this period, weight bearing is limited as well, as per physician recommendations. Early strengthening can include quad sets and OKC hip exercises. Early restricted weight-bearing exercise can be accomplished in an aquatic environment, when incisional healing allows. Please refer to Chapter 19 for more details on aquatic rehabilitation. ROM exercises should focus on attaining flexion and extension within the restrictions. Partial-weightbearing on crutches should progress to full-weightbearing after 6 weeks. Once the brace can be removed, rehabilitation progresses similar to the general progression to regain full ROM and normal muscle strength. Generally, the patient can return to full activity around 3 months.

Not all meniscus tears will require surgery. Some meniscus tears may heal or become asymptomatic without surgical intervention. When a meniscus tear remains symptomatic, surgery is usually recommended. Rehabilitation will vary depending on the course of treatment and type of meniscal injury. Nonoperative rehabilitation aims to reduce swelling, restore full ROM, and normalize gait before returning to normal activities. The specific rehabilitation exercises for nonoperative rehabilitation are similar to those prescribed here for partial meniscectomy.

REHABILITATION PROGRESSION (FOR PARTIAL MENISCECTORY)

Phase I: 1–14 Days

The clinical goals of phase I are to control swelling and inflammation, increase ROM, normalize gait, and improve quadriceps control. The clinician will test bilateral ROM during this phase.

A CryoCuff or other form of cryotherapy is applied six to eight times per day to control pain and swelling. Cold application is particularly important following exercise. Use of a compression garment during the 1st postoperative week will help control swelling. The patient should keep the leg elevated as much as possible the first few days following surgery.

Regaining full extension is a critical factor in this phase. The patient is encouraged to push extension and regain full flexion through towel extensions, prone hangs, and heel slides. Extension can be assisted through a standing knee lock-out with weight shifted to the operated leg.

The patient should begin partial- to full-weightbearing with crutches. Use of crutches can be discontinued once gait is normalized. In most instances, the patient will be full-weightbearing by the end of this phase. The patient may be non-weightbearing for a period of time if an osteochondral lesion is present on a weight-bearing surface.

Quadriceps strengthening exercises are initiated to facilitate early return to normal strength. Strengthening should include straight-leg raises, knee extensions, and calf raises.

Phase II: 2–4 Weeks

Phase II goals include attaining full ROM, normal gait, no swelling, and an early return to agility and sport-specific activities as tolerated. The clinician will again measure ROM.

Cryotherapy should be continued three to four times per day and always after exercise. If the patient does not have full extension or flexion, ROM exercises are continued. Exercises should include unilateral one-quarter squats, unilateral step-downs, unilateral calf raises, and lunges. These exercises should not be performed if pain or crepitus exists.

Bicycle and stair machine workouts can begin in this phase. Initial workouts should be 10–15 minutes in length and progress to 30 minutes with moderate to high resistance. Toward the end of this phase, the patient can perform short sprints in 5-minute intervals. Freestyle and flutter kick swimming can be performed as well, but breaststroke is not encouraged. A jogging to sprinting progression can be performed in chest-deep water.

Once full ROM is regained and the patient has sufficient leg control, weight room activities can be initiated. Exercises include unilateral leg press, unilateral knee extensions, calf raises, and hamstring curls. Once tolerable, agility and sport-specific activities can commence toward the end of this phase.

Phase III: 4 Weeks and On

The focus of phase III is on a functional return to prior activity level. The patient is to maintain full ROM and no swelling. If weakness is noted, strengthening should continue to address the specific deficit. The clinician tests bilateral ROM and isokinetic strength if a specific athletic goal is desired. Implementation of a sport-specific functional progression is appropriate at this time.

GENERAL REHABILITATION PROGRESSION FOLLOWING PATELLOFEMORAL INJURY

Initially, patients with patellofemoral pain should always be treated with a conservative rehabilitation program. The clinician must tailor intervention to address the specific components of the patient's dysfunction. An effective rehabilitation program takes into consideration the anatomy of the involved structures, the biomechanics of the patellofemoral joint as well the proximal and distal joints, the stage of healing, and the patient's response to treatment. An additional discussion of patellofemoral considerations in athletic females is present in Chapter 36. A general three-phase rehabilitation program for patellofemoral injury is presented with specific techniques for defined patellofemoral conditions to follow.

Phase I

Phase I goals are to control pain and inflammation of the involved soft tissue structures, restoration of normal ROM and gait, and patient education. Controlling pain and inflammation allows the patient to progress uninhibited through the rehabilitation process. Restoring full knee ROM and normal gait mechanics is essential for return to typical daily activities and for initiating functional rehabilitation exercise.

Cryotherapy in the form of ice bags or ice massage, three to four times per day, is effective in reducing pain and controlling inflammation. Other physical modalities including ultrasound, iontophoresis, and electrical stimulation may also be effective in controlling patellofemoral symptoms. Physician-prescribed nonsteroidal anti-inflammatory medication can be useful as well. Active and active-assistive ROM exercise, a partial- to full-weightbearing progression, and the use of assistive devices as needed are beneficial in the restoration of knee ROM and normal ambulation. The patient should be educated regarding factors that cause patellofemoral pain and treatment of the dysfunction in order to modify or avoid activities that exacerbate patellofemoral pain as well as self-manage symptoms as they occur.

Phase II

The emphasis of phase II is on flexibility, advanced strengthening, proprioception, and cardiovascular conditioning. Exercise intensity and stresses on the patellofemoral joint should be kept low in an effort to progress through rehabilitation without

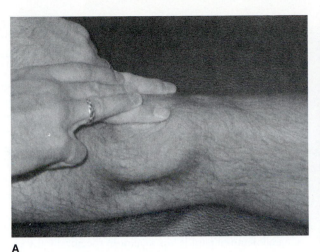
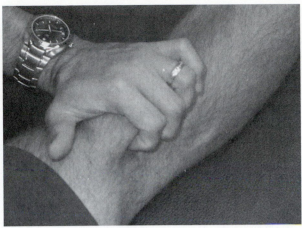

A

B

FIGURE 29-49

Self-mobilization for the patella. **A,** To mobilize the patella for a restricted medial glide, instruct the patient to long sit with knees straight and quadriceps relaxed. With the radial surface of the index finger on the lateral surface of the patella, push the patella medially and apply additional force with the other hand. **B,** To mobilize the patella for a restricted medial tilt, push laterally on the medial edge of the patella with the palmar surface of the hand and grasp the lateral edge of the patella with the fingertips, tilting medially.

increasing symptoms. The clinician should conduct a dynamic biomechanical evaluation once ROM and gait are normal to determine the underlying cause to the dysfunction. By the end of phase II, the patient should have improved flexibility of tightened structures, improved quadriceps strength and proprioception, maintained appropriate level of conditioning, and addressed biomechanical abnormalities.

Flexibility: Flexibility exercises that address deficits in quadriceps, hamstrings, ITB, and gastrocnemius–soleus complex muscle length must be initiated. The frequency and duration of stretching is controversial. Clinically, stretching three sets for 30 seconds is common. Bandy et al.[4,5] have shown that there is no difference in hamstring length when duration is increased from 30 to 60 seconds or when the frequency is increased from one set to three sets.

In addition to muscular flexibility, patellar mobility should be incorporated to address imbalances in the passive soft tissue stabilizers. The patient can be instructed in self-mobilization techniques to correct an abnormal patellar glide or tilt (Fig. 29-49).

OKC and CKC strengthening: Strengthening exercises for patients with patellofemoral dysfunction have shifted from non-weightbearing OKC exercises to more functional CKC exercises. This change has been due to reports that CKC exercise has decreased patellofemoral joint stresses and may be more tolerable for patients with patellofemoral dysfunction.

Steinkamp et al.[85] demonstrated significantly greater knee movement, Fpf, and patellofemoral joint stress with leg extension at 0° and 30° and leg press at 60° and 90°.

Cohen et al.[13] determined that from 20° to 70°, there was no significant difference in patellofemoral contact stress between CKC and the highest load OKC and that OKC exercise appears safe with flexion moments equivalent to 22.5 lbs applied to the ankle from 20° to 90°. Escamilla et al.[22] showed that patellofemoral stress during leg press progressively increases as knee angle increases. During knee extension, the results revealed progressively increasing patellofemoral stress to approximately 60° of knee flexion, and then decreased at higher knee angles. They recommended CKC exercise in a knee range between 0° and 50° and employing lower (0°–30°) or higher (75°–90°) knee angles during OKC exercise.

In 2000, Witvrouw et al.[96] performed the first prospective, randomized study comparing the efficacy of OKC versus CKC in the management of patellofemoral pain. The CKC protocol had a significant improvement in pain and functionality over the OKC group. However, both protocols showed increased quadriceps strength, improved functionality, and decreased pain. As a result of the study, the authors report using both OKC and CKC strengthening exercises in the treatment of patellofemoral pain. In 2004, Witvrouw et al.[95] reported a 5-year follow-up of the patients with patellofemoral pain. The majority of parameters measured revealed no significant difference between both groups and that most of the improvements in strength, functionality, and subjective complaints were maintained over a 5-year period.

Based on current research findings, strengthening of patients with patellofemoral pain should utilize both OKC and CKC exercises. Initially, OKC exercise can be safely performed between 60° and 90° of knee flexion and CKC exercise may be safest from 0° to 50° of knee flexion. In reality, the safe ROM will be different for each patient. The patient and clinician should be conscious of pain, crepitus, and the location of patellar articular surface lesions during exercise. A progression can be utilized that increases repetition, external load, and ROM as well as advancing from bilateral to unilateral activities.

Role of the VMO: For years, clinicians have attempted to isolate the VMO in an effort to counteract the pull of the VL and improve dynamic patellar tracking. To date, contribution and isolation of the VMO remains speculative.

Mirzabeigi et al.[60] studied the electromyographic (EMG) activity of the vastus medialis longus, VMO, vastus intermedius, and VL during nine sets of exercises thought to target VMO recruitment. The results showed that EMG activity of the VMO was not significantly greater than the other muscles tested, suggesting that the VMO cannot be significantly isolated during these exercises. Studies have shown that high levels of EMG activity of the VMO in relation to the VL can be produced during leg press, lateral step-ups, terminal knee extension, quad sets, and hip adduction exercises.[15,82,93]

Recent studies have shifted attention to the timing of VMO activation. Cowan et al.[14] reported a delayed onset of EMG VMO activity in relation to the VL during ascending and descending stair stepping in patients with patellofemoral pain. In contrast, there was no difference in EMG onset for the control group. Cowan et al.[15] also demonstrated that "McConnell"-based physical therapy in subjects with delayed VMO onset during stair stepping was effective in equalizing the EMG onset of the VMO to the VL while ascending stairs, and VMO onset preceded the VL while descending stairs. In turn, subjects reported significant improvements in pain and function.

On the basis of current evidence, exercise that attempts to recruit the VMO does so in a generalized strengthening effect of the entire quadriceps.[60] Quadriceps strengthening has been an emphasized commonality in studies that demonstrate success in treating patients with patellofemoral pain.[8,45,69] In addition, Natri et al.[62] performed a 7-year prospective follow-up study of patients with chronic patellofemoral pain that found extension strength to be a significant predictor of successful outcome.

Distal factors: The role of foot mechanics in patellofemoral joint dysfunction has been theorized for quite some time. Buchbinder et al.[9] proposed that prolonged pronation would internally rotate the lower extremity, producing a medially displaced patella. Tiberio[89] contended that excessive subtalar joint pronation would produce even greater internal rotation of the femur and cause a resultant lateral soft tissue force, increasing lateral patellofemoral contact forces.

As a result, clinicians have attempted to limit the amount of tibial internal rotation along with the coupled femoral internal rotation in an effort to decrease the Q angle and the resultant laterally directed pull of the quadriceps. Klingman et al.[48] reported that a medial-wedge orthosis was capable of producing a mean medial displacement of the patella relative to the femoral trochlear groove of 1.08 mm. Sutlive et al.[87] found that the best

predictors of improvement in patients with patellofemoral pain using an off-the-shelf foot orthosis and modified activity were forefoot valgus alignment of $\geq 2°$, passive great toe extension of $\leq 78°$, or navicular drop of ≤ 3 mm.

A complete lower extremity biomechanical examination in the weight-bearing and non-weightbearing positions is clearly important. The literature supports an association between excessive pronation and lower extremity internal rotation with altered patellofemoral mechanics. Patients demonstrating excessive foot pronation or excessive lower extremity internal rotation may benefit from a foot orthosis intervention as part of a comprehensive rehabilitation program. Chapter 31 discusses examination and prescription of foot orthotics.

Proximal factors: The most recently proposed contributor to patellofemoral pain is hip weakness, specifically the external rotators. Patients with patellofemoral pain who demonstrate a lack of adduction and internal rotation control during weight bearing activities are candidates for hip strengthening. Internal rotation of the femur causes the trochlear groove to rotate underneath the patella, generating increased patellofemoral stress due to the relative lateral position of the patella.[50]

Mascal et al.[57] published a case report on two female patients with patellofemoral pain who did not demonstrate patellar malalignment or maltracking. Subsequent examination revealed substantial hip adduction and internal rotation during gait and a step-down task as well as hip and abdominal weakness. Intervention aimed at these impairments produced significant improvements in pain, gluteal strength, and kinematics. Ireland et al.[43] reported that subjects with patellofemoral pain were 26 percent weaker in hip abduction and 36 percent weaker in hip external rotation compared to a control group.

Clearly, the functional significance of weakened hip musculature can contribute to patellofemoral pain. Also, the clinician must assess the length of the ITB in relation to gluteal muscle strength because of their role in hip internal rotation. Assessment of the hip and pelvis must become a priority in patients with suspected proximal weakness or lack of dynamic pelvic control or further examined in those patients who have failed traditional conservative management of patellofemoral pain.

Proprioception and cardiovascular conditioning: The pain and abnormal tissue stresses present in patellofemoral dysfunction may lead to proprioception deficits. Baker et al.[3] found that joint position sense was significantly decreased in knees with patellofemoral pain compared to the control group, decreased between the symptomatic and asymptomatic knees in the test group, and decreased between the asymptomatic knees in the test group compared to the control group. Whether or not proprioception deficits precede or result from patellofemoral pain, proprioception must be addressed during rehabilitation.

Maintaining cardiovascular conditioning is an important objective when treating a patient with patellofemoral pain. The clinician should strive to provide the patient with alternative training methods that allow pain-free knee ROM and minimize patellofemoral stress for return to prior activity level. Depending on the cause of patellofemoral pain and the tissues involved, options for cardiovascular conditioning include jogging, swimming, bicycling, and using upper body ergometers or other forms of endurance exercise equipment.

Phase III

The goal of phase III is to return the patient to the prior level of activity. A maintenance program of cryotherapy, lower extremity flexibility, and quadriceps strengthening should be continued three times per week to maintain the gains of phase II. Prior to full return to activity, an activity-specific functional progression should be completed with the use of an external support if needed.

Bracing and taping: Many external supports (Fig. 29-50) have been designed to augment the return to pain-free activity through helping to maintain patellar alignment or decrease soft tissue stresses. Patellar braces are typically made of an elastic wrap or neoprene sleeve with various cutouts and pads to help control patellar positioning and tracking. An infrapatellar strap placed around the patellar tendon has been advocated for patellar tendinitis or traction apophysitis and an ITB strap placed around the distal ITB for ITB friction syndrome. These straps apply compression near the site of irritation and act as a "counterforce" to decrease stress at the tendinous insertion. While research on patellar straps is scant, similar braces have been shown to increase pain threshold and affect proprioception in patients with lateral epicondylitis.[63]

Although wearing a brace appears to be effective in reducing pain, radiographic studies show that decreases in pain are not the result of improvement in patellar alignment.[70] Powers et al.[71] found significant reduction in pain immediately upon application of patellar bracing and significantly increased total patellofemoral joint contact area despite no influence on lateral patellar tilt and small but significant changes in lateral patellar displacement. Their results suggest that increases in patellofemoral joint contact area may decrease patellofemoral stress and therefore decrease pain. Powers et al.[72] again supported this theory with a study that showed bracing significantly decreased patellofemoral stress during free and fast walking when compared to the nonbraced condition.

Bracing appears to provide some patients with a decrease in pain, improve patellofemoral joint contact, and allow adequate quadriceps strengthening and exercise progression. The pain reduction secondary to wearing a brace may be the edge a patient needs to continue with rehabilitation exercises and return to sport activity. However, a brace should not be a substitution for a comprehensive rehabilitation program.

A popular adjunct to treating patellofemoral pain is taping (Fig 29-51). In 1986, McConnell[58] published the taping methods for the treatment of patellar chondromalacia. The theory behind the McConnell taping technique is a passive correction of the abnormal glide, tilt, and rotational components of patellar maltracking to allow pain-free rehabilitation and facilitate VMO recruitment.

Much like bracing, numerous studies support that taping provides pain relief. However, alteration in patellar alignment or facilitation of the VMO has also been disputed. Pfeiffer et al.[68] showed that McConnell medial glide taping resulted in significant medial glide of the patellofemoral joint before but not after a running and agility task. Ng and Cheng[64] reported a significant decrease in pain with patellar taping, but also reported a decrease in the relative activity of the VMO. A randomized controlled trial by Wittingham et al.[91] found that the combination of taping and exercise was superior to placebo taping and exercise and exercise alone in treating patients with patellofemoral pain. A multicenter study by Wilson et al.[94] found that patellar taping provided an immediate decrease in pain regardless of how the taping was applied, supporting that it is unlikely that taping works by altering patellar position. Cowan et al.[16] found that individuals receiving therapeutic patellar taping improved in both EMG onset of vasti and pain in a stair-stepping task when compared with placebo taping and no tape.

Clinically and scientifically, taping and bracing both offer significant pain relief in treating patients with patellofemoral pain despite the unknown mechanism by which either works. Whether or not changes occur in vasti recruitment is debatable, but one would expect less muscle inhibition with reduced pain. Evidence has shown that the benefits from external patellar supports probably do not occur from changes in patellar tracking or alignment. Changes in proprioception, increases in patellofemoral joint compression that decreases peak stresses, and shifting contact from sensitive to less irritated areas are more plausible explanations. Regardless of the mechanism by which patients experience relief through these applications, the use of external patellar supports can be a useful adjunct to quadriceps strengthening and exercise progression.

SPECIFIC REHABILITATION TECHNIQUES FOR PATELLOFEMORAL INJURIES

Classification of Patellofemoral and Extensor Mechanism Injuries

Complaints of pain and disability associated with the patellofemoral joint and the extensor mechanism are exceedingly common. The terminology used to describe this anterior knee pain has been a source of some confusion and requires some clarification. Until recently, it was not uncommon for every patient who walked into a clinic complaining of anterior knee pain to be diagnosed as having chondromalacia patella.

Several authors have proposed classification systems for patellofemoral disorders.[24,28,35,41,49,59,92] We have chosen to use the classification system proposed by Wilk et al.[92] because of the comprehensive and clearly defined diagnostic categories. The classification system divides patellofemoral disorders into the following groups: (1) patellar compression syndromes (PCSs), (2) patellar instability, (3) biomechanical dysfunction, (4) direct patellar trauma, (5) soft tissue lesions, (6) overuse

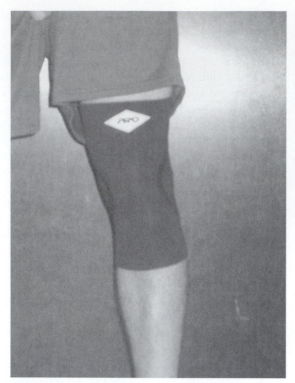

A

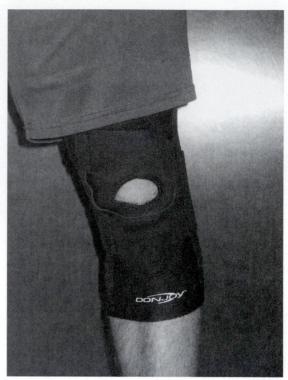

B

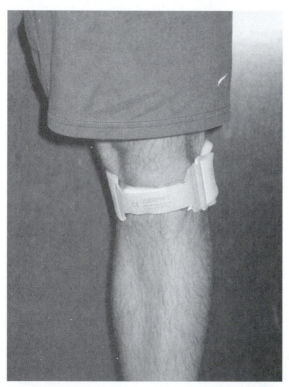

C

FIGURE 29-50

External supports. **A,** Patellar sleeve for increased patellofemoral joint contact area (Pro Orthopedic Devices, Inc., Tucson, AZ). **B,** Patellar sleeve with lateral "J" buttress and straps for patellar subluxation or lateral patellar alignment (dj Orhtopedics, LLC, Vista, CA). **C,** Infrapatellar band for patellar tendinitis and traction apophysitis (Aircast, Summit, NJ).

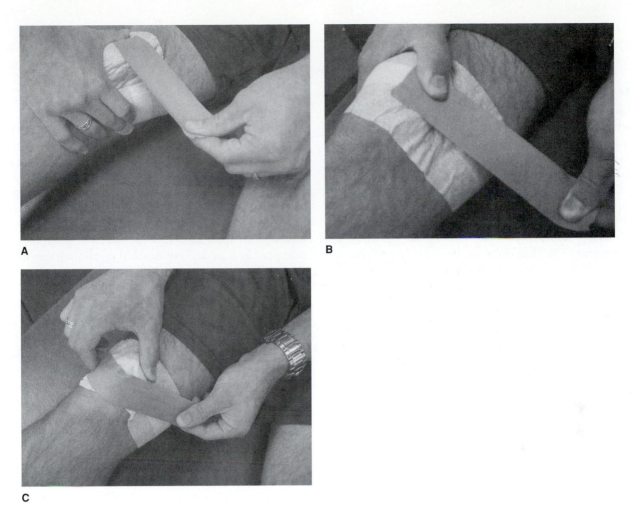

A   **B**   **C**

FIGURE 29-51

Patellofemoral taping. **A,** McConnell technique gliding the patella medially for an abnormal lateral glide. **B,** McConnell technique tilting the patella medially for an abnormal lateral tilt. **C,** McConnell technique internally rotating the patella for an abnormal external rotation.

syndromes, (7) osteochondritis diseases, and (8) neurological disorders. However, the scope of this chapter will not feature management for direct patellar trauma, osteochondritis diseases, or neurological disorders.

In general, the majority of patellofemoral injuries can follow the general patellofemoral rehabilitation progression. When indicated, specific rehabilitation techniques and concerns unique to each disorder will be presented with the corresponding phase. In that case a particular phase is not reported; refer to the general progression.

Patellar Compression Syndromes

PATHOMECHANICS

Patellar compression syndrome is defined as a patella that is overconstrained by the surrounding soft tissue, causing grossly restricting patellar mobility.[92] Typically, PCS occurs on the lateral side but can also occur globally in which case patellar mobility is restricted both medially and laterally. PCS signs and symptoms often include peripatellar pain and crepitus with squatting or stair climbing, synovial irritation, decreased patellar mobility (laterally or globally), patellar malalignment or maltracking, and strength deficit or imbalance.

REHABILITATION PROGRESSION

Phase I

Pain modulation and inflammatory control must begin immediately. Cryotherapy and activity modification should be used to manage these symptoms. Grade I and II patellar mobilizations can be utilized for pain control through large fiber input. In the case of severe lateral compression, patellar taping can be applied to unload the lateral patellofemoral articulation by providing a low-load, long-duration stretch. Patient education becomes critical to modify and avoid painful activities as well as symptom management.

Phase II

The primary focus of phase II is stretching tightened lateral structures. This goal can be accomplished through patellar mobilization, prolonged tape application, and ITB stretching. Inflexibility of the hamstrings, quadriceps, and gastrocnemius should be addressed as well. With global PCS, normal patellar mobility and full knee ROM must be restored before initiating further therapy. Grade III and IV patellar mobilizations should be utilized to address specific limitations. Quadriceps strengthening should be pain free and may be augmented by patellar taping. The clinician must determine appropriate resistance and ROM in which to perform exercises to maintain pain-free strengthening. The focus of strengthening should not be on eliciting activation of the VMO, but rather the quadriceps as a whole. Once normal patellar mobility is restored, the patient can advance to an increased activity progression.

Patellar Instability

PATHOMECHANICS

Patellar instability is the partial or complete lateral displacement of the patella with associated injury to the medial soft tissue structures. Improper patellar tracking leading to patellar subluxation or dislocation may result from a number of different biomechanical factors, including femoral anteversion with increased internal femoral rotation, genu valgum with a concomitant increase in the Q angle, a shallow femoral groove, flat lateral femoral condyles, patella alta, weakness of the vastus medialis muscle relative to the VL, ligamentous laxity with genu recurvatum, excessive external rotation of the tibia, pronated feet, a tight lateral retinaculum, and a patella with a positive lateral tilt.

MECHANISM OF INJURY

The classic noncontact mechanism involves a plant and cut maneuver in which the thigh internally rotates to promote knee valgus. A simultaneous contraction of the quadriceps pulls the patella superiorly, resulting in a lateral patella and creating a force to displace the patella. As a rule, displacement occurs laterally with the patella shifting over the lateral femoral condyle. The patella can also dislocate with contact, forcing the patella laterally. The patient reports a painful giving-way episode. The patient experiences a complete loss of knee function, pain, and swelling, with the patella remaining in an abnormal lateral position. If voluntary relocation does not occur, a physician should immediately reduce the dislocation by applying mild pressure on the patella with the knee extended as much as possible.

A chronically subluxing patella places abnormal stress on the patellofemoral joint and the medial restraints. Pain is a result of swelling, but also results because the medial capsular tissue has been stretched and torn. ROM will be restricted because of the associated swelling. There may also be a palpable tenderness at the attachment site of the medial retinaculum on the adductor tubercle.

REHABILITATION PROGRESSION

Phase I

The goals of phase I are to control pain and inflammation and restore full ROM and normal gait. Acute instability will require immediate cryotherapy and a brief period of immobilization. The patient will require use of crutches and an immobilizer for ambulation until full ROM and normal gait can be attained. Treatment of chronic instability or subluxation will require less drastic efforts to manage pain, inflammation, and effusion compared to acute instability. Nonetheless, irritation can be controlled by icing and avoidance of aggravating activities.

Phase II

The emphasis of phase II is dynamic patellar stabilization through the quadriceps strengthening. If lateral tracking of the patella is involved in the instability, correction of lower extremity alignment or tightened lateral structures must be addressed. Also, if lateral tracking is the result of uncontrolled adduction and internal rotation of the thigh, gluteus medius strengthening must be addressed. Maintaining cardiorespiratory endurance of the lower extremity musculature is also important. As the condition of the knee improves, activities can be gradually advanced.

Phase III

With advanced exercise and a functional progression, the use of a patellar stabilization brace is helpful in maintaining patella stability.

Biomechanical Dysfunction

PATHOMECHANICS

Biomechanical dysfunction is an alteration in the normal biomechanics of the lower extremity. The alteration is often subtle but can have a profound effect via repetition or intense activity. Common areas of biomechanical dysfunction include imbalances of the foot or hip, leg length deficiency, and soft tissue tightness. The proximal and distal factors affecting patellofemoral biomechanics have been previously discussed.

REHABILITATION PROGRESSION

Phase I

Treatment of biomechanical dysfunction of the lower extremity rarely involves focusing on the source of pain. Excessive subtalar joint pronation or other intrinsic imbalance of the foot resulting in altered patellofemoral articulation should be addressed with orthotics. A true or functional limb length discrepancy can cause pronation and other deviation in gait. A lift in the shoe or manual correction may be indicated. Flexibility deficiencies can lead to pronation, increased stress on the extensor mechanism, changes in gait, and lateral displacement of the patella. The clinician should restore any loss of flexibility in the gastrocnemius–soleus complex, quadriceps, hamstrings, ITB, and hip rotators. In addition, weakened gluteal muscles that result in an unstable pelvis and uncontrolled hip adduction and internal rotation during dynamic activities must be functionally strengthened.

Soft Tissue Lesions

PATHOMECHANICS

A soft tissue lesion involves pain and inflammation of the numerous soft tissue structures that surround the knee. Commonly involved tissues include bursa, plica, infrapatellar fat pad, distal ITB, and medial patellofemoral ligament. Soft tissue lesions may be the result of direct trauma, repeated activity, or biomechanical abnormality.

Bursitis in the knee can be acute, chronic, or recurrent and is usually the result of a direct trauma. Although any one of the numerous knee bursae can become inflamed anteriorly, the prepatellar, deep infrapatellar, and suprapatellar bursae have the highest incidence of irritation in sports. Swelling is localized to the location of injury.

The medial patellar plica is the least common but most subject to injury. This band-like tissue can bowstring across the anterior aspect of the medial femoral condyle, impinging between the articular cartilage and the medial patellar facet during knee flexion. The patient may feel or hear a snap and report painful pseudolocking. Injury can also be caused by trauma. Inflammation of the plica leads to fibrosis and thickening with a loss of extensibility. When present, the majority of plicae are pliable and asymptomatic.

The distal ITB is injured while repetitively crossing the lateral femoral condyle during flexion and extension of the knee. Pain will radiate toward the lateral joint line and down toward the proximal tibia, becoming increasingly severe with continued activity. Increased tension of the ITB causing irritation is often the result of leg length discrepancies, tightness in the TFL, hamstrings, and quadriceps, genu varum, excessive pronation, internal tibial torsion, and restricted dorsiflexion.

REHABILITATION PROGRESSION
Phase I

During phase I of the rehabilitation process, iontophoresis and ice massage can be used to control pain and inflammation of numerous soft tissue lesions. Also emphasized are a nonantalgic gait, full ROM, and activity modification. In the case of a chronic bursitis, a compression wrap should be worn continuously. With a chronic ITB syndrome, transverse friction massage can be useful to create a localized inflammation and promote collagen realignment.

Phase II

During phase II, strengthening can begin once inflammation and pain are resolved. In patients with ITB friction syndrome,

caution must be taken with exercise near terminal knee extension where the ITB passes over the lateral femoral condyle. These patients should avoid running hills and stair climbing. Patients with plica syndrome should avoid exercise with full knee flexion such as deep squatting, which can compress an inflamed plica. If the lesion is the result of a biomechanical dysfunction, alignment of the lower extremity must be addressed.

Overuse Syndromes

PATHOMECHANICS

Overuse syndromes are the result of excessive activity or stress to the extensor mechanism and include patellar tendinitis and traction apophysitis. Tendinitis of the extensor mechanism can occur at the superior patellar pole (quadriceps tendinitis), the tibial tubercle, or most commonly at the distal pole of the patella. Patellar tendinitis usually develops in patients involved in activities that require repetitive jumping and is frequently given the title "jumper's knee." Point tenderness on the posterior aspect of the inferior pole of the patella is the hallmark of patellar tendinitis. This condition is typically related to the eccentric shock-absorbing function that the quadriceps provides upon landing from a jump.

Traction apophysitis is a common adolescent condition that results from repeated stress of the patellar tendon at the apophysis of either the tibial tubercle or inferior patellar pole. The condition is characterized by pain and swelling that increases with activity and is relieved with rest. Osgood–Schlatter disease occurs over the tibial tuberosity while Larsen–Johansson disease, although much less common, occurs at the inferior pole of the patella.

REHABILITATION PROGRESSION
Phase I

Ice massage and iontophoresis can be used to control pain and inflammation during this stage of rehabilitation. Avoidance of jumping, kicking, running, and sudden deceleration that can cause undue stress on the extensor mechanism is warranted. Transverse friction massage can be used to facilitate the healing process of patellar tendinitis but should not be performed in conjunction with anti-inflammatory modalities.

Phase II

Eccentric strengthening is a key component in the rehabilitation process of overuse injuries to the extensor mechanism.[84] Eccentric loading moments produce more stress on the patellar tendon than concentric loading.[21] Exercises can be progressed from low velocity to high velocity and bilaterally to unilaterally. Flexibility deficits of the hamstrings and quadriceps must be addressed. The clinician should also take into consideration the ratio of hamstring to quadriceps strengthening, since less than 80 percent has been identified as being associated with overuse knee injuries.[20]

Phase III

The use of a patellar strap can be beneficial to control pain when returning to intense activity. Activities can be progressed if the patient remains pain-free and improvements are maintained. Traction apophysitis is often a self-limiting condition.

REFERENCES

1. Aglietti P, Insall JN, Cerulli G. Patellar pain in incongruence I: Measurements of incongruence. *Clin Orthop* 176:217–224, 1983.

2. Arnoczky SP, Warren RF. Microvasculature of the human meniscus. *Am J Sports Med* 10:90–95, 1982.

3. Baker V, Bennell K, Stillman B, et al. Abnormal knee joint position sense in individuals with patellofemoral pain syndrome. *J Orthop Res* 20:208–214, 2002.

4. Bandy WD, Irion JM. The effect of time on static stretch on the flexibility of the hamstring muscles. *Phys Ther* 79:845–850, 1994.

5. Bandy WD, Irion JM, Briggler M. The effect of time and frequency of static stretching on flexibility of the hamstring muscles. *Phys Ther* 77:1090–1096, 1997.

6. Beynnon BD, Fleming BC, Johnson RJ, et al. ACL strain behavior during rehabilitation exercise in vivo. *Am J Sports Med* 23:24, 1995.

7. Boucher JP, King MA, Lefebvre R, et al. Quadriceps femoris muscle activity in patellofemoral pain syndrome. *Am J Sports Med* 20:527–732, 1992.

8. Brizzini M, Childs JD, Piva SR, et al. Systematic review of the quality of randomized controlled trials for patellofemoral pain syndrome. *J Orthop Sports Phys Ther* 33:4–20, 2003.

9. Buchbinder MR, Napora NJ, Biggs EW. The relationship of abnormal pronation to chondromalacia of the patella in distance runners. *J Am Podiatry Assoc* 69:159–162, 1979.

10. Butler DL, Noyes FR, Grood ES. Ligamentous restraints to anterior-posterior drawer in the human knee: A biomechanical study. *J Bone Joint Surg Am* 62:259–270, 1980.

11. Caborn DN, Johnson BM. The natural history of the anterior cruciate ligament-deficient knee: A review. *Clin Sports Med* 12:625–636, 1993.

12. Cavagna GA, Saibene FP, Margaria R. Mechanical work in running. *J Appl Phys Neuromech Basis Kinesiol* 19:249–256, 1964.

13. Cohen ZA, Roglic H, Grelsamer RP, et al. Patellofemoral stresses during open and closed kinetic chain exercises: An analysis using computer simulation. *Am J Sports Med* 21:480–487, 2001.

14. Cowan SM, Bennell KL, Crossley KM, et al. Delayed onset of electromyographic activity of vastus medialis obliquus relative to vastus lateralis in patients with patellofemoral pain syndrome. *Arch Phys Med Rehabil* 82: 183–189, 2001.

15. Cowan SM, Bennell KL, Crossley KM, et al. Physical therapy alters recruitment of the vasti in patellofemoral pain syndrome. *Med Sci Sports Exerc* 34:1879–1885, 2002.

16. Cowan SM, Bennell KL, Hodges PW. Therapeutic patellar taping changes the timing of vasti muscle activation in people with patellofemoral pain syndrome. *Clin J Sports Med* 12:339–347, 2002.

17. Cox JS. Patellofemoral problems in runners. *Clin Sports Med* 4:699–715.

18. Daniel DM, Stone ML, Dobson BE, et al. Fate of the ACL-injured patient: A prospective outcome study. *Am J Sports Med* 22:632–644, 1994.

19. De Carlo MS, Sell KE. Normative data for range of motion and single-leg hop in high school athletes. *J Sport Rehabil* 6:246–255, 1997.

20. Devan MR, Pescatello LS, Faghri P, et al. A prospective study of overuse knee injuries among female athletes with muscle imbalances and structural abnormalities. *J Athlet Train* 39:263–267, 2004.

21. Elftman H. Biomechanics of muscle with particular application to studies of gait. *J Bone Joint Surg Am* 48:363–377, 1966.

22. Escamilla RF, Fleisig GS, Zheng N, et al. Biomechanics of the knee during closed kinetic chain and open kinetic chain exercises. *Med Sci Sports Exerc* 30:556–569, 1998.

23. Evans NA, Chew HF, Stanish WD. The natural history and tailored treatment of ACL injury. *Phys Sports Med* 29: 19–34, 2001.

24. Ficat RP, Phillippe J, Hungerford DS. Chondromalacia patellae: A system of classification. *Clin Orthop* 144:55–62, 1979.

25. Frank CB, Jackson DW. The science of reconstruction of the anterior cruciate ligament. *J Bone Joint Surg Am* 79: 1556–1576, 1997.

26. Fu FH, Bennett CH, Lattermann C, et al. Current trends in anterior cruciate ligament reconstruction. Part 1: Biology and biomechanics of reconstruction. *Am J Sports Med* 27:821–830, 1999.

27. Fukubayashi T, Kurosawa H. The contact area and pressure distribution pattern of the knee: A study of normal and osteoarthrotic knee joints. *Acta Orthop Scand* 51:871–879, 1980.

28. Fulkerson JP, Kalenak A, Rosenberg TD, et al. Patellofemoral pain. *Instr Course Lect* 41:57–71, 1992.

29. Fullerton LR, Andrews JR. Mechanical block to extension following augmentation of the anterior cruciate ligament: A case report. *Am J Sports Med* 12:166–169, 1984.

30. Geissler W, Whipple T. Intraarticular abnormalities in association with PCL injuries. *Am J Sports Med* 21:846–849, 1993.

31. Girgis FG, Marshall JL, Monajem ARSA. The cruciate ligaments of the knee joint. *Clin Orthop* 106:216–231, 1975.

32. Gollehon DL, Torzilli PA, Warren RF. The role of the posterolateral and cruciate ligaments in the human knee

stability: A biomechanical study. *Trans Orthop Res Soc* 10:270, 1985.

33. Goodfellow J, Hungerford DS, Zindel M. Patello-femoral joint mechanics and pathology. I: Functional anatomy of the patellofemoral joint. *J Bone Joint Surg Br* 58:287–290, 1976.

34. Grana WA, Kriegshauser LA. Scientific basis of extensor mechanism disorders. *Clin Sports Med* 4:247–257, 1985.

35. Grelsamer RP. Classification of patellofemoral disorders. *Am J Knee Surg* 10:96–100, 1997.

36. Grelsamer RP, Klein JR. The biomechanics of the patellofemoral joint. *J Orthop Sports Phys Ther* 28:286–298, 1998.

37. Grood ES, Noyes FR, Butler DL, et al. Ligamentous and capsular restraints preventing straight medial and lateral laxity in intact human cadaver knees. *J Bone Joint Surg Am* 63:1257–1269, 1981.

38. Hawkins RJ, Misamore GW, Merritt TR. Followup of the acute nonoperated isolated anterior cruciate ligament tear. *Am J Sports Med* 14:205–210, 1986.

39. Hughston JC, Eilers AF. The role of the posterior oblique ligament in repairs of acute medial ligament tears of the knee. *J Bone Joint Surg Am* 55:923–940, 1973.

40. Hungerford DS, Barry M. Biomechanics of the patellofemoral joint. *Clin Orthop* 144:9–15, 1979.

41. Insall J. "Chondromalacia patellae": Patellar malalignment syndrome. *Orthop Clin North Am* 10:117–127, 1979.

42. Insall JN, Falvo KA, Wise DW. Chondromalacia patellae: A prospective study. *J Bone Joint Surg Am* 58:1–8, 1976.

43. Ireland ML, Willson JD, Ballantyne BT, et al. Hip strength in females with and without patellofemoral pain. *J Orthop Phys Ther* 11:671–676, 2003.

44. Johnson RJ, Kettelkamp DB, Clark W, et al. Factors effecting late results after meniscectomy. *J Bone Joint Surg Am* 56:719–729, 1974.

45. Kannus P, Natri A, Paakkala T, et al. An outcome study of chronic patellofemoral pain syndrome: Seven-year followup of patient in a randomized, controlled trial. *J Bone Joint Surg Am* 81:355–363, 1999.

46. Kaufer H. Mechanical function of the patella. *J Bone Joint Surg Am* 53:1551–1560, 1971.

47. Kendall FP, McCreary EK, Provance PG. *Muscles: Testing and function*, 4th ed. Baltimore, Williams & Wilkins, 1993.

48. Klingman RE, Liaos SM, Hardin KM. The effect of subtalar joint posting on patellar glide position in subjects with excessive rearfoot pronation. *J Orthop Sports Phys Ther* 25:185–191, 1997.

49. Larson RL, Cabaud HE, Slocum DB, et al. The patellar compression syndrome: Surgical treatment by lateral retinacular release. *Clin Orthop* 134:158–167, 1978.

50. Lee TQ, Morris G, Csintalan RP. The influence of tibial and femoral rotation on patellofemoral contact and pressure. *J Orthop Phys Ther* 11:686–693, 2003.

51. Levine J. Chondromalacia patellae. *Phys Sports Med* 7:41–49, 1979.

52. Levy IM, Torzilli PA, Gould JD, et al. The effect of lateral meniscectomy on motion of the knee. *J Bone Joint Surg Am* 71:401–406, 1989.

53. Levy IM, Torzilli PA, Warren RF. The effect of medial meniscectomy on anterior-posterior motion of the knee. *J Bone Joint Surg Am* 64:883–888, 1982.

54. Lieb FJ, Perry J. Quadriceps function: An anatomical and mechanical study using amputated limbs. *J Bone Joint Surg Am* 50:1535–1548, 1968.

55. Lipke JM, Janecki CJ, Nelson CL, et al. The role of incompetence of the anterior cruciate and lateral ligaments in anterolateral and anteromedial instability: A biomechanical study of cadaver knees. *J Bone Joint Surg Am* 63:954–960, 1981.

56. MacIntyre DL, Robertsone DG. Quadriceps muscle activity in women runners with and without patellofemoral pain syndrome. *Arch Phys Med Rehabil* 73:10–14, 1992.

57. Mascal CL, Landel R, Powers C. Management of patellofemoral pain targeting hip, pelvis, and trunk muscle function: 2 case reports. *J Orthop Sports Phys Ther* 33:647–659, 2003.

58. McConnell J. The management of chonromalacia patellae: A long term solution. *Aust J Physiother* 32:215–223, 1986.

59. Merchant AC. Classification of patellofemoral disorders. *Arthroscopy* 4:235–240, 1988.

60. Mirzabeigi E, Jordan C, Gronley JK, et al. Isolation of the vastus medialis oblique muscle during exercise. *Am J Sports Med* 27:50–53, 1999.

61. Miyasaka KC, Daniel D, Stone M. The incidence of knee ligament injuries in general population. *Am J Knee Surg* 4:3–8, 1991.

62. Natri A, Kannus P, Jarvinen M. Which factors predict the long-term outcome in chronic patellofemoral pain syndrome?: A 7-yr prospective follow-up study. *Med Sci Sports Exerc* 30:1572–1577, 1998.

63. Ng GY, Chan HL. The immediate effects of tension of counterforce forearm brace on neuromuscular performance of wrist extensor muscles in subjects with lateral humeral epicondylosis. *J Orthop Sports Phys Ther* 34:72–78, 2004.

64. Ng GY, Cheng JM. The effect of patellar taping on pain and neuromuscular performance in subjects with patellofemoral pain syndrome. *Clin Rehabil* 16:821–827, 2002.

65. Parolie J, Bergfeld J. Long-term results of non-operative treatment of PCL injuries in the patient. *Am J Sports Med* 14:35–38, 1986.

66. Paulos LE, Wnorowski DC, Greenwald AE. Infrapatellar contracture syndrome: Diagnosis, treatment and long-term follow up. *Am J Sport Med* 22(4):440–449, 1994.

67. Paulos LE, Rusche K, Johnson C, et al. Patellar malalignment: A treatment rationale. *Phys Ther* 60:1624–1632, 1980.

68. Pfeiffer RP, DeBeliso M, Shea KG, et al. Kinematic MRI assessment of McConnell taping before and after exercise. *Am J Sports Med* 32:621–628, 2004.

69. Powers CM, Perry J, Hsu A, et al. Are patellofemoral pain and quadriceps femoris muscle torque associated with locomotor function? *Phys Ther* 77:1063–1078, 1997.

70. Powers CM, Shellock FG, Beering TV, et al. Effect of bracing on patellar kinematics in patients with patellofemoral joint pain. *Med Sci Sports Exerc* 31:1714–1720, 1999.

71. Powers CM, Ward SR, Chan L, et al. The effect of bracing on patella alignment and patellofemoral joint contact area. *Med Sci Sports Exerc* 36:1226–1232, 2004.

72. Powers CM, Ward SR, Chen Y, et al. The effect of bracing on patellofemoral joint stress during free and fast walking. *Am J Sports Med* 32:224–231, 2004.

73. Rivera JE. Open versus closed kinetic chain rehabilitation of the lower extremity: A functional and biomechanical analysis. *J Sports Rehabil* 3:154–167, 1994.

74. Rubinstein RA, Shelbourne KD, Van Meter CD, et al. Effect on knee stability if full hyperextension is restored immediately after autogenous bone-patellar tendon-bone anterior cruciate ligament reconstruction. *Am J Sports Med* 23:365, 1993.

75. Sachs RA, Daniel DM, Stone ML. Patellofemoral problems after ACL reconstruction. *Am J Sport Med* 19:957–964, 1990.

76. Seering WP, Piziali RL, Nagel DA, et al. The function of the primary ligaments of the knee in varus-valgus and axial rotation. *J Biomech* 13:785–794, 1980.

77. Shelbourne KD, Gray T. Results of anterior cruciate ligament reconstruction based on the meniscus and articular cartilage status at the time of surgery: Five- to fifteen-year evaluations. *Am J Sports Med* 28:446–452, 2000.

78. Shelbourne KD, Nitz P. Accelerated rehabilitation after anterior cruciate ligament reconstruction. *Am J Sports Med* 18(3):292–299, 1990.

79. Shelbourne KD, Patel DV. Management of combined injuries of the anterior cruciate and medial collateral ligaments. *J Bone Joint Surg Am* 77:800–806, 1995.

80. Shelbourne KD, Patel DV, Martini DJ. Classification and management of arthrofibrosis of the knee following anterior cruciate ligament reconstruction. *Am J Sports Med* 24:857, 1996.

81. Shelbourne KD, Wilckens JH, Mollabashy A, et al. Arthrofibrosis in acute anterior cruciate ligament reconstruction: The effect of timing of reconstruction and rehabilitation. *Am J Sports Med* 19:332–336, 1991.

82. Simoneau GG, Wilk KE. Electromyographic activity of vastus medialis and lateralis during four exercises [abstract]. *Phys Ther* 73:580, 1993.

83. Souza DR, Gross MT. Comparison of vastus medialis obliquus: Vastus lateralis muscle integrated electromyographic ratios between healthy subjects and patients with patellofemoral pain. *Phys Ther* 71:310–320, 1991.

84. Stanish WD, Rubinovich RM, Curwin S. Eccentric exercise in chronic tendinitis. *Clin Orthop* 208:65–68, 1986.

85. Steinkamp LA, Dillingham MF, Markel MD, et al. Biomechanical considerations in patellofemoral joint rehabilitation. *Am J Sports Med* 21:438–444, 1993.

86. Sullivan D, Levy IM, Heskier S. Medial restraints to anterior-posterior motion of the knee. *J Bone Joint Surg Am* 66:930–936, 1984.

87. Sutlive TG, Mitchell SD, Maxfield SN, et al. Identification of individuals with patellofemoral pain whose symptoms improved after a combined program of foot orthosis use and modified activity: A preliminary investigation. *Phys Ther* 84:49–61, 2004.

88. Terry GC. The anatomy of the extensor mechanism. *Clin Sports Med* 8:163–177, 1989.

89. Tiberio D. The effect of excessive subtalar joint pronation on patellofemoral mechanics: A theoretical model. *J Orthop Sports Phys Ther* 9:160–165, 1999.

90. Tria A, Klein K. *An Illustrated Guide to the Knee.* New York, Churchill Livingstone, 1991.

91. Whittingham M, Palmer S, Macmillan F. Effects of taping on pain and function in patellofemoral pain syndrome: A randomized controlled trial. *J Orthop Sports Phys Ther* 34:504–510, 2004.

92. Wilk KE, Davies GJ, Mangine RE, et al. Patellofemoral disorders: A classification system and clinical guidelines for nonoperative rehabilitation. *J Orthop Sports Phys Ther* 28:307–322, 1998.

93. Wilk KE, Escamilla RF, Fleisig GS, et al. A comparison of tibiofemoral joint forces and electromyographic activity during open and closed kinetic chain exercises. *Am J Sports Med* 24:518–527, 1996.

94. Wilson T, Carter N, Thomas G. A multicenter, single-masked study of medial, neutral, and lateral patellar taping in individuals with patellofemoral pain syndrome. *J Orthop Sports Phys Ther* 33:437–443, 2003.

95. Witvrouw E, Danneels L, Van Tiggelen D, et al. Open versus closed kinetic chain exercises for patellofemoral pain: A 5-year prospective randomized study. *Am J Sports Med* 32:1122–1130, 2004.

96. Witvrouw E, Lysens R, Bellemans J, et al. Open versus closed kinetic chain exercises for patellofemoral pain: A prospective, randomized study. *Am J Sports Med* 28:687–694, 2000.

97. Woo SL, Inoue M, McGurk-Burleson E, et al. Treatment of the medial collateral ligament injury. II: structure and function of canine knees in response to differing treatment regimens. *Am J Sports Med* 15:22–29, 1987.

C H A P T E R 3 0

Rehabilitation of Lower-Leg Injuries

Christopher J. Hirth

O B J E C T I V E S

After completion of this chapter, the therapist should be able to do the following:

- Discuss the functional anatomy and biomechanics of the lower leg during open-chain and weight-bearing activities such as walking and running.
- Identify the various techniques for regaining range of motion, including stretching exercises and joint mobilizations.
- Identify common causes of various lower-leg injuries and provide a rationale for treatment of these injuries.
- Discuss criteria for progression of the rehabilitation program for various lower-leg injuries.
- Describe and explain the rationale for various treatment techniques in the management of lower-leg injuries.
- Discuss the various rehabilitative strengthening techniques, including open- and closed-chain isotonic exercise, balance/proprioceptive exercises, and isokinetic exercise for dysfunction of the lower leg.

FUNCTIONAL ANATOMY AND BIOMECHANICS

The lower leg consists of the tibia and fibula and four muscular compartments that either originate on or traverse various points along these bones. Distally the tibia and fibula articulate with the talus to form the talocrural joint. Because of the close approximation of the talus within the mortise, movement of the leg will be dictated by the foot, especially upon ground contact. This becomes important when examining the effects of repetitive stresses placed upon the leg with excessive compensatory pronation secondary to various structural lower-extremity malalignments.[74,75] Proximally the tibia articulates with the femur to form the tibiofemoral joint as well as serving as an attachment site for the patellar tendon, the distal soft-tissue component of the extensor mechanism. The lower leg serves to transmit ground reaction forces to the knee as well as rotatory forces proximally along the lower extremity that may be a source of pain, especially with weight-bearing activities.[54]

Compartments of the Lower Leg

All muscles work in a functional integrated fashion in which they eccentrically decelerate, isometrically stabilize, and concentrically accelerate during movement.[49] The muscular components of the lower leg are divided anatomically into four compartments. In an open kinetic-chain position, these muscle groups are responsible for movements of the foot primarily in a single plane. When the foot is in contact with the ground, these muscle-tendon units work both concentrically and eccentrically to absorb ground reaction forces, control excessive movements of the foot and ankle to adapt to the terrain, and, ideally, provide a stable base to propel the limb forward during walking and running.

The anterior compartment is primarily responsible for dorsiflexion of the foot in an open kinetic-chain position. Functionally these muscles are active in early and midstance phase of gait, with increased eccentric muscle activity directly after heel strike to control plantarflexion of the foot and pronation of the forefoot.[20] Electromyogram (EMG) studies have noted that the tibialis anterior is active in more than 85 percent of the gait cycle during running.[52]

The deep posterior compartment is made up of the tibialis posterior and the long toe flexors and is responsible for inversion of the foot and ankle in an open kinetic chain. These muscles help control pronation at the subtalar joint (STJ) and internal rotation of the lower leg.[20,52] Along with the soleus, the tibialis posterior will help decelerate the forward momentum of the tibia during midstance phase of gait.

The lateral compartment is made up of the peroneus longus and brevis, which are responsible for eversion of the foot in an open kinetic chain. Functionally the peroneus longus plantarflexes the first ray at heel off, while the peroneus brevis counteracts the supinating forces of the tibialis posterior to provide osseous stability of the subtalar and midtarsal joints during the propulsive phase of gait. This is a prime example of muscles working synergistically to isometrically stabilize during movement. EMG studies of running report an increase in peroneus brevis activity when the pace of running is increased.[52]

The superficial posterior compartment is made up of the gastrocnemius and soleus muscles, which in open kinetic-chain position are responsible primarily for plantarflexion of the foot. Functionally these muscles are responsible for acting eccentrically controlling pronation of the STJ and internal rotation of the leg in the midstance phase of gait and activated concentrically during the push-off phase of gait.[20,52]

REHABILITATION TECHNIQUES FOR SPECIFIC INJURIES

Tibial and Fibular Fractures

PATHOMECHANICS

The tibia and fibula constitute the bony components of the lower leg and are primarily responsible for weight bearing and muscle attachment. The tibia is the most commonly fractured long bone in the body, and fractures are usually the result of either direct trauma to the area or indirect trauma such as a combination rotatory/compressive force. Fractures of the fibula are usually seen in combination with a tibial fracture or as a result of direct trauma to the area. Tibial fractures will present with immediate pain, swelling, and possible deformity and can be open or closed in nature. Fibular fractures alone are usually closed and present with pain on palpation and with ambulation. These fractures should be treated with immediate medical referral and most likely a period of immobilization and restricted weight bearing for weeks to possibly months, depending on the severity and involvement of the injury. Surgery such as open reduction with internal fixation of the bone, usually of the tibia, is common.

INJURY MECHANISM

The two mechanisms of a traumatic lower-leg fracture are either a direct insult to the bone or indirectly through a combined rotatory/compressive force. Direct impact to the long bone, such as from a projectile object or the top of a ski boot, can produce enough damaging force to fracture a bone. Indirect trauma from a combination of rotatory and compressive forces can be manifested when the foot is planted and the proximal segments are rotated with a large compressive force. A fibular fracture may accompany the tibial fracture.

REHABILITATION CONCERNS

Tibial and fibular fractures are usually immobilized and placed on a restricted weight-bearing status for a period of time to facilitate fracture healing. Immobilization and restricted weight bearing of a bone, its proximal and distal joints, and surrounding musculature will lead to functional deficits once the fracture is healed. Depending on the severity of the fracture, there also may be postsurgical considerations such as an incision and hardware within the bone. Complications following immobilization include joint stiffness of any joints immobilized, muscle atrophy of the lower leg and possibly the proximal thigh and hip musculature, as well as an abnormal gait pattern. Bullock-Saxton demonstrated changes in gluteus maximus EMG muscle activation after a severe ankle sprain.[13] Proximal hip muscle weakness is magnified by the immobility and non-weight-bearing action that accompanies lower-leg fractures. It is important that the therapist perform a comprehensive evaluation of the patient to determine all potential rehabilitation problems, including range of motion (ROM), joint mobility, muscle flexibility strength and endurance of the entire involved lower extremity, balance, proprioception, and gait. The therapist must also determine the functional demands that will be placed on the patient upon return to normal activity and set up short- and long-term goals accordingly. Upon cast removal it is important to address ROM deficits. This can be managed with passive ROM (PROM)/active ROM (AROM) exercises in a supportive medium such as a warm whirlpool (Figures 30-1 to 30-4, 30-9, 30-14, 30-15, 30-18, 30-20). Joint stiffness can be addressed via joint mobilization to any joint that was immobilized (Figures 16-61 to 16-68). It is possible to have posttraumatic edema in the foot and ankle after cast removal that can be reduced with massage. Strengthening exercises can help facilitate muscle firing, strength, and endurance (Figures 30-5 to 30-8, 30-10 to 30-13). Balance and proprioception can be improved with single-leg standing activities and balance board activities (Figures 30-22 to 30-25). Cardiovascular endurance can be addressed with pool activities including swimming and pool running with a flotation device, stationary cycling, and the use of an upper-body ergometer (UBE) (Figures 30-16, 30-17, 30-26, 30-27). A stair stepper is also an excellent way to address cardiovascular needs as well as lower-extremity strength, endurance, and weight bearing (Figure 30-17).

Once the patient demonstrates proficiency in static balance activities on various balance modalities, more dynamic neuromuscular control activities can be introduced. Exercise sandals (OPTP, Minneapolis, MN) can be incorporated into rehabilitation as closed kinetic-chain functional exercise that places

TABLE 30-1

Exercise Sandal Progression

1. Walking in place
2. Forward/backward walking—small steps
3. Sidestepping
4. Butt kicks
5. High knees
6. Single-leg stance—10 to 15 seconds
7. Ball catch—sidestepping
8. Sport-specific activity
   - Each activity can be performed for 30–60 seconds with rest between each activity
   - All exercises should be performed with short-foot and good standing posture except where sport-specific activity dictates otherwise

increased proprioceptive demands on the patient. The exercise sandals are wooden sandals with a rubber hemisphere located centrally on the plantar surface (Figure 30-28). Patients can be progressed into the exercise sandals once they demonstrate proficiency in barefoot single-leg stance. Prior to using the exercise sandals the patient is instructed in the short-foot concept—a shortening of the foot in an anterior–posterior direction while the long-toe flexors are relaxed, thus activating the short-toe flexors and foot the intrinsics (Figure 30-36).[36] Clinically the short foot appears to enhance the longitudinal and transverse arches of the foot. Once the patients can perform the short-foot concept in the sandals, they are progressed to walking in place and forward walking with short steps (Figure 30-29). The patient is instructed to assume a good upright posture while training in the sandals. Initially the patient may be limited to 30–60 seconds while acclimating to the proprioceptive demands. Once the patients appear safe with walking in place and small-step forward walking, they can follow a rehabilitation progression (see Table 30-1 and Figures 30-30 to 30-34).

The exercise sandals offer an excellent means of facilitating lower-extremity musculature that can be affected by tibial and fibular fractures. Bullock-Saxton noted increased gluteal muscle activity with exercise sandal training after 1 week.[14] Myers also demonstrated increased gluteal activity, especially with high-knees marching in the exercise sandals.[47] Blackburn has shown increased activity in the lower-leg musculature, specifically the tibialis anterior and peroneus longus, while performing the exercise sandal progression activities.[11] The lower-leg musculature is usually weakened and atrophied, from being so close to the trauma. The exercise sandals offer an excellent means of increasing muscle activation of the lower-leg musculature in a functional weight-bearing manner.

REHABILITATION PROGRESSION

Management of a postimmobilization fracture will require good communication with the physician to determine progression of weight-bearing status, any assistive devices to be used during the rehabilitation process, such as a walker boot, and any other pertinent information that will influence the rehabilitation process. It is important to address ROM deficits immediately with AROM, passive stretching, and skilled joint mobilization. Isometric strengthening can be initiated and progressed to isotonic exercises once ROM has been normalized. After weight-bearing status is determined, gait training to normalize walking should be initiated. Assistive devices should be utilized as needed. Strengthening of the involved lower extremity can be incorporated into the rehabilitation process, especially for the hip and thigh musculature. It is important for the therapist to identify and address this hip muscular weakness early on in rehabilitation through open- and closed-chain strengthening. Balance and proprioceptive exercises can begin once there is full pain-free weight bearing on the involved lower extremity.

As ROM, strength, and walking gait are normalized, the patient can be progressed to a walking/jogging progression and a sport-related functional progression. It must be realized that the rate of rehabilitation progression will depend on the severity of the fracture, any surgical involvement, and length of immobilization. The average healing time for uncomplicated nondisplaced tibial fractures is 10–13 weeks, while for displaced, open, or comminuted tibital fracture, it is 16–26 weeks.[63]

Fibular fractures may be immobilized for 4–6 weeks. Again an open line of communication with the physician is required to facilitate a safe rehabilitation progression for the patient.

CRITERIA FOR FULL RETURN

The following criteria should be met prior to the return to full activity: (1) full ROM and strength, compared to the uninvolved side; (2) normalized walking, jogging, running gait; (3) ability to hop for endurance and 90 percent hop for distance as compared to the uninvolved side, without complaints of pain or observable compensation; and (4) successful completion of an activity-specific functional test.

Tibial and Fibular Stress Fractures

PATHOMECHANICS

Stress fractures of the tibia and fibula are common with physical activity. Studies indicate that stress fractures of the tibia occur at a higher rate than those of the fibula.[7,8,44] Stress fractures in the lower leg are usually the result of the bone's inability to adapt to a repetitive loading response. The bone attempts to adapt to the applied loads initially through osteoclastic activity, which breaks down the bone. Osteoblastic activity, or the laying down of new bone, will soon follow.[51,73] If the applied loads are not reduced during this process, structural irregularities will develop within the bone, which will further reduce the bones' ability to absorb stress and will eventually lead to a stress fracture.[8,26]

Repetitive loading of the lower leg with weight-bearing activity such as running is usually the cause of tibial and fibular stress fractures. Romani reports that repetitive mechanical loading seen with the initiation of a stressful activity may cause an ischemia to the affected bone.[56] He reports that repetitive loading may lead to temporary oxygen debt of the bone, which signals the remodeling process to begin.[56] Also, microdamage to the capillaries further restricts blood flow, leading to more ischemia, which again triggers the remodeling process—leading to a weakened bone and a setup for a stress fracture.[56]

Stress fractures in the tibial shaft mainly occur in the midanterior aspect and the posteromedial aspect.[7,44,53,73] Anterior tibial stress fractures usually present in patients involved in repetitive jumping activities with localized pain directly over the midanterior tibia. The patient will complain of pain with activity that is relieved with rest. The pain can affect activities of daily living (ADLs) if activity is not modified. Vibration testing using a tuning fork will reproduce the symptoms, as will hopping on the involved extremity. A triple-phase technetium[99] bone scan can confirm the diagnosis faster than an X ray, as it can take a minimum of 3 weeks to demonstrate radiographic changes.[51,53,73] Posteromedial tibial pain usually occurs over the distal one-third of the bone with a gradual onset of symptoms.

Focal point tenderness on the bone will help differentiate a stress fracture from medial tibial stress syndrome (MTSS), which is located in the same area but is more diffuse upon palpation. The procedures listed previously will be positive and will implicate the stress fracture as the source of pain. Fibular stress fractures usually occur in the distal one-third of the bone with the same symptomatology as for tibial stress fractures. Although less common, stress fractures of the proximal fibula are noted in the literature.[44,69,82]

INJURY MECHANISM

Anterior tibial stress fractures are prevalent in patients engaging in repetitive physical activities. Authors have noted that the tibia will bow anteriorly with the convexity on the anterior aspect.[18,51,54,73] This places the anterior aspect of the tibia under tension, which is less than ideal for bone healing, which prefers compressive forces. Repetitive stress will place greater tension on this area, which has minimal musculotendinous support and blood supply. Other biomechanical factors may be involved, including excessive compensatory pronation at the STJ to accommodate lower-extremity structural alignments such as forefoot varus, tibial varum, and femoral anteversion. This excessive pronation might not affect the leg during ADLs or with moderate activity, but might become a factor with increases in activity intensity, duration, and frequency, even with sufficient recovery time.[29,73] Increased activity may affect the surrounding muscle-tendon unit's ability to absorb the impact of each applied load, which places more stress on the bone. Stress fractures of the distal posteromedial tibia will also arise from the same problems as listed previously, with the exception of repetitive jumping. Excessive compensatory pronation may play a greater role with this type of injury. This hyperpronation can be accentuated when running on a crowned road, such is the case of the uphill leg.[57] Also, running on a track with a small radius and

tight curves will tend to increase pronatory stresses on the leg that is closer to the inside of the track.[57] Excessive pronation may also play a role with fibular stress fractures. The repeated activity of the ankle everters and calf musculature pulling on the bone may be a source of this type of stress fracture.[51] Training errors of increased duration and intensity along with worn out shoes will only accentuate these problems.[57] Other factors, including menstrual irregularities, diet, bone density, increased hip external rotation, tibial width, and calf girth, have also been identified as contributing to stress fractures.[8,28]

REHABILITATION CONCERNS

Immediate elimination of the offending activity is most important. The patient must be educated on the importance of this to prevent further damage to the bone. Stationary cycling and running in the deep end of the pool with a flotation device can help maintain cardiovascular fitness (Figures 30-16, 30-26). Eyestone et al. have demonstrated a small but statistically significant decrease in maximal aerobic capacity when water running was substituted for regular running.[22] This was also true with using a stationary bike.[22] These authors recommend that intensity, duration, and frequency be equivalent to regular training. Wilder et al. note that water provides a resistance that is proportional to the effort exerted.[78] These authors found that cadence, via a metronome, gave a quantitative external cue that with increased rate showed high correlation with heart rate.[78] Nonimpact activity in the pool or on the bike will help maintain fitness and allow proper bone healing. Proper footware that matches the needs of the foot is also important. For example, a high arched or pes cavus foot type will require a shoe with good shock-absorbing qualities. A pes planus foot type or more pronated foot will require a shoe with good motion control characteristics. A detailed biomechanical examination of the lower extremity both statically and dynamically may reveal problems that require the use of a custom foot orthotic. Stretching and strengthening exercise can be incorporated in the rehabilitation process. The use of ice and electrical stimulation to control pain is also recommended. The utilization of an Aircast with patients who have diagnosed stress fractures has produced positive results.[19] Dickson et al. speculate that the Aircast unloads the tibia and fibula enough to allow healing of the stress fracture with continued participation.[19] Swenson et al. reported that patients with tibial stress fractures who used an Aircast returned to full unrestricted activity in 21 ± 2 days, while patients who used traditional regimen returned in 77 ± 7 days.[72] Fibular and posterior medial tibial stress fractures will usually heal without residual problems if the previously mentioned concerns are addressed. Stress fractures of the mid anterior tibia can take much longer, and residual problems might exist months to years after the initial diagnosis, with attempts at increased activity.[18,21,53,54] Initial treatment may include a short leg cast and non-weightbearing for 6–8 weeks. Batt et al. noted that use of a pneumatic brace in those individuals allowed for return to unrestricted activity, an average of 12 months from presentation.[4] The proposed hypothesis for use of a pneumatic brace is that the elevated osseous hydrostatic and venous blood pressure produce a positive piezoelectric effect that stimulates osteoblastic activity and facilitates fracture healing.[81] Rettig et al. used rest from the offending activity as well as electrical stimulation in the form of a pulsed electromagnetic field for a period of 10–12 hours per day. The authors noted an average of 12.7 months from the onset of symptoms to return to full activity with this regimen.[54] They recommended using this program for 3–6 months before considering surgical intervention.[54] Chang et al. noted good to excellent results with a surgical procedure involving intramedullary nailing of the tibia with individuals with delayed union of this type of stress fracture.[18] Surgical procedures involving bone grafting have also been recommended to improve healing of this type of stress fracture.

REHABILITATION PROGRESSION

After diagnosis of the stress fracture, the patient may be placed on crutches, depending on the amount of discomfort with ambulation. Ice and electrical stimulation can be used to reduce local inflammation and pain. The patients can immediately begin deep-water running with the same parameters as their regular regimen if they are pain-free. Stretching exercises for the gastrocnemius-soleus musculature can be performed two to three times per day (Figure 30-19). Isotonic strengthening exercises with rubber tubing can begin as soon as tolerated on an every-other-day basis, with an increase in repetitions and sets as the therapist sees fit (Figures 30-5 to 30-8). Strengthening of the gastrocnemius can be done initially in an open chain and eventually be progressed to a closed chain (Figure 30-5, 30-12, 30-13). The patient should wear supportive shoes during the day and avoid shoes with a heel, which can cause adaptive shortening of the gastroc-soleus complex and increase strain on the healing bone. Custom foot orthotics can be fabricated for motion control to prevent excessive pronation for those patients that need it. Foot orthotics can also be fabricated for a high arched foot to increase stress distribution throughout the plantar aspect of the whole foot versus the heel and the metatarsal heads. Shock-absorbing materials can augment these orthotics to help reduce ground reaction forces. The exercise sandal progression can also be introduced to help facilitate lower-leg muscle activity and strength (Figure 30-29 to 30-34 and 30-36). As the symptoms subside over a period of 3–4 weeks and X rays confirm that good callus formation is occurring, the athlete may be progressed to a walking/jogging progression on a surface suitable to that athlete's needs. The patient must demonstrate pain-free ambulation prior to initiating a walk/jog program. A quality track or grass surface may be the best choice to begin this progression. The patient may be instructed to jog for 1 minute and then walk for 30 seconds for 10–15 repetitions. This can be performed on an every-other-day basis with high-intensity/long-duration cardiovascular activity occurring daily in the pool or on the bike. The patient should be reminded that the purpose of the walk/jog progression is to provide a gradual increase in stress to the healing bone in a controlled manner. If tolerated, the jogging time can be increased by 30 seconds

every two to three training sessions until the athlete is running 5 minutes without walking. The above progression is a guideline and can be modified based on individual needs.

Romani has developed a three-phase plan for stress fracture management.[56] Phase 1 focuses on decreasing pain and stress to the injured bone while also preventing deconditioning. Phase 2 focuses on increasing strength, balance, and conditioning, and normalizing function, without an increase in pain. After 2 weeks of pain-free exercise in phase 2, running and functional activities of phase 3 are introduced. Phase 3 has functional phases and rest phases. During the functional phase, weeks 1 and 2, running is progressed, while in the third week, or rest phase, running is decreased. This is done to mimic the cyclic fashion of bone growth. During the first 2 weeks, as bone is resorbed, running will promote the formation of trabecular channels; in the third week, while the osteocytes and periosteum are maturing, the impact loading of running is removed.[56] This cyclic progression is continued over several weeks as the patient becomes able to perform activity-specific activities without pain.[56]

CRITERIA FOR NORMAL RETURN

The patient can return to full activity when (1) there is no tenderness to palpation of the affected bone and no pain of the affected area with repeated hopping, (2) plain films demonstrate good bone healing, (3) there has been successful progression of a graded return to running with no increase in symptoms, (4) gastroc-soleus flexibility is within normal limits, (5) hyperpronation has been corrected or shock-absorption problems have been decreased with proper shoes and foot orthotics if indicated, and (6) all muscle strength and muscle length issues of the involved lower extremity have been addressed.

Compartment Syndromes

PATHOMECHANICS AND INJURY MECHANISM

Compartment syndrome is a condition in which increased pressure, within a fixed osseofascial compartment, causes compression of muscular and neurovascular structures within the compartment. As compartment pressures increase, the venous outflow of fluid decreases and eventually stops, which causes further fluid leakage from the capillaries into the compartment. Eventually arterial blood inflow also ceases secondary to rising intracompartmental pressures.[76] Compartment syndrome can be divided into three categories: acute compartment syndrome, acute exertional compartment syndrome, and chronic compartment syndrome (CCS). Acute compartment syndrome occurs secondary to direct trauma to the area and is a medical emergency.[37,70,76] The patient will complain of a deep-seated aching pain, tightness, and swelling of the involved compartment. Reproduction of the pain will occur with passive stretching of the involved muscles. Reduction in pedal pulses and sensory changes of the involved nerve can be present but are not reliable signs.[76,80] Intracompartmental pressure measurements will confirm the diagnosis. Emergency fasciotomy is the definitive treatment. Acute exertional compartment syndrome occurs without any precipitating trauma. Cases have been cited in the literature in which acute compartment syndrome has evolved with minimal to moderate activity. If not diagnosed and treated properly, it can lead to a poor functional outcomes for the patient.[23,80] Again, intracompartmental pressures will confirm the diagnosis, with emergency fasciotomy being the treatment of choice. CCS is activity-related in that the symptoms arise rather consistently at a certain point in the activity. The patient complains of a sensation of pain, tightness, and swelling of the affected compartment, which resolves upon stopping the activity. Studies indicate that the anterior and deep posterior compartments are usually involved.[6,55,61,71,79] Upon presentation of these symptoms, intracompartmental pressure measurements will further define the severity of the condition. Pedowitz et al. have developed modified criteria using a slit catheter measurement of the intracompartmental pressures. These authors consider one or more of the following intramuscular pressure criteria as diagnostic of CCS: (1) preexercise pressure greater than 15 mm Hg, (2) 1 minute postexercise pressure of 30 mm Hg, and (3) a 5-minute postexercise pressure greater than 20 mm Hg.[50]

REHABILITATION CONCERNS

Management of CCS is initially conservative with activity modification, icing, and stretching of the anterior compartment and gastrocnemius-soleus complex (Figure 30-21 to 30-23). A lower-quarter structural examination along with gait analysis might reveal a structural variation that is causing excessive compensatory pronation and might benefit from the use of foot orthotics and proper footwear. These measures will not address the issue of increased compartment pressures with activity, though. Cycling has been shown to be an acceptable alternative in preventing increased anterior compartment pressures when compared to running and can be utilized to maintain cardiovascular fitness.[2] If conservative measures fail, fasciotomy of the affected compartments has produce favorable results in a return to higher level of activity.[55,58,76,79]

The patient should be counseled regarding the outcome expectations after fasciotomy for CCS. Howard reported a clinically significant improvement in 81 percent of the anterior/lateral releases and a 50 percent improvement in deep posterior compartment releases with CCS.[35] Slimmon et al. noted that 58 percent of the subjects responding to a long-term follow-up study for CCS fasciotomy reported exercising at a lower level than before the injury.[64] Micheli et al. noted that female patients may be more prone to this condition and for unclear reasons they did not respond to the fasciotomy as well as their male counterparts.[45]

REHABILITATION PROGRESSION

Following fasciotomy of the CCS, the immediate goals are to decrease postsurgical pain, swelling with RICE (rest, ice, compression, elevation), and assisted ambulation with the use of crutches. After that suture removal and soft-tissue healing of the incision has progressed. AROM and flexibility exercises should be initiated (Figures 30-1 to 30-4, 30-18 to 30-21). Weight bearing will be progressed as ROM improves. Gait training should be incorporated to prevent abnormal movements in the gait pattern secondary to joint and soft-tissue stiffness or muscle guarding. AROM exercises should be progressed to open-chain exercises with rubber tubing (Figure 30-5 to 30-8). Closed kinetic-chain activities can also be initiated to incorporate strength, balance, and proprioception that may have been affected by the surgical procedure (Figure 30-12 to 30-15, 30-22 to 30-25). Lower-extremity structural variations that lead to excessive compensatory pronation during gait should be addressed with foot orthotics and proper shoeware after walking gait has been normalized. These measures should help control excessive movements at the STJ/lower leg and thus theoretically decrease muscular activity of the deep posterior compartment, which is highly active in controlling pronation during running gait.[52] Cardiovascular fitness can be maintained and improved with stationary cycling and running in the deep end of a pool with a flotation device (Figures 30-16, 30-26). When ROM, strength, and walking gait have normalized, a walking/jogging progression can be initiated.

CRITERIA FOR RETURNING TO NORMAL ACTIVITY

The patient may return to normal activity when (1) there is normalized ROM and strength of the involved lower leg, (2) there are no gait deviations with walking, jogging, and running, and (3) the patient has completed a progressive walking/jogging/running program with no complaints of CCS symptoms. It should be noted that patients undergoing anterior compartment fasciotomy may not return to normal activity for 8–12 weeks after surgery, while patients undergoing deep posterior compartment fasciotomy may not return until 3–4 months postsurgery.[39,58]

Muscle Strains

PATHOMECHANICS

The majority of muscle strains in the lower leg occur in the medial head of the gastrocnemius at the musculotendinous junction.[27] The injury is more common in middle-aged patients and occurs in activities requiring ballistic movement such as tennis and basketball. The patient may feel or hear a pop as if being kicked in the back of the leg. Depending on the severity of the strain, the patient may be unable to walk secondary to decreased ankle dorsiflexion in a closed kinetic chain that passively stretches the injured muscle and causes pain during the push-off phase of gait. Palpation will elicit tenderness at the site of the strain and a palpable divot may be present, depending on the severity of the injury and how soon it is evaluated.

INJURY MECHANISM

Strains of the medial head of the gastrocnemius usually occur during sudden ballistic movements. A common scenario is the patient lunging with the knee extended and the ankle dorsiflexed. The ankle plantarflexes, in this case the medial head of the gastrocnemius, are activated to assist in push-off of the foot. The muscle is placed in an elongated position and activated in a very short period of time. This places the musculotendinous junction of the gastrocnemius under excessive tensile stress. The muscle-tendon junction, a transition area of one homogeneous tissue to another, is not able to endure the tensile loads nearly as well as the homogeneous tissue itself, and tearing of the tissue at the junction occurs.

REHABILITATION CONCERNS

The initial management of a gastrocnemius strain is RICE. It is important for the patient to pay special attention to compression and elevation of the lower extremity to avoid edema in the foot and ankle, which can further limit ROM and prolong the rehabilitation process. Gentle stretching of the muscletendon unit should be initiated early in the rehabilitation process (Figure 30-18). Ankle plantarflexor strengthening with rubber tubing can also be initiated when tolerated (Figure 30-5). Weight bearing may be limited to an as-tolerated status with crutches. The foot/ankle will prefer a plantarflexed position, and closed kinetic-chain dorsiflexion of the foot and ankle—which is required during walking—will stress the muscle and cause pain. Pulsed ultrasound can be utilized early in the rehabilitation process and eventually progressed to continuous ultrasound for its thermal effects. A stationary cycle can be used for an active warm-up as well as cardiovascular fitness. A heel lift may be placed in each shoe to gradually increase dorsiflexion of the foot and ankle as the patient is progressed off crutches. Standing, stretching, and strengthening can be added as soft-tissue healing occurs and ROM and strength improve. Eventually the patient can be progressed to a walking/jogging program. It is important that the patient warms up and stretches properly before activity, to prevent reinjury.

REHABILITATION PROGRESSION

Early management of a medial head gastrocnemius strain focuses on reduction of pain and swelling with ice, compression, elevation (ICE), and modified weight bearing. The patient is encouraged to perform gentle towel stretching for the affected muscle group several times per day (Figure 30-18). AROM of the foot and ankle in all planes will also facilitate movement and act to stretch the muscle (Figure 30-1 to 30-4). With mild muscle strains, the patient may be off crutches and performing standing calf stretches and strengthening exercises by about 7–10 days with a normal gait pattern (Figures 30-12, 30-13, 30-19). Moderate to severe strains may take 2–4 weeks before normalization of ROM and gait occur. This is usually due to the excessive edema in the foot and ankle. Strengthening can be progressed from open- to closed-chain activity as soft-tissue healing occurs (Figures 30-14, 30-15, 30-22 to 30-25). As walking gait is normalized, the patient is encouraged to begin a graduated walking program in which distance and speed are modulated throughout the progression. Most soft-tissue injuries demonstrate good healing by 14–21 days postinjury. In the case of mild muscle strain, as the patient becomes more comfortable with jogging and running, plyometric activities can be added to the rehabilitation process. Plyometric activities should be introduced in a controlled fashion with at least 1–2 days of rest between activities to allow for muscle soreness to diminish. As the patient adapts to the plyometric exercises, activity-specific exercises should be added. Care should be taken to save sudden, ballistic activities for when the patient is warmed up and the gastrocnemius is well stretched.

CRITERIA FOR NORMAL RETURN

The patient may return to normal activity when the following criteria have been met: (1) full ROM of the foot and ankle, (2) gastrocnemius strength and endurance that are equal to the uninvolved side, (3) ability to walk, jog, run, and hop on the involved extremity without any compensation, and (4) successful completion of activity-specific functional progression with no residual calf symptoms.

Medial Tibial Stress Syndrome

PATHOMECHANICS

MTSS is a condition that involves increasing pain about the distal two-thirds of the posterior medial aspect of the tibia.[26,66] The soleus and tibialis posterior have been implicated as muscular forces that can stress the fascia and periosteum of the distal tibia during walking/jogging/running activities.[2,25,61] In a cadaveric dissection study, Beck and Osternig implicated the soleus as the major contributor to MTSS and not the tibialis posterior.[5] Magnusson et al. noted reduced bone mineral density at the site of MTSS but could not ascertain whether this was the cause or the result.[41] Bhatt reported abnormal histological appearance of bone and periosteum in long-standing MTSS.[10] Pain is usually diffuse about the distal medial tibia and the surrounding soft tissues and can arise secondary to a combination of training errors, excessive pronation, improper shoeware, and poor conditioning level.[16,62] Initially, the area is diffusely tender and might hurt only after intense activity. As the condition worsens, daily ambulation may be painful and morning pain and stiffness may be present. Rehabilitation of this condition must be comprehensive and address several factors, including musculoskeletal, training, and conditioning, as well as proper shoeware and orthotics intervention.

INJURY MECHANISM

Many sources have linked excessive compensatory pronation as a primary cause of MTSS.[16,25,61,66] Bennett et al. reported that a pronatory foot type was related to MTSS. The authors noted that the combination of the patients gender and navicular drop test measures provided an accurate prediction for the development of MTSS in high-school runners.[9] STJ pronation serves to dissipate ground reaction forces upon foot strike in order to reduce the impact to proximal structures. If pronation is excessive or occurs too quickly or at the wrong time in the stance phase of gait, greater tensile loads will be placed on the muscle-tendon units that assist in controlling this complex triplanar movement.[30,74] Lower-extremity structural variations such as a rearfoot and forefoot varus can cause the STJ to pronate excessively in order to get the medial aspect of the forefoot in contact with the ground for push-off.[66] The magnitude of these forces will increase during running, especially with a rearfoot striker. Training surfaces including embankments and crowned roads can place increased tensile loads on the distal medial tibia; modifications should be made whenever possible.

REHABILITATION CONCERNS

Management of this condition should include physician referral to rule out the possibility of stress fracture via the use of bone scan and plain films. Activity modification along with measures to maintain cardiovascular fitness are set in place immediately.

Correction of abnormal pronation during walking and running can be addressed with antipronation taping and temporary orthotics to determine their effectiveness. Vicenzino et al. reported that these measures were helpful in controlling excessive pronation.[77] If these previously measures are helpful, a custom foot orthotic can be fabricated. Masse' Genova noted that foot orthotics significantly reduced maximum calcaneal eversion and calcaneal eversion at heel rise with abnormal pronaters during treadmill walking.[43] Proper shoeware, especially running shoes with motion control features, can also be very helpful in dealing with MTSS. While the earlier mentioned measures provide passive support to address abnormal pronation, exercise sandals may provide a dynamic approach to managing excessive pronation issues. Michell et al. noted a trend in reduced rearfoot eversion angles in two-dimensional rearfoot kinematics during barefoot treadmill walking with abnormal pronaters who trained in the exercise sandals for 8 weeks.[46] The subjects also demonstrated improved balance in a single-leg stance and subjectively noted improved foot function.[46] These improvements might be due to increased muscle activity of the foot intrinsics via the short-foot concept and increased activity of the lower-leg musculature that may assist in controlling pronation. Also, the exercise sandals appear to place the foot in a more supinated position, which may enhance the cuboid pulley mechanism and its effects on the function of the first ray during the push-off phase of gait.[34] Ice massage to the affected area may help reduce localized pain and inflammation. A flexibility program for the gastrocnemius-soleus musculature should be initiated.

REHABILITATION PROGRESSION

Jogging and activities may need to be completely eliminated for the first 7–10 days after diagnosis. Pool workouts with a flotation device will help maintain cardiovascular fitness during the healing process. Gastrocnemius-soleus flexibility is improved with static stretching (Figure 30-19). Ice and electrical stimulation can be used to reduce inflammation and modulate pain in the early stages. As the condition improves, general strengthening of the ankle musculature with rubber tubing can

be performed along with calf muscle strengthening (Figures 30-5 to 30-8, 30-12, 30-13). These exercises may cause muscle fatigue but should not increase the patient's symptoms. The exercise sandal progression can be introduced to enhance dynamic pronation control at the foot and ankle (Table 30-1) (Figures 30-29 to 30-34, 30-36). An isokinetic strengthening program of the ankle inverters and everters can be utilized to improve strength and has been shown to reduce pronation during treadmill running[24]. As mentioned previously, it is imperative that all structural deviations that cause pronation be addressed with a foot orthotic or at least proper motion-control shoes. As pain to palpation of the distal tibia resolves, the patient should be progressed to a jogging/running program on grass with proper footwear. This may involve beginning with a 10–15-minute run and progressing by 10 percent every week. The patient needs to be compliant with a gradual progression and should be educated to avoid doing too much, too soon, which could lead to a recurrence of the condition or possibly a stress fracture.

CRITERIA FOR RETURNING TO NORMAL ACTIVITY

The patient may return to normal activity when (1) there is minimal to no pain to palpation of the affected area, (2) all causes of excessive pronation have been addressed with an orthotic and proper shoeware, (3) there is sufficient gastrocnemius-soleus musculature flexibility, and (4) the patient has successfully completed the gradual running progression and a activity-specific functional progression without an increase in symptoms.

Achilles Tendinitis

PATHOMECHANICS

Achilles tendinitis is an inflammatory condition that involves the Achilles tendon and/or its tendon sheath, the paratenon. Often there is excessive tensile stress placed on the tendon repetitively, as with running or jumping activities, that overloads the tendon, especially on its medial aspect.[46,60] This condition can be divided into Achilles paratenonitis or peritendinitis, which is an inflammation of the paratenon or tissue that surrounds the tendon, and tendinosis, in which areas of the tendon consist of mucinoid or fatty degeneration with disorganized collagen.[60] The patient often complains of generalized pain and stiffness about the Achilles tendon region, which when localized is usually 2–6 cm proximal to the calcaneal insertion. Uphill running or hill workouts and interval training will usually aggravate the condition. There may be reduced gastrocnemius-soleus muscle flexibility in general that may worsen as the condition progresses and adaptive shortening occurs. Muscle testing of the previously mentioned muscles may be within normal limits, but painful and a true deficit may be observed when performing toe raises to fatigue as compared to the uninvolved extremity.

INJURY MECHANISM

Achilles tendinitis will often present with a gradual onset over a period of time. Initially the patient might ignore the symptoms, which might present at the beginning of activity and resolve as the activity progresses. Symptoms may progress to morning stiffness and discomfort with walking after periods of prolonged sitting. Repetitive weight-bearing activities, such as walking in which the duration and intensity are increased quickly with insufficient recovery time, will worsen the condition. Excessive compensatory pronation of the STJ with concomitant internal rotation of the lower leg secondary to a forefoot varus, tibial varum, or femoral anterversion will increase the tensile load about the medial aspect of the Achilles tendon.[31,60] Decreased gastrocnemius and soleus complex flexibility can also increase STJ pronation to compensate for the decreased closed kinetic-chain dorsiflexion needed during early and midstance phase of running. If the patient continues to train, the tendon will become further inflamed and the gastrocnemius-soleus musculature will become less efficient secondary to pain inhibition. The tendon may be warm and painful to palpation, as well as thickened, which may indicate the chronicity of the condition. Crepitace may be palpated with AROM plantar and dorsiflexion and pain will be elicited with passive dorsiflexion.

REHABILITATION CONCERNS

Achilles tendinitis can be resistant to a quick resolution secondary to the slower healing response of tendinous tissue. It has also been noted that an area of hypovascularity exists within the tendon that may further impede the healing response. It is important to create a proper healing environment by reducing the offending activity and replacing it with an activity that will reduce strain on the tendon. Studies have shown that the achilles tendon force during running approaches six to eight times of body weight.[60] Addressing structural faults that may lead to excessive pronation or supination should be done through proper shoeware and food orthotics as well as flexibility exercises for the gastrocnemius-soleus complex. Soft-tissue manipulation of the gastrocnemius-soleus with a foam roller can be helpful prior to stretching. Modalities such as ice can help reduce pain and inflammation early on, and ultrasound can facilitate an increased blood flow to the tendon in the later stages of rehabilitation. Cross-friction massage may be used to break down adhesions that may have formed during the healing response and further improve the gliding ability of the paratenon. Strengthening of the gastrocnemius-soleus musculature must be progressed carefully so as not to cause a recurrence of the symptoms. Finally, a gradual progression must be made for a safe return to activity to avoid the conditions becoming chronic.

REHABILITATION PROGRESSION

Activity modification is necessary to allow the Achilles tendon to begin the healing process. Swimming, pool running with a flotation device, stationary cycling, and use of an UBE are all possible alternative activities for cardiovascular maintenance (Figures 30-16, 30-26, 30-27). It is important to reduce stresses on the Achilles tendon that may occur with daily ambulation. Proper footwear with a slight hell lift, such as a good shoe, can reduce stress on the tendon during gait. Structural biome-

chanical abnormalities that manifest with excessive pronation or supination should be addressed with a custom foot orthotic. Placing a hell lift in the shoe or building it into the orthotic can reduce stress on the Achilles tendon initially but should be gradually reduced so as not to cause an adaptive shortening of the muscle-tendon unit. Gentle pain-free stretching can be performed several times per day and can be done after an active or passive warm-up with exercise or modalities such as superficial heat or ultrasound (Figures 30-18, 30-19). Open kinetic-chain strengthening with rubber tubing can begin early in the rehabilitation process and should be progressed to closed kinetic-chain strengthening in a concentric and eccentric fashion utilizing the athlete's body weight with modification of sets, repetitions, and speed of exercise to intensify the rehabilitation session (Figures 30-5, 30-12, 30-13). Recent studies have reported excellent results with the use of eccentric training of the gastrocnemius-soleus musculature with chronic Achilles tendinosis over a 12-week period.[1] The patient should be progressed to a regimen of isolated eccentric loading of the Achilles tendon using body weight (Figure 30-35). A walking-jogging progression on a firm but forgiving surface can be initiated when the symptoms have resolved and ROM, strength, endurance, and flexibility have been normalized to the uninvolved extremity. The patient must be reminded that this progression is designed to improve the affected tendon's ability to tolerate stress in a controlled fashion and not to improve fitness level. Studies have shown that cardiovascular fitness can be maintained with biking and swimming.[22] Finally it is important to educate the patient on the nature of the condition in order to set realistic expectations for a safe return without recurrence of the condition.

CRITERIA FOR NORMAL RETURN

The patient may return to normal activity when (1) there has been full resolution of symptoms with ADLs and minimal or no symptoms with sport-related activity, (2) ROM, strength, flexibility, and endurance are equal to the opposite uninvolved extremity, and (3) all contributing biomechanical faults have been corrected during walking and running gait analysis with proper shoeware and/or custom foot orthotics.

Achilles Tendon Rupture

PATHOMECHANICS

The Achilles tendon is the largest tendon in the human body. It serves to transmit force from the gastrocnemius-soleus musculature to the calcaneus. Tension through the achilles tendon at the end of stance phase is estimated at 250 percent of body weight.[60] Rupture of the Achilles tendon usually occurs in an area of 2–6 cm proximal to the calcaneal insertion, which has been implicated as an avascular site prone to degenerative changes.[17,33,38] The injury presents after a sudden plantarflexion of the ankle, as in jumping or accelerating gait. The patient will often feel or hear a pop and note a sensation of being kicked in the back of the leg. Plantarflexion of the ankle will be painful and limited but still possible with the assistance of the tibialis posterior and the peroneals. A palpable defect will be noted along the length of the tendon, and the Thompson test will be positive. The athlete will require the use of crutches to continue ambulation without an obvious limp.

INJURY MECHANISM

Achilles tendon rupture is usually caused by a sudden forceful plantarflexion of the ankle. It has been theorized that the area of rupture has undergone degenerative changes and is more prone to rupture when placed under higher levels of tensile loading.[33,48,59,60] The degenerative changes may be due to excessive compensatory pronation at the STJ to accommodate for structural deviations of the forefoot, rearfoot, and lower leg during walking and running. This pronation can place an increased tensile stress on the medial aspect of the Achilles tendon. Also, a chronically inflexible gastrocnemius-soleus complex will reduce the available amount of dorsiflexion at the ankle joint, and excessive STJ pronation will assist in accommodating this loss. This mechanism may result in tendinitis symptoms that precede the tendon rupture, but this is not always the case. Fatigue of the deconditioned patient or weekend warrior may also contribute to tendon rupture, as well as improper warm-up prior to ballistic activities such as basketball or racquet sports.[32]

REHABILITATION CONCERNS

After an Achilles tendon rupture, the question of surgical repair versus cast immobilization will arise. Cetti et al. report that surgical repair of the tendon is recommended to allow the patient to return to previous levels of activity.[17] Surgical repair of the Achilles tendon may require a period of immobilization for 6–8 weeks to allow for proper tendon healing.[15,33,42] The deleterious effects of this lengthy immobilization include muscle atrophy, joint stiffness including intra-articular adhesions and capsular stiffness of the involved joints, disorganization of the ligament substance, and possible disuse osteoporosis of the bone.[15] Isokinetic strength deficits for the ankle plantarflexors, especially at lower speeds, have been documented with periods of cast immobilization for 6 weeks.[40] Steele et al. noted significant deficits isokinetically of ankle plantarflexor strength after 8 weeks of immobilization.[68] These authors feel that the primary limiting factor that influences functional outcome might be the duration of postsurgical immobilization.[68] Several studies have been done using early controlled ankle motion and progressive weight bearing without immobilization.[3,15,33,42,60,65,67] It is important not only to regain full ROM without harming the repair, but also to regain normal muscle function through controlled progressive strengthening. This can be performed through a variety of exercises, including isometrics, isotonics, and isokinetics (Figures 23-1 to 23-13). Open and closed kinetic-chain activities can be incorporated into the progression to gradually increase weight-bearing stress on the tendon repair as well as to improve proprioception (Figures 23-11, 23-14, 23-15, 23-22 to 23-25). Cardiovascular endurance can be maintained with stationary biking and pool running with a flotation device. Gait

normalization for walking and running can be performed using a treadmill.

REHABILITATION PROGRESSION

It is important for the therapist to have an open line of communication with the physician in charge of the surgical repair. Decisions about length and type of immobilization, weight-bearing progression, allowable ROM, and progressive strengthening should be thoroughly discussed with the physician. Excellent results have been reported with early and controlled mobilization with the use of a splint that allows early plantarflexion ROM and slowly increases ankle dorsiflexion to neutral and full dorsiflexion over a 6–8-week period of time.[15,33] More recent studies have noted excellent functional results with early weight bearing and ROM. Aoki et al. reported a full return to sports activity in 13.1 weeks.[3] Controlled progressive weight bearing based on percentages of the patient's body weight can be done over 6–8 weeks postoperatively, with full weight bearing by the end of this time frame. During the early stages of rehabilitation, ICE is used to decrease swelling. A variety of ROM exercises are done to increase ankle ROM in all planes as well as initiate activation of the surrounding muscles (Figures 30-1 to 30-4, 30-9, 30-10, 30-14, 30-15, 30-18, 30-20). By 4–6 weeks postoperatively, strengthening exercises with rubber tubing can be progressed to closed-chain exercises utilizing a percentage of the patient's body weight with heel raises on a total gym apparatus (Figures 30-5, 30-8, 30-11). It is important to do more concentric than eccentric loading initially, so as not to place excessive stress on the repair. Gradual increases in eccentric loading can occur from 10 to 12 weeks postoperatively. Also at this time, isokinetic exercise can be introduced with submaximal high-speed exercise and be progressed to lower concentric speeds gradually over time. By 3 months, full weight-bearing heel raises can be performed (Figures 30-12, 30-13). At the same time a walking/jogging program can be initiated. Isokinetic strength testing can be done between 3 and 4 months to determine if any deficits in ankle plantarflexor strength exist. The number of single-leg heel raises performed in a specified amount of time as compared to the uninvolved extremity can also be utilized to determine functional plantarflexor strength and endurance. Functional activities can be initiated at 3 months along with a progressive jogging program. A full return to unrestricted activity can begin after 6 months, once the patient successfully meets all predetermined goals.

CRITERIA FOR NORMAL RETURN

The patient can return to normal activity after the following criteria have been met: (1) full AROM of the involved ankle as compared to the uninvolved side, (2) isokinetic strength of the ankle plantarflexors at 90–95 percent of the uninvolved side, (3) 90–95 percent of the number of heel raises throughout the full ROM in a 30-second period as compared to the uninvolved side, and (4) the ability to walk, jog, and run without an observable limp and successful completion of a functional progression without any Achilles tendon irritation.

Retrocalcaneal Bursitis

PATHOMECHANICS

The retrocalcaneal bursae is a disc-shaped piece of synovial of membrane that lies between the Achilles tendon and the superior tuberosity of the calcaneus.[12,60] The patient will report a gradual onset of pain that may be associated with Achilles tendinitis. Careful palpation anterior to the Achilles tendon will rule out involvement of the tendon. Pain is increased with AROM/PROM ankle dorsiflexion and relieved with plantarflexion. Depending on the severity and swelling associated, it may be painful to walk, especially when attempting to attain full closed kinetic-chain ankle dorsiflexion during the midstance phase of gait.

INJURY MECHANISM

Loading the foot and ankle in repeated dorsiflexion, as in uphill running, can be a cause of this condition. When the foot is dorsiflexed, the distance between the posterior/superior calcaneus and the Achilles tendon will be reduced, resulting in a repeated mechanical compression of the retrocalcaneal bursae. Also, structural abnormalities of the foot may lead to excessive compensatory movements at the STJ, which may cause friction of the Achilles tendon on the bursae with running.

REHABILITATION CONCERNS

Because of the close proximity of other structures, it is important to rule out involvement of the calcaneus and Achilles tendon with careful palpation of the area. Rest and activity modification in order to reduce swelling and inflammation is necessary. If walking is painful, crutches with weight bearing as tolerated is recommended for a brief period. Gentle but progressive stretching and strengthening should be added as tolerated, with care being taken not to increase pain with gastrocnemius-soleus stretching (Figures 30-5, 30-12, 30-13, 30-18, 30-19). If excessive compensatory pronation is noted during gait analysis, recommendations on proper footware should be made, especially in regard to the heel counter, and foot orthotics should be considered.

REHABILITATION PROGRESSION

The early management of this condition requires all measures to reduce pain and inflammation including ice, rest from offending activity, proper shoeware, and modified weight bearing with crutches if necessary. Cardiovascular fitness can be maintained with pool running with a flotation device. Gentle stretching of the gastrocnemius-soleus needs to be introduced slowly, because this will tend to increase compression of the retrocalcaneal bursae. As pain resolves and ROM and walking gait are normalized, the athlete may begin a progressive walking/jogging program. The patient can progress back to activity as the condition allows. Heel lifts in both shoes may be necessary in the early return to activity, with gradual weaning away from them as AROM/PROM dorsiflexion improves. The condition may allow full return in 10 days to 2 weeks if treated early enough. If the condition persists, 6–8 weeks of rest, activity modification, and treatment may be needed before a successful result is attained with conservative care.

CRITERIA FOR RETURN TO NORMAL ACTIVITY

The following criteria need to be met before return to normal activity: (1) no observable swelling and minimal to no pain to palpation of the area at rest or after daily activity, (2) full ankle dorsiflexion AROM and normal pain-free strength of the gastrocnemius and soleus musculature, and (3) normal and pain-free walking and running gait.

REHABILITATION TECHNIQUES FOR THE LOWER LEG

Strengthening Techniques

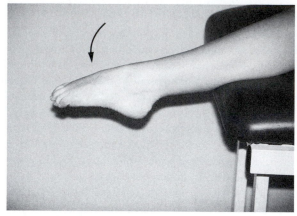

F I G U R E   3 0 - 1

AROM ankle plantarflexion, Used to activate the primary and secondary ankle plantarflexor muscle-tendon units after a period of immobilzation or disuse. This exercise can be performed in a supportive medium such as a whirlpool.

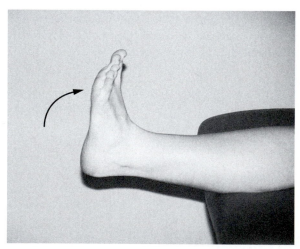

F I G U R E   3 0 - 2

AROM ankle dorsiflexion. Used to activate the tibialis anterior, extensor hallicus longus, and extensor digitorum longus muscle-tendon units after a period of immobilization or disuse.

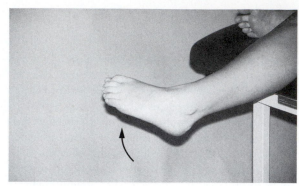

F I G U R E   3 0 - 3

AROM ankle inversion start position/end position. Used to activate the tibialis posterior, flexor hallicus longus, and flexor digitorum longus muscle-tendon units after a period of immobilization or disuse.

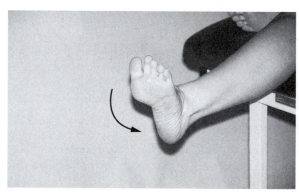

F I G U R E   3 0 - 4

AROM ankle eversion start position/end position. Used to activate the peroneus longus and brevis muscle-tendon units after a period of immobilization or disuse.

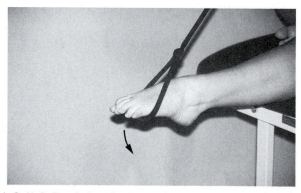

F I G U R E   3 0 - 5

RROM ankle plantarflexion with rubber tubing. Used to strengthen the gastrocnemius, soleus, and secondary ankle plantarflexors, including the peroneals, flexor hallicus longus, flexor digitorum longus, and tibialis posterior, in an open-chain fashion. This exercise will also place a controlled concentric and eccentric load on the Achilles tendon.

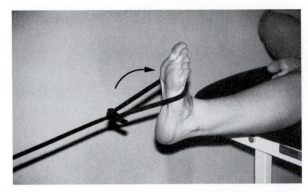

F I G U R E   3 0 - 6

RROM ankle dorsiflexion with rubber tubing. Used to isolate and strengthen the ankle dorsiflexors, including the tibialis anterior, extensor hallicus longus, and extensor digitorum longus, in an open-chain fashion.

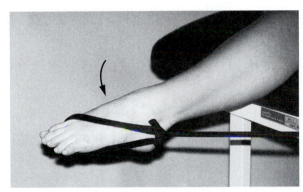

F I G U R E   3 0 - 7

RROM ankle inversion with rubber tubing. Used to isolate and strengthen the ankle inverters, including the tibialis posterior, flexor hallicus longus, and flexor digitorum longus, in an open-chain fashion.

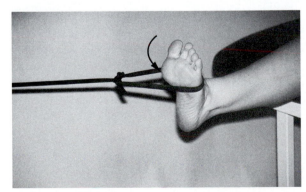

F I G U R E   3 0 - 8

RROM ankle eversion with rubber tubing. Used to isolate and strengthen the ankle everters, including the peroneus longus and peroneus brevis, in an open-chain fashion.

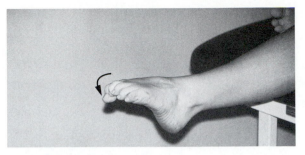

F I G U R E   3 0 - 9

AROM toe flexion/extension. Used to activate the long-toe flexers, extensors, and foot intrinsic musculature. This exercise will also help to improve the tendon-gliding ability of the extensor hallicus longus, extensor digitorum longus, flexor hallicus longus, and flexor digitorum longus tendons after a period of immobilization.

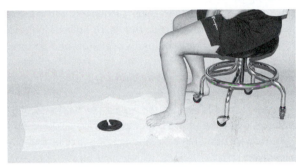

F I G U R E   3 0 - 1 0

Towel-gathering exercise. Used to strengthen the foot intrinsics and long-toe flexor and extensor muscle-tendon units. A weight can be placed on the end of the towel to require more force production by the muscle-tendon unit as ROM and strength improve.

Closed Kinetic-Chain Strengthening Exercises

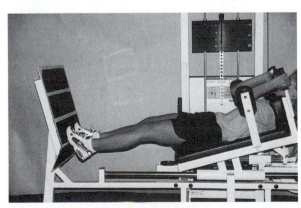

F I G U R E   3 0 - 1 1

Heel raises. Used to strengthen the gastrocnemius musculature and will directly load the Achilles tendon with a percentage of the athlete's body weight depending on the angle of the carriage relative to the ground.

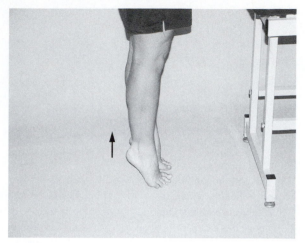

F I G U R E   3 0 - 1 2

Two-legged heel raise. Used to strengthen the gastrocnemius when the knee is extended and the soleus when the knees are flexed. The flexor hallicus longus, flexor digitorum longus, tibialis posterior, and peroneals will also be activated during this activity. The athlete can modify concentric and eccentric activity depending on the type and severity of the condition. For example, if an eccentric load is not desired on the involved side, the athlete can raise up on both feet and lower down on the uninvolved side until eccentric loading is tolerated on the involved side.

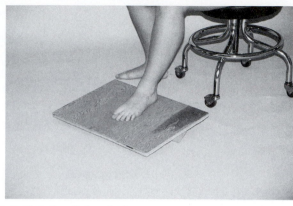

F I G U R E   3 0 - 1 4

Seated closed-chain ankle dorsiflexion/plantarflexion AROM. Used to activate the ankle dorsiflexor/plantarflexor musculature in a closed-chain position.

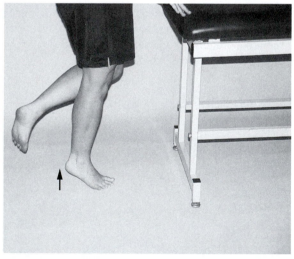

F I G U R E   3 0 - 1 3

One-legged heel raise. Used to strengthen the gastrocnemius and soleus muscles when the knee is extended and flexed, respectively. This can be used as a progression from the two-legged heel raise.

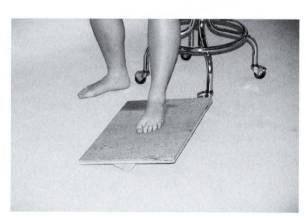

F I G U R E   3 0 - 1 5

Seated closed-chain ankle inversion/eversion AROM. Used to activate the ankle inverter/everter musculature in a closed-chain position.

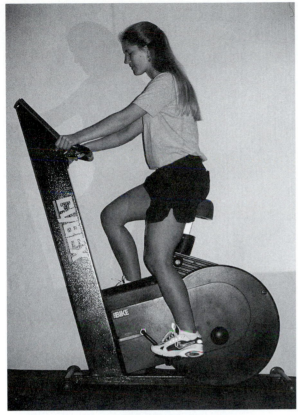

FIGURE 30-16

Stationary cycle. Used to reduce impact weight-bearing forces on the lower extremity while also maintaining cardiovascular fitness levels.

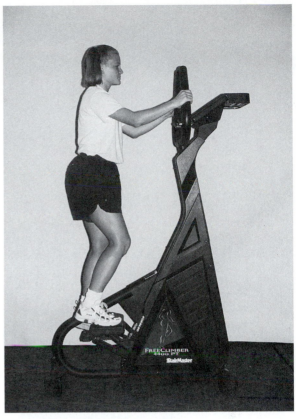

FIGURE 30-17

Stair-stepping machine. Used to progressively load the lower extremity in a closed-kinetic fashion as well as maintain and improve cardiovascular fitness.

Stretching Exercises

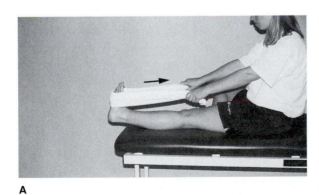

A   **B**

FIGURE 30-18

Ankle plantarflexion towel stretch. Used to stretch the gastrocnemius when the knee is extended and the soleus when the knee is flexed. The Achilles tendon will be stretched with both positions. The athlete can hold the stretch for 20 to 30 seconds.

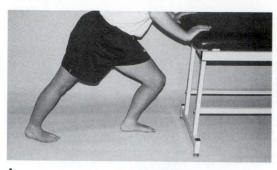

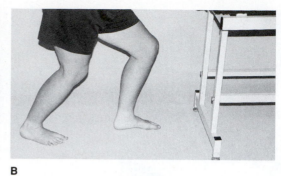

A   B

FIGURE 30-19

A, Standing gastrocnemius stretch. Used to stretch the gastrocnemius muscle. The Achilles tendon will also be stretched. The stretch is held for 20 to 30 seconds. **B,** Standing soleus stretch. Used to stretch the soleus muscle. The Achilles tendon will also be stretched. The stretch is held for 20 to 30 seconds.

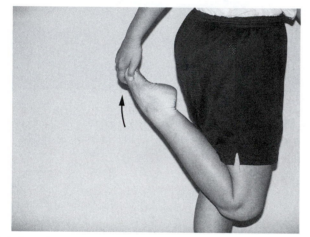

FIGURE 30-20

Standing ankle dorsiflexor stretch. Used to stretch the extensor hallicus longus, extensor digitorum longus, tibialis anterior, and anterior ankle capsule. The stretch is held for 20 to 30 seconds.

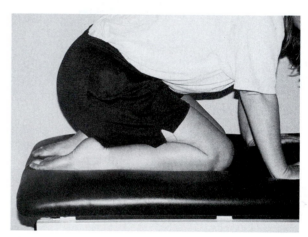

FIGURE 30-21

Kneeling ankle dorsiflexor stretch. Used to stretch the extensor hallicus longus, extensor digitorum longus, tibialis anterior, and anterior ankle capsule. This is an aggressive stretch that can be used in the later stages of rehabilitation to gain end-ROM ankle dorsiflexion.

Exercises to Reestablish Neuromuscular Control

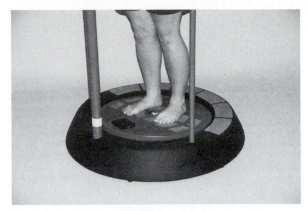

FIGURE   30-22

Standing double-leg balance board activity. Used to activate the lower-leg musculature and improve balance and proprioception in the lower extremity.

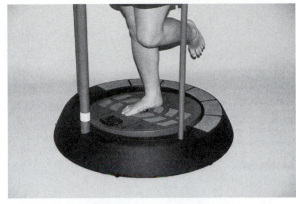

FIGURE   30-23

Standing single-leg balance board activity. Used to activate the lower-leg musculature and improve balance and proprioception in the involved extremity.

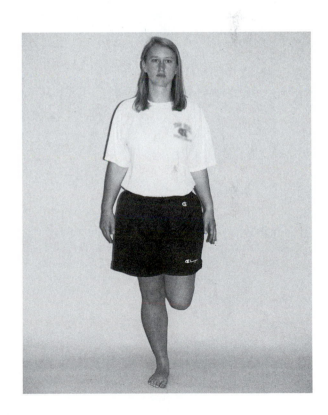

FIGURE   30-24

Static single-leg standing balance progression. Used to improve balance and proprioception of the lower extremity. This activity can be made more difficult with the following progression: (1) single-leg stand, eyes open; (2) single-leg stand, eyes closed; (3) single-leg stand, eyes open, toes extended so only the heel and metatarsal heads are in contact with the ground; (4) single-leg stand, eyes closed, toes extended.

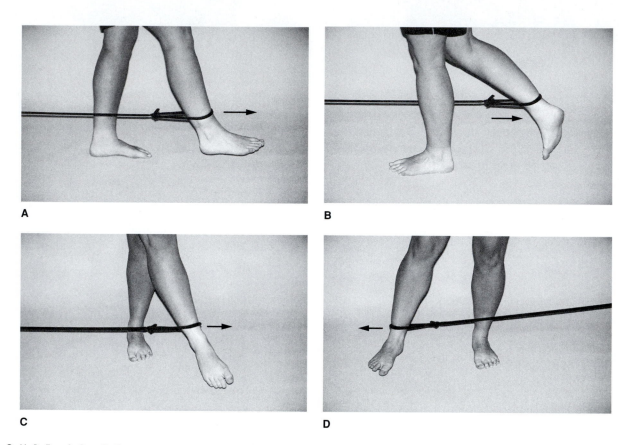

FIGURE 30-25

Single-leg standing rubber-tubing kicks. Used to improve muscle activation of the lower leg to maintain single-leg standing on the involved extremity while kicking against the resistance of the rubber tubing. **A,** Extension. **B,** Flexion. **C,** Adduction. **D,** Abduction.

Exercises to Improve Cardiorespiratory Endurance

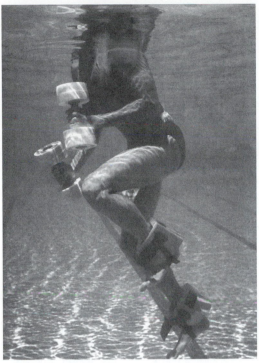

Poor running with flotation device. Used to reduce impact weight-bearing forces on the lower extremity while maintaining cardiovascular fitness level and running form.

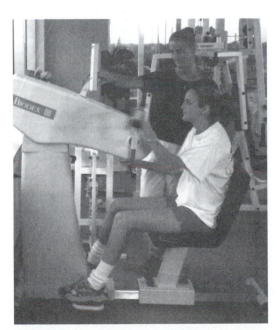

Upper-body ergometer. Used to maintain cardiovascular fitness when lower-extremity ergometer is contraindicated or too difficult for the athlete to use.

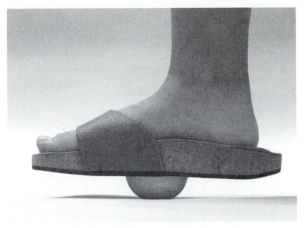

Exercise sandals (OPTP, Minneapolis, MN). Wooden sandals with a rubber hemisphere located centrally on the plantar surface.

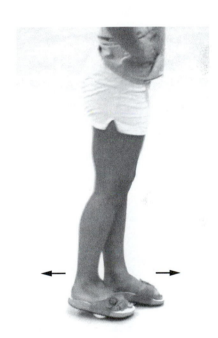

Exercise sandal forward and backward walking. Used to enhance balance and proprioception and increase muscle activity in the foot intrinsics, lower-leg musculature, and gluteals. The patient takes small steps forward and backward.

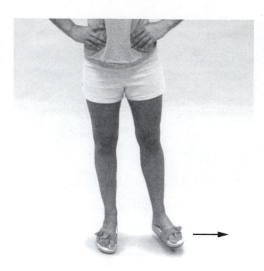

F I G U R E   3 0 - 3 0

Exercise sandals sidestepping. Used to enhance balance and proprioception in the frontal plane. Increases muscle activity of the lower-leg musculature and foot intrinsics. The patient moves directly to the left or right along a straight line with the toes pointed forward.

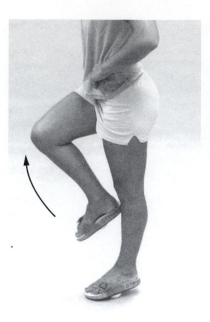

F I G U R E   3 0 - 3 2

Exercise sandals high knees. Used to enhance balance and proprioception and muscle activity of the foot intrinsics, lower-leg musculature, and especially the glueteals. The athlete should maintain an upright posture and avoid trunk flexion with hip flexion. This exercise promotes single-leg stance progression for a short period of time.

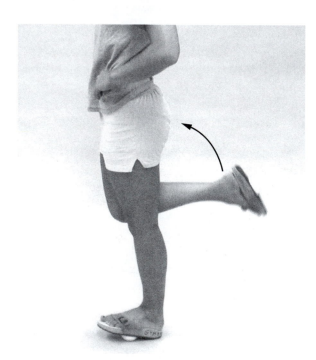

F I G U R E   3 0 - 3 1

Exercise sandals butt kicks. Used to promote balance and proprioception along with increased muscle activity of the foot intrinsics, lower-leg musculature, and gluteals. This exercise enhances single-leg stance in the exercise sandals.

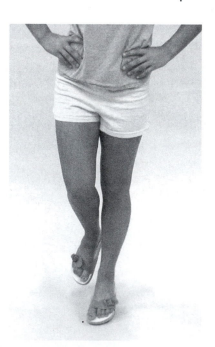

F I G U R E   3 0 - 3 3

Exercise sandals single-leg stance. Used to enhance balance, proprioception, and muscle activity in the entire lower extremity. This exercise is the most demanding in the exercise sandal progression.

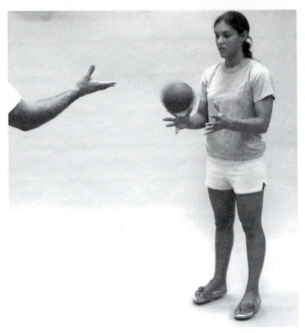

FIGURE 30-34

Exercise sandal ball catch. Used to enhance balance, proprioception, and lower-leg muscle activity. The athlete focuses on catching and throwing the ball to the athletic trainer while moving laterally to the left or right.

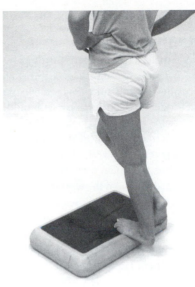

FIGURE 30-35

Achilles tendon eccentric muscle loading. Used to enhance gastrocnemius (knee straight) and soleus (knee bent) strength and Achilles tendon tensile strength. The athletes use the uninvolved side to elevate onto their toes and then place all weight on toes of the involved side to eccentrically lower. Initially the patient lowers to the step and then progresses below the level of the step. Extra weight can be added via a backpack.

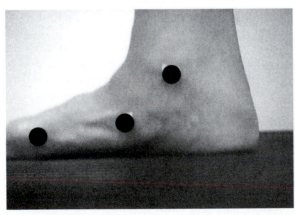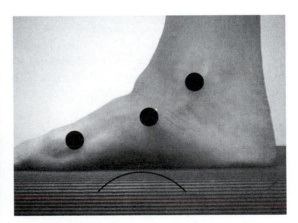

FIGURE 30-36

Short foot concept. Used to enhance and strengthen the foot intrinsic muscles. The athlete is instructed to shorten the foot from front to back while keeping the toes straight. The matatarsal heads should stay in contact with the ground. The athletic trainer can palpate the foot intrinsics and will notice a raised longitudinal arch with a flexible foot type. The shortened foot should be maintained at all times while in the exercise sandals.

Treatment Protocol for Achilles Tendinitis

INJURY SITUATION

A 29-year-old female jogger presents with pain in her right Achilles. She currently has morning stiffness and pain with walking, especially up hills and going down stairs. The patient stands in moderate STJ pronation with mild tibial varum. Her single-leg stance balance is poor, with an increase in STJ pronation and internal rotation of the entire lower extremity. Observation of the tendon reveals slight thickening. Palpation reveals mild crepitus with pain 4 cm proximal to the calcaneal insertion on the medial side of the tendon. ROM testing reveals tightness in both the gastrocnemius-soleus musculature versus the uninvolved side. A 6-in lateral step-down demonstrates restricted closed kinetic-chain ankle dorsiflexion that is painful, with compensation at the hip to get the opposite heel to touch the ground. The patient is able to perform 10 heel raises on the right with pain and 20 on the left without pain. Walking gait reveals increased pronation during the entire stance phase of gait. A 12° forefoot varus is noted on the right with the patient in a prone STJ neutral position.

Phase One—Acute Phase

Goals: Modulate pain, address abnormal pronation, begin appropriate therapeutic exercise.

Estimated length of time (ELT): Day 1–4

Use ice and electrical stimulation to decrease pain. NSAIDs could help reduce inflammation. A foot orthotic could be fabricated to address the excessive pronation, which may be placing increased tensile stress on the medial aspect of the Achilles tendon. A heel lift could be built into the foot orthotic. It might be recommended that the patient wear a motion control running shoe to address pronation and provide a heel life. The patient could begin gentle, pain-free towel stretching for the gastrocnemius-soleus musculature several times per day. Conditioning could be done in a pool or on a bike.

Phase Two—Intermediate Phase

Goals: Increase gastrocnemius-soleus flexibility, gain strength, and improve single-leg stance balance and single-leg stance closed kinetic-chain functional activity.

ELT: Days 5–14

As signs of inflammation decrease, the use of ultrasound could be introduced, first at a pulsed level and then at a continuous level. Stretching could be progressed to standing on a flat surface. Strengthening could be started with isometrics and progressed to open kinetic-chain isotonics with rubber tubing. As the patient improves, standing double-leg heel raises can be introduced. Single-leg stance activity could be added, focusing on control of the lower extremity, especially foot pronation and lower-leg internal rotation. Conditioning at the end of this stage could be upgraded to weight-bearing activity, such as the elliptical trainer with the foot flat on the pedal, avoiding ankle plantarflexion.

Phase Three—Advanced Phase

Goals: Complete elimination of pain and full return to activity.
ELT: Week 3 to full return.

As ROM and strength improve, the patient could be progressed to gastrocnemius-soleus stretching on a slant board and single-leg heel raises, with an increased focus on eccentric loading of the involved side. Dynamic muscle loading via double-leg hopping on a yielding surface such as jumping rope for short periods of time could be added. A running program on a flat, yielding surface such as grass or track could be initiated with good running shoes and the foot orthotic in place. The program should be done every other day to allow the tendon to recover. Achilles taping may be of benefit when the patient returns to training on a daily basis to reduce excess load to the tendon over the next several weeks.

CRITERIA FOR RETURN TO FUNCTION

1. No pain with walking, ADLs, and running.
2. Gastrocnemius-soleus flexibility and strength are equal to the uninvolved extremity.
3. Improved single-leg stance balance, closed kinetic-chain function (step-down, squat, lunge).

Treatment Protocol for MTSS

INJURY SITUATION

A 24-year old female who works as a personal fitness trainer complains of severe discomfort in the medial aspect of the right shin. The patient reports that her shin seemed to ache all the time but the pain became more intense after teaching a cardio class. During palpation, there was severe point tenderness along the medial posterior edge of the tibia approximately 2 inches length, beginning 41/2 inches from the tip of the medial malleolus. Further evaluation showed that the patient had a forefoot varus. X-ray examination showed no indication of stress fracture. The diagnosis was a MTSS (shinsplints) involving the long flexor muscle, the great toe, and the posterior tibial muscle.

Phase One—Acute Phase

Goals: To reduce inflammation, pain, and point tenderness.
ELT: 1–2 weeks.

Initially RICE, NSAIDs, and analgesics should be taken as needed. The patient should be instructed to rest and avoid weight bearing as much as possible. Ice message (7 minutes) should be performed, followed by gentle static stretching to the anterior and posterior muscles two to three times daily. An arch support taping or orthotic device should be fabricated to the arch to correct pronation during weight bearing. Static stretching of the Achilles tendon and anterior part of low leg should be repeated three to four times daily.

Phase Two—Intermediate Phase

Goals: To heal injury, help the patient become symptom free, return to walking, jogging, and finally running.
ELT: 2–3 weeks.

Cold application (5–15 minutes) to shin area before and after walking one time daily. Activity should be stopped if there is shin pain. Ultrasound (0.5–0.075 W/cm^2) (5–10 minutes) one time daily. Transverse friction massage should be given to prevent adhesions. The patient should continue to wear arch taping or orthoses when weight bearing. Ankle ROM exercises plus progressive resistive exercises with rubber tubing to the anterior and posterior leg muscles. Static stretch of lower leg followed by arch and plantarflexion exercises. Towel gathering exercise (10 repetitions, one to three sets); progress from no resistance to 10 lb of resistance daily. Towel scoop exercise (10 repetitions, one to three sets); progress to 10 lb, three times daily. Marble pickup, three times daily. The patient should engage in a program of progressive weight bearing and locomotion within pain-free limits starting with slow heel-toe walking, fast walking, jogging, and finally, running. As pain decreases, activity can increase.

Phase Three—Advaned Phase

Goals: To return to teaching several cardio classes each day.
ELT: 3–6 weeks.

The patient should continue cryokinetics before and after practice. She should continue to wear arch taping or her orthotics to correct for foot pronation. The patient should continue a daily program of lower-leg static stretching after ice application before and after activity. She should engage in a consistent program of ankle ROM exercises and lower-leg progressive resistive exercises 3 days a week.

CRITERIA FOR RETURN TO FUNCTION

1. Leg is symptom free after prolonged activity.
2. The lower leg and ankle have full strength and ROM.
3. Hyperpronation is controlled with an orthotic to prevent reoccurrence.

SUMMARY

- Although some injuries in the region of the lower leg are acute, most injuries result from overuse, most often from walking/jogging/running.
- Tibial fractures can create long-term problems for the athlete if inappropriately managed. Fibular fractures generally require much shorter periods for immobilization. Treatment of these fractures involves immediate medical referral and most likely a period of immobilization and restricted weight bearing.
- Stress fractures in the lower leg are usually the result of the bone's inability to adapt to the repetitive loading response during training and conditioning of the patient and are more likely to occur in the tibia.
- CCSs can occur from acute trauma or repetitive trauma of overuse. They can occur in any of the four compartments, but are most likely in the anterior compartment or deep posterior compartment.

- Rehabilitation of MTSS must be comprehensive and address several factors, including musculoskeletal, training, and conditioning, as well as proper shoes and orthotics intervention.
- Achilles tendinitis will often present with a gradual onset over a period of time and may be resistant to a quick resolution secondary to the slower healing response of tendinous tissue.
- Perhaps the greatest question after an Achilles tendon rupture is whether surgical repair or cast immobilization is the best method of treatment. Regardless of treatment method, the time required for rehabilitation is significant.
- With retrocalcaneal bursitis the patient will report a gradual onset of pain that may be associated with Achilles tendinitis. Treatment should include rest and activity modification in order to reduce swelling and inflammation.

REFERENCES

1. Alfredson H, Pietila T, Jonsson P, et al. Heavy-load eccentric calf muscle training of the treatment of achilles tendinosis. *Am J Sports Med* 26(3):360–366, 1988.
2. Andrish J, Work J. How I manage shin splints. *Phys Sports Med* 18(12):113–114, 1990.
3. Aoki M, Ogiwara N, Ohta T, et al. Early active motion and weightbearing after cross stitch achilles tendon repair. *Am J Sports Med* 26(6):794–800, 1998.
4. Batt M, Kemp S, Kerslake K. Delayed union stress fracture of the tibia: Conservative management. *Br J Sports Med* 35:74–77, 2001.
5. Beck B, Osternig L. Medial tibial stress syndrome. *J Bone Joint Surg* 76-A(7):1057–1061, 1994.
6. Beckham S, Grana W, Buckley P, et al. A comparison of anterior compartment pressures in competitive runners and cyclists. *Am J Sports Med* 21(1):36–40, 1993.
7. Bennell K, Malcolm S, Thomas S, et al. The incidence and distribution of stress fractures in competitive track and field athletes: A twelve-month prospective study. *Am J Sports Med* 24(2):211–217, 1996.
8. Bennell K, Malcolm S, Thomas S, et al. Risk factors for stress fractures in track and filed athletes: A twelve-month prospective study. *Am J Sports Med* 24(6):810–817, 1996.
9. Bennett J, Reinking M, Pleumer B, et al. Factors contributing to the development of medial tibial stress syndrome in high school runners. *J Orthop Sports Phys Ther* 31(9):504–511, 2001.
10. Bhatt R, Lauder I, Allen M, et al. Correlation of bone scintigraphy and histological findings in medial tibial stress syndrome. *Br J Sports Med* 34:49–53, 2000.
11. Blackburn T, Hirth C, Guskiewicz K. EMG comparison of lower leg musculature during functional activities with and without balance shoes. *J Athlet Train* 2002. Review.
12. Bordelon R. The heel. In: DeLee J, Drez D, eds. *Orthopaedic and Sports Medicine: Principles and Practice.* Philadelphia, PA, Saunders, 1994.

13. Bullock-Saxton J. Local sensation changes and altered hip muscle function following severe ankle sprain. *Phys Ther* 74(1):17–31, 1994.

14. Bullock-Saxton J, Janda V, Bullock M. Reflex activation of gluteal muscles in walking. *Spine* 21(6):704–708, 1993.

15. Carter T, Fowler P, Blokker C. Functional postoperative treatment of Achilles tendon repair. *Am J Sports Med* 20(4):459–462, 1992.

16. Case W. Relieving the pain of shin splints. *Phys Sports Med* 22(4):31–32, 1994.

17. Cetti R, Christensen S, Ejsted R, et al. Operative versus nonoperative treatment of Achilles tendon rupture: A prospective randomized study and review of the literature. *Am J Sports Med* 21(6):791–799, 1993.

18. Chang P, Harris R. Intramedullary nailing for chronic tibial stress fractures: A review of five cases. *Am J Sports Med* 24(5):688–692, 1996.

19. Dickson T, Kichline P. Functional management of stress fractures in female athletes using a pneumatic leg brace. *Am J Sports Med* 15(1):86–89, 1987.

20. Donatelli R. Normal anatomy and biomechanics. In: Donatelli R, Wolf S, eds. *The Biomechanics of the Foot and Ankle*, 1st ed. Philadelphia, Pa, Davis, 1990.

21. Ekenman I, Tsai-Fellander L, Westblad P, et al. A study of intrinsic factors in patients with stress fractures of the tibia. *Foot and Ankle* 17(8):477–482, 1996.

22. Eyestone E, Fellingham G, George J, Fisher G. Effect of water running and cycling on maximum oxygen consumption and 2-mile run performance. *Am J Sports Med* 21(1):41–44, 1993.

23. Fehlandt A, Micheli L. Acute exertional anterior compartment syndrome in an adolescent female. *Med Sci Sports Exerc* 27(1):3–7, 1995.

24. Feltner M, Macrae H, Macrae P, et al. Strength training effects on rearfoot motion in running. *Medicine and Science in Sports and Exercise* 26(8):102–7, 1994.

25. Fick D, Albright J, Murray B. Relieving painful shin splints. *Phys Sports Med* 20(12):105–113, 1992.

26. Fredericson M, Bergman A, Hoffman K, Dillingham M. Tibial stress reaction in runners: A correlation of clinical symptoms and scintigraphy with a new magnetic resonance imaging grading system. *Am J Sports Med* 23(4):472–481, 1995.

27. Garrick J, Couzens G. Tennis leg: How I manage gastrocnemius strains. *Phys Sports Med* 20(5):203–207, 1992.

28. Giladi M, Milgrom C, Simkin A, et al. Stress fractures: Identifiable risk factors. *Am J Sports Med* 19(6):647–652, 1991.

29. Goldberg B, Pecora C. Stress fractures: A risk of increased training in freshmen. *Phys Sports Med* 22(3):68–78, 1994.

30. Gross M. Lower quarter screening for skeletal malalignment: Suggestions for orthotics and shoeware. *J Orthop Sports Phys Ther* 21(6):389–405, 1995.

31. Gross M. Chronic tendinitis: Pathomechanics of injury factors affecting the healing response and treatment. *J Orthop Sports Phys Ther* 16(6):248–261, 1992.

32. Hamel R. Achilles tendon ruptures: Making the diagnosis. *Phys Sports Med* 20(9):189–200, 1992.

33. Heinrichs K, Haney C. Rehabilitation of the surgically repaired Achilles tendon using a dorsal functional orthosis: A preliminary report. *J Sport Rehabil* 3:292–303, 1994.

34. Hirth C. Rehabilitation strategies in the management of foot and ankle dysfunction: Research and practical applications. Paper presented at the National Athletic Trainers Association 52nd Annual Meeting and Clinical Symposium, Los Angeles, CA, 19–23 June, 2001.

35. Howard J, Mohtadi N, Wiley J. Evaluation of outcomes in patients following surgical treatment of chronic exertional compartment syndrome in the leg. *Clin J Sports Med* 10(3):176–184, 2000.

36. Janda V, VaVrova M. *Sensory Motor Stimulation* [Video]. Brisbane, Australia, Body Control Systems, 1990.

37. Kaper B, Carr C, Shirreffs T. Compartment syndrome after arthroscopic surgery of knee: A report of two cases managed nonoperatively. *Am J Sports Med* 25(1):123–125, 1997.

38. Karjalainen P, Aronen H, Pihlajamaki H, et al. Magnetic resonance imaging during healing of surgically repaired Achilles tendon ruptures. *Am J Sports Med* 25(2):164–171, 1997.

39. Kohn H. Shin pain and compartment syndromes in running. In: Guten G, ed. *Running Injuries*. Philadelphia, Pa, Saunders, 1997.

40. Leppilahti J, Siira P, Vanharanta H, et al. Isokinetic evaluation of calf muscle performance after Achilles rupture repair. *Int J Sports Med* 17(8):619–623, 1996.

41. Magnusson H, Westlin N, Nyqvist F, et al. Abnormally decreased regional bone density in athletes with medial tibial stress syndrome. *Am J Sports Med* 29(6):712–715, 2001.

42. Mandelbaum B, Myerson M, Forster R. Achilles tendon ruptures: A new method of repair, early range of motion, and functional rehabilitation. *Am J Sports Med* 23(4):392–395, 1995.

43. Masse' Genova J, Gross M. Effect of foot orthotics in calcaneal eversion during standing and treadmill walking for subjects with abnormal pronation. *J Orthop Sports Phys Ther* 30(11):664–675, 2000.

44. Matheson G, Clement B, McKenzie C, et al. Stress fractures in athletes. A study of 320 cases. *Am J Sports Med* 15(1):46–58, 1987.

45. Micheli L, Solomon K, Solomon R, et al. Surgical treatment for chronic lower leg compartment syndrome in young female athletes. *Am J Sports Med* 27:197–201, 1999.

46. Michell T, Guskiewicz K, Hirth C, et al. Effects of training in exercise sandals on 2-D rearfoot motion and postural sway in abnormal pronaters. Undergraduate honors thesis, University of North Carolina, Chapel Hill, 2000.

47. Myers R, Padua D, Prentice W, et al. Electromyographic analysis of the gluteal musculature during closed kinetic chain exercises. Masters thesis, University of North Carolina, Chapel Hill, 2002.

48. Myerson M, McGarvey W. Instructional course lectures, The American Academy of Orthopaedic Surgeons: Disorders of the insertion of the achilles tendon and achilles tendinitis. *J Bone Joint Surg* 80:1814–1824, 1998.

49. National Academy of Sports Medicine. *Performance Enhancement Specialist Online Manual.* Callabassus, CA, Author, 2002.

50. Pedowitz R, Hargens A, Mubarek S, et al. Modified criteria for the objective diagnosis of chronic compartment syndrome of the leg. *Am J Sports Med* 18(1):35–40, 1990.

51. Puddu G, Cerullo G, Selvanetti A, DePaulis F. Stress fractures. In: Harries M, Williams C, Stanish W, Micheli L, eds. *Oxford Textbook of Sports Medicine.* New York, Oxford University Press, 1994.

52. Reber L, Perry J, Pink M. Muscular control of the ankle in running. *Am J Sports Med* 21(6):805–810, 1993.

53. Reeder M, Dick B, Atkins J, et al. Stress fractures: Current concepts of diagnosis and treatment. *Sports Med* 22(3):198–212, 1996.

54. Rettig A, Shelbourne K, McCarrol J, et al. The natural history and treatment of delayed union stress fractures of the anterior cortex of the tibia. *Am J Sports Med* 16(3):250–255, 1988.

55. Rettig A, McCarroll J, Hahn R. Chronic compartment syndrome: Surgical intervention in 12 cases. *Phys Sports Med* 19(4):63–70, 1991.

56. Romani W. Mechanisms and management of stress fractures in physically active persons. *J Athlet Train* 37(3):306–314, 2002.

57. Sallade J, Koch S. Training errors in long distance runners. *J Athlet Train* 27(1):50–53, 1992.

58. Schepsis A, Martini D, Corbett M. Surgical management of exertional compartment syndrome of the lower leg: Long term followup. *Am J Sports Med* 21(6):811–817, 1993.

59. Schepsis A, Wagner C, Leach R. Surgical management of Achilles tendon overuse injuries: A long-term follow-up study. *Am J Sports Med* 22(5):611–619, 1994.

60. Schepsis A, Jones H, Haas H. Achilles tendon disorders in athletes. *Am J Sports Med* 30(2):287–305, 2002.

61. Schon L, Baxter D, Clanton T. Chronic exercise-induced leg pain in active people: More than just shin splints. *Phys Sports Med* 20(1):100–114, 1992.

62. Shwayhat A, Linenger J, Hofher L, et al. Profiles of exercise history and overuse injuries among United States Navy Sea, Air, and Land (SEAL) recruits. *Am J Sports Med* 22(6):835–840, 1994.

63. Simon R. The tibial and fibular shaft. In: Simon R, Koenigshnecht S, eds. *Emergency Orthopedics: The Extremities,* 3rd ed. Norwalk, CT, Appleton-Lange, 1995.

64. Slimmon D, Bennell K, Bruker P, et al. Long-term outcome of fasciotomy with partial fasciectomy for chronic exertional compartment syndrome of the lower leg. *Am J Sports Med* 30:581–588, 2002.

65. Solveborn S, Moberg A. Immediate free ankle motion after surgical repair of acute Achilles tendon ruptures. *Am J Sports Med* 22(5):607–610, 1994.

66. Sommer H, Vallentyne S. Effect of foot posture on the incidence of medial tibial stress syndrome. *Med Sci Sport Exerc* 27(6):800–804, 1995.

67. Speck M, Klaue K. Early full weightbearing and functional treatment after surgical repair of acute achilles tendon rupture. *Am J Sports Med* 26:789–793, 1998.

68. Steele G, Harter R, Ting A. Comparison of functional ability following percutaneous and open surgical repairs by acutely ruptured tendons. *J Sports Rehabil* (2):115–127, 1993.

69. Strudwick W, Stuart G. Proximal fibular stress fracture in an aerobic dancer. A case report. *Am J Sports Med* 20(4):481–482, 1992.

70. Stuart M, Karaharju T. Acute compartment syndrome: Recognizing the progressive signs and symptoms. *Phys Sports Med* 22(3):91–95, 1994.

71. Styf J, Nakhostine M, Gershuni D. Functional knee braces increase intramuscular pressures in the anterior compartment of the leg. *Am J Sports Med* 20(1):46–49, 1992.

72. Swenson E, DeHaven K, Sebastianelli J, et al. The effect of a pneumatic leg brace on return to play in athletes with tibial stress fractures. *Am J Sports Med* 25(3):322–338, 1997.

73. Taube R, Wadsworth L. Managing tibial stress fractures. *Phys Sports Med* 21(4):123–130, 1993.

74. Tiberio D. Pathomechanics of structural foot deformities. *Phys Ther* 68(12):1840–1849, 1988.

75. Tiberio D. The effect of excessive subtalar joint pronation on patellofemoral mechanics: A theoretical model. *J Orthop Sports Phys Ther* 9(4):160–165, 1987.

76. Vincent N. Compartment syndromes. In: Harries M, Williams C, Stanish W, Micheli L, eds. *Oxford Text-Book of Sports Medicine.* New York, Oxford University Press, 1994.

77. Vincenzino B, Griffiths S, Griffiths L, et al. Effect of antipronation tape and temporary orthotics on vertical navicular height before and after exercise. *J Orthop Sports Phys Ther* 30(6):333–339, 2000.

78. Wilder R, Brennan D, Schotte D. A standard measure for exercise prescription for aqua running. *Am J Sports Med* 21(1):45–48, 1993.

79. Wiley J, Clement D, Doyle D, et al. A primary care perspective of chronic compartment syndrome of the leg. *Phys Sports Med* 15(3):111–120, 1987.

80. Willy C, Becker B, Evers H. Unusual development of acute exertional compartment syndrome due to delayed diagnosis: A case report. *Int J Sports Med* 17(6):458–461, 1996.

81. Whitelaw G, Wetzler M, Levy A, et al. A pneumatic leg brace for the treatment of tibial stress fractures. *Clin Orthop* 270:301–305, 1991.

82. Yasuda T, Miyazaki K, Tada K, et al. Stress fracture of the right distal femur following bilateral fractures of the proximal fibulas: A case report. *Am J Sports Med* 20(6):771–774, 1992.

CHAPTER 31

Rehabilitation of the Ankle and Foot

Scott Miller, Skip Hunter, and William E. Prentice

OBJECTIVES

After completing this chapter, the therapist should be able to do the following:

- Discuss the biomechanics and functional anatomy of the foot and ankle.
- Discuss the various injuries that occur at the ankle and foot.
- Discuss the various treatment options for rehabilitating the ankle and foot.
- Discuss the various functional exercises and appropriate progressions.
- Discuss the effect of first ray position, forefoot varus, forefoot valgus, and calcaneal varus on the foot and lower extremity.
- Describe a biomechanical examination of the foot.
- Describe techniques for orthosis fabrication.
- Identify specific pathomechanics and/or pathology associated with the foot and ankle and the appropriate treatment options.

FUNCTIONAL ANATOMY AND BIOMECHANICS

Talocrural Joint

The ankle or talocrural joint is a hinge joint formed by articular facets on the distal tibia, the medial malleolus, and the lateral malleolus, which articulate with the talus. The talus is the second largest tarsal bone and main weight-bearing bone of the articulation linking the lower leg to the foot. The relatively square shape of the talus allows the ankle only two movements about the transverse axis: plantarflexion and dorsiflexion. Because the talus is wider on the anterior aspect than posteriorly, the most stable position of the ankle is dorsiflexion as the talus fits tighter between the malleoli. By contrast, as the ankle moves into plantarflexion, the wider portion of the tibia is brought into contact with the narrower posterior aspect of the talus, creating a less stable position than dorsiflexion.[5]

The lateral malleolus of the fibula extends further distally so that the bony stability of the lateral aspect of the ankle is more stable than the medial. Motion at the talocrural joint ranges from 20° of dorsiflexion to 50° of plantarflexion, depending on the patient. A normal foot requires 20° of plantarflexion and 10° of dorsiflexion for walking and up to 25° for running with the knee extended for a normal gait.[2,3]

TALOCRURAL JOINT LIGAMENTS

The ligamentous support of the ankle consists of the articular capsule, three lateral ligaments, two ligaments that connect the tibia and fibula, and the medial or deltoid ligament (Fig. 31-1). The three lateral ligaments include the anterior talofibular, posterior talofibular, and calcaneofibular ligaments. The anterior and posterior tibiofibular ligaments bridge the tibia and fibula and form the distal portion of the interosseous membrane. The thick deltoid ligament provides primary resistance to foot eversion. A thin articular capsule encases the ankle joint.

TALOCRURAL JOINT MUSCLES

The muscles passing posterior to the lateral malleolus will produce ankle plantarflexion along with toe flexion. Anterior muscles serve to dorsiflex the ankle and to produce toe extension. The anterior muscles include the extensor hallucis longus, the extensor digitorum longus, the peroneus tertius, and the tibialis anterior. The posterior muscle group falls into three layers: at the superficial layer is the gastrocnemius; the middle layer includes the soleus and the plantaris; and the deep layer contains the tibialis posterior, flexor digitorum longus, and flexor hallucis longus.[5]

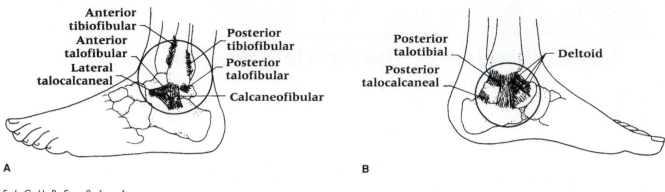

FIGURE 31-1

Ligaments of the talocrural joint. **A,** Lateral aspect. **B,** Medial aspect.

Subtalar Joint

The subtalar joint (STJ) consists of the articulation between the talus and the calcaneus (Fig. 31-2).[80] Supination and pronation, are normal movements that occur at the STJ. These movements are triplanar movements, that is, movements that occur in all three planes simultaneously.[23,61,69] In nonweight bearing, pronation is the composite motion of abduction, dorsiflexion, and calcaneal eversion. Supination is the composite motion of adduction, plantarflexion, and calcaneal inversion.[2,23,61,91,98]

In weight bearing, the STJ also acts as a torque convertor to translate the pronation or supination into leg rotation.[2,91,98] STJ pronation creates tibial internal rotation with the knee unlocking, while supination facilitates tibial external rotation with the knee extending. The movements of the talus during pronation and supination have profound effects on the lower extremity both proximally and distally.

EFFECTS OF REARFOOT AND FOREFOOT ALIGNMENT AND MOBILITY ON STJ POSITION

The evaluation of rearfoot and forefoot alignment and mobility to determine if there are primary abnormalities of the foot is essential in the treatment of any lower-extremity overuse injury.

This assessment is performed in a subtalar joint neutral (STJN) position, most commonly with the patient in a prone position. Once STJN is attained, the evaluator looks for deviations from intrinsic normalcy, which can be described as the bisection of the calcaneus (posteriorly) being parallel with the bisection of the lower third of the lower leg between the tibia and fibula. Next, the posterior bisection of the calcaneus is perpendicular to the line bisecting the second through fifth metatarsal heads. Finally, metatarsal's two through five should be in the same plane as the first metatarsal.[2,3]

When alignment abnormalities are present in the forefoot or rearfoot, compensation for these alignment faults occur. Compensation can be defined as the movement of one body part in order to neutralize the effects of a movement or alignment of another body part. Normal compensation allows for normal function of the foot and ankle. However, excessive compensation occurs when the motion of the foot and ankle surpasses the tolerance of the supportive tissues, which can result in soft-tissue damage.

Compensation can take place at either the rearfoot or the forefoot. Rearfoot compensation occurs when the STJ pronates or supinates to get the plantar surface of the calcaneus flat on the ground. Forefoot compensation occurs when the STJ and

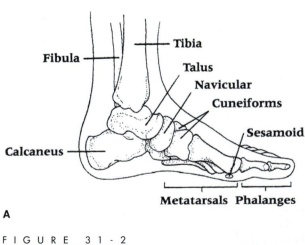

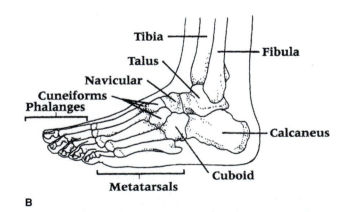

FIGURE 31-2

Bones of the foot. **A,** Medial aspect. **B,** Lateral aspect.

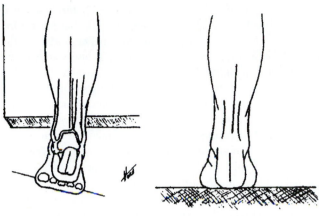

FIGURE   31-3

Compensated subtalar or calcaneal varus. Comparing non-weightbearing neutral to weight-bearing resting position. Figure used with permission of Brian Hoke, American Physical Rehabilitation Network.

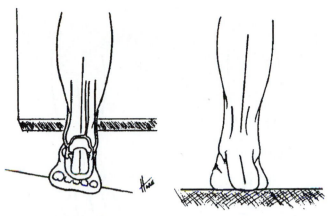

FIGURE   31-5

Compensated forefoot varus. Comparing non-weightbearing neutral to weight-bearing resting position. Figure used with permission of Brian Hoke, American Physical Rehabilitation Network.

midtarsal joint (MTJ) pronate or supinate to get the metatarsal heads flat on the ground. A foot is described as uncompensated when the rearfoot or forefoot does not reach flat contact to the ground, usually due to lack of STJ motion or extreme abnormal alignment in the lower extremity.[2,3]

Compensated subtalar (calcaneal) varus is present when the calcaneus is inverted and the forefoot is in neutral in a non-weightbearing position. In weight bearing, compensation is then noted with increased STJ pronation bringing the plantar surface of the calcaneus flat to the ground (Fig. 31-3). Uncompensated subtalar (calcaneal) varus is evident when there is insufficient motion of the STJ to compensate for the deformity and the calcaneus remains inverted (Fig. 31-4).[2,3]

Compensated forefoot varus is present when the calcaneus is neutral and the forefoot is in a varus position (first metatarsal more cephalad as compared to the fifth) in a non-weightbearing

position. In weight bearing, compensation occurs secondary to increased STJ pronation bringing the forefoot into contact with the ground (Fig. 31-5). Typically, this compensation involves excessive forefoot mobility and the STJ remains pronated throughout stance phase. Uncompensated forefoot varus is evident when there is insufficient motion at the STJ, MTJ, or first ray to bring the forefoot into contact with the ground (Fig. 31-6).[2,3]

Compensated forefoot valgus is present when the calcaneus is neutral and the forefoot is in a valgus position (first metatarsal more caudal as compared to the fifth) in a non-weightbearing position. In weight bearing, compensation occurs when the calcaneus moves into an inverted position (Fig. 31-7). In this condition, there is often decreased mobility of the first ray and the STJ resupinates before the foot flat phase of stance due to the premature loading of the medial forefoot.[2,3]

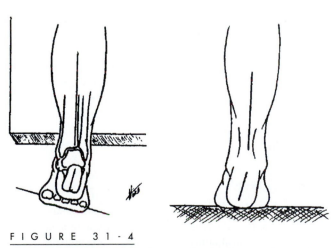

FIGURE   31-4

Uncompensated subtalar or calcaneal varus. Comparing non-weightbearing neutral to weight bearing resting position. Figure used with permission of Brian Hoke, American Physical Rehabilitation Network.

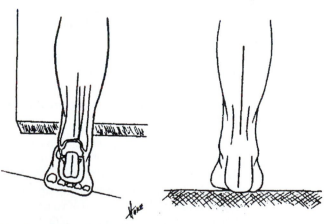

FIGURE   31-6

Uncompensated forefoot varus. Comparing non-weightbearing neutral to weight-bearing resting position. Figure used with permission of Brian Hoke, American Physical Rehabilitation Network.

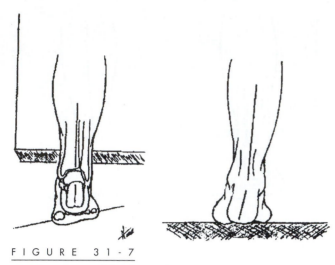

F I G U R E   3 1 - 7

Compensated forefoot valgus. Comparing non-weightbearing neutral to weight-bearing resting position. Figure used with permission of Brian Hoke, American Physical Rehabilitation Network.

It is less typical, but not uncommon to have combinations of subtalar varus with either a forefoot varus or valgus. Mobility of the rearfoot, forefoot, and first ray play a key role in whether compensation is noted or not.

Midtarsal Joint

The MTJ consists of two distinct joints with two different axes that function simultaneously: the calcaneocuboid laterally and the talocalcaneonavicular joints medially.[2,3] The MTJ depends mainly on ligamentous and muscular tension to maintain position and integrity. The midtarsal region comprises two joint axes: an oblique and a longitudinal. The axes can undergo independent motion in a non-weightbearing position; however, the movement of the axes in a weight bearing position are controlled by the STJ. This is considered a constrained system and the stability of the MTJ is directly related to the position of the STJ. Furthermore, as the MTJ becomes more or less mobile, it has an overall direct effect on the distal portion of the foot due to the articulations at the tarsometatarsal joint.[64]

EFFECTS OF MTJ POSITION DURING PRONATION

During pronation, the talus adducts and plantar flexes and makes the joint articulations of the MTJ more congruous. The planes of the oblique and longitudinal axes of the talocalcaneonavicular and calcaneocuboid joints become more parallel, thus allowing increased mobility so the foot becomes more supple. The resulting foot is in a loose pack position and often referred to as a "loose bag of bones."[23,80] This normal effect of the MTJ allows the foot to accommodate to both even and uneven surfaces.

As more motion occurs at the MTJ, the lesser tarsal bones, particularly the first metatarsal and first cuneiform, become more mobile. These bones comprise a functional unit known

as the first ray. With pronation of the MTJ, the first ray is more mobile because of its articulations with that joint. One of the original descriptions was Morton's paper describing the now classic Morton's toe.[65] The first ray is also stabilized by the attachment of the long peroneal tendon, which attaches to the base of the first metatarsal. The long peroneal tendon passes posteriorly around the base of the lateral malleolus and then through a notch in the cuboid to cross the foot to the first metatarsal. The cuboid functions as a pulley to increase the mechanical advantage of the peroneal tendon. Stability of the cuboid is essential in this process. In the pronated position, the cuboid loses much of its mechanical advantage as a pulley; therefore the peroneal tendon no longer stabilizes the first ray effectively. This condition creates hypermobility of the first ray and increases pressure on the other metatarsals.

EFFECTS OF MTJ POSITION DURING SUPINATION

During supination, the talus abducts and dorsi flexes, which raises the level of the talonavicular joint superior to that of the calcaneocuboid joint and allows less congruency of both joint articulations.[79] The planes of the oblique and longitudinal axes of the joints become more oblique or nonparallel. This position of the axes causes increased stability of the foot, making the foot more rigid and tight. Because less movement occurs at the calcaneocuboid joint, the cuboid becomes hypomobile. The long peroneal tendon has a greater amount of tension because the cuboid has less mobility and thus will not allow hypermobility of the first ray. In this case the majority of the weight is borne by the first and fifth metatarsals. This normal effect of the MTJ allows the foot to become a more rigid lever for more efficient push off during late stance phase.

Tarsometatarsal Joint

The tarsometatarsal joint comprises the four proximal tarsal bones of the first, second, and third cuneiforms and the cuboid articulating distally with the bases of the five metatarsal bones. The articulating bones of the tarsometatarsal joint allow for accommodation of rotational forces introduced to the midfoot and forefoot region when the foot is engaged in weight-bearing activities. The tarsometatarsal joints move as a unit and work in unison with the midtarsal and STJs, and it is often difficult to distinguish the individual contributions to the overall movement pattern of the foot.[60] Also known as Lisfranc's joint, the tarsometatarsal joint provides a locking device that enhances foot stability.

Metatarsal Joints

Together with subtalar, talonavicular, and tarsometatarsal interrelationships, foot stabilization depends on the interaction between the metatarsal joints. The first ray moves independently from the other metatarsal bones. As a main functional weight bearing unit, the first ray is necessary for body propulsion. Stabilization depends on the peroneus longus muscle, which attaches on the medial aspect of the first ray. As with the other segments of the foot, stability of the first metatarsal bone depends on the relative position of the subtalar and talonavicular joints. Control of the first ray with orthotic therapy has shown to be effective in the management of lower-extremity overuse injuries.[2]

The fifth metatarsal bone, like the first metatarsal bone, moves independently. With plantarflexion, the first metatarsal moves into abduction and eversion while the fifth moves into adduction and inversion. Conversely, with dorsiflexion, the first metatarsal moves into adduction and inversion while the fifth moves into abduction and eversion.[2,40]

The second ray is the most stable of the five rays due to the secure connection with the tarsals. The second ray functions as the pivot point, as the other rays undergo a torsional twist during the motions of foot pronation and supination.[60]

Biomechanics of Normal Gait

The functions of the foot during the gait cycle are adaptation, shock absorption, rigid support for leverage, and torque conversion. The action of the lower extremity during gait can be divided into two phases. The first is the stance, or support phase, which starts with the initial contact at heel strike and ends at toe-off. Stance phase can be subdivided into three defined events: contact, mid-stance, and propulsion. The second is the swing or recovery phase (Fig. 31-8). This represents the time immediately after toe-off in which the leg is moved from behind the body to a position in front of the body in preparation for heel strike.[2,3]

There are distinct differences in the gait cycle of an individual who is walking, jogging, or running. These differences include speed, vertical ground reaction force (GRF), and stance time. Speed of gait can be defined for various forms of gait, including walking 15–30 minute/mile pace (2–4 mph), jogging

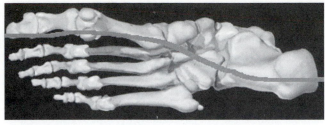

FIGURE 31-9

Center of weightbearing forces. (Adapted from American Physical Rehabilitation Network, 2000.)

7–14 minute/mile pace (5–9 mph), and running 6 minute/mile pace or faster (10+ mph).[3]

There is variability in GRF data between the left and right foot of an individual, as well as between individuals. Generally speaking, with walking, peak GRF at initial contact is less than body weight (BW) and exceeds BW near the end of contact. Peak GRF then diminishes at midstance but exceeds BW to the highest peak value during propulsion. During jogging, peak GRF at initial contact is 1.5–2 times BW, which increases to approximately two to three times BW during propulsion. With running, there is no peak GRF at initial contact, but a single peak of two to three times BW occurs during propulsion, which is actually less than jogging (Fig. 31-9).[3]

The time an individual spends in each phase depends on whether they are walking, jogging, or running. One complete gait cycle is defined as initial contact of left foot through the initial contact of the left foot again. The duration of the gait cycle is approximately 1.0 second for walking, 0.7 seconds for jogging, and 0.6 seconds for running. The start of the gait cycle is described by heel strike during walking, and either heel, midfoot, or forefoot strike with jogging or running. The part of the foot that strikes during jogging or running depends on the speed of the activity. With walking, there is a period of time called the *double limb support phase* in which there is an overlap between stance phase of one limb and stance phase of the opposite limb. This phase constitutes the first 12 percent and the last 12 percent of each stance phase. During jogging and running, there is no double limb support phase. There is actually a *nonsupportive or float phase* with running and jogging. The duration of stance is also reduced as an individual progresses from walking to running, with walking stance duration approximately 0.6 seconds; jogging 0.23 seconds; and running 0.17 seconds. When comparing walking to running, the ratio of stance to swing changes with the percentage of stance phase diminishing and the percentage of swing phase increasing.[3]

The foot's function during the support phase of running is twofold. At heel strike, the foot acts as a shock absorber to the impact forces and then adapts to the uneven surfaces. At push-off, the foot functions as a rigid lever to transmit the explosive force from the lower extremity to the running surface.

In a heel-strike running gait, initial contact of the foot is on the lateral aspect of the calcaneus with the STJ in supination.[8] Associated with this supination of the STJ is an obligatory

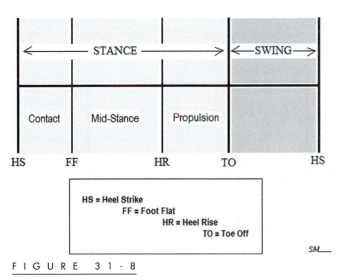

FIGURE 31-8

Gait cycle. (Adapted from American Physical Rehabilitation Network, 2000.)

external rotation of the tibia. As the foot is loaded, the STJ moves into a pronated position until the forefoot is in contact with the running surface. The change in subtalar motion occurs between initial heel strike and 20 percent into the support phase of running. As pronation occurs at the STJ, there is obligatory internal rotation of the tibia. Transverse plane rotation occurs at the knee joint because of this tibial rotation.[8] Pronation of the foot unlocks the MTJ and allows the foot to assist in shock absorption and to adapt to uneven surfaces. It is important during initial impact to reduce the GRFs and to distribute the load evenly on many different anatomic structures throughout the foot and leg. Pronation is normal and allows for this distribution of forces to as many structures as possible to avoid excessive loading on just a few structures. The STJ remains in a pronated position until 55–85 percent of the support phase with maximum pronation is concurrent with the body's center of gravity passing over the base of support.[5] Maximal pronation is 6°–8° for walking and 9°–12° for running.[3]

The foot begins to resupinate and will approach the neutral subtalar position at 70–90 percent of the support phase. In supination, the MTJs are locked and the foot becomes stable and rigid to prepare for push-off. This rigid position allows the foot to exert a great amount of force from the lower extremity to the running surface.[46]

Pathomechanics of Gait Associated with Primary Abnormalities of the Foot

STJ motion can be analyzed throughout the entire phase of gait with significant differences noted with the previously described abnormalities of the forefoot and rearfoot, most effectively through slow motion video analysis. Having an understanding of these differences will assist in proper treatment and management of lower-extremity overuse injuries. STJ is evaluated during the contact, midstance, and propulsion stages of stance phase.

With intrinsic normalcy (Fig. 31-10), during contact the STJ is slightly supinated at heel strike and pronates to 3°–5° of pronation by foot flat. During midstance, the STJ resupinates

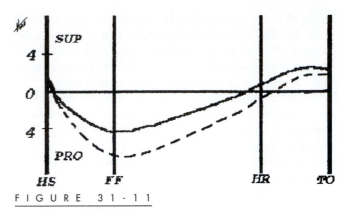

F I G U R E   3 1 - 1 1

Subtalar joint motion analysis. Compensated subtalar or calcaneal varus. Figure used with permission from Brian Hoke, American Physical Rehabilitation Network.

to neutral or slight supination by heel rise. During propulsion, the STJ continues to supinate to toe off.[2,3]

With compensated subtalar varus (Fig. 31-11), during contact the calcaneus is inverted more than normal at initial heel strike, thus the STJ must excessively pronate to compensate for this abnormality. During midstance, the STJ will resupinate as the weight shifts from the heel; however there is a lag as compared to normal as heel rise approaches. Because of this lag, there is associated delayed tibial external rotation. During propulsion, the STJ continues to toe off.[2,3]

With uncompensated subtalar varus (Fig. 31-12), during contact the calcaneus is again inverted more than normal at heel strike; however in this situation the STJ motion is insufficient to compensate for the deformity. The calcaneus remains inverted throughout midstance and propulsion toward toe off. Weight-bearing is more lateral than normal during midstance but will shift medially as the heel rises.[2,3]

With compensated forefoot varus (Fig. 31-13), during contact the STJ reacts the same as in intrinsic normalcy. However, during midstance, the STJ continues to pronate to compensate for the forefoot alignment. Due to the continued pronation, this mechanism unlocks the MTJ creating excessive forefoot mobility at heel rise. During propulsion, the STJ remains

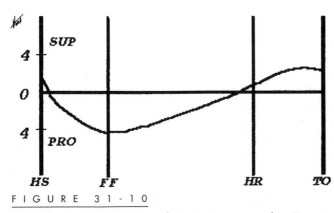

F I G U R E   3 1 - 1 0

Subtalar joint motion analysis. Intrinsic normalcy. Figure used with permission from Brian Hoke, American Physical Rehabilitation Network.

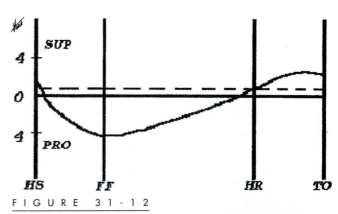

F I G U R E   3 1 - 1 2

Subtalar joint motion analysis. Uncompensated subtalar or calcaneal varus. Figure used with permission from Brian Hoke, American Physical Rehabilitation Network.

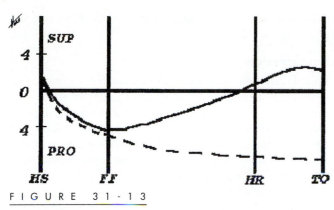

F I G U R E   3 1 - 1 3

Subtalar joint motion analysis. Compensated forefoot varus. Figure used with permission from Brian Hoke, American Physical Rehabilitation Network.

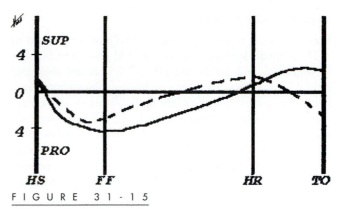

F I G U R E   3 1 - 1 5

Subtalar joint motion analysis. Compensated forefoot valgus. Figure used with permission from Brian Hoke, American Physical Rehabilitation Network.

pronated throughout the remainder of stance. This is described as either late pronation or delayed resupination, and typically there is associated excessive tibial internal rotation.[2,3]

With uncompensated forefoot varus (Fig. 31-14), during contact the STJ is slightly supinated at heel strike, however usually pronates less that the normal 3°–5°. During midstance, the STJ motion is insufficient to compensate for the forefoot alignment and weightbearing stays on the lateral forefoot. During propulsion, there is a small amount of continued pronation at the STJ and no resupination as the foot approaches toe off. These individuals are classified as neither an overpronator nor supinator, just lacking sufficient motion at the STJ.[2,3]

Finally, with compensated forefoot valgus (Fig. 31-15), during contact the STJ pronates, but this motion may be limited to premature loading of the first ray. As a result, during midstance, the STJ rapidly resupinates due to the influence of the normal or rigid first ray. During propulsion, when the heel begins to rise, potential STJ pronation occurs to achieve the necessary weight shift from the lateral aspect of the stance foot to the contralateral limb. This is typically observed when the foot snaps back into pronation late in the stance phase.[2,3]

| REHABILITATION TECHNIQUES FOR SPECIFIC INJURIES

ANKLE SPRAINS

PATHOMECHANICS AND INJURY MECHANISM

Ankle sprains are among the more common musculoskeletal injuries.[10,21,100] Injuries to the ligaments of the ankle may be classified either according to their location or by the mechanism of injury.

Inversion Sprains

An inversion ankle sprain is the most common and often results in injury to the lateral ligaments. The anterior talofibular ligament is the weakest of the three lateral ligaments. Its major function is to stop forward subluxation of the talus. It is injured in an inverted, plantar flexed, and internally rotated position.[48,93] The calcaneofibular and posterior talofibular ligaments are also likely to be injured in inversion sprains as the force of inversion is increased. Increased inversion force is needed to tear the calcaneofibular ligament. Because the posterior talofibular ligament prevents posterior subluxation of the talus, its injuries are severe, such as complete dislocations.[11] The deltoid ligament may also be contused in inversion sprains due to impingement between the fibular malleolus and the calcaneous.

Eversion Sprains

The eversion ankle sprain is less common than the inversion ankle sprain, largely because of the bony and ligamentous anatomy. As mentioned previously, the fibular malleolus extends further inferiorly than does the tibial malleolus. This, combined with the strength of the thick deltoid ligament, prevents excessive eversion. More often, eversion injuries may involve an avulsion fracture of the tibia before the deltoid ligament tears.[16] Despite the fact that eversion sprains are less common, the severity is such that these sprains may take longer to heal than inversion sprains.[71]

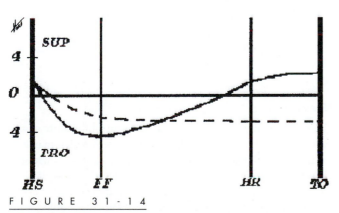

F I G U R E   3 1 - 1 4

Subtalar joint motion analysis. Uncompensated forefoot varus. Figure used with permission from Brian Hoke, American Physical Rehabilitation Network.

Syndesmodic Sprains

Isolated injuries to the distal tibiofemoral joint are referred to as syndesmodic sprains. The anterior and posterior tibiofibular ligaments are found between the distal tibia and fibula and extend up the lower leg as the interosseous ligament or syndesmodic ligament. Sprains of the ligaments are more common than has been realized in the past. These ligaments are torn with increased external rotational or forced dorsiflexion and are often injured in conjunction with a severe sprain of the medial and lateral ligament complexes.[92] Initial rupture of the ligaments occurs distally at the tibiofibular ligament above the ankle mortise. As the force of disruption is increased, the interosseous ligament is torn more proximally. Sprains of the syndesmodic ligaments are extremely hard to treat and often take months to heal. Treatments for this problem are essentially the same as for medial or lateral sprains, with the difference being an extended period of immobilization. Rehabilitation will likely require a longer period of time than for the inversion or eversion sprains.

Severity of the Sprain

There are several factors involved with the severity of an ankle sprain, including previous history, intrinsic and extrinsic abnormalities, velocity, and mechanism of injury. In a grade I sprain, there is some stretching or perhaps tearing of the ligamentous fibers, with little or no joint instability. Mild pain, little swelling, and joint stiffness may be apparent. With a grade II sprain, there is some tearing and separation of the ligamentous fibers and moderate instability of the joint. Moderate to severe pain, swelling, and joint stiffness should be expected.

Grade III sprains involve total rupture of the ligament, manifested primarily by gross instability of the joint. Severe pain may be present initially, followed by little or no pain due to total disruption of nerve fibers. Swelling may be profuse, and thus the joint tends to become very stiff some hours after the injury. A grade III sprain with marked instability usually requires some form of immobilization lasting several weeks. Frequently the force producing the ligament injury is so great that other ligaments or structures surrounding the joint may also be injured. With cases in which there is injury to multiple ligaments, surgical repair or reconstruction may be necessary to correct instability.

REHABILITATION CONCERNS

During the initial phase of ankle rehabilitation, the major goals are reduction of post-injury swelling, bleeding, and pain, and protection of the already healing ligament. As is the case in all acute musculoskeletal injuries, initial treatment efforts should be directed toward limiting the amount of swelling.[74] This is perhaps more true in the case of ankle sprains than with any other injury. Controlling initial swelling is the single most important treatment measure that can be taken during the entire rehabilitation process. Limiting the amount of acute swelling can significantly reduce the time required for rehabilitation. Initial management includes compression, ice, elevation, rest, and protection.

Compression

Immediately following injury and evaluation, a compression wrap should be applied to the sprained ankle. An elastic bandage should be firmly and evenly applied, wrapping distal to proximal. It is also recommended that the elastic bandage be wet to facilitate the passage of cold. To add more compression, a horseshoe-shaped felt pad may be inserted under the wrap over the area of maximum swelling.

Following initial treatment, open Gibney taping may be applied under an elastic wrap to provide additional compression and support. Care should be taken not to compartmentalize this treatment by placing tape across the top and bottom of the open area of the open Gibney (Fig. 31-16). Uneven pressure or uncovered areas over any part of the extremity may allow the swelling to accumulate.

Other devices are available that apply external compression to the ankle to control or reduce swelling. External compression should be used both initially and throughout the rehabilitative process. Most of these devices use either air or cold water within an enclosed bag to provide pressure to reduce swelling. One commonly used device is the intermittent compression unit, such as a Jobst pump or Cryo-cuff (Fig. 31-17).

Ice

The use of ice on acute injuries has been well documented in the literature. Initially, ice and compression should be used together, because this treatment regimen is more effective than ice alone.[87] The initial use of ice is indicated for constricting superficial blood flow to prevent hemorrhage as well as in reducing the hypoxic response to injury by decreasing cellular metabolism. Long-term benefits may be from reduction of pain and guarding.[5] Garrick suggests the use of ice for a minimum of 20 minutes once every 4 waking hours.[30] Ice should not be used longer than 30 minutes, especially over superficial nerves such as the peroneal and ulnar nerves. Prolonged use of ice in such areas may produce transient nerve palsy.[25]

Current literature suggests that ice can be used during all phases of rehabilitation[51] but is most effective if used immediately after injury.[74] Ice can certainly do no harm if used properly, but heat, if applied too soon after injury, may lead to increased swelling. Often the switch from ice to heat cannot be made for days or weeks.

Elevation

Elevation is an essential part of edema control. Pressure in any vessel below the level of the heart is increased, which may lead to increased edema.[17] Elevation allows gravity to work with the lymphatic system rather than against it. Elevation decreases hydrostatic pressure to decrease fluid loss and also assists venous and lymphatic return through gravity.[74] Patients should be encouraged to maintain an elevated position as often as possible, particularly during the first 24–48 hours following injury. An

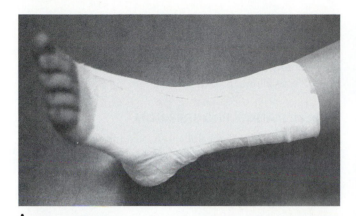

A

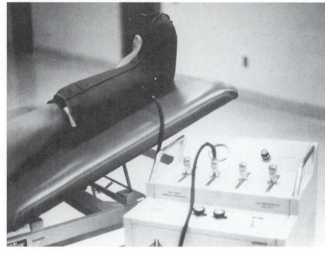

A

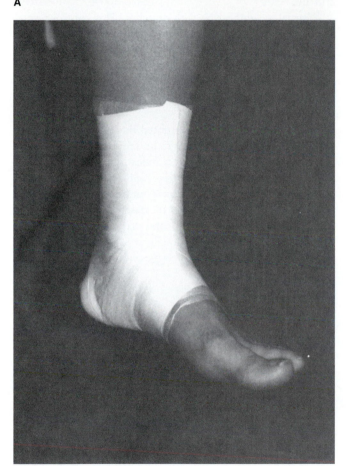

B

FIGURE   31-16

A, Correctly done open Gibney tape. **B,** Closed-basket weave tape.

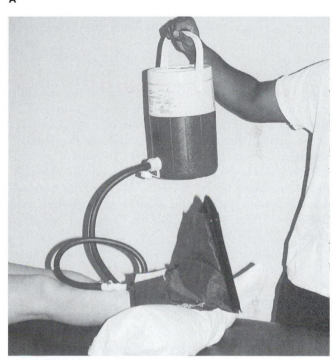

B

FIGURE   31-17

A, Jobst intermittent air compression device. **B,** Cryo-cuff.

attempt should be made to treat in the elevated position rather than the gravity-dependent position. Any treatment done in the dependent position will allow edema to increase.[74,85]

Rest

It is important to allow the inflammatory process to run its course during the first 24–48 hours before incorporating aggressive exercise techniques. However, rest does not mean that the injured patient does nothing. Contralateral exercises may be performed to obtain cross-transfer effects on the muscles of the injured side.[50] Isometric exercises may be performed very early in dorsiflexion, plantarflexion, inversion, and eversion (see Exercises 31-1 to 31-4). These types of exercises may be performed to prevent atrophy without fear of further injury to the ligament. Active plantarflexion and dorsiflexion may be initiated early because they also do not endanger the healing ligament as long as they are done in a pain-free range. Active

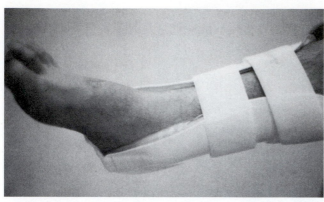

FIGURE   31-18
Commercially available Aircast ankle stirrup.

plantarflexion and dorsiflexion can be done while the patient is iced and elevated. Inversion and eversion are to be avoided, because they might initiate bleeding and further traumatize ligaments.

Protection

Several appliances are available to accomplish this early protected motion. Quillen[75] recommends the ankle stirrup, which allows motion in the sagittal plane while limiting movement of the frontal plane and thus avoids stressing the ligaments through inversion and eversion (Fig. 31-18). Several commercially available braces accomplish this goal and also apply cushioned pressure to help with edema.[88] When a commercially available product is not feasible, a similar protective device may be fashioned from thermoplastic materials such as Hexalite® or Orthoplast® (Fig. 31-19).

The open Gibney taping technique also provides early medial and lateral protection while allowing plantarflexion and dorsiflexion, in addition to being an excellent mechanism of edema control (Fig. 31-16).

Gross et al. compared the effectiveness of a number of commercial ankle orthoses and taping in restricting eversion and inversion. All of these support systems significantly reduced

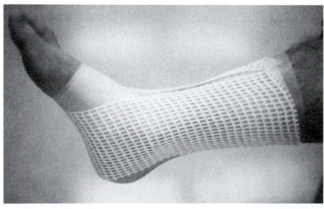

FIGURE   31-19
Molded Hexalite ankle stirrup.

inversion and eversion immediately after initial application and following an exercise bout when compared to preapplication measures. Of the support systems tested, taping provided the least amount of support after exercise.[38] Early application of these devices allows for early ambulation.

REHABILITATION PROGRESSION

In the early phase of rehabilitation, vigorous exercise is discouraged. The injured ligament must be maintained in a stable position so that healing can occur. Thus, during the period of maximum protection following injury, the patient should be either non-weightbearing or perhaps partial weight bearing on crutches.

Partial weightbearing with crutches helps control several complications to healing. Muscle atrophy, proprioceptive loss, and circulatory stasis are all reduced when even limited weight-bearing is allowed. Weight-bearing also inhibits contracture of the tendons, which may lead to tendinitis. For these reasons, early ambulation, even if only touchdown weightbearing, is essential.[56]

It has been clearly demonstrated that a healing ligament needs a certain amount of stress to heal properly. The literature suggests that early limited stress following the initial period of inflammation may promote faster and stronger healing.[11,68] These studies found that protected motion facilitated proper collagen reorientation and thus increased the strength of the healing ligament. Once swelling and pain decrease, indicating that ligaments have healed enough to tolerate limited stress, rehabilitation can become more aggressive.

Range of Motion

In the early stages of the rehabilitation, inversion and eversion should be minimized. Light joint mobilization concentrating on dorsiflexion and plantarflexion should be started first.[55] Range of motion (ROM) can be improved by manual joint mobilization techniques (see Exercises 31-31 to 31-35). It can also be improved through exercises such as towel stretching for the plantarflexors (see Exercise 31-27) and standing or kneeling stretches for the dorsiflexors (see Exercise 31-29). Patients are encouraged to do these exercises slowly, without pain, and to use high repetitions (2–3 sets of 30–40 repetitions).

As tenderness over the ligament decreases, inversion-eversion exercises may be initiated in conjunction with plantarflexion and dorsiflexion exercises. Early exercises include pulling a towel from one side to the other by alternatively inverting and everting the foot (see Exercise 31-12 B) and alphabet drawing in an ice bath, which should be done in capital letters to ensure that full range is used.

Exercises performed on a BAPS® (Board Spectrum Therapy Products, Inc.) board, Fitter® Rocker board, Fitter® Wobble board, or BOB® may be beneficial for ROM as well as a beginning exercise for regaining neuromuscular control.[94] These exercises typically should first be performed in a seated position, progressing to partial and then full weightbearing.

Initially the patient should start in the seated position with Fitter® Rocker board in the plantarflexion-dorsiflexion direction. As pain decreases and ligament healing progresses, the board may be turned in the inversion-eversion direction (see Exercises 31-25A and B). As the patient performs these movements easily, the patient could start weight bearing active-assisted ROM in the plantarflexion-dorsiflexion direction with the BOB® (see Exercise 31-11). A seated BAPS® board or Fitter® Wobble board may be used for full ROM exercises, including clock-wise and counter clock-wise directions (see Exercise 31-45A). When seated exercises are performed with ease, progression to partial weight-bearing exercises should be initiated, utilizing a leg press machine or Total Gym®. Finally, progression to full weight-bearing exercises is initiated, focusing on ROM and balance retraining (see Exercises 31-45B and C).

Vigorous pain-free heel cord stretching for the gastrocnemius and soleus should be initiated as soon as possible, utilizing either static or dynamic multiplanar techniques (see Exercises 31-26, 31-28, and 31-11). McCluskey et al.[58] found that the heel cord acts as a bowstring when tight and may increase the chance of ankle sprains.

Strengthening

Isometrics may be done in the four major ankle motion planes, frontal and sagittal (see Exercises 31-1 to 31-4). They may be accompanied early in the rehabilitative phase by plantarflexion and dorsiflexion isotonic exercises, which do not endanger the healing ligaments (see Exercises 31-7, 31-8, and 31-10). As the ligaments heal and ROM increases, strengthening exercises may be initiated in all planes of motion (see Exercises 31-5 and 31-6). Care must be taken when exercising the ankle in inversion and eversion to avoid tibial rotation as a substitute movement.

During the early stages of rehabilitation, foot intrinsic strengthening exercises are recommended, including towel curls (see Exercise 31-12A) and arch raises (see Exercises 31-13A–D).

Pain should be the basic guideline for deciding when to start inversion-eversion isotonic exercises. Light resistance with high repetitions has fewer detrimental effects on the ligaments (2–4 sets of 15–25 repetitions). Resistive tubing exercises, ankle weights around the foot, or a multidirectional Elgin ankle exerciser (see Exercise 31-9) are excellent methods of strengthening inversion and eversion. Tubing has advantages in that it may be used both eccentrically and concentrically.

Isokinetics have advantages in that more functional speeds may be obtained (see Exercises 31-19 and 31-20). Proprioceptive neuromuscular facilitation strengthening exercises, which isolate the desired motions at the talocrural joint, can also be used (see Exercises 31-21 to 31-24).

Proprioception and Neuromuscular Control

The role of proprioception in repeated ankle trauma has been questioned.[15,26,29,66] The literature suggests that proprioception is certainly a factor in recurrent ankle sprains. Rebman[77] reported that 83 percent of patients experienced a reduction in chronic ankle sprains after a program of proprioceptive ex-

ercises. Glencross and Thornton[36] found that the greater the ligamentous disruption, the greater the proprioceptive loss.

Early weightbearing has previously been mentioned as a method of reducing proprioceptive loss. During the early rehabilitation phase, standing on both feet with side-to-side and heel-to-toes weight shifting is recommended, as well as double-limb stance with eyes closed. Next progression would be single-leg stance on a stable surface starting with eyes open working toward eyes closed including performing this with additional weight shifting toward the heel (see Exercises 31-43A–D). This exercise series can be progressed to single-limb stance on unstable surfaces, which should be done initially with support from the hands, using such commercial devices as foam rollers, Fitter Wobble board, Fitter Rocker board, Dyna Disc® (a registered trademark of Exertools), BOSU® (a registered trademark of DW Fitness LLC) Balance Trainer, or KAT® system. Once the patient demonstrates good control on a specific device, the patient can progress to free standing and controlling the board through all ranges (see Exercises 31-44A–D). To further challenge the patient's neuromuscular control and incorporate more functional activities, perturbations can be introduced via the upper extremities using tubing, medicine balls, or the Body Blade® while in a single-limb stance position (see Exercises 31-46A–E).

Other closed-kinetic chain (CKC) exercises may be functionally beneficial. Leg press (see Exercise 31-48), mini-form squats (see Exercise 31-50A), or mini-lunges (see Exercise 31-51) are each examples of CKC exercises. Initially, start any of the CKC exercises in double-limb stance and progress to single limb (see Exercise 31-49) or on unstable surfaces (see Exercise 31-50 B). Single-leg standing kicks using abduction, adduction, extension, and flexion of the uninvolved side, while weightbearing on the affected side, will increase both strength and proprioception. This may be accomplished either by free standing (see Exercise 31-47) or while having the patient stand on an unstable surface.

Additional information on impaired neuromuscular control and reactive neuromuscular training can be referenced in Chapter 11.

Proximal Stability

The focus of this chapter is on the foot and ankle. However, it is essential that when managing a patient with foot and ankle pathology or pathomechanics, that proximal stability is addressed, specifically that of the knee, hip, and trunk musculature. As already discussed, ROM, strength, flexibility, and neuromuscular control are all key components. More detailed information is available in several previous chapters, including Chapters 17 and 18.

To further expand on strengthening exercises, when a patient has weight-bearing restrictions, initiating mat table exercises for proximal trunk and hip stability early in the rehabilitation process are recommended. For example, exercises for gluteus medius, hip lateral rotators, trunk extensors, and gluteus maximus can be initiated against gravity, against resistance or using an exercise ball (see Exercises 31-57A–B, 31-58A–C). Once weight bearing is progressed to full and pain-free, then a more functional program can be implemented.

Finally, it is important when managing a patient with a proximal movement-related dysfunction or diagnosis, to examine the foot and ankle. It is well accepted that when the foot comes into contact with the ground, there is a biomechanical influence up the kinetic chain.[2,3] Thus, the assumption can be made that overuse injuries involving knees, hips, or back could be related to foot or ankle pathomechanics.

Cardiorespiratory Endurance

Cardiorespiratory conditioning should be maintained during the entire rehabilitation process. A stationary bike, NuStep (a registered trademark of NuStep Inc.) , or elliptical trainer are all appropriate forms of no impact, partial to full-weightbearing activities as long as pain-free motion is achieved (see Exercises 31-54 to 31-56). An upper-extremity ergometer or Airdyne (a registered trademark of Schwinn Fitness) bike with the hands (see Exercise 31-53) provides excellent cardiovascular exercise without placing stress on the lower extremities. Pool activities such as running using a float vest or swimming are also good cardiovascular exercises (see Exercise 31-52). Further information on aquatic therapy in rehabilitation is available in Chapter 19.

Functional Progressions

Functional progressions may be as complex or simple as needed. The more severe the injury, the greater the need for a detailed functional progression. The typical progression begins early in the rehabilitation process as the patient becomes partial weight-bearing. Full weightbearing activities should be started when ambulation can be performed without a limp. Running may be initiated as soon as ambulation is pain-free. Pain-free hopping on the affected side may also be a guideline to determine when running is appropriate.

Exercising in a pool allows for early running. The patient is placed in the pool in a swim vest that supports the body in water. The patient then runs in place without touching the bottom of the pool. Proper running form should be stressed. Eventually the patient is moved into shallow water so that more weight is placed on the ankle.

Progression is then to running on a smooth, flat surface, ideally a track. Initially the patient should jog straight and walk the curves, and then progress to jogging the entire track. Initially, a time-based progression is easier for the patient to follow as they may start a low as 5 minutes of running for the first time. For the first 4 weeks, the patient may increase the running time after two successful runs at the allowed time. It is also important during the first 4 weeks to run every other day with a rest day in between. Rest does not necessarily mean doing nothing. It is recommended that cross-training takes place on the off days as previously described in the Cardiorespiratory Endurance section. After 4 weeks of pain-free running, the patient is then allowed to start running 2 days in a row with a day off in between. General guidelines for return to running include 10–15 percent increase in total mileage or time per week. Once a pain-free running base has been reestablished, speed may be increased to a sprint in a straight line.

Movement in directions other than straight planes is necessary for return to sport. The cutting sequence should begin with circles of diminishing diameter. Cones may be set up for the patient to run figure-8s as the next cutting progression. The crossover or side step is next.[4] The patient sprints to a predesignated spot and cuts or sidesteps abruptly. When this progression is accomplished, the cut should be done without warning on the command of another person. Jumping and hopping exercises should be started on both legs simultaneously, and gradually reduced to only the injured side.

The patient may perform at different levels for each of these functional sequences. One functional sequence may be done at half speed while another is done at full speed. An example of this is the patient who is running full speed on straights of the track while doing figure-8s at only half speed. Once the upper levels of all the sequences are reached, the patient may return to limited practice, which may include early teaching and fundamental drills.

It has been estimated that 30–40 percent of all inversion injuries result in reinjury.[26,43,44,57,82] In the past, patients were simply allowed to return to their normal activities once the pain was low enough to tolerate the activity. The contemporary rehabilitative process should include a gradual progression of functional activities that slowly increase the stress on the ligaments.[49]

It is common practice that some type of ankle support be worn initially. It appears that ankle taping does have a stabilizing effect on unstable ankles,[31,95] without interfering with motor performance.[27,58] McCluskey et al.[58] suggest taping the ankle and also taping the shoe onto the foot to make the shoe and ankle function as one unit. High-topped footwear may further stabilize the ankle.[39] An Aircast or some other supportive ankle brace can also be worn for support as a substitute for taping (Fig. 31-18).

Subluxation and Dislocation of the Peroneal Tendons

PATHOMECHANICS

The peroneus brevis and longus tendons pass posterior to the fibula in the peroneal groove under the superior peroneal retinaculum. Peroneal tendon dislocation may occur because of rupture of the superior retinaculum or because the retinaculum strips the periosteum away from the lateral malleolus, creating laxity in the retinaculum. It appears that there is no anatomic correlation between peroneal groove size or shape and instability of the peroneal tendons.[47] An avulsion fracture of the lateral ridge of the distal fibula may also occur with a subluxation or dislocation of the peroneal tendons.

INJURY MECHANISM

Subluxation of peroneal tendons can occur from any mechanism causing sudden and forceful contraction of the peroneal muscles that involves dorsiflexion and eversion of the foot.[47] This forces the tendons anteriorly, rupturing the retinaculum and potentially causing an avulsion fracture of the lateral malleolus. The patient will often hear or feel a "pop." In differentiating peroneal subluxation from a lateral ligament sprain or tear, there will be tenderness over the peroneal tendons and swelling and ecchymosis in the retromalleolar area. During active eversion, the subluxation of the peroneal tendons may be observed and palpated. This is easier to observe when acute symptoms have subsided. The patient will typically complain of chronic "giving way" or "popping." If the tendon is dislocated on initial evaluation, it should be reduced using gentle inversion and plantarflexion with pressure on the peroneal tendon.[47]

REHABILITATION CONCERNS AND PROGRESSION

Following reduction, the patient should be initially placed in a compression dressing with a felt pad cut in the shape of a keyhole strapped over the lateral malleolus, placing gentle pressure on the peroneal tendons. Once the acute symptoms abate, the patient should be placed in a short leg cast in slight plantarflexion and non-weightbearing for 5–6 weeks (Fig. 31-20). Aggressive ankle rehabilitation, as previously described, is initiated after cast removal.

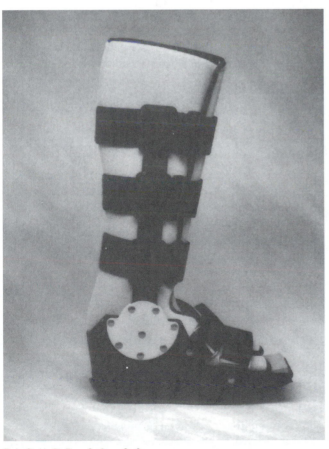

FIGURE 31-20

Short-leg walking cast.

In the case of an avulsion injury or when this becomes a chronic problem, conservative treatment is unlikely to be successful and surgery is needed to prevent the problem from recurring. A number of surgical procedures have been recommended, including repair or reconstruction of the superior peroneal retinaculum, deepening of the peroneal groove, or rerouting the tendon. Following surgery, the patient should be placed in a non-weightbearing short-leg cast for about 4 weeks. The course of rehabilitation is similar to that described for ankle fractures with increased emphasis on strengthening of the peroneal tendons in eversion.[47]

The patient may require approximately 10–12 weeks for rehabilitation.

Tendinopathy

PATHOMECHANICS AND INJURY MECHANISM

Inflammation of the tendons surrounding the ankle joint is common. The tendons most often involved are the posterior tibialis tendon behind the medial malleolus, the anterior tibialis under the extensor retinaculum on the dorsal surface of the ankle, and the peroneal tendons both behind the lateral malleolus and at the base of the fifth metatarsal.[92]

Tendinitis or tendinopathy of these tendons may result from one specific cause or from a collection of mechanisms, including faulty foot mechanics, which will be discussed later in this chapter; inappropriate or poor footwear that can create faulty foot mechanics; acute trauma to the tendon; tightness in the heel cord complex; or training errors in the athletic population. Training errors would include training at intensities that are too high or too often, changing training surfaces, or changes in activities within the training program.[92]

Patients who develop a tendinopathy are likely to complain of pain both with active movement and passive stretching; swelling around the area of the tendon due to inflammation of the tendon and the tendon sheath; crepitus on movement; and stiffness and pain following periods of inactivity but particularly in the morning.

REHABILITATION CONCERNS AND PROGRESSION

In the early stages of rehabilitation, exercises are used to produce increased circulation and thus increased lymphatic flow. This will not only facilitate removal of fluid and the by-products of the inflammatory process, but will also increase nutrition to the healing tendon. In addition, exercise should also be used to limit atrophy, which may occur with disuse, and to minimize loss of strength, proprioception, and neuromuscular control.

Techniques should be incorporated into rehabilitation that act to reduce or eliminate inflammation, including rest, using therapeutic modalities (ice, ultrasound, iontophoresis, or diathermy), and use of anti-inflammatory medications as prescribed by a physician.

If faulty foot mechanics are a cause of tendinitis, it may be helpful to construct an appropriate orthotic device to correct the foot and ankle biomechanics. Taping of the foot may also be helpful in temporarily reducing stress on the tendons.

In many instances, if the mechanism causing the irritation and inflammation of the tendon is removed, and the inflammatory process runs its normal course, the tendinopathy will often resolve within 10 days to 2 weeks. This is particularly true if rest and treatment are begun as soon as the symptoms begin. Unfortunately, as is most often the case, if treatment does not begin until the symptoms have been present for several weeks or even months, the tendinopathy will take much longer to resolve. This is due to the fact that because of long-standing inflammation, the tendon thickens and the period of time required for that tendon to remodel is significantly greater.

In our experience, it is better to allow the patient to rest for a sufficient period of time so that tendon healing can take place. With tendinopathy, an aggressive approach that does not allow the tendon to first eliminate the inflammatory response and then to begin tissue realignment and remodeling will not allow the tendon to heal. This may potentially exacerbate the existing inflammation and cause chronic inflammation. Thus, the rehabilitation progression must be slow and controlled, with full return when the patient is free of tendon pain.

Ankle Fractures and Dislocation

PATHOMECHANICS AND INJURY MECHANISM

When dealing with fractures of the ankle or tibial and fibular malleoli, the therapist must always be cautious about suspecting an ankle sprain when a fracture actually exists. A fracture of the malleoli will generally result in immediate swelling. Ankle fractures can occur from several mechanisms that are similar to those seen for ankle sprains. In an inversion injury, medial malleolar fractures are often accompanied by a sprain of the lateral ligaments of the ankle. A fracture of the lateral malleolus is often more likely to occur than a sprain if an eversion force is applied to the ankle. This is due to the fact that the lateral malleolus extends as far as the distal aspect of the talus. With a fracture of the lateral malleolus, however, there may also be a sprain of the deltoid ligament. Fractures result from either avulsion or compression forces. With avulsion injuries, it is often the injured ligaments that prolong the rehabilitation period.[37]

Osteochondral fractures are sometimes seen in the talus. These fractures may also be referred to as dome fractures of the talus. Generally, they will be either nondisplaced or compression fractures.[37]

While sprains and fractures are very common, dislocations in the ankle and foot are rare. They most often occur in conjunction with fractures and require open reduction and internal fixation.[81]

REHABILITATION CONCERNS

Generally, non-displaced ankle fractures should be managed with rest and protection until the fracture has healed, while displaced fractures are treated with open reduction and internal fixation. Non-displaced fractures are treated by casting the limb in a short-leg walking cast for 6 weeks with early weight bearing. The course of rehabilitation following this period of immobilization is generally the same as for ankle sprains. Following surgery for displaced or unstable fractures, the patient may be placed in a removable walking cast; however it is essential to closely monitor the rehabilitation process to make certain that the patient is compliant.[37]

If an osteochondral fracture is displaced and there is a fragment, surgery is required to remove the fragment. In other cases, if the fragment has not healed within a year, surgery may be considered to remove the fragment.[37]

REHABILITATION PROGRESSION

Following open reduction and internal fixation, a posterior splint with the ankle in neutral should be applied, and the patient should be nonweight bearing for about 2 weeks. During this period efforts should be directed at controlling swelling and wound management.

At 2–3 weeks, the patient may be placed in a short-leg walking brace (Fig. 31-20), which allows for partial weight-bearing, for 6 weeks. Active ROM (AROM) plantarflexion and dorsiflexion exercises can begin and should be done two or three times a day, along with general strengthening exercises for the rest of the lower extremity.

At 6 weeks, the patient can be weightbearing in the walking brace and this should continue for 2–4 weeks more. Isometric exercises (see Exercises 31-1 to 31-4) can be performed initially without the brace, progressing to isotonic strengthening exercises (see Exercises 31-5 to 31-8, 31-10), which concentrate on eccentrics. Stretching exercises can also be incorporated (see Exercises 31-11, 31-25 to 31-29). If there are specific joint restrictions at the ankle and foot, mobilization techniques by a therapist may be used to reduce capsular tightness (see Exercises 31-31 to 31-42).

Exercises to regain proprioception and neuromuscular control, as previously described in the Ankle Sprains Section, can be progress from sitting to standing and from stable to unstable surfaces as tolerated (see Exercises 31-25, 31-43 to 31-47). As strength and neuromuscular control continue to increase, more functional, CKC-strengthening activities can begin (see Exercises 31-14 to 31-18 and 31-48 to 31-51).

Excessive Pronation and Supination

PATHOMECHANICS AND INJURY MECHANISM

Often when we hear the terms "pronation" or "supination," we automatically think of some pathological condition related to gait. It must be reemphasized that pronation and supination of the foot and STJ are normal movements that occur during the support phase of gait. However, if pronation or supination is excessive, delayed, or prolonged, overuse injuries may develop. Excessive or prolonged supination or pronation at the STJ is likely to result from some structural or functional deformity

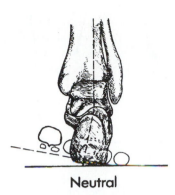
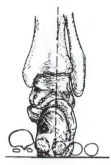

Neutral   Weight-bearing

FIGURE   31-21

Subtalar or calcaneal varus. Comparing weightbearing neutral and resting positions.

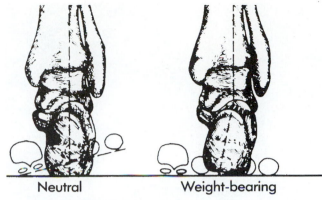

Neutral   Weight-bearing

FIGURE   31-23

Forefoot valgus. Comparing weightbearing neutral and resting positions.

in the foot or leg. The structural deformity forces the STJ to compensate in a manner that will allow the weightbearing surfaces of the foot to make stable contact with the ground and get into a weightbearing position. Thus, excessive pronation or supination is a compensation for an existing structural deformity. Three of the most common structural deformities of the foot as previously described are subtalar or calcaneal varus (Fig. 31-21), forefoot varus (Fig. 31-22), and forefoot valgus (Fig. 31-23).

Structural calcaneal varus and forefoot varus deformities are usually associated with excessive pronation. A structural forefoot valgus usually causes excessive supination. The deformities usually exist in one plane, but the triplane STJ will interfere with the normal functions of the foot and make it more difficult to act as a shock absorber, adapt to uneven surfaces, and act as a rigid lever for push off. The compensation rather than the deformity itself usually causes overuse injuries.

Excessive, delayed, or prolonged pronation of the STJ during the support phase of running is one of the major causes of stress injuries. Overload of specific structures results when excessive pronation is produced in the support phase or when pronation is prolonged into the propulsive phase of running.

Excessive pronation during the support phase will cause compensatory STJ motion such that the MTJ remains unlocked, resulting in an excessively loose foot. There is also an increase in tibial rotation, which forces the knee joint to absorb more transverse rotation motion. Delayed or late pronation of the STJ is when the motion initially is not excessive, but because of the continued pronation during stance phase, a similar result exists as with excessive pronation. Prolonged pronation of the STJ will not allow the foot to resupinate in time to provide a rigid lever for push off, resulting in a less powerful and efficient force. Thus, various foot and leg problems will occur with excessive, delayed, or prolonged pronation during the support phase, including callus formation under the second metatarsal, stress fractures of the second metatarsal, bunions due to hypermobility of the first ray, plantar fasciitis, posterior tibial tendinitis, Achilles tendinitis, tibial stress syndrome, iliotibial band friction syndrome, or medial knee pain.

Several extrinsic keys may be observed that indicate pronation.[80] Excessive eversion of the calcaneus during the stance phase indicates pronation (Fig. 31-24). Excessive or

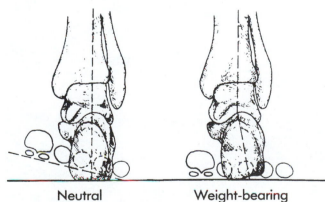

Neutral   Weight-bearing

FIGURE   31-22

Forefoot varus. Comparing weightbearing neutral and resting positions.

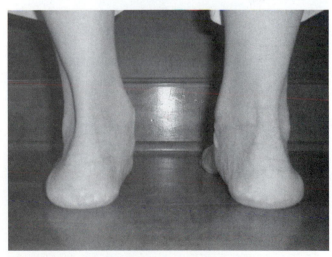

FIGURE   31-24

Eversion of the calcaneus, indicating pronation.

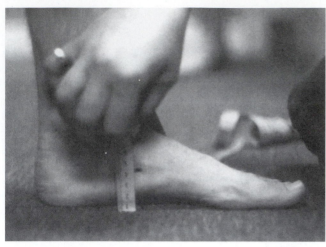

FIGURE   31-25

Measurement of the navicular differential.

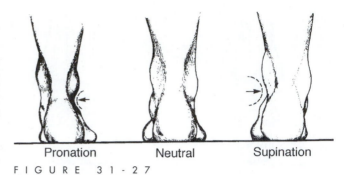

Pronation   Neutral   Supination

FIGURE   31-27

Concavity below the lateral malleolus, indicating pronation. Concavity below the medial malleolus, indicating supination.

prolonged internal rotation of the tibia is another sign of pronation. This internal rotation may cause increased symptoms in the shin or knee. A lowering of the medial arch accompanies pronation. It may be measured as the navicular differential[59]—the difference between the height of the navicular tuberosity from the floor in a non-weightbearing position versus a weightbearing position (Fig. 31-25). As previously discussed, the talus plantar flexes and adducts with pronation. It may be seen as a medial bulging of the talar head (Fig. 31-26). This same talar adduction causes increased concavity below the lateral malleolus in a posterior view while the calcaneus everts (Fig. 31-27).[61]

At heel strike in prolonged or excessive supination, compensatory movement at the STJ will not allow the MTJ to unlock, causing the foot to remain excessively rigid. Thus, the foot cannot absorb the GRFs as efficiently. Excessive supination limits tibial internal rotation. Injuries typically associated with

excessive supination include fifth metatarsal stress fractures, Achilles tendinopathy, inversion ankle sprains, tibial stress syndrome, peroneal tendinitis, iliotibial band friction syndrome, or trochanteric bursitis.

Structural deformities originating outside the foot also require compensation by the foot for a proper weightbearing position to be attained. Tibial varum is the common bow-leg deformity.[61] The distal tibia is medial to the proximal tibia (Fig. 31-28).[23] This measurement is taken weightbearing with the foot in neutral position.[41] The angle of deviation of the distal tibia from a perpendicular line from the calcaneal midline is considered tibial varum.[33] Tibial varum increases pronation to allow proper foot function.[12] At heel strike the calcaneus must evert to attain a perpendicular position.[91]

Ankle joint equinus is another extrinsic deformity that may require abnormal compensation. It may be considered an

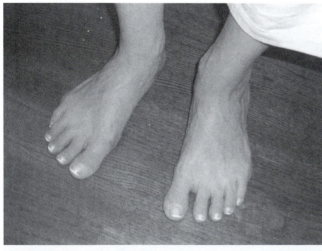

FIGURE   31-26

Medial bulge of the talar head of the left foot, indicating pronation.

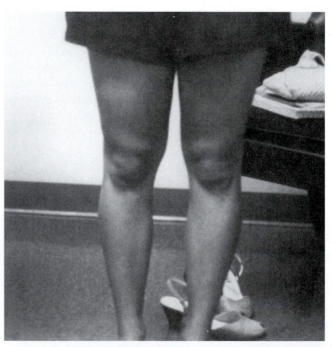

FIGURE   31-28

Tibial varum or bow-leg deformity.

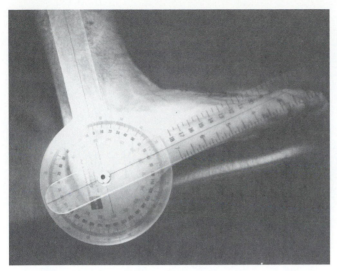

FIGURE 31-29

Dorsiflexion of 10° is necessary for normal walking gait.

extrinsic or intrinsic problem, but is typically a result of loss of talocrural joint ROM into dorsiflexion. The key compensator is the oblique MTJ. If the MTJ is hypermobile or unstable, there will be increased dorsiflexion and forefoot abduction at the MTJ. If the MTJ is hypomobile or stable, there will be early heel rise during propulsion with continued forced pronation.

During normal gait, the tibia must move anterior to the talar dome. Approximately 10° of dorsiflexion for walking and 15°–20° for running is required for this movement (Fig. 31-29).[61] Lack of dorsiflexion may cause compensatory pronation of the foot with resultant foot and lower-extremity pain. Often this lack of dorsiflexion results from tightness of the posterior leg muscles. Other causes include forefoot equinus, in which the plane of the forefoot is below the plane of the rearfoot.[61] It occurs in many high-arched feet. This deformity requires more ankle dorsiflexion. When enough dorsiflexion is not available at the ankle, the additional movement is required at other sites, such as dorsiflexion of the MTJ and rotation of the leg.

REHABILITATION CONCERNS

In individuals who excessively pronate or supinate, the goal of treatment is quite simply to correct the faulty biomechanics that occur due to the existing structural deformity. An accurate biomechanical analysis of the foot and lower extremity should identify those deformities that require abnormal compensatory movements. In the majority of cases, faulty biomechanics can be corrected by constructing an appropriate orthotic device.

Despite arguments in the literature, the authors have found orthotic therapy to be of tremendous value in the treatment of many lower-extremity problems. This view is supported in the literature by several clinical studies. Donatelli[23] found that 96 percent of patients reported pain relief from orthotics and 52 percent would not leave home without the devices in their shoes. McPoil et al. found that orthotics were an important treatment for valgus forefoot deformities only.[60] Riegler reported that 80

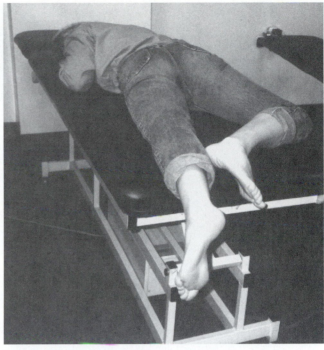

FIGURE 31-30

Examination position for STJN position.

percent of patients experienced at least a 50 percent improvement with orthotics.[78] This same study reported improvements in sports performance with orthotics. Hunt reported decreased muscular activity with orthotics.[41]

The process for evaluating the foot biomechanically, constructing an orthotic device, and selecting the appropriate footwear is given in detail in next section.

Examination

The first step in the evaluation process is to establish a position of STJN. The patient should be prone with the distal third of the leg hanging off the end of the table (Fig. 31-30). A line should be drawn bisecting the posterior lower leg and posterior calcaneus (Fig. 31-31).[92] With the patient still prone and the left foot as the example, the therapist palpates the talus with the right hand while the forefoot is inverted or everted using the left hand. One finger should palpate the talus near the anterior aspect of the fibula and the thumb near the anterior portion of the medial malleolus (Fig. 31-32). The position at which the talus is equally prominent on both sides is considered neutral subtalar position.[45] Root et al.[80] describe this as the position of the STJ where it is neither pronated or supinated. It is the standard position in which the foot should be placed to examine deformities.[69] In this position, the lines on the lower leg and calcaneus should form a straight line. Any variance is considered to be a rearfoot valgus or varus deformity. The most common deformity of the foot is a rearfoot varus deformity.[63] A varus deviation of 2°–3° is normal.[97]

Another method of determining STJN position involves using the lines that were drawn on the leg and back of the

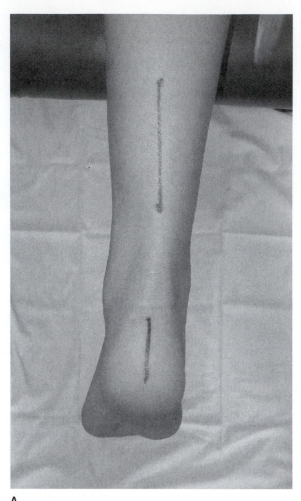

A

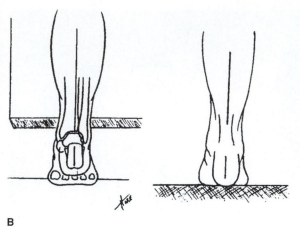

B

FIGURE 31-31

A, Line bisecting the posterior leg and calcaneus. **B,** Comparing non-weightbearing neutral to weightbearing resting position. Figure used with permission from Brian Hoke, American Physical Rehabilitation Network.

heel in a different manner. With the patient prone, the calcaneus is moved into full eversion and inversion, with angle measurements taken at the end range of each position. Neutral position is then considered to be two-thirds of the total STJ ROM away from maximum inversion or one-third of the total STJ motion away from maximum eversion. For example, from a neutral position, if the foot inverts 27° and everts 3°, the total STJ ROM equals 30°. Thus, the position at which this foot is neither pronated nor supinated is that point at which the calcaneus is inverted 7°, which is calculated by subtracting 20° (two-thirds of 30°) from maximal inversion (27°). The normal foot pronates 6°–8° from neutral.[80]

Once the STJ is placed in a neutral position, mild dorsiflexion should be applied to the forefoot at the fifth metatarsophalangeal joint while observing the metatarsal heads (specifically 2nd to 5th) in relation to the plantar surface of the calcaneus. First metatarsal position is evaluated independently of the other metatarsals. Forefoot varus is an osseous deformity in which the

medial metatarsal heads are inverted in relation to the plane of the calcaneus (Fig. 31-22). Forefoot varus is the most common cause of excessive pronation, according to Subotnick.[89] Forefoot valgus is a position in which the lateral metatarsals are everted in relation to the rearfoot (Fig. 31-23). These forefoot deformities benign in a non-weightbearing position, but in stance the foot or metatarsal heads must somehow get to the floor to bear weight. This compensated movement is accomplished by the talus rolling down and in and the calcaneus everting for a forefoot varus. For the forefoot valgus, the calcaneus inverts and the talus abducts and dorsiflexes. McPoil et al.[63] report that forefoot valgus is the most common forefoot deformity in their sample group.

In a calcaneal varus deformity, when the foot is in STJN position nonweight bearing, the calcaneus is in an inverted position; however, the metatarsals are still in a relative perpendicular position to the calcaneus. To get to foot flat in weightbearing, the STJ must pronate (Fig. 31-21). Minimal osseous deformities

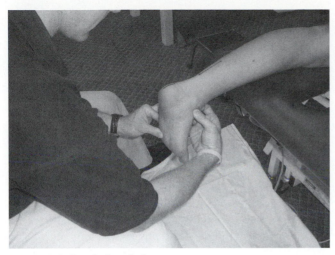

FIGURE 31-32

Palpation of the talus to determine STJN position.

of the forefoot have little effect on the function of the foot. When either forefoot varus or valgus is too large, the foot compensates through abnormal movements to bear weight.

Further consideration for the position and mobility of the first ray is necessary. The first ray in relationship to the remainder of the metatarsals can either be dorsiflexed, neutral, or plantarflexed. Clinically, a neutral or plantarflexed first ray is most commonly seen. Mobility of the first ray is an important predictor in pathomechanics and injury mechanism.[2,3] For example, a rigid plantarflexed first ray will respond differently in weightbearing than a mobile plantarflexed first ray. This distinction in mobility is important when making recommendations for orthosis fabrication in regard to forefoot correction. With a flexible first ray, a medial post may be used directly under the first ray only. With a more rigid first ray, medial posting material will extend more laterally to encompass additional metatarsals (Fig. 31-33). Further discussion on specific orthotic construction is there in a later section.

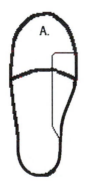 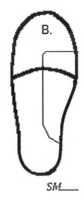

A. Flexible 1st Ray Correction   B. Rigid 1st Ray Correction

FIGURE 31-33

First ray correction for a foot orthosis.

Stress Fractures in the Foot

PATHOMECHANICS AND INJURY MECHANISM

The most common stress fractures in the foot involve the navicular, second metatarsal (March fracture), and diaphysis of the fifth metatarsal (Jones fracture). Navicular and second metatarsal stress fractures are likely to occur with excessive foot pronation, while fifth metatarsal stress fractures tend to occur in a more rigid pes cavus foot.

Navicular Stress Fractures

Individuals who excessively pronate during running gait are likely to develop a stress fracture of the navicular. This is attributed most commonly to individuals with either a compensated calcaneal and/or forefoot varus. Due to the compensatory movement and increased stress at the talonavicular joint of the tarsal bones, it is most likely to have a stress fracture.

Second Metatarsal Stress Fractures

Second metatarsal stress fractures occur most often in running and jumping sports. As is the case with other injuries in the foot associated with overuse, the most common causes include calcaneal varus and/or forefoot varus structural deformities in the foot that result in excessive pronation, flexible first ray, training errors, changes in training surfaces, and wearing inappropriate shoes. The base of the second metatarsal extends proximally into the distal row of tarsal bones and is held rigid and stable by the bony architecture and ligament support. In addition, the second metatarsal is particularly subjected to increased stress with excessive pronation, which causes a hypermobile foot. In addition, if the second metatarsal is longer than the first, as seen with a Morton's toe, it is theoretically subjected to greater bone stress during running. A bone scan, as opposed to a standard radiograph, is frequently necessary for diagnosis.

Fifth Metatarsal Stress Fractures

Fifth metatarsal stress fractures can occur from overuse, acute inversion, or high-velocity rotational forces. A Jones fracture occurs at the diaphysis of the fifth metatarsal most often as a sequela of a stress fracture.[81] The patient will complain of a sharp pain on the lateral border of the foot and will usually report hearing a "pop." Because of documented poor blood supply and a history of delayed healing, a Jones fracture may result in nonunion, requiring an extended period of rehabilitation. A common foot type seen with this injury is more of a supinatory foot, or those patients with a forefoot valgus or a rigid plantarflexed first ray. The patient spends more time laterally, thus increasing stresses to the fifth metatarsal.

REHABILITATION CONCERNS

Rehabilitation efforts for stress fractures should focus on determining the precipitating cause or causes and alleviating them. Second metatarsal stress fractures tend to do well with modified rest and non-weightbearing exercises, such as pool running (see Exercise 31-52), upper-body ergometer (see Exercise 31-53), stationary bike (see Exercise 31-54), or NuStep® (see Exercise 31-55) to maintain the patient's cardiorespiratory fitness for 2–4 weeks. An elliptical trainer may be utilized to transition the patient from non-weightbearing activity to non-impact weightbearing exercise. This is followed by a progressive return to full-impact activities of running and jumping functional activities over a 2- to 3-week period potentially using appropriately constructed orthoses and modified footwear. Stress fractures of both the navicular of the proximal shaft of the fifth metatarsal usually require more aggressive treatment, requiring non-weightbearing short-leg casts for 6–8 weeks for nondisplaced fractures. With cases of delayed union, non-union, or especially displaced fractures, both the Jones and navicular fractures require internal fixation, with or without bone grafting. In the highly active patient, immediate internal fixation should be recommended.

Plantar Fasciitis/Fasciosis

PATHOMECHANICS

Heel pain is a very common problem that may be attributed to several etiologies, including heel spurs, plantar fascia irritation (acute or chronic), and bursitis. Plantar fasciitis is a "catch-all term" that is commonly used to describe pain in the proximal arch and heel. However, when truly defining whether someone has plantar fasciitis, it is important to consider the absence or presence of inflammation. If histological findings indicate the presence of inflammation, then the diagnosis of plantar fasciitis is appropriate and subsequent treatment appropriate for acute inflammation should be considered. However, if findings include myxoid degeneration with fragmentation and degeneration of the plantar fascia, as well as bone marrow vascular ectasia, the diagnosis can be made of degenerative fasciosis without inflammation, not fasciitis.[53] Thus, treatment intervention should be varied chronic versus acute conditions.

The plantar fascia (plantar aponeurosis) runs the length of the sole of the foot. It is a broad band of dense connective tissue that is attached proximally to the medial surface of the calcaneus. It fans out distally, with fibers and their various small branches attaching to the metatarsophalangeal articulations and merging into the capsular ligaments. Other fibers, arising from well within the aponeurosis, pass between the intrinsic muscles of the foot and the long flexor tendons of the sole and attach themselves to the deep fascia below the bones. The function of the plantar aponeurosis is to assist in maintaining the stability of the foot and in securing or bracing the longitudinal arch.[92]

Tension develops in the plantar fascia both during extension of the toes and depression of the longitudinal arch as the result of weightbearing. When the weight is principally on the heel, as in ordinary standing, the tension exerted on the fascia is negligible. However, when the weight is shifted to the ball of the foot (on the heads of the metatarsals), fascial tension is increased. In running, because the push-off phase involves both a forceful extension of the toes and a powerful push-off

thrust off the metatarsal heads, fascial tension is increased to approximately twice the BW.

Patients who have a mild pes cavus foot type are particularly prone to fascial strain. Modern street shoes, by nature of their design, take on the characteristics of splints and tend to restrict foot action to such an extent that the arch may become somewhat rigid. This occurs because of shortening of the ligaments and other mild abnormalities. The patient, when changing from dress shoes to softer, more flexible athletic shoes, often develops irritation of the plantar fascia. Trauma may also result from poor running technique or improper running footwear. Excessive lumbar lordosis—a condition in which an increased forward tilt of the pelvis produces an unfavorable angle of foot strike when there is considerable force exerted on the ball of the foot—can also contribute to this problem.

INJURY MECHANISM

A number of anatomic and biomechanical conditions have been studied as possible causes of plantar fasciitis. They include leg-length discrepancy, excessive pronation of the STJ, inflexibility of the longitudinal arch, and tightness of the gastrocnemius–soleus unit. Wearing shoes without sufficient arch support, a lengthened stride during running, and running on soft surfaces are also potential causes of plantar fasciitis.

The patient complains of pain in the anteromedial aspect of the heel, usually at the attachment of the plantar fascia to the calcaneus, which eventually moves more centrally into the central portion of the plantar fascia. This pain is particularly troublesome upon arising in the morning or upon bearing weight after sitting for a prolonged period of time. However, the pain typically decreases after a few steps. Pain also will be intensified when the toes and forefoot are forcibly dorsiflexed, particularly with terminal stance phase in weightbearing.

REHABILITATION CONCERNS

With respect to the treatment of heel pain or plantar fasciitis/fasciosis, research has not indicated any consensus on a specific treatment regimen that has proven to resolve heel pain with any statistical significance. However, Gill[35] states that there is agreement that nonsurgical treatment is ultimately effective in approximately 90 percent of patients. Despite the uncertainty in the literature regarding a specific treatment, there are several different interventions that have proven to be beneficial in the acute and chronic management of heel pain.

Orthotic therapy is very useful in the treatment of this problem. The authors have found that semiflexible orthoses addressing the patient's specific biomechanical and structural concerns, in combination with exercises, can significantly reduce the pain level of these patients (Fig. 31-34).

A semiflexible orthosis tends to be more effective than a rigid orthotic device, particularly in a more active patient or athlete, because it allows for forefoot and rearfoot correction for decreasing pathomechanical compensation with appropriate shock absorption. An extra-deep heel cup could also be built into the orthosis to provide improved calcaneal and subsequent

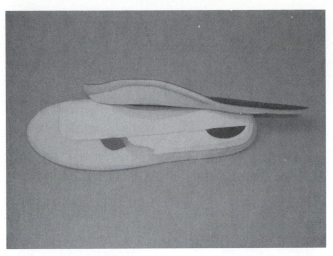

FIGURE 31-34
Semiflexible full-length custom orthosis.

STJ control. The orthosis should be worn at all times, especially upon arising from bed in the morning. The patient should be encouraged to wear a supportive shoe with the prescribed orthosis, rather than ambulating barefooted.[13] When soft orthoses are not feasible, longitudinal arch taping may reduce the symptoms. A simple arch taping or alternative taping technique often allows pain-free ambulation.[101] For those patients who have a distended calcaneal fat pad, the use of a heel cup will help to reapproximate the lateral margins of the fat pad under the calcaneous, reestablishing the natural cushion under the area of irritation.

The use of low-dye longitudinal arch taping to unload the plantar aponeursosis or a night splint to maintain a position of static stretch has also been recommended (Fig. 31-35A and B). In some cases, it may be necessary to use a short-leg walking cast for 4–6 weeks.

Pain-free heel cord stretching should be used, along with an exercise to stretch the plantar fascia in the arch (see Exercises 31-30B and C) if these tissues are tight. During the acute phase or if there is pain with passive stretching of heel cords or

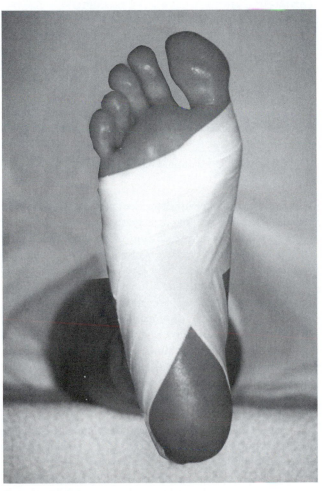

A

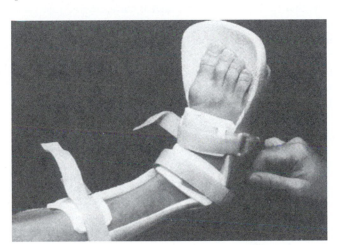

B

FIGURE 31-35
A, Low-dye arch taping. B, Night splint.

plantar fascia, dynamic stretching can be done (See Exercises 31-28). Exercises or manual therapy techniques that help to increase dorsiflexion of the great toe also may be of benefit to this problem (see Exercises 31-26 and 31-30A). Passive stretching should be performed using the principle of a low load, prolonged stretch and done at least three times a day.[83] Effective stretching is most effective with "consistency versus intensity."

As for the use of anti-inflammatory intervention, it is important to consider the stage of healing (acute versus chronic). In the acute phase, nonsteroidal anti-inflammatory medications may be beneficial. Steroidal injection may be warranted at some point if symptoms fail to resolve, although review of the literature is inconclusive as to the efficacy of injections for long-term benefits.[1,28,32,52,53,62,70,71,73,84] Concerns regarding the use of steroidal injection for management of heel pain or plantar fasciitis or fasciosis include the potential for calcaneal fat pad deterioration, plantar fascia rupture, decreased plantar fascia tension, reduced arch height, ineffectiveness of subsequent extracorporeal shock wave therapy (ESWT), and the potential development of several other foot problems.[1,52,70,71,84] Lemont[53] suggests that treatment regimens, such as corticosteroid injections into the plantar fascia, should be reevaluated in the absence of inflammation.

Other possible interventions include ultrasound, iontophoresis with acetic acid or dexamethasone, ESWT, or surgery. Preliminary research in the literature has shown that ESWT has been successful in managing plantar fasciosis.[62,71,76]

Management of plantar fasciitis will generally require an extended period of treatment. It is not uncommon for symptoms to persist for as long as 8–12 weeks. Persistence on the part of the patient in doing the recommended stretching and foot intrinsic strengthening exercises is critical, along with addressing any biomechanical or structural concerns. As with many of the foot and ankle injuries cited in this chapter, orthotic therapy, activity modification, appropriate footwear, and addressing any proximal neuromusculoskeletal concerns are also keys to successfully managing plantar fasciitis or fasciosis.

Cuboid Subluxation

PATHOMECHANICS AND INJURY MECHANISM

A condition that often mimics plantar fasciitis is cuboid subluxation. Pronation and trauma have been reported to be prominent causes of this syndrome.[99] Displacement of the cuboid causes pain along the fourth and fifth metatarsals, as well as directly over the cuboid. The primary reason for pain is the stress placed on the long peroneal muscle when the foot is in pronation. In this position, the long peroneal muscle allows the cuboid bone to move downward and medially. This problem often refers pain to the heel area as well. Many times this pain is increased upon arising after a prolonged non-weightbearing period.

REHABILITATION CONSIDERATIONS

Dramatic treatment results may be obtained by manipulation technique to restore the cuboid to its natural position. The

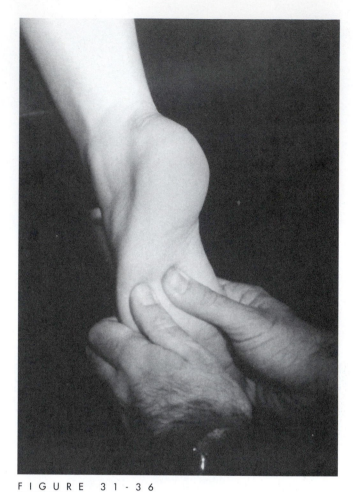

F I G U R E   3 1 - 3 6

Prone position for cuboid manipulation.

manipulation is done with the patient prone (Fig. 31-36). The plantar aspect of the forefoot is grasped by the thumbs with the fingers supporting the dorsum of the foot. The thumbs should be over the cuboid. The manipulation should be a thrust downward to move the cuboid into its more dorsal position. Often a pop is felt as the cuboid moves back into place. Once the cuboid is manipulated, an orthosis or taping technique is required to support it in its proper position.

If manipulation is successful, quite often the patient can return to normal function immediately with little or no pain. It should be recommended that the patient wears an appropriately constructed orthosis to reduce the chances of recurrence, along with specific foot intrinsic strengthening exercises (see Exercise 31-13).

Peelen describes an alternate way of manipulating a subluxated cuboid using a specific sequence for mobilizing the other bones of the foot first in order to effectively remobilize the cuboid. He states that it is rare that only or two bones of the foot are dysfunctional in isolation. By first mobilizing the talus, calcaneus, navicular, cuneiforms, and metatarsals, the necessary space to reduce the cuboid under the distal lip of the calcaneus is achieved.[72]

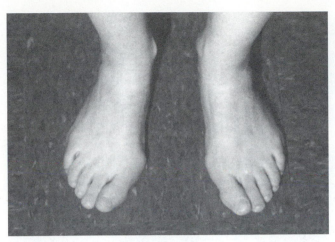

FIGURE 31-37

Hallux valgus deformity with a bunion.

Hallux Valgus Deformity (Bunions)

PATHOMECHANICS AND INJURY MECHANISM

A bunion is a deformity of the head of the first metatarsal in which the large toe assumes a valgus position (Fig. 31-37). A bunion is commonly associated with a structural forefoot varus or flexible first ray. The result of the outward splaying of the first ray is an increased pressure on the first metatarsal head. The bursa over the first metatarsophalangeal joint becomes inflamed and eventually thickens. The joint becomes enlarged and the great toe becomes malaligned, moving laterally toward the second toe, sometimes to such an extent that it eventually overlaps the second toe. This type of bunion may also be associated with a depressed or flattened transverse arch. Often the bunion occurs from wearing shoes that are pointed, too narrow, too short, or having high heels.

A bunion is one of the most frequent painful deformities of the great toe. As the bunion is developing, there is typically associated tenderness, swelling, and enlargement with calcification of the head of the first metatarsal. Shoes that fit poorly can increase the irritation and pain of the bunion.

REHABILITATION CONCERNS

Prevention is the key; however if the condition progresses, a custom orthosis is recommended to help normalize foot mechanics. Often an orthotic designed to correct a structural forefoot varus or flexible first ray can help increase stability and significantly reduce the symptoms and progression of a bunion. Shoe selection may also play an important role in the treatment of bunions. Shoes of the proper width cause less mechanical irritation to the bunion. Local therapy, including moist heat, soaks, iontophoresis, or ultrasound, may alleviate some of the acute symptoms of a bunion. Protective devices such as wedges, pads, and tape can also be used. Surgery to correct the hallux valgus deformity is very common during the later stages of this condition, but the potential of postoperative stiffness or loss of motion is a concern.

Morton's Neuroma

PATHOMECHANICS AND INJURY MECHANISM

A neuroma is a mass occurring about the nerve sheath of the common plantar nerve while it divides into the two digital branches to adjacent toes. It occurs most commonly between the metatarsal heads and is the most common nerve problem of the lower extremity. A Morton's neuroma is located between the third and fourth metatarsal heads where the nerve is the thickest, receiving both branches from the medial and lateral plantar nerves. The patient complains of severe intermittent pain radiating from the distal metatarsal heads to the tips of the toes and is often relieved when non-weightbearing. Irritation increases with the collapse of the transverse arch of the foot, putting the transverse metatarsal ligaments under stretch and thus compressing the common digital nerve and vessels. Excessive foot pronation can also be a predisposing factor, with more metatarsal shearing forces occurring with the prolonged forefoot abduction.

The patient complains of a burning paresthesia in the forefoot that is often localized to the third web space and radiating to the toes.[91] Hyperextension of the toes on weightbearing—as in squatting, stair climbing, or running—can increase the symptoms. Wearing shoes with a narrow toe box or high heels can increase the symptoms. If there is prolonged nerve irritation, the pain can become constant. A bone scan is often necessary to rule out a metatarsal stress fracture.

REHABILITATION CONCERNS

Orthotic therapy is essential to reduce the shearing movements of the metatarsal heads. To reduce this shearing effect, often either a metatarsal bar is placed just proximal to the metatarsal heads or a teardrop-shaped pad is placed between the heads of the third and fourth metatarsals in an attempt to have these splay apart with weightbearing (Fig. 31-38). The goal of the orthosis is to decrease pressure on the affected area (Fig. 31-39).

Therapeutic modalities such as ultrasound or iontophoresis can be used to help reduce inflammation. Shoe selection also plays an important role in treatment of neuromas. Narrow shoes, particularly women's shoes that are pointed in the toe area and certain men's boots, may squeeze the metatarsal heads together and exacerbate the problem. A shoe that is wide in the toe-box area should be selected. A straight-laced shoe often provides increased space in the toe box.[86] Firm-soled, inflexible shoes (such as clogs) can assist in managing this problem by inhibiting hyperextension of the toes during gait. Often, appropriate soft orthotic padding or a gel pad will markedly reduce pain. On a rare occasion surgical excision may be required.

Turf Toe

PATHOMECHANICS AND INJURY MECHANISM

Turf toe is a hyperextension injury that usually occurs in the athletic population and results in a sprain of the metatarsophalangeal joint of the great toe, either from repetitive overuse or

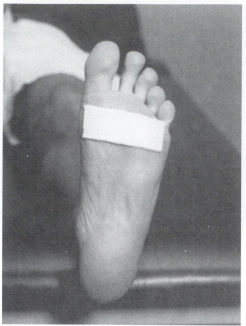
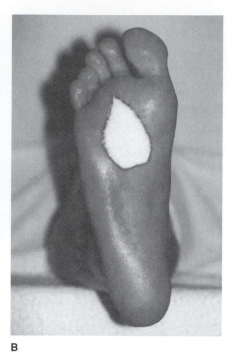

FIGURE 31-38

A, Metatarsal bar.
B, Teardrop pad.

A   B

trauma.[96] Typically, this injury occurs on unyielding synthetic turf, although it can occur on grass or hard court surfaces as well. Many of these injuries occur because artificial turf shoes often are more flexible and allow more dorsiflexion of the great toe.

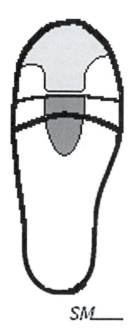

*SM*___

■ **Metatarsal pad**
■ **Metatarsal cut out area**

FIGURE 31-39

Foot orthosis correction for Morton's neuroma or metatarsalgia.

REHABILITATION CONCERNS

Some shoe companies have addressed this problem by adding steel or other materials to the forefoot of their turf shoes to stiffen them. Flat insoles that have thin sheets of steel under the forefoot are also available. When commercially made products are not available, a thin, flat piece of Orthoplast® may be placed under the shoe insole or may be molded to the foot.[96] Taping the toe to prevent dorsiflexion may be done separately or with one of the shoe-stiffening suggestions (Fig. 31-40).

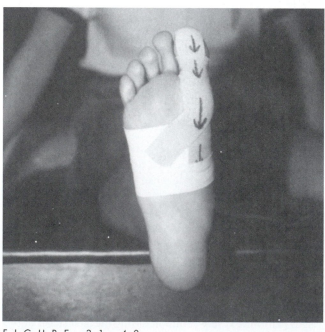

FIGURE 31-40

Turf toe taping.

Modalities of choice include ice, iontophoresis, or ultrasound. One of the key components for the acute management for turf toe is rest and protection.

In less-severe cases, patient can continue normal activities with the addition of a rigid insole. With more severe sprains, 3–4 weeks may be required for pain to reduce to the point where the patient can push off on the great toe.

Tarsal Tunnel Syndrome

PATHOMECHANICS AND INJURY MECHANISM

The tarsal tunnel is a loosely defined area about the medial malleolus that is bordered by the retinaculum, which binds the tibial nerve.[34] Overpronation, overuse conditions, and trauma may cause neurovascular problems in the ankle and foot. Symptoms may vary with pain, numbness, and paresthesia reported along the medial ankle and into the sole of the foot.[9] Tenderness may be present over the tibial nerve area behind the medial malleolus.

REHABILITATION CONCERNS

Neutral foot control with a custom orthosis may alleviate symptoms in less involved cases. Surgery is often performed if symptoms do not respond to conservative treatment or if weakness occurs in the flexors of the toes.[9]

Rehabilitation Techniques Summary

The ankle and foot can be a complicated and confusing region to manage with success. Thus, with any ankle or foot injury, it is important to "treat what you find," and evaluate "above and below" the joint. Furthermore, address any imbalances in strength, flexibility, mobility, or neuromuscular control both proximally and distally, as well as biomechanical and gait considerations. Finally, help the patient to help themselves with the skills and knowledge available to reach their functional goals.

ORTHOSIS AND FOOTWEAR RECOMMENDATIONS

Philosophy of Orthotic Therapy

Almost all problems of the lower extremity have been treated by orthotic therapy. The use of an orthosis (commonly referred to as "orthotic") for control of foot deformities has been recommended by various health care professionals for many years.[7,18,20,34,45,79,89,91,98] The normal foot functions most efficiently when no deformities are present that predispose it to injury or exacerbation of existing injuries. Orthoses are used to control abnormal compensatory movements of the foot by "bringing the floor to the foot."[42]

The foot functions most efficiently in an STJN position. By providing support so that the foot does not have to move abnormally, an orthosis should help prevent compensatory problems.

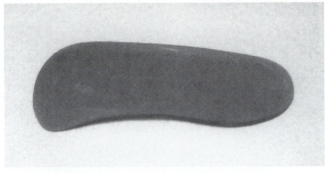

Hard orthosis.

For problems that have already occurred, the orthosis provides a platform of support so that soft tissues can heal properly without undue stress. In summary, the goal is to create a biomechanically balanced kinetic chain by using a device capable of controlling motion pathology in the foot and leg by maintaining the foot in or close to STJN position. Basically there are two types of orthoses:

• Biomechanical orthosis—a hard device (Fig. 31-41) or semiflexible device (Figs. 31-34 and 31-42) capable of controlling movement-related pathology by attempting to guide the foot into functioning at or near STJN. This device consists of a shell (or module) that is either rigid or flexible with noncompressible posting (wedges) angled in degrees that will address both forefoot and rearfoot deformities (Fig. 31-43). The rigid style shell is fabricated from carbon graphite, acrylic rohadur, or (polyethylene) hard plastic. The control acquired is high, while shock absorption is sacrificed somewhat. The flexible shell is fabricated from thermoplastic, rubber, or leather (Fig. 31-44) and is the preferred device for the more active or sports-specific patient. The semirigid device takes advantage of various types of materials that provide both shock absorption and motion control under increased loading while retaining their original shape. The rigid devices take the opposite approach and are designed to firmly restrain foot motion and alter its position with nonyielding materials. Both the

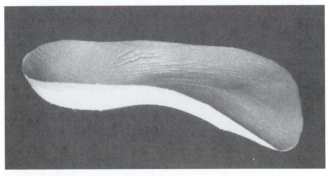

Semiflexible ³/₄ length custom orthosis.

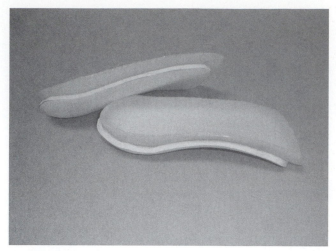

FIGURE   31-43

Foot orthosis semiflexible shell with noncompressible posting attached underneath.

rigid and flexible shells are molded from a neutral cast and allow control for most overuse symptoms.[2,3,42,54,91]

• Accommodative orthosis—a device that does not attempt to establish foot function around the STJN but instead allows the foot to compensate. These devices are designed for patients who are deemed to be poor candidates for biomechanical control due to congenital malformations, restricted motions at foot or leg, neuromuscular dysfunctions, insensitive feet, illness, or physiologic old age. The materials used to fabricate the shell are softer that will yield to foot forces rather than resist them. Compressible wedges are used to bias the foot.[2,3]

Although not considered a true orthosis, often times pads and soft, flexible felt or gel supports (Figs. 31-45 and 31-46) can be readily fabricated for situations when shoe space is com-

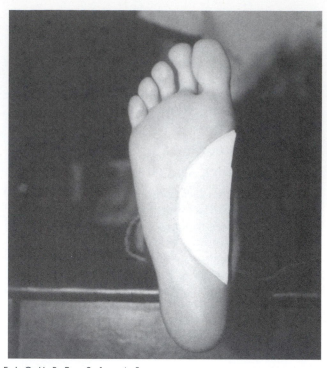

FIGURE   31-45

Felt pads.

promised (e.g., running spikes) or when shoes are not worn (e.g., ballet dancing). This type of foot correction is advocated for mild overuse syndromes.

Negative Foot Impression

Some therapists will make a negative impression of the patient's foot using a foam box or slipper casting using plaster strips

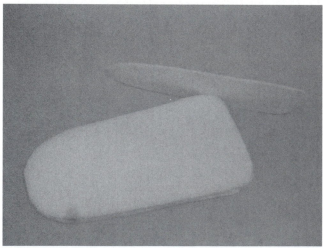

FIGURE   31-44

Polyethylene shell (Distributed by JMS Plastics Supply, Inc.)

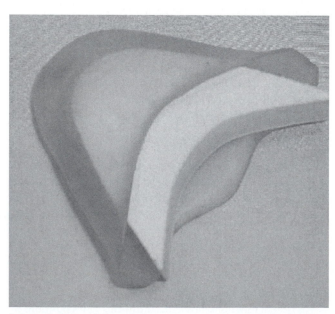

FIGURE   31-46

Gel toe cap for ballet dancers.

or a commercial casting product. This negative impression is mailed to an orthotic laboratory, where it is fabricated utilizing therapist recommendations or laboratory discretion. Others like to complete the entire orthosis from start to finish, which requires a much more skilled evaluator and technician, as well as the necessary equipment and supplies. There are obvious cost advantages and disadvantages to in-office fabrication.

No matter which method is chosen, the first step is the fabrication of the negative impression, which is done with the patient in a STJN. If using the foam-box impression method, the patient is placed in a seated position with the knee directly over the foot. The patient's foot is gently placed on the foam box. The therapist will then place the foot in an STJN position. While maintaining this semi-weightbearing alignment, the therapist will apply a downward force through the knee and the forefoot toward the floor until the heel is seated in the foam. Finally, the toes are seated into the foam avoiding overcompression of the foam. The foot is carefully removed from the foam box by lifting the heel first. This is then repeated on the contralateral side (Fig. 31-47).

The other method of developing the negative mold is using the slipper cast technique. Once STJN is found in a nonweightbearing position, three layers of plaster splints are applied to the plantar surface and sides of the foot (Fig. 31-48).

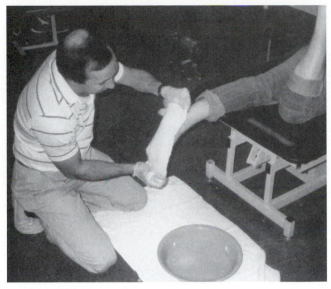

FIGURE   31-48

Three layers of plaster form neutral mold.

STJN position is maintained as pressure is applied on the fifth metatarsal area in a dorsiflexion direction until the MTJ is locked (Fig. 31-49). This position is held until the plaster dries. At this point the plaster cast may be sent out to have the orthosis fabricated by the lab or ready for the next step by the therapist (Fig. 31-50). If it is mailed out, the appropriate measurements of forefoot and rearfoot positions should be sent, along with any extrinsic measurements.

The next step is making the positive mold (Fig. 31-51) by pouring plaster of Paris into the cast or foam-box impression (Fig. 31-52). When working with the cast molds, the inside of the plaster should be liberally lined with talc or powder.

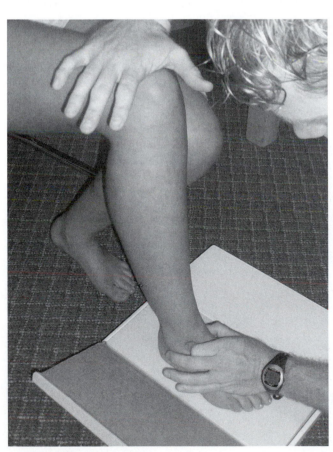

FIGURE   31-47

Foam-box impression.

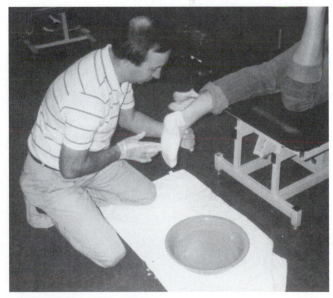

FIGURE   31-49

Mild pressure over the fifth metatarsal to lock the MTJ.

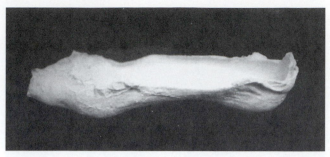

FIGURE 31-50

Neutral mold.

No special preparation is required when using the foam-box impressions.

Orthosis Materials and Fabrication

Many different materials may be used in the fabrication of a custom orthosis, including the shell (or module), top covers, posting materials, or any type of additional padding or inserts (e.g., gel heel insert). The specific type of materials used by a therapist or orthotist depends on the preference of that individual. Considerations should include long-term goal of the device, what material has proven to be successful, availability of the material, and ease of working with the material. Other considerations include color, stiffness (durometer), durability, and shock absorption.

One author uses 1/8-in. Aliplast® covering (Alimed Inc., Boston) with a 1/4-in. Plastazote® underneath. A rectangular piece of each material large enough to completely encompass the lower third of the mold is cut. These two pieces are placed in a convection oven (Fig. 31-53) at approximately 275°F. At this temperature, the two materials bond together and become moldable in about 5–7 minutes. At this time the materials are

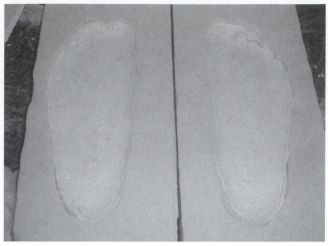

FIGURE 31-52

Positive mold from foam-box impression.

removed from the oven and placed on the positive mold (Fig. 31-54). Ideally, a form or vacuum press should be used to form the orthosis to the mold.[42]

If the patient is present and once cooled, the uncut orthosis is placed under the foot while the patient sits in a chair (Fig. 31-55). Excess material is then trimmed from the sides of the orthosis with scissors. Any material that can be seen protruding from either side of the foot should be trimmed (Fig. 31-56) to provide the proper width of the orthosis. The length should be trimmed so that the end of the orthosis bisects the metatarsal heads (Fig. 31-57). This style is slightly longer than traditional sulcus length orthosis, but one author has found that this length provides better comfort.[42]

Next, a third layer of medial Plastazote® may be glued to the arch to fill that area to the floor. Grinding begins with the sides of the orthosis, which should be ground so that the sides are slightly beveled inward (Fig. 31-58) to allow better shoe fit. The bottom of the orthosis is leveled so that the surface is perpendicular

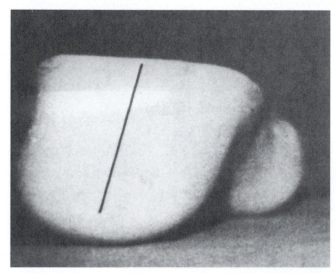

FIGURE 31-51

Positive mold.

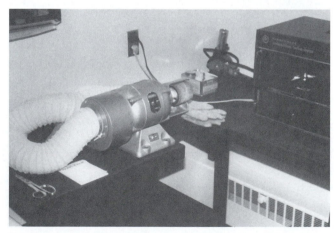

FIGURE 31-53

Convection oven and grinder.

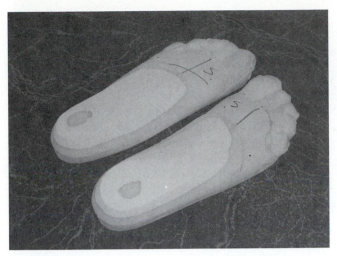

FIGURE 31-54

Materials placed on positive impression.

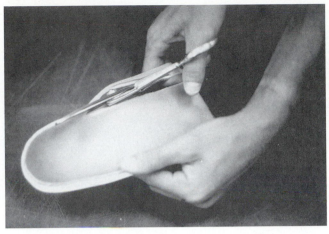

FIGURE 31-56

Trim excess material from orthosis.

to the bisection of the calcaneus (Fig. 31-59). Grinding is continued until very little Plastazote® remains under the Aliplast® at the heel. The forefoot is posted by selectively attaching and/or grinding Plastazote® just proximal to the metatarsal heads. Forefoot varus is posted by grinding more laterally than medially. Forefoot valgus requires grinding more medially than laterally. With the metatarsal length orthosis, the final step is to grind the distal portion of the orthosis so that only a very thin piece of Aliplast® is under the area where the orthosis ends. This prevents discomfort under the forefoot where the orthosis stops. If the patient feels that this area is a problem and the metatarsal length device has already been fabricated, a full insole of Spenco® or other material may be used to cover the orthosis to the end of the shoe to eliminate the drop-off sometimes felt as the orthosis ends.

Another author has developed a measurement system in conjunction with an orthotic laboratory (Biocorrect Custom Foot Orthotics Laboratory, Kentwood, MI) to determine the amount of forefoot and rearfoot posting required for the needed biomechanical corrections. Having already performed the lower leg and calcaneal bisection and the non-weightbearing assessment, weight-bearing measurements are taken using an inclinometer in an STJN position, resting position, and end-range dorsiflexed position of 25° (Fig. 31-60A and B). The end-range measurements are then used to prescribe the recommended rearfoot posting (0°–3° maximum) and forefoot posting (0°–6°

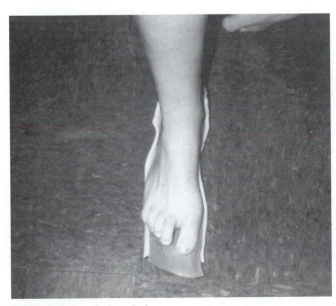

FIGURE 31-55

Orthosis mold under the foot with patient sitting.

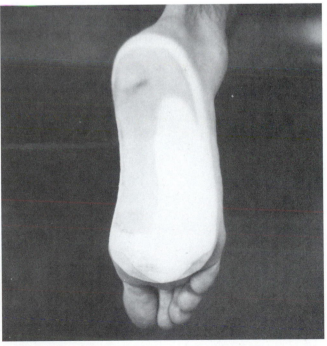

FIGURE 31-57

The metatarsal length orthosis should bisect the metatarsal heads.

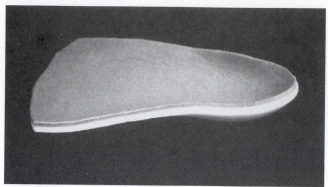

F I G U R E   3 1 - 5 8

Sides of the orthotic should be leveled inward.

maximum). When making recommendations to an orthotics laboratory, other considerations need to be made including materials used for shells, posting, top covers, length of orthosis, cutouts, deep heel cups, gel heel inserts, metatarsal pads or bars, or external flanges. The length of an orthosis can be described as either full, sulcus, or metatarsal length device. A full-length device starts at the calcaneus and extends past the distal phalanges. A metatarsal length device extends distal to the metatarsal phalangeal joints, whereas the sulcus length device stops just proximal to the metatarsal phalangeal joints. An external flange, not routinely used, is an extension of the shell and rearfoot posting to provide additional motion or position control. Finally, the thickness of the orthosis needs to be considered depending on its use and the footwear into which the device is going to be placed.

In the majority of cases, a full-length orthosis that allows for forefoot and first ray correction along with the standard rearfoot correction is suggested. Exact corrections will be determined depending on the patient's biomechanical issues.

Biocorrect Custom Foot Orthotics Laboratory recommends a high-density (1–3 mm) polyethylene shell (Fig. 31-44),

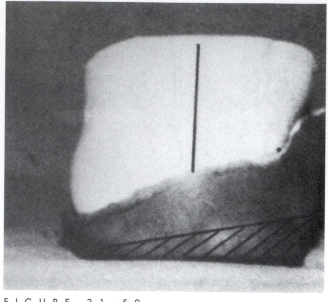

F I G U R E   3 1 - 5 9

Bottom of orthosis leveled to be perpendicular with calcaneal bisection.

which is light weight and high-impact resilient (JMS Plastics Supply Inc., Neptune, NJ). Various top covers (ACOR Inc., Cleveland, OH) are available using 1/8-in. Vinair®, leather, or Neosponge® in combination with 1/16–3/16 in. P-Cell or Microcell Puff® ethylene vinyl acetate (EVA) material for additional shock absorption (Fig. 31-61). A firmer EVA (45–50 durometer) material (JMS Plastics Supply Inc.) is used for the extrinsic forefoot/rearfoot posting and arch support (Fig. 31-62).

The process is essentially the same as previously described, except the patient does not need to be present to determine the necessary forefoot, rearfoot, or first ray corrections. These prescribed corrections have already been established during the

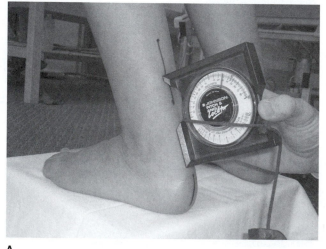

A

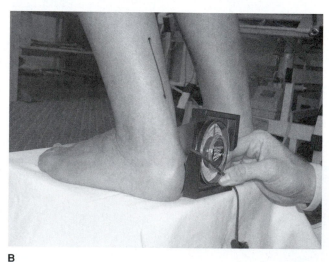

B

F I G U R E   3 1 - 6 0

A, End-range dorsiflexion (25°). **B,** Rear foot measurement with inclinometer.

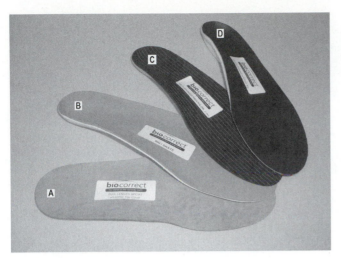

FIGURE 31-61

Various top cover materials. **A,** Leather top cover.
B, Microcell Puff® top cover. **C,** Neosponge® top cover.
D, Vinair® top cover.

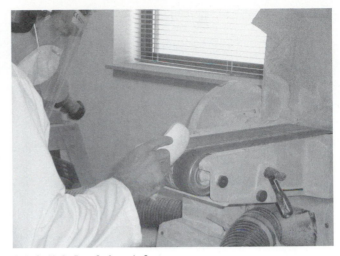

FIGURE 31-63

Final grinding of orthosis.

evaluation process. Once all of the specific materials have been attached or glued to the shell, the necessary grinding will take place to complete the finished orthosis (Fig. 31-63).

Time must be allowed for proper break-in. The patient should wear the orthosis for 3–4 hours the first day, 6–8 hours the next day, and then all day on the third day. Physical activities should be started with the orthosis only after it has been worn all day for several days.[40]

Sometimes corrections or adjustments are necessary to the orthosis. Orthotic therapy is "an art and a science," so it is important to be able to make corrections or adjustments quickly and easily. This may influence a clinician as to whether they choose an out-of-state versus a local laboratory, or make the investment of having a full or partial in-house laboratory.

Shoe Selection

Shoes are one of the biggest considerations in treating a foot problem successfully.[90] Even a properly made orthosis is less effective if placed in a poorly constructed shoe or an inappropriate shoe for the patient.

As noted, pronation is usually a problem of hypermobility. Thus, pronatory foot types need stability and firmness to reduce excess movement. Research indicates that forefoot compression of the outer sole of the shoe may actually increase pronation versus a barefoot condition.[6] The ideal shoe for a pronated foot is less flexible with good rearfoot control. Conversely, supinated feet are usually more rigid. Shoes with adequate cushion and flexibility benefit this type of foot.

Several construction factors may influence the firmness and stability of a shoe. The basic form upon which a shoe is built is called the last (Fig. 31-64).[3,6] The upper is fitted onto a last in several ways. Each method has its own flexibility and control

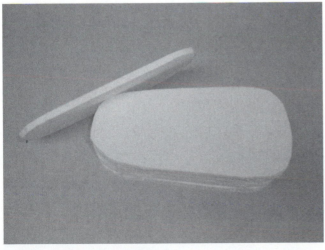

FIGURE 31-62

Firmer EVA for posting (Distributed by JMS Plastics Supply, Inc.)

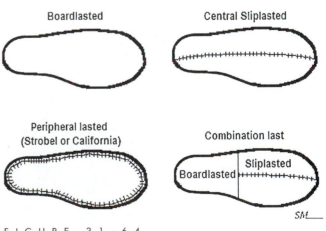

FIGURE 31-64

Shoe last construction.

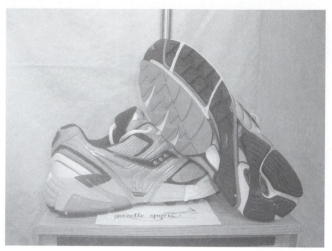

FIGURE 31-65

Motion control shoe (Saucony Grid Stabil MC).

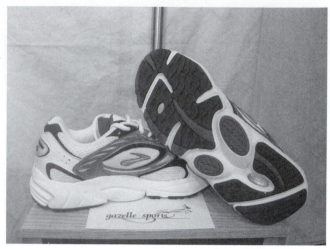

FIGURE 31-67

Stable cushion shoe (Brooks Dyad 3).

characteristics. A central sliplasted shoe is sewn together like a moccasin and is very flexible. A peripheral (Strobel or California) lasted shoe has similar characteristics as the central slip, except the stitching is along the outside of the shoe. Board-lasting provides a piece of fiberboard upon which the upper is attached, which provides a very firm, inflexible base for the shoe. A combination-lasted shoe is boarded in the back half of the shoe and slip-lasted in the front, which provides rear-foot stability with forefoot mobility. The shape of the last may also be used to assist with shoe selection. The three different types of shapes are straight lasted, curved lasted, and semicurved lasted and are usually consistent with the construction of a shoe. The shape and the construction of the last are typically consistent with one another. Most patients with excessive pronation perform better in a straight-lasted shoe,[3,6] that is, a shoe in which the forefoot does not curve inward in relation to the rear-foot.

In comparing all of the dress and athletic shoes available to the consumer, running shoes have the greatest investment in money and resources by the manufactures for research and development with respect to controlling the motion of the foot. Thus, when it comes to providing a patient with specific footwear recommendations, running shoes have the largest selection of options to choose from. There are several different categories of running shoes, some for training and others for performance. Within each category, there are several different brands with their own unique cushioning and control systems. The categories can be defined as motion control (Fig. 31-65), stability (Fig. 31-66), stable cushion (Fig. 31-67), cushion (Fig. 31-68), light-weight trainer (Fig. 31-69),

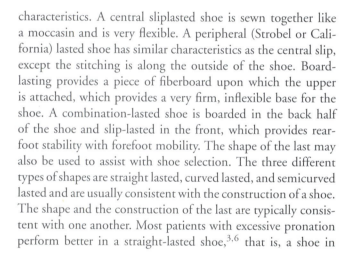

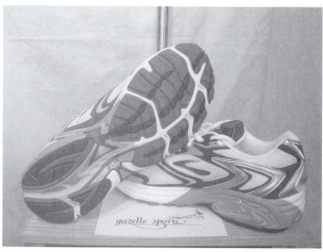

FIGURE 31-66

Stability shoe (Brooks Adreneline GTS).

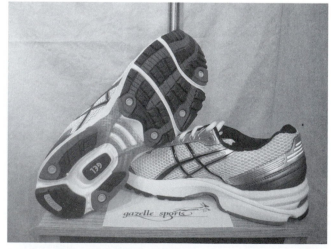

FIGURE 31-68

Cushion shoe (Asics Gel Cumulus VII).

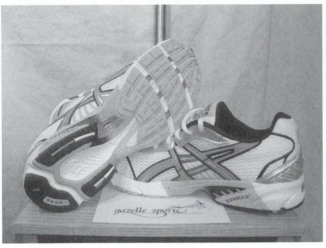

F I G U R E   3 1 - 6 9

Light-weight trainer/performance shoe (Asics Gel DS Trainer).

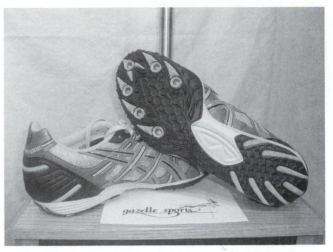

F I G U R E   3 1 - 7 1

Cross country spike (Asics Gel Dirt Dog Spike).

ultra-light-weight trainer (Fig. 31-70), cross country spikes (Fig. 31-71), and trail runner (Fig. 31-72).

Midsole design also affects the stability of a shoe. The midsole separates the upper from the outsole.[3,14] EVA is one of the most commonly used materials in the midsole.[3,71] Often, denser EVA, which is colored differently to show that it is denser, is placed under the medial aspect of the foot to control pronation. Also, in an effort to control rearfoot movement, many shoe manufacturers have reinforced the heel counter both internally and externally, often in the form of extra plastic along the outside of the heel counter (Figs. 31-65 and 31-66).[3,59] Other factors that may affect the performance of a shoe are the outsole contour and composition, lacing systems, and forefoot wedges (for specific details, refer to Table 31-1).

Shoe Wear Evaluation

Shoe wear patterns can sometimes give the therapist helpful information about the patient's biomechanical considerations and potential movement dysfunctions. Patients with excessive pronation often wear out the front of the running shoe under the second metatarsal (Fig. 31-73). Shoe wear patterns are commonly misinterpreted by patients who think they must be pronators because they wear out the back outside edges of their heels. Actually, most people who wear out the back outside edges of their shoes are consistent with lateral heel strike at initial contact. Just before heel strike, the anterior tibial muscle fires to prevent the foot from slapping forward. The anterior tibialis muscle not only dorsiflexes the foot but also slightly

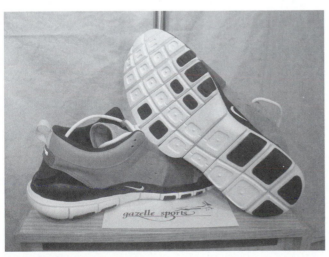

F I G U R E   3 1 - 7 0

Ultra-light-weight trainer (Nike Free Trainer 5.0).

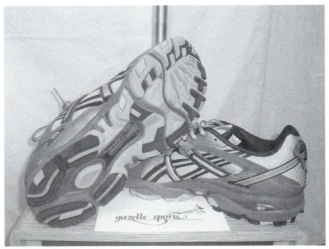

F I G U R E   3 1 - 7 2

Trail running shoe (Asics Gel Eagle Trail IV).

T A B L E   3 1 - 1

Classification and Characteristics of Running Shoe Types

MOTION CONTROL SHOE
- Indications: Moderate to severe over-pronator
- Straighter last shape
- Board or combination last construction*
- Midsole materials (EVA or PU) depend on BW
- Firmer medial midsole or stabilization device
- Reinforced and/or extended heel counter
- Will sometimes use higher medial side versus lateral side (wedge) for increased early motion control

STABILITY SHOE
- Indications: Neutral to mild over-pronator
- Semicurved last shape
- Combination or peripheral last construction
- Midsole materials (EVA or PU) dependent on BW
- Firmness of medial midsole or stabilization device dependent of range of stability shoe. Lower-end stability shoes have no stabilization device
- Firm heel counter

STABLE CUSHION SHOE
- Indication: Neutral to supinatory foot that is unstable
- Newer *transition* shoe that bridges the gap between cushion and stability mostly with the geometry of the shoe
- Straighter last shoe
- Midsole materials (EVA or PU) dependent on BW, but usually lean to lighter-weight EVA
- Single density midsole
- May utilize stability pillars (e.g., Brooks Dyad series)
- Firmer heel counter

CUSHION SHOE
- Indication: Supinatory foot
- Typically more curve last shape
- Central or peripheral slip last construction
- Midsole materials (EVA or PU) dependent on BW, but usually lean to lighter-weight EVA
- Single density midsole
- Midsole cushioning units (rearfoot and forefoot)

*Board last combination primarily used with older running shoes and basketball shoes. Combination last primarily used with newer running shoes.
SOURCE: Gazelle Sports, Grand Rapids, Michigan

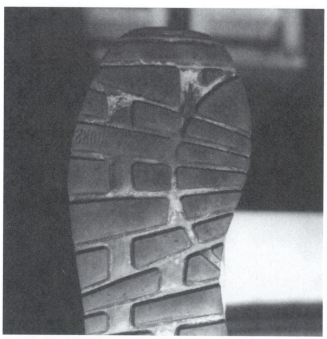

F I G U R E   3 1 - 7 3

Front forefoot of a running shoe showing the typical wear pattern of a pronator.

inverts it, hence the wear pattern on the back edge of the shoe. For those runners who are midfoot to forefoot strikers, typically less lateral heel wear is evident. The key to inspection of wear patterns on shoes is observation of the heel counter and the forefoot.

Another evaluation technique for footwear is to determine if the patient is placing an exceptional amount of torsional torque on the shoe, specifically through the midfoot region. By simply placing the shoe on a flat surface, and pushing down on the front of the toe box in the center, observe the natural movement pattern of the shoe. If the shoe veers medially or laterally, this is indicative of increased torsion on the shoe. This may indicate that a more stable shoe is required to counteract the force, or an orthosis is necessary to create improved balance throughout stance phase.

EXERCISES

REHABILITATION TECHNIQUES

Strengthening Exercises

ISOMETRIC STRENGTHENING EXERCISES

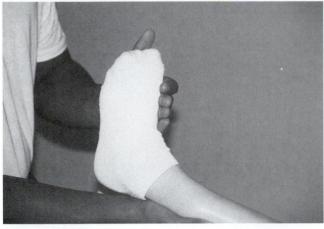

EXERCISE 31-1

Isometric inversion against a stable object. Used to strengthen the posterior tibialis, flexor digitorum longus, and flexor hallucis longus.

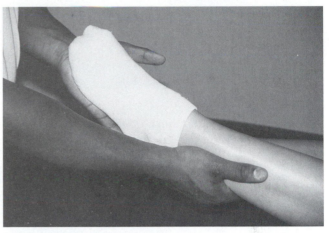

EXERCISE 31-3

Isometric plantarflexion against a stable object. Used to strengthen the gastrocnemius, soleus, posterior tibialis, flexor digitorum longus, flexor hallucis longus, and plantaris.

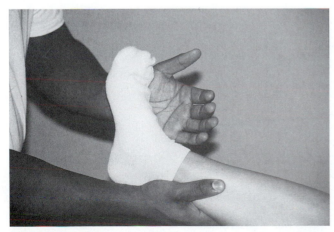

EXERCISE 31-2

Isometric eversion against a stable object. Used to strengthen the peroneus longus, brevis, tertius, and extensor digitorum longus.

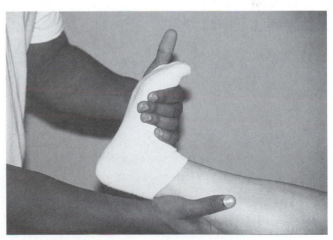

EXERCISE 31-4

Isometric dorsiflexion against a stable object. Used to strengthen the anterior tibialis and peroneus tertius.

ISOTONIC OPEN-CHAIN STRENGTHENING EXERCISES

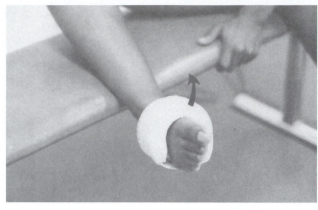

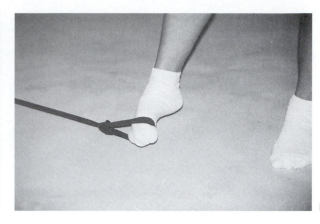

A

B

EXERCISE 31-5

Inversion exercise. **A,** Using a weight cuff. **B,** Using resistive tubing. Used to strengthen the posterior tibialis, flexor digitorum longus, and flexor hallucis longus.

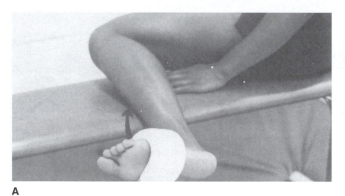

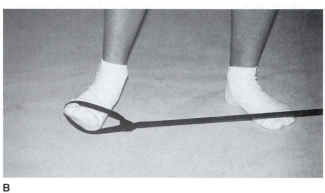

A

B

EXERCISE 31-6

Eversion exercise. **A,** Using a weight cuff. **B,** Using resistive tubing. Used to strengthen the peroneus longus, brevis, tertius, and extensor digitorum longus.

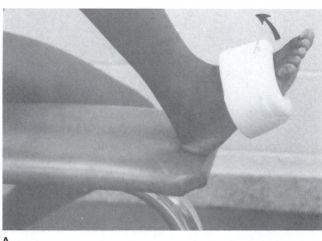

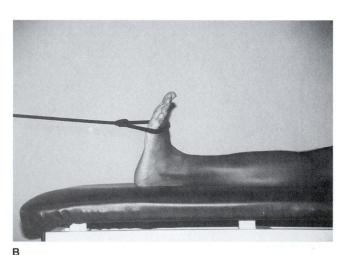

A

B

EXERCISE 31-7

Dorsiflexion exercise. **A,** Using a weight cuff. **B,** Using resistive tubing. Used to strengthen the anterior tibialis and peroneus tertius.

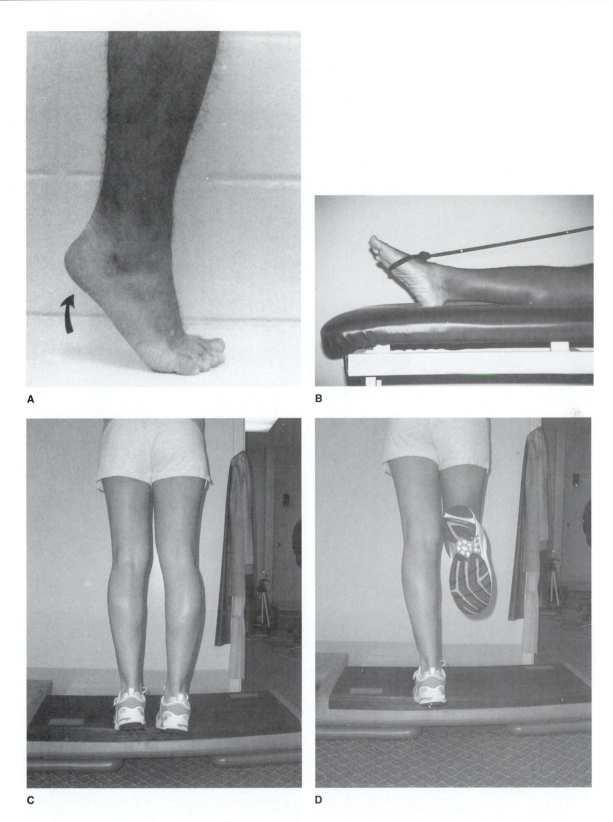

EXERCISE 31-8

Plantarflexion exercise. **A,** Concentric against gravity. **B,** Using surgical tubing.
C, Eccentric-Stage 1. **D,** Eccentric-Stage 2. Used to strengthen the gastrocnemius,
soleus, posterior tibialis, flexor digitorum longus, flexor hallucis longus, and plantaris.

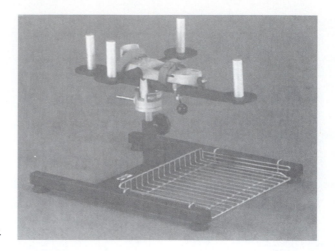

EXERCISE   31-9

Multidirectional Elgin ankle exerciser.

EXERCISE   31-10

Isolated toe raises. **A,** Toe raises with extended knee strengthens the gastrocnemius. **B,** Toe raises with flexed knee strengthens the soleus.

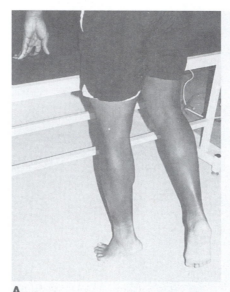

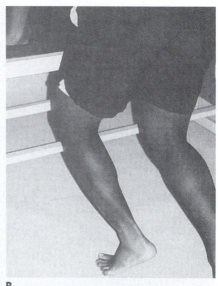

A   **B**

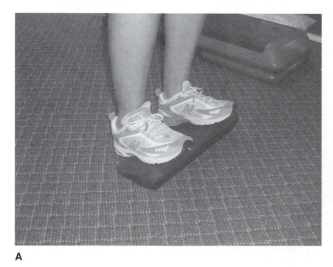

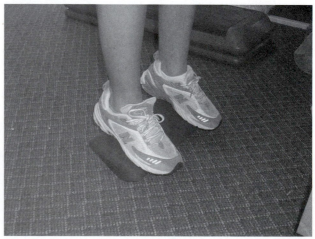

A   **B**

EXERCISE   31-11

Active-assisted plantarflexion using the BOB®. **A,** Starting position. **B,** Finishing position. Can also use as a static stretch by holding end range positions.

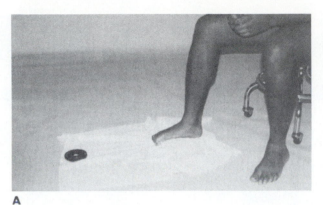
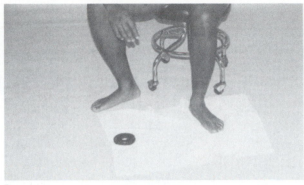

A   B

EXERCISE 3 1 - 1 2

Towel gathering exercise. **A,** Toe flexion. Used to strengthen the flexor digitorum longus and brevis, lumbricales, and flexor hallucis longus. **B,** Inversion/eversion exercises. Used to strengthen the posterior tibialis, flexor digitorum longus, flexor hallucis longus, peroneus longus, brevis, tertius, and extensor digitorum longus.

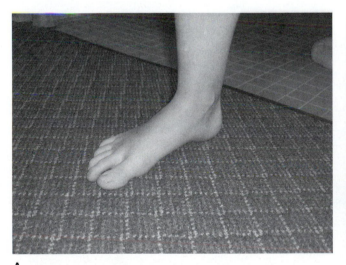
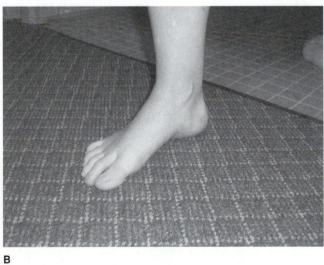

A   B

EXERCISE 3 1 - 1 3

Foot intrinsic strengthening. **A,** Starting position. **B,** Arch raises in sitting. **C,** Arch raises in double-limb stance. **D,** Arch raises in single-limb stance.

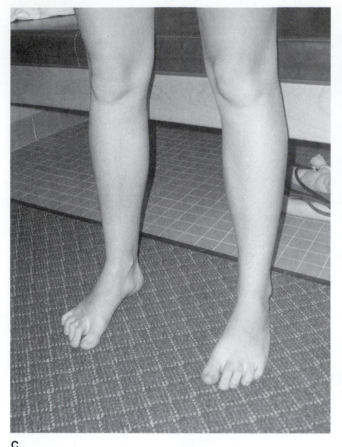

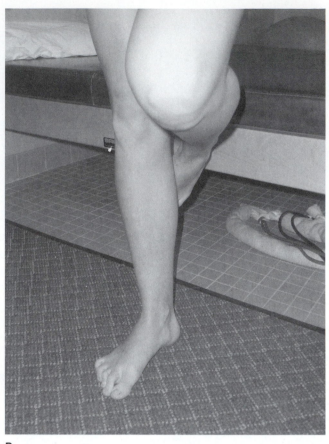

C

D

E X E R C I S E   3 1 - 1 3

(Continued)

CLOSED-CHAIN STRENGTHENING EXERCISES

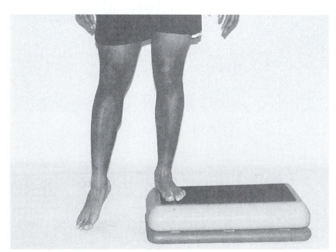

E X E R C I S E   3 1 - 1 4

Lateral step-ups.

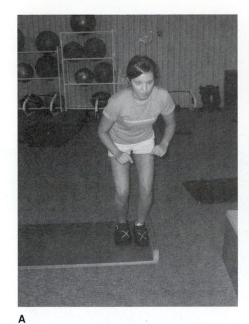

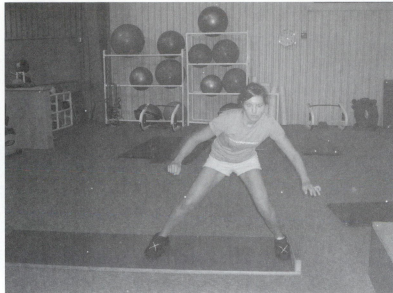

A   **B**

EXERCISE   31-15

Slide board exercises. **A,** Starting position. **B,** Push off.

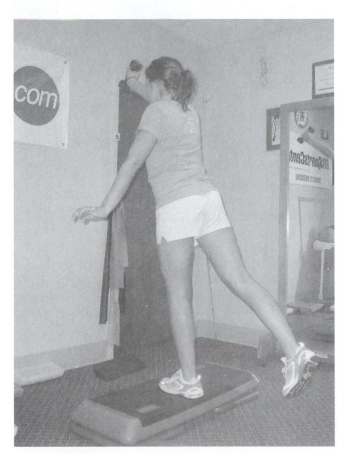

EXERCISE   31-17

Forward step-up with alternate arm raise using a dumbbell. Used for cross-over strengthening of gluteus maximus and contralateral dorsal musculature associated with thoracolumbar fascia. Can also be used in conjunction with biofeedback for proper recruitment.

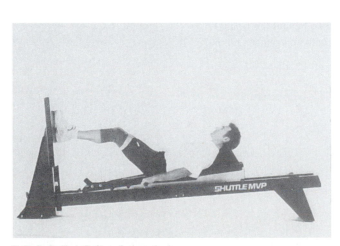

EXERCISE   31-16

Shuttle exercise machine.

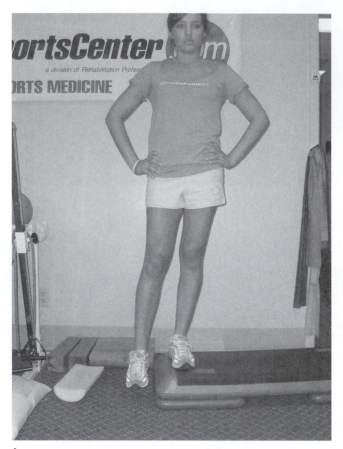

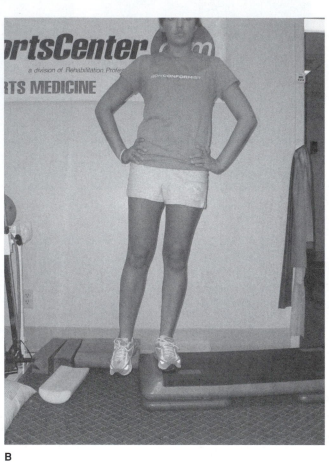

A

B

EXERCISE 31-18

Hip hiking. **A,** Starting position. **B,** Finishing position. Used to strengthen gluteus medius. Can also be used as a neuromuscular retraining exercise having the patient stop when pelvis is level or in conjunction with a biofeedback unit over gluteus medius for proper recruitment.

ISOKINETIC STRENGTHENING EXERCISES

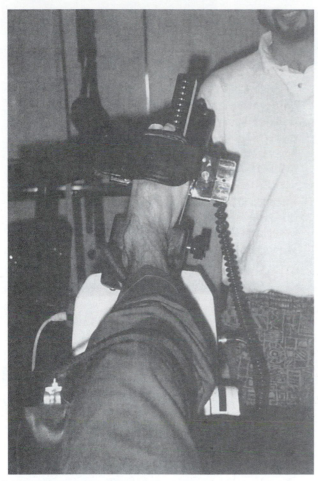

EXERCISE   31-19

Isokinetic inversion/eversion exercise. Used to improve the strength and endurance of the ankle inverters and everters in an open chain. Also can provide an objective measurement of muscular torque production.

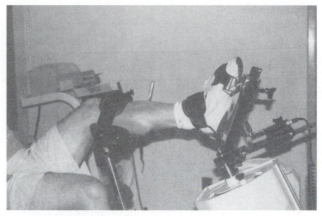

EXERCISE   31-20

Isokinetic plantarflexion/dorsiflexion exercise. Used to improve the strength and endurance of the ankle dorsiflexors and plantarflexors in an open chain. Also can provide an objective measurement of torque production.

PROPRIOCEPTIVE NEUROMUSCULAR FACILITATION STRENGTHENING EXERCISES

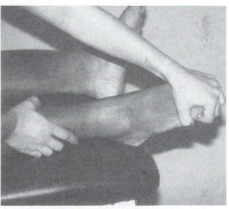

A

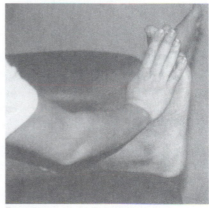

B

EXERCISE   31-21

D1 pattern moving into flexion. **A,** Starting position: ankle plantar flexed, foot everted, toes flexed.
B, Terminal position: ankle dorsiflexed, foot inverted, toes extended.

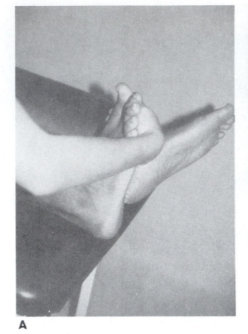

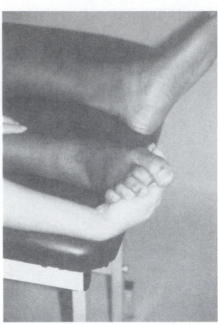

EXERCISE 31-22

D1 pattern moving into extension. **A,** Starting position: ankle dorsiflexed, foot inverted, toes extended. **B,** Terminal position: ankle plantar flexed, foot everted, toes flexed.

A

B

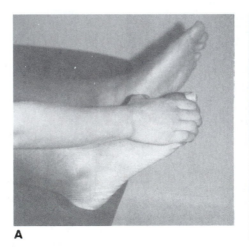

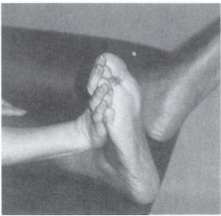

EXERCISE 31-23

D2 pattern moving into flexion. **A,** Starting position: ankle plantar flexed, foot inverted, toes flexed. **B,** Terminal position: ankle dorsiflexed, foot everted, toes extended.

A

B

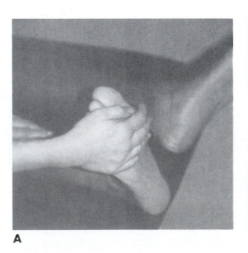

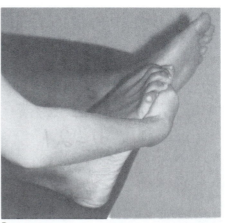

EXERCISE 31-24

D2 pattern moving into extension. **A,** Starting position: ankle dorsiflexed, foot everted, toes extended. **B,** Terminal position: ankle plantar flexed, foot inverted, toes flexed.

A

B

Stretching Exercises

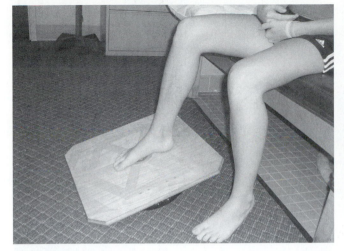

A

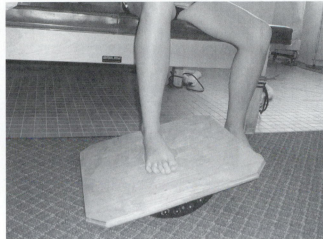

B

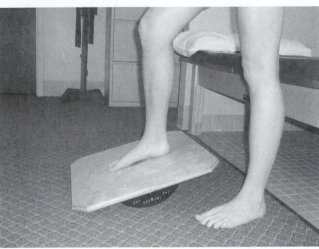

C

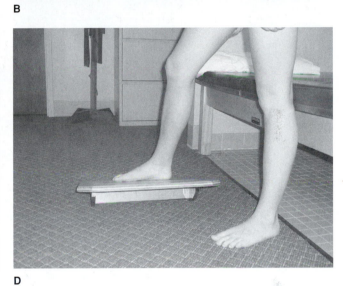

D

E X E R C I S E   3 1 - 2 5

Fitter® Rocker board exercises are an AROM exercise, useful in regaining normal ankle motion and early neuromuscular retraining. **A,** Seated plantarflexion—dorsiflexion. **B,** Seated inversion—eversion. **C,** Standing plantarflexion—dorsiflexion. **D,** Standing inversion—eversion.

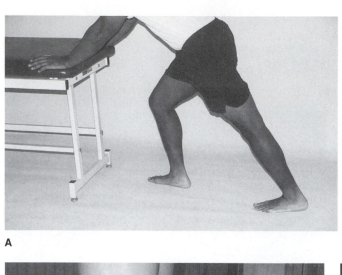

A

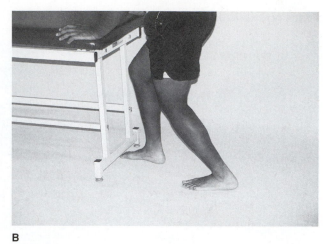

B

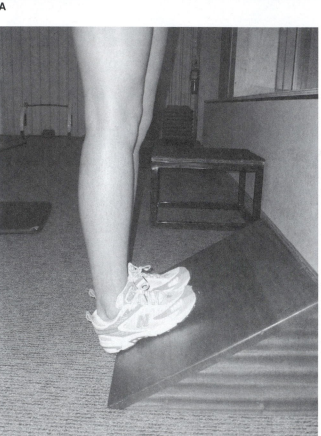

C

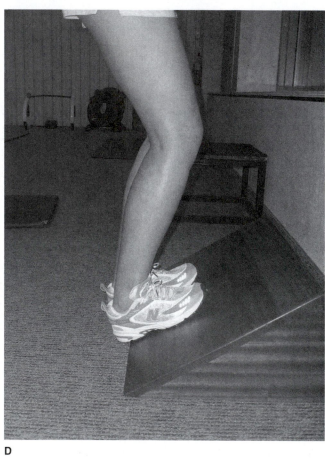

D

E X E R C I S E   3 1 - 2 6

Standing heel cord stretch. **A,** Gastrocnemius. **B,** Soleus. **C,** Gastrocnemius stretch using a slant board. **D,** Soleus stretch using a slant board.

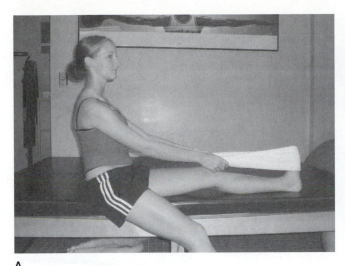

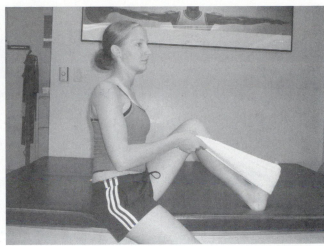

A   B

EXERCISE 31-27

Seated heel cord stretch using a towel. **A,** Gastrocnemius. **B,** Soleus.

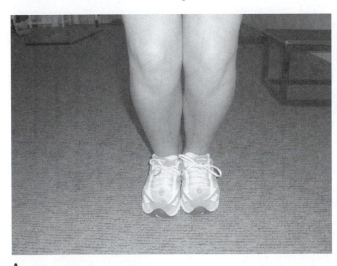

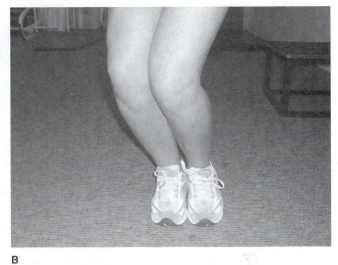

A   B

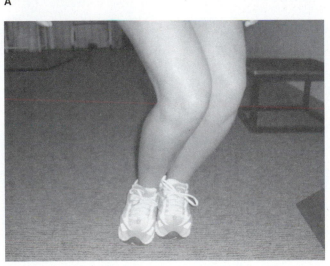

C

EXERCISE 31-28

Dynamic heel cord stretch. **A,** Position 1. **B,** Position 2. **C,** Position 3.

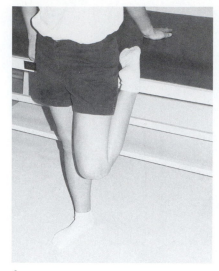

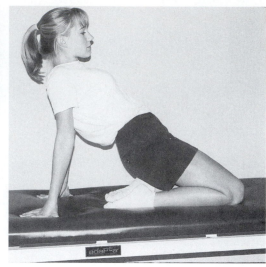

E X E R C I S E 3 1 - 2 9

Ankle dorsiflexors stretch for the anterior tibialis. **A,** Standing. **B,** Kneeling.

A

B

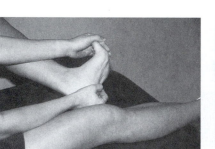

A

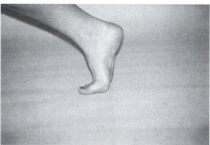

B

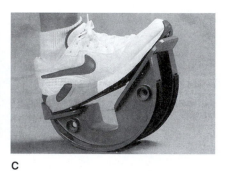

C

E X E R C I S E 3 1 - 3 0

Plantar fascia stretches. **A,** Manual. **B,** Floor stretch. **C,** Prostretch.

Joint Mobilizations

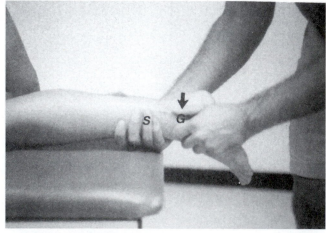

E X E R C I S E 3 1 - 3 1

Distal anterior and posterior fibular glides. Anterior and posterior glides of the fibula may be done distally. The tibia should be stabilized, and the fibular malleolus is mobilized in an anterior or posterior direction.

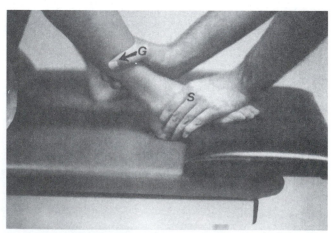

E X E R C I S E 3 1 - 3 2

Posterior tibial glides. Posterior tibial glides increase plantarflexion. The foot should be stabilized, and pressure on the anterior tibia produces a posterior glide.

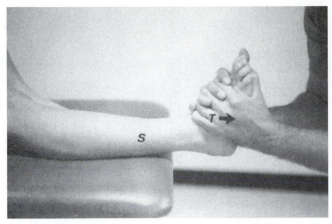

EXERCISE 31-33

Talocrural joint traction. Talocrural joint traction is performed using the patient's BW to stabilize the lower leg and applying traction to the midtarsal portion of the foot. Traction reduces pain and increases dorsiflexion and plantarflexion.

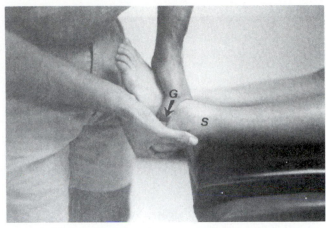

EXERCISE 31-35

Posterior talar glides. Posterior talar glides may be used for increasing dorsiflexion. With the patient supine, the tibia is stabilized on the table, and pressure is applied to the anterior aspect of the talus to glide it posteriorly.

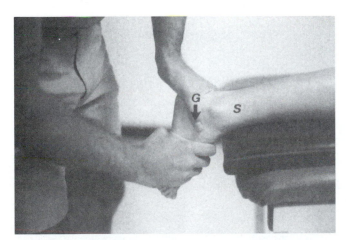

EXERCISE 31-34

Anterior talar glides. Plantarflexion may also be increased by using an anterior talar glide. With the patient prone, the tibia is stabilized on the table and pressure is applied to the posterior aspect of the talus to glide it anteriorly.

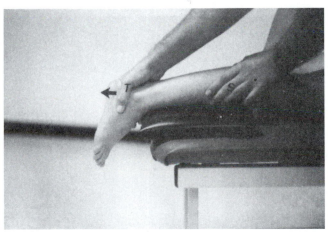

EXERCISE 31-36

STJ traction. STJ traction reduces pain and increases inversion and eversion. The lower leg is stabilized on the table, and traction is applied by grasping the posterior aspect of the calcaneus.

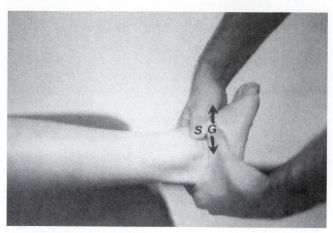

E X E R C I S E   3 1 - 3 7

STJ medial and lateral glides. STJ medial and lateral glides increase eversion and inversion. The talus must be stabilized while the calcaneus is mobilized medially to increase inversion and laterally to increase eversion.

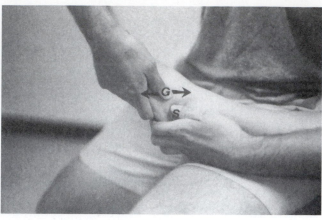

E X E R C I S E   3 1 - 3 9

Anterior/posterior cuboid metatarsal glides. Anterior/posterior cuboid metatarsal glides are done with one hand stabilizing the cuboid and the other gliding the base of the fifth metatarsal. They are used for increasing mobility of the fifth metatarsal.

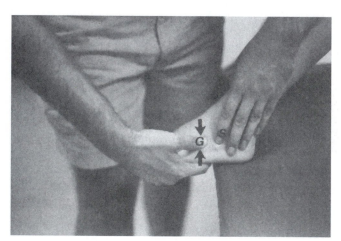

E X E R C I S E   3 1 - 3 8

Anterior/posterior calcaneocuboid glides. Anterior/posterior calcaneocuboid glides may be used for increasing adduction and abduction. The calcaneus should be stabilized while the cuboid is mobilized.

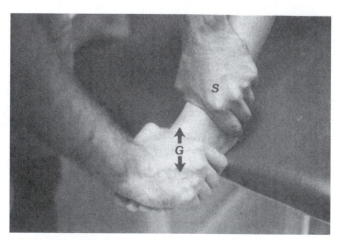

E X E R C I S E   3 1 - 4 0

Anterior/posterior carpometacarpal glides. Anterior/posterior carpometacarpal glides decrease hypomobility of the metacarpals.

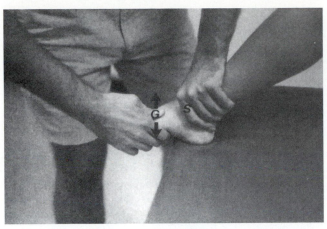

EXERCISE 31-41

Anterior/posterior talonavicular glides.
Anterior/posterior talonavicular glides also increase
adduction and abduction. One hand stabilizes the talus
while the other mobilizes the navicular bone.

Exercises to Reestablish Neuromuscular Control

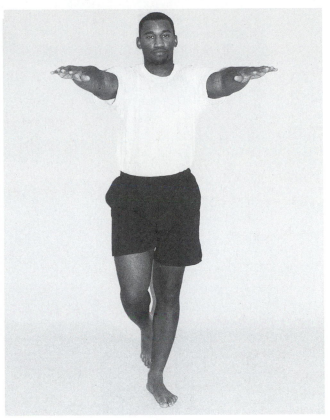

EXERCISE 31-43

Static single-leg standing balance progression. Used to
improve balance and proprioception of the lower
extremity. This activity can be made more difficult with
the following progression: **A,** single-leg standing with
eyes open; **B,** single-leg standing with eyes closed; **C,**
single-leg standing with eyes open and toes extended so
only the heel and metatarsal heads are in contact with
the ground; and **D,** single leg standing with eyes closed
and toes extended.

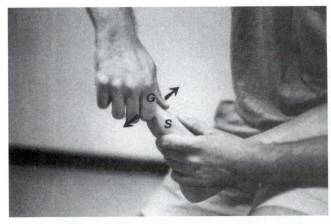

EXERCISE 31-42

Anterior/posterior metacarpophalangeal glides. With
anterior/posterior metacarpophalangeal glides, the
anterior glides increase extension, and posterior glides
increase flexion. Mobilizations are accomplished by
isolating individual segments.

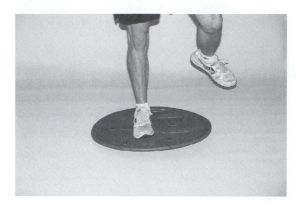

A

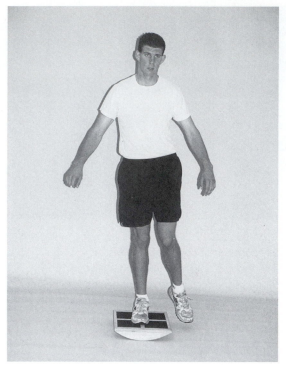

B

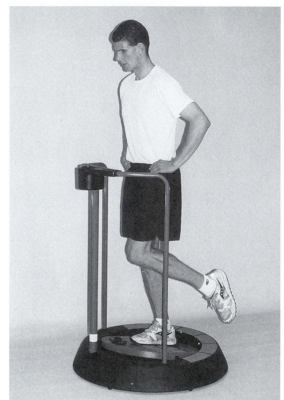

C

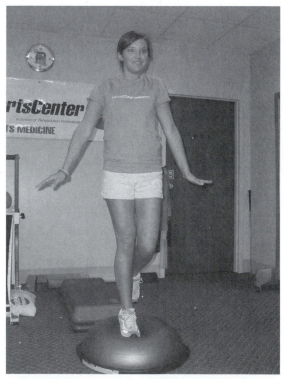

D

E X E R C I S E   3 1 - 4 4

Standing single leg balance board activity. Used to activate the lower-leg musculature
and improve balance and proprioception of the involved extremity. **A,** Wedge board.
B, BAPS® board. **C,** KAT® system. **D,** BOSU® ball.

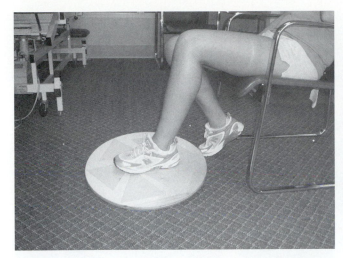

A

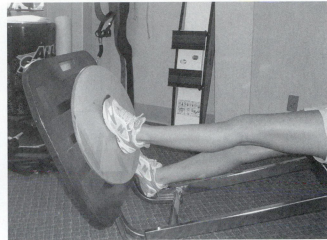

B

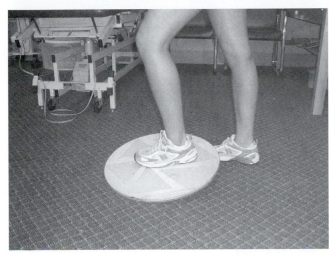

C

E X E R C I S E   3 1 - 4 5

Fine motor-control activity using the Fitter® wobble board for weightbearing progressions. **A,** Seated. **B,** Total Gym®. **C,** Standing.

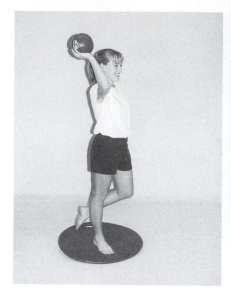

A

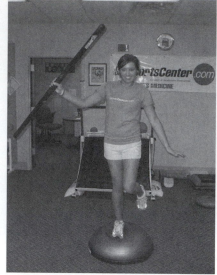

B

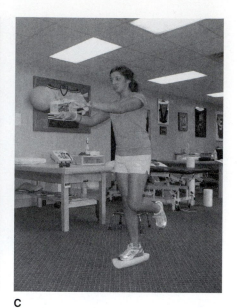

C

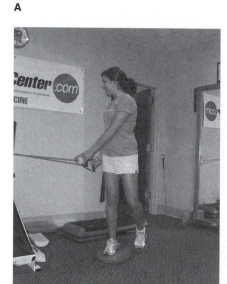

D

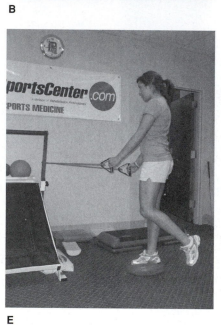

E

EXERCISE   31-46

Single-leg stance on an unstable surface while performing functional activities.
A, Single-limb stance on BAPS® board with medicine ball. **B,** Single-limb stance on
BOSU® ball with Body Blade®. **C,** Single-limb stance on $1/2$ foam roller with plyoback
medicine ball toss. **D,** Single-limb stance on Dyna Disc® with tubing self-perturbations
(forward). **E,** Single-limb stance on Dyna Disc® with tubing self-perturbations (sideways).

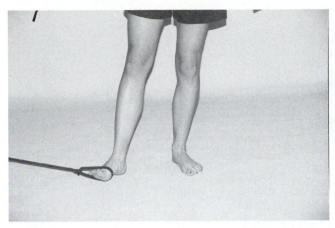

EXERCISE 31-47

Single-limb stance tubing kicks. Resisted kicks with the tubing around the uninvolved side while weight bearing on the involved side will challenge neuromuscular control.

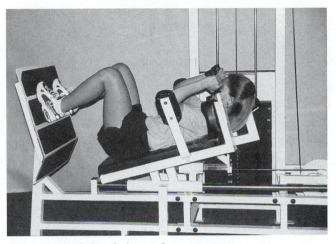

EXERCISE 31-48

Double leg press.

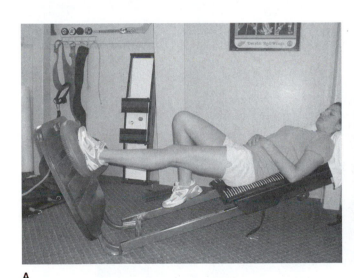

A   B

EXERCISE 31-49

Single-leg press on Total Gym® using a Dyna Disc®. **A,** Starting position. **B,** Finishing position.

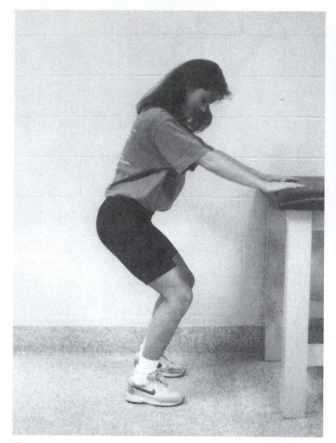

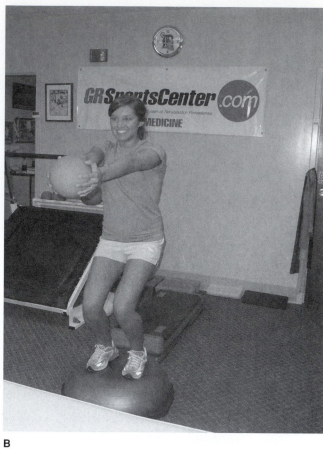

A

B

EXERCISE 31-50

A, Mini-form squats. **B,** Mini-form squat on BOSU® ball with overhead medicine ball lift to increase difficulty due to perturbation offered by the upper-extremity movement and weighted medicine ball.

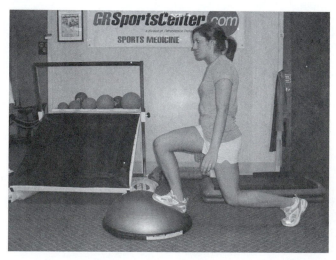

EXERCISE 31-51

Mini-lunge to unstable surface (BOSU® ball).

Exercises to Improve Cardiorespiratory Endurance

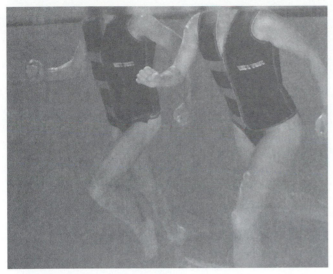

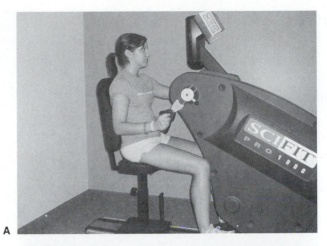

A

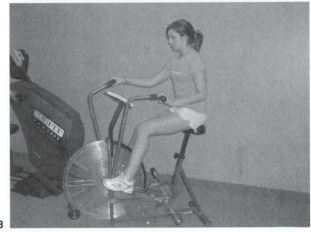

B

EXERCISE 31-52

Pool running with flotation device. Used to reduce the impact of weight-bearing forces on the lower extremity while maintaining cardiovascular fitness level and running form.

EXERCISE 31-53

Upper-body ergometer. **A,** SCIFIT PRO1000®. **B,** Airdyne® with arms only. Used to maintain cardiovascular fitness when lower-extremity ergometer is contraindicated or too difficult for the patient to use.

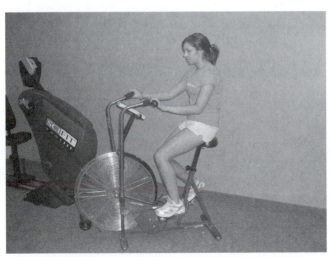

EXERCISE 31-54

Airdyne® stationary exercise bike. Used to maintain cardiovascular fitness when lower-extremity weight bearing is difficult.

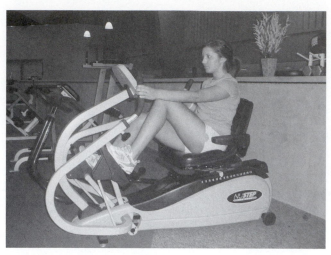

E X E R C I S E   3 1 - 5 5

NuStep® upper- and lower-extremity ergometer. Used to maintain cardiovascular fitness when lower-extremity weight bearing or use of a stationary bike is difficult or contraindicated.

Exercises for Initial Hip Strengthening

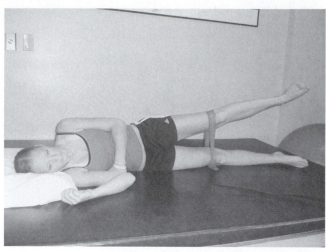

A

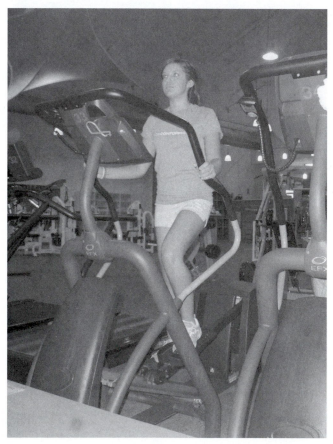

E X E R C I S E   3 1 - 5 6

Elliptical trainer. Used to maintain cardiovascular fitness when weight bearing, no impact activity is recommended.

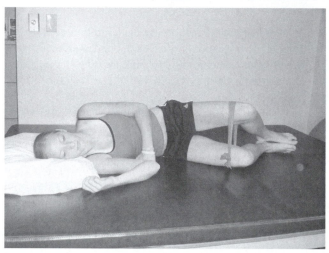

B

E X E R C I S E   3 1 - 5 7

A, Hip abduction (gluteus medius) with resistive band. **B,** Hip lateral rotators with resistive band. Recommended exercises before initiating functional exercises in weight bearing.

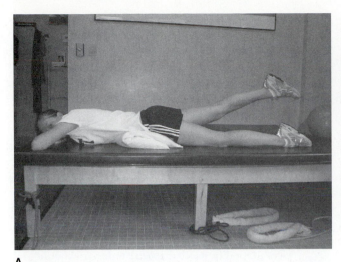

A

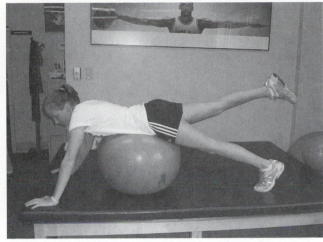

B

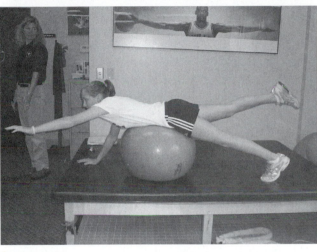

C

E X E R C I S E   3 1 - 5 8

Trunk and hip extensor progression. **A,** Prone hip extension against gravity. **B,** Prone hip extension over exercise ball. **C,** Prone alternate arm and leg raise over exercise ball. Recommended exercises before initiating functional exercises in weight bearing.

SUMMARY

- The movements that take place at the talocrural joint are ankle plantarflexion and dorsiflexion. Inversion and eversion occur at the STJ.
- The position of the STJ determines whether the MTJs will be hypermobile or hypomobile. Dysfunction at either joint may have a profound effect on the foot and lower extremity.
- Ankle sprains are very common. Inversion sprains usually involve the lateral ligaments of the ankle, and eversion sprains frequently involve the medial ligaments of the ankle. Rotational injuries often involve the tibiofibular and syndesmodic ligaments and may be very severe.
- The early phase of treatment of ankle sprains includes use of ice, compression, elevation, rest, and protection, all of which are critical components in preventing swelling.

- Early weightbearing following ankle sprain is beneficial to the healing process. Rehabilitation may become more aggressive following the acute inflammatory response phase of healing.
- Non-displaced ankle fractures should be managed with rest and protection until the fracture has healed, while displaced fractures are treated with open reduction and internal fixation.
- Subluxation of peroneal tendons can occur from any mechanism causing sudden and forceful contraction of the peroneal muscles that involves dorsiflexion and eversion of the foot. In the case of an avulsion injury or when this becomes a chronic problem, conservative treatment is unlikely to be successful and surgery is needed to prevent the problem from recurring.

- Tendinitis in the posterior tibialis, anterior tibialis, and the peroneal tendons may result from one specific cause or from a collection of mechanisms. Techniques should be incorporated into rehabilitation that acts to reduce or eliminate inflammation, including rest, using therapeutic modalities (ice, ultrasound, iontophoresis), and using anti-inflammatory medications as prescribed by a physician.
- Excessive or prolonged supination or pronation at the STJ is likely to result from some structural or functional deformity, including forefoot varus, a forefoot valgus, or a rearfoot varus, which forces the STJ to compensate in a manner that will allow the weightbearing surfaces of the foot to make stable contact with the ground and get into a weightbearing position.
- Orthotics are used to control abnormal compensatory movements of the foot by "bringing the floor to the foot." By providing support so that the foot does not have to move abnormally, an orthotic should help prevent compensatory problems.
- Shoe selection is an important parameter in the treatment of foot problems. The type of foot will dictate specific shoe features.
- The most common stress fractures in the foot involve the navicular, second metatarsal (March fracture), and diaphysis of the fifth metatarsal (Jones fracture). Navicular and second metatarsal stress fractures are likely to occur with excessive foot pronation, while fifth metatarsal stress fractures tend to occur in a more rigid pes cavus foot.
- A number of anatomic and biomechanical conditions have been studied as possible causes of plantar fasciitis. There is pain in the anterior medial heel, usually at the attachment of the plantar fascia to the calcaneus. Orthotics in combination with stretching exercises can significantly reduce pain.
- Subluxation of the cuboid will create symptoms similar to plantar fasciitis and can be corrected with manipulation.
- A bunion is a deformity of the head of the first metatarsal in which the large toe assumes a valgus position that is commonly associated with a structural forefoot varus in which the first ray tends to splay outward, putting pressure on the first metatarsal head.
- In treating a Morton's neuroma, a metatarsal bar is placed just proximal to the metatarsal heads or a teardrop-shaped pad is placed between the heads of the third and fourth metatarsals in an attempt to have these splay apart with weight bearing.
- Turf toe is a hyperextension injury resulting in a sprain of the metatarsophalangeal joint of the great toe.

REFERENCES

1. Acevedo JI, Beskin JL. Complications of plantar fascia rupture associated with corticosteroid injection. *Foot Ankle Int* 2:91–97, 1998.

2. American Physical Rehabilitation Network. When the feet hit the ground . . . everything changes. Program outline and prepared notes—a basic manual. Sylvania, OH, 2000.

3. American Physical Rehabilitation Network. When the feet hit the ground . . . take the next step. Program outline and prepared notes—an advanced manual. Sylvania, OH, 1994.

4. Andrews JR, McClod W, Ward T, et al. The cutting mechanism. *Am J Sports Med* 5:111–121, 1977.

5. Arnheim D, Prentice W. *Principles of Athletic Training*. New York, McGraw-Hill, 2000.

6. Baer T. Designing for the long run. *Mech Eng* 6:67–75, 1984.

7. Bates BT, Osternig L, Mason B, et al. Foot orthotic devices to modify selected aspects of lower extremity mechanics. *Am J Sports Med* 7:338, 1979.

8. Baxter D. *The Foot and Ankle in Sport*. St. Louis, MO, Mosby, 1995.

9. Birnham JS. The Musculoskeletal Manual. New York, Academic Press, 1982.

10. Bosien WR, Staples OS, Russell SW. Residual disability following acute ankle sprains. *J Bone Joint Surg Am* 37:1237, 1955.

11. Bostrum L. Treatment and prognosis in recent ligament ruptures. *Acta Chir Scand* 132:537–550, 1966.

12. Brody DM. Techniques in the evaluation and treatment of the injured runner. *Orthop Clin North Am* 13:541, 1982.

13. Brotzman B, Brasel J. Foot and ankle rehabilitation. In: Brotzman B, ed. *Clinical Orthopaedic Rehabilitation*. St. Louis, MO, Mosby, 1996.

14. Brunwich T, Wischnia B. Battle of the midsoles. *Runner's World*, April 1987, p. 47.

15. Burgess PR, Wei J. Signalling of kinesthetic information by peripheral sensory receptors. *Annu Rev Neurosci* 5:171–187, 1982.

16. Calliet R. *Foot and Ankle Pain*. Philadelphia, Pa, sDavis, 1968.

17. Canoy WF. *Review of Medical Physiology*, 7th ed. Los Altos, Lange, 1975.

18. Cavanaugh PR. An evaluation of the effects of orthotics force distribution and rearfoot movement during running. Paper presented at meeting of American Orthopedic Society for Sports Medicine, Lake Placid, 1978.

19. Choi J. Acute conditions: Incidence and associated disability. *Vital Health Stat* 120:10, 1978.

20. Collona P. Fabrication of a custom molded orthotic using an intrinsic posting technique for a forefoot varus deformity. *Phys Ther Forum* 8:3, 1989.

21. Cutler JM. Lateral ligamentous injuries of the ankle. In: Hamilton WC, ed. *Lateral Ligamentous Injuries of the Ankle*. New York, Springer-Verlag, 1984.

22. Delacerda FG. A study of anatomical factors involved

in shinsplints. *J Orthop Sports Phys Ther* 2:55–59, 1980.

23. Donatelli R. Normal biomechanics of the foot and ankle. *J Orthop Sports Phys Ther* 7:91–95, 1985.

24. Donatelli R, Hurlbert C, Conaway D, et al. Biomechanical foot orthotics: A retrospective study. *J Orthop Sports Phys Ther* 10:205–212, 1988.

25. Drez D, Faust D, Evans P. Cryotherapy and nerve palsy. *Am J Sports Med* 9:256–257, 1981.

26. Freeman M, Dean M, Hanhan I. The etiology and prevention of functional instability at the foot. *J Bone Joint Surg Br* 47:678–685, 1965.

27. Fumich RM, Ellison A, Guerin G, et al. The measured effect of taping on combined foot and ankle motion before and after exercise. *Am J Sports Med* 9:165–169, 1981.

28. Fury JG. Plantar fasciitis. The painful heel syndrome. *J Bone Joint Surg Am* 5:672–673, 1975.

29. Garn SN, Newton RA. Kinesthetic awareness in subjects with multiple ankle sprains. *J Am Phys Ther Assoc* 68:1667–1671, 1988.

30. Garrick JG, When can I . . . ? A practical approach to rehabilitation illustrated by treatment of an ankle injury. *Am J Sports Med* 9:67–68, 1981.

31. Garrick JG, Requa RK. Role of external supports in the prevention of ankle sprains. *Med Sci Sports Exerc* 5:200, 1977.

32. Gene H, Saracoglu M, Nacir B, et al. Long-term ultrasonographic follow-up of plantar fasciitis patients treated with steroid injection. *Joint Bone Spine* 72(1):61, 2005.

33. Giallonardo LM. Clinical evaluation of foot and ankle dysfunction. *Phys Ther* 68:1850–1856, 1988.

34. Gill E. Orthotics. *Runner's World.* February 1985, 55–57.

35. Gill LH. Plantar fasciitis: Diagnosis and conservative management. *J Am Acad Orthop Surg* 2:109–117, 1997.

36. Glencross D, Thornton E. Position sense following joint injury. *J Sport Med Phys Fitness* 21:23–27, 1981.

37. Glick J, Sampson T. Ankle and foot fractures in athletics. In: Nicholas J, Hershman E, eds. *The Lower Extremity and Spine in Sports Medicine.* St. Louis, MO, Mosby, 1996.

38. Gross M, Lapp A, Davis M. Comparison of Swed-O-Universal ankle support and Aircast Sport Stirrup orthoses and ankle tape in restricting eversion—inversion before and after exercise. *J Orthop Sports Phys Ther* 13:11–19, 1991.

39. Hirata I. Proper playing conditions. *J Sports Med* 4:228–234, 1974.

40. Hoppenfield S. *Physical Examination of the Spine and Extremities.* New York, Appleton-Century-Crofts, 1976.

41. Hunt G. Examination of lower extremity dysfunction. In: Gould J, Davies G, eds. *Orthopedic and Sports Physical Therapy*, Vol. 2. St. Louis, MO, Mosby, 1985.

42. Hunter S, Dolan M, Davis M. *Foot Orthotics in Therapy and Sports.* Champaign, IL, Human Kinetics, 1996.

43. Isakov E, Mizrahi J, Solzi P, et al. Response of the peroneal muscles to sudden inversion of the ankle during standing. *Int J Sports Biomech* 2:100–109, 1986.

44. Itay S. Clinical and functional status following lateral ankle sprains: Follow-up of 90 young adults treated conservatively. *Orthop Rev* 11:73–76, 1982.

45. James SL. Chondromalacia of the patella in the adolescent. In: Kennedy SC, ed. *The Injured Adolescent.* Baltimore, MD, Lippincott Williams & Wilkins, 1979.

46. James SL, Bates BT, Osternig LR. Injuries to runners. *Am J Sports Med* 6:43, 1978.

47. Jones D, Singer K. Soft-tissue conditions of the foot and ankle. In: Nicholas J, Hershman E, eds. *The Lower Extremity and Spine in Sports Medicine.* St. Louis, MO, Mosby, 1996.

48. Kelikian H, Kelikian AS. *Disorders of the Ankle.* Philadelphia, PA, Saunders, 1985.

49. Kergerris S. The construction and implementation of functional progressions as a component of athletic rehabilitation. *J Orthop Sports Phys Ther* 5:14–19, 1983.

50. Klein KK. A study of cross transfer of muscular strength and endurance resulting from progressive resistive exercises following surgery. *J Assoc Phys Mental Rehabil* 9:5, 1955.

51. Kowal MA. Review of physiologic effects of cryotherapy. *J Orthop Sports Phys Ther* 5:66–73, 1983.

52. Leach R, Jones R, Silva T. Rupture of the plantar fascia in athletes. *J Bone Joint Surg Am.* 4:44–46, 1978.

53. Lemont H, Ammirati KM, Usen N. Plantar fasciitis: a degenerative process (fasciosis) without inflammation. *J Am Podiatr Med Assoc* 3:234–237, 2003.

54. Loudin J, Bell S. The foot and ankle: An overview of arthrokinematics and selected joint techniques. *J Athl Train* 31:173–178, 1996.

55. Mandelbaum BR, Finerman G, Grant T, et al. Collegiate football players with recurrent ankle sprains. *Phys Sports Med* 15:57–61, 1987.

56. Mayhew JL, Riner WF. Effects of ankle wrapping on motor performance. *Athl Train* 3:128–130, 1974.

57. McCluskey GM, Blackburn TA, Lewis T. Prevention of ankle sprains. *Am J Sports Med* 4:151–157, 1976.

58. McPoil TG. Footwear. *Phys Ther* 68:1857–1865, 1988.

59. McPoil TG, Adrian M, Pidcoe P. Effects of foot orthoses on center of pressure patterns in women. *Phys Ther* 69:149–154, 1989.

60. McPoil TG, Brocato RS. The foot and ankle: Biomechanical evaluation and treatment. In: Gould J, Davies G, eds. *Orthopedic and Sports Physical Therapy.* St. Louis, MO, Mosby, 1985.

61. McPoil TG, Knecht HG, Schmit D. A survey of foot types in normal females between the ages of 18 and 30 years. *J Orthop Sports Phys Ther* 9:406–409, 1988.

62. Melegati G, Tornese D, Bandi M, et al. The influence of local steroid injections, body weight and the length of symptoms in the treatment of painful subcalcaneal spurs with extracorporeal shock wave therapy. *Clin Rehabil* 7:789–94, 2002.

63. Morris JM. Biomechanics of the foot and ankle. *Clin Orthop* 122:10–17, 1977.

64. Morton DJ. Foot disorders in general practice. *JAMA* 109:1112–1119, 1937.

65. Nawoczenski DA, Owen M, Ecker M, et al. Objective evaluation of peroneal response to sudden inversion stress. *J Orthop Sports Phys Ther* 7:107–119, 1985.

66. Nicholas JA, Hershman EB. The lower extremity and spine in sports medicine. St. Louis, MO, Mosby, 1990.

67. Noyes FR. Functional properties of knee ligaments and alterations induced by immobilization: A correlative biomechanical and histological study in primates. *Clin Orthop* 123:210–243, 1977.

68. Oatis CA. Biomechanics of the foot and ankle under static conditions. *Phys Ther* 68:1815–1821, 1988.

69. Ogden J, Alvarez RG, Cross GL, et al. Plantar fasciopathy and orthotripsy: The effect of prior contisone injection. *Foot Ankle Int* 3:231–233, 2005.

70. Ogden J, Alvarez RG, Levitt, RL, et al. Electrohydraulic high-energy shock-wave treatment for chronic plantar fasciitis. *J Bone Joint Surg Am* 10:2216–2228, 2004.

71. Pagliano JN. Athletic footwear. *Sports Med Digest* 10:1–2, 1988.

72. Peeland A. The relationship of pedal osseous malalignment to pain in other body segments. *Current Podiatric Medicine* May, 1998.

73. Porter MD, Shadbolt B. Intralesional corticosteroid injection versus extracorporeal shock wave therapy for plantar fasciopathy. *Clin J Sport Med* 3:119–124, 2005.

74. Prentice W. *Therapeutic Modalities in Sports Medicine.* Dubuque, WCB/McGraw-Hill, 1999.

75. Quillen S. Alternative management protocol for lateral ankle sprains. *J Orthop Sports Phys Ther* 12:187–190, 1980.

76. Rajkumar P, Schmitgen GF. Shock waves do more than just crush stones: Extracorporeal shockwave therapy in plantar fasciitis. *Int J Clin Pract* 10:735–737, 2002.

77. Rebman LW. Ankle injuries: Clinical observations. *J Orthop Sports Phys Ther* 8:153–156, 1986.

78. Riegler HF. Orthotic devices for the foot. *Orthop Rev* 16: 293–303, 1987.

79. Rogers MM, LeVeau BF. Effectiveness of foot orthotic devices used to modify pronation in runners. *J Orthop Sports Phys Ther* 4:86–90, 1982.

80. Root ML, Orien WP, Weed JH. Normal and abnormal functions of the foot. Los Angeles, Clinical Biomechanics, 1977.

81. Sammarco JG. *Rehabilitation of the Foot and Ankle.* St. Louis, MO, Mosby, 1995.

82. Sammarco JG. Biomechanics of foot and ankle injuries. *Athl Train* 10:96, 1975.

83. Sapega AA, Quedenfeld TC, Moyer RA, et al. Biophysical factors in range-of-motion exercise. *Phys Sports Med* 12:57–64, 1981.

84. Sellman JR. Plantar fascia ruptures associated with corticosteroid injection. *Foot Ankle Int* 7:376–381, 1994.

85. Sims D. Effects of positioning on ankle edema. *J Orthop Sports Phys Ther* 8:30–33, 1986.

86. Sims DS, Cavanaugh PR, Ulbrecht JS. Risk factors in the diabetic foot. *Phys Ther* 68:1887–1901, 1988.

87. Sloan JP, Guddings P, Hain R. Effects of cold and compression on edema. *Phys Sports Med* 16:116–120, 1988.

88. Stover CN, York JM. Air stirrup management of ankle injuries in the patient. *Am J Sports Med* 8:360–365, 1980.

89. Subotnick SI. The flat foot. *Phys Sports Med* 9:85–91, 1981.

90. Subotnick SI. *The Running Foot Doctor.* Mt. Vias, CA, World, 1977.

91. Subotnick SI, Newell SG. *Podiatric Sports Medicine.* Mt. Kisko, NY, Futura, 1975.

92. Tiberio D. Pathomechanics of structural foot deformities. *Phys Ther* 68:1840–1849, 1988.

93. Tippett SR. A case study: The need for evaluation and reevaluation of acute ankle sprains. *J Orthop Sports Phys Ther* 4:44, 1982.

94. Tropp H, Askling C, Gillquist J. Prevention of ankle sprains. *Am J Sports Med* 13:259–266, 1985.

95. Vaes P, DeBoeck H, Handleberg F, et al. Comparative radiologic study of the influence of ankle joint bandages on ankle stability. *Am J Sports Med* 13:46–49, 1985.

96. Visnich AL. A playing orthoses for "turf toe." *Athl Train* 22:215, 1987.

97. Vogelbach WD, Combs LC. A biomechanical approach to the management of chronic lower extremity pathologies as they relate to excessive pronation. *Athl Train* 22:6–16, 1987.

98. Williams JGP. The foot and chondromalacia—A case of biomechanical uncertainty. *J Orthop Sports Phys Ther* 2:50–51, 1980.

99. Woods A, Smith W. Cuboid syndrome and the techniques used for treatment. *Athl Train* 18:64–65, 1983.

100. Yablon IG, Segal D, Leach RE. *Ankle Injuries.* New York, Churchill Livingstone, 1983. Zylks DR. Alternative taping for plantar fasciitis. *Athl Train* 22:317, 1987.

REHABILITATION PROTOCOLS

Achilles Tendon Repair Program*

Surgical indications: Rupture of the Achilles tendon from the insertion on the calcaneus.

Surgical interventions: Surgical fixation of the Achilles tendon to the anatomical insertion on the calcaneus.

ACUTE PHASE

Beginning of Week 3 Postoperatively

1. Weight-bearing status: Nonweight bearing
2. Patient education in protection of surgical site
3. ROM exercises:
   a. Out-of-splint AROM
   b. Plantarflexion and/or dorsiflexion (two sets of five repetitions three times per day)
4. Strengthening:
   a. Initiate non-weightbearing proximal strengthening activities for lower extremities and core stabilizers (3 sets of 15 repetitions)
5. Proprioceptive/neuromuscular re-education exercises:
   a. Seated rocker board for plantarflexion and dorsiflexion

Week 4 Postoperatively

1. Weight-bearing status: Nonweight bearing
2. ROM exercises:
   a. Out-of-splint AROM
   b. Plantarflexion and/or dorsiflexion (2 sets of 20 repetitions)
   c. Inversion and/or eversion (2 sets of 20 repetitions)
   d. Circumduction in both directions (2 sets of 20 repetitions)
3. Strengthening exercises:
   a. Isometric inversion and/or eversion in neutral (2 sets of 20 repetitions)
   b. Toe curls with towel and weight
   c. Continue with non-weightbearing proximal strengthening for lower extremities and core stabilizers (3 sets of 15 repetitions)
4. Proprioceptive/neuromuscular re-education exercises:
   a. Seated rocker board for plantarflexion-dorsiflexion and inversion-eversion
   b. Seated wobble board for clockwise and counterclockwise circumduction
5. Physical therapy adjuncts:
   a. Gentle manual mobilization of scar tissue
   b. Cryotherapy with caution of any open areas

Week 5 Postoperatively

1. Weight-bearing status: Progressive partial-weight bearing in walker splint
2. ROM exercises:
   a. Previous AROM exercises continued
   b. Begin gentle passive stretching into dorsiflexion with towel
3. Strengthening exercises:
   a. Isometric inversion and/or eversion (2 sets of 20 repetitions)
   b. Isometric plantarflexion (initially 2 sets of 10 repetitions, progressing to 2 sets of 20 repetitions over the course of the week)
   c. Theraband inversion and/or eversion (2 sets of 10 repetitions)
   d. Theraband plantarflexion and/or dorsiflexion (2 sets of 10 repetitions)
   e. Continue with proximal strengthening for lower extremity and core stabilizers in non- or partial-weight bearing in walker splint (3 sets of 15 repetitions)
4. Proprioceptive/neuromuscular re-education exercises:
   a. Standing rocker board for plantarflexion-dorsiflexion and inversion-eversion maintaining weight-bearing restrictions
   b. Standing wobble board for clockwise and counterclockwise circumduction maintaining weight-bearing restrictions
5. Conditioning activities:
   a. Stationary bicycling begins, 7–12 minutes, minimal resistance
   b. Water therapy can begin under total buoyant conditions with use of a floatation device (Aqua-jogger vest)
   c. In the water, ankle ROM and running/walking activities can be initiated
6. Physical therapy adjuncts:
   a. Manual mobilization of scar and cyrotherapy continues
   b. Manual mobilization of ankle and foot joints (if necessary)
   c. Gentle passive manual stretching (unless patient already has 10° of dorsiflexion)

INTERMEDIATE PHASE

Weeks 6–8 Postoperatively

1. Weight-bearing status: Progressive partial- to full-weight bearing by week 7 or 8
2. ROM exercises:
   a. Previous ROM exercises decreased to one set of 10 repetitions each direction
   b. Passive stretching continues into dorsiflexion with progressively greater efforts (knee in full extension and flexed to 35°–40°)
   c. Begin standing calf stretch with full extension and flexed at week 7

---

*The Achilles Tendon Repair Program modified and used with permission from Orthopaedic Associates of Grand Rapids, P.C. (Grand Rapids, MI).

3. Strengthening exercises:
   a. Decrease isometrics to one set of 10 repetitions for inversion and/or eversion and plantarflexion
   b. Progress Theraband resistance for inversion, eversion, plantarflexion, and dorsiflexion (3 sets of 20 repetitions)
   c. Continue with proximal lower-extremity and core-stability exercises progressing to full-weight bearing after week 7.
4. Conditioning exercises:
   a. Stationary bicycling to 20 minutes with minimal resistance
   b. Water therapy exercises continue in totally buoyant state
5. Proprioceptive/neuromuscular re-education exercises:
   a. Continue with previous wobble board and rocker board exercises
   b. *Once full-weight bearing achieved*, can initiate single-leg balance activities on stable surfaces
6. Physical therapy adjuncts:
   a. Gentle cross-fiber massage to Achilles tendon to release adhesions between tendon and peritendon soft-tissue structures
   b. Continue with previous manual therapy techniques if needed
   c. Cryotherapy continues; ultrasound and electrical stimulation may be added for chronic swelling or excessive scar formation

ADVANCED PHASE
Weeks 8–14 Postoperatively

1. Weight-bearing status: Full-weight bearing with heel lift (high top shoes)
2. ROM exercises:
   a. Further progressed with standing calf stretch
   b. Add dynamic heel cord stretching in multiple planes
3. Strengthening exercises:
   a. Discontinue isometric exercises
   b. Continue with progressive resistance Theraband ankle strengthening in all directions
   c. Begin double-leg heel raises (plantarflexion) with BW as tolerated
   d. Continue with proximal lower-extremity and core-stability exercises in full-weight bearing
4. Proprioceptive/neuromuscular re-education exercises:
   a. Initiate single leg balance activities on unstable surfaces, including rocker board, wobble board, foam rollers, Dyna Disc, BOSU Balance Trainer, or KAT system as tolerated
   b. Progress single-leg balance activities on unstable surfaces with perturbations by therapist or using medicine balls, dumb bell weights, Theratubing, or Body Blade

5. Conditioning activities:
   a. Stationary cycling
   b. Treadmill walking
   c. StairMaster
   d. Elliptical trainer
   e. NuStep
   f. Water therapy exercises in chest-deep water
6. Therapy adjunct:
   a. Previously described if needed

RETURN TO FUNCTION PHASE
Weeks 14 and Beyond Postoperatively

1. Strengthening exercises:
   a. Heel raises should progress to use additional weight at least as great as BW, and in the case of athletes, up to 1.5 times BW
   b. Initiate single-leg heel raises as tolerated, possibly eccentric first, the progressing to concentric
   c. Progress functional strengthening exercises specific to athletic activity as patient tolerates
2. Conditioning activities:
   a. Progress to jogging on trampoline and then to treadmill running via a walk-run program
   b. Eventually perform steady-state outdoor running up to 20 minutes before adding figure-8 or cutting drills
   c. Water therapy exercises performed in shallow (waist deep) water
   d. In the water, begin to include hopping, bounding, and jumping drills
3. Goals:
   a. The completely rehabilitated Achilles tendon repair allows 15°–20° of dorsiflexion and the ankle. This must be maintained with regular stretching of the gastrocnemius-soleus group. Caution must be considered not to *over-stretch* the Achilles tendon. Do not want to continue manual or passive stretching once 20° of dorsiflexion is achieved
   b. Strength and endurance are developed to preinjury levels, and continued strength and flexibility work is advised
   c. Once return to sporting activities allowed, patient can complete functional sports-specific drills without pain or compensation

Modified Brostrom Ankle Rehabilitation Program*

Surgical indications: Chronic lateral ankle instability.
Surgical interventions: A lateral incision is made to the ankle region, at which time the capsule and lateral ligament

---

*The Modified Brostrom Ankle Rehabilitation Program modified and used with permission from Orthopaedic Associates of Grand Rapids, P.C. (Grand Rapids, MI).

structures, including the anterior talofibular and calcane-ofibular ligaments are tightened. Surgery may also include Os Calcis osteotomy.

ACUTE PHASE
Weeks 0–6 Postoperatively

Prior to Start of Physical Therapy

1. Weight-bearing status: Nonweight bearing progressing to full-weight bearing (depends on the physician orders)
2. Patient education in protection of surgical site

INTERMEDIATE PHASE
Weeks 6–8 Postoperatively

1. Weight-bearing status: Full-weight bearing
2. ROM exercises: *Protect inversion. Do not stretch out repair*
   a. Out-of-splint AROM
   b. Plantarflexion and/or dorsiflexion (2 sets of 20 repetitions)
   c. Eversion and limited inversion (2 sets of 20 repetitions)
   d. Circumduction in both directions (2 sets of 20 repetitions)
3. Strengthening exercises:
   a. Ankle isometrics in all directions or light manual resistance (2 sets of 20 repetitions)
   b. Initiate proximal lower-extremity strengthening activities for lower extremity and core stabilizers (3 sets of 15 repetitions)
4. Stretching exercises:
   a. Pain-free gastrocnemius-soleus stretching (30 second hold ×3 sets)
5. Proprioceptive/neuromuscular re-education exercises:
   a. Seated rocker board for plantarflexion and dorsiflexion
   b. Seated rocker board for eversion and limited inversion
   c. Seated wobble board for clockwise and counterclockwise circumduction
   d. Single-leg balance activities on stable surface progressing to perturbations by therapist or using medicine balls, dumb bell weights, Theratubing or, Body Blade
6. Physical therapy adjuncts:
   a. Gentle manual mobilization of scar tissue
   b. Manual therapy for joint mobility protecting surgical site (if needed)
   c. Modalities for pain and swelling control
   d. Gait training
7. Conditioning exercises:
   a. Stationary bicycling to 20 minutes, minimal resistance
   b. Water therapy can begin under total buoyant conditions with use of a floatation device (Aqua-jogger vest)
   c. In the water, ankle ROM and running/walking activities can be initiated

ADVANCED PHASE
Weeks 8–14 Postoperatively

1. Weight-bearing status: Full-weight bearing
2. ROM exercises:
   a. As needed. *Do not stretch out repair*
3. Strengthening exercises:
   a. Concentric/eccentric strengthening in both open- and closed-kinetic chain positions
   b. Discontinue isometric exercises
   c. Initiate isokinetic strengthening (50 percent maximum effort)
   d. Continue with proximal lower-extremity and core-stability exercises in full-weight bearing
4. Proprioceptive/neuromuscular re-education exercises:
   a. Initiate single-leg balance activities on unstable surfaces, including rocker board, wobble board, foam rollers, Dyna Disc, BOSU Balance Trainer, or KAT system as tolerated
   b. Progress single-leg balance activities on unstable surfaces with perturbations by therapist or using medicine balls, dumb bell weights, Theratubing or, Body Blade
5. Conditioning activities:
   a. Stationary cycling
   b. Treadmill walking
   c. Straight line running progression program
   d. StairMaster
   e. Elliptical trainer
   f. NuStep
   g. Water therapy exercises in chest-deep water
6. Therapy adjunct:
   a. Previously described if needed

RETURN TO FUNCTION PHASE
Weeks 14 and Beyond Postoperatively

1. Strengthening exercises:
   a. Progress functional strengthening exercises specific to athletic activity as patient tolerates
2. Conditioning activities:
   a. Progress straight line running program to 20 minutes before adding figure-8 or cutting drills
   b. Water therapy exercises performed in shallow (waist deep) water
   c. In the water, begin to include hopping, bounding, and jumping drills
3. Goals:
   a. The completely rehabilitated Modified Brostrom procedure allows for full ankle ROM maintaining protection into inversion not to *over-stretch* the repair.
   b. Strength and endurance are developed to preinjury levels, and continued strength and flexibility work is advised
   c. Return to sporting activities allowed once patient can complete functional sports specific drills without pain or compensation

Rehabilitation of Injuries to the Spine

Daniel N. Hooker and William E. Prentice

O B J E C T I V E S

After completing this chapter, the therapist should be able to do the following:

- Discuss the functional anatomy and biomechanics of the spine.
- Describe the difference between spinal segmental stabilization and core stabilization.
- Explain the rationale for using the different positioning exercises for treating pain in the spine.
- Conduct a thorough evaluation of the back before developing a rehabilitation plan.
- Compare and contrast the importance of using either joint mobilization or core stabilization exercises for treating spine patients.
- Differentiate between the acute versus reinjury versus chronic stage models for treating low back pain.
- Explain the eclectic approach for rehabilitation of back pain in the athletic population.
- Describe basic- and advanced-level training in the reinjury stage of treatment.
- Discuss the rehabilitation approach to conditions of the thoracic spine.
- Incorporate the rehabilitation approach to specific conditions affecting the low back.
- Discuss the rehabilitation approach to conditions of the cervical spine.

FUNCTIONAL ANATOMY AND BIOMECHANICS

From a biomechanical perspective, the spine is one of the most complex regions of the body with numerous bones, joints, ligaments, and muscles, all of which are collectively involved in spinal movement. The proximity to and relationship of the spinal cord, the nerve roots, and the peripheral nerves to the vertebral column adds to the complexity of this region. Injury to the cervical spine has potentially life-threatening implications, and low back pain is one of the most common ailments known to humans.

The 33 vertebrae of the spine are divided into five regions: cervical, thoracic, lumbar, sacral, and coccygeal. Between each of the cervical, thoracic, and lumbar vertebrae lie fibrocartilaginous intervertebral disks that act as important shock absorbers for the spine.

The design of the spine allows a high degree of flexibility forward and laterally and limited mobility backward. The movements of the vertebral column are flexion and extension, right and left lateral flexion, and rotation to the left and right. The degree of movement differs in the various regions of the vertebral column. The cervical and lumbar regions allow extension, flexion, and rotation around a central axis. Although the thoracic vertebrae have minimal movement, their combined movement between the first and twelfth thoracic vertebrae can account for 20°–30° of flexion and extension.

As the spinal vertebrae progress downward from the cervical region, they grow increasingly larger to accommodate the upright posture of the body, as well as to contribute to weight bearing. The shape of the vertebrae is irregular, but the vertebrae possess certain characteristics that are common to all. Each vertebra consists of a neural arch through which the spinal cord passes and several projecting processes that serve as attachments for muscles and ligaments. Each neural arch has two pedicles and two laminae. The pedicles are bony processes that project backward from the body of the vertebrae and connect with the laminae. The laminae are flat bony processes occurring on either side of the neural arch that project backward and inward from the pedicles. With the exception of the first and second cervical vertebrae, each vertebra has a spinous and transverse process for muscular and ligamentous attachment, and all vertebrae have an articular process.

Intervertebral articulations are between vertebral bodies and vertebral arches. Articulation between the bodies is of the symphysial type. Besides motion at articulations between the bodies of the vertebrae, movement takes place at four articular processes that derive from the pedicles and laminae. The direction of movement of each vertebra is somewhat dependent on the direction in which the articular facets face. The sacrum articulates with the ilium to form the sacroiliac joint, which has a synovium and is lubricated by synovial fluid.

Ligaments

The major ligaments that join the various vertebral parts are the anterior longitudinal, the posterior longitudinal, and the supraspinous. The anterior longitudinal ligament is a wide, strong band that extends the full length of the anterior surface of the vertebral bodies. The posterior longitudinal ligament is contained within the vertebral canal and extends the full length of the posterior aspect of the bodies of the vertebrae. Ligaments connect one lamina to another. The interspinous, supraspinous, and intertransverse ligaments stabilize the transverse and spinous processes, extending between adjacent vertebrae. The sacroiliac joint is maintained by the extremely strong dorsal sacral ligaments. The sacrotuberous and the sacrospinous ligaments attach the sacrum to the ischium.

Muscle Actions

The muscles that extend the spine and rotate the vertebral column can be classified as either superficial or deep. The superficial muscles extend from the vertebrae to ribs. The erector spinae is a group of superficial paired muscles that is made up of three columns or bands, the longissimus group, the iliocostalis group, and the spinalis group. Each of these groups is further divided into regions, the cervicis region in the neck, the thoracis region in the middle back, and the lumborum region in the low back. Generally the erector spinae muscles extend the spine. The deep muscles attach one vertebra to another and function to extend and rotate the spine. The deep muscles include the interspinales, multifidus, rotators, thoracis, and the semispinalis cervicis.

Flexion of the cervical region is produced primarily by the sternocleidomastoid muscles and the scalene muscle group on the anterior aspect of the neck. The scalenes flex the head and stabilize the cervical spine as the sternocleidomastoids flex the neck. The upper trapezius, semispinalis capitis, splenius capitis, and splenius cervicis muscles extend the neck. Lateral flexion of the neck is accomplished by all of the muscles on one side of the vertebral column contracting unilaterally. Rotation is produced when the sternocleidomastoid, the scalenes, the semispinalis cervicis, and the upper trapezius on the side opposite to the direction of rotation contract in addition to a contraction of the splenius capitus, splenius cervicis, and longissimus capitus on the same side of the direction of rotation.

Flexion of the trunk primarily involves lengthening of the deep and superficial back muscles and contraction of the abdominal muscles (rectus abdominus, internal oblique, external oblique) and hip flexors (rectus femoris, iliopsoas, tensor faciae lata, sartorius). Seventy-five percent of flexion occurs at the lumbosacral junction (L5-S1), whereas 15–70 percent occurs between L4 and L5. The rest of the lumbar vertebrae execute 5–10 percent of flexion.[8] Extension involves lengthening of the abdominal muscles and contraction of the erector spinae and the gluteus maximus, which extends the hip. Trunk rotation is produced by the external obliques and the internal obliques. Lateral flexion is produced primarily by the quadratus lumborum muscle, along with the obliques, latissimus dorsi, iliopsoas, and the rectus abdominus on the side of the direction of movement.

Spinal segment stability is produced by the deep muscles of the spine (multifidi, medial quadratus lumborum, iliocostalis lumborum, interspinales, intertransversarii) working in concert with the transversus abdominis and internal abdominal oblique (Fig. 32-1). Their location is close to the center of rotation of the spinal segment and their short muscle lengths are ideal for controlling each spinal segment. The transversus abdominis, because of its pull on the thoracolumbar fascia, and its ability to create increased intra-abdominal pressure, is a major partner in spinal segment stability (Fig. 32-2). The transversus abdominis contraction also narrows the abdominal cavity, which creates increased intra-abdominal pressure. This combination creates

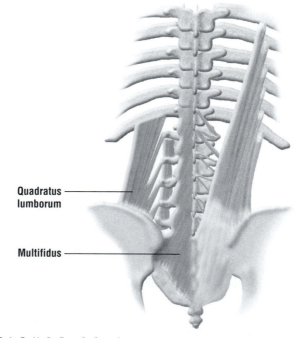

F I G U R E   3 2 - 1

Muscles of the low back. The multifidus and the quadratus lumborum muscles.

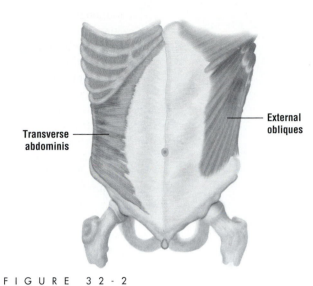

FIGURE 32-2

The transverse abdominis and external oblique muscles.

a rigid cylinder and in concert with the deep spinal muscles provides significant segmental stability to the lumbar spine and pelvis.[14,27–29,44–46,48,51–53]

Spinal Cord

The spinal cord is that portion of the central nervous system that is contained within the vertebral canal of the spinal column. Thirty-one pairs of spinal nerves extend from the sides of the spinal cord, coursing downward and outward through the intervertebral foramen passing near the articular facets of the vertebrae. Any abnormal movement of these facets, such as in a dislocation or a fracture, may expose the spinal nerves to injury. Injuries that occur below the third lumbar vertebra usually result in nerve root damage but do not cause spinal cord damage.

The spinal nerve roots combine to form a network of nerves, or a plexus. There are five nerve plexuses: cervical, brachial, lumbar, sacral, and coccygeal.

THE IMPORTANCE OF EVALUATION IN TREATING BACK PAIN

In many instances after referral for medical evaluation, the patient returns to the therapist with a diagnosis of low back pain. Even though this is a correct diagnosis, it does not offer the specificity needed to help direct the treatment planning. The therapist planning the treatment would be better served with a more specific diagnosis such as spondylolysis, disk herniation, quadratus lumborum strain, piriformis syndrome, or sacroiliac ligament sprain.

Regardless of the diagnosis or the specificity of the diagnosis, the importance of a thorough evaluation of the athlete's

back pain is critical to good care. The therapist should become an expert on this individual patient's back. Taking the time to perform a comprehensive evaluation will pay great rewards in the success of treatment and rehabilitation. The evaluation has six major purposes:

1. To clearly locate areas and tissues that might be part of the problem. The therapist should use this information to direct treatments and exercises.[23,28,41]

2. To establish the baseline measurements used to assess progress and guide the treatment progression and help the therapist make specific judgments on the progression of or changes in specific exercises. The improvement in these measurements also guides the return to activity and provides one measure of the success of the rehabilitation plan.[31,37,54]

3. To provide some provocative guidance to help the athlete probe the limits of their condition, help them better understand their problem, present limitations, and understand the management of their injury problem.[31,37,54]

4. To establish confidence in the athletic trainer. This increases the placebo effect of the athletic trainer–athletic interaction.[69,70]

5. To decrease the anxiety of the patient. This increases the patient's comfort, which will increase their compliance with the rehabilitation plan; a more positive environment is created, and the therapist and patient avoid the "no one knows what is wrong with me" trap.[11]

6. To provide information for making judgments on pads, braces, and corsets.

Table 32-1 provides a detailed scheme for evaluation of back pain.

REHABILITATION TECHNIQUES FOR THE LOW BACK

Positioning and Pain-Relieving Exercises

Most patients with back pain have some fluctuation of their symptoms in response to certain postures and activities. The therapist logically treats this patient by reinforcing pain-reducing postures and motions and by starting specific exercises aimed at specific muscle groups or specific ranges of motion. A general rule to follow in making these decisions is as follows: *any movement that causes the back pain to radiate or spread over a larger area should not be included during this early phase of treatment.* Movements that centralize or diminish the pain are correct movements to include at this time.[4,41] Including some exercise during initial pain management generally has a positive effect on the patient. The exercise encourages them to be active in the rehabilitation plan and helps them to regain lumbar movement.[18,70]

When a patient relieves pain through exercise and attention to proper postural control, he/she is much more likely to adopt

T A B L E   3 2 - 1

Lumbar and Sacroiliac Joint Objective Examination

1. *Standing position*
    a. Posture—alignment
    b. Gait
        i.   Patient's trunk frequently bent laterally or hips shifted to one side
        ii. Walks with difficulty or limps
    c. Alignment and symmetry
        i.   Level of malleoli
        ii.   Level of popliteal crease
        iii. Trochanteric levels
        iv.   PSIS and ASIS levels
        v.   Levels of iliac crests
        Recent studies have raised the concern that these clinical assessments of alignment are not valid because of the small movements available at the sacroiliac joints. These tests should be used as a small part of the overall evaluation and not as stand-alone tests. In sacroiliac dysfunction, the ASIS, PSIS, and iliac crests may not appear to be in the same horizontal plane.
    d. Lumbar spine active movements
        i.   With sacroiliac dysfunction, the patient will experience exacerbation of pain with side bending toward the painful side
        ii. Often a lumbar lesion is present along with a sacroiliac dysfunction
    e. Single-leg standing backward bending is a provocation test and can provoke pain in cases of spondylolysis or spondylolisthesis

2. *Sitting position*
    a. Lumbar spine rotation
    b. Passive hip internal rotation and external rotation
        i.   Piriformis muscle irritation would be provoked by internal rotation and could be present from sacroiliac joint dysfunctions or myofascial pain from overuse of this muscle
        ii. Limited range of motion of the hip can be a red flag for hip problems
    c. Sitting knee extension produces some stretch to the long neutral structures
    d. Slump sit is used to evaluate lumbar flexibility and neutral tension

3. *Supine position*
    a. Hip external rotation in a resting position may indicate piriformis muscle tightness
    b. Palpation of the transversus abdominis, as the athlete is directed to contract, can help in the assessment of spinal segment control. Can the patient isolate this contraction from the other abdominal muscles?
    c. Palpation of the symphysis pubis for tenderness. Some sacroiliac problems create pain and tenderness in this area. Sometimes the presenting subjective symptoms mimic adductor or groin strain but the objective evaluation does not show pain or weakness on muscle contraction or muscle tenderness that would support this assessment
    d. Straight-leg raise
        i.   Interpretation of straight-leg raise: pain provoked before
             • 30°—hip problem or very inflamed nerve
             • 30°–60°—sciatic nerve involvement
             • 70°–90°—sacroiliac joint involvement
             • Neck flexion—exacerbates symptoms—disk or root irritation
             • Ankle dorsiflexion or Lasegue's sign—exacerbated symptoms usually indicate sciatic nerve or root irritation
    e. Sacroiliac loading test (compression, distraction, posterior shear)—pain provoked by physical stress through the sacroiliac joints can be helpful in assessing for sacroiliac joint dysfunction
    f. FABER (flexion, abduction, external rotation), also known as Patrick's test—at end range assesses irritability of the sacroiliac joint; hip muscle tightness can also be assessed using this test
    g. FADIR (flexion, adduction, internal rotation) produces some stretch on the iliolumbar ligament

Continued

(Continued)

 h. Bilateral knees to chest—will usually exacerbate lumbar spine symptoms as the sacroiliac joints move with the sacrum in this maneuver

 i. Single knee to chest can provoke pain from a variety of sources from sacroiliac joint to lumbar spine muscles and ligaments; make the patients be specific about their pain location and quality

4. *Side-lying position*

 a. Anterior and posterior iliac rotation—pain on movement indicates irritation of the sacroiliac joints; may also be used as a joint mobilization to ease pain

 b. Iliotibial band length—long-standing sacroiliac joint problems sometimes create tightness of the iliotibial band

 c. Quadratus lumborum stretch and palpation

 d. Hip abduction and piriformis muscle test
     Pain provocation with any of this test indicates primary myofascial pain problems or secondary tightness, weakness, and pain from muscle guarding associated with different pathologies.

5. *Prone position*

 a. Palpation

   i.   Well-localized tenderness medial to or around the PSIS indicates sacroiliac dysfunction

   ii. Tenderness lateral and superior to the PSIS indicates gluteus medius irritation or myofascial trigger point

   iii. Gluteus maximus area—sacrotuberous and sacrospinous ligaments are in this area, as well as piriformis muscle and sciatic nerve. Changes in tension and tenderness can help make the evaluation more specific

   iv. Tenderness or alignment from S-1 to T-10 implicates some lumbar problems

 b. Anterior–posterior or rotational prevocational stresses can be applied to the spinous processes

 c. Sacral provocation stress test—pain from anterior–posterior pressure at the center of the sacral base and/or on each side of the sacrum just medial to the PSIS may be indicative of sacroiliac joint dysfunction

 d. Hip extension–knee flexion stretch will provoke the L3 nerve root and create a nerve quality pain down the anterolateral thigh

 e. Anterior rotation stress to the sacroiliac joint can be delivered by using passive hip extension and PSIS pressure; pain would be indicative of sacroiliac dysfunction

6. *Manual muscle test*
   If the lumbar spine or posterior hip musculature is strained, active movement against gravity and/or resistance should provoke a pain complaint similar to patients' subjective description of their problem

 a. Hip extension

 b. Hip internal rotation

 c. Hip external rotation

 d. Hip flexion

 e. Hip adduction

 f. Trunk extension—arm and shoulder extension

 g. Trunk extension—arm, shoulder, and neck extension

 h. Trunk extension—resisted

 i. Multifidus activation and control

 j. Spinal segment coactivation of transversus abdominis and multifidi[16,31,37,53,54]

these procedures into a daily routine. Patient whose pain is relieved via some other passive procedure, and then is taught exercises, will not be able to readily see the connection between relief and exercise.[4,14,30,44,53]

The types of exercises that may be included in initial pain management include the following:

- Spinal segment control, transverse abdominis, and multifidus coactivation
- Lateral shift corrections
- Extension exercises
- Flexion exercises
- Postural traction positions

SPINAL SEGMENT CONTROL EXERCISE

In devising exercise plans to address the different clinical problems of the lumbo-pelvic-hip complex, *the use of core-stabilizing exercises is a must for every problem for recovery, maintenance, and prevention of reinjury.* Clinically, the core stabilization rehabilitation exercise sequence begins with relearning the muscle activation patterns necessary for segmental spinal stabilization.

This beginning exercise plan is based on the work of Richardson, Jull, Hodges, and Hides.[27–29,30,46,52,53]

The first step in segmental spinal stabilization is to reestablish separate control of the transversus abdominis and the lumbar multifidii (Figs. 32-1 and 32-2). The control and activation of these deep muscles should be separated from the control and activation of the global or superficial muscles of the core. Once the patients have mastered the behavior of coactivation of the transversus abdominis and multifidii to create and maintain a corset-like control and stabilization of the spinal segments, they may then progress to using the global muscles in the core stabilization sequence and more functional activities. Segmental spinal stabilization is the basic building block of core stabilization exercises and should be an automatic behavior to be used in every subsequent exercise and activity.[27,28,30,44,45]

The basic exercise that the patient must master is coactivation of the transversus abdominis and multifidii, isolating them from the global trunk muscles. This contraction should be of sufficient magnitude to create a small increase in the intra-abdominal pressure. This is a simple concept, but these muscle contractions are normally under subconscious automatic control; and in patients with low back pain, the subconscious control of timing and firing patterns become disturbed and the patient loses spinal segmental control.[28] To regain this vital skill and return the subconscious timing and firing patterns of these muscles, the patient will need individual instruction and testing to prove that he/she has mastered the conscious control of each muscle individually and in a coactivation pattern. The next step is to incorporate this coactivation pattern into functional exercise and other activities. The success of this exercise is dependent upon this muscular coactivation becoming a habitual postural control movement under both conscious and subconscious control.

A muscle contraction of 10–15 percent of the maximum voluntary contraction of the multifidus and the transversus abdominis is all that is necessary to create segmental spinal stability. Contraction levels greater than 20 percent of maximum voluntary contraction will cause overflow of activity to the more global muscles and negate the exercise's intent of isolating control of the transversus abdominis and multifidii.[30] Precision of contraction and control is the intent of these exercises; the ultimate goal is a change in the patient's behavior. As this behavior is incorporated into more daily activities and exercise, the strength and endurance of these muscle groups will also improve and the core system will work more effectively and efficiently.[30,44,45,52,53]

Transversus Abdominis Behavior Exercise Plan

1. Test the patient's ability to consciously contract and control the transversus abdominis in isolation from the other abdominal muscles. The therapist can assess the contraction through observation and palpation. The patient is positioned in a comfortable relaxed posture: stomach-lying, back-lying, side-lying, or hand-knee position. The best palpation location is medial to the anterior superior iliac spine

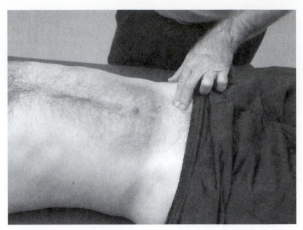

F I G U R E   3 2 - 3

Palpation location to feel for isolated transversus abdominis contraction.

(ASIS) about 1.5 in. (Fig. 32-3). The internal abdominal oblique has more vertical fibers and is closest to the ASIS, whereas the transversus fibers run horizontal from ilia to ilia. The therapist monitors the muscle with light palpation and instructs the patient to contract the muscle, feeling for the transversus drawing together across the abdomen. As the contraction increases, the internal oblique fibers and external oblique fibers will start to fire. If the patients cannot separate the firing of the transversus from the other groups and/or cannot maintain the separate contraction for 5–10 seconds, they will need individual instruction with various forms of feedback to regain control of this muscle behavior. In patients with low back pain, transversus contraction usually becomes more phasic and fires only in combination with the obliques or rectus.[30,53]

2. The patients are positioned in a comfortable pain-free position and instructed to breathe in and out gently, stop the breathing, and slowly, gently contract and hold the contraction of their transversus—and then resume normal light breathing while trying to maintain the contraction. Changes in body position (positions of choice are prone, side-lying, supine, or quadriped), verbal cues, and visual and tactile feedback will speed and enhance the learning process (Figs. 32-4A and B). The use of imaging ultrasound to visualize the contractions of these muscles is a unique new idea for biofeedback in isolating and bringing these muscle contractions under cognitive control.[30,53]

3. The lumbar multifidii contractions are taught with tactile pressure over the muscle bellies next to the spinous processes (Fig. 32-5). The patient is asked to contract the muscle so that the muscle swells up directly under the finger pressure. The feeling should be a deep tension. A rapid superficial contraction or a contraction that brings in the global muscles is not acceptable, and continued trial and error with feedback is used until the desired contraction and control are achieved.[30,53]

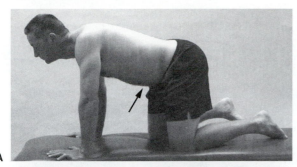

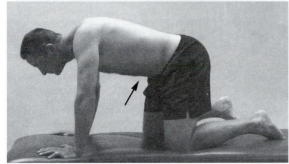

FIGURE 32-4

The quadriped position can be used to demonstrate and practice the isolated transversus abdominis contraction. The patients are instructed to **A,** let their belly sag, and then **B,** slowly and gently contract their pelvic floor muscles and practice holding this position for 10 seconds.

4. As soon as cognitive control of the transversus and multifidii is achieved, more functional positions and exercises aimed at coactivation of both muscles are begun. The therapist should attempt to have the patient use the transversus and multifidii coactivation in a comfortable neutral

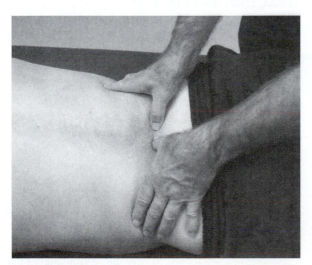

FIGURE 32-5

Palpation location to feel for isolated lumbar multifidii contractions.

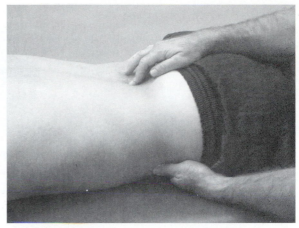

FIGURE 32-6

Palpation location to feel contractions and to give the patients feedback on their ability to perform a coactivation segmental spinal stabilization contraction.

lumbopelvic position with restoration of a normal lordotic curve so that the muscle coactivation strategies can start to be incorporated into the athlete's daily life (Fig. 32-6). Repetition improves the effectiveness of this contraction, and as it is used more, the cognitive control becomes less and the subconscious pattern of segmental spinal stabilization returns to normal.[30,53]

5. Incorporating the coactivation back into activities is the next step and is accomplished by graduating the exercises to include increases in stress and control. Supine-lying with simple leg and arm movements is a good starting point. Using a pressure biofeedback unit for this phase will help the athletes measure their ability to use the coactivation contraction effectively during increased exercise. The pressure bladder or blood pressure cuff is inflated to a pressure about 40 mm Hg. As the patient coactivates the transversus abdominis and multifidi, the pressure reading should stay the same or decrease slightly and remain at that level throughout the increased movement exercises (Figs. 32-7A and B). This is an indirect measure of the spinal segment stabilization, but gives the athletes an outside feedback source to keep them more focused on the exercise.[30,53]

6. This can be followed with trunk inclination exercises in which the patients maintain a neutral lumbopelvic position and incline their trunk in different positions away from the vertical alignment and hold in positions of forward-lean to side-lean for specific time periods (Figs. 32-8A and B and 32-9A and B). This is first done in the sitting position. As control, strength, and endurance increase, the positions can become more exaggerated and the holding times longer.

7. Return the patient to a structured progressive resistive core exercise program (see Chapter 18). The incorporation of the segmental spinal stabilization coactivation contraction as the precursor to each exercise is the goal at this point in returning the patient back to functional activity.

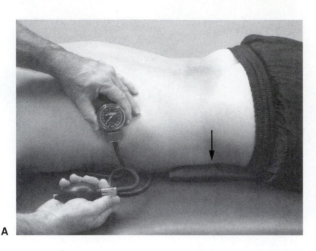
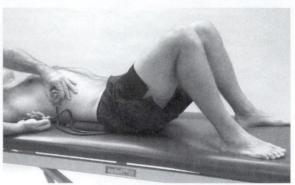

FIGURE 32-7

Pressure gauge biofeedback can be used as an indirect method of measuring correct activation of the spinal segment stabilization coactivation contraction. The pressure bladder or blood pressure cuff is inflated to 40 mm Hg pressure and placed under the patient's **A,** abdomen, or **B,** bank. The patient is instructed to contract the transversus in a way that does not make the pressure in the cuff start to rise or fall.

8. The therapist should teach this technique both as an exercise and as a behavior. The exercises should be taught and monitored in an individual session with opportunity for feedback and correction. The patients must also use this skill in the functional things they do every day. The patients are asked to trigger this spinal segment control skill in response to daily tasks, postures, pains, and certain movements (Figs. 32-10A and B). As their pain is controlled,

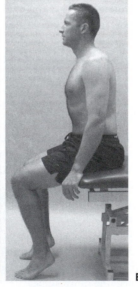

FIGURE 32-8

Trunk inclination exercise. The patient finds a comfortable neutral spine position and coactivates his/her transversus abdominis and lumbar multifidii to provide the segmental spinal stabilization.

the coactivation contraction should be incorporated into activities of daily living.

Segmental spinal stabilization is complementary for all forms of treatment and different pathologies. This exercise program can be incorporated and started at the same time as other therapies. The different forms of therapy summate, and the patient improves more quickly and maintains the gains in range and strength achieved with other therapies. Spinal segment control may also decrease pain and give the athlete a measure of control to use in minimizing painful stress through the injured tissues.

LATERAL SHIFT CORRECTIONS

Lateral shift corrections and extension exercises probably should be discussed together because the indications for use are similar, and extension exercises will immediately follow the lateral shift corrections.

The indications for the use of lateral shift corrections are as follows:

- Subjectively, the patient complains of unilateral pain reference in the lumbar or hip area.
- The typical posture is scoliotic with a hip shift and reduced lumbar lordosis.
- Walking and movements are very guarded and robotic.
- Forward bending is extremely limited and increases the pain.
- Backward bending is limited.
- Side bending toward the painful side is minimal to impossible.
- Side bending away from the painful side is usually reasonable to normal.

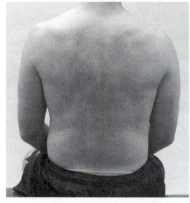
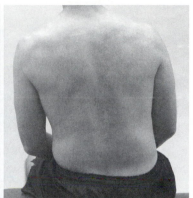

FIGURE 32-9

The patient challenges his/her spinal segment control by leaning away from the vertical position while holding the neutral spine position for 10 seconds.

A **B**

- A test correction of the hip shift either reduces the pain or causes the pain to centralize.
- The neurological examination may or may not elicit the following positive findings:
  1. Straight-leg raising may be limited and painful, or it could be unaffected.
  2. Sensation may be dull, anesthetic, or unaffected.
  3. Manual muscle test may indicate unilateral weakness of specific movements, or the movements may be strong and painless.
  4. Reflexes may be diminished or unaffected.[4,41]

The patient will be assisted by the therapist with the initial lateral shift correction. The patient is then instructed in the techniques of self-correction. The lateral shift correction is designed to guide the patient back to a more symmetrical posture. The therapist's pressure should be firm and steady and more guiding than forcing. The use of a mirror to provide visual feedback is recommended for both the therapist-assisted and self-corrected maneuvers. The specific technique guide for therapist-assisted lateral shift correction is as follows (Fig. 32-11):

1. Preset the patient by explaining the correction maneuver and the roles of the patient and the therapist.
   a. The patient is to keep the shoulders level and avoid the urge to side bend.

   b. The patient should allow the hips to move under the trunk and should not resist the pressure from the therapist but allow the hips to shift with the pressure.
   c. The patient should keep the therapist informed about the behavior of the back pain.
   d. The patient should keep the feet stationary and not move after the hip shift correction until the standing extension part of the correction is completed.
   e. The patient should practice the standing extension exercise as part of this initial explanation.
2. The therapist should stand on the patient's side that is opposite his/her hip shift. The patient's feet should be a comfortable distance apart, and the therapist should have a comfortable stride stance aligned slightly behind the patient.
3. Padding should be placed around the patient's elbow, on the side next to the therapist to provide comfortable contact between the patient and the therapist.
4. The therapist should contact the patient's elbow with the shoulder and chest, with the head aligned along the patient's back. The therapist's arms should reach around the patient's waist and apply pressure between the iliac crest and the greater trochanter (Fig. 32-11).
5. The therapist should gradually guide the patient's hips toward him/her. If the pain increases, the therapist should ease the pressure and maintain a more comfortable posture

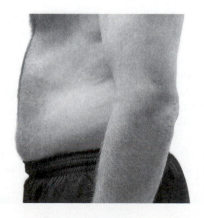
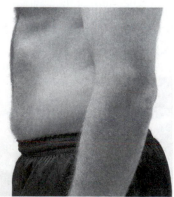

FIGURE 32-10

The patient is instructed to become posture savvy by frequently using the coactivation contraction throughout their day. The coactivation thereby becomes a subconscious movement pattern the athletes incorporate into all they do.

A **B**

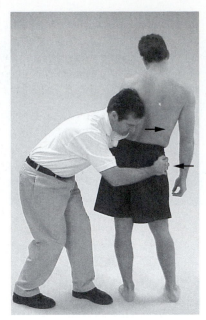

F I G U R E   3 2 - 1 1

Lateral shift correction exercise. Emphasis is on pulling the hips, not on pushing the ribs.

for 10–20 seconds, and then again pull gently. If the pain increases again, the therapist should again lessen the pull and allow comfort, then instruct the patient to actively extend gently, pushing the back into and matching the resistance supplied by the therapist. The goal for this maneuver is an overcorrection of the scoliosis, reversing its direction.

6. Once the corrected or overcorrected posture is achieved, the therapist should maintain this posture for 1–2 minutes. This procedure may take 2–3 minutes to complete, and the first attempt may be less than a total success. Repeated efforts 3–4 minutes apart should be attempted during the first treatment effort before the therapist stops the treatment for that episode.

7. The therapist gradually releases pressure on the hip while the patient does a standing extension movement (see Fig. 32-16). The patient should complete approximately six repetitions of the standing extension movement, holding each for 15–20 seconds.

8. Once the patient moves the feet and walks even a short distance, the lateral hip shift usually will recur, but to a lesser degree. The patient then should be taught the self-correction maneuver (Fig. 32-12). The patient should stand in front of a mirror and place one hand on the hip where the therapist's hands were and the other hand on the lower ribs where the therapist's shoulder was.

9. The patient then guides the hip under the trunk, watching the mirror to keep the shoulders level and trying to achieve a corrected or overcorrected posture. He/she should hold this posture for 30–45 seconds and then follow with several

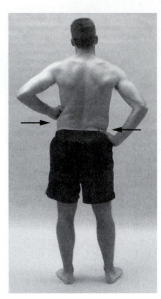

F I G U R E   3 2 - 1 2

Hip shift self-correction. The patients can use a mirror for visual feedback as they apply the gentle guiding force to correct their hip shift posture. The patients use one hand to stabilize themselves at the rib level and use the other hand to guide the hips across to correct their alignment. This position is held for 30–45 seconds, and then the athlete is instructed to go into the standing extension position for five to six repetitions, holding the position for 20–30 seconds.

standing extension movements as described in step 7 (Fig. 32-12).[4,41]

EXTENSION EXERCISES

The indications for the use of extension exercise are as follows:

*   Subjectively, back pain is diminished with lying down and is increased with sitting. The location of the pain may be unilateral, bilateral, or central, and there may or may not be radiating pain into either or both legs.
*   Forward bending is extremely limited and increases the pain, or the pain reference location enlarges as the athlete bends forward.
*   Backward bending can be limited, but the movement centralizes or diminishes the pain.
*   The neurological examination is the same as outlined for lateral shift correction.[4,41,42]

The efficacy of extension exercise is theorized to be from one or a combination of the following effects:

*   A reduction in the neural tension
*   A reduction of the load on the disk, which in turn decreases disk pressure
*   Increases in the strength and endurance of the extensor muscles

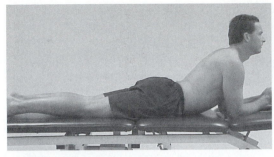

FIGURE 32-13

Prone extension on elbows.

- Proprioceptive interference with pain perception as the exercises allow self-mobilization of the spinal joints

Hip shift posture has previously been theoretically correlated to the anatomical location of the disk bulge or nucleus pulposus herniation. Creating a centralizing movement of the nucleus pulposus has been the theoretical emphasis of hip shift correction and extension exercise. This theory has good logic, but research on this phenomenon has not been supportive.[49] However, in explaining the exercises to the patient, the use of this theory may help increase the patient's motivation and compliance with the exercise plan.

End-range hyperextension exercise should be used cautiously when the patient has facet joint degeneration or impingement of the vertebral foramen borders on neural structures. Also, spondylolysis and spondylolisthesis problems should be approached cautiously with any end-range movement exercise using either flexion or hyperextension.

Figures 32-13 to 32-20 are examples of extension exercises. These examples are not exhaustive but are representative of most of the exercises used clinically.

The order in which exercises are presented is not significant. Instead, each therapist should base the starting exercises on the evaluative findings. Jackson, in a review of back exercise, stated, "no support was found for the use of a preprogrammed flexion regimen that includes exercises of little value or potential harm and is not specific to the current needs of the patient, as determined by a thorough back evaluation." The review also

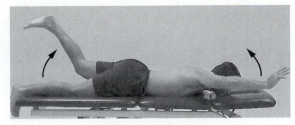

FIGURE 32-15

Alternate arm and leg extension.

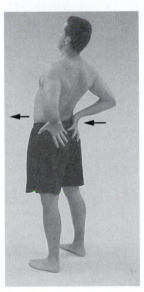

FIGURE 32-16

Standing extension.

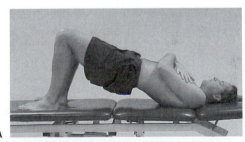

A

B

FIGURE 32-17

Supine hip extension—butt-lift or bridge. **A,** Double-leg support. **B,** Single-leg support.

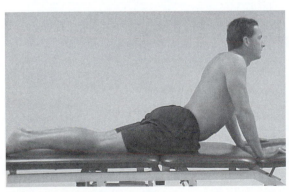

FIGURE 32-14

Prone extension on hands.

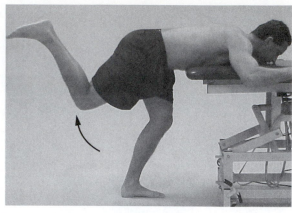 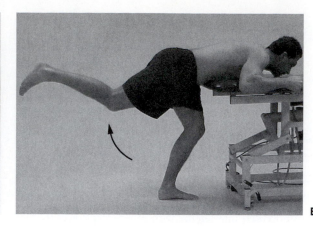

F I G U R E   3 2 - 1 8

Prone single-leg hip extension. **A,** Knee flexed. **B,** Knee extended.

included a report of Kendall and Jenkin's study, which stated that one-third of the patients for whom hyperextension exercises had been prescribed worsened.[23]

FLEXION EXERCISES

The indications for the use of flexion exercises are as follows:

- Subjectively, back pain is diminished with sitting and is increased with lying down or standing. Pain is also increased with walking.
- Repeated or sustained forward bending eases the pain.
- The patients' lordotic curve does not reverse as they forward bend.
- The end range of sustained backward bending is painful or increases the pain.
- Abdominal tone and strength are poor.

In his approach, Saal elaborates on the thought that "No one should continue with one particular type of exercise regimen during the entire treatment program."[56] We concur with this and believe that starting with one type of exercise should not preclude rapidly adding other exercises as the athlete's pain resolves and other movements become more comfortable.

The efficacy of flexion exercise is theorized to derive from one or a combination of the following effects:

- A reduction in the articular stresses on the facet joints
- Stretching to the thoracolumbar fascia and musculature
- Opening of the intervertebral foramen
- Relief of the stenosis of the spinal canal
- Improvement of the stabilizing effect of the abdominal musculature
- Increasing the intra-abdominal pressure because of increased abdominal muscle strength and tone
- Proprioceptive interference with pain perception as the exercises allow self-mobilization of the spinal joints[33]

Flexion exercises should be used cautiously or avoided in most cases of acute disk prolapse and when a laterally shifted posture is present. In patients recovering from disk-related back pain, flexion exercise should not be commenced immediately after a flat-lying rest interval longer than 30 minutes. The disk can become more hydrated in this amount of time, and the patient would be more susceptible to pain with postures that increase disk pressures. Other, less stressful exercises should be initiated first and flexion exercise done later in the exercise program.[4,42]

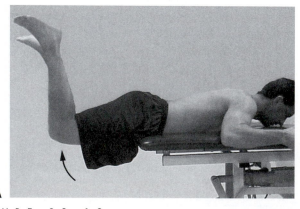 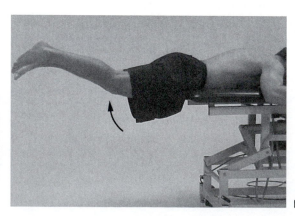

F I G U R E   3 2 - 1 9

Prone double-leg hip extension **A,** Knees flexed. **B,** Knees extended.

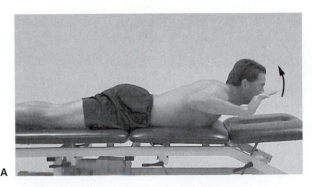

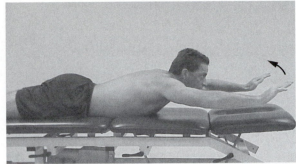

FIGURE 32-20

Trunk extension—prone. **A,** Hands near head. **B,** Arms extended—superman position.

Figures 32-21 to 32-31 show examples of flexion exercises. Again these examples are not exhaustive but are representative of the exercises used clinically.

Joint Mobilizations

The indications for the use of joint mobilizations are as follows:

- Subjectively, the patient's pain is centered around a specific joint area and increases with activity and decreases with rest.
- The accessory motion available at individual spinal segments is diminished.
- Passive range of motion is diminished.
- Active range of motion is diminished.
- There may be muscular tightness or increased fascial tension in the area of the pain.
- Back movements are asymmetrical when comparing right and left rotation or side bending.
- Forward and backward bending may steer away from the midline.

The efficacy of mobilization is theorized to be from one or a combination of the following effects:

- Tight structures can be stretched to increase the range of motion.

- The joint involved is stimulated by the movement to more normal mechanics, and irritation is reduced because of better nutrient waste exchange.
- Proprioceptive interference occurs with pain perception as the joint movement stimulates normal neural firing whose perception supersedes nociceptive perception.

Mobilization techniques are multidimensional and are easily adapted to any back pain problem. The mobilizations can be active or passive or assisted by the therapist. All ranges (flexion, extension, side bending, rotation, and accessory) can be incorporated within the exercise plan. The mobilizations can be carried out according to Maitland's grades of oscillation as discussed in Chapter 16. The magnitude of the forces applied can range from grade 1 to grade 4 depending on levels of pain. The theory, technique, and application of the therapist-assisted mobilizations are best gained through guided study with an expert practitioner.[37]

Figures 32-30 to 32-39 show the various self-mobilization exercises.

Figures 16-35 to 16-45 show joint mobilizations that can be used by the therapist.

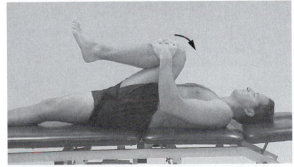

FIGURE 32-21

Single knee to chest. **A,** Stretch holding 15–20 seconds. **B,** Same as step 2.

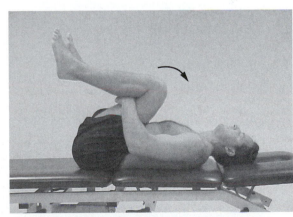

FIGURE 32-22

Double knee to chest. **A,** Stretching—holding posture 15–20 seconds. **B,** Mobilizing—using a rhythmic rocking motion within a pain-free range of motion.

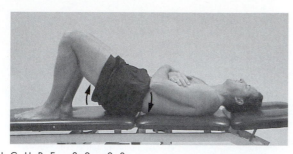

F I G U R E   3 2 - 2 3

Posterior pelvic tilt.

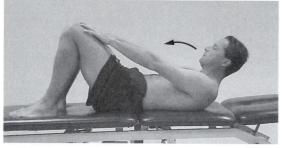

F I G U R E   3 2 - 2 4

Partial sit-up.

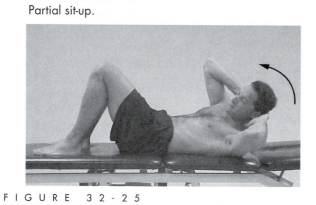

F I G U R E   3 2 - 2 5

Rotation partial sit-up.

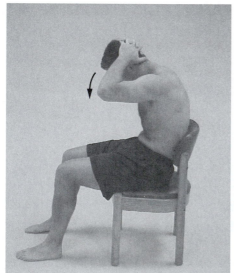

F I G U R E   3 2 - 2 6

Slump sit stretch position.

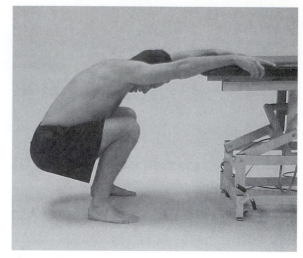

F I G U R E   3 2 - 2 7

Flat-footed squat stretch.

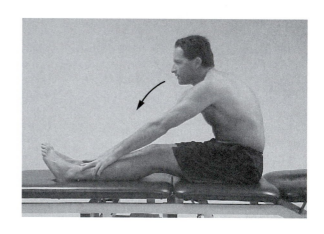

F I G U R E   3 2 - 2 8

Hamstring stretch.

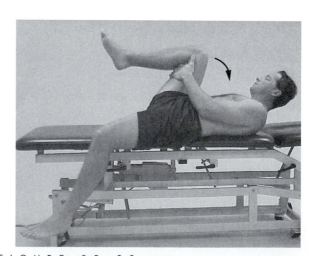

F I G U R E   3 2 - 2 9

Hip flexor stretch.

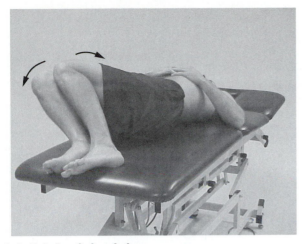

FIGURE 32-30

Knee rocking side to side.

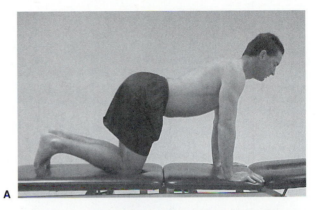

A

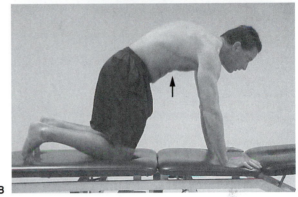

B

FIGURE 32-33

Pelvic tilt or pelvic rock. **A,** Swayback horse. **B,** Scared cat.

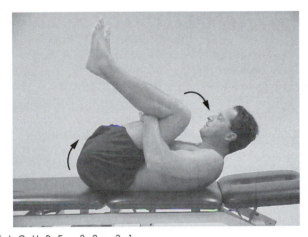

FIGURE 32-31

Knees toward chest rock.

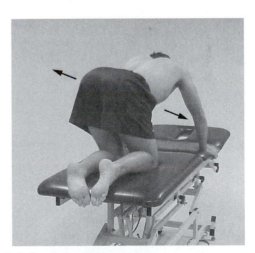

FIGURE 32-34

Kneeling—dog-tail wags.

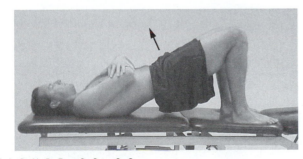

FIGURE 32-32

Supine hip-lift-bridge-rock.

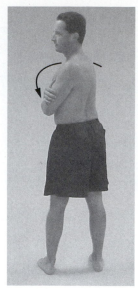

Sitting or standing rotation.

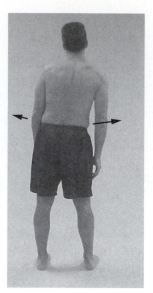

F I G U R E   3 2 - 3 7

Standing hip shift side to side.

REHABILITATION TECHNIQUES FOR LOW BACK PAIN

Low Back Pain

PATHOMECHANICS

In most cases, low back pain does not have serious or long-lasting pathology. It is generally accepted that the soft tissues (ligament, fascia, and muscle) can be the initial pain source. The patient's response to the injury and to the provocative stresses of evaluation is usually proportional to the time since the injury and the magnitude of the physical trauma of the injury. The soft tissues of the lumbar region should react according to the biological process of healing, and the time lines for healing should be like those for other body parts. There is little substantiation that injury to the low back should cause a pain syndrome that lasts longer than 6–8 weeks.[11,56]

INJURY MECHANISM

Back pain can result from one or a combination of the following problems: muscle strain, piriformis muscle or quadratus

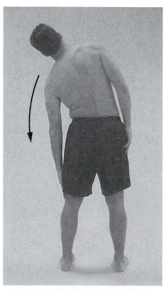

F I G U R E   3 2 - 3 6

Sitting or standing side bending.

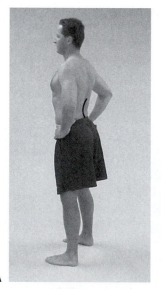
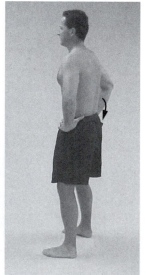

A   B

F I G U R E   3 2 - 3 8

Standing pelvic rock. **A,** Butt out. **B,** Tail tuck.

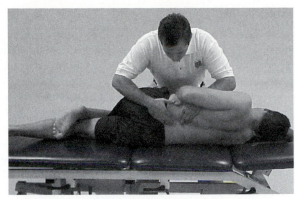

FIGURE 32-39

Various side-lying and back-lying positions can be used to both stretch and mobilize specific joint in the lumbar area.

lumborum myofascial pain or strain, myofascial trigger points, lumbar facet joint sprains, hypermobility syndromes, disk-related back problems, or sacroiliac joint dysfunction.

REHABILITATION CONCERNS

Acute versus Chronic Low Back Pain

The low back pain that most often occurs is an acute, painful experience rarely lasting longer than 3 weeks. As with many injuries, therapists often go through exercise or treatment fads in trying to rehabilitate the patient with low back pain. The latest fad might involve flexion exercise, extension exercise, joint mobilization, dynamic muscular stabilization, abdominal bracing, myofascial release, electrical stimulation protocols, and so on. To keep perspective, as therapists select exercises and modalities, they should keep in mind that 90 percent of people with back pain get resolution of the symptoms in 6 weeks, regardless of the care administered.[56,70]

There are patients who have pain persisting beyond 6 weeks. This group of patients will generally have a history of reinjury or exacerbation of previous injury. They describe a low back pain that is similar to their previous back pain experience.

These patients are experiencing an exacerbation or reinjury of previously injured tissues by continuing to apply stresses that may have created their original injury. This group of patients needs a more specific and formal treatment and rehabilitation program.[11,56]

There are also people who have chronic low back pain. This is a very small percentage of the population suffering from low back pain. The difference between the patient with an acute injury or reinjury and a person with chronic pain has been defined by Waddell. He states, "Chronic pain becomes a completely different clinical syndrome from acute pain."[70] Acute and chronic pain not only are different in time scale but are fundamentally different in kind. Acute and experimental pains bear a relatively straightforward relationship to peripheral stimulus, nociception, and tissue damage.

There may be some understandable anxiety about the meaning and consequences of the pain, but acute pain, disability, and illness behavior are generally proportionate to the physical findings. Pharmacological, physical, and even surgical treatments directed to the underlying physical disorder are generally highly effective in relieving acute pain. Chronic pain, disability, and illness behavior, in contrast, become increasingly dissociated from their original physical basis, and there may be little objective evidence of any remaining nociceptive stimulus. Instead, chronic pain and disability become increasingly associated with emotional distress, depression, failed treatment, and adoption of a sick role. Chronic pain progressively becomes a self-sustaining condition that is resistant to traditional medical management. Physical treatment directed to a supposed but unidentified and possibly nonexistent nociceptive source is not only understandably unsuccessful but may also cause additional physical damage. Failed treatment may both reinforce and aggravate pain, distress, disability, and illness behavior.[70]

REHABILITATION PROGRESSION

A discussion of the rehabilitation progression for the patient with low back pain can be much more specific and meaningful if treatment plans are lumped into two stages. Stage I (acute stage) treatment consists mainly of the modality treatment and pain-relieving exercises. Stage II treatment involves treating patients with a reinjury or exacerbation of a previous problem. The treatment plan in stage II goes beyond pain relief, strengthening, stretching, and mobilization to include trunk stabilization and movement training sequences and to provide a specific, guided program to return the patient to functional activity.[56]

Stage I (Acute Stage) Treatment

Modulating pain should be the initial focus of the therapist. Progressing rapidly from pain management to specific rehabilitation should be a primary goal of the acute stage of the rehabilitation plan. The most common treatment for pain relief in the acute stage is to use ice for analgesia. Rest, but not total bed rest, is used to allow the injured tissues to begin the healing process without the stresses that created the injury.[12]

Along with rest, during the initial treatment stage, the patient should be taught to increase comfort by using the *appropriate* body positioning techniques, described previously, which may involve (1) lateral shift corrections (Fig. 32-11), (2) extension exercises (Figs. 32-13 to 32-20), (3) flexion exercises (Figs. 32-21 to 32-31), or (4) self-mobilization exercises (see Figs. 16-46 and 16-47). Segmental spinal stabilization exercise should be initiated concurrently with these other exercises. Outside support, in the form of corsets and the use of props or pillows to enhance comfortable positions, also needs to be included in the initial pain management phase of treatment.[56,70] The patient should also be taught to avoid positions and movements that increase any sharp, painful episodes. The limits of these movements and positions that provide comfort should be the initial focus of any exercises.

The patient should be encouraged to move through this stage quickly and return to activity as soon as range, strength, and comfort will allow. The addition of a supportive corset during this stage should be based mostly on patient comfort. We suggest using an electric approach to the selection of the exercises, mixing the various protocols described according to the findings of the patient's evaluation. Rarely will a patient present with classic signs and symptoms that will dictate using one variety of exercise.

Stage II (Reinjury Stage) Treatment

In the reinjury or chronic stage of back rehabilitation, the goals of the treatment and training should again be based on a thorough evaluation of the patient. Identifying the causes of the patients' back problem and recurrences is very important in the management of their rehabilitation and prevention of reinjury. A goal for this stage of care is to make the patients responsible for the management of their back problem. Th therapist should identify specific problems and corrections that will help the patients better understand the mechanisms and management of their problem.[56]

Specific goals and exercises should be identified about the following:

- Which structures to stretch
- Which structures to strengthen
- Incorporating segmental spinal stabilization and abdominal bracing into the patient's daily life and exercise routine
- Progression of core stabilization exercises
- Which movements need a motor learning approach to control faulty mechanics[56]

Stretching

The therapist and the patient need to plan specific exercises to stretch restricted groups, maintain flexibility in normal muscle groups, and identify hypermobility that may be a part of the problem. In planning, instructing, and monitoring each exercise, adequate thought and good instruction must be used to ensure that the intended structures get stretched and areas of hypermobility are protected from overstretching.[23] Inadequate stabilization will lead to exercise movements that are so general that the exercise will encourage hyperflexibility at already hypermobile areas. Lack of proper stabilization during stretching may help perpetuate a structural problem that will continue to add to the patient's back pain.

In the therapist's evaluation of the patient with back pain, the following muscle groups should be assessed for flexibility.[31]

- Hip flexors
- Hamstrings
- Low back extensors
- Lumbar rotators
- Lumbar lateral flexors
- Hip adductors
- Hip abductors
- Hip rotators

Strengthening

There are numerous techniques for strengthening the muscles of the trunk and hip. Muscles are perhaps best strengthened by using techniques of progressive overload to achieve specific adaptation to imposed demands (SAID principle). The overload can take the form of increased weight load, increased holding time, increased repetition load, or increased stretch load to accomplish physiologic changes in muscle strength, muscle endurance, or flexibility of a body part.[13]

The treatment plan should call for an exercise that the athlete can easily accomplish successfully. Rapidly but gradually, the overload should push the patient to challenge the muscle group needing strengthening. The therapist and the patient should monitor continuously for increases in the patient's pain or recurrences of previous symptoms. If those changes occur, the exercises should be modified, delayed, or eliminated from the rehabilitation plan.[33,56]

Core Stabilization

Core stabilization training, dynamic abdominal bracing, and finding neutral position all describe a technique used to increase the stability of the trunk (see Chapter 18). This increased stability will enable the patient to maintain the spine and pelvis in the most comfortable and acceptable mechanical position that will control the forces of repetitive microtrauma and protect the structures of the back from further damage. Core muscular control is one key to giving the patients the ability to stabilize their trunk and control their posture. Abdominal strengthening routines are rigorous, and the patient must complete them with vigor. However, in their functional activities, the patients need to take advantage of their abdominal strength to stabilize the trunk and protect the back.[23,38,58]

Richardson et al. focus attention on motor control of the transversus abdominis and lumbar multifidii in various positions.[28,56] Once this control is established, different positions and movements are added. As the vigor of the exercise is progressively increased, the patient will incorporate the more global muscles in stabilizing his/her core (see Chapter 18). Then the patient moves into the functional exercise progression with the spinal segment stabilization as the base movement in core stabilization, which is needed to perform functionally.[56] The concept of increasing trunk stability with muscle contractions that support and limit the extremes of spinal movement is important.

Basic functional training. The patients must be constantly committed to improving body mechanics and trunk control in all postures in their activities of daily living. The therapist needs to evaluate the patients' daily patterns and give them instruction, practice, and monitoring on the best and least stressful body mechanics in as many activities as possible.

The basic program follows the developmental sequence of posture control, starting with supine and prone extremity movement while actively stabilizing the trunk. The patient is then progressed to all fours, kneeling, and standing (Fig. 32-40).

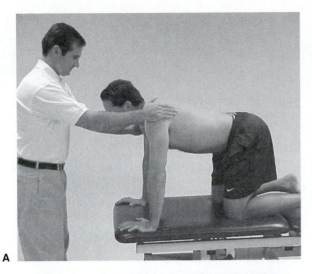

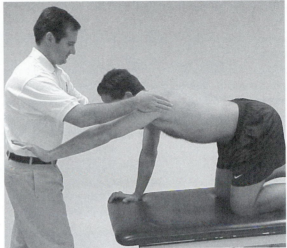

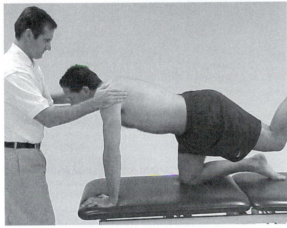

FIGURE 32-40

Weight shifting and stabilization exercises should progress from **A,** quadriped to **B,** triped to **C,** biped.

Emphasis on trunk control and stability is maintained as the patient works through this exercise sequence.[23,40,56]

The most critical aspect for developing motor control is repetition of exercise. However, variability in positioning, speed of movement, and changes in movement patterns must also be incorporated. The variability of the exercise will allow the patients to generalize their newly learned trunk control to the constant changes necessary in their movements. The basic exercise, transversus abdominis and lumbar multifidii coactivation, is the key. Incorporating this stabilization contraction into various activities helps reinforce trunk stabilization and returns trunk control a subconscious automatic response.

The use of augmented feedback (EMG, palpation, ultrasound imagery, pressure gauges) of the transversus abdominus and lumbar multifidii contractions may be needed early in the exercise plan to help maximize the results of each exercise session supervised by the therapist. The therapist should have the patient internalize this feedback as quickly as possible to make the athlete apparatus-free and more functional. With augmented feedback, it is recommended that the patient be rapidly and progressively weaned from dependency on external feedback.

Advanced functional training. Each activity that the patient is involved in becomes part of the advanced exercise rehabilitation plan. The usual place to start is with the patient's strength and conditioning program. Each step of the program is monitored, and emphasis is placed on spinal segmental stabilization for even the simple task of putting the weights on a bar or getting on and off of exercise equipment. Each exercise in their strength and conditioning program should be retaught, and the patients are made aware of their best mechanical position and the proper stabilizing muscular contraction. The strength program is patient specific, attempting to strengthen weak areas and improve strength in muscle groups needed for better function.[56]

The patients should be taught to start their stabilizing contractions before starting any movement. This presets their posture and stabilization awareness before their movement takes place. As the movement occurs, they will become less aware of the stabilization contraction as they attempt to complete an exercise.

They might revert to old postures and habits, so feedback is important.

Each patient is different, not only with the individual back problem but also with the abilities to gain motor skill. Athletes differ in degree of control and in the speed at which they acquire these new skills of core stabilization.

Reducing stress to the back by using braces, orthotics, shoes, or comfortable supportive furniture (beds, desks, or chairs) is essential to help the patients minimize chronic or overload stresses to their back. The stabilization exercise should also be incorporated into their activities of daily living.[45] The use of a low back corset or brace may also make the patient more comfortable (Fig. 32-56).

CRITERIA FOR NORMAL RETURN

For most low back problems the stage I treatment and exercise programs will get the patients back into their activities quickly. If the pain or dysfunction is pronounced or the problem becomes recurrent, an in-depth evaluation and treatment using stage I and stage II exercise protocols will be necessary. The team approach, with patient, doctor, and physical therapist working together, will provide the comprehensive approach needed to manage the patient's back problem. Close attention to and emphasis on the patient's progress will provide both the patient and the therapist with the encouragement to continue this program.

Muscular Strains

INJURY MECHANISM

Evaluative findings include a history of sudden or chronic stress that initiates pain in a muscular area during the workout. There are three points on the physical examination that must be positive to indicate the muscle as the primary problem. There will be tenderness to palpation in the muscular area; the muscular pain will be provoked with contraction and with stretch of the involved muscle.

REHABILITATION PROGRESSION

The treatment should include the standard protection, ice, and compression. Ice may be applied in the form of ice massage or ice bags, depending on the area involved. An elastic wrap or corset would protect and compress the back musculature. Additional modalities would include pulsed ultrasound for a biostimulative effect and electrical stimulation for pain relief and muscle reeducation. The exercises used in rehabilitation should make the involved muscle contract and stretch, starting with very mild exercise and progressively increasing the intensity and repetition loads. In general this would include active extension exercises such as hip lifts (Figs. 32-17 to 32-19), alternate arm and leg, hip extension (Fig. 32-15), trunk extension

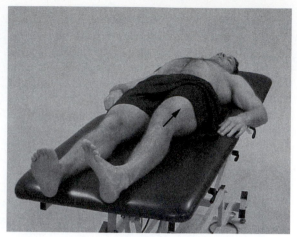

FIGURE 32-41

Back-lying—hip-hike shifting.

(Fig. 32-20), and quadratus hip shift exercises (Figs. 32-41 to 32-43). A good series of abdominal spinal segmental stabilization and core stabilization exercises would also be helpful (Figs. 32-23 and 32-24). Stretching exercises might include the following: knee to chest (Figs. 32-21 and 32-22), side-lying leg hang to stretch the hip flexors (Fig. 32-29), slump sitting (Fig. 32-26), and knee rocking side to side (Fig. 32-30).

CRITERIA FOR RETURN TO NORMAL

Initially, the patients may wish to continue to use a brace or corset, but they should be encouraged to do away with the corset as their back strengthens and their performance returns to normal.[13,33]

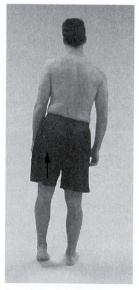

FIGURE 32-42

Standing hip hike.

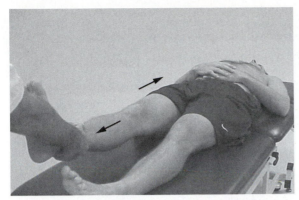

FIGURE 32-43

Back-lying—hip hike resisted.

Piriformis Muscle Strain

PATHOMECHANICS

Piriformis syndrome was discussed in detail in Chapter 28. The piriformis muscle refers pain to the posterior sacroiliac region, to the buttocks, and sometimes down the posterior or posterolateral thigh. The pain is usually described as a deep ache that can get more intense with exercise and with sitting with the hips flexed, adducted, and medially rotated. The pain gets sharper and more intense with activities that require decelerating medial hip and leg rotation during weight bearing.[5]

Tenderness to palpation has a characteristic pattern, with tenderness medial and proximal to the greater trochanter and just lateral to the posterior superior iliac spine (PSIS). Isometric abduction in the sitting position produces pain in the posterior hip buttock area, and the movement will be weak or hesitant. Passive hip internal rotation in the sitting position will also bring on posterior hip and buttock pain.[47]

REHABILITATION PROGRESSION

Rehabilitation exercises should include both strengthening and stretching.[5,47] Strengthening exercises should include prone-lying hip internal rotation with elastic resistance (Fig. 32-44), hip-lift bridges (Fig. 32-45), hand-knee position fire hydrant exercise (Fig. 32-46), side-lying hip abduction straight leg raises (Fig. 32-47), and prone hip extension exercise (Fig. 32-48).

Stretching exercises for the piriformis include back-lying legs-crossed hip abduction stretch (Fig. 32-49), back-lying with the involved leg crossed over the uninvolved leg, ankle to knee position, pulling the uninvolved knee toward the chest to create the stretch (Fig. 32-50), contract-relax-stretch with elbow pressure to the muscle insertion during the relaxation phase (Figs. 32-51A and B).[34,61,64] This can also be done in the sitting position with the same mechanics, but the patient leans over at the waist and brings the chest toward the knee.

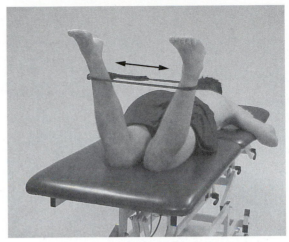

FIGURE 32-44

Prone-lying hip internal rotation with elastic resistance.

Quadratus Lumborum Strain

PATHOMECHANICS

Pain from the quadratus lumborum muscle is described as an aching, sharp pain located in the flank, in the lateral back area, and near the posterior sacroiliac region and upper buttocks. The patient usually describes pain or moving from sitting to standing, standing for long periods, coughing, sneezing, and walking. Activities requiring trunk rotation or side bending aggravate the pain. The muscle is tender to palpation near the origin along the lower ribs and along the insertion on the iliac crest. Pain will be aggravated on side bending, and the pain will usually be localized to one side. For example, with a right quadratus problem, side bending right and left would provoke only right-side pain. Supine hip-hiking movements would also provoke the pain.

REHABILITATION PROGRESSION

Rehabilitation strengthening exercise should include back-lying hip-hike shifting (Fig. 32-54), standing with one leg on elevated surface and the other free to move below that level, hip-hike on the free side (Fig. 32-55), and back-lying hip-hike resisted by pulling on the involved leg (Fig. 32-43).

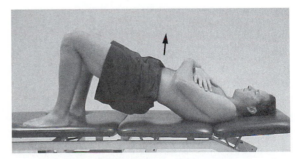

FIGURE 32-45

Hip-lift bridges.

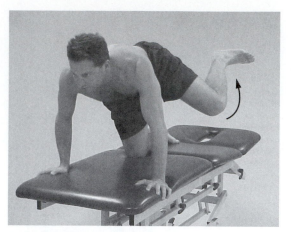

F I G U R E   3 2 - 4 6

Hand-knee position—fire hydrant exercise.

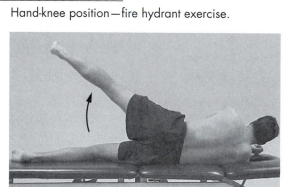

F I G U R E   3 2 - 4 7

Side-lying hip abduction straight-leg raises.

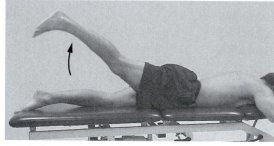

F I G U R E   3 2 - 4 8

Prone hip extension exercise.

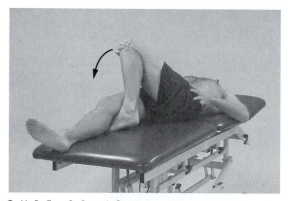

F I G U R E   3 2 - 4 9

Back-lying legs-crossed hip adduction stretch.

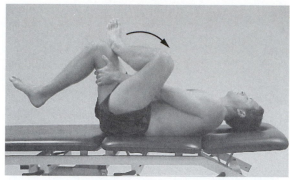

F I G U R E   3 2 - 5 0

Self piriformis stretch.

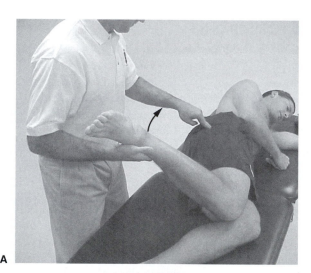

A

B

F I G U R E   3 2 - 5 1

Piriformis stretch using elbow pressure. **A,** Start-contract.
B, Relaxation-stretch.

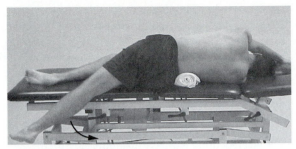

FIGURE 32-52

Side-lying stretch over pillow roll.

Stretching exercises should include side-lying over a pillow roll leg-hand stretch (Fig. 32-52), supine self-stretch with legs crossed (Fig. 32-53), hip-hike exercise with hand pressure to increase stretch (Fig. 32-54), and standing one leg on a small book stretch (Fig. 32-55).[71]

Myofascial Pain and Trigger Points

PATHOMECHANICS AND INJURY MECHANISM

The above examples of muscle-oriented back pain in both the piriformis and quadratus lumborum could also have a myofascial origin. The major component in successfully changing myofascial pain is stretching the muscle back to a normal resting length. The muscle irritation and congestion that create the trigger points are relieved, and normal blood flow resumes, further reducing the irritants in the area. Stretching through a painful trigger point is difficult.

A variety of comfort and counterirritant modalities can be used preliminary to, during, and after the stretching to enhance the effect of the exercise. Some of the methods used successfully are dry needling, local anesthetic injection, ice massage, friction massage, acupressure massage, ultrasound electrical stimulation, extracorporal shock wave therapy, and cold sprays.[32]

The indications for treating low back pain with myofascial stretching and treatment techniques are as follows[32]:

1. Subjectively, muscle soreness and fatigue from repetitive motions are common antecedent mechanisms. Patients are also susceptible as fatigue and stress overload specific muscle groups. There may be a history of sudden onset during

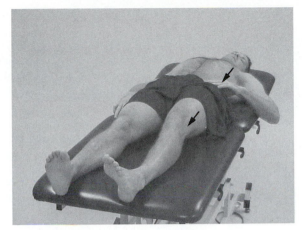

FIGURE 32-54

Hip-hike exercise with hand pressure.

or shortly after an acute overload stress, or there may be a gradual onset with repetitive or postural overload of the affected muscle.

The pain may be an incapacitating event in the case of acute onset, but it may also be a nagging, aggravating type of pain with an intensity that varies from an awareness of discomfort to a severe unrelenting type of pain. The pain location is usually a referred pain area remote from the actual myofascial trigger point. These trigger points can be present but quiescent until they are activated by overload, fatigue, trauma, or chilling. These points are called *latent trigger points*. This deep, aching pain can be specifically localized, but the athlete is not sensitive to palpation in these areas. This pain can often be reproduced by maintaining pressure on a hypersensitive myofascial trigger point.

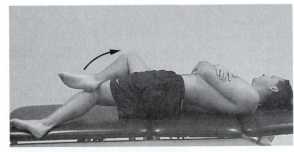

FIGURE 32-53

Supine self-stretch—legs crossed.

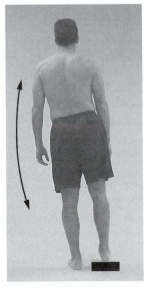

FIGURE 32-55

Standing one-leg-up stretch.

2. Passive or active stretching of the affected myofascial structure increases pain.

3. The stretch range of muscle is restricted.

4. The pain is increased when the muscle is contracted against a fixed resistance or the muscle is allowed to contract into a very shortened range. The pain in this case is described as a muscle cramping pain.

5. The muscle may be slightly weak.

6. Trigger points may be located within a taut band of the muscle. If taut bands are found during palpation, explore them for local hypersensitive areas.

7. Pressure on the hypersensitive area will often cause a "jump sign"; as the therapist strums the sensitive area, the patient's muscle involuntarily jumps in response.

8. The primary muscle groups that create low back pain in athletes are the quadratus lumborum and the piriformis muscles.[34,61,62,64]

Travell and Simons have devoted two volumes to the causes and treatment of various myofascial pains.[61,62] They have done a very thorough job of describing the symptoms and signs of each area of the body, and they give very specific guidance on exercises and positioning in their treatment protocols.

REHABILITATION TECHNIQUE

Myofascial trigger points may be treated using the following steps:

1. Position the patient comfortably but in a position that will lend him/her to stretching the involved muscle group.

2. Caution the patient to use mild progressive stretches rather than sudden, sharp, hard stretches.

3. Hot pack the area for 10 minutes, and follow with an ultrasound and electrical stimulation treatment over the affected muscle.

4. Use an ice cup, and use two to three slow strokes starting at the trigger point and moving in one direction toward their pain reference area and over the full length of the muscle.

5. Begin stretching well within the patient's comfort. A stretch should be maintained for a minimum of 15 seconds. The stretch should be released until the patient is comfortable again. The next stretch repetition should then be progressively more intense if tolerated, and the position of the stretch should also be varied slightly. Repeat the stretch four to six times.

6. Hot pack the area, and have the patient go through some active stretches of the muscle.

7. Refer to Travell and Simons' manual for specific references on other muscle groups.[34,61,62]

8. Active release and position release techniques are used to treat and resolve trigger points (see Chapter 15). Therapeutic eccentric active massage has shown some clinical success. In this technique, the muscle for fascia associated with the identified trigger point is actively contracted to its shortest possible length. Using a small amount of lubricant, the active trigger point is compressed with a firm steady pressure. The therapist provides resistance to the shortened movement, and the patient is instructed to continue to resist but also allow the eccentric lengthening of the muscle to occur in a smooth, controlled manner. As the muscle lengthens under the compressive massage, the trigger point is compressed and the irritants in the area are dispersed over a greater area. This helps the pain decease, and the muscle begins to function more normally.

The first repetition is usually uncomfortable for the patient. Subsequent repetitions are more comfortable and the patient can control the contraction better. Six to eight repetitions are used for each trigger point treated. This technique is empirically based, and research studies are needed to establish their validity.

Lumbar Facet Joint Sprains

PATHOMECHANICS AND INJURY MECHANISM

Sprains may occur in any of the ligaments in the lumbar spine. However, the most common sprain involves lumbar facet joints. Facet joint sprain typically occurs when bending forward and twisting while lifting or moving some object. The patients will report a sudden acute episode that caused the problem, or they will give a history of a chronic repetitive stress that caused the gradual onset of a pain that got progressively worse with continuing activity. The pain is local to the structure that has been injured, and the patient can clearly localize the area. The pain is described as a sore pain that gets sharper in response to certain movements or postures. The pain is located centrally or just lateral to the spinous process areas and is deep.

Local symptoms will occur in response to movements, and the athlete will usually limit the movement in those ranges that are painful. When the vertebra is moved passively with a posteroanterior or rotational pressure through the spinous process, the pain may be provoked.

REHABILITATION PROGRESSION

The treatment should include the standard protection, ice, and compression as mentioned previously. Both pulsed ultrasound and electrical stimulation could also be used similarly to the treatment of muscle strains but localized to the specific joint area.

Joint mobilization using posterior–anterior glides (see Fig. 16-36) and rotational glides (see Figs. 16-38 and 16-39) should help reduce pain and increase joint nutrition. The patient should be instructed in segmental spinal stabilization exercises using transversus abdominis and lumbar multifidii coactivation and good postural control (Figs. 32-3 to 32-10). Strengthening exercises for abdominals (Figs. 32-23 to 32-25) and back extensors (Figs. 32-17 to 32-20) should initially be limited to a pain-free range. Stretching in all ranges should start well within a comfort range and gradually increase until trunk movements reach normal ranges. Patients should be supported with a corset or range-limiting brace, which should be used only temporarily until normal strength, muscle control, and pain-free range are achieved.[13,36,37,66,67] It is important to guard against the development of postural changes that might occur in response to pain.

Hypermobility Syndromes (Spondylolysis/Spondylolisthesis)

PATHOMECHANICS

Hypermobility of the low back may be attributed to spondylolysis or spondylolisthesis. Spondylolysis involves a degeneration of the vertebrae and, more commonly, a defect in the pars interarticularis of the articular processes of the vertebrae.[43] It is often attributed to a congenital weakness, with the defect occurring as a stress fracture. Spondylolysis might produce no symptoms unless a disk herniation occurs or there is sudden trauma such as hyperextension. Commonly spondylolysis begins unilaterally. However, if it extends bilaterally, there may be some slipping of one vertebra on the one below it.[26]

A spondylolisthesis is considered to be a complication of spondylolysis often resulting in hypermobility of a vertebral segment.[15] Spondylolisthesis has the highest incidence with L5 slipping on S1.[43]

INJURY MECHANISM

Movements that characteristically hyperextend the spine are most likely to cause this condition.[43]

REHABILITATION CONCERNS

The patients usually have a relatively long history of feeling "something go" in their back. They complain of a low back pain described as a persistent ache across the back (belt type). This pain does not usually interfere with their workout performance but is usually worse when fatigued or after sitting in a slumped posture for an extended time. The patients may also complain of a tired feeling in the low back. They describe the need to move frequently and get temporary relief of pain through self-manipulation. They often describe self-manipulative behavior more than 10 times a day. Their pain is relieved by rest, and they do not usually feel the pain during exercise. On physical examination, the patient usually will have full and painless trunk movements, but there may be a wiggle or hesitation in forward bending at the midrange. On backward bending, their movement may appear to hinge at one spinal segment. When extremes of range are maintained for 15–30 seconds, the patient feels a lumbosacral ache. On return from forward bending, the patient will use thigh climbing to regain the neutral position. On palpation there may be tenderness localized to one spinal segment.[43,50]

REHABILITATION PROGRESSION

Patients with this problem will fall into the reinjury stage of back pain and may require extensive treatment to regain stability of the trunk. The patient's pain should be treated symptomatically. Initially, bracing and occasionally bed rest for 1–3 days will help reduce pain. The major focus in rehabilitation should be

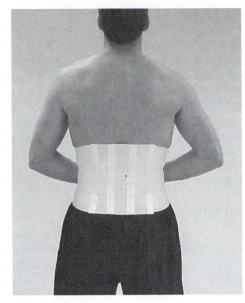

FIGURE 32-56

A lower-lumbar corset or brace.

on segmental spinal stabilization exercises that control or stabilize the hypermobile segment (Figs. 32-3 to 32-10). Progressive trunk-strengthening exercises, especially through the midrange, should be incorporated. Core stabilization exercises that concentrate on transversus abdominis behavior and endurance should also be used (see Chapter 18).[27,28,30,39,46,48,51–53] The patient should avoid manipulation and self-manipulation as well as stretching and flexibility exercises. Corsets and braces are beneficial if the patient uses them only for support during higher-level activities and for short (1–2 hour) periods to help with pain relief and fatigue (Fig. 32-56).[23,56] Hypermobility of a lumbar vertebrae may make the patient more susceptible to lumbar muscle strains and ligament sprains. Thus it may be necessary for the patient to avoid vigorous activity. The use of a low back corset or brace might also make the patient more comfortable (Fig. 32-56).[26]

Disk-Related Back Pain

PATHOMECHANICS

The lumbar disks are subject to constant abnormal stresses stemming from faulty body mechanics, trauma, or both, which, over a period of time, can cause degeneration, tears, and cracks in the annulus fibrosus.[9] The disk, most often injured, lies between the L4 and L5 vertebrae. The L5-S1 disk is the second most commonly affected.[63]

INJURY MECHANISM

The mechanism of a disk injury is the same as that for the lumbosacral sprain—forward bending and twisting that places abnormal strain on the lumbar region. The movement that produces herniation or bulging of the nucleus pulposus may be minimal, and associated pain may be significant. Besides injuring soft tissues, such a stress may herniate an already degenerated disk by causing the nucleus pulposus to protrude into or through the annulus fibrosis. As the disk progressively degenerates, a prolapsed disk may develop in which the nucleus moves completely through the annulus. If the nucleus moves into the spinal canal and comes in contact with a nerve root, this is referred to as extruded disk. This protrusion of the nucleus pulposus may place pressure on the spinal cord or spinal nerves, causing radiating pains similar to those of sciatica, as occurs in piriformis syndrome. If the material of the nucleus separates from the disk and begins to migrate, a sequestrated disk exists.[63]

REHABILITATION CONCERNS

The patients will report a centrally located pain that radiates unilaterally or spreads across the back. They may describe a sudden or gradual onset that becomes particularly severe after they have rested and then tried to resume their activities. They may complain of tingling or numb feelings in a dermatomal pattern or sciatic radiation. Forward bending and sitting postures increase their pain. The patient's symptoms are usually worse in the morning on first arising and get better through the day. Coughing and sneezing may increase their pain.[63]

On physical examination, the patient will have a hip shifted, forward bent posture. On active movements, side bending toward the hip shift is painful and limited. Side bending away from the shift is more mobile and does not provoke the pain. Forward bending is very limited and painful, and guarding is very apparent. On palpation, there may be tenderness around the painful area. Posteroanterior pressure over the involved segment increases the pain. Passive straight-leg raising will increase the back or leg pain during the first 30° of hip flexion. Bilateral knee-to-chest movement will increase the back pain. Neurological testing (strength, sensory reflex) may be positive for differences between right and left.[63]

REHABILITATION PROGRESSION

The patient should be treated initially with pain-reducing modalities (ice, electrical stimulation, rest). The therapist should then use the lateral shift correction (Fig. 32-11), followed by a gentle extension exercise (Fig. 32-16). The patient is then sent home with the following rest and home exercise program.

The patient must commit to resting in a flat-lying position three to four times a day for 20–30 minutes. During that time the patient can use some prone press-up extension exercises, holding the stretched position for 15–20 seconds for each repetition (Figs. 32-13 and 32-14). Another recommended pain-relieving position is the 90/90 position—90° of hip flexion and 90° of knee flexion (Fig. 32-57). Both of these exercises provide very mild traction to the lumbar spine, which enhances the centralization and nourishment effect of the flat-lying position on the disk, which in turn leads to decreased pain and increased function. Segmental spinal stabilization exercises can also be incorporated into the rest positions and may be used concurrently with other modalities (Figs. 32-3 to 32-10).[68]

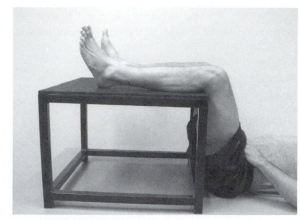

F I G U R E   3 2 - 5 7

The 90/90 position. The patient is positioned back-lying with hips flexed to 90° and knees supported at 90° by stool or pillows.

The goal is to reduce the disk protrusion and restore normal posture. When posture, pain, and segmental spinal control return to normal, the core stabilization exercises should be emphasized and progressed. The patient may recover easily from the first episode, but if repeated episodes occur, then the patient should also start on the reinjury stage of back rehabilitation.

When the patient changes positions—sit to stand or lying to stand—he/she should do a lateral shift self-correction (Figs. 32-12 and 32-16), followed by a segmental spinal coactivation contraction (Figs. 32-8 to 32-10). Some gentle flexion exercises, low back corsets, and heat wraps may make the athlete more comfortable.

If the desk is extruded or sequestrated, about the only thing that can be done is to modulate pain with electrical stimulation. Flexion exercises and lying supine in a flexed position may help with comfort. The use of a low back corset or brace may also make the patient more comfortable (Fig. 32-56). Sometimes the symptoms will resolve with time. But if there are signs of nerve damage, surgery may be necessary.[68]

Sacroiliac Joint Dysfunction

PATHOMECHANICS AND INJURY MECHANISM

A sprain of the sacroiliac joint may result from twisting with both feet on the ground, stumbling forward, falling backward, stepping too far down and landing heavily on one leg, or forward bending with the knees locked during lifting.[36] Activities involving unilateral forceful movements are the usual activities associated with the onset of pain. Any of these mechanisms can produce stretching and irritation of the sacroiliac, sacrotuberous, or sacrospinous ligaments.[39]

REHABILITATION CONCERNS

The patient will report a dull, achy back pain near or medial to the PSIS, with some associated muscle guarding. The pain may radiate into the buttocks or posterolateral thigh. The patient may describe a heaviness, dullness, or deadness in the leg or referred pain to the groin, adductor, or hamstring on the same side. The pain may be more noticeable during the stance phase of walking and on stair climbing.[72]

Side bending toward the painful side will increase the pain. Straight-leg raising will increase pain in the sacroiliac joint area after 45° of motion. On palpation, there may be tenderness over the PSIS, medial to the PSIS, in the muscles of the buttocks, and anteriorly over the pubic symphysis. The back musculature will have increased tone on one side.[16,31,54]

If a sacroiliac joint is stressed and reaches an end-range position in rotation, the joint can become dysfunctional as pain, mechanical form closure locking, and/or muscle guarding create hypomobility at the joint. This hypomobility is usually temporary, and often spontaneous repositioning will occur. This allows the pain to go away and muscle guarding to disappear. With the joint back to normal alignment, function returns to normal.[31,54]

When normal alignment does not spontaneously return, treatment efforts should initially mobilize the joints and then work on spinal segment stabilization to maintain and improve sacroiliac joint stability. These exercises, along with core stability training are the key to preventing recurrences. The therapist should consider sacroiliac dysfunction as a problem with pelvic stability rather than mobility.[31,52]

REHABILITATION PROGRESSION

Recent studies of sacroiliac joint testing cast severe doubt on our ability to recognize the postural asymmetries that have been associated with directionally specific techniques.[16,31,54] The treatment of sacroiliac dysfunction has been grounded in the empiricism of doing techniques that reduce pain. Postural asymmetries have given the therapist a starting point for directional specific techniques, but the instruction in deciding on appropriate technique is to try one and, if the outcome is not satisfactory, move on to the next technique, which may be biomechanically opposite to the first technique.[13,39] Empirically, these mobilizations have been used for many years and have demonstrated a good effect on sacroiliac dysfunctions with an asymmetry of the pelvis and pain. Each technique will have about the same effect on the pelvis and sacroiliac joints because the joints are part of an arch, and forces at any point in the arch can be translated throughout the structure to affect each joint. These stretches should be used only at the beginning stage of treatment to free the joint from the initial hypomobility.[72]

A posterior innominate rotation may be used to treat sacroiliac dysfunction (Fig. 32-58). The patient is positioned with legs and trunk moved toward the side of the low ASIS. This locks the lumbar spine so that the mobilization will affect the sacroiliac joint. The therapist stands on the side away from the low ASIS and rotates the patient's trunk toward the therapist. The patient is instructed to breathe and relax as the therapist overpressures the rotation to take up the slack. The lower hand contacts the low ASIS and mobilizes the innominate into posterior rotation.[50]

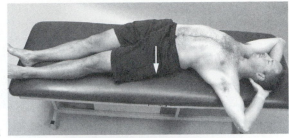

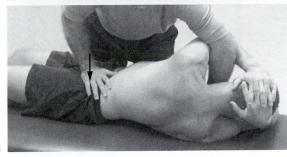

FIGURE 32-58

Posterior innominate rotation. **A,** Starting position. **B,** Mobilization position.

The therapist should also mobilize the sacroiliac joint using stretching positions 1 and 2 or the anterior–posterior sacroiliac joint rotation stretch to correct the postural asymmetry (Figs. 32-59 and 32-60).[7–9,22,71] The stretch exercise should be done in two or three bouts a day, three or four repetitions each time, holding the stretch position for 20–30 seconds. Spinal segment stability exercises are utilized after each stretching about (Figs. 32-4 to 32-10).[52] The stretches should not be continued longer than 2 or 3 days. The spinal segmental stabilization exercises are continued to try to create the behaviors that stabilize the sacroiliac joints and strengthen the muscles that support the joint. The exercises should be progressed to include more core stabilization and functional training, leading to return to sports. Corsets and pelvic stabilizing belts are also helpful during higher-level activities and/or if the patient is having problems with recurrences (Fig. 32-56).[50]

Sacroilic stretch positions 1 and 2 that will help realign patients' pelvis when they are having sacroiliac dysfunction. Position-1 (Fig. 32-59) and position-2 (Fig. 32-60) stretches can be done in both right side-lying and left side-lying positions. The starting position of the position-1 stretch is side-lying with the upper hip flexed 70°–80° and the knee flexed about 90° (Fig. 32-59). The patient's trunk is then rotated toward the upper side as far as is comfortable. The patient is instructed to lift the top leg into hip abduction and internal rotation, and resist the athletic trainer for 5 seconds. The patient is instructed to breathe and exhale as the therapist gently overpressures the trunk rotation. The patient is then instructed to relax the hip and leg and allow the leg to drop toward the floor. As the patient relaxes, the therapist applies a gentle overpressure to the foot and takes up the slack as the patient allows the hip and leg to drop further to the floor.

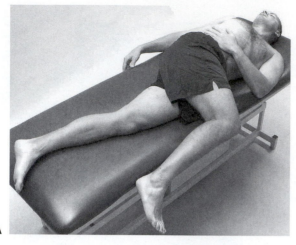
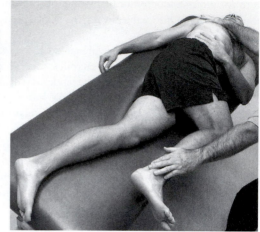
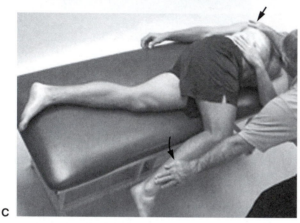

FIGURE 32-59

Sacroiliac stretch position 1. **A,** Starting position. **B,** Position for isometric resistance.
C, Stretch position.

In the position-2 stretch (Fig. 32-60), the patient is positioned on either the right or left side. The patient is side-lying with the trunk rotated so that the lower arm is behind the hip and the upper arm is able to reach off the table toward the floor. Both knees and hips are flexed to approximately 90°. The patient's knees are supported on the therapist's thigh. The therapist also supports the feet in this stage of the stretch.

Before beginning the stretch component of the position-2 stretches, the therapist provides isometric resistance to lifting both legs toward the ceiling, holding the contraction for 5 seconds. The patient is instructed to exhale while relaxing the legs and allowing them to drop toward the floor. The therapist adds a light pressure to the feet and shoulder blade area to guide the stretch and take up slack. The therapist holds the patient in a comfortable maximum stretch for 20–30 seconds.

Rehabilitation Techniques for Thoracic Spine Conditions

Injuries to the thoracic region of the spine have a much lower rate in incidence than do injuries to the cervical, lumbar, and sacral regions. This lower rate of acute injury is due primarily to the articulation of the thoracic vertebrae with the ribs, which acts to stabilize and limit motion of the vertebrae. However,

there are two conditions that affect the thoracic region of the spine and thus posture that should be discussed: Scheuermann's kyphosis and scoliosis.

Scheuermann's Kyphosis

Kyphosis refers to the natural sagittal plane curve of the thoracic spine, which normally has a forward curve of 20°–40°. If the thoracic curve is more than 40°–50°, it is considered excessive. This is an abnormal spinal deformity. There are many possible causes of excessive kyphosis, including posture, healed vertebral fractures, osteoporosis, rheumatoid arthritis, or Scheuermann's disease.[19]

PATHOMECHANICS

Scheuermann's disease occurs during growth in the adolescent.[73] In lay terms this deformity has been described as "hunchback" posture. In this condition the thoracic curve is usually 45°–75°. This is due to vertebral wedging of greater than 5° of three or more adjacent vertebrae. In patients with Scheuermann's disease, the anterior longitudinal ligament is thickened. Tightness of this ligament may affect the growth of the vertebra during childhood, leading to too much growth in the posterior

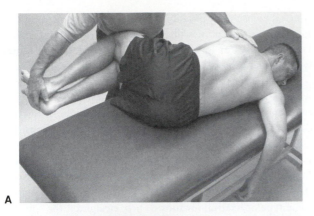

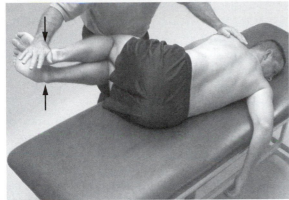

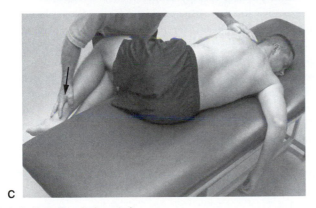

FIGURE 32-60

Sacroiliac stretch position 2. **A,** Starting position. **B,** Position for isometric resistance. **C,** Stretch position.

portion of the vertebrae and too little anteriorly, which produces a wedged vertebra. Problems with the mechanics of the spine, muscle imbalances, and avascular necrosis may also play a role in the development of kyphosis. Wedging of the vertebrae in this triangular shape causes an excessive curve in the spine. In addition, Schmorl's nodes can also develop, where the disc between the affected vertebra herniates through the bone at the bottom and the top of that vertebra's endplate.[73] Males are twice as likely to develop this type of kyphosis as females and there also seems to be a high genetic predisposition to this disease.[19,21]

REHABILITATION CONCERNS

Symptoms of Scheuermann's disease generally develop around puberty, between the ages of 10 and 15. When the problem

actually begins is hard to determine because X-rays will not show the changes until the patient is around 10 or 11. The disease is often discovered when parents notice the onset of poor posture, or slouching, in their child. Alternatively, the adolescent might experience fatigue and some pain in the mid-back. The pain is rarely disabling or severe at this point, unless the deformity is severe. The onset of excessive kyphosis is generally slow. With Scheuermann's disease, there is generally a rigid deformity or curvature. It worsens with flexion and partially corrects with extension. Pain typically increases with time and length of the deformity. About one-third of patients with Scheuermann's kyphosis will also have scoliosis. As the patient ages, arthritic changes may appear on the X-rays.

If the kyphosis is less than 75°, the deformity will usually be treated without surgery. The usual option is casting, or bracing.[21] The brace will be successful in straightening the spine only in patients who are still growing. The brace is designed to hold the spine in a straighter, upright posture. The goal of bracing is to try to "guide" the growth of the vertebrae to straighten the spine. This is thought to work by taking pressure off the anterior potion of the vertebra, and allowing the anterior bone growth to catch up with the posterior growth. In older patients, a brace may be used to support the spine and relieve pain, but it will not actually change the curve. Though many braces are available, the Milwaukee brace is the most commonly used. The brace will include lateral pads to keep the shoulders pulled back and a chin extension. The brace is usually effective in adolescents with curves of less than 75°. If the patient wears the brace 16 hours each day, there is often correction of the deformity within 2 years.[25]

Surgery for the correction of Scheuermann's kyphosis typically consists of a fusion of the abnormal vertebrae. The operation has two phases—one operation is done on the front of the spine and another on the back of the spine. A posterior-only fusion is rare because of the rigidity of the curves. In the operation, the spine is fused anteriorly and posteriorly with surgical implants.[19,25]

REHABILITATION PROGRESSION

In nonoperative cases exercises are used in combination with a brace. Extension exercises for the upper back (Figs. 32-13 to 32-20) can improve posture and prevent the spine from slouching forward. Hamstring stretches (Fig. 32-28) and pelvic tilt exercises (Fig. 32-33) improve posture by preventing extra lordosis in the low back. Pain should also be addressed by applying heat, cold, ultrasound, and massage treatments. Adults who have had kyphosis for many years (and the resulting low back pain from too much lordosis) benefit from postural exercises to reduce the lumbar curve, followed by core stabilization exercises to help them keep better posture.[19]

Rehabilitation after surgery is more complex. In-hospital treatment sessions should help patients learn to move and do routine activities of daily living without putting extra strain on the back. Patients should wear a back brace or support belt. They should be cautious about overdoing activities in the first few weeks after surgery. Many patients wait up to 3 months before beginning a rehabilitation program after fusion surgery for Scheuermann's disease. Exercises should include both flexion and extension activities and should particularly concentrate on core stabilization. Treatment should last for 8–12 weeks. Full recovery may take up to 8 months.[21]

Scoliosis

PATHOMECHANICS

A scoliosis is an abnormal curve that occurs in the coronal or frontal plane in the thoracic spine or in the lumbar spine, or in both regions simultaneously. The curves can range from as minor as 10° to severe cases of more than 100°. The most common type of scoliosis called *idiopathic adolescent scoliosis* is first observed and treated in childhood or adolescence at the growth spurt of puberty.[55] Idiopathic adolescent scoliosis is generally treated with a brace, or in severe cases, surgery at the end of the teenager's growth spurt.[10]

A condition called *adult scoliosis* develops after puberty.[6] Adult scoliosis can be the result of untreated or unrecognized childhood scoliosis, or it can actually arise during adulthood. Sometimes adult scoliosis is the result of changes in the spine due to aging and degeneration of the spine. The causes of scoliosis that begins in adulthood are usually very different from the childhood types.

The cause of scoliosis can be either functional or structural. *Functional scoliosis* results from extraspinous factors such as leg length discrepancy or pelvic obliquity. This type of scoliosis corrects itself once the underlying problem is eliminated. *Structural scoliosis* is a fixed deformity that results from, paralytic, congenital, or most often idiopathic conditions.[24]

REHABILITATION CONCERNS

Initially, the majority of cases of scoliosis are painless. Patients with scoliosis seek medical attention when they note a problem with how the back looks or some asymmetrical abnormalities including one shoulder or hip that is higher than the other and sticks out further; a "rib hump" appears when scoliosis causes the chest to twist, causing a hump on one side of the back as the ribs stick out further when bending forward; or, one arm hanging longer than the other because of a tilt in the upper body. As the condition progresses, back pain can develop. The deformity may cause pressure on nerves leading to weakness, numbness, loss of coordination, and pain in the lower extremities. If the chest is deformed due to the scoliosis, the lungs and heart may be affected leading to breathing problems and fatigue. Bracing is usually considered with curves between 25° and 40°, particularly if the patient is still growing and the curve is likely to get bigger.[55]

Adult scoliosis has a variety of treatment options. Whenever possible, the first choice of treatment for adult scoliosis is always going to be conservative. Spinal surgery will always be the last choice of treatment because of the risks involved. Conservative treatment that is commonly recommended includes medications, exercise, and certain types of braces to support the spine. The use of a spinal brace may provide some pain relief. However, in adults, it will not cause the spine to straighten. Usually, curves of less then 40° will be treated nonsurgically while curves over 40° might be recommended for surgery.[6]

The most common reason for surgery is pain relief. Surgery will nearly always be recommended for curves above 60°, as the twisting of the torso can lead to more serious lung and heart conditions. Generally, the only cases where surgery is considered are severe cases that lead to continual physical pain, difficulty in breathing, significant disfigurement, or continued progression of the curve. The goal is to first straighten the spine and then fuse the vertebrae together. Nearly all surgeries will use some type of fixation, or rods to help straighten the spine and hold the vertebrae in place while the fusion heals and becomes solid.[6,24]

Curves above 100° are rare, but they can be life-threatening if the spine twists the body so much that the heart and lungs do not function properly.

REHABILITATION PROGRESSION

A well-designed exercise program can provide pain relief in many patients. Initially, the best treatment for patients having spinal fusion surgery will be walking as much as possible to regain strength and facilitate healing. The goal will be to increase walking distance each day. It is not advisable for patients to begin physical therapy sooner than 6 weeks after surgery as excessive and premature exercise may impede healing. After approximately 6 weeks, the patient can begin general conditioning, extremity strengthening and stretching, and learning correct body mechanics to maintain erect posture that counteracts the effects of the scoliosis. Patients are usually able to return to activities of daily living within 3 months following spinal fusion surgery. Rehabilitation after spinal fusion surgery should usually continue for approximately 6 months. Even after full recovery and rehabilitation from spinal fusion surgery for scoliosis, patients should avoid high-contact sports. They may pursue other activities such as tennis, hiking, and swimming.[6,25]

REHABILITATION TECHNIQUES FOR THE CERVICAL SPINE

Acute Facet Joint Lock

PATHOMECHANICS

Acute cervical joint lock is a very common condition, more frequently called wryneck or stiff neck. The athlete usually complains of pain on one side of the neck following a sudden backward bending, side bending, and/or rotation of the neck. Pain can also occur after holding the head in an unusual position over a period of time, as when awakening from sleep. This problem can also occasionally follow exposure to a cold draft of air. There is no report of other acute trauma that could have produced the pain. This usually occurs when a small piece of synovial membrane lining the joint capsule or a meniscoid body is impinged or trapped within a facet joint in the cervical

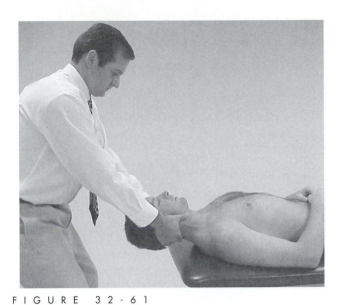

F I G U R E   3 2 - 6 1

Cervical traction.

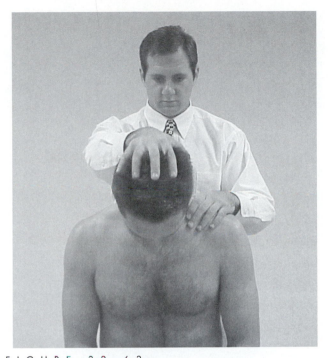

F I G U R E   3 2 - 6 3

Manually assisted flexion stretching exercise.

vertebrae. During inspection, there is palpable point tenderness and marked muscle guarding. The patient will report that the neck is "locked." Side bending and rotation are painful when moving in the direction opposite to the side on which there is locking. Other movements are relatively painless.[60]

REHABILITATION PROGRESSION

Various therapeutic modalities may be used to modulate pain in an attempt to break a pain-spasm-pain cycle. Joint mobilizations involving gentle traction (Fig. 32-61), rotation (see Fig. 16-32), and lateral bending (see Fig. 16-33), first in the pain-free direction and then in the direction of pain, can help reduce the guarding. Occasionally pain will be relieved almost immediately following mobilization. If not, it may be helpful to wear a soft cervical collar to provide for comfort (Fig. 32-62). This muscle guarding will generally last for 2 or 3 days as the athlete progressively regains motion.

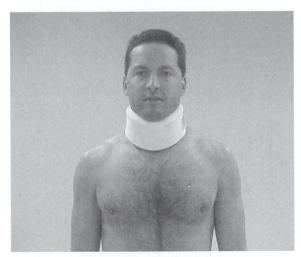

F I G U R E   3 2 - 6 2

The use of a soft or hard collar can increase comfort.

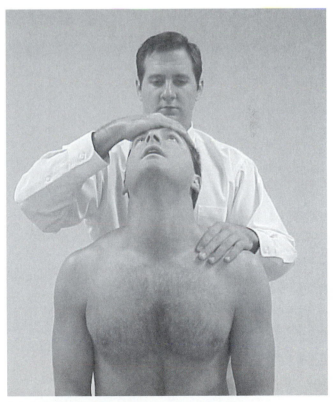

F I G U R E   3 2 - 6 4

Manually assisted extension stretching exercise.

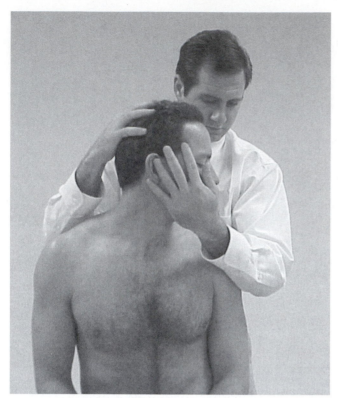

F I G U R E   3 2 - 6 5

Manually assisted rotation stretching exercise.

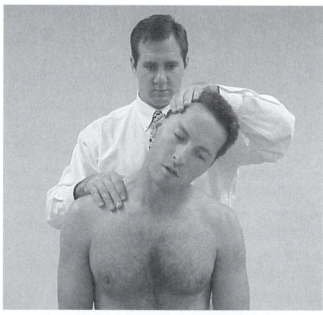

F I G U R E   3 2 - 6 6

Manually assisted side-bending stretching exercise.

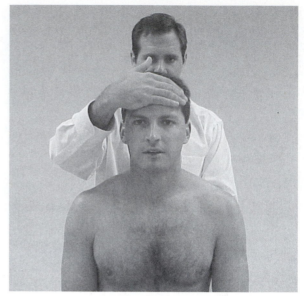

F I G U R E   3 2 - 6 7

Manually resisted flexion strengthening exercise.

Cervical Sprain

PATHOMECHANICS AND INJURY MECHANISM

A cervical sprain usually results from a moderate to severe trauma. More commonly the head snaps suddenly, while unprepared. Frequently muscle strains occur with ligament sprains. A sprain of the neck can produce tears in the major supporting tissue of the anterior or posterior longitudinal ligaments, the interspinous ligament, and the supraspinous ligament. There may be palpable tenderness over the transverse and spinous processes that serve as sites of attachment for the ligaments.[74]

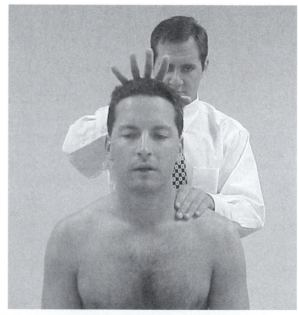

F I G U R E   3 2 - 6 8

Manually resisted extension strengthening exercise.

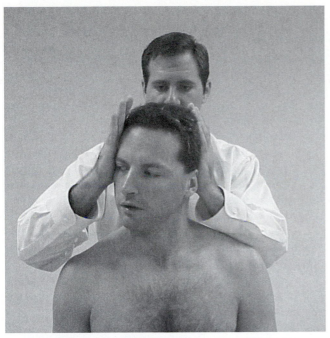

FIGURE 32-69

Manually resisted rotation strengthening exercise.

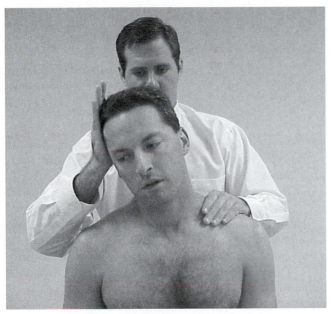

FIGURE 32-70

Manually resisted side-bending strengthening exercise.

The sprain displays all the signs of the facet joint lock, but the movement restriction is much greater and can potentially involve more than one vertebral segment. The main difference between the two is that acute joint lock can usually be dealt within a very short period of time but a sprain will require a significantly longer period for rehabilitation. Pain may not be significant initially but always appears the day after the trauma.

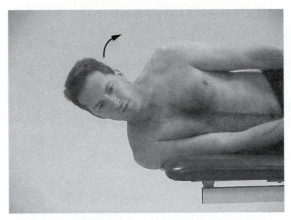

FIGURE 32-71

Gravity-resisted cervical stabilization exercise done on a treatment table with the head maintaining a static position. May be done side-lying (right and left), prone, and supine.

Pain stems from the inflammation of injured tissue and a protective muscle guarding that restricts motion.[74]

REHABILITATION PROGRESSION

As soon as possible the patient should have a physician evaluation to rule out the possibility of fracture, dislocation, disk injury, or injury to the spinal cord or nerve root. A soft cervical collar may be applied to reduce muscle guarding (Fig. 32-62). Ice and electrical stimulation are used for 48–72 hours, while the injury is in the acute stage of healing. In a patient with a severe injury, the physician may prescribe 2–3 days of bed rest, along with analgesics and anti-inflammatory medication. Range-of-motion exercises through a pain-free range should begin as soon as possible, including flexion (Fig. 32-63), extension (Fig. 32-64), rotation (Fig. 32-65), and side bending (Fig. 32-66). It has been demonstrated that using early ROM exercises, as opposed to long periods of immobility, tends to reduce the likelihood of neck hypomobility when the healing process is complete.[46] It is important to regain motion as soon as possible.

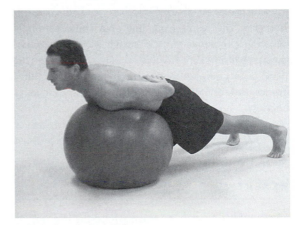

FIGURE 32-72

Cervical stabilization exercises done on a Swiss ball.

However, it is critical to understand that a sprain, particularly one that involves a complete ligament tear, causes hypermobility. Thus strengthening exercises (Figs. 32-67 to 32-70) along with stabilization exercises (Figs. 32-71 and 32-72) should also be incorporated into the rehabilitation program.[74]

Mechanical traction may also be prescribed to relieve pain and muscle guarding (Figs. 32-71 and 32-72).

SUMMARY

- The low back pain that patients most often experience is an acute, painful experience of relatively short duration that seldom causes significant time loss from practice or competition.
- Regardless of the diagnosis or the specificity of the diagnosis, a thorough evaluation of the patient's back pain is critical to good care.
- Back rehabilitation may be classified as a two-stage approach. Stage I (acute stage) treatment consists mainly of the modality treatment and pain-relieving exercises. Stage II treatment involves treating patients with a reinjury or exacerbation of a previous problem.
- Segmental spinal stabilization and core exercise should be included in the exercise plan of every patient with back pain.
- The types of exercises that may be included in the initial pain management phase include the following: lateral shift corrections, extensions exercises, flexion exercises, mobilization exercises, and myofascial stretching exercises.
- It is suggested that the therapist use an eclectic approach to the selection of exercises, mixing the various protocols described according to the findings of the patient's evaluation.
- Specific goals and exercises included in stage II should address which structures to stretch, which structures to strengthen, incorporating segmental spinal stabilization into the athlete's daily life and exercise routine, and which movements need a motor learning approach to control faulty mechanics.
- The rehabilitation program should include functional training, which may be divided into basic and advanced phases.
- Back pain can result from one or a combination of the following problems: muscle strain, piriformis muscle or quadratus lumborum myofascial pain or strain, myofascial trigger points, lumbar facet joint sprains, hypermobility syndromes, disk-related back problems, or sacroiliac joint dysfunction.
- Cervical pain can result from muscle strains, acute cervical joint lock, ligament sprains, and various other problems.

REFERENCES

1. Adams MA, May S, Freeman BJC, Morrison HP, Dolan P. Effects of backward bending on lumbar intervertebral discs. *Spine* 25(4):431–437, 2000.

2. Beattie P. The use of an electric approach for the treatment of low back pain: A case study. *Phys Ther* 72(12):923–928, 1992.

3. Binkley J, Finch E, Hall J, et al. Diagnostic classification of patients with low back pain: Report on a survey of physical therapy experts. *Phys Ther* 73(3):138–155, 1993.

4. Bittinger J. *Management of the Lumbar Pain Syndromes.* Course Notes, 1980.

5. Broadhurst N. Piriformis syndrome: Correlation of muscle morphology with symptoms and signs. *Arch Phys Med Rehabil* 85(12):2036–2039, 2004.

6. Cheng J, Rainville J. Effect of spine rehabilitation in adult scoliosis patients with back pain (poster session). *Am J Phys Med Rehabil* 81(7):536, 2002.

7. Cibulka M. The treatment of the sacroiliac joint component to low back pain: A case report. *Phys Ther* 72(12):917–922, 1992.

8. Cibulka M, Delitto A, Koldehoff R. Changes in innominate tilt after manipulation of the sacroiliac joint in patients with low back pain: An experimental study. *Phys Ther* 68(9):1359–1370, 1988.

9. Cibulka M, Rose S, Delitto A, et al. Hamstring muscle strain treated by mobilizing the sacroiliac joint. *Phys Ther* 66(8):1220–1223, 1986.

10. Correia K. Treatment of musculoskeletal and balance impairments in adolescent idiopathic scoliosis. *J Orthop Sports Phys Ther* 35 (1):A51, 2005.

11. DeRosa C, Porterfield J. A physical therapy model for the treatment of low back pain. *Phys Ther* 72(4):261–272, 1992.

12. Deyo R, Diehl A, Rosenthal M. How many days of bed rest for acute low back pain? A randomized clinical trial. *N Engl J Med* 315:1064–1070, 1986.

13. Donley P. Rehabilitation of low back pain in athletes: The 1976 Schering symposium on low back problems. *Athlet Train* 12(2):65–69, 1977.

14. Ebenbichler GR, Oddsson LI, Kollmitzer J, Erim Z. Sensory-motor control of the lower back: Implications for rehabilitation. *Med Sci Sport Exerc* 33(11):1889–1898, 2001.

15. Erhard R, Bowling R. The recognition and management of the pelvic component of low back and sciatic pain. *Am Phys Ther Assoc* 2(3):4–13, 1979.

16. Freburger JK, Riddle DL. Using published evidence to guide the examination of the sacroiliac joint region. *Phys Ther* 81(5):1135–1143, 2001.

17. Friberg O. Clinical symptoms and biomechanics of lumbar spine and hip joint in leg length inequality. *Spine* 8(6):643–650, 1983.

18. Frymoyer J. Back pain and sciatica: Medical progress. *N Engl J Med* 318(5):291–300, 1988.

19. Gavin T. The etiology and natural history of Scheuermann's kyphosis. *J Prosthet Orthot* 15(4 Suppl):S11–S14, 2003.

20. George SZ. Characteristics of patients with lower

extremity symptoms treated with slump stretching: A case study. *J Orthop Sports Phys Ther* 32(8):391–398, 2002.

21. Gomez M, Flanagan P, Gavin T. An alternative bracing approach to Scheuermann's disease: A case study. *J Prosthet Orthot* 14(3):109–112, 2002.

22. Grieve G. The sacro-iliac joint. *Physiotherapy* 62:384–400, 1976.

23. Grieve G. Lumbar instability: Congress lecture. *Physiotherapy* 68(1):2–9, 1982.

24. Hawes M. *Scoliosis and the Human Spine.* Tucson, AZ, Willowship Press, 2002.

25. Hentges C. The team approach to the orthotic treatment of idiopathic scoliosis and Scheuermann's kyphosis. *J Prosthet Orthot* 15(4 Suppl):S49–S52, 2003.

26. Herman M. Spondylolysis and spondylolisthesis in the child and adolescent athlete. *Orthop Clin N Am* 34(3):461–467, 2003.

27. Hides JA, Richardson CA, Jull GA. Multifidus muscle recovery is not automatic after resolution of acute, first-episode low back pain. *Spine* 21(23):2763–2769, 1996.

28. Hodges PW, Richardson CA. Inefficient muscular stabilization of the lumber spine associated with low back pain. *Spine* 21(22):2640–2650, 1996.

29. Hodges PW, Richardson CA. Contraction of the abdominal muscles associated with movement of the lower limb. *Phys Ther* 77(2):132–144, 1997.

30. Hodges PW. *Science of Stability: Clinical Application to Assessment and Treatment of Segmental Spinal Stabilization for Low Back Pain.* Course Handbook and Course Notes, September 29, Northeast Seminars, Durham, NC, 2002.

31. Hooker DN. Evaluation of the lumbar spine and sacroiliac joint: What, why, and how? Paper presented at the N.A.T.A. National Convention, Los Angeles, 2001.

32. Huguenin L. Myofascial trigger points: The current evidence. *Phys Ther Sport* 5(1):2–12, 2004.

33. Jackson C, Brown M. Analysis of current approaches and a practical guide to prescription of exercise. *Clin Orthop Rel Res* 179:46–54, 1983.

34. Lewit K, Simons D. Myofascial pain: Relief by post-isometric relaxation. *Arch Phys Med Rehabil* 65(8):452–456, 1984.

35. Lindstrom I, Ohlund C, Eek C, et al. The effect of graded activity on patients with subacute low back pain: A randomized prospective clinical study with an operant-conditioning behavioral approach. *Phys Ther* 72(4):279–290, 1992.

36. Maigne R. Low back pain of thoracolumbar origin. *Arch Phys Med Rehabil* 61(9):391–395, 1980.

37. Maitland G. *Vertebral Manipulation,* 5th ed. London, Butterworth, 1990.

38. Mapa B. An Australian programme for management of low back problems. *Physiotherapy* 66(4):108–111, 1980.

39. McGrath M. Clinical considerations of sacroiliac joint anatomy: A review of function, motion and pain. *J Osteopath Med* 7(1):16–24, 2004.

40. McGraw M. *The Neuro-Muscular Maturation of the Human Infant.* New York, Hafner, 1966.

41. McKenzie R. Manual correction of sciatic scoliosis. *N Z Med J* 76(484):194–199, 1972.

42. McKenzie R. *The Lumbar Spine: Mechanical Diagnosis and Therapy, Spinal Publications.* New Zealand, Lower Hutt, 1981.

43. McNeely M. A systematic review of physiotherapy for spondylolysis and spondylolisthesis. *Man Ther* 8(2):80–91, 2003.

44. Norris CM. Spinal stabilization. *Physiotherapy* 81(2):61–79, 1995.

45. Norris CM. Spinal stabilization. *Physiotherapy* 81(3):127–146, 1995.

46. O'Sullivan PB, Twomey LT, Allison GT. Evaluation of specific stabilizing exercise in the treatment of chronic low back pain with radiologic diagnosis of spondylolysis or spondylolisthesis. *Spine* 22(24):2959–2967, 1997.

47. Papadopoulos E. Piriformis syndrome. *Orthopedics* 27(8):797–799, 2004.

48. Pizzutillo PD, Hummer CD. Nonoperative treatment for painful adolescent spondylolysis or spondylolisthesis. *J Pediatr Orthop* 9(5):538–540, 1994.

49. Porter R, Miller C. Back pain and trunk list. *Spine* 11(6):596–600, 1986.

50. Prather H. Sacroiliac joint pain: Practical management. *Clin J Sport Med* 13(4):252–255, 2003.

51. Rantanen J, Hurme M, Falck B, et al. The lumbar multifidus muscle five years after surgery for a lumbar intervertebral disc herniation. *Spine* 18(5):568–574, 1993.

52. Richardson CA, Snijders CJ, Hides JA, Damen L, Pas MS, Storm J. The relationship between the transversus abdominis muscles, sacroiliac joint mechanics, and low back pain. *Spine* 27(4):399–405, 2002.

53. Richardson C, Jull G, Hodges P, Hides J. *Therapeutic Exercise for Spinal Segmental Stabilization in Low Back Pain.* Sydney, Churchill Livingstone, 1999.

54. Riddle D, Freburger J. Evaluation of presence of sacroiliac joint region dysfunction using a combination of tests: A multicenter intertester reliability study. *Phys Ther* 82(8):772–781, 2002.

55. Rooney R. Idiopathic scoliosis in children: An update on screening and bracing. *J Musculoskeletal Med* 21(5):268–270 and 273–275, 2004.

56. Saal J. Rehabilitation of football players with lumbar spine injury. *Physician Sports Med* 16(9):61–68, 1988.

57. Saal J. Rehabilitation of football players with lumbar spine injury. *Physician Sports Med* 16(10):117–125, 1988.

58. Saal J. Dynamic muscular stabilization in the nonoperative treatment of lumbar pain syndromes. *Orthop Rev* 19(8):691–700, 1990.

59. Saal JA, Saal JS. Nonoperative treatment of herniated lumbar intervertebral disk with radiculopathy: An outcome study. *Spine* 14(4):431–437, 1989.

60. Saunders D. *Evaluation, Treatment, and Prevention of Musculoskeletal Disorders.* Bloomington, MN, Educational Opportunities, 2004.

61. Simons D, Travell J. *Myofascial Pain and Dysfunction: The Lower Extremities.* Baltimore, Lippincott Williams & Wilkins, 1998.

62. Simons D, Travell J. *Myofascial Pain and Dysfunction: The Trigger Point Manual.* Baltimore, Lippincott Williams & Wilkins, 1998.

63. Solomon J. Discogenic low back pain. *Crit Rev Phys Rehabil Med* 16(3):177–210, 2004.

64. Steiner C, Staubs C, Ganon M, et al. Piriformis syndrome: Pathogenesis, diagnosis, and treatment. *J Am Orthop Acad* 87(4):318–323, 1987.

65. Tenhula J, Rose S, Delitto A. Association between direction of lateral lumbar shift, movement tests, and side of symptoms in patients with low back pain syndrome. *Phys Ther* 70(8):480–486, 1990.

66. Threlkeld A. The effects of manual therapy on connective tissue. *Phys Ther* 72(12):893–902, 1992.

67. Twomey L. A rationale for treatment of back pain and joint pain by manual therapy. *Phys Ther* 72(12):885–892, 1992.

68. Verrills P. Interventions in chronic low back pain. *Aust Fam Physician* 33(6):421–426 and 447–448, 2004.

69. Waddell G. Clinical assessment of lumbar impairment. *Clin Orthop Relat Res* 221:110–120, 1987.

70. Waddell G. A new clinical model for the treatment of low-back pain. *Spine* 12(7):632–644, 1987.

71. Walker J. The sacroiliac joint: A critical review. *Phys Ther* 72(12):903–916, 1992.

72. Warren P. Management of a patient with sacroiliac joint dysfunction: A correlation of hip range of motion asymmetry with sitting and standing postural habits. *J Man Manipulative Ther* 11(3):153–159, 2003.

73. Wood K. Spinal deformity in the adolescent athlete. *Clin Sports Medicine* 21(1):77–92, 2002.

74. Zmurko M. Cervical sprains, disc herniations, minor fractures, and other cervical injuries in the athlete. *Clin Sports Med* 22(3):513–521, 2003.

TREATMENT PROTOCOL TO CORRECT SACROILIAC DYSFUNCTION

INJURY SITUATION: A 47-year-old male was crossing an intersection when he stepped off the curb onto his left foot and misjudged the height. He felt immediate sharp pain in his low back. He was referred to physical therapy for evaluation and treatment. The patient complained of mild pain and a stiff-tight feeling in his left groin area, with hip flexion and adduction, increasing his discomfort. His previous medical history was unremarkable for hip, sacroiliac, or muscle problems, and he was in excellent physical condition with no other injuries at this time.

Functionally, the patient walked with a reduced stride length on the left, which produced a mild limp. Walking produced some mild left groin pain, and stair climbing increased this pain in his left groin. Range of motion was assessed. Lumbar spine range was full in all ranges, but side-bending left and backward bending created pain in the left sacroiliac region. Holding the backward bent position created some left groin pain similar in nature to the pain that occurred initially. Passive hip range of motion was full in all ranges, with mild groin pain provoked on the end range of flexion, abduction, and internal rotation. On manual muscle test, hip flexion and abduction were strong but produced pain in the left groin similar in nature to the presenting pain. Right and left straight-leg raise tests were positive for left groin pain. Bilateral knees-to-chest test was full-range and painless, as were the stress test of iliac approximation, iliac rotation, and posterior–anterior spring test. On palpation, there was mild tenderness along the left sacroiliac joint and over the left gluteus medius just lateral to the PSIS. The hip abductors, hip flexors, and hamstring muscles were nontender but had increased tone.

Phase One—Acute Phase

GOALS: modulate the pain, stretch, and strengthen the sacroiliac joint to return them to a more symmetric position.

Estimated length of time (ELT): days 1–3

The patient was treated with stretching to bring his sacroiliac joints into symmetric positions. Spinal segment stabilization was initiated along with beginning core stabilization exercises (hip-lift bridges, isometric hip adduction ball squeezes). The left groin and sacroiliac area were treated with ice. The patient was instructed to repeat stretching and the strengthening exercises three times a day. He was also given analgesic medicine to make him more comfortable.

On day 2, stretching was continued and the stretching exercise load was increased by adding repetitions. A stretching program was begun for the hip abductors, hip internal rotators, hip flexors, and hamstrings. His usual weight-lifting session was modified to a non-weightbearing program. His conditioning workout was done on the exercise bike and in the pool. Hot packs were applied to the adductor area preliminary to the exercise and stretching programs. The sacroiliac area was treated with ice and electrical stimulation at a moderate sensory intensity.

On day 3, stretching was discontinued. Strengthening was increased with the addition of elastic resistance to hip abduction and adduction. Functional exercises were initiated, including line walking, minisquats, side shuffle with tubing resistance. Modalities remained the same.

Phase Two—Intermediate Phase

GOALS: increase spinal segment awareness, core stabilization strength, return to functional exercises, and return to practice and play status.

ELT: days 4–7

Pain modalities were continued. Stretching exercises to the left hip abductors, flexors, and internal rotators were continued. Strengthening exercises continued with increased repetitions, resistance, and difficulty. Hot packs and electrical stimulation were continued, as were the spinal segment and core stabilization exercises.

Phase Three—Advanced Phase

GOALS: maintain spinal segment strength, increase core strength, and return to normal exercise routines.

ELT: day 8 to 6 weeks postinjury

Pain modalities should be used if needed. Tight muscle groups should continue to be stretched two or three times a day. Strengthening routines should become more challenging but not more time-consuming.

Criteria for Return to Function

1. The patient demonstrates that he can perform functional activities and activities of daily living with no noticeable compensatory movements.

TREATMENT OF DISK-RELATED BACK PAIN

INJURY SITUATION: A 31-year-old mother was attempting to put her 2-year-old daughter in the child restraint seat of her minivan. After picking the child up, she bent forward and twisted to get the child into the seat and felt immediate intense pain in her low back and down the back of her right leg. Her right leg gave way and she collapsed to the floor with back and right leg pain. She was referred to a physical therapist for evaluation and treatment by a family practice physician.

Functionally she was very guarded and stiff looking. On forward bending, she was very guarded and used compensating movement patterns to move from sit to stand or standing to lying down. Lumbar spine forward bending and right straight-leg raising provoked central back pain that radiated into her right posterior thigh. Backward bending provoked central pain and was restricted at 50 percent of normal range. Sitting knee extension movement with the right leg provoked central pain and posterior thigh pain when the knee flexion angle reached 60°. Dorsiflexion at the ankle and chin to chest movement increased this pain. Posterior–anterior mobilizations to the sacrum and the L5 spinous process increased central back pain and caused some shooting pain down the right leg. On manual muscle test, trunk extension was strong and painless. Left hip extension and left hip internal rotation and external rotation were strong but provoked right posterior leg pain. A sensory check demonstrated normal feeling over both lower extremities. On palpation, she was nontender over all major structures.

Phase One—Acute Phase

GOALS: decrease pain, encourage rest, maintain spinal segment stability, and create safe, pain-free movement behaviors that minimize the stress on the disk complex.

ELT: days 1–3

The patient was treated with 3 days of relative bed rest. She was encouraged to work on spinal segment stability exercises, knees toward chest, and knee rocking mobilizations while in a flat-lying position (supine, side-lying, or prone). Multiple bouts of the 90/90 position and prone-on-elbows position were used for their positional traction benefit. Activities of daily living were kept to a necessary level—remain at home, avoid sitting posture. Standing and walking for brief periods (less than 10 minutes) were allowed. The physician prescribed analgesic and anti-inflammatory medications.

Phase Two—Intermediate Phase

GOALS: decrease pain, encourage motion. Encourage rest positions that enhance centralization of the disk nucleus and provide optimum nourishment for the disk complex.

ELT: day 4 to week 4

After 3 days, the patient was encouraged to come to the physical therapy clinic for treatment, once a day. The above activities were preceded with the comfort modalities of hot packs and electrical stimulation. Spinal segment stabilization was reassessed, and the patient started on the beginning-level core stability exercises. The patient was instructed to be flat lying for 20–30 minutes four times daily and to continue to minimize time spent in sitting postures. At 1 week, the patient was encouraged to walk for conditioning and movement purposes, starting with 10 minutes and working up to 30 minutes. The walking was followed by flat-lying and positional traction periods of 20–30 minutes. The core stability exercises were gradually progressed to continue to challenge strength and endurance as the pain became more manageable. At 3 weeks, more functional exercises were included. Squats, balance activities, and light weight lifting (no axial loading) were begun. Flat-lying postures, four times daily, were encouraged. At 4 weeks, the patient was instructed to gradually increase sitting times, guided by comfort.

Phase Three—Advanced Phase

GOALS: maximize core stability strength and endurance, retrain functional movement patterns to include spinal segment and core stability, return normal flexibility and strength to lower extremities, and encourage good mechanics in activities of daily living.

ELT: week 5 to 6 months

The patient was reevaluated, and specific flexibility and strengthening problems were identified. Tight muscle groups were stretched three or four times a day, weak muscle groups were isolated and progressively strengthened. Spinal segment stability and core stability were stressed with more challenging exercises. Normal strength and conditioning exercises were encouraged, but technique was monitored closely and the patient was encouraged to use spinal segment stability coactivation patterns in every exercise. Functional activities of daily living drills were begun, with the patient being encouraged to incorporate spinal segment coactivation patterns into her motor planning for each drill.

Criteria for Return to Function

1. The patient demonstrates good spinal segment control in the physical therapy clinic

2. The patient has normal flexibility and strength in her lower extremities.

3. Functional performance test scores are at least 90 percent of previous baseline scores.

4. The patient tolerates 1–1.5 hours of exercise with no system.

5. The patient demonstrates in exercises that she can perform the activities of daily living with no noticeable compensatory movement patterns.

PART 5

Special Considerations for Specific Patient Populations

CHAPTER 33

Rehabilitation Considerations for the Geriatric Patient

Jolene L. Bennett and Michael J. Shoemaker

OBJECTIVES

After completing this chapter, the therapist should be able to do the following:

- Describe the facets of the normal aging process in terms of successful aging.
- Identify and apply common principles for managing older patients with orthopedic disorders.
- Describe system changes that occur predictably with aging, inactivity, and disease.
- Describe musculoskeletal injuries common to the geriatric population and the related treatment principles.
- Discuss and describe key elements of the history and physical examination for the rehabilitation of the older patient that may differ from younger patient populations.
- Understand the importance of rehabilitation for targeted functional outcomes and maintenance of functional independence in the geriatric population.

INTRODUCTION

Rehabilitative care of older adults has evolved into a specialty area of practice for many clinicians. Geriatrics, or the care of the elderly, is based on the recognition that the aging process causes the body to respond differently to injury, disease, and medical care than when patients were younger. The field of geriatrics continues to gain attention due to the rapid growth of this segment of the population and its predicted socioeconomic impact in the present century.

Traditionally, demographers have used the age of 65 to delineate an individual reaching "old age." Reasons for this delineation include established social practices, such as retirement from work, and the onset of benefits such as Social Security and Medicare. This segment of the population is growing steadily, both in absolute numbers and in proportion to the total population. A tremendous increase in the number of individuals reaching old age is projected during the next 40–50 years. In 1900, there were three million persons aged 65 years and older in the United States, representing 4 percent of the total population. In 1988, the number of persons aged 65 years and older grew to 31.6 million or 12.7 percent of the total population.[65]

It is estimated that in 2020, 51 million individuals will be over the age of 65, representing 17.3 percent of the population. This dramatic growth is a result of the large cohorts born during the post-World War II "baby boom" that will be reaching old age, and the improved survivorship in all age cohorts, especially those regarded as the oldest-old at 100+ years. Since the mid-nineteenth century, life expectancy in the United States has nearly doubled, from 40 years to almost 80 years, due to both medical and scientific breakthroughs and improved health habits. Of this 65 and older category, it is estimated that 48 percent are actually over 75 years old. The number of elders aged 85 or older is predicted to triple in number by 2040.[5] As a result of this growth, the definition of old age is being redefined to better differentiate this large segment of the population (Table 33-1).

Orthopedic rehabilitation for older adults is a rapidly expanding area of practice for physical therapists. The ability to move is a prerequisite to functional independence, and functional independence is considered to be a large contributor to quality of life with aging. Pain and musculoskeletal impairments can lead to disability among older Americans, and at least 39 percent of Medicare enrollees have at least one health-related activity of daily living (ADL) disability.[12] As the rehabilitative

TABLE 33-1

Chronological Age Descriptions

DESCRIPTION	AGE RANGE (YEARS)
Infant	0–2
Child	3–12
Adolescent	13–17
Young adult	18–24
Adult	25–44
Middle age	45–64
Young-old	65–74
Old	75–84
Old-old	85–99
Oldest-old	100+

specialists for movement dysfunction, physical therapists have a critical role in helping older adults age successfully.

Orthopedic care of older adults requires the clinician to utilize a unique perspective that is different from that used when caring for younger adults. Older adults often have multiple comorbidities that require careful consideration to provide safe and effective care. Additionally, the impact of pain and musculoskeletal impairment on function is often underreported and incorrectly attributed to normal aging. This chapter will provide a perspective with which to view the elderly patient/client, in addition to specific considerations for the orthopedic rehabilitation of older adults.

GERIATRIC PRINCIPLES OF AGING

Reduced Reserve Capacity

Although several theories of aging have been postulated, it is commonly accepted that nearly all body systems demonstrate age-related changes, resulting in a reduced physiologic reserve and reduced capacity to respond to stress. Thus, older persons may require greater time to recover from exercise or acute medical illness, or they may be more susceptible to a decline in functional status. As physiologic reserve decreases, it is apparent that there is a threshold below which a decline in function becomes evident.[13] For example, combined quadriceps strength of approximately 300 N is required to perform a sit-to-stand without the use of the upper extremities.[23] Strength below this threshold results in impaired functional performance in sit-to-stand activities such as toileting. Another example can be found with peak oxygen consumption, where $20 \ mL \cdot kg^{-1} \cdot min^{-1}$ is the threshold, below which decline in functional status in community ambulation becomes evident.[18]

Function as the Sum of Multisystem Deficits

Given that a marked loss of physiologic reserve can result in functional loss, partial loss of physiologic reserve in multiple systems may also result in a change in functional status, and may be evident before a person presents to a clinician with a complaint of functional limitation or disability.[13] Preclinical disability is a clinically detectable decline in physical function, characterized by increased time to complete a task, modification of a task, or a decreased frequency of task performance.[25,26] Therefore, a patient/client may report that he/she only goes shopping once every 2 weeks because it is starting to take too long, or that she occasionally must use the powered cart. Such a patient might demonstrate a mild decline in gait speed and Timed Up and Go (TUG).[51] Yet this particular patient/client may not recognize this as a change in functional status or see the potential for continued decline in function over time if no intervention is received.

Heterogeneity of Aging

The overall aging process is heterogeneous; and chronological age does not necessarily correlate with physiologic age.[13,41] The effect of chronic illnesses, lifestyle choices, and acute illnesses have a much greater impact on function than chronological age alone. Therefore, rehabilitation potential should be determined using a variety of factors, which include the need to differentiate between the effects of aging, inactivity, and disease on function.

Differentiation between the Effects of Aging, Inactivity, and Disease

The diagnostic process used by physical therapists includes confirming or refuting hypotheses used to explain why a particular patient/client presents with a movement dysfunction. In the elderly, the history and physical examination must differentiate between the effects of aging, inactivity, and disease on the underlying impairments and functional limitations that result in movement dysfunction.[41] Mild impairments in range of motion (ROM) may be due to increased stiffness associated with aging that occurs in the tendinous or ligamentous structures around a joint. They may also be due to chronic inactivity and reduced demand on a particular joint for full ROM. It is also possible that an acute immobilization contributed to the disuse of a particular joint. And of course, ROM impairments may be due to a pathological process within the joint or of periarticular tissues. In the elderly, pronounced effects of aging, increased likelihood of multiple disease states, and greater susceptibility to the effects of inactivity all require careful differentiation of these factors. In short, examination of the elderly often requires greater attention by the physical therapist than examination of average aged adults.

The Impact of Social, Emotional, and Financial Resources on the Effects of Aging, Inactivity, and Disease on Function and Quality of Life

A common definition of frailty is a state of reduced physiologic reserve associated with an increased susceptibility to functional limitations and disability. However, frailty has also been defined as vulnerability to dependence in psychological, social, physical, cultural, or economic ways.[8] An older patient with severe rheumatoid arthritis who has a healthy spouse may be able to cope well with a change in functional status. Likewise a patient who has the financial resources to make home modifications or purchase adaptive equipment will be impacted in his/her quality of life much differently than if that same individual did not have those same resources. History taking must consider both human and financial resources to determine how each individual's quality of life is affected by the movement dysfunction. Likewise, the treatment plan and goals may need to be modified, and appropriate referrals to other health care practitioners and community resources may need to be provided.

Tertiary Prevention as a Part of Routine Clinical Decision Making

Given that as age advances, there is increasing likelihood of a number of comorbid diseases that may contribute directly or indirectly to movement dysfunction. Tertiary prevention is defined as limiting the degree of disability and promoting rehabilitation and restoration of function in patients with chronic and irreversible diseases. When managing elderly patients/clients in the orthopedic setting, consideration needs to be given to the multitude of ways by which chronic diseases impact function, beyond the most immediate, overt impairments and functional limitations.[41] This can include counseling on maintaining or increasing activity levels and establishing exercise programs that have components that address aerobic capacity, balance, and functional mobility skills. Additionally, by screening for common patterns of functional decline, appropriate referrals may be made to address currently undiagnosed medical problems and movement dysfunctions.

SYSTEM CHANGES WITH AGING, INACTIVITY, AND DISEASE

Cardiovascular System

With age, there is a decrease in maximal heart rate, a mild decrease in stroke volume, and reduced arteriovenous O_2 difference which contribute to a reduction in maximal oxygen consumption by approximately 5–15 percent per decade after age 25.[52] Activity level, however, can either mitigate or exacerbate this loss. Elderly subjects have demonstrated comparable gains in maximal oxygen consumption when placed on an exercise or training program with younger subjects. Acute inactivity, such as that which occurs with hospitalization, can account for drastic reductions in $\dot{V}O_{2max}$. Increased blood viscosity (due to fluid loss and subsequent increase in hematocrit) and venous stasis increase the risk of thromboembolic disease. Cardiac diseases such as coronary artery disease and the sequelae of myocardial infarction and cardiomyopathy will greatly reduce $\dot{V}O_{2max}$.

Peripheral arterial vascular disease can substantially reduce walking tolerance through muscle ischemia and claudication pain.[52]

The impact of these changes on function is of great concern. First, with a reduction in activity tolerance, there is a tendency in the elderly for further activity curtailment, resulting in further deconditioning and exacerbation of disease. Patients with recent hospitalizations may also sustain significant declines in their function. Up to 35 percent of elderly patients admitted to an acute care experience a decline in ADLs by discharge.[16] Those patients/clients with cardiovascular disease and a history of inactivity are at a much greater risk of an adverse event during exercise, and therefore careful consideration, screening, and monitoring must occur to ensure safety with a rehabilitation program.

In a direct access environment, physical therapists must be able to screen for risk factors of cardiovascular disease, take and interpret a cardiovascular history, and safely account for cardiac disease by modifying exercise programs, and make appropriate referrals to other practitioners. Because of the high prevalence of cardiovascular disease in older adults, it is essential that physical therapists in orthopedic practice screen for and assess cardiovascular comorbidities in each patient/client encounter. Table 33-2 highlights modifiable and nonmodifiable risk factors for cardiovascular disease. The American Heart Association has guidelines for risk classification and vital sign monitoring during exercise, and should be strongly considered when initiating or progressing exercise in an older adult with known risk factors for cardiovascular disease[24] (Table 33-3).

Deep vein thrombosis is another potentially fatal cardiovascular disease that requires consideration of the orthopedic physical therapist. Patients undergoing orthopedic surgery with subsequent immobilization of a limb are at particularly high risk. The popular Homan's sign is of little clinical value, as it has been demonstrated to have sensitivity of less than 50 percent. Wells and colleagues[54,68] have developed clinical decision rules that can be particularly useful in assessing likelihood of the presence of deep vein thrombosis (Table 33-4).

TABLE 33-2

Risk Factors for Cardiovascular Disease

Modifiable risk factors
  Smoking
  Hypertension
  Hyperlipidemia
  Physical inactivity

Nonmodifiable risk factors
  Age
  Family history
  Male gender

Other risk factors
  Diabetes mellitus
  Obesity
  Stress

T A B L E   3 3 - 3

Risk Classification for Exercise Training and Vital Sign Monitoring

AMERICAN HEART ASSOCIATION RISK CLASSIFICATION	STRESS TEST OR PHYSICIAN CLEARANCE	VITAL SIGN MONITORING
A1: • nonelderly with no symptoms or risk factors	No	At rest during initial exam
A2: • elderly patients with less than two cardiovascular risk factors	Yes	At rest and during exercise on initial exam only
A3: • elderly patients with more than two risk factors	Yes	At rest and during exercise on initial exam; consider periodic monitoring
B: • known cardiovascular disease but stable, and without resting ischemia or angina • history of mild heart failure; compensated, stable • appropriate vital sign response with activity • only mild dyspnea, fatigue or palpitations with normal, higher level activities (New York Heart Class I–II)	Yes	At rest and during exercise until safety established, and whenever intensity is increased
C: • inappropriate vital sign response to activity/exercise • moderate to significant dyspnea, fatigue, or palpitations with low levels of activity (New York Heart Class III–IV) • known ischemia during exercise testing	Yes	At rest and during exercise throughout the episode of care
D: • unstable ischemia/angina at rest • severe valvular stenosis or regurgitation • heart failure that is not compensated • uncontrolled arrhythmias	Yes	Exercise for conditioning purposes not recommended. Monitor vital signs at rest and during changes in functional activity level.

Adapted from Brooks.[6]

Pulmonary System

Age-related changes in the pulmonary system include reduced chest wall compliance, decreased lung elasticity, and increased peripheral chemoreceptor sensitivity to respond to respiratory acidosis.[52] These changes, however, do not account for limitations in exercise tolerance. Therefore, dyspnea not explained by previous medical history, especially in the absence of a recent cardiac work-up, requires physician referral.

Inactivity, especially bed rest, can have significant impacts on pulmonary function, primarily due to mismatches in ventilation and perfusion, reduced alveolar ventilation, and increased susceptibility to airway closure and secretion retention.

Pulmonary diseases are most responsible for ventilatory limitations on exercise tolerance in the elderly. Diseases such as asthma, emphysema, and chronic bronchitis comprise the diagnoses known as chronic obstructive pulmonary diseases. Restrictive diseases, including pulmonary fibrosis, may also account for dyspnea and limited exercise tolerance in the elderly.

The impact of these age, inactivity, and disease-related changes in the pulmonary system on function often result in the downward spiral of activity curtailment and further deconditioning due to dyspnea. These patients may also have complaints about fatigue. Patients with pulmonary disease are also more susceptible to recurrent infections and disease exacerbation, leading to frequent hospitalization and the functional declines associated with it.

Because cardiac disease is frequently found as a comorbidity in patients with lung disease, the previous discussion regarding risk factors and monitoring is applicable. Additionally, positioning during physical therapy interventions is a consideration, as the supine position without an elevated head can result in dyspnea. Because of a significant reduction in exercise tolerance, frequent rest breaks, as well as cueing to increase respiratory depth and decrease respiratory rate may be needed. Breath holding should be avoided, and coordination of breathing with movement should be encouraged. For example, expiraton with bending forward, and inspiration with thoracic extension and reaching overhead.

T A B L E 3 3 - 4

Clinical Decision Rule Developed by Wells and Colleagues to Predict Likelihood of Peripheral Deep Vein Thrombosis

Active cancer (within 6 months of diagnosis or palliative care)	1
Paralysis, paresis, or recent Plaster immobilization of lower extremity	1
Recently bedridden ≥3 days or major surgery within 4 weeks of application of clinical decision rule	1
Localized tenderness along distribution of the deep venous system[a]	1
Entire lower-extremity swelling	1
Calf swelling ≥3 cm compared with asymptomatic lower extremity[b]	1
Pitting edema (greater in the symptomatic lower extremity)	1
Collateral superficial veins (nonvaricose)	1
Alternative diagnosis as likely or greater than that of deep vein thrombosis[c]	2

Score interpretation:

0: probability of proximal lower-extermity deep vein thrombosis (PDVT) of 3 %(95% confidence interval [CI]_1.7%–5.9%),

1 or 2: probability of PDVT of 17% (95% CI_12%–23%)

3: probability of PDVT of 75% (95%CI_63%–84%)

[a]Tenderness along the deep venous system is assessed by firm palpation in the center of the posterior calf, the popliteal space, and along the area of the femoral vein in the anterior thigh and groin.

[b]Measured 10 cm below tibial tuberosity.

[c]Most common alternative diagnoses are cellulitis, calf strain, and postoperative swelling.

Sensory Systems

Maintaining an upright posture requires adequate sensory input regarding the body's position in space. Somatosensation, vision, and vestibular information comprise the three main sensory systems involved in balance and postural control. Because falls pose such a significant concern for the elderly, and because falls often result in orthopedic injuries, understanding how age and disease can impact these sensory systems is important for physical therapists managing elderly patients with orthopedic dysfunction.

Age-related changes in somatosensation include diminished touch, vibration, and proprioception senses.[17] Age-related changes in vision include decreased visual acuity, contrast sensitivity, dark adaptation, and depth perception.[17] Age-related changes in the vestibular system include reduced sensory hair cells and neurons, which reduces sensitivity to movement and position.[17] Any of these changes alone should not account for clinically significant declines in performance. However, when combined with either significant age-related changes in multi-

ple systems or disease in one or more of the sensory systems, these changes can contribute to impaired balance and increased fall risk.

Somatosensory diseases such as peripheral polyneuropathy associated with diabetes can contribute to increased fall risk and decreased stability, especially on unlevel surfaces and when walking in dark or low-light conditions. Common diseases affecting vision include macular degeneration, cataracts, and glaucoma. Reduced visual function results in difficulty maintaining balance on unlevel surfaces, and can markedly impair the ability to maintain balance in the presence of vestibular disease. Vestibular diseases such as vestibular neuritis, Meniere's disease, and perilymphatic fistula will greatly reduce the ability to maintain balance and stability in low-light conditions, unlevel surfaces, or in the presence of impaired vision or somatosensation. If the treatment room has windows, make sure the sunlight is not directly in the patient's eyes. The patient should sit with the back to the window and the clinician should have the daylight shining on the face to enhance the visual field for the patient.

Screening for sensory impairment contributions to impaired balance is necessary to develop optimal compensatory strategies, designing an appropriate balance retraining program, or to facilitate referral to a specialized balance center or other appropriate practitioner.

Auditory changes with age include high-frequency hearing loss, reduced speech discrimination, and reduced filtering of background noise.[17] A variety of disease processes can further reduce conductive and/or sensorineural hearing function. Clinicians need to make an extra effort to speak directly to the patient/client, annunciate clearly, vary the volume of speech as necessary, reduce background noise, and utilize visual and tactile cues to augment communication.

DEMENTIA AND DEPRESSION

Dementia

Age-related declines in cognitive function are relatively minimal compared to changes that occur due to pathology such as Alzheimer's and vascular dementia. Acute changes in cognitive function (delirium) do have an element of reversibility, but can often contribute to additional, persistent changes.[41]

The functional impact of cognitive decline is great, and leads to increasing dependence on others to remain in the community, and is highly associated with nursing home placement. Additionally, cognitive-related ADL changes and loss of function are diagnostic features of dementia.[19]

Detection of cognitive decline and initiation of referral for further work-up is important so that reversible causes can be ruled out, patient/caregiver education can begin, and referral to appropriate resources can be made to minimize the impact on function. Of particular concern to the orthopedic physical therapist is to ensure that instruction in precautions and home exercise programs be simplified in a way to ensure retention

TABLE 33-5

Strategies for Providing Intervention to Cognitively Impaired Elderly

- Simplify—instructions, cues (verbal, and tactile), programs, environment.
- Explain—in simple terms, in a consistent manner, with frequent repetition.
- Slow down—speech, pace of session.
- Avoid change—maintain consistency of therapist, environment, program.
- Educate and support the family—include family, if willing, in education on treatment plan, and home exercise programs. Also be ready to confront denial in the patient and family about the patient's cognitive impairments. Encourage seeking out support groups, respite care, etc.

Adapted from Lewis CB, Bottomly JM.[41]

and follow-through.[41] Table 33-5 provides strategies to help with this.

Depression

Up to 18 percent of older adults experience depression, and depression is closely associated with physical disability, chronic pain, and cognitive decline.[29] It is essential that symptoms of depression be recognized, and that appropriate referrals be made, especially given the multiple treatment options that are available, including medication, psychotherapy, and family therapy. In the elderly, depression is primarily manifested as physical rather than emotional symptoms.[47] This places the physical therapist in a key position to help with early detection of symptoms of depression and the subsequent need for referral.

The impact of depression on function cannot be overstated. Those with persistent symptoms of depression have been shown to have up to a fivefold increase in functional disability over time, and depression has been shown to negatively impact rehabilitation gains and functional status during inpatient rehabilitation.[39,67] Depression can also impact cognitive functioning, and is considered to be a cause of reversible dementia.

Physical therapists may suspect depression in patients/clients with overt or preclinical functional decline, especially in the absence of any change in medical status. Symptoms of depression may also be suspected in patients who are having trouble with concentration, retention of home exercise programs, or other signs of cognitive decline. Additionally, probing questions about stressors, changes, or losses may help with determining whether depressive symptoms are contributing to the observed cognitive and functional decline.

MUSCULOSKELETAL SYSTEM

The biological and mechanical behaviors of all of the musculoskeletal soft tissues—including skeletal muscle, articular cartilage, intervertebral disks, tendons, ligaments, and joint capsules—are altered with age.

Skeletal Muscle

Loss of skeletal muscle mass with age is well documented. Muscle size decreases an average of 30–40 percent over one's lifetime and affects the lower extremities more than the upper extremities.[28] This decrease in muscle mass is a direct result of a reduction in both muscle fiber size and number that occurs with advancing age and is largely attributed to progressive inactivity and sedentary lifestyles.[28] Fiber loss appears to be more accelerated in type II muscle fibers, which decrease from an average of 60 percent in sedentary young men to below 30 percent after the age of 80.[37] Type II fibers have approximately twice the intrinsic strength per unit area and twice the velocity of contraction of type I fibers. Type II fibers are used primarily in activities requiring power such as sprinting or strength training and are not stimulated by normal ADLs.

Strength Changes

With reduced muscle mass comes a reduction in muscle force production, strength, and aerobic fitness—frequently hallmarks of advancing age. Strength loss may begin slowly around the age of 50 and becomes more rapid with advancing age. Strength loss correlates with mass loss until advanced age, at which time fiber atrophy may not account fully for the observed strength loss, suggesting a possible neural influence. Loss of muscle strength with age is attributed to muscle fiber loss, muscle fiber atrophy, and denervated muscle fibers.[50]

Strength Training

Exercise intensity has been shown to be the most important variable for improving strength and function in the elderly.[9] High-intensity strength training (60–80 percent of one's one-repetition max) has been shown to be safe and results in significant gains in muscle strength, size, and functional mobility even in the most frail elderly.[9] Improvements in lower-extremity strength positively impact mobility and independence with ADLs. Sedentary individuals should begin exercise programs at lower initial levels and progressively increase intensity as tolerance allows. Individuals with arthritic joints may not tolerate large compressive forces across the joints and will require modifications in exercise position and intensity. It is also important to incorporate exercises that work on retraining the easily atrophied type II fibers. Exercises incorporating quicker, more explosive actions are also necessary to prepare the elderly patients for real-life situations such as tripping on an obstacle and losing their balance. These explosive and reactive-type exercises must be modified for each patient's level of function and progress as tolerated, taking safety into consideration with each task.

ARTICULAR CARTILAGE

Morphological changes in articular cartilage with age include a reduced number of chondrocytes, decreased rates of collagen and elastin synthesis, altered composition of fibril types, and reduced water content. Dehydrated cartilage may have a reduced ability to dissipate forces across the joint, leading to increased susceptibility to mechanical failure.[1] With aging and increased wear and tear, cartilage may break down, beginning with fibrillation and eventually leading to sclerosis of subchondral bone and continued cartilage degeneration. Some degree of mechanical breakdown seems to be part of the normal aging process, but severe destruction of cartilage and subchondral bone involvement leads to osteoarthritis (OA), which is the most common form of joint disease in the United States. OA can lead to significant impairments in joint function and marked disability, leading to eventual joint replacement. Rehabilitation efforts should include reduction of pain, elimination of joint stress, maintenance of joint ROM, maintenance of strength and endurance, and improvement in functional independence.[49]

TENDON, LIGAMENT, AND JOINT CAPSULE

The most prevalent symptom of changes in periarticular connective tissue is loss of extensibility and subsequent reduction in joint motion. Changes in structure and function may occur as a result of normal aging and from disuse and inactivity. In addition, the tensile properties of some ligament–bone complexes show a decline in tensile stiffness and ultimate load to failure with increasing age.[69] Degenerative changes in dense fibrous tissues may result in spontaneous or low-energy-level ruptures of the rotator cuff of the shoulder, the long head of the biceps, the posterior tibial tendon, patellar ligament, and Achilles tendon; they also may lead to sprains of joint capsules and ligaments, including those of the spine. Care should be taken with explosive, high-energy activities and loading of joints in the older individual, especially when initiating an exercise program in a previously sedentary person.

BONE

Bone mineral density is defined as bone mineral content relative to the area or volume of bone in the site of measurement and is expressed as $g \cdot cm^{-2}$, with $2 \ g \cdot cm^{-2}$ considered a normal value. Strength of bone and ability to withstand compressive and tensile forces is related to bone mineral density. Bone mineral density reductions are known to occur with age and disuse, as are the strength properties of bone. Throughout life, women may lose as much as 35–40 percent of cortical bone and 50–60 percent of trabecular bone.[20] Men lose slightly less bone with age. Reduction of bone mineral density below $1 \ g \cdot cm^{-2}$ is considered below the fracture threshold and increases the risk of osteoporotic-related fractures.

OSTEOPOROSIS

Osteoporosis is a generalized disease of bone in which there is a marked decrease in the amount of bone. The World Health Organization defines osteoporosis as a decrease in bone mineral density of more than 2.5 standard deviations below the mean as compared to young normals. Postmenopausal osteoporosis is caused by a decrease in estrogen and results in rapid bone loss 5–7 years following the onset of menopause. Women in this group have a high incidence of vertebral body fractures with subsequent postural changes, loss of body height, and often-persistent pain and loss of function. Advancing age is among the risk factors for developing osteoporosis (Table 33-6). Age-related osteoporosis occurs equally in men and women ages 70 and greater and manifests mainly in hip and vertebral fractures. Fractures of the proximal humerus, proximal tibia, pelvis, and metatarsal bones are also common. It may be prudent to assume that even

TABLE 33-6

Osteoporosis Risk Factors

- Age (over 50 years)
- Genetic factors
    Sex (women > men)
    Race (white > black)
    Family history
    Body type (small frame > large frame)
- Postmenopause
- Nutritional factors
    Low body weight
    Low dietary intake of calcium
    High alcohol consumption
    Eating disorders
    High caffeine consumption
- Lifestyle factors
    Immobilization/inactivity
    Cigarette smoking
- Medical factors
    Early menopause
    Medication use: corticosteroids, antacids, anticoagulants
    Menstrual cycle disorders

asymptomatic older adults may have a reduction in bone mineral density, as reduced bone mineral density of as much as 30 percent may be present before being evident on plain film X-ray. Exercise and mechanical stress to the bone, along with estrogen replacement and increased calcium consumption, have been well documented as preventative for the development and progression of osteoporosis.[36] Weight-bearing and strengthening exercises have been shown to maintain bone density and reduce the incidence of osteoporosis-related fractures.[36] A consistently sustained program of walking may be adequate for the lower extremities and spine, but upper-extremity exercises should also be given. For the older individual, safety and fall prevention during exercise are important concerns. The therapist should be creative in designing exercises that stress the skeletal system while ensuring safety of the patient.

Many patients who receive physical therapy have medical conditions that require long-term corticosteroid use. Corticosteroids assist in the management of inflammatory and autoimmune illnesses. Unfortunately, long-term corticosteroid use results in a significant decrease in bone density. Bone density for patients treated with corticosteroids for periods of 5 years is 20–40 percent less than density for nontreated control subjects.[53] Clinicians need to be aware of their patients' use of corticosteroids because exercise and activity protocols for these patients may need to be modified in order to prevent fractures from occurring.

AGING SPINE

As noted above, the bone density changes of the spine are significant and are a normal part of aging. Other structures which undergo significant aging changes within the spine include the ligaments of the spine, the intervertebral discs, and the zygapophyseal joints. As noted above, the aging ligaments of the spine are no different than other ligaments in the body and they also diminish in tensile strength. This loss in tensile strength combined with loss of trunk musculature strength may lead into spinal instability. The ligamentum flavum thickens with aging and it has been demonstrated that there is a 50 percent increase in thickness in persons over 60 years of age.[64] The thickened ligamentum flavum occupies valuable space within the spinal canal, and with extension of the spine this ligament can cause spinal cord compression since it causes narrowing of the canal. This spinal canal narrowing is also exacerbated in the elderly patient by the usual aging process of osteophyte development. Lumbar stenosis is a common diagnosis among the elderly. The intervertebral disc also undergoes significant changes with aging. The greatest changes occur at the nucleus pulposus and the transitional region between the nucleus pulposus and the annulus fibrosis. Dehydration of the nucleus pulposus starts to occur by the age of 40 and the gelatinous nucleus pulposus becomes firm. The disc becomes stiffer and this stiffness plays a role in the decreased overall spinal ROM noted in the elderly. With aging, fissures and cracks begin to appear in the disc and

disc herniation may progress with increased flexion loads to the spine while performing ADLs with poor body mechanics and sustained sitting postures which are normal with the older patient. The aging discs' ability to distribute force is also altered with these physiologic changes and thus more load is placed on the vertebral body's, zygapophyseal joints, and spinal ligaments. The zygapophyseal joints undergo a degenerative process that is typical of synovial joints and particular degeneration of the articular cartilage is noted in the cervical and lumbar spine.[43] Spinal disorders may progress into decreased mobility due to pain and lower-extremity weakness, and with decreased mobility comes the other functional deficits noted in previous sections. It is important for the physical therapist to thoroughly evaluate the aging client to determine if the pain is due to musculoskeletal, neurogenic, vascular, or systemic dysfunction. The aging process causes dysfunctions in all these systems and any of these systems may be the cause of spine pain. The treatment program must look at the total body and include lower-extremity strengthening and flexibility exercise to provide a foundation that allows the aging client to perform proper body mechanics. Trunk stabilization exercises must also be incorporated but the clinician may need to alter the position of treatment to accommodate areas of weakness or stiffness in the elderly patient.

FRACTURES IN THE ELDERLY

Fractures are a common occurrence in older adults and are of both medical and socioeconomic importance. Approximately 250,000 individuals over the age of 65 experience a hip fracture in the United States each year.[62] Hip fractures alone have an associated mortality rate as high as 50 percent. Other common fracture sites include the proximal humerus, distal radius, and vertebrae. There are many reasons for the increased incidence of fractures in the elderly, but the two primary risk factors are osteoporosis and falls. Therefore, interventions for fractures in the elderly should also include measures to prevent osteoporosis and reduce the risk for falls. Once a fracture has occurred, the clinician must work toward the restoration of preinjury levels of function, mobility, and self-care.

Fractures of the Proximal Humerus

Fractures of the proximal humerus account for approximately 4–5 percent of all fractures.[3] Their incidence rises dramatically beyond the fifth decade and occurs more frequently among women than among men. Existing osteoporosis is a major risk factor for proximal humeral fractures in the senior population. The most common mechanism of injury is a fall on an outstretched hand from standing height or less. Fractures of the proximal humerus sustained in this manner are usually through the surgical neck and are nondisplaced or minimally displaced. When the mechanism involves a direct blow to the shoulder (as in a fall to the side without a protective response), the fracture pattern is usually much more complex.

Neer Classification of Proximal Humerus Fractures

CATEGORY	DESCRIPTION
1-Part	Nondisplaced or minimally displaced
2-Part	1 Part displaced >1 cm or angulated > 45°
3-Part	2 Parts displaced and/or angulated from each other, and from the remaining part
4-Part	4 Parts displaced and/or angulated from each other
Fracture dislocation	Displacement of the humeral head from the joint space with fracture

CLASSIFICATION

About 85 percent of fractures at the proximal humerus are nondisplaced or minimally displaced.[14] The remaining 15 percent exhibit various fracture patterns. Neer developed the most commonly used classification system for these fractures (Table 33-7). The Neer system classifies fractures according to the number of parts or fracture fragments and the degree of angulation (or malalignment) of the parts. To be classified as displaced or angulated, the part must be displaced at least 1 cm or angulated at least 45°.[15] The four important parts that may be displaced or angulated are the head (at the level of the surgical neck or anatomic neck), the greater and lesser tuberosities, and the shaft. When either of the tuberosities fracture, the pull of the attached muscles likely will cause displacement of the fracture's fragments. Fractures at the level of the anatomic neck frequently cause interruption of blood supply to the humeral head and may result in avascular osteonecrosis.

TREATMENT

Many methods of treatment of proximal humeral fractures have been proposed through the years. The disability that results from proximal humeral fracture is usually the result of lost ROM and the development of a frozen shoulder. Shoulder ROM can be lost by angular deformity of the proximal humerus, injury to the rotator cuff, or the development of arthrofibrosis secondary to prolonged immobilization.[15] The treatment goal for patients with a proximal humeral fracture is a united fracture with pain-free function. To achieve this goal, reasonable restoration of the normal anatomy and early rehabilitation are needed. Fortunately, the majority of proximal humeral fractures are nondisplaced or minimally displaced and can be satisfactorily treated with conservative measures. The arm is immobilized with a sling until pain and discomfort decrease. Active exercises for the elbow, wrist, and fingers should begin immediately to avoid stiffness and disability in these noninjured joints. Initial immobilization and early motion has been continually described as having a high degree of success because most proximal humeral fractures are minimally displaced. Because adhesive capsulitis is a frequent complication after fractures of the proximal humerus, early motion exercises should begin as soon as tolerated. Typically, active-assisted exercises can begin about 1 week after the injury. The patient should wear the sling during periods of activity (such as walking) or when sleeping until the soft callus has stabilized the fracture fragments (usually 3–4 weeks after injury). The patient may remove the sling while exercising or when inactive (such as resting in a chair). Attention should also be given to scapular stabilization exercises. The function of these muscles is important for normal scapulohumeral rhythm. As the fracture healing approaches a clinical union, strengthening exercise with external resistance should be added to the overall program (Table 33-8).

Displaced Fractures

Displaced fractures are difficult to treat by closed reduction. Even if closed reduction of the "two-part" and more severe fracture is successful, the rehabilitation program may need to be scaled back to avoid redisplacement. This becomes even more true if the pull of the muscle attachments displaced one of the

Exercise Guidelines for Proximal Humeral Fracture

PROBLEM	EXERCISE	TIME LINE
Maintain or improve ROM	Assisted ROM (wand, wall climbs, pendulum) Passive Overhead stretching (overhead pulley)	End of inflammatory stage (usually 1 week)
Restore strength	Submaximal isometrics	No risk of fragment displacement, usually immediate
	Full active ROM against gravity	X-ray evidence of union, usually 6 weeks
	External resistance/isotonics	Ability to perform full active ROM against gravity, X-ray evidence of union, usually 6 weeks
Maximize function	Touch top of head, back of neck, low back	Assisted—evidence of callus
		Unassisted—X-ray evidence of union, usually 6 weeks

tuberosities. Fractures classified as two-part and above have a greater likelihood of operative reduction and internal fixation (ORIF) to achieve stable fixation.

For patients undergoing open reduction with internal fixation, the postoperative goals remain the same as with nondisplaced fractures: early return to function and avoiding the development of adhesive capsulitis. Because of the numerous types of fracture patterns and different surgical fixations, exercise guidelines must be individual and modified as needed. In some cases, the surgeon will be confident that the internal fixation is stable and the patient may progress through the exercise program more rapidly. In other cases, the rehabilitation program will be slower secondary to comminution, osteoporosis, or damage to the vascular supply. Each of these may compromise stability and/or delay healing.

Fractures of the Distal Radius

Fractures of the distal radius are one of the most common fractures encountered in orthopedics. These fractures constitute 15 percent of all fractures that result in emergency room visits.[21] The elderly have an increased number of distal radius fractures for two reasons. The first is related to the fragility of the bone, secondary to postmenopausal osteoporosis. The second is related to the increased incidence of falls in the elderly as compared to younger individuals. As with proximal humeral fractures in older persons, the usual mechanism of injury is a fall on an outstretched arm.

CLASSIFICATION

No universally accepted classification of distal radius fractures has been developed to date. In order to be considered a distal radius fracture, the fracture must have occurred within 3 cm of the radiocarpal joint.[45] The Colles' fracture is the most common type of distal radius fracture and is by definition a dorsally angulated and displaced fracture of the radial metaphysis within 2 cm of the articular surface.[21] Comminution of the fracture is most common in the elderly. Because of the fracture fragment displacement, the majority of these fractures require some type of reduction to ensure anatomic alignment. Most Colles' fractures are managed by closed reduction and cast fixation. Open reduction with internal fixation, external fixators, or percutaneous pins and plaster may be used for severe cases with displacement. A Smith's fracture, conversely, is a volar angulated and displaced metaphyseal fracture that may be intra-articular, extra-articular, or part of a fracture dislocation.[21] This type of fracture usually occurs from a fall onto the dorsum of the hand. A Smith's fracture is often very unstable and may result in significant disability after it has healed. Carpal tunnel syndrome and reflex sympathetic dystrophy are potential complications of Smith's fracture.

TREATMENT

General principles for exercise and treatment are similar for both types of distal radial fracture. Nondisplaced fractures are treated nonoperatively. A short arm cast is usually applied and

the fracture immobilized for 3–4 weeks. If at that time there is radiographic evidence of healing and the fracture site is minimally tender, a removable splint is applied until the area is nontender. Overall, the most important rehabilitation consideration is early ROM. Full active ROM exercises for all nonimmobilized joints of the upper extremity should begin as soon as the fracture has been stabilized. This is most important for the glenohumeral joint in order to prevent the development of adhesive capsulitis. Although the cast should end at the proximal palmar crease to allow motion of the metacarpophalangeal (MCP) joints, sometimes the cast nevertheless limits motion. Therefore, it is important to move the MCP joints as much as the cast will allow. The patient should also perform active exercises of the remaining thumb and finger joints. Strict compliance with active ROM exercises several times a day will minimize loss of function during the immobilization period.

Typically, all immobilization is removed at about 6 weeks postinjury and ROM and strengthening exercises for the immobilized joints are initiated at this time. Emphasis should be on restoring motion in wrist extension, forearm supination, thumb opposition, and finger MCP joint flexion. Restoring wrist extensor and grip strength exercises is very important to restore function of the hand and wrist.

With displaced fractures, surgical fixation is usually required. Types of surgical fixation include pins in plaster, percutaneous pinning, external fixation, and open reduction with internal fixation. Postreduction care will parallel that of nondisplaced fractures.

Fractures of the Proximal Femur

Fractures of the proximal femur are common problems for the older population and are one of the most potentially devastating injuries in the elderly. The incidence of hip fracture increases after the age of 50 and then doubles for each decade beyond 50 years of age.[35] More than 200,000 hip fractures occur in the United States each year, and the current mortality rate 1 year after hip fracture in elderly patients ranges from 12 to 36 percent.[35] Mortality is higher than for age-matched individuals without hip fractures, with the highest mortality rates occurring in institutionalized patients. After 1 year, mortality rates return to those for age- and sex-matched controls.[35]

Osteoporosis is a common predisposing factor for hip fractures. As many as 7 percent of hip fractures may occur spontaneously.[35] The most common mechanism for injury is a fall producing a direct blow over the greater trochanter. Following fracture, disability and functional dependence are common. Therefore, the overall goal of the treatment is to return the patient to the preinjury level of function.

CLASSIFICATION

The three common classifications of femoral neck fractures are those based on (1) anatomic location of the fracture, (2) direction of the fracture angle, and (3) displacement of the fracture fragments. With regard to anatomic location, surgeons divide fractures of the proximal femur into three groups. Femoral neck fractures are located from just below the articular surface to just superior to the intertrochanteric area. Intertrochanteric fractures are located between the greater and lesser trochanters. Subtrochanteric fractures occur in the proximal shaft below the level of the lesser trochanters. For patients over the age of 65, 95 percent of hip fractures are in the femoral neck or the intertrochanteric regions.[35]

TREATMENT

It is generally accepted that surgical management, followed by early mobilization, is the treatment of choice for hip fractures in the elderly. Historically, nonoperative management resulted in an excessive rate of medical morbidity and mortality as well as malunion and nonunion in displaced fractures. The overall goal of treatment for fracture of the proximal femur is to return the patient to the preinjury level of function as quickly and as safely as possible. Age, cognitive impairment, and coexisting morbidities may impact the level of independence the patient is able to achieve. The therapist should develop the postoperative care on an individual basis in consultation with the physician. Because of the high degree of variability in fracture patterns and postoperative fracture stability, ongoing communication is essential to developing a safe and effective rehabilitation program.

Physical therapy should begin on the first postoperative day. Patients who receive more than one physical therapy treatment session per day are more likely to regain functional independence and return home.[32] The treatment program should include ROM and strengthening exercises, training in transfers and gait with an assistive device, and training in functional activities such as ADLs. The exercise program should increase in intensity and difficulty until the day of discharge. Some surgeons have recommended restricted weight bearing until the fracture has healed, whereas others have shown that unrestricted weight bearing can be started immediately without detrimental effects in the presence of stable internal fixation. Biomechanical data have shown that non-weightbearing ambulation places significant stresses across the hip as a result of muscular contraction at the hip and knee.[35] Gait training with an assistive device should begin on the first postoperative day. Distance should be advanced and stair training introduced over the next couple of days. Ideally, the patient should be able to ambulate well enough to negotiate the indoor home environment by the time of discharge. Weight bearing as tolerated with a walker is appropriate for the majority of femoral neck and intertrochanteric fracture patients treated with ORIF or prosthetic replacement.

Cemented fixation of prosthetic replacements allows immediate full-weightbearing, whereas biological growth fixation may delay full-weightbearing for 6–12 weeks. Biological growth fixation is thought to have a lower fixation failure rate than cemented fixation and is preferable in younger, more active individuals. For older individuals who are at risk for greater morbidity and mortality after fracture, the early weight-bearing status afforded by cemented fixation may be desirable. Because there is a greater likelihood of instability and healing complica-

tions with subtrochanteric fractures, patients with these types of fractures may require a longer period of protected weight bearing. The patient should advance to a cane and eventually eliminate the assistive devices when fracture healing and safety considerations permit.

During the first few weeks of fracture healing, emphasis should focus on active or active-assistive ROM exercises with gravity eliminated, progressing to full active motion exercises against gravity as soon as allowed by adequate fracture healing. It is important that the patient begin the exercise program as tolerated on the first postoperative day. The exercise program should be designed to help prepare the patient for functional activities. Patients should perform the exercises in the supine, sitting, and standing positions. It is important for the patient to be able to move the operated limb through a full ROM against gravity in order to perform simple ADLs, such as bed mobility and transfers. In most cases following ORIF, there is no restriction of the ROM activities. In contrast, patients who undergo prosthetic replacement of the femoral head will likely be restricted in the amounts of hip flexion ($<90°$), adduction ($0°$), and internal rotation ($0°$) allowed in the early postoperative period because of hip dislocation risk. Exercises should progress in intensity each day until the patient can move and control the limb independently. After some healing has occurred (3–4 weeks), external resistance may be added, provided the patient's strength is good enough to achieve full ROM against gravity without assistance. Pain during resistance exercise may indicate that the exercise is too intensive and should be monitored by the therapist. Restoring hip-abductor and knee-extensor strength are critical for ambulatory function after hip fracture and should receive particular attention.

Fractures of the Spine

Compression fractures of the vertebrae are a common result of osteoporosis, leading to significant pain and functional limitation for seniors. Each year in the United States, an estimated 538,000 vertebral fractures occur in elderly patients with osteoporosis.[42] The rate of vertebral fractures rises sharply with advancing age. At age 70, for every 100 people, there are 20 vertebral fractures each year, and 90 percent of the population has vertebral body compression on plain film radiographs by age 75 years.[42]

Vertebral fractures in this group often result from relatively minor trauma. Osteoporotic compression fractures can be the result of a fall, but often occur spontaneously or in association with normal functional activities such as bending forward. There is a sudden onset of pain in the back and sometimes along the distribution of intercostal nerves. Because the fracture does not damage the posterior and middle columns of the vertebrae, there is no neurological deficit. These fractures are sometimes called anterior wedge fractures because the anterior vertebral body collapses to form a triangular or trapezoidal shape. They are associated with an increase of kyphosis at the level of the fracture and a shortening in the height of the individual.

TREATMENT

The management of spinal fractures is guided by the same principal considerations that guide the management of spinal disorders in general: stability, deformity, and integrity of the neural elements.[42] Osteoporotic compression fractures take from 3 to 6 months to heal, but delayed union may result from interrupted vascular supply or from general poor health and old age.[59] The anterior wedge deformity most often persists, even if the bone heals. Initially there is severe pain associated with muscle spasm. The treatment program should be designed to provide symptomatic relief, restore mobility, and provide education in body mechanics to prevent further trauma and deformity. Therapists should teach patients to avoid flexion postures and to logroll onto their sides before sitting up. External supports such as corsets or braces help to maintain posture and relieve pain but many times are poorly tolerated by elderly individuals.

As soon as patients can tolerate movement (usually within 2 weeks), they should be taught how to arise and ambulate without flexing the spine. Patients should always keep the spine erect, avoiding flexion and rotation. Bending the knees should replace bending at the waist, and turning the whole body should replace twisting at the spine. Patients may use assistive devices for ambulation if needed, but this may encourage flexion postures. Safety and fall prevention are paramount and should determine progression to ambulation without an assistive device.

Sinaki and Mikkelsen advocate extension exercises to minimize the possibility of sustaining more compression fractures in the future. Flexion exercises greatly increased the frequency of additional compression fractures.[59] Extension exercises reverse kyphotic postures, unload the anterior vertebral bodies, and strengthen the erector spinae muscles.[59] The exercise program should be graded according to the stage of healing and the patient's symptoms. Initial exercises should consist of gentle elevation and retraction of the scapula while supine and sitting to reverse the kyphotic posture. Have the patient take a deep breath to elevate the ribcage while elevating and retracting the scapula. As symptoms allow, instruct the patient to raise the arms overhead in conjunction with scapular elevation and deep breathing. The patient should next gradually progress to the prone-lying posture. When prone lying is tolerated and is relatively asymptomatic (usually 4–6 weeks), erector spinae strengthening exercises should be added to the program. With the patient prone lying with the arms at the sides, have the patient raise the head and shoulders off the supporting surface without using the arms to push up. Intensity of exercise can be increased gradually by moving the arms from the sides to overhead. Eventually, the patient can advance to exercising on all fours by raising alternate arms and legs off of the supporting surface.

Recent medical advances in treating thoracic compression fractures include the minimally invasive procedure called balloon kyphoplasty. The goal of this procedure is to restore vertebral body height by filling in the compressed body of the vertebrae and alleviate pain quickly. The procedure consists of a small incision made on the posterior aspect of the spine through which a narrow tube is placed. Using fluoroscopy to guide the tube into the vertebral fracture site, the narrow tube serves as the working channel. A special balloon is inserted through the tube into the compressed vertebral site and is inflated. As the balloon inflates, it elevates the fracture, returning the vertebral body to a more normal position. It creates an inner cavity inside the vertebral body. The balloon is then deflated and removed. A pasty cement like substance is then inserted through the channel and fills in the cavity within the vertebral body. The substance hardens quickly and stabilizes the fracture and sustains the vertebral height. This procedure is performed under local anesthesia, and the patient usually goes home within 24 hours of the procedure, barring no complications. The patient is advised to resume normal ADLs but to refrain from strenuous activities especially lifting for 6 weeks. This procedure may not be appropriate for all patients with compression fractures, and more research is needed to determine the outcomes and long-term effects of balloon kyphoplasty.[7] As noted above, trunk strengthening exercises and postural training is essential in restoring function and further fracture prevention and should be a part of the follow-up care for this procedure.

TOTAL JOINT ARTHROPLASTY

Hip, knee, and shoulder arthroplasty are increasingly common procedures. Replacement of damaged cartilage surfaces with artificial weight bearing materials has enabled surgeons to dramatically improve function and relieve pain in many patients. OA is the precursor to most total joint replacements and it is estimated that prevalence of OA in the United States will increase from 43 million in 1997 to 60 million in 2020.[11] Medical advances have allowed total joint replacements of the hip and knee to become much less invasive in the past few years and depending on the type of fixation, either cemented or noncemented, immediate weight bearing of some degree is possible. The large volumes of information on this topic does not allow for an in-depth discussion on this topic to occur in this chapter. Consensus in the research does indicate that therapeutic exercise is the treatment modality of choice for preoperative and the postoperative care following total joint arthroplasties.[49]

SPECIAL CONSIDERATIONS

Polypharmacy

Older persons are more likely to have a number of medical problems and to be taking many medications. The excessive use of medication in the elderly is known as polypharmacy. Patients may take different medications prescribed by different physicians. It has been reported that 87 percent of older patients are taking at least one prescription medication and three over-the-counter drugs each day.[46] There is a linear relationship between the number of drugs taken and the increased potential for adverse drug reactions.[30] Approximately 19 percent of hospital admissions of older persons are attributable to drug reactions.[30] Increased sensitivity to drug effects can be due to changes in drug absorption with age, the number of drugs taken simultaneously, or failure of health care providers to take into account the proper way to prescribe and administer drugs to geriatric patients.

Although there are many potential adverse outcomes of polypharmacy, some are of particular interest here. The effects of drugs—particularly benzodiazepines, barbiturates, and antidepressants—are among the risk factors associated with falls. Even if the individual does not suffer a serious fall, the threat of a fall is often enough to cause one to limit activity, which results in deconditioning and functional decline. Delirium, a temporary change in attention and consciousness, may be mistaken for dementia (a permanent loss of intellectual abilities), when in fact it may be due to drug sensitivity. Confusion is especially common when drug reactions occur in someone with preexisting mild dementia. A person suffering from a mild adverse drug reaction that goes undetected for months may experience a gradual reduction in self-care skills and independence. Patients experiencing musculoskeletal complaints often are chronic users of nonsteroidal anti-inflammatory drugs, which can cause gastric bleeding. Narcotics may result in oversedation and loss of functional ability.[41]

All medications taken by the elderly population should be regularly checked by their primary physician. The physician needs to know what drugs the patient is taking so that he/she can eliminate duplications and generally be aware of and avoid adverse effects of drug interactions. A thorough history of the older adult seeking rehabilitation services should include a list of current medications. One should consider adverse reactions when evaluating acute changes in functional ability and mentation. Patients and families should be instructed to keep all medications in the original containers, never mix several drugs in one bottle, and throw away what is no longer in use.

CONSIDERATIONS FOR THE GERIATRIC HISTORY AND PHYSICAL EXAMINATION

When conducting a history for the elderly patient/client in an orthopedic setting, there are several considerations that must be made. Table 33-9 provides an overview of some of the additional questions that incorporate the concepts discussed previously. It is important to gain insight into whether or not the patient/client has experienced a decline in function. If so, it is important to further determine the time line of this decline and what precipitating factors may have contributed, including the presenting orthopedic problem. Other cognitive or psychosocial factors may be responsible for or have contributed to the decline, and referral to another practitioner may be indicated. Screening for signs of preclinical decline is needed if the patient/client does not report any frank decline in function. It is helpful to include family members or caregivers in the history, as they may have other observations about the patient/client's functional status.

Inquiring about the patient/client's home environment and barriers to independence and safety should be done with respect to the presenting problem and overall functional status. Additionally, assistive device use should be determined. It is helpful to differentiate between devices that were prescribed by an appropriately trained clinician versus those that are borrowed from family or friends. Often times, those devices that are borrowed from friends or family are not optimal for the individual patient's need, and may even increase risk of injury.

Obtaining a patient's fall history is an essential element to the geriatric history, especially for those orthopedic problems that are the result of a fall or that may contribute to impaired balance and gait disturbances. Orthopedic foot problems, lower-extremity weakness, and gait disturbances are consistently found to increase fall risk. Persons with one or more falls in the preceding 6 months are at an elevated risk for future falls.[56,57] Asking

---

TABLE 33-9

Additional Data to be Collected during the History and Systems Review

- Determine not only recent prior level of function, but also how level of function has changed over the past several years. Try to identify time line and precipitating events for change in function.
- Functional status with respect to basic ADLs and instrumental ADLs. If assistance is required, who provides that assistance.
- What activities take longer to perform, are done less frequently, or have to do differently than previously (signs of preclinical decline).
- If the patient's family member or caregiver is available, solicit both the patient's and family/caregiver's perception and observations about past and current level of function.
- Ask about home environment and what barriers to improved level of function exist.
- Assistive device use. Distinguish between devices owned versus borrowed, and who prescribed the device.
- Community resources used to assist with ADLs.
- Caregiver ability and availability.
- Fall history and ability to rise from the floor.
- Medications: medications associated with high fall risk, medications associated with extrapyramidal symptoms (EPS), pain management.

about ability to rise from the floor without assistance is not only an indicator about general mobility, but can also predict the need for instruction in floor transfers.[63]

Finally, a review of medications associated with increased fall risk should be conducted. Medications associated with increased fall risk include anti-Parkinson, anticonvulsant, antihypertensive, and antidepressant (especially tricyclic antidepressants) medications.[22,38]

The physical examination for various orthopedic problems may not be significantly different in an elderly patient/client; however, the instruments or tests used to assess function are different. It is particularly helpful to use tests that not only attempt to quantify function, but also (1) provide some age- or population-related norms or averages, and/or (2) provide a threshold to use as a reference for detecting clinically significant limitations. This allows the differentiation between normal age-related changes versus clinically significant changes associated with either inactivity and/or disease processes. Other findings from the history and physical exam will then help with determining the contributions from each. Performance-based functional tests are commonly used and are useful in assessing different areas of functional mobility and independence. Table 33-10 provides a summary of age-related norms for these tests.

The TUG measures the time it takes to stand from a standard armchair, walk 3 m, return to the chair, and sit. Thresholds to distinguish between levels of independence with ADLs include independence (<20 seconds), assistance with ADLs (>30 seconds), and varying levels of independence (20–29 seconds).[51] The TUG has also been used to assess fall risk, but has not consistently demonstrated to be sensitive in detecting fallers.

The Timed Chair Rise is a measure of functional mobility and lower-body strength. Several versions of the test have been studied, including the time required to perform five sit-to-stand repetitions (17-in. high armless chair, no use of the upper extremities), or how many repetitions can be performed in 30 seconds.[34]

The 6-minute walk test has been used as a measure of exercise tolerance and endurance. In candidates awaiting heart transplantation, distances less than 300 m are associated with a significantly higher risk of death or pretransplant hospitalization within 6 months.[10]

Comfortable gait speed is a measure of walking ability and balance. Gait speeds of less than $0.56 \text{ m} \cdot \text{s}^{-1}$ in frail elderly have an increased risk of recurrent falls,[66] and speeds less than $0.6 \text{ m} \cdot \text{s}^{-1}$ are strongly associated with poorer health status.[60]

T A B L E   3 3 - 1 0

Age-Related Normative Values for Functional Performance Measures

	AGE MEAN (SD) [SE]		
	60–69	70–79	80–89
Timed up and go (sec)			
Male	8 (2)	9 (3)	10 (1)
Female	8 (2)	9 (2)	11 (3)
Combined	7.24 [.17]	8.54 [.17]	
30-sec timed chair rise (repetitions)			
Male	15.8 (4.4)	14.3 (4.2)	11.8 (4.3)
Female	14 (3.75)	12.7 (3.7)	10.8 (4.1)
Combined	14 (2.4)	12.9 (3.0)	11.9 (3.6)
5-repetitions timed chair rise (sec)			
Male	12.7 [.24]	13.4 [.29]	14.7 [.25]
Female	13.2 [.22]	14.2 [.29]	16.58 [.30]
6-min walk test (m)			
Male	572 (92)	527 (85)	417 (73)
Female	538 (92)	471 (75)	392 (85)
Male	597 (90)	534 (104)	457 (120)
Female	536 (85)	483 (97)	406 (113)
Comfortable gait speed (m/sec)			
Male	1.59 (.24)	1.38 (.23)	1.21 (.18)
Female	1.44 (.25)	1.33 (.22)	1.15 (.21)

The information in this table is compiled from Refs. 33, 34, 48, 55, and 61.

The physical performance test (PPT) is a measure of basic ADL and instrumental ADL, where higher scores indicate higher levels of function. It exists as a 7-item (PPT-7) and 9-item (PPT-9) versions. PPT-7 cutoff scores of 15 demonstrated 78 and 71 percent sensitivity and specificity for recurrent falls,[66] and PPT-7 scores between 20 and 23 were consistent with declines in walking ability.[4] As a measure of frailty, PPT-9 scores are as follows: not frail (32–36 points), mildly frail (25–31 points), or moderately frail (17–24 points).[8]

Community ambulation has been defined by (1) the ability to ambulate 332 m continuously, negotiate a 7–8-in. curb, climb three steps and ramp without a rail, and walk at a gait speed of at least $1.16 \text{ m} \cdot \text{s}^{-1}$ to cross a street.[40] Shumway-Cook et al.[58] have further described how individual-related factors interact with environmental demands such as gait speed requirements, carrying a load, uneven terrain, and postural transitions to contribute to mobility disability. Therefore, consideration of a variety of functional gait tasks must be considered in determining the extent of functional limitation and designing rehabilitation programs for orthopedic-related limitations in mobility.

Other objective testing during the evaluation of the elderly patient may also reveal general patterns such as significant postural changes, decreases in joint ROM in all peripheral joints and the spine, and overall decrease in muscular strength throughout the body. All of these changes have a strong ability to impact overall physiologic capabilities of the elderly client but do not necessarily mean functional loss or cessation of activity. The objective findings during the evaluation will lead the clinicians in their treatment plan and allow them to prioritize the treatment goals.

An example of how a neurological comorbidity of an elderly patient plays a role in the rehabilitation of a typical orthopedic condition is as follows. A 75-year-old male presents to an outpatient orthopedic clinic with a diagnosis of adhesive capsulitis of the shoulder. The patient reports that the mechanism of injury was when he stumbled on a throw rug at home and fell onto the floor with the force directly on his shoulder. This injury occurred approximately 4 weeks prior and now his shoulder is stiff, painful, and weak. The patient's primary complaint is that he cannot move his arm enough to put on his shirt without help from his wife, reach his back pocket, or put on his seat belt. The patient reports he had a contusion in the deltoid region that has now resolved and he had X-rays and an MRI that ruled out any fractures or rotator cuff tears. His medical history includes an 11-year history of Parkinson's disease with no other remarkable comorbidities noted.

Based on the subjective patient's history the physical therapist has two different issues that must be evaluated. The patient has the orthopedic injury that started as a hematoma and has developed into a soft tissue restriction due to patient-induced immobilization secondary to pain and fear of hurting his shoulder more with activity. Another issue the clinician must take into consideration is the effect of Parkinson's disease on the patient's balance and gait, which may have been the underlying cause of the fall. The examination process must evaluate both the movement dysfunction of the shoulder and also the balance and dynamic gait deficits that are present due to the 11-year history of Parkinson's. Comprehensive treatment of this patient would include treating the shoulder dysfunction and also developing an exercise program and patient education plan, taking into consideration the neurological issues associated with Parkinson's. Other issues to consider while treating this patient would be the postural changes that have occurred with this long history of Parkinson's and its effect on various treatment positions such as supine, side-lying, and prone. The forward head and thoracic kyphosis that typically accompany this neurological condition must be accommodated with pillows to facilitate a comfortable treatment posture when lying on the treatment table. It is also important to monitor when the patient takes the medication (usually Levodopa) to control his Parkinson's tremors and rigidity. It would be advantageous to perform the joint and soft tissue mobilizations along with the active exercises during the time frame when the body is at its most relaxed state. The clinician will have difficulty making therapeutic gains and could put the patient at risk of injury if he/she performs manual therapy techniques to the shoulder when the rigidity of the muscles is at its highest. The patients should be able to tell the clinician at which time in their medication cycle they feel their muscles are the most relaxed, and that would be the desirable time for treatment.

The above example illustrates the challenges present when treating the elderly patient in an orthopedic setting. Rarely, will an elderly patient present with a "simple" orthopedic injury that is not compounded with other comorbidities. The physical therapist must look at the big picture and evaluate multiple systems and determine what functional deficits are present at the orthopedic injury site (such as shoulder in above example) and how the aging process on the entire body may affect the overall functional status of the patient. Treatment plans must incorporate exercises for both local and global deficits detected in the evaluation process.

Patient Education

The key to successful treatment of any dysfunction is the ability and desire of the patients to follow through with the prescribed exercise program given to them by the treating clinician. Through years of experience in treating the elderly patient the authors of this chapter have found that using an analogy of a car and comparing it to the aging process of the human body is an excellent way to educate the patient. We all desire to drive a luxury automobile that is powerful, smooth, efficient, quiet, and reliable. This can also be said about our human body. As we age, individual systems of the body, not unlike those of the automobile, can become deficient and affect the overall performance of the entire car. An example of this may be when the strength and flexibility of the lower extremities are diminished (i.e., worn shocks and suspension system of the car), the articular surfaces of the joints may be more susceptible to

T A B L E   3 3 - 1 1

Patient Education Using the Car Analogy

CAR SYSTEM	BODY SYSTEM
Shock and suspension system	Muscle strength and flexibility
Tires	Articular cartilage and joints
Engine	Cardiovascular and muscular endurance
Air filter and exhaust system	Pulmonary system
Car frame	Skeletal system
Fluids (gas, oil, coolant, etc.)	Hydration and nutrition

degeneration and damage (wear and tear on the tires). Similar examples can be found using this human body and car analogy. See Table 33-11.

EXERCISE TRAINING GUIDELINES FOR OLDER ADULTS

The deleterious effects of immobility are well documented. Because of the summative effects of aging on multiple systems, fatigue, reduction in sensory information, fear of falling, and effects of accumulated disease processes, many older adults experience a gradual reduction in activity level over time. This decreased activity or a state of hypokinesia sets up a vicious cycle of disuse and loss of function. Loss of muscle mass, demineralization of bone, diminished cardiopulmonary function, and loss of neuromotor control have been directly related to lack of physical activity. Disuse exacerbates the aging process and negatively impacts physiologic reserve in the face of disease and injury. Participation in a regular exercise program has proven to be an effective intervention/modality to reduce or prevent functional declines associated with aging (Table 33-12). Regular exercise can also provide a number of psychological benefits related to preserved cognitive function, alleviation of depression

symptoms, and behavior and an improved concept of personal control and self-efficacy.

Participation in a regular exercise program is an effective intervention/modality to reduce/prevent a number of functional declines associated with aging. Older individuals well into eighth and ninth decades of life respond to both endurance and strength training. Regular exercise and physical activity contribute to a healthier, independent lifestyle with associated improved functional capacity and quality of life. Rehabilitation following injury or illness should include education regarding the benefits of physical activity and instruction for the implementation of and safe participation in a lifelong exercise program.

The American College of Sports Medicine has established guidelines for exercise testing and participation for older individuals. Prior to the initiation of any exercise program, it is recommended that all individuals undergo a physical examination and a diagnostic exercise workup. A proper warm-up routine is essential for all individuals engaged in an exercise program. The warm-up routine should involve some gentle stretching exercises that may last from 5 to 15 minutes. Some stretching activities and a cool-down period at the conclusion of the exercise program are also recommended. The intensity level is recommended to be 20–30 minutes, a minimum of

T A B L E   3 3 - 1 2

Summary of the Physiologic Benefits of Physical Activity for Older Persons

- *Aerobic/cardiovascular endurance.* Substantial improvements in almost all aspects of cardiovascular functioning have been observed following appropriate physical training.
- *Muscle strength.* Individuals of all ages can benefit from muscle strengthening exercises. Resistance training can have a significant impact on the maintenance of independence in old age.
- *Flexibility.* Exercises that incorporate movement throughout the range of motion assist in the preservation and restoration of flexibility.
- *Balance/coordination.* Regular activity helps prevent and/or postpone the age-associated declines in balance and coordination that are risk factors for falls.
- *Velocity of movement.* Behavioral slowing is a characteristic of advancing age. Individuals who are regularly active can often postpone these age-related declines.

SOURCE: World Health Organization, 1997.

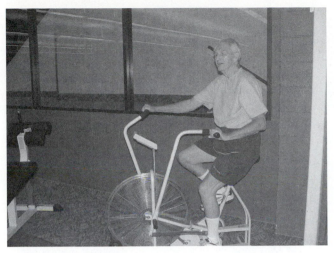

FIGURE 33-1

The airdyne bicycle, an excellent choice for aerobic exercise in the geriatric population.

three times per week, at light to moderate intensity levels to optimize health. Walking, running, swimming, and cycling are large-muscle rhythmic aerobic forms of exercise and minimize the risk of musculoskeletal injuries (Figs. 33-1 and 33-2).[2]

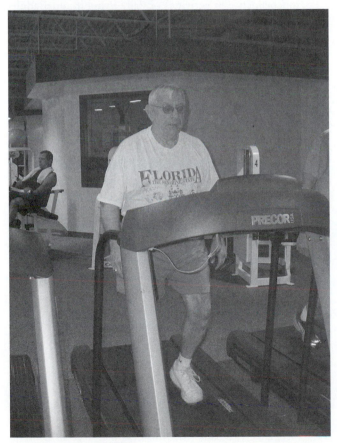

FIGURE 33-2

The treadmill, an alternate choice for aerobic training in the geriatric population.

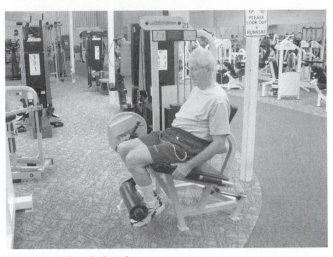

FIGURE 33-3

A senior performing resistance training for the lower extremities. Caution must be used to promote proper technique and avoid irritation to the joints.

For resistance training, exercise should be performed with proper body mechanics and should include large-muscle groups (Figs. 33-3 and 33-4). Attention should focus closely on the quality of movement rather than the quantity. Each exercise should be performed slowly and through a full ROM if possible. Once muscle fatigue occurs, the movement pattern becomes poor, the smoothness of motion is reduced, and the ROM is decreased, thereby reducing the training effect. Quick or ballistic movements should be avoided. It is best to use several sets of exercise (usually a minimum of three) consisting of 7–10 repetitions. If the intent of the exercise program is to build muscular endurance and not muscle mass, the number of repetitions must be increased to 20 or more.[2]

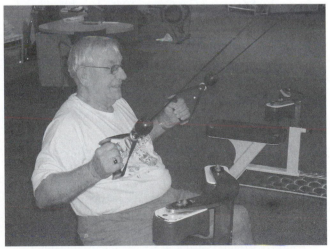

FIGURE 33-4

A senior performing resistance training for the upper extremities. Caution must be used to promote proper technique, and avoid substitution and joint irritation.

SUMMARY

- The field of geriatrics will continue to grow as the population ages. As life expectancy increases, rehabilitation of the physically disabled elderly will become an increasingly essential component of overall geriatric care.
- The aging process affects multiple systems in the body and has a direct impact on the rehabilitation of acute and chronic musculoskeletal conditions common in the elderly.
- Orthopedic conditions are commonly experienced by the older population. Fractures commonly occur and are often the result of osteoporosis and falls. When articular cartilage damage is severe or there is chronic joint pain, hip, knee, and shoulder arthroplasty are increasingly common procedures specifically designed to provide patients with dramatically improved lifestyle and function.
- Examination and evaluation of older adults must focus on determining the relative contributions from aging, inactivity, and disease on reduced physical functioning.
- Emphasis in the rehabilitation program should be placed upon the importance of physical activity in preventing injury and minimizing functional decline. Rehabilitation providers must be aware of the special needs that this population has in order to facilitate the development of effective rehabilitation interventions.

REFERENCES

1. Abyad A, Boyer JT. Arthritis and aging. *Curr Opin Rheumatol* 4:153–159, 1992.
2. American College of Sports Medicine. *Guidelines for Exercise Testing and Prescription*, 5th ed. Baltimore, Williams & Wilkins, 1995, pp. 1–373.
3. Bigliani LU, Craig EV, Butters KP. Fractures of the shoulder. In: Rockwood CA, Green DP, Bucholz RW, eds. *Fractures in Adults*. Philadelphia, Lippincott, 1991.
4. Brach JS, VanSwearingen JM. Identifying early decline of physical function in performance-based and self-report measures. *Phys Ther* 82:320–328, 2002.
5. Brock DB, Guralnik JM, Brody JA. Demography and epidemiology of aging in the United States. In: Schneider EL, Rowe JW, eds. *Handbook of the Biology of Aging*, 3rd ed. San Diego, Academic Press, 1990.
6. Brooks G. Physical therapy associated with primary prevention, risk reduction, and deconditioning. In: DeTurk WE, Cahalin LP, Guccione AA, eds. *Cardiovascular and Pulmonary Physical Therapy*. New York, McGraw-Hill, 2004.
7. Brown CW, Wong DC. Description of kyphoplasty surgery, 2005. Available at www.spine-health.com.
8. Brown M, Sinacore DR, Ehsani AA, Binder EF, Holloszy JO, Kohrt WM. Physical and performance measures for the identification of mild to moderate frailty. *J Gerontol A Biol Sci Med Sci* 55(6):M350–M355, 2000.
9. Buchner DM. Understanding variability in studies of strength training in older adults: A meta-analytic perspective. *Top Geriatr Rehabil* 8:1–21, 1993.
10. Cahalin LP. The six-minute walk test predicts peak oxygen uptake and survival in patients with advanced heart failure. *Chest* 110:325–332, 1996.
11. Centers for Disease Control and Prevention. Arthritis prevalence and activity limitations—United States. *Morb Mortal Wkly Rep* 43:433–438, 1994.
12. Chan L, Tsai JC, Want CH. Disability and health care costs in the medicare population. *Arch Phys Med Rehabil* 83:1196–1201, 2002.
13. Chandler JM, Duncan PW. Balance and falls in the elderly: Issues in evaluation and treatment. In: Guccione AA, ed. *Geriatric Physical Therapy*. St. Louis, MO, Mosby, 1993.
14. Connolly JF. Fractures of the upper end of the humerus. In: Connolly JF, ed. *Deplama's Management of Fractures and Dislocations: An Atlas*, 3rd ed. Philadelphia, WB Suanders, 1981, pp. 686–738.
15. Cornell CN, Schneider K. Proximal humerus. In: Koval KJ, Zuckerman JD, eds. *Fractures in the Elderly*. Philadelphia, Lippincott, 1998.
16. Covinsky KE, Palmer RM, Fortinsky RH, et al. Loss of independence in activities of daily living in older adults hospitalized with medical illnesses: Increased vulnerability with age. *J Am Geriatr Soc* 51:451–458, 2003.
17. Craik RL. Sensorimotor changes and adaptation in the older adult. In: Guccione AA, ed. *Geriatric Physical Therapy*. St. Louis, MO, Mosby, 1993.
18. Cress ME, Meyer M. Maximal voluntary and functional performance levels needed for independence in adults aged 65 to 97 years. *Phys Ther* 83:37–48, 2003.
19. Daiello LA, Micca JL, Newsome RJ. Optimal care of the patient with dementia: From independent living to assisted living. Paper presented at the American Society of Consultant Pharmacists Annual Meeting and Exhibition, Anaheim, CA, 2002.
20. Deal CL. Osteoporosis: Prevention, diagnosis, and management. *Am J Med* 102:35S–39S, 1997.
21. Dinowitz MI, Koval KJ. Distal radius. In: Koval KJ, Zuckerman JD, eds. *Fractures in the Elderly*. Philadelphia, Lippincott, 1998.
22. Ensrud KE, Blackwell TL, Mangione CM, et al. Central nervous system—active medications and risk for falls in older women. *J Am Geriatr Soc* 50(10):1629–1637, 2002.
23. Eriksrud O, Bohannon RW. Relationship of knee extension force to independence in sit-to-stand performance in patients receiving acute rehabilitation. *Phys Ther* 83:544–551, 2003.
24. Fletcher GF, Balady GJ, Amsterdam EA, et al. Exercise standards for testing and training: A statement for healthcare professionals from the American Heart Association. *Circulation* 104:1694–1740, 2001.

25. Fried LP, Starer DJ, King DE, Lodder F. Preclinical disability: Hypotheses about the bottom of the iceberg. *J Aging Health* 3:285–300, 1991.

26. Fried LP, VanDoorn C, O'Leary JR, Tinetti ME, Drickamer MA. Preclinical mobility predicts incident mobility disability in older women. *J Gerontol A Biol Med Sci* 55:M43–M52, 2000.

27. Friedland R, Summer L. Demography is not destiny. *Washington DC: National Academy on an Aging Society*, 1999.

28. Gallagher D, Visser M, DeMeersman RE. et al. Appendicular skeletal muscle mass: Effects of age, gender, and ethnicity. *J Appl Physiol* 83:229–239, 1997.

29. Greerlings SW, Twish JW, Beekman AT, et al. Longitudinal relationship between pain and depression in older adults: Sex, age, and physical disability. *Soc Psychiatry Psychiatr Epidemiol* 37:23–30, 2002.

30. Grymonpre RE, Mitenko PA, Sitar DS, et al. Drug associated hospital admissions in older medical patients. *J Am Geriatr Soc* 36:1092–1098, 1998.

31. Harda ND, Chiu V, Stewart AL. Mobility-related function in older adults: Assessment with a 6 minute walk test. *Arch Phys Med Rehabil* 80:837–841, 1999.

32. Hoenig H, Rubenstein LV, Sloane R, et al. What is the role of timing on the surgical and rehabilitative care of community dwelling older persons with acute hip fracture? *Arch Intern Med* 157:513–520, 1997.

33. Isles RC, Low Choy NL, Steer M, Nitz JC. Normal values of balance tests in women aged 20–80. *J Am Geriatr Soc* 52:1367–1372, 2004.

34. Jones CJ, Rikli RE, Beam WC. A 30-s chair-stand test as a measure of lower body strength in community-residing older adults. *Res Q Exerc Sport* 70:113–117, 1999.

35. Koval KJ, Zuckerman JD. Hip. In: Koval KJ, Zuckerman JD, eds. *Fractures in the Elderly.* Philadelphia, Lippincott, 1998.

36. Lane JM. Osteoporosis: Medical prevention and treatment. *Spine* 22:32–37, 1997.

37. Larsson L, Sjodin B, Karlsson J. Histochemical and biochemical changes in human skeletal muscle with age in sedentary males, age 22–65 years. *Acta Physiol Scand* 103:31–39, 1978.

38. Leipzig RM, Cumming RG, Tinetti ME. Drugs and falls in older people: A systematic review and meta-analysis. *J Am Geriatr Soc* 47(1):30–50, 1999.

39. Lenze EJ, Schulz R, Martire LM, et al. The course of functional decline in older people with persistently elevated depressive symptoms: Longitudinal findings from the Cardiovascular Health Study. *J Am Geriatr Soc* 53:569–575, 2005.

40. Lerner-Frankiel MB, Vargas S, Brown MB, et al. Functional community ambulation: What are your criteria? *Clin Manage Phys Ther* 6:12–15, 1986.

41. Lewis CB, Bottomly JM. *Geriatric Physical Therapy: A Clinical Approach.* Norwalk, CT, Appleton & Lange, 1994.

42. Main WK, Cammisa FP, O'Leary PF. The Spine. In: Koval KJ, Zuckerman JD, eds. *Fractures in the Elderly.* Philadelphia, Lippincott, 1998.

43. McKenzie R, May S. *The Lumbar Spine Mechanical Diagnosis and Therapy*, Vol. 1. Waikane, New Zealand Spinal Publications, 2004.

44. McKinnis LN. Thoracic spine, sternum and ribs. In: McKinnis LN, ed. *Fundamentals of Orthopedic Radiology.* Philadelphia, FA Davis, 1997, pp. 135–176.

45. Melton LJ, Thamer M, Ran NF, et al. Fractures attributable to osteoporosis: Report from the National Osteoporosis Foundation. *J Bone Miner Res* 12:16–23, 1997.

46. Moellar JF, Mathiowetz NA. Prescribed medicines: A summary of use and expenditures for Medicare beneficiaries. Rockville, MD, U.S. Department of Health and Human Services, 1989, pub. no. PHC 89-3448.

47. Mulsant BH, Ganguli M. Epidemiology and diagnosis of depression in late life. *J Clin Psychiatry* 60(Suppl 20):9–15, 1999.

48. Ostechega Y, Harris TB, Hirsch R, et al. Reliability and prevalence of physical performance examination assessing mobility and balance in older persons in the US: Data from the Third National Health and Nutrition Examination Survey. *J Am Geriatr Soc* 48:1136–1141, 2000.

49. Ottawa Panel Evidence-Based Clinical Practice Guidelines for Therapeutic Exercises and Manual Therapy in the Management of Osteoarthritis. *Phys Ther* 85:907–971, 2005.

50. Phillips SK, Bruce SA, Newton D, et al. The weakness of old age is not due to failure of muscle activation. *J Gerontol* 47:M45–M49, 1992.

51. Podsiadlo D, Richardson S. The timed up and go: A test of basic mobility in frail elderly persons. *J Am Geriatr Soc* 43:17–23, 1995.

52. Protas EJ. Physiological change and adaptation to exercise in the older adult. In: Guccione AA, ed. *Geriatric Physical Therapy.* St. Louis, MO, Mosby, 1993.

53. Reid IR. Glucocorticoid-induced osteoporosis: Assessment and treatment. *J Clin Densiometry* 1:65–73, 1998.

54. Riddle DL, Wells PS. Diagnosis of lower-extremity deep vein thrombosis in outpatients. *Phys Ther* 84:729–735, 2004.

55. Rikli RE, Jones CJ. Functional fitness normative scores for community-residing older adults, aged 60–94. *J Aging and Phys Activity* 7:162–181, 1999.

56. Schmid MA. Reducing patient falls: A research-based comprehensive fall prevention program. *Mil Med* 155:202–207, 1990.

57. Shumway-Cook A, Baldwin M, Polissar NL, et al. Predicting the probability of falls in community-dwelling older adults. *Phys Ther* 77:812–819, 1997.

58. Shumway-Cook A, Patla AE, Stewart A, et al. Environmental demands associated with community mobility in older adults with and without mobility disabilities. *Phys Ther* 82:670–681, 2002.

59. Sinaki M, Mikkelsen BA. Postmenopausal spinal osteoporosis: Flexion versus extension exercises. *Arch Phys Med Rehabil* 65:593–596, 1984.

60. Studenski S, Perera S, Wallace D, et al. Physical performance measures in the clinical setting. *J Am Geriatr Soc* 51:314–322, 2003.

61. Steffen TM, Hacker TA, Mollinger L. Age and gender related test performance in community-dwelling elderly people: Six minute walk test, berg balance scale, timed up and go, and gait speeds. *Phys Ther* 82:128–137, 2002.

62. Tibbitts GM. Patients who fall: How to predict and prevent injuries. *Geriatrics* 51:24–31, 1996.

63. Tinetti ME, Liu WL, Claus EB. Predictors and prognosis of inability to get up after falls among elderly persons. *JAMA* 269:65–70, 1993.

64. Twomey L, Taylor J. Age changes in the lumbar spine and intervertebral canals. *Paraplegia* 26:238–249, 1988.

65. U.S. Bureau of the Census. Population estimates by age, sex, race, and Hispanic origin: 1980–1988. Current Population Reports, series P-25, no. 1045. Washington, DC, U.S. Government Printing Office, 1990.

66. VanSwearingen JM, Paschal KA, Bonino P, et al. Assessing recurrent fall risk of community-dwelling, frail older veterans using specific tests of mobility and the physical performance test of function. *J Gerontol A Biol Sci Med Sci* 53:M457–M464, 1998.

67. Webber AP, Martin JL, Harker JO, et al. Depression in older patients admitted for postacute nursing home rehabilitation. *J Am Geriatr Soc* 53:1017–1022, 2005.

68. Wells PS, Hirsch J, Anderson DR, et al. A simple clinical model for the diagnosis of deep vein thrombosis combined with impedence plethysmography: Potential for an improvement in the diagnostic process. *J Intern Med* 243:15–23, 1998.

69. Woo SL, Hollis JM, Adams DJ, et al. Tensile properties of the human femur-anterior cruciate ligament-tibia complex. The effects of specimen age and orientation. *Am J Sports Med* 19:217–225, 1991.

CHAPTER 34

Considerations for the Pediatric Patient

Steven R. Tippett

OBJECTIVES

After completing this chapter, the therapist should be able to do the following:

- Describe common macrotraumatic and microtraumatic musculoskeletal injuries occurring in the skeletally immature patient.
- Describe selected congenital, acquired, and musculoskeletal pathologies seen in active skeletally immature patients.
- Apply basic rehabilitation principles governing the care and prevention of macrotraumatic and microtraumatic musculoskeletal injuries in the skeletally immature patient.
- Differentiate between categories of growth plate fractures.
- Describe physiologic considerations unique to the active skeletally immature patient.
- Describe special psychological considerations for the skeletally immature athlete.
- Describe participation guidelines for the skeletally immature athlete.

Although the physical and psychological demands placed upon the young patient can be almost as rigorous as the demands placed upon an adult, young minds and bodies are often not suited to accept these demands. Growing musculoskeletal tissue is innately predisposed to specific injuries that vary greatly from the injuries sustained by their skeletally mature counterparts. This chapter briefly describes common macrotraumatic and microtraumatic injuries sustained by the young patient along with basic principles that govern the treatment of these injuries. Macrotraumatic injuries occur as a result of a single, supramaximal loading of bone, ligament, muscle, or tendon. Common youth macrotraumatic injuries that will be discussed include epiphyseal and avulsion fractures. Microtraumatic injuries, on the other hand, result from submaximal loading that occurs in a cyclic and repetitive fashion. Common microtraumatic injuries that occur in the immature musculoskeletal system that will be presented include osteochondroses and traction apophysites. Special concerns unique to the immature musculoskeletal system that do not fall neatly into the macrotraumatic or microtraumatic categories will also be presented in this chapter. Finally, physiologic and psychological issues unique to the youth patient will also be presented.

MACROTRAUMATIC MUSCULOSKELETAL INJURIES

Epiphyseal Fractures

Growing bone is the weak musculoskeletal link in the young athlete. Physical demands resulting in muscle strain or ligament sprain in the skeletally mature patient may result in epiphyseal plate injury in the young patient. The epiphyseal plate or growth plate is divided into zones differentiated from one another via structure and function. Beginning at the growth area of long bone and progressing in the direction of mature long bone, the four regions of the growth plate include the reserve zone, proliferative zone, hypertrophic zone, and bony metaphysis. The reserve zone produces and stores matrix, while the proliferative zone also produces matrix and is the site for longitudinal bone cell growth. The hypertrophic zone is subdivided into the maturation zone, degenerative zone, and zone of provisional calcification. It is within the hypertrophic zone that matrix is prepared for calcification, and it is here that the matrix is ultimately calcified.[18]

It is difficult to predict the collective strength of the entire growth plate due to varying amounts and composition of matrix, along with varying cellular architecture and density.[18] Injury to the growth plate can occur when stress or tensile loads placed upon bone exceed mechanical strength of the growth plate-metaphysis complex. Two factors that impact epiphyseal plate injury are (1) the ability of the growth plate to resist failure and (2) the forces applied to bone or the stresses induced in the growth plate. Based upon results from animal studies, it has been determined that the weakest region of the growth plate is the hypertrophic zone. The hypertrophic zone is susceptible to injury because of the low volume of bone matrix and high amount of developing immature cells in this region.[18]

The majority of epiphyseal fractures are due to high-velocity injuries. Although growth plate fractures certainly result from youth sporting activities, a detailed description of all epiphyseal plate fractures is beyond the scope of this chapter. A brief description of the Salter-Harris classification of growth plate fractures along with some of the more common epiphyseal plate fractures in sports, however, is warranted.

The Salter-Harris classification of growth plate fracture consists of five types of fractures and is based upon the relationship of the fracture line to the growing cells of the epiphyseal plate as well as the mechanism of injury (Fig. 34-1). Type I fractures are due to shearing forces in which there is complete separation of the epiphysis without fracture through bone. These fractures are most commonly seen in the very young people when the epiphyseal plate is relatively thick. Type II fractures are the most common type of growth plate fractures and result from shearing and bending forces. In the type II fracture, the line of separation traverses a variable distance along the epiphyseal plate and then makes its way through a segment of the bony metaphysis that results in a triangular-shaped metaphyseal fragment. Type II fractures usually occur in an older child who has a thin epiphyseal plate. Type III fractures usually result from shearing forces and result in intra-articular fractures from the joint surface to the deep zone of the growth plate and then along the growth plate to its periphery. Type IV fractures are intra-articular and also result from shearing forces. These fractures extend from the joint surface through the epiphysis across the entire thickness of the growth plate and then through a segment of the bony metaphysis. Type V fractures are due to a crushing mechanism and relatively uncommon.[34]

Salter-Harris type III fractures warrant special mention. These fractures are typically limited to the distal tibial epiphysis.[34] Injury to the proximal tibial epiphysis or distal femoral epiphysis may result from valgus loading of the knee, which is frequently encountered in contact and collision sports. The clinician cannot rely solely on radiographic examination to confirm this type of injury. In a series of six high school athletes (five playing football, one playing soccer), all injured by a valgus load, routine anterior-posterior and lateral X rays did not demonstrate Salter-Harris type III fractures of the distal femoral epiphysis. Oblique X rays with femoral rotation, cross-table lateral views demonstrating fat in the joint, or aspiration

of a hemarthrosis with fat in the aspirate, will help confirm growth plate fracture with an intra-articular component.[46] A thorough ligamentous examination with careful palpation skills is required to help differentiate joint line opening from epiphyseal plate opening.

Other common epiphyseal fractures seen in children involve the medial epicondyle and the bones of the hand. The medial epicondyle epiphyseal fracture is the most common elbow fracture seen in the young patient. From a macrotraumatic standpoint, epiphyseal fracture of the medial epicondyle is frequently the childhood counterpart of elbow dislocation in the adult and is typically caused by hyperextension and valgus loading.[1] Epiphyseal plate fractures of the medial epicondyle are typically Salter-Harris type I or II, although types III and IV injuries have also been reported. Medial epicondyle fractures typically result in the epicondyle being displaced inferiorly and possibly trapped in the elbow joint.[31] As the medial epicondyle serves as the attachment of the elbow and wrist flexors, avulsion fractures of the medial epicondyle also occur and will be discussed later in this chapter.

Epiphyseal fractures in children are more common in the hand than in other long bones of the upper extremity.[38] As a result, care must be taken by the parent, coach, or health care professional not to simply disregard finger injuries as simply a "jammed finger." Growth plate fractures in the hand usually involve the proximal and middle phalanges of the border digits. The most common epiphyseal plate fracture in the skeletally immature hand is a Salter-Harris type II at the base of the proximal phalanx of the little finger.[38]

The term "Little League shoulder" is used to describe an epiphyseal fracture of the proximal humeral epiphysis that typically occurs in the young baseball pitcher.[11] Although this injury can be macrotraumatic in nature (i.e., as a result of one specific throw), the condition is thought to be due to repetitive microtrauma. Fractures of the proximal humeral epiphysis are usually Salter-Harris type I or II. Radiographs demonstrate widening of the proximal humeral physis, and to a lesser degree may demonstrate lateral metaphyseal fragmentation, along with demineralization or sclerosis of the proximal humeral metaphysis. Avoiding all throwing until the patient is asymptomatic is vital in the treatment of this condition. Most patients are able to safely return to throwing with symptoms despite abnormal radiographs.[12]

Avulsion Fractures

As in the case with growing bone, much of the information regarding growing muscle is also based on animal studies. Although the physiology of the growth plate allows for bone growth, muscle does not inherently possess a specific structural site to allow for adaptation. It is clear that muscle adaptation does occur in order to accommodate for skeletal growth or as a response to therapeutic stretching exercise following periods of immobilization with muscle tissue in a shortened position. Based upon animal studies, it appears that a change in muscle

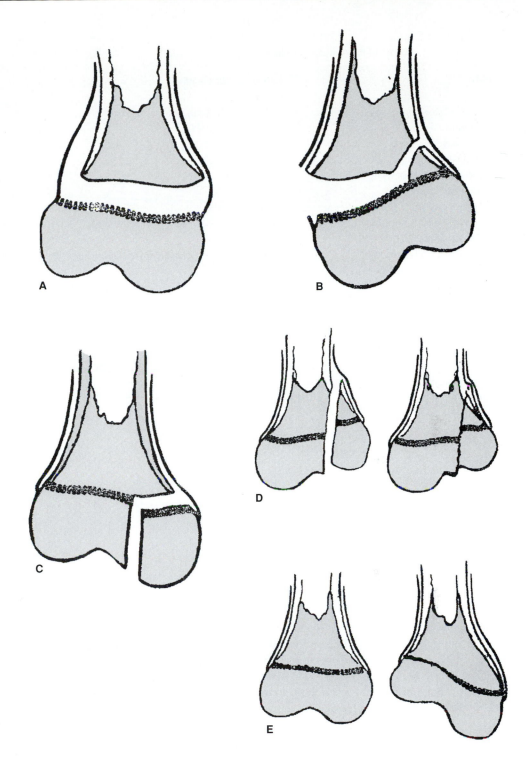

FIGURE 34-1

Growth plate fractures according to the Salter-Harris classification. **A,** Type I. **B,** Type II. **C,** Type III. **D,** Type IV. **E,** Type V.

length results from changes within the actual muscle belly itself and/or an increase in tendon length. In the skeletally immature animal model, change in muscle length occurs via changes in the length of both muscle and tendon. Research involving mature animals, on the other hand, indicates an increase in muscle length that occurs primarily through elongation of the muscle belly.[14]

When changes in muscle length do not match the changes in long-bone growth, tensile loads placed within the muscle predispose the youngster to injury. Contractile unit injury from voluntary contraction or passive stretch can be exacerbated due to inadequate muscle length. Injuries can range from various degrees of muscle strain to situations where the bony attachment of the muscle fails prior to muscle damage. Common sites of avulsion fracture in the lower extremity include the anterior superior iliac spine (ASIS), anterior inferior iliac spine (AIIS), ischial tuberosity, and the base of the fifth metatarsal. As forces across the joints of the lower extremity due to running,

TABLE 34-1

Maturation of Bones of the Arm and Shoulder

BONE	MATURATION TIMETABLE
Clavicle, sternal epiphysis	Closure 18th–24th yr.
Acromion	Closure 18th–19th yr.
Coracoid	Closure 18th–21st yr.
Subcoracoid	Closure 18th–21st yr.
Scapula, vertebral margin and inferior angle	Closure 20th–21st yr.
Glenoid cavity	Closure 19th yr.
Humerus, head, center, and lesser tuberosities	Fuse together 4th–6th yr.; fuse to shaft 19th–21st yr. (males), 18th–20th yr. (females)
Humerus, capitulum, lateral epicondyle, and trochlea	Fuse together at puberty; fuse to shaft at 17th yr. in males, 14th yr. in females
Olecranon	Closure 15th–17th yr. in males, 14th–15th yr. in females
Radius, head	Closure 13th–17th yr. in males, 14th–15th yr. in females
Radial tuberosity	Closure 14th–18th yr.
Ulna, distal epiphysis	Closure 19th yr. in males, 17th yr. in females
Styloid of ulna	Closure 18th–20th yr.
Radius, distal epiphysis	Closure 19th yr. in males, 17th yr. in females
Styloid process, radius	Closure variable
Lunate	Appears 4th yr.
Navicular	Appears 6th yr.
Pisiform	Appears 12th yr.
Triquetrum	Appears 1st–2nd yr.
Hamate	Appears 6th mo.
Capitate	Appears 6th mo.
Trapezoid	Appears 4th yr.
Trapezium	Closure 5th yr.
Metacarpal I epiphysis	Closure 14th–21st yr.
Metacarpals II–IV, epiphysis	Closure 14th–21st yr.
Proximal phalanx I, epiphysis	Closure 14th–21st yr.
Distal phalanx I, epiphysis	Closure 14th–21st yr.

jumping, and kicking exceed most forces across the upper extremity, avulsion fractures of the lower extremity outnumber avulsion fractures of the upper extremity. Stresses across the shoulder and elbow of the young throwing athlete, however, are sufficient enough to result in avulsion of the medial humeral epicondyle and proximal humerus.

LOWER EXTREMITY

Anterior Superior Iliac Spine

Avulsion of the ASIS is caused by a contraction or stretch of the sartorius. The sartorius is the longest muscle in the body and crosses the anterior hip and proximal medial knee joints. The growth center at the ASIS appears between the ages of 13 and 15 years and fuses to the pelvis between the ages of 21 and 25 years (Table 34-1 and Fig. 34-2).[29] Excessive force from the pulling of the sartorius with the hip in extension and knee in flexion may result in an avulsion of the ASIS. Positions of

hip extension combined with knee flexion seen in the trail leg during sprinting and hurdling can predispose these athletes to ASIS avulsion fracture. When the growth center does avulse from the bony origin on the pelvis, displacement of the avulsed fragment is uncommon.[37]

Anterior Inferior Iliac Spine

Avulsion of the AIIS is caused by a stretch or contraction of the rectus femoris. The AIIS serves as the site of the direct (anterior, or straight) head of the rectus femoris. As in the case with ASIS avulsions, activities involving hyperextension of the hip combined with knee flexion can also result in AIIS avulsion. The growth center at the AIIS appears between the ages of 13 and 15 years and fuses at approximately 16–18 years.[29] Due to earlier ossification, avulsion fractures at the AIIS are less frequent than avulsion fractures involving the ASIS. Athletes involved in running, jumping, and kicking sports usually sustain

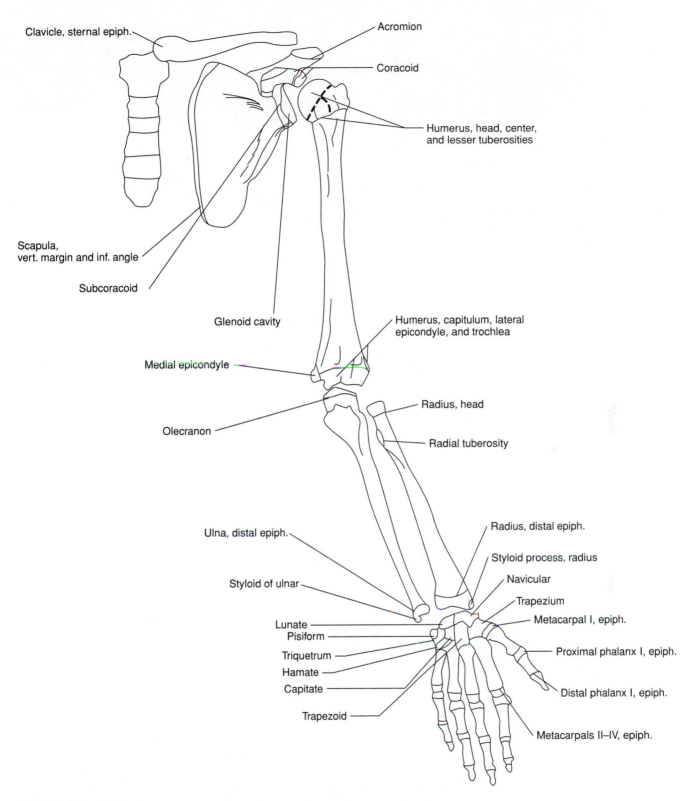

Clavicle, sternal epiph.

Acromion

Coracoid

Humerus, head, center, and lesser tuberosities

Scapula, vert. margin and inf. angle

Subcoracoid

Glenoid cavity

Humerus, capitulum, lateral epicondyle, and trochlea

Medial epicondyle

Olecranon

Radius, head

Radial tuberosity

Ulna, distal epiph.

Radius, distal epiph.

Styloid process, radius

Navicular

Styloid of ulnar

Trapezium

Metacarpal I, epiph.

Lunate
Pisiform
Triquetrum
Hamate
Capitate

Proximal phalanx I, epiph.

Distal phalanx I, epiph.

Trapezoid

Metacarpals II–IV, epiph.

FIGURE 34-2

A, Upper-extremity ossification and epiphyseal plate closure. **B,** Lower-extremity ossification and epiphyseal plate closure.

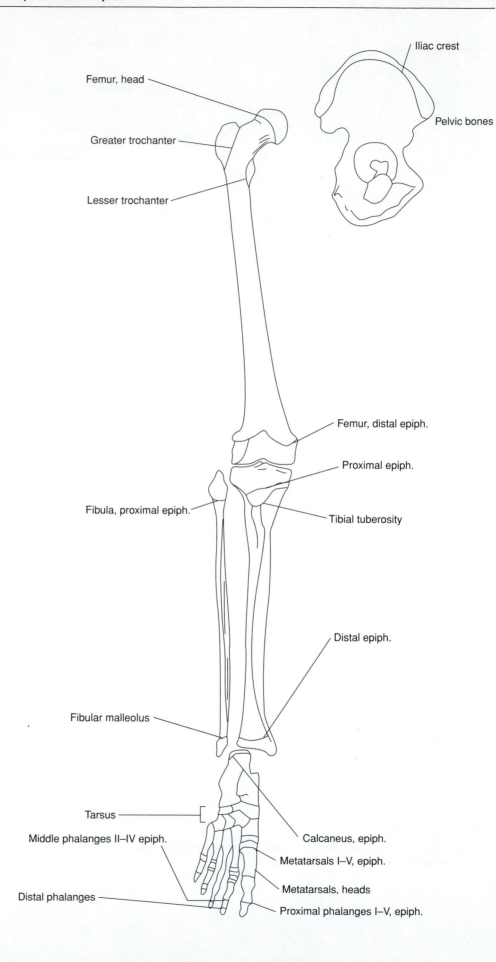

Femur, head

Greater trochanter

Lesser trochanter

Iliac crest

Pelvic bones

Femur, distal epiph.

Proximal epiph.

Fibula, proximal epiph.

Tibial tuberosity

Distal epiph.

Fibular malleolus

Tarsus

Middle phalanges II–IV epiph.

Distal phalanges

Calcaneus, epiph.

Metatarsals I–V, epiph.

Metatarsals, heads

Proximal phalanges I–V, epiph.

FIGURE   34-2

(Continued)

AIIS avulsion fractures.[29] When avulsion occurs, displacement of the bony muscle origin is rare because the tensor fascia lata, inguinal ligament, and an intact reflected (posterior) head of the rectus femoris (which originates at the superior rim of the acetabulum) all serve to prevent significant AIIS displacement.[37]

With both ASIS and AIIS avulsion fractures, the youngster is typically able to remember a specific event and usually unable to continue participation.[5] The patient demonstrates weakness of the involved muscle as evidenced by resisted hip flexion. In the avulsed ASIS, resisted hip flexion with the external rotation may be useful in the physical assessment. Point tenderness of the ASIS or AIIS is virtually always present. Swelling, if present, may be minimal, and there is minimal if any ecchymosis noted. Transfers from sit to supine are usually guarded and may require assistance from the patient's upper extremities or the contralateral lower extremity. Assuming a prone position may be uncomfortable. Passive stretch into complete knee flexion may or may not produce pain. Passive stretch of the hip into extension with simultaneous knee flexion may increase symptoms. Gait is typically antalgic with increased trunk flexion during stance, decreased hip flexion during swing-through, and decreased hip extension during late stance.[44]

Peroneals

Inversion ankle sprains are sustained frequently by patients of all ages in a wide variety of sport and nonsport-related activities. As the patient inverts the ankle, stresses can be placed through the evertor muscle group, either by passive stretch and/or active contraction to pull the foot back into eversion. Excessive forces generated by the peroneus brevis may result in avulsion of its insertion at the base of the fifth metatarsal. Avulsion fracture of the base of the fifth metatarsal typically results in point tenderness along with weakness of resisted ankle eversion, especially when resisted at the athlete's available end-range inversion. Resisted eversion may or may not cause pain. Passive inversion of the ankle typically increases pain at the bony insertion. Swelling may be present, but occurs distal to the traditional location of swelling seen in ankle sprains. Ecchymosis, if present, typically does not arise until a few days following injury.[44]

Ischial Tuberosity

Avulsion of the hamstring origin at the ischial apophysis was first described in the middle 1850s, and it occurs with greater frequency than avulsions on the anterior aspect of the pelvis.[37] Growth centers in this region appear between the ages of 15 and 17 years and fuse to the ilia between the ages of 19 and 25 years.[29,37] Athletes with an avulsion fracture of the ischial tuberosity typically demonstrate discomfort with prolonged sitting. Assessment of hamstring length at 90° of hip flexion will often show inadequate flexibility bilaterally, with more limitation on the involved side that is usually accompanied by pain. There may or may not be weakness with resisted knee flexion, but there is usually weakness noted with resisted or nonresisted

prone active hip extension. There is typically minimal if any ecchymosis in the area, and swelling is usually not apparent.[44]

UPPER EXTREMITY

A medial epicondyle epiphyseal fracture is the most common elbow fracture seen in the young patient.[1] As discussed previously, this injury may occur as a result of a macrotraumatic hyperextension or valgus injury. The medial epicondyle serves as the attachment site of the forearm flexor/pronator group, and as such can also be a location for avulsion fracture. This type of injury is typically due to valgus loading during the acceleration phase of the throwing mechanism. Avulsion of the triceps attachment at the olecranon has also been reported. This condition has been seen to result in separated ossification centers that persist into adulthood with subsequent olecranon nonunion.[19]

Treatment Principles

Conservative treatment of all avulsion fractures mimics that of a severe muscle strain. In fractures involving the lower extremity, assisted gait is a must until weight-bearing activities are pain free and without substitution. Compression of the area in the form of elastic wraps or neoprene sleeves may provide warmth and minimize discomfort experienced with activities of daily living and early rehabilitation efforts. Modalities to minimize pain and facilitate healing are indicated early in the treatment regimen. Once inflammation from the initial injury has subsided, gentle single-joint stretching exercises can begin. Two-joint stretching exercises should begin only after one-joint stretches are pain free. Submaximal single-joint strengthening exercises can begin when pain free. Strengthening efforts should be preceded by warm-up activities, and strengthening exercises should also be followed by stretching of the involved muscle. When isolated two-joint strengthening efforts are tolerated without difficulty, the young athlete can be allowed to return to a functional progression program.[44] Avulsion injuries of the upper extremity must be treated with rest until the youngster is asymptomatic. A gradual return to throwing sports through a supervised functional progression program is vital.

MICROTRAUMATIC INJURIES

Apophysitis

The apophysis of growing bone differs from the epiphysis of skeletally immature bone. The apophysis is an independent center of ossification that does not contribute to the longitudinal length of a long bone. An apophysis, however, does contribute to the structure and form of mature long bone by serving as a site of tendinous or ligamentous attachment. It is the role of the apophysis as the site for tendinous attachment that enters the picture of overuse injuries seen in the growing patient. At skeletal maturity, the apophysis fuses to its site of attachment to its respective long bone. Prior to skeletal maturity, however, traction placed upon an apophysis from an inflexible musculotendinous unit may result in apophyseal inflammation and delayed fusion to the long bone. Traction apophysitis commonly occurs at the tibial tubercle, calcaneus, and iliac crest.

LOWER EXTREMITY

Repetitive loading activities of the lower extremities in combination with muscle-tendon length insufficiency can yield traction forces through apophyseal centers that result in inflammation of the apophysis. Young patients involved in running, jumping, and kicking activities are inherently predisposed to large traction forces through apophyseal centers, especially during a growth spurt. These traction apophysites are typically self-limiting, but cases that do not respond to traditional conservative measures may require short-term immobilization to assist in eliminating pain and inflammation.

Calcaneal Apophysitis (Sever's Disease)

Sever's disease is a traction apophysitis of the growth center of the calcaneus. Sever's disease typically affects youngsters 8–13 years of age, with the peak incidence occurring at 11 years in young females and at 12 years in young males.[24,28] Sever's disease frequently affects youngsters involved in outdoor fall sports following a dry summer that results in dry, hard ground. Soccer, football, and even band participants, especially early in the season, are commonly diagnosed with Sever's disease.[44] Young soccer players who routinely participate on artificial surfaces may also experience symptoms consistent with Sever's disease.[24] Spikes or other shoes lacking in adequate shock absorption and forefoot support, or shoes with broken-down heel counters, contribute to the incidence of Sever's disease.

Sever's disease is characterized by pain and point tenderness at the posterior calcaneus near the insertion of the Achilles tendon. Local signs of inflammation may be present in acute cases. Swelling at the calcaneal apophysis may also be present, but this is an exception rather than the rule. Patients with tight calves, internal tibial torsion, forefoot varus, a dorsally mobile first ray, weak dorsiflexors, and genu varus may be more susceptible to Sever's disease.

Treatment of Sever's disease should focus on establishing normal flexibility of the gastrocnemius-soleus group (Figs. 34-3 and 34-4). Calf stretching should include exercises with the knee extended and the knee flexed. Just as importantly, stretching in a weight-bearing position should be performed with the correction of any rearfoot to lower leg or forefoot to rearfoot abnormality. Orthotic intervention may be a consideration in the treatment of Sever's disease and may range from temporary heel lifts or heel cups to more sophisticated custom-fit orthotics to correct biomechanical abnormalities. Dorsiflexion strengthening exercises along with foot intrinsic strengthening may also help manage symptoms.[44]

Tibial Tubercle Apophysitis (Osgood-Schlatters Disease)

Initially described in 1903, Osgood-Schlatters disease (OSD) is commonly seen in active and nonactive youngsters alike.[22] Like all traction apophysitises, the condition is usually self-limiting, but due to its prevalence and the ominous name, parents and young patients may mistakenly expect a poor prognosis. This is not to downplay the potential long-standing problems that can arise when the condition is not adequately diagnosed and treated.

Development of the tibial apophysis begins as a cartilaginous outgrowth. Secondary ossification centers appear with subsequent progression to an epiphyseal phase when the proximal tibial physis closes and the tibial apophysis fuses to the tibia.[16] Calcification of the apophysis begins distally at the average age of 9 years in females and at 11 years in males. Fusion of the apophysis to the tibia can take place via several ossification centers and occurs on average at 12 years in females and 13 years in males.[22] There is a normal transition from distal fibrocartilage to proximal fibrous tissue at the tibial apophysis. Fibrous tissue is more readily able to withstand the high tensile loads involved with athletic activities than is the weaker cartilage of the secondary ossification center. Microavulsions can occur through the area of bone and cartilage at the secondary ossification center, resulting in the potential for the development of separate ossicles, which can be a source of prolonged pain or reinjury.[22] Complications of OSD are few, but in addition to the formation of an accessory ossicle, patellar subluxation (secondary to patella alta), patella baja, nonunion of the tibial tubercle, and genu recurvatum have been reported.[20,23,50]

The diagnosis of OSD is not a clinical challenge. Symptoms are typically unilateral, although up to 25 percent of cases can be bilateral in nature.[16] There may or may not be a history of injury. Traditional literature reveals that OSD affects more young males than females; however, recent evidence suggests no significant difference between male and female involvement.[41] The youngster typically complains of aching around the tibial tubercle that is increased during or following jumping, climbing, or kneeling activities. The tibial tubercle may be reddened, raised, or tender to palpation. Symptoms are usually confined to the tibial tubercle and typically not present at the superior or inferior patellar poles or the patellar tendon; however, patellofemoral tenderness may be present.[39] Tenderness at the cartilaginous junction of the patella and patellar tendon at the inferior patellar pole is indicative of Sinding-Larsen-Johannson disease.[40] Findings on X ray (especially if only performed unilaterally) are often misleading, as it is difficult to differentiate between abnormal fragmentation from normal centers of ossification. Radiographs, however, may reveal soft-tissue swelling. Some athletes with OSD also have patella alta, and some authors have noted a link between patients with OSD and Severs disease.[22]

Treatment of Osgood-Schlatter's disease should emphasize a judicious stretching program. Inadequate quadriceps flexibility is virtually always present. The shortened muscle group combined with the ballistic nature of quadriceps activity in jumping sports are at the heart of OSD. Overzealous stretching of the quadriceps, however, may increase the pull on the tibial tubercle and only serve to increase symptoms. Stretching

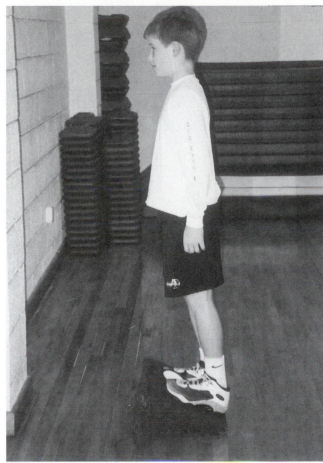

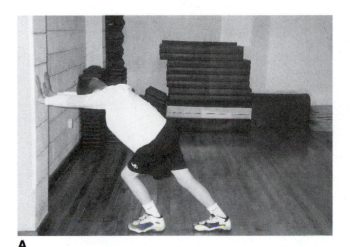

A   B

FIGURE 34-3

A, Front knee should be flexed for soleus stretching, back knee should be straight for gastrocnemius stretching, and heels should remain on the floor. **B,** Standing on a slantboard (see also Fig. 34-4) at the point of a discernable stretch for 10 minutes can be incorporated into a home stretching program.

of the quadriceps should begin prone, stressing an increase in quadriceps length at the knee joint only. A bolster under the hips may be required to place the muscle on slack at the hip joint. All stretching must be accompanied by a pull within the quadriceps muscle belly, not at the tibial tubercle. Two-joint stretching exercises should be instituted when adequate muscle length is established at the knee without an increase in tibial tubercle tenderness (Fig. 34-5). Quadriceps weakness is frequently not a major concern in this patient population; many of these youngsters have excellent quadriceps recruitment with no atrophy. Chronic cases, however, will result in quadriceps atrophy. Pain-free isometrics or low-load and high-repetition knee extension exercise may be incorporated if quadriceps atrophy is noted. Progressive resistive exercises of the quadriceps must be used judiciously, as they may only serve to increase pain at the tibial tubercle. As tight hamstrings require increased quadriceps force to overcome the tight posterior structures, hamstring exercises must be included in the comprehensive program to

manage OSD (Figs. 34-6 and 34-7). If competing in a contact or collision sport, young athletes with OSD should be fit with a protective pad to minimize the risks of blunt trauma to the area. When the tibial tubercle area is inflamed, even when the athlete is not participating, protective padding should also be considered to minimize the incidence of inadvertent blunt trauma encountered in activities of daily living.[44]

Iliac Apophysitis

Iliac apophysitis is a condition typically seen in the older youngster involved in running sports. Active patients between the ages of 14 and 16 years are usually the prime candidates for iliac apophysitis.[13] The ossification center of the iliac crest appears anterolaterally and advances posteriorly until it reaches the posterior iliac spine. The average age of closure is 16 years in boys and 14 years in girls, but closure may be delayed up to 4 additional years.[28] The gluteus medius originates on the ilium just inferior to the iliac crest and is another muscle that

SLANT BOARD DIAGRAM

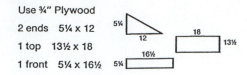

Use ¾" Plywood
2 ends   5¼ x 12
1 top   13½ x 18
1 front 5¼ x 16½

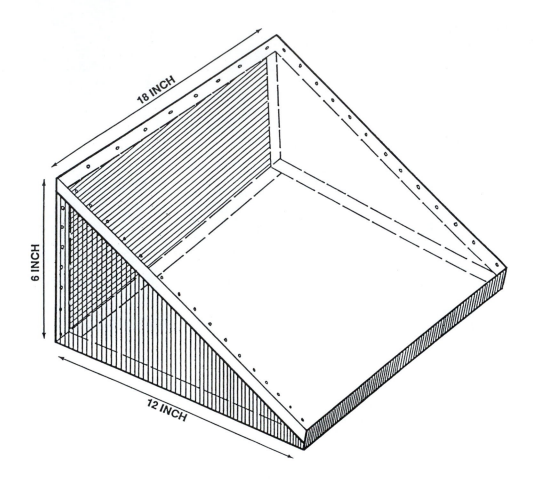

FIGURE 34-4

Directions for fabricating
a slantboard to facilitate
gastrocnemius-soleus
stretching.

may contribute to iliac apophysitis. The gluteus medius helps
to maintain pelvic symmetry for single-leg stance activities during running and hopping. Inflammation of the iliac apophysis
is thought to be due to a repetitive pull of the abdominal musculature at its insertion on the iliac crest.[37] During physical
activities, the abdominal muscles serve as trunk stabilizers and
accessory muscles of respiration. Although most commonly seen
as an overuse apophysitis, incomplete avulsion fractures of the
iliac apophysis have been reported from sudden contraction of
the abdominals with a quick change in direction while running.

Patients who experience iliac apophysitis usually demonstrate exquisite point tenderness along the iliac crest, which is
typically unilateral and located along the anterior one-half of the
iliac crest. Seated or standing lateral trunk flexion away from the
side of involvement is usually uncomfortable. Weakness or pain
with resisted hip abduction, oblique abdominal muscular activ-

ity, and pain or compensation with hopping on the involved leg
may also be present. A complete lower-extremity biomechanical examination may be indicated to determine structural or
compensatory leg length inequality that may contribute to iliac
apophysitis.

Treatment of iliac apophysitis should center on regaining
normal flexibility of the iliotibial band (ITB), the abdominals,
and gluteus medius. The patient at the outset of a flexibility program typically tolerates two-joint stretching of the ITB
with the knee extended (see Fig. 34-8). The traditional Ober
test position, along with variations, are efficient stretching activities but often accompanied by substitution of excessive hip
flexion, trunk flexion, or rotation. Seated lateral flexion away
from the side of involvement, progressed to standing lateral flexion, which is then progressed to standing lateral flexion with
arms extended overhead, is a good stretching progression. Prone

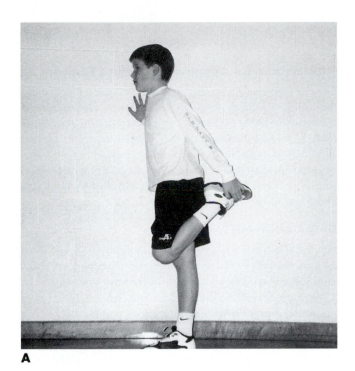
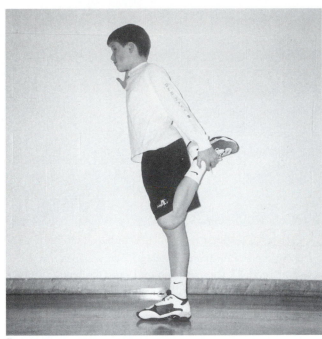

A   **B**

FIGURE   34 - 5

Quadriceps stretching. **A,** Proper technique. **B,** Improper technique with excessive trunk flexion.

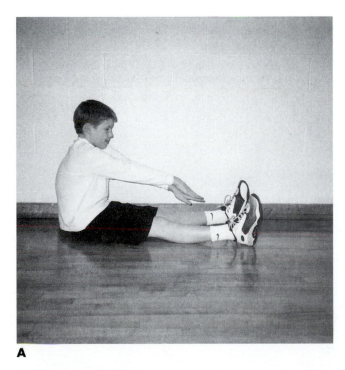
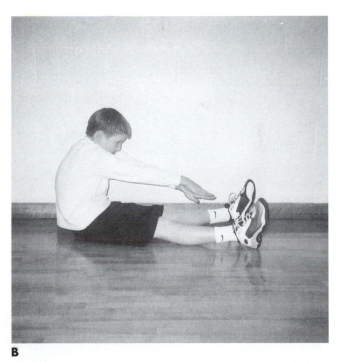

A   **B**

FIGURE   34 - 6

Long-sitting hamstring stretching. **A,** Proper technique. **B,** Improper technique with excessive thoracolumbar flexion.

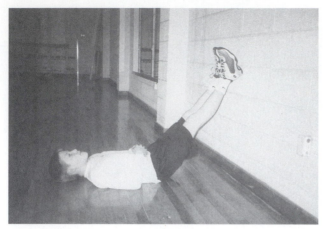

FIGURE 34-7

Wall stretch hamstring stretching. The youngster should maintain full knee extension and keep the buttocks on the floor. As hamstring flexibility improves, the youngster should ultimately be able to place the heels, backs of the knees, and buttocks against the wall.

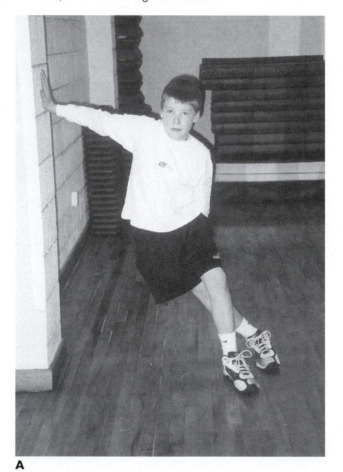

press-ups with rotation and lateral flexion may also be incorporated into the stretching program.[44]

Fifth Metatarsal Apophysitis (Iselin's Disease)

Out of many traction apophysites that affect the young patient, Iselin's disease is the most rarely encountered. The insertion of the peroneus brevis may be irritated by activities requiring fine foot control as in the case of dancers and gymnasts. Patients with abnormal relationships between the forefoot and rearfoot may be predisposed to Iselin's disease. A tight gastrocnemius-soleus complex or weak dorsiflexors may also contribute to apophysitis at the base of the fifth metatarsal.[28]

UPPER EXTREMITY

Because the stresses placed across an apophysis of the lower extremity usually exceed those placed across the upper extremity, most cases of apophysitis affect the legs of the growing patient. There are a few cases of upper-extremity apophysitis that do occur and warrant brief attention at this point. As previously noted, the elbow is subjected to large valgus forces during the acceleration phase of the throwing mechanism. In the skeletally mature patient, these valgus forces can result in medial elbow laxity. In the skeletally immature patient, these valgus forces may result in an apophysitis of the medial epicondyle. Stretching and strengthening of the forearm and wrist musculature may be beneficial in minimizing the chances for upper-extremity overuse injuries in the growing patients. Abnormal throwing mechanics may contribute to youth upper-extremity overuse injury; however, the vast majority of injuries are due to training errors. The most frequently committed training error is the amount of pitching that a youngster is allowed to perform. In order to minimize the risk of overuse injury, the athlete must adhere to common-sense guidelines regarding the amount of

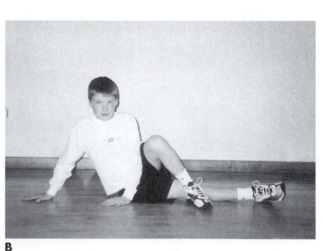

A   **B**

FIGURE 34-8

A, Standing ITB stretching. The uninvolved leg is crossed over in front of the involved leg and the youngster dips the hips toward the wall. **B,** Side-lying ITB stretching. Lying on the involved side with feet, hips, and shoulders in a straight alignment, the athlete pushes up onto extended elbows.

TABLE 34-2

Maturation of Bones of the Leg and Hip

BONE	MATURATION TIMETABLE
Pelvic bones	Fuse at puberty
Iliac crest	Closure 20th yr.
Femur, head	Closure 17th–18th yr. in males, 16th–17th yr. in females
Greater trochanter	Closure 16th–17th yr.
Lesser trochanter	Closure 16th–17th yr.
Femur, distal epiphysis	Closure 18th–19th yr. in males, 17th yr. in females
Proximal epiphysis	Closure 18th–19th yr. in males, 16th–17th yr. in females
Tibial tuberosity	Closure 19th yr.
Fibula, proximal epiphysis	Closure 18th–20th yr. in males, 16th–18th yr. in females
Fibular malleolus	Closure 17th–18th yr.
Distal epiphysis	Closure 17th–18th yr.
Calcaneus, epiphysis	Closure 12th–22nd yr.
Tarsus	Completion variable
Metatarsals I–V, epiphysis	Closure 18th yr. in males, 16th yr. in females
Metatarsals, heads	Closure 14th–21st yr.
Proximal phalanges I–V, epiphysis	Closure 18th yr.
Middle phalanges, II–V, epiphysis	Closure 18th yr.
Distal phalanges	Closure 18th yr., beginning proximally

pitching. Little League baseball and softball have established guidelines that govern the amount of pitching that a youngster can perform.[25]

While these guidelines are an important step in preventing upper-extremity overuse injury, they are only part of the story. Many youngsters participate in organized baseball programs that are not officially affiliated with Little League. These youngsters may not have guidelines to regulate how much an individual can pitch. These guidelines also do not apply to batting practice and often are not considered when youngsters pitch in tournament play. Finally, the number of innings may not be the best indicator to use, as an inning in baseball played by 9- to 12-year olds ranges from 4 to 50 pitches per inning, and the number of pitches per pitching outing ranges from 4 to 100.[2]

SPINE

Most spine injuries involve the muscles, ligaments, and intervertebral disks. These injuries are usually self-limiting and rarely result in significant neurologic compromise.[43] Two conditions of the osseous structures of the spine, however, do involve the young patient: spondylolysis and spondylolisthesis. Spondylolysis is a bony defect in the pars interarticularis, a portion of the neural arch located between the superior and inferior articular facets. Physical forces encountered by youngsters involved in physical activities play a significant role in the development of spondylolysis. Activities that involve repetitive loading, especially with the lumbar spine in extension/hyperextension, such as ballet, gymnastics, diving, football, weight lifting, and wrestling, have been implicated in spondylolysis. Spondylolysis originates in children between

the ages of 5 and 10 years and most frequently occurs at the fifth lumbar vertebra, with the fourth lumbar vertebra being involved second most frequently.[42] Many youngsters with sponylolysis remain asymptomatic for long periods of time and are not diagnosed until later in their skeletal development. X rays from the lateral and oblique views are required in order to visualize the fracture in its entirety along the longitudinal plane. Positive X-ray findings include asymmetry of the neural arch, inferior apophyseal joint, and posterior elements with rotation of the spinous process away from a unilateral spondylolytic lesion. CT scan and bone scan with single photon emission computed tomography (SPECT) can aid in the radiological diagnosis and staging of spondylolysis.[27] A common finding in patients with spondylolysis (symptomatic or asymptomatic) is hamstring spasm.[42] The etiology of this hamstring spasm is felt to be due to either a postural reflex to stabilize the L5-S1 segment or to nerve root irritation.[27,42]

Spondylolisthesis is a condition in which a vertebra slips anterior to the vertebra immediately below it. Spondylolisthesis most frequently takes place between the fifth lumbar and first sacral vertebrae, although the condition can occur at more than one spinal segment. The superior border of the inferior vertebra is divided into quarters, and the slip is described in terms of the width that the superior vertebra slips anteriorly in relation to the vertebra below it. A grade one spondylolisthesis is an anterior slip of 25 percent or less of the vertebral width; a grade two slip is up to 50 percent of the vertebral width; a grade three spondylolisthesis is a slip up to 75 percent of the vertebral width; and a grade four is a complete anterior slip. Spondylolisthesis is classified as degenerative, traumatic, pathologic, or isthmic. It is the isthmic classification that typically involves the young patient. In the isthmic category of spondylolisthesis, it is debatable whether a bilateral spondylolysis is a precursor for slippage and resultant instability of a spinal segment.

Treatment of spondylolysis and spondylolisthesis centers on healing of the bony defect and decreasing the patient's symptoms. Treatment depends upon the physician's personal preference and ranges from relative rest without a brace to 23 hours of bracing. When bracing is used, the brace is typically a rigid custom-fit lumbar spinal orthosis designed to keep the youngster out of extension. In addition to activity modification, hamstring stretching is an integral part of the treatment program.

SPECIAL CONSIDERATIONS

Musculoskeletal Considerations

Some conditions involving the young patient may actually be congenital in nature, but do not cause symptoms until the youngster becomes physically active in youth sports or physical education classes. Conditions such as these have unknown etiologies; some clearly have genetic predispositions, while others may be traced to excessive activity. Musculoskeletal conditions that will be discussed include tarsal coalition, Legg-Calvé-Perthes disease (LCPD), slipped capital femoral epiphysis (SCFE), osteochondroses, and patellofemoral pain syndrome.

TARSAL COALITION

Persistent ankle and foot pain in the young patient in conjunction with recurrent ankle sprains could possibly be due to an underlying tarsal coalition. A tarsal coalition is an abnormal fusion between tarsal bones in the rearfoot or midfoot due to a failure of bony segmentation. The most common tarsal coalitions occur between the calcaneus and navicular, the talus and the navicular, or the talus and calcaneus. Most tarsal coalitions present clinically in patients between the ages of 8 to 16 years, with anywhere from 50 to 60 percent of tarsal coalitions occurring bilaterally. There is familial predisposition in some cases of tarsal coalition.[24] As coalitions can be fibrous, cartilaginous, or osseous, X rays of the foot are many times interpreted as being unremarkable. Bone scan and CT scan may be of benefit in those cases where X rays fail to demonstrate pathological findings. Stretching and strengthening of extrinsic and intrinsic ankle musculature may help to minimize motion and strength losses. A custom-made or off-the-shelf orthosis may also help to minimize symptoms.[36]

LEGG-CALVÉ-PERTHES DISEASE

Legg-Calvé-Perthes disease is an avascular necrosis of the femoral head thought to be due to an occlusion of the blood supply to the femoral head from excessive fluid pressure resulting from an inflammatory or traumatic synovial effusion of the hip joint. LCPD typically involves active youngsters between the ages of 3 and 11 years and is found four times more frequently in young boys than young girls. LCPD is usually unilateral, although 15 percent of youngsters have bilateral involvement.[34] Youngsters diagnosed with LCPD may or may not be able to recall a history of trauma, but LCPD should be ruled out in any male athlete younger than 12 years of age with long-standing groin or knee pain worsened by a weight-bearing position. Young patients usually will present with a limp and a compensated or uncompensated gluteus medius gait. It should be noted that it is not unusual for the youngster to have no complaints of hip pain. Pain, when present, is usually in the groin and very frequently referred to the knee. In fact, LCPD can be misdiagnosed as patellofemoral pain.[45]

SLIPPED CAPITAL FEMORAL EPIPHYSIS

Slipped capital femoral epiphysis, although rare, is a condition that may not manifest itself until a youngster becomes involved in sports activities. SCFE involves boys twice as often as girls and typically occurs between 10 and 15 years of age during a period of rapid growth.[37] A suspected causative factor is a potential hormonal imbalance; therefore SCFE should be suspected in youngsters who are tall and thin or short and obese who complain of long-standing thigh, groin, or knee pain. Progressive cases of SCFE may result in a varus deformity with concomitant external rotation.

There are also other conditions that may result in groin pain or pain around the pelvis that may be manifested after a macrotraumatic event. Musculoskeletal conditions include hernia, avulsion fracture of the lesser trochanter, iliopectineal bursitis/tendinitis (snapping hip), abdominal muscle strain, congenital dislocation of the hip, septic arthritis, and toxic synovitis. Nonmusculoskeletal differential diagnoses as a source of acute or persistent hip pain include leukemia and neuroblastoma.[48] Other potential causes of hip pain are bone tumor, appendicitis, pelvic inflammatory disease, hemophilia, arterial insufficiency, and sickle cell anemia.[15]

OSTEOCHONDROSES

Osteochondrosis and osteochondritis are two distinctly different pathologic entities. Osteochondrosis is typically a self-limiting disorder that involves a secondary epiphyseal center or pressure epiphysis at the end of a long bone or a primary epiphyseal center of a small bone.[34] Osteochondrosis involves degeneration or avascular necrosis with resultant regeneration or recalcification and typically does not demonstrate bony fragmentation.[6,34] Osteochondritis, on the other hand, is an inflammation of the subchondral bone and articular cartilage. Osteochondritis dissecans involves resultant fragmentation of articular cartilage within the joint. Many of the osteochondroses have their origins in chronic, repetitive trauma. The pathology and subsequent prognosis of osteochondrosis and osteochondritis of immature bone differ from that of mature bone.

Juvenile osteochondritis dissecans (JOCD) of the knee can be a devastating condition if not diagnosed and treated early. Although ischemia, genetic predisposition, and abnormal ossification are theoretical causes of JOCD,[17] growing evidence suggests that microtrauma to the immature knee over the course of months and years is the primary cause of JOCD.[7,9] The majority of JOCD lesions involve the medial femoral condyle, and most lesions occur on the weight-bearing surface. The site of JOCD pathology is subchondral bone, not articular cartilage.[9] Many lesions go undiagnosed or misdiagnosed. In a series of 192 patients, 80 percent of patients had symptoms for more than 15 months and 90 percent of patients had symptoms for greater than 8 months.[7] Symptoms center around an insidious onset of knee pain, with or without effusion, and knee pain that is increased with weight-bearing activities and typically reduced with rest. Youngsters with JOCD are usually involved in year-round physical activity, or participate in more than one sport with little if any rest between sporting seasons. Successful treatment is based upon accurate diagnosis, staging of the activity of the lesion, the ability of the lesion to heal, and subsequent nonoperative or operative intervention. Conservative treatment centers around minimizing weight-bearing and shear forces, activity modification, stretching of inflexible hamstrings and calves that serve to increase joint reaction forces, and appropriate quadriceps strengthening exercises initiated and progressed on an individual basis.

Another common site of osteochondrosis involves the elbow of a growing patient. Osteochondrosis of the capitellum of the elbow is called Panner's disease. Panner's disease is typically seen in young throwing athletes who complain of chronic dull aching in the elbow joint. Point tenderness at the lateral elbow is common, as is a subtle loss of elbow extension.[6] As the condition progresses the loss of extension can be more pronounced and accompanied by a loss of pronation and supination as well. Initially, rest and activity modification is important and should be followed by a range of motion and strengthening program along with a supervised functional progression program to return to throwing.

PATELLOFEMORAL PAIN

Patellofemoral pain is frequently encountered in many physical therapy clinics. Symptoms in youngsters are comparable to their adult counterparts. Dull peripatellar aching, pain with stairs or prolonged sitting, giving way of the knee, and pseudo-locking episodes in extension are classic signs of patellofemoral involvement. Treatment is symptomatic and should include pain-free quadriceps strengthening; hamstring, calf, and ITB stretching; correction of biomechanical abnormalities; activity modification; bracing; and screening for signs of hyperelasticity that may indicate patellofemoral joint instability.

GROWING PAINS

Prior to closing out the description of various microtaumatic concerns in the youngster, the clinician should also be made aware of the significance of the diagnosis of growing pains. It is not uncommon for the physical therapist to receive a referral to address various musculoskeletal issues in a growing child with the chief complaint of pain. The referring practitioner may lack sufficient knowledge in musculoskeletal examination principles to provide an adequate clinical impression. Since the presenting chief complaint in an active child can be pain, a clinical diagnosis of growing pains is made. Growing pains is a misnomer as the process of growing should not be painful and the majority of children who truly have growing pains do not experience symptoms during growth spurts. The diagnosis of growing pains should never be taken at face value by the therapist.

When present, growing pains are typically seen in younger children. Pain is usually in the thighs, calves, or shins and is bilateral. Pain is usually present during the evening or at night, and there is usually no morning stiffness. The youngster does not typically limp on the involved lower extremity. In cases where pain is located in areas other than the lower extremities, when pain is accompanied by morning stiffness, a limp, malaise, recurrent fever, and/or night sweats, further examination is indicated as opposed to accepting the clinical impression of growing pains at face value.

Physiologic Considerations

The youngster's cardiovascular response to exercise is related to the size of the youngster.[49] Children demonstrate a double sigmoid growth pattern from birth to adulthood. There is a rapid gain in growth in infancy and early childhood that slows down during middle childhood. The second rapid increase in growth occurs during adolescence. The peak height velocity is defined as the maximum rate of growth in stature and occurs in girls from 10.5 to 13 years but may start as early as 9 years or as late as 15 years. Peak height velocity of boys occurs from 12.5 to 15 years but may start as early as 10 years or as late as 16 years.[35]

As the youngster's heart is smaller than that of the mature adult, the capacity as a reservoir for blood is also smaller in the child's heart. Children, therefore, have a lower stroke volume at all levels of exercise.[49] The exercising youngster compensates for this lower stroke volume with an increased heart rate. As is seen in the adult, the youngster's systolic blood pressure rises during exercise, but the child's elevation in systolic blood pressure is less than that seen in the adult.[49] The red blood cell count for young boys and girls are similar with comparable abilities to carry oxygen to exercising organs. After menarche, however, females demonstrate lower blood volume and fewer red blood cells with a resultant decreased oxygen carrying capacity. Young girls, therefore, typically demonstrate a mean blood pressure lower than that seen in young boys.[35]

As the child's thoracic cavity is smaller than that of the mature adult, the child demonstrates a smaller vital capacity than the adult and also shows an elevated respiration rate as compared to the mature adult.[4,49] As the child matures, the ability to perform work (both aerobic and anaerobic) increases.[4,49] After menarche, girls have a slightly lower oxygen uptake per kilogram of body weight but are similar to boys per kilogram of lean body weight.[21] The maximum oxygen uptake is similar in young boys and girls until approximately 12 years of age. Males continue to demonstrate an increase until 16–18 years, with females failing to show significant gains after 12–14 years of age.[3,33] Young boys and girls have similar proportions of slow-twitch and fast-twitch muscle fiber. Strength differences between the genders are minimal when strength is expressed relative to fat-free weight.[47] Both young boys and young girls have been shown to be able to safely participate in strength-training programs.[8,26]

Independent of gender, the young athlete typically does not tolerate prolonged periods of heat exposure; therefore, care must be taken when the youngster participates in sports in a hot and humid environment. A child has a greater surface area-to-mass ratio than the typical adult, resulting in a greater transfer of heat into their young bodies. The child also has a higher production of metabolic heat per kilogram of body weight as compared to adult counterparts, which serves to further challenge the young thermoregulatory system.[4,49]

Psychological Considerations

To this point, the chapter has presented many physical and physiologic characteristics that constitute the unique challenges to evaluating and treating youth injuries. Before concluding this chapter, however, one other vital area must also be discussed and that is the unique psychological demands placed upon young athletes, especially those involved in intense competition and training.

There are many benefits of physical activity in the youngster (Table 34-3).[10] There are many differences, however, between free-flowing play and organized sports. Organized sports, fortunately or unfortunately, carry the obligatory win or lose connotations of competition and also involve adults who coach and train the youngster as well as adults who interpret and enforce the rules that govern competition. The adverse effect of adult influences upon the young athlete is but one potential negative psychological aspect of youth sport participation.

Participation in organized sport can be taken to an extreme. Intensive participation can be described in terms of frequency and/or intensity. Examples of intensive participation include the ice skater or gymnast who trains daily for hours and competes all year round for years on end. Other examples include the multisport athlete who trains and competes on a daily basis all year round. This intensive participation places significant physical demands on the body, demands that may result in serious overuse or stress-failure injury. Just as the young body grows to accept greater physical demands, so does the young mind. Intensive participation places many demands on the youngster, some of which may be unrealistic. As this relates to intense competition, research demonstrates that a child's cognitive ability to develop a mature understanding of the competition process does not occur until the age of 12. It is not until between the ages of 10 and 12 years that children develop the capacity to comprehend more than just one other viewpoint. Finally, after the age of 12 years the youngster can readily adopt a team perspective.[30]

TABLE 34-3

Benefits of Physical Activity in Children

PHYSICAL

Increased maximal aerobic power and general stamina
Control of body mass and fat reduction
Increased muscle strength and endurance
Increased range of motion
Decreased blood lipid levels
Improved ventilatory efficiency
Increased oxygen consumption

PSYCHOLOGICAL

Feelings of competency and mastery
Personal self-esteem
Engaging in enjoyable behavior
Achieving desired goals
Gaining admiration of others
Safe training in risk-taking behavior
Satisfaction in achievement
Feeling of working toward a goal
Peer group interaction
Awareness of, and adherence to, rules
Personal role definition

The negative psychological aspects of intense youth sport participation can be found in Table 35-4. Psychological issues may also enter the picture when rehabilitating youth sport participants involved in intense competition and training. Risk factors for psychological complications in the injured child include stress in the family, high-achieving siblings, over- or underinvolved parent(s), a paradoxical lack of leisure in athletic activity, self-esteem that is reliant on athletic prowess, and a narrow range of interests beyond athletics.[32]

This chapter has provided an overview of the unique physical and psychological issues that affect youth sport participants.

TABLE 34-4

Potential Negative Aspects of Intensive Youth Sport Participation

- Children are not permitted to be children.
- Children are denied important social contacts and experiences.
- Children are victims of a disrupted family life.
- Children may experience impaired intellectual development.
- Children are exposed to excessive psychological/physiologic stress.
- Children may become so involved with sport that they become detached from society.
- Children may face a type of abandonment upon completion of their athletic career.

The rehabilitation professional evaluating and treating the young athlete must be cognizant of these unique features. Evaluation and treatment principles must reflect the special circumstances that present in the youth athlete.

REFERENCES

1. Andrish JT. Upper extremity injuries in the skeletally immature athlete. In: Nicholas JA, Hershman EB, eds. *The Upper Extremity in Sports Medicine*. St. Louis, MO, Mosby, 1990, p. 673.

2. Axe MJ, Snyder-Mackler L, Konin JG, Strube MJ. Development of a distance-based interval throwing program for Little League-aged athletes. *Am J Sports Med* 24:594, 1996.

3. Bar-Or O. The prepubescent female. In: Shangold M, Mirkin G, eds. *Women and Exercise*, 2nd ed. Philadelphia, PA, Davis, 1994.

4. Bar-Or O. *Pediatric Sports Medicine for the Practitioner: From Physiologic Principles to Clinical Applications*. New York, Springer-Verlag, 1983.

5. Best TM. Muscle-tendon injuries in young athletes. *Clin Sports Med* 14:669, 1995.

6. Bianco AJ. Osteochondritis dissecans. In: Morrey BF, ed. *The Elbow and Its Disorders*. Philadelphia, PA, Saunders, 1985, p. 254.

7. Cahill BR. Treatment of juvenile osteochondritis of the knee. *Sports Med Arthroscopy Rev* 2:65, 1994.

8. Cahill BR, moderator. Proceedings of the conference on strength training and the pubescent. Chicago, American Orthopaedic Society for Sports Medicine, 1988.

9. Cahill BR. Treatment of juvenile osteochondritis dissecans and osteochondritis dissecans of the knee. *Clin Sports Med* 4:367, 1985.

10. Cahill BR, Pearl AJ. *Intensive Participation in Children's Sports*. Champaign, IL, Human Kinetics, 1993.

11. Cahill BR, Tullos HS, Fain RH. Little League shoulder. *Sports Med* 2:150, 1974.

12. Carson WC, Gasser SI. Little Leaguer's shoulder: A report of 23 cases. *Am J Sports Med* 26:575, 1998.

13. Clancy WG. Running. In: Reider B, ed. *Sports Medicine: The School-Aged Athlete*. Philadelphia, PA, Saunders, 1991, p. 632.

14. Garrett WE, Best TM. Anatomy, physiology, and mechanics of skeletal muscle. In: Simon SS, ed. *Ortho-paedic Basic Science*. Rosemont, IL, American Academy of Orthopaedic Surgeons, 1994.

15. Goodman CG, Snyder TE. *Differential Diagnosis in Physical Therapy*, 2nd ed. Philadelphia, PA, Saunders, 1995.

16. Graf BK, Fujisaki CK, Reider B. Disorders of the patellar tendon. In: Reider B, ed. *Sports Medicine: The School-Aged Athlete*. Philadelphia, PA, Saunders, 1991, p. 355.

17. Graf BK, Lange RH. Osteochondritis dissecans. In: Reider B, ed. *Sports Medicine: The School-Aged Athlete*. Philadelphia, PA, Saunders, 1991.

18. Iannotti JP, Goldstein S, Kuhn J, et al. Growth plate and bone development. In: Simon SS, ed. *Orthopaedic Basic Science*. Rosemont, IL, American Academy of Orthopaedic Surgeons, 1994.

19. Ireland ML, Andrews JR. Shoulder and elbow injuries in the young athlete. *Clin Sports Med* 7:473, 1988.

20. Jakob RP, Von Gumppenberg S, Engelhardt P. Does Osgood–Schlatter disease influence the position of the patella? *J Bone Joint Surg Br* 63:579, 1981.

21. Kemper HC. Exercise and training in childhood and adolescence. In: Torg JS, Welsh RP, Shephard RJ, eds. *Current Therapy in Sports Medicines* 2. Toronto, Decker, 1990.

22. Kujala UM, Kvist M, Heinonen O. Osgood–Schlatter's disease in adolescent athletes: Retrospective study of incidence and duration. *Am J Sports Med* 13:239, 1985.

23. Lancourt JE, Cristini JA. Patella alta and patella infera: Their etiological role in patellar dislocation, chondromalacia, and apophysitis of the tibial tubercle. *J Bone Joint Surg Am* 57:1112, 1975.

24. Larkin J, Brage M. Ankle, hindfoot, and midfoot injuries. In: Reider B, ed. *Sports Medicine: The School-Aged Athlete*. Philadelphia, PA, Saunders, 1991, p. 365.

25. Little League Baseball, Inc. Williamsport, PA.

26. National Strength and Conditioning Association. Position paper on prepubescent strength training. *Natl Strength Train J* 7:27, 1985.

27. O'Leary PF, Boiardo RA. The diagnosis and treatment of injuries of the spine in athletes. In: Nicholas JA, Hershman EB, eds. *The Lower Extremity and Spine in Sports Medicine*, 3rd ed. St. Louis, MO, Mosby, 1995, p. 1171.

28. Outerbridge AR, Micheli LJ. Overuse injuries in the young athlete. *Clin Sports Med* 14:503, 1995.

29. Paletta GA, Andrish JT. Injuries about the hip and pelvis in the young athlete. *Clin Sports Med* 14:59, 1995.

30. Passer MW. Determinants and consequences of children's competitive stress. In: Smoll FL, Magill RA, Ash MJ, eds. *Children in Sport*, 3rd ed. Champaign, IL, Human Kinetics, 1988.

31. Peterson HA. Physeal fractures. In: Morrey BF, ed. *The Elbow and Its Disorders*. Philadelphia, PA, Saunders, 1985, p. 222.

32. Pillemer FG, Micheli LJ. Psychological considerations in youth sports. *Clin Sports Med* 7:679, 1988.

33. Roemmich JN, Rogol AD. Physiology of growth and development: Its relationship to performance in the young athlete. *Clin Sports Med* 14:483, 1995.

34. Salter RB. *Textbook of Disorders and Injuries of the Musculoskeletal System*, 2nd ed. Baltimore, MD, Lippincott Williams & Wilkins, 1983.

35. Sanborn CF, Jankowski CM. Physiological considerations for women in sport. *Clin Sports Med* 13:315, 1994.

36. Santopietro FJ. Foot and foot-related injuries in the young athlete. *Clin Sports Med* 7:563, 1988.

37. Sim FH, Rock MG, Scott SG. Pelvis and hip injuries in athletes: Anatomy and function. In: Nicholas JA, Hershman EB, eds. *The Lower Extremity and Spine in Sports Medicine*, 3rd ed. St. Louis, MO, Mosby, 1995, p. 1025.

38. Simmons BP, Lovallo JL. Hand and wrist injuries in children. *Clin Sports Med* 7:495, 1988.

39. Smith AD, Tao SS. Knee injuries in young athletes. *Clin Sports Med* 14:650, 1995.

40. Stanitski CL. Anterior knee pain syndrome in the adolescent. *J Bone Joint Surg Am* 75:1407, 1993.

41. Stanitski CL. Combating overuse injuries: A focus on children and adolescents. *Phys Sports Med* 21:87, 1993.

42. Stinson JT. Spondylolysis and spondylolisthesis in the athlete. *Clin Sports Med* 12:517, 1993.

43. Tall RL, DeVault W. Spinal injury in sport: Epidemiologic considerations. *Clin Sports Med* 12:441, 1993.

44. Tippett SR. Lower extremity injuries in the young athlete. *Orthop Phys Ther Clin North Am* 6:471, 1997.

45. Tippett SR. Referred knee pain in a young athlete: A case study. *J Orthop Sports Phys Ther* 19:117, 1994.

46. Torg JS, Pavlov H, Morris VB. Salter–Harris type-III fracture of the medial femoral condyle occurring in the adolescent athlete. *J Bone Joint Surg Am* 63:586–591, 1981.

47. Van De Loo DA, Johnson MD. The young female athlete. *Clin Sports Med* 14:687, 1995.

48. Waters PM, Millis MB. Hip and pelvic injuries in the young athlete. *Clin Sports Med* 7:513, 1988.

49. Woodall WR, Weber MD. Exercise response and thermoregulation. *Orthop Phys Ther Clin North Am* 7:1, 1998.

50. Zimbler S, Merkow S. Genu recurvatum: A possible complication after Osgood–Schlatter disease. *J Bone Joint Surg Am* 66:1129, 1984.

C H A P T E R 3 5

Considerations for Treating Amputees

Robert Gailey

O B J E C T I V E S

After completing this chapter, the therapist should be able to do the following:

- Perform a postsurgical evaluation of the lower-limb amputee.
- Instruct the amputee on the care of the stump and prepare the limb for prosthetic fitting.
- Design a preprosthetic training plan for the care of the lower-limb amputee.
- Identify different designs of lower-limb prosthetics and discuss the functions of their principal components.
- Instruct the lower-limb amputee on the use of a prosthesis.
- Instruct the lower-limb amputee on the fundamentals of running.
- Identify different designs of upper-limb prosthetics and discuss the functions of their principal components.
- Design a prosthetic training plan for the care of the upper-limb amputee.

The prosthetist and the physical therapist, as members of the rehabilitation team, often develop a very close relationship when working together with lower-limb amputees. The prosthetist is responsible for fabricating and modifying the specific socket design and providing prosthetic components that will best suit the lifestyle of a particular individual. The physical therapist's role is fourfold: First, the amputee must be properly evaluated to assess impairment, functional limitation, disability, or other health-related conditions in order to formulate an appropriate and focused rehabilitation program that will physically prepare him/her for prosthetic gait training. Second, the amputee must be educated about residual limb care, prior to being fitted with the prosthesis, in addition to learning how to use and care for the prosthesis. Third, the amputee must be reeducated in the biomechanics of gait, while learning how to use a prosthesis. Once success is achieved with ambulation and the functional activities of that individual's daily routine, the amputee may look forward to resuming a productive life. Finally, the therapist should introduce the amputee to higher levels of activity beyond just learning to walk. The amputee may not be ready to participate in recreational activities immediately; however, providing the names of support groups and disabled recreational organizations can furnish the necessary information for the individual to seek involvement when ready.

EVALUATION OF THE AMPUTEE

Assessment of the amputee is extremely important and performed on a continual basis. The Amputee Assessment and Progress Form (Fig. 35-1) outlines the essential items necessary for a complete evaluation. The following section will briefly describe some of the procedures and findings specific to the amputee, and the formulation of his/her individual rehabilitation program.

Past Medical History

A complete medical history should be taken from the client to provide the therapist with information that may be pertinent to the rehabilitation program.

Past Social History

Poor diet, the use of tobacco and alcohol, and lack of exercise often contribute to poor health and possibly, the ill effects that lead to amputation. Reinforcement of positive behaviors throughout rehabilitation can only help encourage clients to make better choices.

Amputee Acute Assessment and Progress Form

Admitting Diagnosis _____ **Admission Date** _____

Precautions _____

Surgical Procedure _____

Past Medical History _____

_____

Past Social History _____

_____

Fall History _____

_____

Current Medications _____

_____

Subjective Comments _____

_____

Mental Status

    Person/Place/Time _____

Observation/Inspection

    <u>Amputated Limb</u>

        Skin color _____

        Edema _____

        Temperature _____

        Pulses _____

    <u>Sound Limb</u>

        Skin color _____

        Edema _____

        Temperature _____

        Pulses _____

        Open lesions/ulcers _____

            Location _____

            Size/Description _____

Vital Signs

Date	_____	_____	_____	_____
Blood pressure	_____	_____	_____	_____
Heart rate	_____	_____	_____	_____

F I G U R E   3 5 - 1

Amputee acute assessment and progress form. (Reproduced, with permission, from
Advanced Rehabilitation Therapy, Inc., Miami, FL.)

Upper Extremity Screening

	Strength		ROM	
	Right	Left	Right	Left
Shoulder				
Abduction	_____	_____	_____	_____
Adduction	_____	_____	_____	_____
Int. Rotation	_____	_____	_____	_____
Ext. Rotation	_____	_____	_____	_____
Elbow				
Flexion	_____	_____	_____	_____
Extension	_____	_____	_____	_____
Wrist				
Flexion	_____	_____	_____	_____
Extension	_____	_____	_____	_____
Grasp	_____	_____	_____	_____

Upper Extremity Screening

	Strength		ROM	
	Right	Left	Right	Left
Hip				
Flexion	_____	_____	_____	_____
Extension	_____	_____	_____	_____
Abduction	_____	_____	_____	_____
Adduction	_____	_____	_____	_____
Int. Rotation	_____	_____	_____	_____
Ext. Rotation	_____	_____	_____	_____
Knee				
Flexion	_____	_____	_____	_____
Extension	_____	_____	_____	_____
Ankle				
Plantarflexion	_____	_____	_____	_____
Dorsiflexion	_____	_____	_____	_____

Sensation

	Sharp/Dull		Light Touch		Proprioception		Vibration	
	Rt.	Lt.	Rt.	Lt.	Rt.	Lt.	Rt.	Lt.
L1	_____	_____	_____	_____	_____	_____	_____	_____
L2	_____	_____	_____	_____	_____	_____	_____	_____
L3	_____	_____	_____	_____	_____	_____	_____	_____
L4	_____	_____	_____	_____	_____	_____	_____	_____
L5	_____	_____	_____	_____	_____	_____	_____	_____
S1	_____	_____	_____	_____	_____	_____	_____	_____
S2	_____	_____	_____	_____	_____	_____	_____	_____

Deep Tendon Reflexes

	Right	Left		Right	Left
Triceps	_____	_____	Patella	_____	_____
Brachial	_____	_____	Achilles	_____	_____

Balance

	Unsteady	Steady with support	Steady Independent
Sitting eyes open	_____	_____	_____
Sitting eyes closed	_____	_____	_____
Sitting reach	_____	_____	_____
Sitting nudge	_____	_____	_____
Standing eyes open	_____	_____	_____
Standing eyes closed	_____	_____	_____
Standing reach	_____	_____	_____
Standing nudge	_____	_____	_____

FIGURE 35-1

(Continued)

Bed Mobility and Transfers

	Assist × 2	Assist × 1	Standby	Independent
Bridging	_____	_____	_____	_____
Rolling	_____	_____	_____	_____
Supine to sit	_____	_____	_____	_____
Bed to Chair	_____	_____	_____	_____
Sit to Stand	_____	_____	_____	_____
Bed to Toilet	_____	_____	_____	_____

Ambulation

Assistive Device	WC _____	Walker _____	Crutches _____	Loft Strands _____	Cane _____
Date	_____	_____	_____	_____	_____
Distance	_____	_____	_____	_____	_____
Time	_____	_____	_____	_____	_____

Compression Therapy

Wrap _____   Elastic Sleeve _____   Shrinker _____

Education

	Presented	Remembered
Positioning	_____	_____
Residual Limb Care	_____	_____
Skin Care	_____	_____
Sound Foot Care	_____	_____
Footwear	_____	_____
Home Exercise	_____	_____
Medication	_____	_____
Nutrition	_____	_____

Additional Identified Problems

1) _____
2) _____
3) _____
4) _____

Assessment

_____
_____
_____
_____
_____
_____

Plan

Goals	Action
1) _____	_____
2) _____	_____
3) _____	_____
4) _____	_____
5) _____	_____
6) _____	_____

Clinician _____   Date _____

F I G U R E   3 5 - 1

(Continued)

Fall History

Assessment of falls is paramount especially with elder amputees when determining their prosthetic candidacy. Preventing falls that could lead to additional health problems is important, especially as amputees attempt to gain confidence in using their prosthesis.

Mental Status

The therapist should be concerned with assessing the client's potential to perform activities such as donning and doffing the prosthesis, stump sock regulation, bed positioning, skin care, safe ambulation, and other functional activities.

Observation/Inspection

Inspection of the skin of both the intact limb and residual limb should include the following:

1. Skin color. Increased redness is indicative of infection, inflammation, or irritation. Blanching white suggests lack of circulation. Dark blackish color could indicate gangrene.
2. Edema. Swelling may relate to venous insufficiency, diet, or poor residual limb-wrapping technique.
3. Temperature. Increased warmth indicates infection or inflammation. Coolness demonstrates lack of circulation.
4. Pulses. Decreased pulses relate to poor circulation.
5. Lesions and ulcers. Any lesion or ulcer should be reported, treated, and monitored immediately.

Strength

Functional strength of the major muscle groups should be assessed through manual muscle testing of all extremities, including the residual limb and the trunk. This will help determine the client's potential skill level to perform activities such as transfers, wheelchair management, and ambulation, with and without the prosthesis.

Range of Motion

A functional assessment of gross upper-limb and sound lower-limb motions should be made. A measurement of the stump's range of motion (ROM) should be recorded for future reference. Contractures are a complication that can greatly hinder the amputee's ability to ambulate efficiently using a prosthesis; thus, extra care should be taken to avoid this situation. The most common contracture for the transfemoral amputee is hip flexion, external rotation, and abduction, and knee flexion is the most frequently seen contracture for the transtibial amputee.

Sensation

The evaluation of the amputee's sensation can provide insight into possible insensitivity of the residual limb and/or sound

limb. This may affect proprioceptive feedback for balance and single limb stance, which in turn can lead to gait difficulties. The client must be made aware that decreased pain, temperature, and light touch sensation can increase the potential for injury and tissue breakdown to the intact foot, or residual limb.

Balance/Coordination

The ability to maintain adequate sitting and standing balance demonstrates the amputee's control of the center of gravity over the base of support (BOS). The ease of movement and the refinement of motor skills relates to coordination. Both balance and coordination are required for weight shifting from one limb to another in sitting and standing and during dynamic activities such as walking.

Bed Mobility/Transfer

Bed mobility skills are essential for maintaining correct bed positioning and preventing contractures, and in avoiding excessive friction of the sheets against the suture line or frail skin of the insensitive foot. Adequate bed mobility is a splinter skill for higher-level skills such as, bed to wheelchair transfers, and, if the client is unable to perform these skills independently, assistance must be provided to prevent injury. More functional transfers such as toilet, shower, and car transfers must also be assessed before discharge to more completely determine the client's level of independence.

Ambulation with Assistive Devices without a Prosthesis

The selection of an assistive device should meet with the amputee's level of skill, keeping in mind that with time the assistive device may change. For example, initially an individual may require a walker, but with proper training forearm crutches may prove more beneficial as a long-term assistive device. The primary means of mobility for a large majority of amputees, either temporarily or permanently, will be a wheelchair. The energy conservation of the wheelchair over prosthetic ambulation is considerable for some levels of amputation, and therefore use of a wheelchair should be positively introduced to those amputees, without implication of failure if used more for mobility than the prosthesis.

Residual Limb Wrapping

Early wrapping of the residual limb can have a number of positive effects. It can decrease edema, increase circulation, assist in shaping, help counteract contractures, provide skin protection, reduce redundant tissue problems, reduce phantom limb pain/sensation, and desensitize local stump pain. Controversy does exist around the use of traditional ace wrapping versus the use of stump shrinkers. Currently, many institutions prefer commercial shrinkers for their ease of donning. Advocates of ace wrapping express that more control over the pressure gradient, and tissue shaping, is provided. Regardless of the individual preference, application must be performed correctly to prevent circulation constriction, poor stump shaping, and edema.

EDUCATION

The importance of educating the client in the self-care, management of the postsurgical residual limb, and preservation of the intact foot cannot be overstated. The following items are included in the evaluation process as a reminder that each topic must be presented to the client as early as feasible during rehabilitation.

Limb Management

POSITIONING

Prevention of decreased ROM and contractures is a major concern to all involved; therefore, proper limb positioning becomes important. The transfemoral amputee should place a pillow laterally along the residual limb to maintain neutral rotation with no abduction, when in a supine position. If the prone position is tolerable during the day or evening, then a pillow is placed under the residual limb to maintain hip extension. Transtibial amputees should avoid knee flexion for prolonged periods of time. A stump board will help maintain knee extension when using a wheelchair. All amputees must be made aware that continual sitting in a wheelchair without any effort to promote hip extension may lead to limited motion during prosthetic ambulation.

SKIN CARE

Every client should be instructed to visually inspect the residual limb on a daily basis or after any strenuous activity. More frequent inspection of the residual limb should be routine in the initial months of prosthetic training. A hand mirror may be used to view the posterior residual limb and the plantar surface of the foot. Reddened areas should be monitored very closely as potential sites for abrasions. If a skin abrasion occurs, the client must understand that in most cases the prosthesis should not be worn until healing occurs.

RESIDUAL LIMB AND SOUND FOOT CARE

It is important that the client understands the care of the residual limb and sound limb. For example, the dysvascular client's prosthetic gait training could be delayed 3–4 weeks if an abrasion should occur. The client must be taught the difference between weight bearing and pressure sensitive areas when inspecting the skin. Preservation of the sound limb foot, in many cases, permits continued bipedal ambulation and delays further medical complications. One reason for this concern is that the sound limb routinely compensates for the amputee's inability to maintain equal weight distribution between limbs, resulting in altered gait mechanics. Two effects on the sound side limb

raise concern: (1) the force being placed on the weight-bearing surfaces of the foot and (2) the change in ground reaction forces throughout the skeletal structures of the limb during ambulation, with or without an assistive device. Increased forces placed on the intact limb can be of considerable concern during ambulation since the foot often presents with neuropathic symptoms and is vulnerable to soft tissue injury brought about by altered biomechanics.

Footwear

The need for appropriate footwear is extremely important, especially for the dysvascular amputee. Shoes should be made of soft leather or some other yielding lightweight material. A blucher-style closure for easier donning is suggested with an enlarged toe box, flat block heels, nonskid outer soles, and possibly a lateral toe flair for increased stability. Custom orthotic inserts are an excellent idea for every amputee to accommodate for the changes in weight-bearing forces and to maintain the arches of the foot. Shoes should be inspected daily for foreign objects inside the shoes, and for tacks or nails that may have penetrated the soles.

Home Exercise

Providing instruction for home exercise should be initiated from the time of discharge from the hospital. Typically, three exercises should be prescribed, with the selection of the exercises designed to prepare or augment prosthetic gait training.

PREPROSTHETIC EXERCISE

Dynamic Stump Exercises

Eisert and Otester first described dynamic stump exercises in 1954.[1] Since then, these antigravity exercises have been the most favorable method of strengthening the stump. Dynamic stump exercises require little in the way of equipment. A towel roll and step stool is all that is required. These exercises offer additional benefits aside from strengthening, such as desensitization, bed mobility, and joint ROM. The exercises are relatively easy to learn and can be performed independently, permitting the therapist to spend client contact time on other more advanced skills.

Incorporating isometric contractions at the peak of the isotonic movement will help to maximize strength increases. A period of a 10-second contraction followed by 10 seconds of relaxation for 10 repetitions gives the client an easy pneumonic to remember, the "rule of ten." The rationale behind a 10-second contraction is that a maximal isometric contraction can be maintained for 6 seconds; however, there is a 2-second rise time and a 2-second fall time. Thus, 2-second rise time plus 6-second maximal contraction plus 2-second fall = 10 seconds total time for each repetition.[2] Figure 35-2 demonstrates the

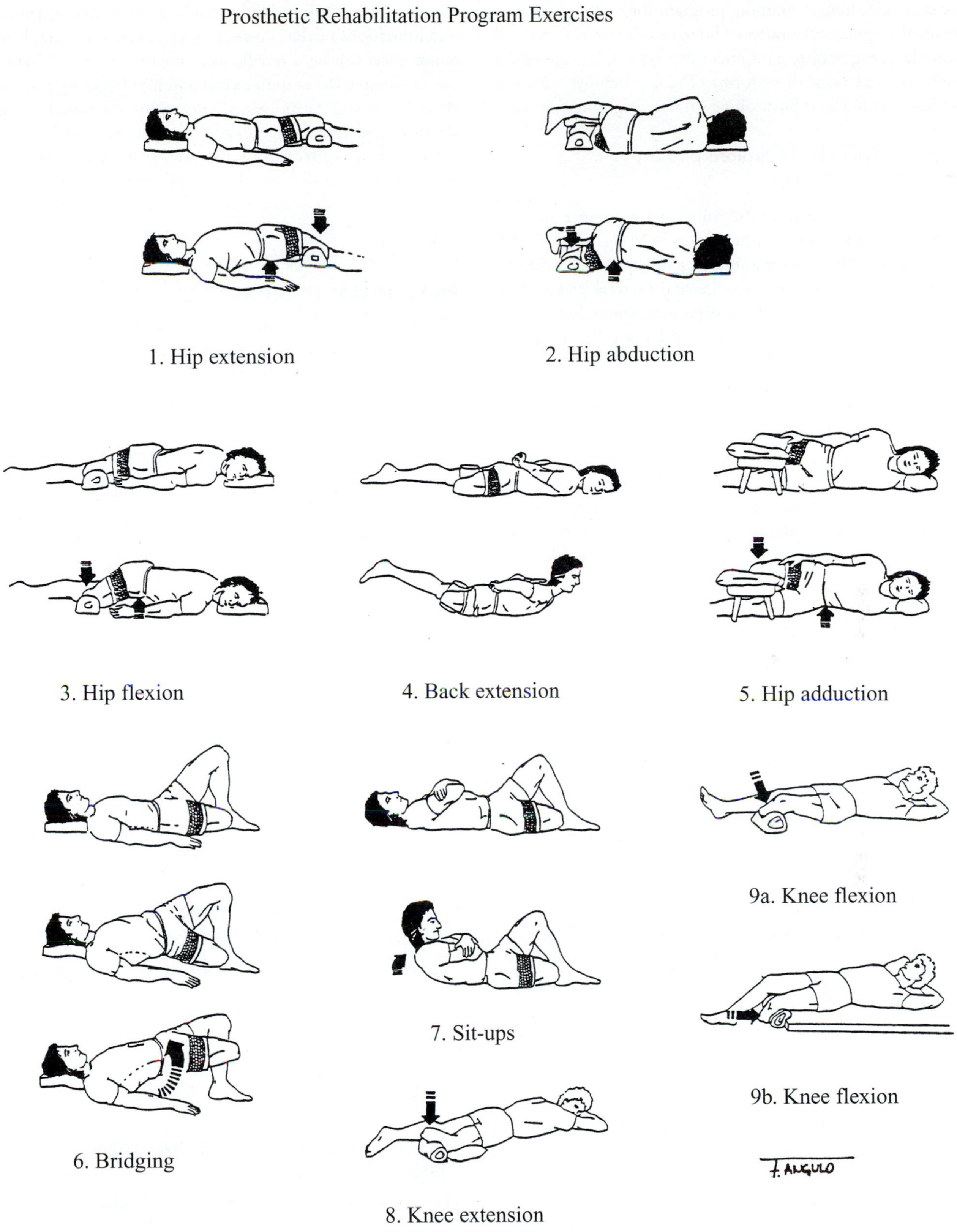

Prosthetic Rehabilitation Program Exercises

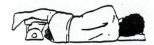
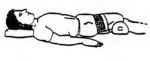
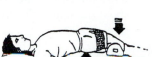
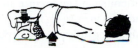

1. Hip extension   2. Hip abduction

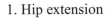
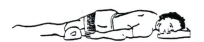
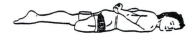
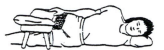
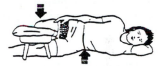
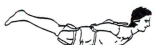
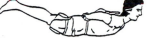
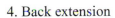

3. Hip flexion   4. Back extension   5. Hip adduction

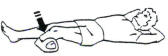

9a. Knee flexion

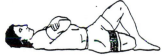

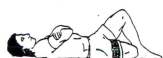
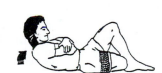

7. Sit-ups

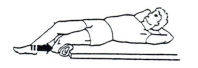

9b. Knee flexion

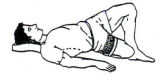
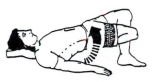

6. Bridging

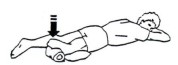

8. Knee extension

F. ANGULO

FIGURE 35-2

Dynamic stump strengthening exercises. (Reproduced, with permission, from Advanced Rehabilitation Therapy, Inc., Miami, FL.)

basic dynamic strength-training program for transfemoral and transtibial amputees. Amputees who have access to isotonic and isokinetic strengthening equipment can take advantage of the benefits derived from these forms of strengthening, with few modifications in client positioning on the weight machines.

General Activities and Cardiorespiratory Endurance Conditioning

Often, decreased general conditioning and endurance are contributory factors leading to difficulties in learning functional activities and prosthetic gait training. Regardless of age or present physical condition, a progressive general exercise prescription can be written for every client, beginning immediately after surgery, through the preprosthetic period and to be continued as part of the daily routine.

The list of possible general strengthening/endurance exercise activities is vast: cuff weights in bed, wheelchair propulsion for a predetermined distance, ambulation with assistive device prior to the prosthesis, lower- or upper-extremity ergometer, wheelchair aerobics, swimming, aquatic therapy, lower- and upper-body strengthening at the local fitness center, any sport or recreational activity of interest. The amputee should select one or more of these activities and begin participation to tolerance, progressing to 1 hour or more a day.

Coordination and Balance Exercises

In preparation for ambulation without a prosthesis, all amputees must learn to compensate for the loss of weight of the amputated limb by balancing the center of mass (COM) over the sound limb. Preparing the amputee to control the COM can begin as early as long sitting on a mat table and moving objects from one side of the body to the other. As the amputee progresses with trunk strength, raising him/her to high kneeling on a bolster will increase the difficulty of the exercise and improve motor patterning. Finally, single-limb balance must be learned initially to provide confidence during stand pivot transfers, ambulation with assistive devices, and eventually hopping, depending on the amputee's level of skill. After receiving the prosthesis, the same exercises may be continued in standing and the amputee should have greater success after progressing through this series of postures.

Exercises that can be performed with this postural progression include moving objects from side to side, progressing the weight of side-to-side objects (e.g., cups, 1-kg balls, to medicine balls), diagonal patterns with a stretch cord, and playing catch. Additionally, the surface that the amputee is sitting or standing on can be altered from a noncompliant to compliant surface (Fig. 35-3).

LEVELS OF LOWER-LIMB AMPUTATIONS AND PROSTHETIC COMPONENTS

Prosthetic components have advanced tremendously over the years, affording the amputee more comfortable and respon-

sive prosthetic choices. Understanding the mechanical abilities and limitations of the prosthetic components for each level of amputation can be a terrific asset for the clinician, especially when assessing the amputee's gait and in instructing functional skills. Knowing the nomenclature and terms associated with the prosthesis can assist in gaining the patient's confidence and enable the therapist to communicate with the prosthetist and rehabilitation team more clearly and with a greater sense of comprehension about the amputee's rehabilitation program.

Partial Foot Amputations

PHALANGEAL (PARTIAL TOE)

The phalangeal amputation is the excision of any part of one or more toes and typically, a prosthesis is not necessary unless the foot is at risk for deformity or further injury as a result of absent digits.

TRANSPHALANGEAL (TOE DISARTICULATION)

The disarticulation amputation at the metatarsophalangeal joint of one or more toes. The prosthetic options vary depending on the number of digits involved. If one to three toes are involved, not including the first ray, a simple toe filler can be placed in the shoe, such as lamb's wool, sponge rubber, or foam filler. When the first digit or great toe is involved, a steel shank spring can be used in the sole of the shoe to assist with push-off, in addition to the toe filler, if needed. In the event that all the toes have been removed, an insole with a metatarsal support is used to relieve weight from the metatarsal heads and a cavus support is provided for the high arch that often results from the lack of stretch to the plantar structures.

The following foot amputations identify the site of the surgical procedure (Fig. 35-4). Examples follow of prosthetic devices that could be employed to improve the amputee's overall functional ability.

METATARSAL RAY RESECTION (PARTIAL RAY RESECTION)

The resection of the third, fourth, and fifth metatarsals and digits.

TRANSMETATARSAL

Amputation through the midsection of all metatarsals.

TARSOMETATARSAL DISARTICULATION (LISFRANC OR MIDFOOT)

The disarticulation of all five metatarsals and the digits.

MIDTARSAL DISARTICULATION (CHOPART)

A disarticulation through the midtarsal joint, leaving only the calcaneous and talus.

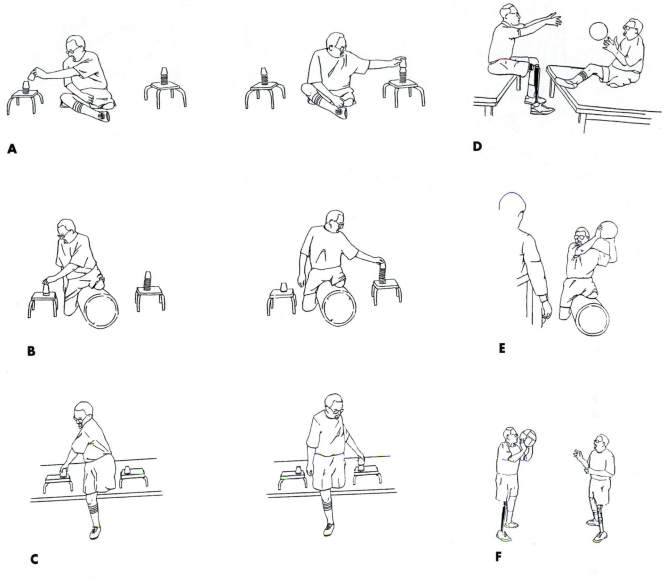

A

D

B

E

C

F

FIGURE 35-3

Weight shifting and balance progression exercises. Two examples would be moving a cup from one side to the other. **A,** Sitting, **B,** kneeling, and **C,** standing or catching a ball; **D,** sitting, **E,** kneeling, **F,** standing. (Reproduced, with permission, from Advanced Rehabilitation Therapy, Inc., Miami, FL.)

PROSTHETIC DEVICES

Custom-Molded Insole with Toe Filler

A simple foam filler with plastic insert for transverse arch of the foot and a heel counter for rear foot stability is widely accepted by many clients who do not experience foot or equinus deformity. To provide a smooth transition throughout the stance phase of gait, a rigid footplate is placed within the shoe or prosthesis, with a rocker bottom under the shoe.

Rigid Plate

To prevent the potential equinus deformity that can occur in the absence of the foot and the shortening of the gastrocnemius and soleus muscles, an ankle-foot orthosis-type appliance is coupled with a toe filler. A plate supports the residual foot and attaches to a shell that is formed around the calf, and the toe filler is fixed to the footplate.

Slipper-Type Elastomer Prosthesis

A more cosmetic approach is the slipper-type elastomer prosthesis, where semiflexible urethane elastomers are modeled to provide a foot-shaped prosthesis with a soft socket that conforms to the residual foot. The footplate and toe filler are incorporated into the slipper-type elastomer prosthesis design.[1]

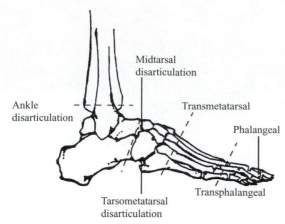

FIGURE 35-4

Surgical sites for partial foot amputations. (Reproduced, with permission, from Advanced Rehabilitation Therapy, Inc., Miami, FL.)

Syme Ankle Disarticulation

This amputation is not a true disarticulation of the ankle, as the removal of the malleoli and distal tibial/fibular flares occurs to create a smooth bony distal end with the attachment of the heel pad to the distal end of the tibia.

Veterans Administration Prosthetic Center Syme Prosthesis

A medial window or cutout at the distal end of the socket provides an opening for ease of donning for the bulbous end pad created by the anatomical heel pad. Velcro straps typically secure the removable door piece to the prosthesis. The device is usually fabricated with a prosthetic foot designed specifically for a Syme prosthesis (Fig. 35-5).

Elastic-Liner Syme Prosthesis

The inner liner is an expandable wall that permits the bulbous distal end of the stump to pass down and sit snugly within the socket as the flexible Silastic elastomer walls envelop the limb for a total contact fit, which prevents swelling. The absence of doors and windows on the socket's exterior provides a more cosmetic and stronger prosthesis. This prosthetic approach cannot be used with extremely bulbous or sensitive stumps.

Transtibial (Below Knee)

The most common surgery is the posterior flap procedure where approximately 40 percent of the tibia and fibula are retained, and the gastrocnemius and soleus muscles are wrapped around the distal end of the limb and sutured anteriorly (Fig. 35-6).

Knee Disarticulation

A number of surgical procedures exist for the knee disarticulation process, mostly describing the flap or how the muscles

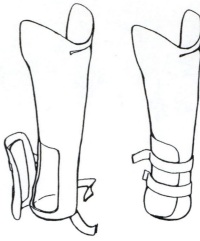

FIGURE 35-5

Veterans Administration Prosthetic Center Syme prosthesis. The medical window provides an opening for ease of donning. (Reproduced, with permission, from Advanced Rehabilitation Therapy, Inc., Miami, FL.)

are secured. Today, most procedures require the shaping of the distal femur, squaring the condyles for an even weight-bearing surface.

Transfemoral (Above Knee)

Once again, many procedures exist for a transfemoral amputation; however, one procedure, the myocutaneous flap, attempts

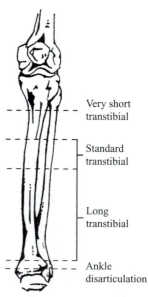

FIGURE 35-6

Surgical sites for transtibial amputations. (Reproduced, with permission, from Advanced Rehabilitation Therapy, Inc., Miami, FL.)

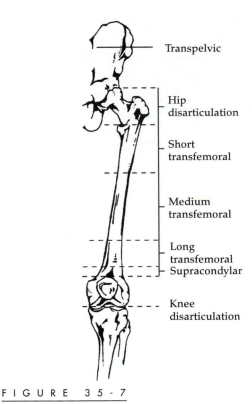

FIGURE 3 5 - 7

Surgical sites for femoral and pelvic amputations. (Reproduced, with permission, from Advanced Rehabilitation Therapy, Inc., Miami, FL.)

to maintain femoral adduction by performing a myodesis (the surgical attachment of muscle to bone), suturing the adductor magnus to the lateral femur, and wrapping the quadriceps muscle over the adductor magnus and suturing it to the posterior femur.[6]

Hip Disarticulation

A disarticulation of the femur and the pelvis resulting in a myoplasty (the surgical attachment of muscle to muscle) of the surrounding musculature (Fig. 35-7).

Prosthetic Devices

The selection of prosthetic components for the major amputations is very similar. Socket designs are fabricated and the number of prosthetic joints is determined according to the level of amputation; however, for the most part, the prosthetist can select from a wide variety of components to construct a prosthesis for each individual's needs. The following components and socket designs are described generically, with some isolated specific brand names discussed when necessary. There are literally hundreds of specific components, variations, and combinations of prosthetic design beyond what is presented here; however, the majority of components and socket designs are represented generically.

Foot-Ankle Assembly

The function of the foot-ankle assembly is threefold: (1) it provides a BOS during standing and in the stance phase of gait, (2) the heel provides shock attenuation at initial contact as the foot moves into plantarflexion, and (3) the forefoot is designed to simulate metatarsophalangeal joint hyperextension during late stance. All foot motions occur passively, in response to the load applied by the amputee. Foot-ankle assemblies are divided into two general categories.

ARTICULATED FOOT-ANKLE ASSEMBLIES

Articulated foot-ankle assemblies provide motion at the level of the anatomical ankle in one or more planes.

Single-Axis Foot

Allows dorsiflexion (5°–7°) and plantarflexion (15°), which are limited by rubber bumpers or spring systems. Single-axis feet offer adjustable plantar and dorsiflexion for greater ROM than nonarticulated foot-ankle designs, allowing foot-flat on low-grade ramps and terrain, but may not conform to steep ramps. Some limitations include no medial/lateral or rotary movements are permitted, parts can be noisy as wear and fatigue occurs over time.

Multiple-Axis Foot

In addition to sagittal motions, the lateral and rotary movements increase the foot-ankle assembly's ability to absorb the impact of uneven terrain, while reducing the torsional forces transmitted through the limb to the stump/socket interface. Although a large variety of excellent multiple-axis foot designs are commercially available, some can be bulky, maintenance and adjustments are frequent, and the additional components may increase the overall weight (Fig. 35-8).

Multiflex Ankle

The ball and snubber, or universal joint design, allows full ROM including inversion, eversion, some rotation, in addition to plantarflexion and dorsiflexion. The rotational component has the ability to absorb some of the torsional forces placed on the prosthesis. Thus, the foot is capable of adjusting to a wide variety of terrains. The keel is produced from a carbon-reinforced plastic (Fig. 35-9).

Tru-Step Foot

Designed to mimic the anatomical foot and ankle. Eight motions are possible: plantarflexion, dorsiflexion, inversion, eversion, adduction, abduction, supination, and pronation. It features a three-point weight transfer system and shock-absorbing heel to reduce ground reaction forces and provide stability. The three bumpers within the system can be changed by the prosthetist to provide the correct resistance for a smooth gait (Fig. 35-10).

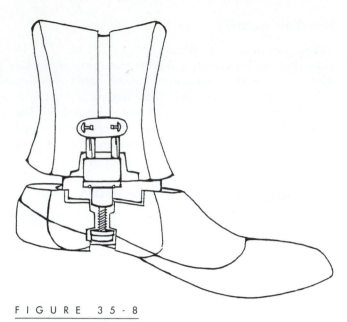

FIGURE 35-8

Multiple-axis foot. (Reproduced, with permission, from Advanced Rehabilitation Therapy, Inc., Miami, FL.)

Elation Foot

The foot functions as a dynamic response system with a single carbon fiber deflector plate, and the single-axis ankle has adjustable bumpers that control plantarflexion and dorsiflexion. What makes the system unique is an innovative heel height adjustment at the ankle. A simple push of a release button allows for easy adjustment of up to 10° of dorsiflexion for ascending, or 25° of plantarflexion for descending ramps or hills. The plantarflexion adjustment is most commonly used for heel height adjustment, particularly for women who enjoy the option of wearing both flat and high-heel shoes (Fig. 35-11).

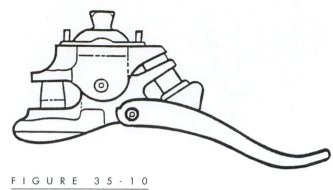

FIGURE 35-10

Tru-Step foot. (Reproduced, with permission, from Advanced Rehabilitation Therapy, Inc., Miami, FL.)

NONARTICULATED FOOT-ANKLE ASSEMBLIES

Nonarticulated foot-ankle assemblies have continuous external surfaces from the sole of the foot to the shank of the prosthesis. There is no articulated joint, and plantarflexion during early stance is achieved with the compression of a cushion heel or the deflection of flexible heel.

Solid Ankle Cushioned Heel Foot

As the most prescribed prosthetic foot worldwide, the molded heel cushion, made of a high density foam rubber, forms the foot and ankle into one component. At heel strike, the rubber heel wedge compresses for shock attenuation. There are no moving parts, thus no maintenance and no noise. The lightweight design offers good absorption of ground reaction forces, smooth transition of weight over the rubber forefoot, and provides resistance to toe extension during the late stance phase of gait. The limitations include limited adjustment of plantarflexion/dorsiflexion, compression of the heel makes walking up inclines difficult, limited motion for active people, and the materials wear (Fig. 35-12).

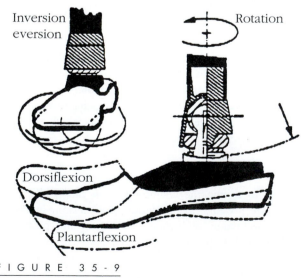

FIGURE 35-9

Endolite Multiflex ankle. (Reproduced, with permission, from Advanced Rehabilitation Therapy, Inc., Miami, FL.)

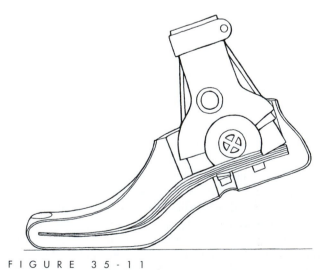

FIGURE 35-11

Elation foot. (Reproduced, with permission, from Advanced Rehabilitation Therapy, Inc., Miami, FL.)

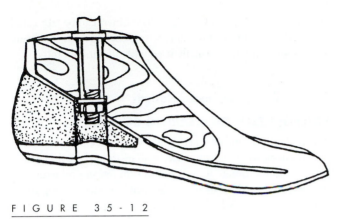

Solid ankle cushioned heel foot. (Reproduced, with permission, from Advanced Rehabilitation Therapy, Inc., Miami, FL.)

Stationary Attachment Flexible Endoskeletal II Foot

Fashioned after the human foot, the stationary attachment flexible endoskeletal II foot bolt block articulates with a rigid polyurethane elastomer keel section at a 45° angle in the sagittal plane to stimulate the human subtalar joint. Two bands made of Dacron polyester fiber further mimic the anatomical foot. The long plantar ligament band provides stability, while the plantar fascia band is designed to tighten, providing a semirigid lever for a smooth transition at toe-off. The flexible keel permits adaptation to various terrains but it is not considered to be a dynamic response foot.

Seattle Foot

Designed for the more active individual, the Seattle foot was the first to provide dynamic keel or deflector plate capabilities. The keel is made of Delrin (acetal polymer), a plastic that deflects during midstance to terminal stance, thus "storing energy," and provides "spring" or "push-off" during toe-off. Two additional innovations made this foot very popular upon release in the early 1980s. The external foam covering is reinforced with Kevlar and has the appearance of an anatomical-looking foot. The second is the cleft between the second and great toe, permitting the wearing of beach thongs. The Seattle Lite foot is one-third lighter than the original foot because the bolt block has been decreased significantly. This permits use by the Symes amputee and adaptation to other ankle units. Currently, the Seattle Lite foot is becoming more popular than the original foot.

Carbon Copy II

Carbon Copy II is a solid ankle design with a heel polyurethane foam cushion. The keel is a unique dual-deflection plate structure made of a carbon composite, which provides two-stage resistance at terminal stance. In normal walking, the thin primary deflection plate provides gentle energy return, while the auxiliary deflection plate provides additional push-off during

higher cadence activities such as running. The Carbon Copy II Light foot has recessed the bolt block and keel to permit the use of hybrid ankle systems, to fit Symes amputees and to reduce the weight of the foot.

Flex Foot

The Modular III is a lightweight graphite composite foot designed with a keel consisting of two leaf springs, one arising from the heel and the other from the toe, both bound individually at the ankle. The Flex foot uses the entire distance from the socket, not just the length of the keel, to "store energy" within the anterior deflector plate. As a result, the Flex foot has been identified as the foot with the greatest energy return of the dynamic response feet. The "split toe" in the footplate enables the foot to function uniformly with the toe deflection on uneven terrain, including the capabilities of inversion and eversion. The Ceterus foot offers greater shock attenuation with the addition of a urethane tube and rubber sole designed to absorb ground reaction forces during ambulation (Fig. 35-13).

Sprint Flex

The Flex foot design is also widely known as being popular with athletes. Although many variations of the foot are designed for amputees of all activity levels, the Sprint Flex is specifically designed for sprinting or long-distance running in a single direction (Fig. 35-14).

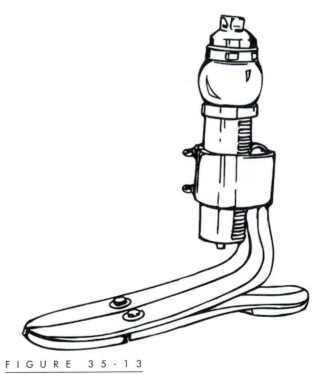

Ceterus. (Reproduced, with permission, from Advanced Rehabilitation Therapy, Inc., Miami, FL.)

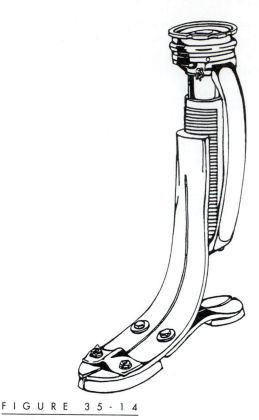

FIGURE 35-14

Flex foot. (Reproduced, with permission, from Advanced Rehabilitation Therapy, Inc., Miami, FL.)

Shanks

The area between the knee and foot is commonly referred to as the shank. There are two basic structural designs of the shank that determine the general structural classification of a prosthesis:

1. The *exoskeletal design* (crustacean), where the exterior of the structure provides the required support for the weight of the body. Thermosetting plastic and wood are the common materials used to fabricate exoskeletal prostheses.
2. The *endoskeletal design* has an internal skeleton or pylon that supports the load with an outer covering, usually made of foam to give the shank a cosmetic shape. The *pylon* is a narrow vertical support typically made of metal or plastic tubing connecting the socket to the foot-ankle assembly. The endoskeletal design has become more popular over the years because it is typically lighter and allows the prosthetist to remove the cosmetic cover to make adjustments to the internal components.

Sockets

There are two general classifications of sockets: One is the hard socket, where there is direct contact between socket's inner surface and stump. The second is the soft socket, which incorporates the use of a liner as a cushion between the socket and stump

and in some cases provides suspension. Liners can be fabricated with pelite, silicone, or urethane. Stump socks do not constitute a soft socket and are normally used with all hard sockets.

Transtibial Amputee Socket Designs

PATELLAR TENDON-BEARING SOCKETS

The socket is a total contact design which refers to the closed distal end, creating a totally closed system around the skin which offers a more intimate fit and avoids skin lesion problems that can occur when the soft tissues are not completely supported. The anterior wall is high enough to encompass the distal half of the patella, while the posterior wall rises slightly higher than the knee joint line. The posterior wall provides an anterior force to maintain the patella on the patellar bar (a small bulge in the socket), and it is also contoured with socket reliefs to prevent excessive pressure on the hamstrings. The medial and lateral walls are slightly higher than the anterior wall, adding stability, but for the most part, stability in the mediolateral plane is provided by the amputee's own knee. The patellar bar allows for weight to be borne on the patellar tendon; however, the weight bearing is also shared by the tibial flares. The patellar tendon-bearing (PTB) socket often requires cuff straps or other forms of suspension.

Two variations for the PTB are the PTB-supracondylar (PTB-SC) and the PTB–supracondylar/suprapatellar (PTB-SC/SP) socket. Both designs incorporate higher medial and lateral walls to encompass both femoral condyles to increase medial and lateral stability of the knee. The PTB-SC/SP raises the anterior wall to cover all of the patella, with the suprapatellar area of the socket being contoured inward to create a "quadricep bar," resulting in additional suspension and resistance to recurvatum, in the case of very short residual limbs or unstable knees, respectively. The posterior wall remains unchanged in both socket variations (Fig. 35-15).

TRANSTIBIAL AMPUTEE SUCTION SOCKET DESIGNS

Because many of the suction sockets use the same proximal brim design such as PTB or PTB-SC, but use suction, a form of suspension, there is some gray area as to whether these sockets are a particular brim shape using a suction suspension, or whether they constitute a separate category of socket design. Regardless of how they are categorized, they are very popular and warrant discussion.

Many sockets today are designed for a suction suspension, which means creating a vacuum between both a flexible roll-on sleeve and the skin, between the sleeve and the socket, or both, in order to hold the socket on the residual limb. The sleeves are made from silicon, urethane, or other composite gel materials, for the purpose of suspension, and in some cases act as soft liners to reduce pressure to bony prominences. All of the sleeves are rolled on over the residual limb, creating a sealed airless environment to keep the sleeve on the limb. The socket

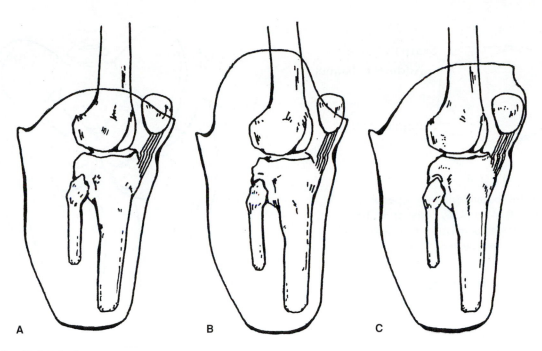

FIGURE 35-15

Comparison between the **A,** PTB socket brim, **B,** the PTB-SC socket brim, and **C,** the PTB SC/SP socket brim. (Reproduced, with permission, from Advanced Rehabilitation Therapy, Inc., Miami, FL.)

is connected to the sleeve by a pin and lock system or one-way valve system. Pin and lock systems use a small pin screwed into a hard cup at the end of the sleeve. When the sleeve-covered limb is placed completely into the socket, a locking mechanism at the distal socket receives the pin, locking the sleeve securely to the socket. A release pin is found on the exterior of the socket, or the sleeve can be removed.

Suction sockets use a one-way valve system that permits the expulsion of air out of the socket but does not permit air to return back into the socket. So when the sleeve-covered residual limb is fully donned into the socket and the air is evacuated, because the volume of the limb takes all the space, a vacuum is formed. To seal the top of the socket, an external suspension sleeve that covers the socket is rolled over the thigh, whereby, an airtight suspension system is formed, and the prosthesis is suspended. Residual limb socks may be worn over the internal sleeves for volume control. The benefits of these suction systems include secure suspension, reduced pistoning, reduced friction, and the elimination of straps, cuffs, or sleeves.

TRANSTIBIAL AMPUTEE SUSPENSION SYSTEMS

Methods for keeping the socket on the body for transtibial amputees are numerous, and there is no one method that works for all amputees. As a result, prosthetists have a wide variety of suspension techniques to meet the specific needs of each individual. Frequently, more than one suspension system may be employed: a primary method that is chiefly responsible for suspending the socket, a secondary system to provide an added sense of security, or improved suspension during higher-level

activities. Common suspension methods include the external suspension sleeve, medial wedge, lateral wedge, suction, removable medial brim, supracondylar cuff, thigh corset or thigh lacer, inverted Y strap, and waist belt.

Transfemoral Amputee Socket Designs

QUADRILATERAL SOCKET

The quadrilateral design is characterized by a series of reliefs or depressions in the socket designed to reduce pressure on relatively firm tissue, tendons, muscles, and bone and bulges, and prominent buildups of materials intended to press on soft areas to provide load sharing. The socket should have total contact between the socket and residual limb with a wider medial–lateral than anterior–posterior dimension. The basic concept of the quadrilateral socket is that the body sits on top of the socket and that all the soft tissue and bony prominences are accounted for with appropriate placement of the reliefs and bulges.

Some of the structural characteristics of the socket design consist of an ischial seat or a thickening on the medial part of posterior brim, where the majority weight-bearing area is intended via the ischial tuberosity. The medial brim is the same height as posterior brim, or slightly lower, so the socket should not press on the pubic ramus. The anterior wall is 2.5 in. higher than the medial wall with the prominent Scarpa's bulge, maintaining the ischial tuberosity on the ischial seat by providing counterpressure against the posterior wall. The lateral wall is higher than the anterior wall and set in 10° of adduction (Fig. 35-16).

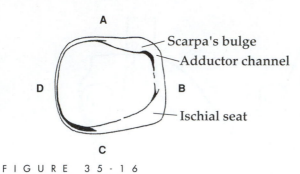

FIGURE   35-16

Quadrilateral socket design—a superior view.
A, Anterior. **B,** Medial. **C,** Posterior. **D,** Lateral.
(Reproduced, with permission, from Advanced
Rehabilitation Therapy, Inc., Miami, FL.)

ISCHIAL CONTAINMENT SOCKET

Characterized by the encapsulation of the ischial tuberosity
within the socket, and greater adduction of the femur, creating
a narrow medial–lateral dimension within the ischial containment socket, the design permits the pelvis and the socket to act
as one for greater prosthetic control. Additionally, by adducting the femur, the muscles would theoretically be placed in an
optimal length–tension position for better quality of muscular contraction. Because of the vast number of socket designs
and names assigned to ischial containment sockets, a generic
description will be presented here.

The structural characteristics of the ischial containment
socket create a high posterior wall where the ischial tuberosity
is enclosed within the socket, and the gluteus maximus muscle
is pocketed by the socket within a gluteal channel, applying a
stretch to the hamstrings. The medial wall slants upward, en-
capsulating the ischial ramus with a counterpressure provided
by the lateral wall. The anterior wall provides a counterpressure
for the posterior wall. The lateral wall rises superiorly above
the greater trochanter with femoral adduction (10°–15°) maintained by a force applied through the greater trochanter and the
length of the shaft of the femur, with a counterforce is applied
at the ischial ramus. The weight should be distributed evenly
throughout the lateral limb (Fig. 35-17).

The materials that sockets are currently constructed from
enable prosthetists to design prostheses that have proximal
brims that rise so high. The copolymer plastics, which are very
flexible, permit greater sitting comfort and increased expand-
ability of muscles as they contract.

Transfemoral Amputee Suspension Systems

Suction is used with a well-shaped, fairly strong residual limb,
and usually, for younger and active amputees who wear no
stump socks and have the required ability to don and doff the
prosthesis. The suspension systems described for the transtibial
sockets apply for the transfemoral sockets. One other form of
suction, used only with transfemoral amputees, is a technique

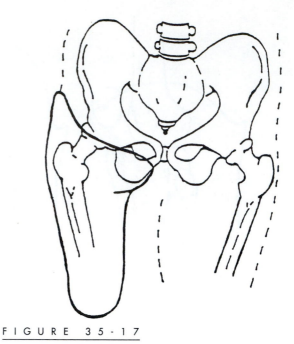

FIGURE   35-17

Ischial containment socket anterior view. (Reproduced,
with permission, from Advanced Rehabilitation Therapy,
Inc., Miami, FL.)

referred to as partial suction. In partial suction, stump socks are
used but there is still a close fit. Because the suction is not complete, it does not fully suspend the prosthesis; therefore, a secondary suspension system such as a Silesian bandage or a pelvic
belt must be incorporated into the design. Suspension methods
include the Silesian bandage, pelvic belt, neoprene belt, and
internal suction sleeve.

Prosthetic Knee Units

Prosthetic knee units provide stability during early stance
through mid-stance, and controlled flexion and extension to
allow the foot to clear the floor and advance the limb during
swing. The speed of the lower leg as it extends should be damp-
ened to control walking cadence and decrease terminal impact
when the knee movement hits the extension stop. Additionally,
flexion for sitting, kneeling, and related activities should not be
restricted.

Because there are so many knee systems available today,
it would be difficult to describe the various knee systems in
detail; however, understanding the three major mechanisms of
knee units—the knee axis, swing phase control mechanism,
and stance phase control mechanism—affords a good general
understanding of prosthetic knees and how they function.

KNEE AXIS

There are two classifications of knee axes, single and polycentric. The single axis works like a hinge joint to maintain a
single stationary axis point which either end may move around.
This is the most common type of axis used in prosthetics. The

polycentric axis is any knee unit with more than one axis. Traditionally, this type of knee axis was referred to as the four-bar linkage system, because there were four connecting rods or bars that created the knee joint mechanism. Today, this is no longer true because of some additional designs that are considered polycentric but do not use the four-bar system. The advantages to this knee axis design include an instantaneous center of rotation as the shank moves about the knee's axis. As a result, during sitting the shank moves under the distal end of the socket, preventing the prosthetic knee from protruding too far in front of the contralateral anatomical knee. During ambulation, as the shank moves posteriorly to the knee's center, greater toe clearance is permitted during swing.

SWING PHASE CONTROL MECHANISMS

Three general classifications of swing phase control mechanisms are available: mechanical constant friction, pneumatic or air control knee mechanism, and hydraulic or fluid control knee mechanisms. Extension-assist bias systems are designed to provide assistance with extension and do not constitute a category of swing phase control because these systems are used to aid with friction control knee systems.

Mechanical Constant Friction

The swing resistance is generated by a friction system that creates a drag on the prosthetic shank, or controls the speed of walking. The amount of resistance does not vary during the swing phase regardless of the angle of knee flexion or the cadence speed. The advantages of friction systems are that they are the simplest of knee units, typically lightweight, durable with few mechanical parts, and are relatively low in cost. The main disadvantage is the inability to vary the speed of cadence.

Pneumatic Control Knee Mechanism

Pneumatic units are air-filled cylinders that provide cadence response utilizing the spring action of a compressible medium, air. When the knee is flexed, the piston rod compresses the air, storing energy. As the knee moves into extension during late swing, the energy is returned, assisting with extension. To prevent an abnormal speed of return or terminal impact, a portion of the air is leaked off. The adjustment screw controls resistance. If the needle completely blocks the port at the top of the cylinder, no air is allowed to enter, and the knee is locked in extension. If the port is completely open, there is little resistance. A second adjustment screw can control extension in many manufacturers' designs. The key advantage to this system is the cadence responsive function that is generally lighter weight than most hydraulic systems and is easier to maintain than many hydraulic units. The disadvantages when compared to friction units are the increased maintenance, increased weigh, and increased expense.

Hydraulic Control Knee Mechanisms

The physical law that liquids are essentially incompressible is the fundamental principle behind the hydraulic units. When the knee flexes, the piston rod is pushed into the oil-filled cylinder, forcing the oil through one or more chambers, thus regulating the speed of movement. The degree of resistance can be controlled by an adjustment screw, which varies the cross-sectional area of the chamber(s). If the amputee has a slow or weak gait, a greater cross-sectional area is created as the chambers open and in turn the resistance is lowered. With a faster walking speed, the cross-sectional area is decreased, the resistance increased, and speed of the limb accommodates accordingly. As the knee swings into extension, the piston rod returns to the top of the cylinder, collecting the oil as it passes each chamber.

The major advantages of hydraulic systems are the cadence responsive function and the ability of most designs to withstand greater forces than pneumatic units. In general, the disadvantages are cost, weight, mechanical failure, and maintenance, which are overshadowed by the advantage of variable cadence without manual adjustment in those amputees who can walk at a variety of speeds.

Extension-Bias Assists

Although not really a knee design classification, the extension-bias assist units help advance the limb or extend the knee during swing. Two basic types are available, internal and external. With the internal unit, a spring provides assistance with extension once knee flexion is completed during ambulation. If the knee flexion is greater than $60°$, the knee will remain flexed as in sitting. With the external unit, an adjustable (or nonadjustable) elastic strap is attached to the socket anteriorly, descending to the anterior shank. As the knee is flexed, the strap is stretched. Once an extension force is initiated, the strap shortens. The strap, unless adjusted, will remain stretched during flexion as in sitting. The external types frequently provide a greater extension force than the internal type.

STANCE PHASE CONTROL MECHANISMS

Stance control can be established individually or in combination through five mechanisms: alignment, manual lock, friction brakes, fluid resistance, and polycentric linkage.

Alignment

All knee units require that the trochanter-knee-ankle or weight line pass anterior to the axis, creating an extension moment and, in turn, knee stability. There is one exception to this rule: the Total Knee requires that the weight line pass posteriorly to the knee axis. (The Total Knee is described in the subsequent "Polycentric Axis Knee Unit" section.)

Manual Locks

Designed to prevent any knee motion once engaged, manual locks are available with one of two basic lock systems: manually operated, where a small lever or ring and cable system is accessible for the amputee to engage or disengage as needed; or spring loaded, which engages automatically when the knee is extended.

Weight-Activated Friction Knee

With a weight-activated friction knee, the knee unit functions as a constant friction knee during swing phase; however, during weight bearing in the stance phase, a housing with a high coefficient of friction presses against the knee mechanism and prevents knee flexion. The "flexion stop," or brake mechanism, can be adjusted to the amputee's body weight. There are a variety of weight-activated friction or "safety" knees, all of which generally prevent flexion from the point of full extension to 25° of flexion, decreasing the risk of buckling during initial contact to loading response.

Hydraulic Swing-N-Stance Control Units

The same hydraulic principles apply as described in the swing phase, but there is an additional advantage with stance control. As weight is applied when the knee is in full extension and up to 25° of flexion, increased resistance is employed from the cylinder, as too rapid a fluid flow results in the immediate closing of valves that stop fluid flow, preventing the knee from buckling and allowing the amputee to regain balance.

Polycentric Axis Knee Unit

The polycentric knee system was historically considered only for knee disarticulation amputees; recently, however, greater acceptance for the general transfemoral amputee population has been observed. Prescription criteria for this system currently extend to (1) knee disarticulations, (2) short transfemoral amputees with less than 50 percent femur length, (3) amputees with weak hip extensors, and (4) amputees requiring greater stability.

One key advantage to the polycentric knee axis design in stance is that because there is no one center of rotation, there exists a greater zone of stability. In other words, in a single-axis system, the weight line is either anterior, creating a stable knee, or posterior, resulting in an unstable knee. In the polycentric design, the area between the anterior and posterior bars is the zone of stability, or the area where the knee is neither too stable nor too unstable. The other key advantage for stability is the raised functional knee center as the point where it takes the least amount of effort or force to control flexion and extension of the knee unit, which is moved proximally and posteriorly as a result of the four-bar linkage system. As a result, the easiest point for controlling the prosthetic knee within the socket is brought up to the level of the residual limb in very short limbs.

The Total Knee is also a polycentric knee, but does not have a four-bar linkage design and the weight-line characteristics vary from all other traditional knees. Because of its popularity the Total Knee warrants description for therapist who will work with this knee unit. This knee design offers a seven-axis system with a unique geometric locking and unlocking action. When the knee moves into extension during terminal swing, the knee is locked; as the body weight is shifted onto the prosthetic limb during loading response, the weight line moves posterior to the axis, flexing the knee to 15° as the anatomical knee would

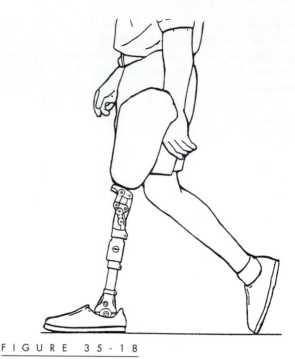

FIGURE 35-18

Total Knee polycentric knee design. (Reproduced, with permission, from Advanced Rehabilitation Therapy, Inc., Miami, FL.)

flex. As the body weight moves over the prosthesis to terminal stance, the weight line moves anterior, releasing the locking mechanism and permitting free and easy knee flexion as the limb moves into swing phase. The cadence is controlled by a rack-and-pinion design where a piston drives the hydraulic fluid. Coupled with the dual flexion adjustment, the knee permits independent flexion control from 0° to 60° and 60° to 160° of knee flexion, reducing excessive heel rise and creating a smooth gait (Fig. 35-18).

Microprocessor Knees

Microprocessor knee systems use one or a combination of force-sensing strain gauge and/or angle sensor to determine phase of gait and walking speed coupled with a single chip electronic central processing unit (CPU) or microprocessor designed to control the flow of the medium that controls swing speed or applies the stance control mechanism. Algorithms are written for the software to continuously adjust the swing and stance control rate for the amputee's activity. The prosthetist has the ability to adjust the primary knee setting with a PC-based computer or personal digital assistant (PDA). As the amputee walks, sits, or negotiates ramps and stairs, the CPU controls the rate of flow for the medium within the set parameters, providing either stance control or swing resistance for a symmetrical gait. The speed of the CPUs or the number of electronic data readings per second varies from 50 to 1000 Hz. One of the central issues a clinician should become familiar with microprocessor knees is actuator speed or the time from when a change in force is recognized on the prosthetic limb to when the knee control

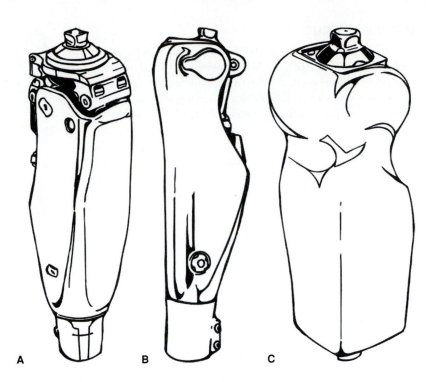

FIGURE 35-19

Microprocessor knees. **A,** Adaptive Knee (Endolite). **B,** C-Leg (Otto Bock). **C,** Rheo Knee (Össur). (Reproduced, with permission, from Advanced Rehabilitation Therapy, Inc., Miami, FL.)

A   **B**   **C**

responds to the forces. CPU speed only accounts for the time that it takes the microprocessor to read the information and not the time that it takes for the knee to adapt to the forces. Currently, actuator speed is not available for all knees, so we look at the CPU speed, programming methods, and the medium that controls knee movement. The following highlight some of the knees currently available.

Adaptive knee (Endolite): microprocessor 62.5 Hz, wireless programming, uses pneumatic swing control and hydraulic stance control (Fig. 35-19A).

C-leg (Otto Bock): microprocessor 50 Hz, PC-based software hard-wire or wireless programming, uses hydraulic swing and stance control (Fig. 35-19B).

Rheo Knee (Össur): microprocessor 1000 Hz, PDA-based software hard-wire programming, uses magnetorheological fluid for swing and stance control (Fig. 35-19C).

Freedom knee (Freedom Innovations): microprocessor 1000 Hz, PDA-based software, PDA-based wireless programming, uses hydraulic swing and stance control.

Hip Disarticulation and Transpelvic Socket Designs

Hip disarticulation and transpelvic socket designs are somewhat similar, with the absence of bony structure making stability more difficult in the transpelvic socket. The essential concept of all the current socket designs is the encapsulation of the ischium and ascending ramus, and additionally, the soft tissues of the remaining musculature, extending to the gluteal fold, must be encased within the socket to create a pseudohydrostatic environment for the tissues and viscera. The socket extends around both iliac crests, compressing the tissues snuggly and providing

a stable environment within the socket. The major difficulty is finding the balance between a well-fitting functional socket and patient comfort, both in standing and sitting. The flexible thermoplastics, silicones, and urethane materials have created a much more comfortable environment within the socket, while lighter weight rigid materials help to maintain the much-needed external stability. As a result of the material advances, it appears that many more high-level amputees are using prostheses today than ever before.

Hip Joints

CANADIAN HIP JOINT

The Canadian hip joint is a single axis joint that remains in extension during stance and flexes during swing. The hip joint is attached to the socket anteriorly to keep the weight line posterior to the knee access for stance phase stability. At preswing the amputee posteriorly rotates the pelvis with a brief thrusting motion to flex both the knee and hip to clear the ground and move into swing phase. One of the inherent limitations of the Canadian design is that the prosthesis must be significantly short (1 cm+) to avoid forcing the amputee to vault for toe clearance.

HIP FLEXION BIAS SYSTEM

A coil spring is compressed during midstance and released during preswing, thrusting the prosthetic thigh forward. The benefit of this design is the elimination of the excessive pelvic rocking that is required with traditional hip joint designs. The amputee has a much more natural gait, providing he/she fully loads the spring and rapidly transfers the weight to the sound limb, allowing the limb to thrust forward smoothly.

LITTIG HIP STRUT

A carbon composite strut in the shape of a band connects to the socket and the knee unit. As body weight is placed over the strut, it deflects or bends, and then as the body weight is reduced during preswing and the limb moves into swing, the strut recoils or thrusts the prosthetic limb forward. The thickness and length of the hip strut vary according to the height and weight of the amputee. The need for excessive pelvic motion is eliminated as the amputee once again must confidently transfer the body weight on and off the prosthesis as appropriate.

PROSTHETIC GAIT TRAINING*

Orientation to Center of Gravity and Base of Support

Orientation of the COM over the BOS in order to maintain balance requires that the amputee become familiar with these terms and aware of their relationship. The body's COM is located 2 in. anterior to the second sacral vertebrae, and the average person stands with the feet 2–4 in. (5–10 cm) apart, both varying according to body height.[7,8] Various methods of proprioceptive and visual feedback may be employed to promote the amputee's ability to maximize the displacement of the COM over the BOS. The amputee must learn to displace the COM forward and backward, as well as from side to side (Fig. 35-20). These exercises vary little from the traditional weight-shifting exercises, with the one exception that the concentration is placed on the movement of the COM over the BOS, rather than weight bearing into the prosthesis. Increased weight bearing will be a direct result of improved COM displacement, and will establish a firm foundation for actual weight shifting during ambulation.

Single-Limb Standing

Single-limb balance over the prosthetic limb, while advancing the sound limb, should be practiced in a controlled manner so that when called on to do so in a dynamic situation such as walking, this skill can be employed with relatively little difficulty. The stool-stepping exercise is an excellent method through which this skill may be learned. Have the amputee stand in the parallel bars with the sound limb in front of a 4- to 8-in. stool (or block), height depending on level of ability. Then ask him/her to step slowly onto the stool with the sound limb while using bilateral upper-limb support on the parallel bars. To further increase this weight-bearing skill, ask the client to remove the sound side hand from the parallel bars, and eventually the other hand. Initially, the speed of the sound leg will increase when upper-limb support is removed, but with practice the speed will become slower and more controlled, promoting increased weight bearing on the prosthesis (Fig. 35-21).

---

*The following amputation rehabilitation program is adapted, with permission, from Gailey RS, Gailey AM. *Prosthetic Gait Training Program for Lower Extremity Amputees.* Miami, FL, Advanced Rehabilitation Therapy Inc., 1989.[4]

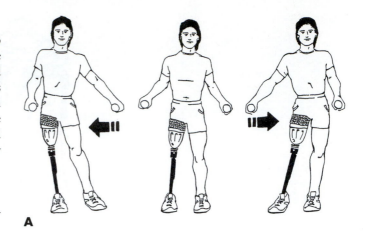

A

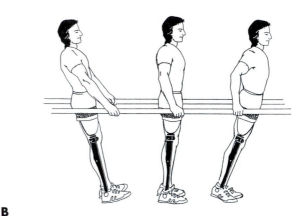

B

F I G U R E   3 5 - 2 0

A, Lateral weight shifting and balance orientation. **B,** Sagittal weight shifting and balance orientation. (Reproduced, with permission, from Advanced Rehabilitation Therapy, Inc., Miami, FL.)

The amputee's ability to control sound limb advancement is directly related to the ability to control prosthetic limb stance. The following are three contributing factors that may help the amputee achieve adequate balance over the prosthetic limb. The first is control of the musculature of the residual limb side to maintain balance over the prosthesis. Second, the client must learn to utilize the available sensation within the residual limb/socket interface, such as proprioception, in order to control the prosthesis. Third, the amputee must visualize the prosthetic foot and its relationship to the ground. New amputees will have difficulty understanding this concept at first, but will gain a greater appreciation as time goes on.

Gait Training Skills

SOUND AND PROSTHETIC LIMB TRAINING

Another component in adjusting to the amputation of a limb is the restoration of the gait biomechanics that were unique to a particular person prior to the amputation. That is to say, not everyone has the same gait pattern. Prosthetic developments in

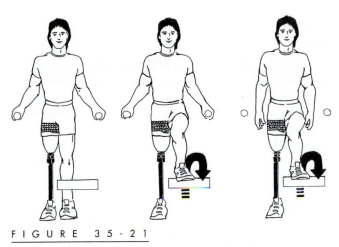

FIGURE   35-21

Stool-stepping exercise. (Reproduced, with permission, from Advanced Rehabilitation Therapy, Inc., Miami, FL.)

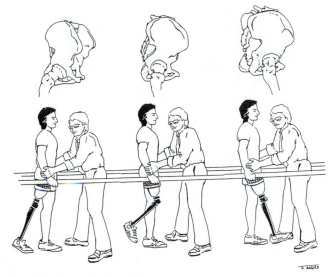

FIGURE   35-22

Resistive gait training techniques are proprioceptive neuromuscular facilitation techniques to assist and establish a normalized gait pattern. (Reproduced, with permission, from Advanced Rehabilitation Therapy, Inc., Miami, FL.)

the last decade have provided limbs that replicate the mechanics of the human leg closely. Therefore, the goal of gait training should be the restoration of function to the remaining joints of the amputated limb. Prosthetic gait training should not alter the amputee's gait mechanics for the prosthesis, but instead, the mechanics of the prosthesis should be designed around the amputee's individual gait.

PELVIC MOTIONS

The pelvis and the body's COM, as a unit, moves in four directions: displaces vertically, shifts laterally, tilts horizontally, and rotates transversely. Each of these motions can directly affect the amputee's gait, resulting in gait deviations or in a rise in energy expenditure during ambulation. If restoration of function to the remaining joints of the amputated limb is the goal of gait training, then the pelvic motions play a decisive role in determining the final outcome of an individual's gait pattern.

Normalization of trunk, pelvic, and extremity biomechanics can be taught to the amputee in a systematic way. First, independent movements of the various joint and muscle groups are developed. Second, the independent movements are incorporated into functional movement patterns of the gait cycle. Finally, all component movement patterns are integrated to produce a smooth normalized gait.

Resistive gait training techniques can be employed to restore the correct pelvic motion. The amputee places his/her prosthetic limb behind the sound limb while holding on to the P-bars with both hands. The therapist blocks the prosthetic foot to prevent forward movement of the prosthesis. Rhythmic initiation is employed, giving the amputee the feeling of rotating the pelvis forwardly as passive flexion of the prosthetic knee occurs. As the amputee becomes comfortable with the motion, he/she can begin to move the pelvis actively, eventually progressing to resistive movements when the therapist deems appropriate (Fig. 35-22).

Once the amputee and therapist are satisfied with the pelvic motions, the swing phase of gait can be instructed. The amputee

is now ready to step forward and backward with the prosthetic limb. Attention must be given to the pelvic motions: the line of progression of the prosthesis remains constant without circumducting, and that heel contact occurs within boundaries of the BOS. As the amputee improves, release the sound side hand from the parallel bars and eventually both hands. There should be little, if any, loss of efficiency with the motion; but if there is, revert to the previous splinter skill.

Return to sound limb stepping with both hands on the P-bars. Observe that the mechanics are correct and that the sound foot is not crossing midline as heel strike occurs. When ready, have the amputee remove the sound side hand from the P-bars. At this time, there may be an increase in the speed of the step, a decrease in step length and/or lateral leaning of the trunk. This is a direct result of the inability to weight bear or balance over the prosthesis. Cue the amputee in remembering the skills learned while performing the stool-stepping exercise as previously described.

When each of the skills described are developed to an acceptable level of competency, the amputee is ready to combine the individual skills, and actually begin walking with the prosthesis. Initially, begin in the P-bars with the therapist and amputee facing each other, the therapist's hands on the amputee's anterior superior iliac spine and the amputee holding onto the P-bars. As the amputee ambulates within the P-bars, the therapist applies slight resistance through the hips, providing proprioceptive feedback for the pelvis and involved musculature of the lower limb.

When both the therapist and the amputee are comfortable with the gait demonstrated in the P-bars, the same procedure as described above is practiced out of the P-bars, with the amputee

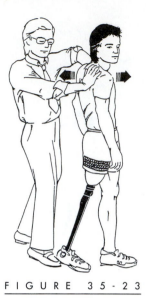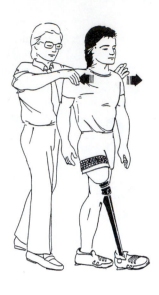

F I G U R E   3 5 - 2 3

Passive trunk rotation will assist in restoring arm swing for improved balance, symmetry of gait, and momentum. (Reproduced, with permission, from Advanced Rehabilitation Therapy, Inc., Miami, FL.)

initially using the therapist's shoulders as support and progressing to both hands free when appropriate. The therapist may or may not continue to provide proprioceptive input to the pelvis.

Trunk rotation and arm swing are the final components needed to restore the complete biomechanics of gait. During human locomotion, the trunk and upper limbs rotate opposite to the pelvic girdle and lower limbs. Trunk rotation is necessary for balance, momentum, and symmetry of gait. Many amputees have decreased trunk rotation and arm swing, especially on the prosthetic side. This may be the result of fear of displacing their COM too far forward or backward over the prosthesis (Fig. 35-23).

Instructing trunk rotation and arm swing is easily accomplished by utilizing rhythmic initiation, or passively cueing the trunk as the amputee walks. The therapist stands behind the amputee with one hand on either shoulder. As the amputee walks, the therapist gently rotates the trunk. When the left leg steps forward, the right shoulder is rotated forward, and vice versa. Once the amputee feels comfortable with the motion, he/she can actively take over the motion.

Both amputees who will be independent ambulators and those who will require an assistive device can benefit to varying degrees from the above systematic rehabilitation program. Most clients can be progressed to the point of ambulating out of the P-bars. At that time, the amputee must practice ambulating with the chosen assistive device, maintaining pelvic rotation, adequate BOS, equal stance time and equal stride length—all of which can have a direct influence on the energy cost of walking. Trunk rotation would be absent with amputees utilizing a walker as an assistive device; however, those ambulating with crutches or a cane should be able to incorporate trunk rotation into their gait.

Advanced Gait Training Activities

STAIRS

Ascending and descending stairs is most safely and comfortably performed one-step at a time (step-*by*-step). A few exceptional transfemoral amputees can descend stairs step-*over*-step, or by the "jack knifing" method and even fewer yet, very strong amputees, can ascend stairs step-over-step. Most transtibial amputees have the option of either method, while hip disarticulation and hemipelvectomy amputees are limited to the step-by-step method.

CURBS

The methods described for stairs are identical for curbs. Depending on the level of skill, the amputee can step up or down curbs with either leg.

UNEVEN SURFACES

A good practice with gait training is to have the amputee ambulate over a variety of surfaces including concrete, grass, gravel, uneven terrain, and varied carpet heights. Initially, the new amputee will have difficulty in recognizing the different surfaces, secondary to the loss of proprioception. To promote an increased awareness, spending time on different surfaces and becoming visually aware of the changes help to initiate this learning process. Additionally, the amputee must realize that in some instances, it is important that he/she observe the terrain ahead to avoid any slippery surfaces or potholes that might result in a fall.

RAMPS AND HILLS

Ascending inclines presents a problem for all amputees because of the lack of dorsiflexion present within most prosthetic foot/ankle assemblies. For most amputees, descending inclines is even more difficult than ascending, primarily because of the lack of plantarflexion in the foot–ankle assembly. Transtibial amputees, and prosthetic wearers with knee joints, have the added dilemma of the weight line falling posterior to the knee joint, resulting in a flexion moment.

When ascending an incline, the body weight should be slightly more forward than normal to obtain maximal dorsiflexion with articulating foot–ankle assemblies, and to keep the knee in extension. Depending on the grade of the incline, pelvic rotation with additional acceleration may be required in order to achieve maximal knee flexion during swing.

Descent of an incline usually occurs at a more rapid pace than normal because of the lack of plantarflexion, resulting in decreased stance time on the prosthetic limb. Amputees with prosthetic knees must exert a greater than normal force on the posterior wall of the socket to maintain knee extension.

Most amputees find it easier to ascend and descend inclines with short but equal strides. They prefer this method since it simulates a more normal appearance as opposed to the sidestepping or zigzag method.

When ascending and descending hills, the amputee will find sidestepping to be the most efficient means. The sound limb should lead, providing the power to lift the body to the next level, while the prosthetic limb remains slightly posterior to keep the weight line anterior to the knee and acts as a firm base. During descents, the prosthetic limb leads but remains slightly posterior to the sound limb. The prosthetic knee remains in extension, again acting as a form of support so that the sound limb may lower the body.

BRAIDING

Braiding may be taught either in the P-bars or in an open area depending upon the person's ability. Simple braiding is one leg crossing in front of the other. As the amputee's skill improves, the crossing leg can alternate, first in front of and then behind the other leg. When ability improves, the speed of movement should increase. With increased speed, the arms will be required to assist with balance, and likewise, trunk rotation will increase, further emphasizing the need for independent movement between the trunk and pelvis.

FALLING

Falling, or lowering oneself to the floor is an important skill to learn not only for safety reasons, but also as a means to perform floor level activities. During falling, the amputee must first discard any assistive device to avoid injury. He/she should land on the hands, with the elbows slightly flexed to dampen the force, and decrease the possibility of injury. As the elbows flex, the amputee should roll to one side, further decreasing the impact of the fall.

Lowering the body to the floor in a controlled manner is initiated by squatting with the sound limb, followed by gently leaning forward onto the slightly flexed upper extremities. From this position, the amputee has the choice of remaining in quadruped or assuming a sitting posture.

FLOOR TO STANDING

Many techniques exist for teaching the amputee how to rise from the floor to a standing position. The fundamental principle is to have the amputee use the assistive device for balance and the sound limb for power as the body begins to rise. Depending on the type of amputation and the level of skill, the amputee and therapist must work closely together to determine the most efficient and safe manner to successfully master this task.

RUNNING SKILLS[†]

For most amputees, running is the single most commonly given reason for limiting participation in recreational activities—and yet, it is the most wanted skill. Many amputees who do not have a strong desire to run for sport or leisure do have an interest in

---

[†]The following running program is adapted, with permission, from Gailey RS. *The Essentials of Lower Limb Amputee Running and Sports Training.* Miami, FL, Advanced Rehabilitation Therapy Inc., 2004.[5]

learning how to run for the simple peace of mind of knowing that they could move quickly to avoid a threatening situation. Rarely, if ever, is running taught in the rehabilitation setting. Running, as with all gait training and advanced skills, takes time and practice to master. If the amputee is exposed to the basic skills of running during rehabilitation, then the individual may make the decision to pursue running in the future.

The Syme and transtibial amputee does have the ability to achieve the same running biomechanics as able-bodied runners if emphasis is placed on the following:

1. At ground contact, the prosthetic limb hip should be flexed moving toward extension, the knee should be flexed, and the prosthetic foot dorsiflexed. The knee flexion not only permits greater shock absorption but, in addition, creates a backward force between the ground and the foot to provide additional forward momentum.

2. As the center of gravity is transferred over the prosthesis during the stance phase, the ipsilateral arm should be fully forward (shoulder flexed to 60°–90°), while at the same time the contralateral arm is backward (shoulder extended). Extreme arm movement can be difficult for the amputee concerned with maintaining balance.

3. The hip, during late midstance to toe-off, should be forcefully driving downward and backward through the prosthesis as the knee extends. If the prosthetic foot is "dynamic elastic response," the force produced by the hip extension should deflect the keel so that the prosthetic foot will provide additional push-off.

4. Forward swing and the float phase is a period when the hip should be rapidly flexing, elevating the thigh. The arms should again be opposing the advancing lower limb, with the ipsilateral arm backward and the contralateral arm forward.

5. During foot descent, the hip should be flexed and beginning to extend as the knee is rapidly extending and reaching forward for a full stride.

Transfemoral and knee disarticulation amputees traditionally run with a period of double support on the sound limb during the running cycle, commonly referred to as the "hop-skip" running gait pattern. The typical running gait cycle begins with a long stride with the prosthetic leg, followed by a shorter stride with the sound leg. In order to give the prosthetic leg sufficient time to advance, the sound leg takes a small hop as the prosthetic limb clears the ground and moves forward to complete the stride. The speed that a transfemoral amputee runner may achieve will be hampered, because every time either foot makes contact with the ground, the foot's forces are traveling forward, and therefore, the reaction force of the ground must be in a backward or opposite direction. The result is that each time the foot contacts the ground, forward momentum is decelerated. In other words, with every stride the amputee is slowing down when running with the hop-skip gait.

The ability to run "leg-over-leg" has been achieved by a number of transfemoral amputees who have developed this technique through training and working with knowledgeable coaches. The transfemoral amputee takes a full stride with the prosthetic leg, followed by a typically shorter stride with the sound leg. With training, equal stride length and stance time may be achieved. This running pattern is a more natural gait where the double support phase of the sound limb is eliminated, and both legs may maintain forward momentum. Initially, other problems that may occur include excessive vaulting off the sound limb to insure ground clearance of the prosthetic limb, decreased pelvic and trunk rotation, decreased and asymmetrical arm swing, and excessive trunk extension. Again with training, many of these deviations will decrease and possibly be eliminated.

The transfemoral amputee has an additional consideration when learning to run. To date, no knee system permits flexion during the prosthetic support phase, resulting in the stump having to absorb the ground reaction forces during initial ground contact. Other problems with present knee units that transfemoral amputees must contend with are maintaining cadence speed during swing. Hydraulic knee units offer the ability to adjust the hydraulic resistance during knee flexion and extension. During running, less resistance in extension permits faster knee extension, while increased resistance in flexion increases the amount of time until full knee flexion is achieved, allowing the same-side hip time to reach greater flexion, producing a more powerful stride. Seasoned runners often reduce both knee extension and flexion hydraulic resistance, permitting the prosthetic knee timing and mechanics to match the speed and ROM of the sound limb. As the runner's technique progresses and the level of competition elevates, it is important that the prosthesis be fine-tuned to match the athlete's abilities.

The leg-over-leg running style does permit the transfemoral amputee to run faster, for short distances, but at a greater metabolic cost. While leg-over-leg is preferred, the hop-skip method is often more easily taught and less physically demanding on the amputee. If the sole purpose of instructing running is to permit the individual to move quickly in a safe manner, the hop-skip method is most frequently suggested (Fig. 35-24).

RECREATIONAL ACTIVITIES

By definition, recreation is any play or amusement used for the refreshment of the body or mind. That is to say, the term recreational activities need not exclusively mean athletics such as running or team sports. In fact, many people enjoy recreational activities such as gardening, shuffleboard, or playing cards as a means of socializing or relaxing. A comprehensive rehabilitation program should include educating the amputee on how he/she can return to those activities that he/she finds pleasurable. For example, the therapist can teach the physical splinter skills such as weight shifting necessary to help the amputee participate in shuffleboard, or various methods of kneeling for gardening. In addition, there are many national and local recreational organizations and support groups, which provide clinics, coaching, or another amputee who can teach from experience how to perform various higher-level recreational skills. Providing the amputee with information on how to contact these groups is the first step to mainstreaming the client back into a lifestyle complete with recreational skills as well as activities of daily living.

UPPER-LIMB PROSTHETIC REHABILITATION

Levels of Upper-Limb Amputation

The classification for upper-limb amputees is based on the anatomical location of the amputation or surgical site (Fig. 35-25). When an amputation occurs to the digits of the hand, prosthetic fitting is most frequently for cosmetic rather than functional purposes. In some instances, custom-made prostheses are fabricated for functional purposes, especially when ROM or strength has been severely affected. The acceptance of upper-limb prosthetic devices varies depending on the age, gender, culture, activity level, and "gadget tolerance" of the amputee. Many amputees prefer to learn how to adapt with the sound arm and use the stump of the amputated side as an assist. Youngsters adapt very well without the use of a prosthesis, whereas adults who lose an upper extremity prefer to

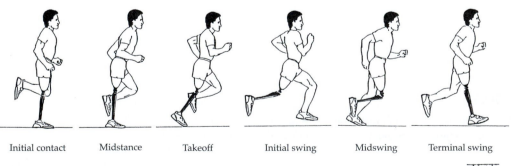

Initial contact   Midstance   Takeoff   Initial swing   Midswing   Terminal swing

F I G U R E   3 5 - 2 4

Transfemoral amputee running. (Reproduced, with permission, from Advanced Rehabilitation Therapy, Inc., Miami, FL.)

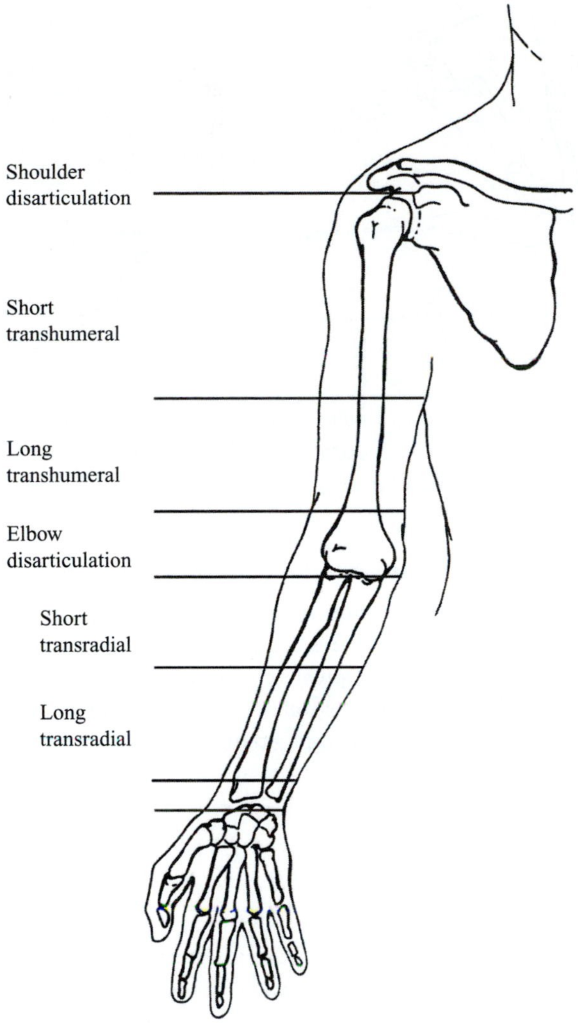
Shoulder disarticulation
Short transhumeral
Long transhumeral
Elbow disarticulation
Short transradial
Long transradial

FIGURE 35-25

Surgical sites for upper limb amputations. (Reproduced, with permission, from Advanced Rehabilitation Therapy, Inc., Miami, FL.)

use a prosthesis for both aesthetic and functional reasons. This section will review the common components of an upper-limb prosthesis and outline the rehabilitation progression.

Terminal Devices

HOOKS

The most common terminal device (TD) used is the split-hook type. By allowing the amputee to open and close the hook, objects can be grasped between the "finger" of the hook (each side of the metal hook is referred to as a finger). The fingers of the hook have the ability for carrying, holding, or pushing objects (Fig. 35-26).

Voluntary-Opening Hooks

The amputee exerts a force on the control cable of a voluntary-opening hook to open the fingers of the hook against the force of the rubber bands, which act as a spring to close the fingers and provide prehension, or pinch force. The force is approximately 1.5 lbs per rubber band. The standard hook is used for general use and activities, while the farmer's hook is often prescribed for heavier work-related activities, and for carrying loads.

Voluntary-Closing Hooks

The less commonly seen voluntary-closing hook permits the amputee more precise ability to close the device because the amputee powers the closing by use of cable control. Prehension force ranges from 0.5 to 25 lbs. A self-locking mechanism automatically locks the hook in a grasp position. This TD is preferred for control of fine work without great exertion.

HANDS

More cosmetically appealing to some amputees, the prosthetic hand has become more popular over the years; however, it is not considered to be as functional as the hook. Many amputees

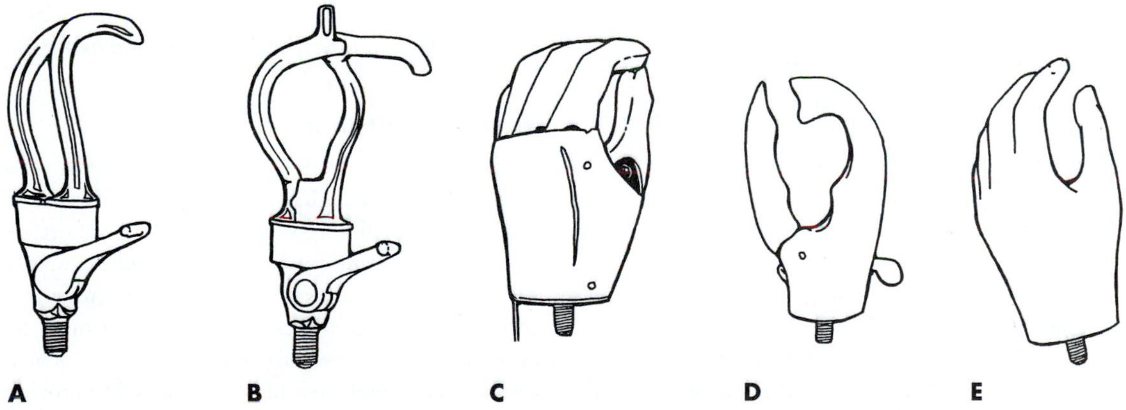
A
B
C
D
E

FIGURE 35-26

Terminal devices. Hooks: **A,** Standard voluntary opening (VO) hook. **B,** Farmer VO hook. **C,** Voluntary-closing hook. Hands: **D,** VO hand. **E,** Passive or cosmetic hand. (Reproduced, with permission, from Advanced Rehabilitation Therapy, Inc., Miami, FL.)

use a hand on an interchangeable basis with a hook TD (see Fig. 35-26).

Voluntary-Opening Hands

Operation of the hand voluntary-opening hand is the same as the voluntary-opening hook; however, the fingers form the "three-jaw-chuck" pinch with the index and middle finger joining the thumb. The mechanics of the hand and fingers vary a little between the different manufacturers in that some hands offer multiple locking positions, different grips, and some vary the number of moveable fingers.

Passive or Cosmetic Hands

The passive hand has no functional mechanism and is intended purely for cosmetic effect. Many people will change to a cosmetic hand for formal dress or occasions where appearance exceeds the need for function.

WRIST UNITS

Wrist units are used for attaching the TD to the forearm and provide TD rotation (pronation/supination). Wrist units can be either constant-friction controlled or locking. TD rotation is performed passively by the sound hand or by pushing the TD against an object. Quick-change wrist units permit easy removal and replacement of the TD, offering the amputee a variety of TDs, depending on the activity.

Wrist flexion units are very practical adaptations, permitting easier control for midline activities such as eating, grooming, and dressing. Bilateral upper-limb amputees find that one, if not both, wrist unit must flex to perform everyday activities independently. There are two types of wrist flexion units, internal and external. The internal units combine a constant-friction wrist and a wrist-flexion unit that has locking settings of $0°$, $30°$, or $50°$ of flexion. The external units are designed for manual positioning of the TD in either flexion or full extension.

TRANSRADIAL SOCKETS
Split Socket

Typically used with very short transradial amputee (TRA), split sockets are used with step-up hinges because elbow flexion is often limited. The step-up gear ratio is 2:1, which permits $2°$ of forearm shell movement for every degree of elbow flexion (Fig. 35-27).

Munster Socket

Often referred to as the self-suspending socket, the Munster socket was designed for short TRA. The extremely narrow anterior–posterior dimension suspends the socket on the residual limb. The disadvantage of this socket is that the proximity of the anterior trim line frequently prevents full elbow flexion, and the forearm shell is typical preflexed, limiting the appearance of full extension. When a manual TD is used, a harness is used to power the TD (figure-9). If a myoelectric control system is used, no other suspension device is necessary (Fig. 35-28).

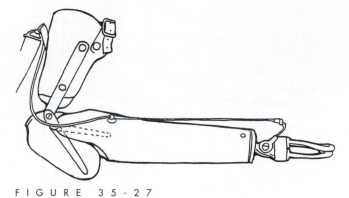

FIGURE 35-27

Split socket design with triceps pad and a standard hook terminal device. (Reproduced, with permission, from Advanced Rehabilitation Therapy, Inc., Miami, FL.)

Northwestern University Supracondylar Socket

Because of the ROM limitations associated with the Munster socket, the Northwestern University supracondylar design has become the most popular self-suspending socket design, where the medial and lateral walls of the socket narrow over the humeral epicondyles, suspending the prosthesis very adequately without any loss of ROM in the sagittal plane or the need to preflex the forearm shell (Fig. 35-29).

HINGES

Transradial hinges connect the socket to a triceps cuff, or pad on the posterior upper arm, and assist with suspension and stability. Selection of the hinge type depends on the site of amputation and the residual function.

Flexible Elbow Hinges

Constructed of flexible materials such as Dacron webbing fabric, leather, or lightweight metals, flexible elbow hinges assist with suspension of the forearm shell and permit rotational motion of the forearm in long TRA and wrist disarticulations.

Rigid Elbow Hinges

Constructed of more rigid metals and composite plastics, rigid hinges are used for midforearm to short TRA with normal elbow ROM. Rigid hinges are also used with short TRA because little supination and pronation is available anatomically; also a smaller stump requires greater stability in order to better control the prosthesis. Because of the limited motion, pronation and supination are performed at the shoulder. The three major categories are single-axis hinges, designed to provide rotational stability between the socket and forearm; polycentric hinges, used with short TRA and designed to help to increase elbow flexion by reducing the bunching of soft tissue in the cubital fossa; and step-up hinges, used with the split socket and offering the 2:1 ratio of elbow motion to forearm movement.

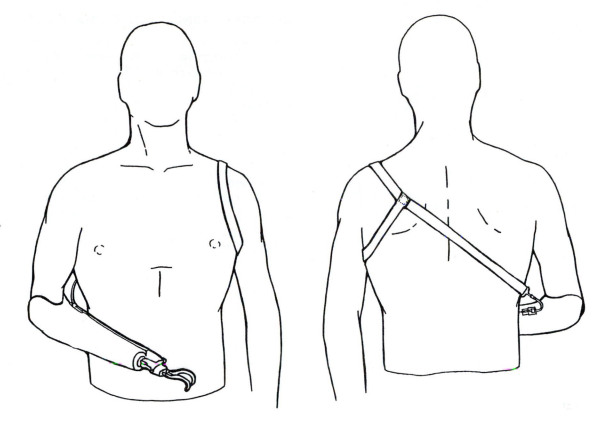

FIGURE 35-28

Munster socket with figure-9 harness. (Reproduced, with permission, from Advanced Rehabilitation Therapy, Inc., Miami, FL.)

TRANSRADIAL HARNESS AND CONTROLS

The function of the harness is to suspend the prosthesis from the shoulder so that the socket is held firmly in place on the stump. Movement of the scapulothoracic region, scapular abduction or

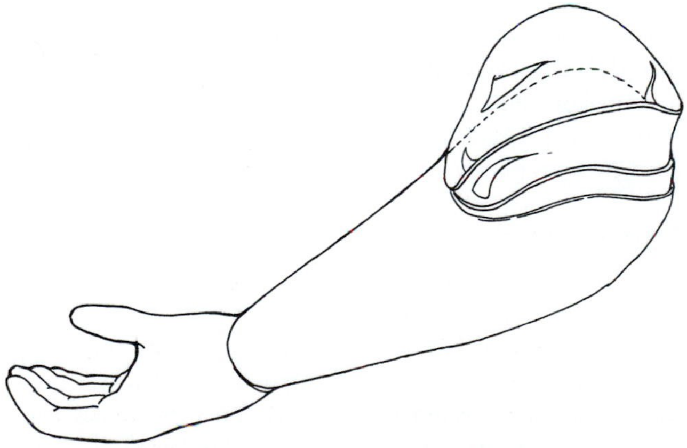

FIGURE 35-29

Northwestern University supracondylar socket. (Reproduced, with permission, from Advanced Rehabilitation Therapy, Inc., Miami, FL.)

protraction, and shoulder flexion increase pull on the control cable or create excursion, which in turn controls the TD or elbow joint as the amputee wishes. The harness is adjusted, so the movements required by the shoulder or scapula are small and go relatively unnoticed.

Figure-8 Harness

The figure-8 is the most commonly used harness. The axilla loop acts as a reaction point for the transmission of body forces to the TD. The anterior support strap and inverted-Y suspensor strap accept the major portion of the axial load (Fig. 35-30).

Chest-Strap Harness with Shoulder Saddle

Used when the amputee cannot tolerate an axilla loop, or if greater suspension is required for heavy lifting; the chest-strap harness is not appropriate for women as it has a tendency to rotate up on the chest when excessive forces are applied to the control cable (Fig. 35-31).

Figure-9 Harness

Typically employed with a self-suspending prosthesis, the figure-9 harness consists of an axilla loop and a control attachment strap. The advantage over conventional harnesses is the greater

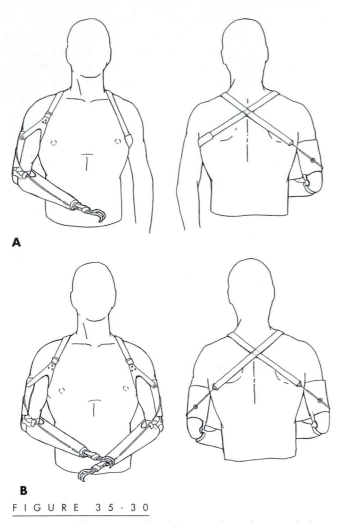

A

B

FIGURE 35-30

Figure-8 harness used with **A,** a unilateral transradial amputee and **B,** a bilateral transradial amputee. (Reproduced, with permission, from Advanced Rehabilitation Therapy, Inc., Miami, FL.)

freedom and comfort by eliminating the usual front support strap and triceps pad (see Fig. 35-28).

ELBOW UNITS

External Elbow Units

External elbows are used with an elbow-disarticulation prosthesis with an outside-locking hinge system. For cosmetic and mechanical reasons it is not possible to use the standard internal elbow unit (Fig. 35-32).

Internal Elbow Units

Transhumeral amputees with at least 2 in. of the distal humerus removed have the space required to accommodate an inside-locking elbow unit. The elbow can be locked in 11 different positions of flexion. Moreover, the friction turntable offers the ability to manually rotate the prosthetic forearm, substituting for humeral internal and external rotation.

SHOULDER HARNESS AND CONTROL CABLES

Most shoulder systems are designed to meet the individual needs of the user. A combination of chest, waist, and abdominal straps are necessary for adequate stabilization of the prosthesis and control of the joints and TD. The harness and control cables usually include a waistband with a strap connected to the elbow-lock control cable. The most commonly control motions are shoulder-girdle flexion for elbow flexion and use of the TD, with shoulder elevation for elbow locking and unlocking.

If the amputee cannot successfully operate the prosthesis with the basic harness, three additions may be helpful: (1) an excursion amplifier will increase excursion with less force produced by the body, (2) an axilla loop that operates as described previously, and (3) a shoulder sling with an axilla that provides a wider area through which the extreme tip of the shoulder swings when the scapulae are abducted, allowing greater excursion.

MYOELECTRIC UPPER-LIMB COMPONENTS

Myoelectric Hands

Myoelectric TDs—hands—typically offer palmar pinch or three-jaw-chuck closure, although TDs can be hooks as well. The average prehension force is about 11 lbs, with heavy-duty TDs having 13–20 lbs of pinch. The average opening speed ranges from 10 cm/sec to 25 cm/sec for heavy-duty TDs.

Electric Greifer

The Greifer myoelectric TD is available in only one size with two fingers and is not very cosmetic; however, it offers 31.5 lbs of grip force, greatest amount of any myoelectric TD. The Greifer is often selected by amputees who need a powerful hand for work situations such as manual labor or other activities that require maximum grip strength (Fig. 35-33).

SensorHand

Myoelectric prosthetics have been rejected by some wearers because the speed of hand movement is relatively slow as compared to the human hand. The SensorHand opens and closes with a range of speed of 1.5–30 cm/sec, which is considerably faster than the other myoelectric hands. Additionally, there is a proportional prehension force of 0–22 force pounds, referred to as Autograsp, that keeps objects from slipping, by monitoring and changing grip force as needed (Fig. 35-34).

Myoelectric Elbow

Myoelectric elbows are designed to control elbow flexion and extension, with surface electrodes, over specific muscle groups; typically, a contraction of the biceps for flexion and triceps for extension with transhumeral amputees, or pectoralis major for flexion and infraspinatus for extension with shoulder disarticulation amputees. Once in position, the elbow is locked and the same muscle can operate the TD. The range of motion varies from 0° to 135° or 15° to 150°, depending on the specific elbow. Myoelectric elbows operate at speeds of 100°–125°/second, with a maximum lift capacity of 2.5–4 ft-lbs with

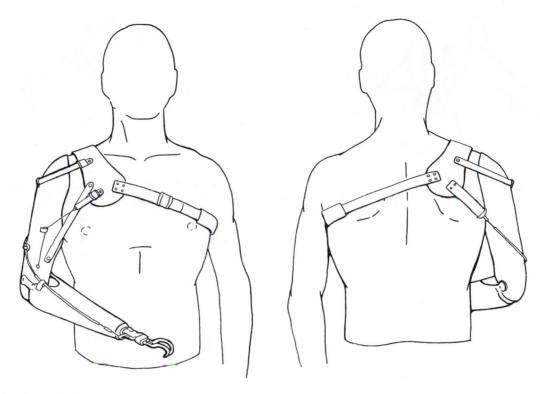

Chest-strap harness with shoulder saddle used with a transhumeral amputee.
(Reproduced, with permission, from Advanced Rehabilitation Therapy, Inc., Miami, FL.)

a passive (locked) lift capacity of 50 ft-lbs. Elbow flexion can be locked at a wide variety of flexion angles to allow the amputee to position the prosthetic hand to perform activities comfortably. Humeral internal and external rotation is manually performed with a friction control located within the prosthetic elbow.

UTAH ARM

The Utah arm uses microprocessor technology to allow the amputee to fine-tune adjustments for proportional control of

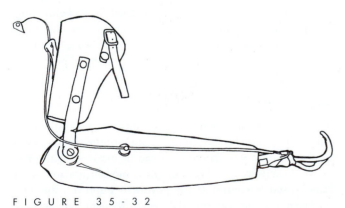

External elbow unit or outside locking hinges used with an elbow-disarticulation prosthesis. (Reproduced, with permission, from Advanced Rehabilitation Therapy, Inc., Miami, FL.)

the elbow, hand, and wrist. Therefore, movements can be slow or fast in an effort to create more natural arm movements. A variety of combination of elbows, wrists, and hands are available.

HYBRID PROSTHESES

A hybrid prosthesis is a combination of body-powered prosthetic components combined with myoelectric components. Hybrid upper-limb prosthesis is a common option with higher-level transhumeral, shoulder disarticulation, and bilateral upper-limb amputees.

Prosthetic Training

COMPRESSION WRAPPING

Compression wrapping with elastic bandages or the use of elastic shrinkers will reduce postoperative swelling. The amputee typically needs assistance wrapping, although the use of shrinkers does provide a certain degree of independence for those individuals able to properly don the shrinkers. The reduction in edema is necessary prior to casting for the prosthesis.

DESENSITIZATION

Residual upper limbs are frequently highly sensitive postsurgically and must become tolerant to touch and pressure. A progression of contact with soft materials such as cotton or lambs wool, progressing to burlap-type materials often assists with the

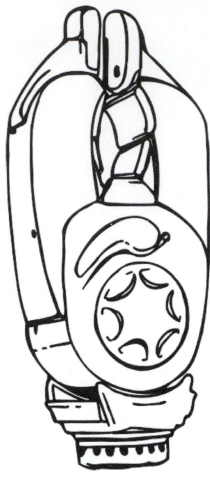

F I G U R E   3 5 - 3 3

Electric Greifer terminal device. (Reproduced, with permission, from Advanced Rehabilitation Therapy, Inc., Miami, FL.)

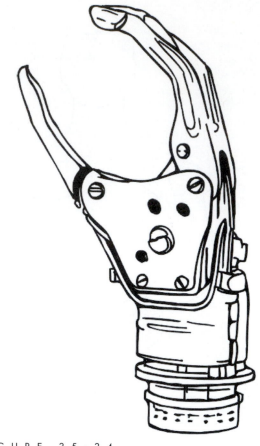

F I G U R E   3 5 - 3 4

SensorHand. (Reproduced, with permission, from Advanced Rehabilitation Therapy, Inc., Miami, FL.)

desensitization process. Rubbing, tapping, and performing resistive exercises with the residual limb also assist in preparing the limb for prosthetic fitting.

RANGE OF MOTION

Stretching and ROM exercises are extremely important postsurgically. Because an elbow or shoulder contracture can happen relatively quickly, the amputee must be taught to perform a simple independent stretching program daily to prevent loss of ROM. It is also imperative that the scapulothoracic region be stretched to ensure the mobility of the scapula so that full excursion may take place to control the prosthesis.

STRENGTH TRAINING

Selected strengthening exercises must be performed to increase the strength of the residual musculature. Traditional isometric exercises, progressing to isotonics with cuff weights, can be performed initially. As strength improves, simple adaptations with traditional weight machines may be made for the amputee. Some amputees find it comfortable to continue weight training

with the use of their prosthesis to maintain general fitness after rehabilitation.

CHANGE OF HAND DOMINANCE

In many instances the amputated limb was the dominant hand. Therefore, it becomes necessary to change hand dominance for the majority of activities such as writing, eating, and grooming. The prosthetic arm becomes the assistive limb. For adults this can become a challenging and frustrating experience. The therapist must choose simple splinter skills to start and progress to more complex skills as appropriate.

PROSTHETIC TRAINING

The amputee must learn how to don and doff the prosthesis independently and check the fit. Operation of the prosthesis can take some time and patience but can be mastered with practice and everyday use. Typically, gross movements are taught initially and as control of the prosthesis improves, fine motor movements are introduced. Gross movements taught begin with dressing and light work activities such as light housework and cleaning activities. Learning hygiene and feeding skills require greater dexterity as both gross and fine motor skills are required. Skills such as tying shoes and fastening buttons can be very challenging. During the initial training period, the use of Velcro with some items can reduce the frustration level and permit the amputee to focus on other activities. As the skill level improves, and depending on the amputee's dedication to mastering prosthetic skills, even minute tasks can be performed by the accomplished prosthetic user. Returning the amputee to leisure and recreational activities that they enjoyed prior to the amputation is also paramount to a successful rehabilitation program. It is important that the amputee learn the correct terminology for the parts of the prosthesis and how to care for it by cleaning and simple maintenance of parts.

SUMMARY

- The physical therapist must work closely with the rehabilitation team to provide comprehensive care for the amputee.
- The therapist must carefully assess the amputee to ensure that rehabilitation goals for the amputee are designed to meet the patient's specific needs.
- Provide amputees with an individualized program that must be constructed according to the level of ability and skill of each patient.
- Understanding the function, fitting, and care of the prosthesis is important in the instruction of prosthetic use and will assist the amputee in obtaining the goal, maximizing prosthetic control.
- Establishing long-term goals that will return the amputee to preamputation lifestyle is essential for a complete rehabilita-

tion program. Recreational activities can assist the amputee in the process and restore the sense of being a productive member of society with the ability to live a life with choices.

REFERENCES

1. Condie D, Stills M. Prosthetic and orthotic management. In: Bowker JH, Michael JW, eds. *Atlas of Limb Prosthetics: Surgical, Prosthetic, and Rehabilitation Principles.* St. Louis, MO, Mosby, 1992, p. 410.
2. Davis GJ. *A Compendium of Isokinetics in Clinical Usages and Rehabilitation Techniques,* 2nd ed. La Crosse, WI, S&S Publishing, 1985.
3. Eisert O, Tester OW. Dynamic exercises for lower extremity amputees. *Arch Phys Med Rehabil* 35:695–704, 1954.
4. Gailey RS, Gailey AM. *Prosthetic Gait Training Program for Lower Extremity Amputees.* Miami, FL, Advanced Rehabilitation Therapy Inc., 1989.
5. Gailey RS. *The Essentials of Lower Limb Amputee Running and Sports Training.* Miami, FL, Advanced Rehabilitation Therapy Inc., 2004.
6. Gottschalk F, Kourosh S, Stills M, et al. Does socket configuration influence the position of the femur in above-knee amputation? *J Prosthet Orthot* 2:94–102, 1989.
7. Murray MP. Gait as a total pattern of movement. *Am J Phys Med* 16:290–333, 1967.
8. Peizer E, Wright DW, Mason C. Human locomotion. *Bull Prosthet Res* 10:48–105, 1969.

Considerations for the Physically Active Female

Barbara J. Hoogenboom, Teresa L. Schuemann, and Robyn K. Smith

O B J E C T I V E S

After completing this chapter, the therapist should be able to do the following:

- Recognize/identify general anatomic, physiologic, and neuromuscular differences that exist between genders.
- Develop an understanding of common gender differences that predispose the female athlete to development of patellofemoral dysfunction.
- Identify characteristics that may contribute to increased susceptibility of the female to anterior cruciate ligament (ACL) injury, including mechanism of injury, intrinsic factors, extrinsic factors, and combined factors.
- Identify typical muscular activation and timing patterns, as well as the kinematics and joint position of the lower extremity during performance of physical tasks by females.
- Educate physically active females, coaches, and other sports medicine personnel regarding prevention of ACL injuries including proper cutting and jumping techniques, and neuromuscular re-education/strengthening of the lower extremity.
- Prescribe a lower extremity reactive neuromuscular training exercise program for the physically active female to aid in ACL injury prevention.
- Identify possible sequelae to ACL injury and rehabilitation.
- Utilize the concept of "envelope of function" to minimize adverse effects of musculoskeletal injury and subsequent rehabilitation.
- Understand the importance of incorporating core strengthening into an exercise program of the physically active female.
- Identify the potential stresses and risks that occur in the shoulder joint complex due to softball windmill pitching.
- Prescribe an exercise program specific to the windmill softball pitcher.
- Understand the potential stresses to the shoulder complex during free-style swimming and identify which musculature is at greatest risk for fatigue and subsequent impingement.
- Develop a comprehensive rehabilitation program for the swimmer with a shoulder injury.
- Develop a general understanding of most common injuries sustained by female gymnasts and identify potential risks involved in the excessive training at an early age common among female gymnasts.

- Acknowledge the implications that excessive, early training may have on hormonal and growth processes in the young female athlete.
- Describe the components of the female triad to enable prevention, identification, and treatment of these components as a member of a multidisciplinary medical team.
- Educate physically active females in proper exercise guidelines when planning for, during, and after pregnancy with a thorough knowledge of the physiologic changes that occur during this unique time.

INTRODUCTION

The visibility of the athletic female, which has grown dramatically over the past century, is now established throughout the world. At the beginning of the century, in 1902, the modern Olympic Games were founded, but women were excluded from participation. At that time, women's sports were considered to be "against the laws of nature."[202] In 1972, Title IX of the Educational Assistance Act was passed. This was a pivotal point in the history of the United States in female participation in sports and exercise. Title IX states that "no person in the U.S. shall, on the basis of sex, be excluded from participation in, be denied the benefits of, or be subject to discrimination under any educational program of action receiving federal financial assistance" (Ref. 202, p. 841). After Title IX, a 600 percent increase was seen in all levels of women's athletic participation.[201] Women and girls of all ages and abilities are participating in sports in record high numbers. In fact, 43 percent of collegiate athletes[5] and approximately 40 percent of Olympic athletes[3] were female in 2003–2004.

Participation in sports by girls and women continues to grow. The National Federation of State High School Associations (NHFS) has collected data on sports participation across the United States since 1971.[6] In its 2003–2004 school year report, the NFHS reports 6,903,552 prep/scholastic athletes (both male and female), the greatest number of participants ever. Likewise, the total number of females participating set an all time high with 2,865,299 participants.[6] Basketball remains the most popular prep sport for girls in the United States, and in 2004, had 457,986 participants. Volleyball (almost 400,000 participants) and soccer (309,000 participants) are ranked third and fifth, respectively.[6]

Studies by the National Collegiate Athletic Association (NCAA) describe a 10 percent increase in participation across athletic programs for women from 1989 to 1993.[24] Between 1989 and 1995, the number of intercollegiate female soccer participants increased by 50 percent while male participants increased only by 9 percent .[6] The NCAA reports that greater than 100,000 women participate in intercollegiate sports each year.[125] In its report on the 1998–1999 season, the NCAA reported an increase in women's sports participation by 9.3 percent to a total of 145,832 participants.[5] In the 2003–2004 participation report, 162,752 women participated in collegiate sports (42.8 percent of all participants). Currently, women in a wide variety of sports, played at many levels, are offered the opportunity not only to participate, but also to gain mone-

tary reimbursement (scholarship and professional salaries) and improved media acclaim. As participation and notoriety has increased, so has the need to understand the injuries being sustained by female athletes.

With the increase in women's participation in sport came an increased injury incidence among female athletes.[40] It was common, even 15–20 years ago, for a female athlete to receive different treatment than a male with an identical injury. For example, women runners who complained of tendonitis were often told to stop running, whereas men were given a specific treatment protocol that combined rest with activity. This is no longer common place. No longer are male athletes predominant recipients of rehabilitation. Active females are being rehabilitated as frequently as active males. There has been some suggestion that females are more susceptible to athletic injury than males[171]; however, more current literature states that injury patterns are more sport-specific than gender-specific.[202,234] Nonetheless, there are several types of injuries, which seem to be more prevalent in the female athlete. Such injuries are of increasing concern to the sports medicine specialist.

One heavily researched area in the sports medicine arena is the increased rate of anterior cruciate ligament (ACL) injury among females when compared to males.[202,253] Female athletes have a four- to six-time higher incidence of ACL injuries compared to their male counterparts.[129] Other injuries found to be frequent among female athletes include patellofemoral pain syndrome, spondylosis and spondylolithesis, stress fractures, bunions, and shoulder pain.[16,30,40,78,83,153,217,245] The reasons for the high frequencies of these types of injuries in females remain elusive but have been receiving more attention in the last decade. The media, medical, and rehabilitation communities have brought female ACL injuries and the female athlete triad to the forefront of attention. A discussion regarding basic gender differences will serve as a basis for further discussion of injuries common to representative, individual sports as well as other considerations regarding the active female.

GENDER DIFFERENCES

Physiologic Strength Differences

Gender differences between females and males are evident in strength, aerobic capacity, and endurance. These differences become pronounced after puberty. Prepubertal boys and girls have similar strength, and when corrected for lean body mass, and their $\dot{V}O_2$ max is also similar.[235,241] Endurance performance is just slightly better in boys than girls before puberty. However, these differences may be due to social rather than biological constraints, including the possibility of fewer role models for girls, less opportunities, and different training programs.[202,241]

At puberty, these gender-related discrepancies are exaggerated, due to anatomical and physiologic differences. Skeletal muscle physiology in men and women does not differ significantly. Testosterone and androstenedione are the androgenic hormones that are most important in muscle fiber development. There is a variance in resting testosterone levels, but the average for females is between $1/10$ and $1/2$ the blood levels of males. Therefore men have greater potential for strength and power development related to testosterone levels alone. When considering estrogen levels, women have higher levels than men, and this hormone interferes with muscular development due to its role in increasing body fat stores. After puberty, women typically have less lean body mass than men, especially in the lower body due to increased estrogen levels and subsequent fat body mass increases.[86] Average body fat for a sedentary college-age woman is 23–27 percent, while for a college-age man it is 15–18 percent. It is typical for some athletes to demonstrate lower body fat percentages especially runners, gymnasts, and ballet dancers. These two physiologic hormonal differences (body fat and blood hormone levels) help to explain why muscle mass is predictably lower in women than men.[86,258]

Strength can be examined in two different ways. Absolute strength is the maximum amount of weight one can lift (i.e., 50 lbs). Relative strength relates this maximal amount to an individual's muscle mass (i.e., 80 lbs of muscle mass can lift 50 lbs).[136] Men appear to demonstrate larger *absolute* strength gains due to larger cross sectional muscle fiber size. However, the actual number of muscle fibers is similar between genders. When examining *relative* gains in strength, studies have shown that women and men achieve similar results while undergoing identical weight training programs.[136,190] "Because muscle cross-sectional area (muscle fiber size multiplied by the number of muscle fibers) is directly related to the ability to produce force, individuals who have larger muscles are able to lift more weight" (Ref. 190, p. 4). See Table 36-1 for examples of this conclusion.

When comparing strength to lean body mass (body weight without fat) or cross-sectional area, women are about equal to men and are equally capable of developing strength *relative* to total muscle mass.[190] Gender is irrelevant in the ability of a muscle to produce force.[190] Holloway and Baechle[136] were unable to show significant gender differences in adaptations to resistance training, except for the amount of muscle hypertrophy. Absolute strength gains are due to the combination of muscle hypertrophy and neuromuscular recruitment. When diet is unchanged during a resistance training program, the average woman responds with a decrease in intramuscular and subcutaneous fat stores, and little change in limb circumference (less hypertrophy than males) mostly due to lower testosterone levels and smaller muscle fiber size.[136,190,202] True muscle hypertrophy is less visible in females, but improved muscular definition is evident.[190]

In 2004, Dore et al.[86] found that males and females exhibited similar cycling peak power (CPP) until age 14. At age 14, loosely considered to be the transition to puberty, males demonstrated higher CPP. Males had higher lean leg volume (LLV) than females. As age increased, where there were similar LLV, males still showed greater CPP. Conclusions were twofold: (1) the sex-related difference can be explained by the difference in body composition, specifically lower limb fat increase in girls whereas boys experience increased lean body mass; and (2) the question of the possibility that differences in neuromuscular activation exist, which could play a role in peak muscle performance.[86] Neuromuscular differences will be examined more thoroughly later in this chapter.

So far, no evidence exists to suggest that women should undergo strength training any differently than men. "Assuming equal nutrition, the rate and degree of improvement in strength should be equal between genders. Significant gains in muscle strength and endurance can be achieved by use of a training program 3 to 4 days a week" (Ref. 190, p. 5). Once either gender has reached a high level of competitiveness and muscularity, changes in muscle mass and fiber content is minimal.[17] However, women do show lower proportions of their total lean body mass in their upper body contributing to gender strength differences that are greater in the upper body than in the lower body. Nevertheless, hypertrophy and absolute strength differs in genders due to the physiologic changes that occur at puberty.[190]

Anatomical Differences

Anatomical differences bring reason for variance in strength as well. Men and women's bodies respond differently to similar

---

TABLE 36-1

Relative Versus Absolute Strength in Female Versus Male Athletes

Female soccer player 125 lbs	With 15% body fat = 106 lbs lean body mass Absolute strength = 150 lbs squat Relative strength = 150/106 = 1.4
Male soccer player 155 lbs	with 12% body fat = 136.5 lbs lean body mass Absolute strength = 185 lbs squat Relative strength = 185/136.5 = 1.4

Note: Equal *relative strength* but greater *absolute strength* in the male soccer player.

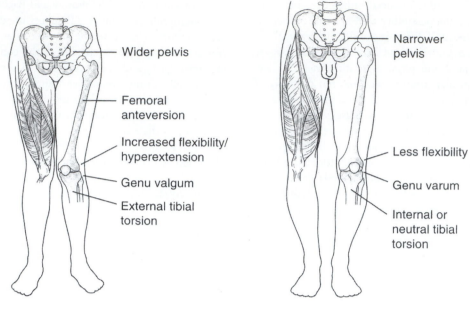

FIGURE 36-1

Structural differences between men and women. Women (left) typically exhibit a wider pelvis, femoral anteversion greater tibial external rotation, and genu valgum. (Reproduced from: Griffin LY. *Rehabilitation of the Injured Knee.* St. Louis: Mosby—Year Book, 1995, with permission from Elsevier.)

weight training programs due to anatomical differences. These differences include: women are 3–4 in. shorter; are 25–30 lbs lighter; have 10–15 lbs (8–10 percent) more body fat; have 40–45 less pounds of fat-free weight (bone, muscle, organs); have less muscle mass supported by narrower shoulders; and shorter extremities.[190] "All these factors, combined give men a mechanical advantage over women which enables them to handle more weight and generate more power" (Ref. 190, p. 3). Broader shoulders tend to benefit males in developing muscular strength in the upper body, whereas wider pelvises seem to benefit females in developing lower body strength. Men with broader shoulders have a higher center of gravity than women with wider pelvises giving them a mechanical advantage to gain upper-body mass.[190] Thus, as previously stated, the largest difference in absolute strength is found to be greater in the upper body as compared to the lower body.[136]

Structural differences have been noted between genders in both the upper and lower extremities. In the upper body, structural differences include narrower shoulders, shorter arm lengths, decreased muscle fiber and total muscle cross-sectional area, and according to some authors, increased carrying angle of the forearm.[190,235] When examining structural differences of the lower extremity between genders, multiple factors affect alignment. Women have greater amounts of static external knee rotation, greater active internal hip rotation, greater interacetablular distance, and increased hip width when normalized to femoral length than men.[63] These factors have been shown to contribute to greater knee valgus (genu valgum) angles in women. The structural combination of increased hip adduc-

tion, femoral anteversion, and genu valgum may explain the larger Q-angle and rotational positioning of the lower extremity in women than men (Figs. 36-1 and 36-2). The average Q-angle for men is 13° and women is 18°,[59] but measurement of the Q-angle is examiner dependent and can be erratic. Lower extremity structural differences may play a factor in lower-extremity injuries in the active female.[63] Structural differences related to ACL injury will be discussed in greater detail later in this chapter.

Patellofemoral Dysfunction

As previously mentioned, the larger Q-angle found in females has been identified as a predisposing factor to patellofemoral dysfunction which plagues many active females regardless of sport or age. Anterior knee pain is one of the most common sources of complaint among female athletes.[38] Most patellofemoral dysfunction can be categorized as mechanical or inflammatory with the rare exceptions of tumors, regional pain syndrome, and referred pain patterns.[142] For the active female, patellofemoral dysfunction should be thoroughly evaluated to determine instability, malalignment, tracking abnormalities or compression forces contributing to the anterior knee discomfort. Appropriate patellar mobility should include sufficient superior glide with active quadriceps contraction as well as equal medial and lateral glide.[223] Increased patellar lateral glide indicates abnormal laxity and instability when correlated with a positive apprehension test that simulates instances of patellar subluxation or dislocation.[142,223] Patellar instability is

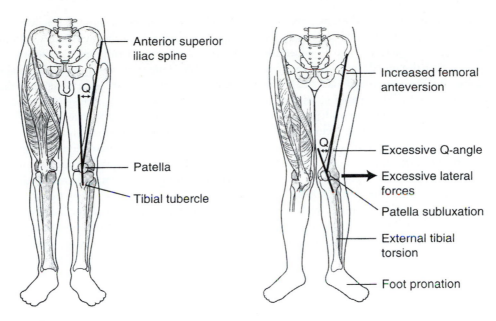

F I G U R E   3 6 - 2

Gender differences in Q-angle. Women (right) exhibit greater Q-angle, increased external tibial torsion, and femoral anteversion. (Reproduced from: Griffin LY, *Rehabilitation of the Injured Knee*. St. Louis: Mosby—Year Book, 1995, with permission from Elsevier.)

a mechanical cause of anterior knee pain and occurs more frequently in females than males.[142] The active female is more susceptible to patellar instability secondary to the anatomical alignment and muscular strength differences already described. Treatment of patellar instability and patellofemoral diagnoses have been discussed in Chapter 29.

Alignment observation should include not only Q-angle measurements but also determination of tibial torsion, foot position, and leg length discrepancies. Malalignment may include superior or inferior position of the patella, medial or lateral patellar glide, rotation or tilt. Abnormal positions of the patella may include one or a combination of these factors.[185] Common patellar malalignment patterns include "Grasshopper" or "squinting" patella. A complete evaluation of muscular balance including both flexibility and strength will direct treatment to minimize these malalignment patterns.[184] Patellar taping provides proprioceptive input to improve patellar tracking and has been shown to provide symptomatic relief in many patients which allows for a conservative rehabilitation program to be completed.[184]

A static Q-angle measurement is not as helpful as the same measurement before and during an activity such as a mini-squat to determine if the Q-angle increases causing abnormal patellar tracking or patellofemoral compression.[142] Patellar tracking should be assessed to ensure normal position of the patella within the trochlear groove throughout knee motion. An example of abnormal patellar tracking is a "J" sign, when the examiner observes the patella jump laterally when the knee is moving into extension at approximately 30° and is associated with

patellofemoral symptoms.[173,223] Conservative management of patellar tracking abnormalities, especially in the adolescent female athlete, should be the rule[142] and should be addressed systematically after a thorough evaluation of the muscle imbalance for flexibility and strength. Neuromuscular training to address recruitment patterns, proprioception, core stability, and balance deficits are elaborated upon later in this chapter. Techniques to be discussed have applicability with the rehabilitation program for most mechanical causes of anterior knee pain.

This discussion of patellofemoral dysfunction illustrates the increased predisposition to this injury complaint of the physically active female based on the gender differences in anatomical and strength differences. A subsequent review of the neuromuscular differences precedes the discussion of another widespread knee injury that is more common in female than male athletes.

Neuromuscular Differences

When comparing genders, research supports differences in dynamic neuromuscular control of lower limb biomechanics.[125,126,129,207,277] Neuromuscular control is a combination of proprioception and the muscular systems' response to the proprioceptive input. Imbalances in quadriceps to hamstring ratios, differences in jump-landing positions, weakness in proximal hip musculature, higher landing forces, and lower gluteus maximus electromyographic (EMG) activity during landing are all reported in females when compared to males.[128,140,277] Noyes et al.[207] conducted a drop jump test on male and female athletes that measured the distance between the hips, knees, and ankles in the coronal plane during landing. Findings revealed no significant difference between male and female subjects in mean knee and ankle separation distance during the landing and takeoff phases. Significant differences between male and female athletes were shown in knee and ankle separation during the prelanding phase only (three phases include take off, prelanding, landing). However, after a 6-week Sportsmetrics neuromuscular training program[128] (Appendix A), female athletes had statistically greater knee and ankle separation distances than those of males in all three phases of the jump-land sequence.[207]

Hewett et al.[126] went beyond the coronal plane and measured a drop jump-landing task in females with three-dimensional (3D) motion analysis. Data was gathered on athletes prior to sports participation. Athletes that had injured their ACL demonstrated significantly higher knee abduction angles (knee valgus) at initial contact and increased maximal limb displacement than those who were uninjured. Peak vertical ground reaction force corresponded with knee abduction angle. The greater the abduction angle, the greater the ground reaction force in ACL-injured athletes but not in uninjured athletes. Athletes who sustained ACL injuries "demonstrated significant increases in dynamic lower extremity valgus and knee abduction loading before sustaining their injuries compared to uninjured controls" (Ref. 126, p. 497). Maximum knee flexion angle at landing was 10.5° less in injured compared to noninjured athletes. These differences suggest decreased neuromuscular control or alternative strategies for function in the lower extremity as evidenced by biomechanical differences observed.[126]

Coactivation of the quadriceps and hamstrings is reported to protect the knee joint against not only excessive anterior shear forces, but also against knee abduction and dynamic lower-extremity valgus forces.[32] Female athletes have lower hamstring to quadriceps strength ratios than males during isokinetic testing at 300°/second.[125] When the hamstrings are under-recruited, insufficient quadriceps activation can result. This insufficiency may directly limit the potential for muscular co-contraction, which aids in protecting ligaments.[126] It has been postulated that males may use a protective mechanism involving the hamstrings, considered to resist anterior tibial translation, to counteract high-peak landing forces. Females tend to contract their quadriceps first in response to an anterior tibial translation, which provides additional anterior translation, whereas males responded by contracting their hamstrings first, thereby limiting the anterior translation. With these findings, it is suggested that females tend to be "ligament-dominant" in their joint strategies, whereas males demonstrate more "muscle-dominant" joint strategies.[129]

Greater knee abduction angles during jump-stop unanticipated cutting activity were also described by Ford et al.[103] Females demonstrated greater knee abduction angles (knee valgus) at initial contact than their male counterparts. Greater knee abduction angles support the concept of ligament dominance rather than muscular control to absorb the ground reaction force during sporting maneuvers. In such a movement strategy,

the athlete is allowing the ground reaction force to control the direction of motion of the knee joint which in turn causes the ligaments to take up a disproportionate amount of force.[103]

Proximal hip musculature activation is also found to differ between genders. Zazuulak et al.[277] reported that female athletes demonstrated less activity of the gluteus maximus compared to males during the landing phase of a single-leg drop jump. Decreased activation of proximal hip stabilizers may contribute to the valgus landing position observed in female athletes. Greater rectus femoris activity was also observed in females compared to males during the precontact period of the jump. This is postulated to place an increased anterior sheer force on the tibia during landing. The authors concluded that these two findings together may contribute to altered kinetic energy absorption during landing, as well as causing increased ground reaction forces and high valgus torques contributing to knee injury.[277]

Female sex hormones may also have significant effects on neuromuscular control. Estrogen has both direct and indirect affects on the neuromuscular system. During the ovulatory phase, there is a slowing of muscle relaxation. Throughout the menstrual cycle, estrogen levels fluctuate radically. Fluctuating hormone status has profound effects on muscle function, tendon and ligament strength, and on the central nervous system.[129] Hormonal influences on neuromuscular control will be discussed further in the ACL section of this chapter. Clearly, neuromuscular patterning and performance is affected by many factors.

ANTERIOR CRUCIATE LIGAMENT INJURIES

With higher participation rates of females at all levels, increased sport-related injuries would be expected; however, what was unexpected was the disproportionate number of knee ligament injuries that occurred. The most serious injury that has risen to the forefront of attention is injury to the ACL of females. A pattern of disproportionately high ACL injury rates in females, compared to their male athlete counterparts, was identified. For example, during the 1989–1990 intercollegiate basketball season, the NCAA Injury Surveillance System data showed that female athletes injured their ACLs 7.8 times more often than males.[216] Sports that appear to have high risk, at all levels of play, involve jumping, rapid deceleration, and cutting maneuvers. Sports such as soccer, basketball, volleyball, team handball, and gymnastics have been identified as high-risk sports for the female athlete.[24,25,42,101,128,166,175,211,232,278] In fact, more than 30,000 serious knee injuries are projected to occur in the United States, in female athletes at the intercollegiate and high-school levels yearly.[125]

The costs of ACL injuries are dramatic, not only financially (medical and rehabilitation services), but also in terms of long-term consequences, such as concurrent injury (such as articular cartilage or meniscus), lost playing time, lost scholarships, and increased potential for long-term posttraumatic degeneration and disability.[109,116,271] According to Ireland,[145] even in the era

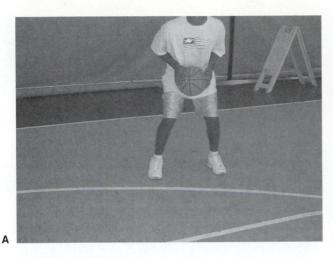 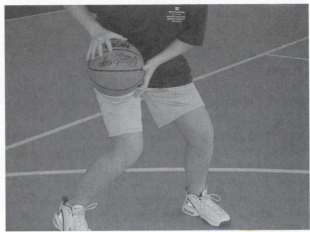

A   B

FIGURE 36-3

Male (left) versus female (right) position for stop and pass or shoot. Note neutral lower extremity positioning, in male (left).

where prevention has been deemed important, females continue to experience a higher rate of injury to the ACL than their male counterparts. What is especially troubling is that even as years have passed and female athletes begin sports play earlier, train harder, and receive improved training and coaching, their injury rate has not declined.[145] Therefore, the focus of the late 1990s to the present has shifted from reporting injury statistics and hypothesizing about potential causes to an era of prevention. Prevention of ACL injuries in the female athlete has become a priority for the sports medicine, rehabilitation, and research communities.

Mechanisms of Injury

As more women and girls participate in sports, much attention has been given to understanding the mechanisms of ACL injuries. Many authors have described two mechanisms of injury: contact and noncontact.[24,25,141,207] Approximately 30 percent of all ACL injuries are classified as contact injuries, and the remaining 70 percent are not related to direct contact and classified as noncontact.[116] Some authors have reported that as many as 75 percent of sports-related injuries to the ACL are via noncontact mechanisms.[208] Contact injuries are easily discerned from the clinical history surrounding the injury and are typical to contact sports like football and rugby. In contrast, the mechanisms and activities that are involved in noncontact ACL injuries are less apparent and vary between sports. Sports that are at high risk for and incur many noncontact ACL injuries, are those classified as noncontact or collision sports such as basketball, soccer, volleyball, gymnastics, and team handball.[23,25,29,108,145,265]

Early writing by Henning in the late 1980s influenced much of the current thinking about the mechanisms of noncontact ACL injuries.[116] After studying injuries incurred by female basketball players over a 10-year time span, Henning concluded that the three most common mechanisms of injury were[116]

- Planting and cutting (29 percent of all injuries) (Fig. 36-3A and B)
- Straight-knee landings (28 percent of all injuries) (Fig. 36-4)
- One-step stop with the knee hyperextended (26 percent of all injuries)

Henning concluded that prevention and skill development (especially in the female athlete) must incorporate the *opposite* of the previously mentioned motor behaviors, including

- The accelerated rounded turn off a bent knee
- Bent knee landings (Fig. 36-5)
- Three-step stop

These motor behaviors are addressed more thoroughly later in the chapter in the section on prevention and training.

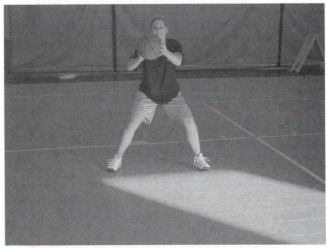

FIGURE 36-4

Landing from a rebound with straight legs and wide base of support.

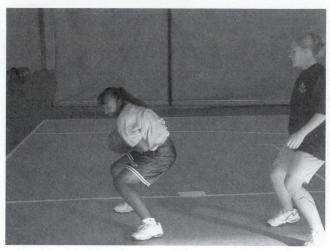

FIGURE 36-5

Proper position for bent-knee landing after a basketball rebound.

Subsequently, many mechanisms have been described for contributing to noncontact injuries, including sudden forceful twisting motions with the foot planted,[188] planting/sidestepping/cutting maneuvers,[75] "out of control play" (Ref. 116, p. 142), landing,[47,101] and deceleration maneuvers.[116] Video analysis of ACL injuries which occurred during the play of basketball and soccer demonstrated that women were injured most commonly when landing from a jump and when they suddenly stopped running.[116] It is very interesting to note that women and girls have been shown to perform landing and cutting activities with more erect posture than men and therefore place themselves at greater risk for ACL injury.[116] Video analysis of actual ACL injuries has demonstrated that the position of the lower limb at the time of injury is often knee flexion less than 30°, a position of knee valgus, and external rotation of the foot relative to the knee (Fig. 36-6).[47,116]

Postural and positional variations in motor skills, when combined with greater valgus alignment and increased quadriceps activation, may further increase the possibility of injury for the female athlete.[128] Total positional control of the lower extremity is important, both in terms of flexion/extension and varus/valgus (Fig. 36-7A and B). Low flexion angles (commonly described as less than 45° flexion) increase the anterior strain on the ACL when active quadriceps contractions occur. The quads act as the ACL antagonist and add to the anterior/posterior straight plane load sustained by the ACL. Likewise, increased varus/valgus positioning of the lower extremity adds torque to the knee which challenges the ACL in its derotational function. Factors to explain the position of the lower extremities of females during landing may include deficits in muscle strength and endurance as well as neuromuscular skill factors.

Finally, related to impact during landing, current research suggests that strategies differ in females as compared to males. This may be due to biomechanical factors, poorer muscle strength and/or neuromuscular control, or insufficient strate-

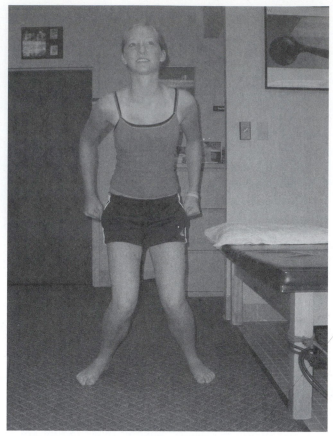

FIGURE 36-6

Typical position of ACL injury. Note that knee valgus, foot external rotation, knee flexion are less than 30°.

gies for shock absorption, as previously discussed.[164] Dufek and Bates[92] examined the relationship between landing forces and injury stating that many injuries that occur during jumping sports occur during landing. Male athletes appear to employ different mechanisms to compensate for high landing forces than females.[125,128] Markolf et al.[181] demonstrated that muscular contraction can decrease both the varus and valgus laxity of the knee when landing. Jumping and landing will be addressed in greater detail in a later section.

In summary, although women do sustain contact mechanism ACL injuries, the vast majority appears to occur by noncontact mechanisms. According to the Hunt Valley Consensus conference.[116] "The common at-risk situation for non-contact ACL injuries appears to be deceleration, which occurs when the athlete cuts, changes direction, or lands from a jump (Ref. 116, p. 149)."

Although many studies offer strong support for noncontact mechanisms of injury as prevalent in the female athlete,[25,115,175,199,200,262] Ireland maintains that the "true incidence of non-contact ACL injuries and the actual numbers of athletes affected are difficult to determine" (Ref. 145, p. 150). The discrepancy between ACL injury rates by sex and mechanism of injury, at all levels of sport participation, remains a

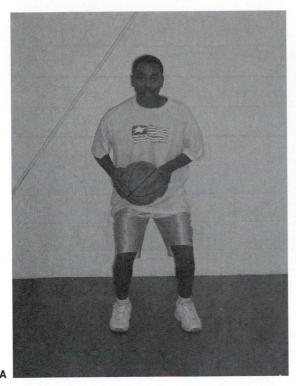
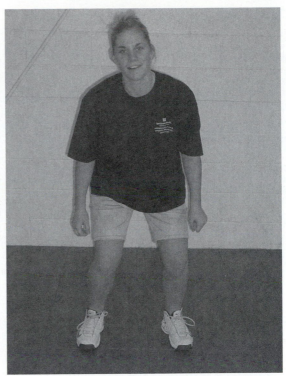

A   B

FIGURE 36-7

Typical male (left) versus female (right) posture and position with motor skills. Note the valgus alignment at the knee, in the female athlete (R).

hot topic in sports medicine. Fortunately, neuromuscular control, balance, and motor skill training all appear to be critical modifiable factors associated with injury prevention.

Factors Related to ACL Injury in the Female Athlete

Why women continue to sustain two to eight times more ACL injuries than their male counterparts continues to be an unanswered question for researchers in many disciplines. Clearly, injuries to the ACL occur due to complex interactions of anatomical, biomechanical, neuromuscular, hormonal, and environmental factors. Various factors have been suggested to explain these differences and are categorized by many authors as intrinsic (factors that are not controllable) and extrinsic (factors that are controllable).[22,24,115,121,141,145] More recently, a third category of factors, described as "both" or partially controllable has been described by Ireland (Table 36-2).[145]

INTRINSIC FACTORS

Intrinsic or noncontrollable factors have been described as hormonal effects of estrogen, inherent ligamentous laxity present in females, and other anthropometric differences in men and women such as lower-extremity alignment, notch width, and ACL size.

Investigation regarding notch width and ACL size has demonstrated females to have smaller notches and smaller ACLs

than males[22,139,252,262]; however the evidence correlating this with injury is contradictory.[129] Regardless, there is little or no opportunity for reasonable intervention, and these areas have been researched less in the last several years. Likewise, although laxity is greater in females than in males,[233] there is conflicting evidence regarding the relationship of laxity to injury. Exercise-induced laxity that occurs after 30 minutes of athletic activity may play a role in ligament injury and relate to neuromuscular protective training.[255] Finally, investigations of Q-angle in relationship to injury demonstrate that injury rate differences between males and females could not be accounted for by the differences in anatomy.[115] Newer investigations are focusing on the thigh/foot angle, which may correlate with increased risk of injury to the ACL, but at present "there is insufficient data to relate lower extremity anatomic alignment to ACL injury" (Ref. 116, p. 148).

Much current research is being dedicated to understanding the interaction between female sex hormones and ACL injuries. Because the female sex hormones estrogen, progesterone, and relaxin are cyclical and affect ligaments, they may play a role in fluctuation in both strength and laxity of the ACL.[129,271] Conflicting research evidence exists as to what portion of the menstrual cycle is the most "risky,"[25,26,270,271] and whether the effects of hormones (estrogen, especially) may be greater than just on the ligament itself and may extend to changes in motor skill.[129,224] Originally, the ovulatory phase was described

Summary of Factors Suggested to Contribute to ACL Injury in Female Athletes

INTRINSIC FACTORS	EXTRINSIC FACTORS	COMBINED FACTORS
Lower-extremity alignment • Q-angle/pelvic width • Varus/valgus of the knee (see Figures 36-2 and 36-10) • Foot alignment	Strength Endurance Shoes/footwear Motivation	Proprioception • Balance • Position sense Neuromuscular control Muscular firing order
Hyperextension		Kinematics of movement (See Figs. 36-3B, 36-4, and 36-8)
Physiologic rotatory laxity ACL size Notch size and shape		Acquired skills • Sport-specific motor programs
Hormonal influences Inherited skills/coordination		

as the time during which most injuries occurred.[271] More recently, Slauterbeck and Hardy[247] found that many injuries occurred around menses. In their most recent work, Wojtys et al.[270] described that more ACL injuries than expected (43 percent) occurred during the ovulatory phase (in all females) and fewer injuries than expected occurred during the luteal phase (34 percent). The distribution of injury by phases was different for those women who were taking oral contraceptives, with only a trend toward more injuries in the ovulatory phase (29 percent), and fewer injuries than expected during the follicular phase (14 percent), demonstrating the potential for some protection offered by use of oral contraceptives. Möller-Neilson and Hammer[193] also reported decreased injury rates in women who used oral contraceptives.

The effects of hormones may extend beyond their affect on the ACL itself. Evidence suggests that the neuromuscular system may be significantly affected by the fluctuating milieu of female sex hormones.[129] Estrogen may have effects on neuromuscular patterning and performance throughout the menstrual cycle, but seems to decrease motor skills in the premenstrual phase.[224]

Clearly, the relationship between female hormones and ACL injuries must continue to be investigated, not only in terms of susceptibility of ligaments to injury but also in terms of mechanism and location of action. It is not clear whether hormones influence muscle function and motor skills,[224] the neuromuscular system,[129,168,218] or cerebral/central nervous system function.[160,224,270] Interestingly, over the last several decades, suggestions for control of intrinsic factors have been given, such as notchplasty and hormonal manipulation for protection of the ACL in females. These examples were not received by the medical community with much zeal and were never accepted as likely interventions. Most in sports medicine agree that in order

to reduce the number of ACL injuries sustained by the female athlete, attention must be paid to factors that are modifiable,[145] such as extrinsic or combination factors.

EXTRINSIC FACTORS

Extrinsic or controllable factors are parameters such as leg strength (both total absolute strength and hamstrings/quadriceps ratios), muscle recruitment order, muscle reaction time, playing style, training/preparation, coaching/conditioning, skill acquisition, and surfaces of play.[141,145,272]

Generation of muscular force is a key element in providing dynamic stability about joints. The inability to control external forces may result in injury to the static structures providing stability to that joint. The inherent physiologic differences in muscle mass and hormonal levels of testosterone between males and females make it predictable that males will always be stronger than females. If body mass is accounted for and subjects of similar activity levels are compared does this inequality still exist?

Huston and Wojtys[140] tested this hypothesis using isokinetic testing and concluded that athletic females and a control group of females were both statistically weaker in quadriceps and hamstrings muscle strength at 60°/second, as compared to their male counterparts. Other researchers have also documented that women have less muscle strength in the quadriceps and hamstrings than men, even when normalized for body weight.[119] Anderson et al.[22] also tested the quadriceps and hamstrings isokinetically at 60°/second and 240°/second and found similar results. With corrections for body mass, the male athletes generated greater peak torque, greater work, and average power outputs than the female athletes for both quadriceps and hamstrings ($p < 0.05$).[22] Knapik et al.[153] determined that female athletes with one hamstring muscle group more than

15 percent weaker than the other were 2.5 times more likely to sustain a lower-extremity injury. They also reported that this side-to-side imbalance in hamstring strength existed in 20–30 percent of female athletes.

Previous research illustrates the importance of hamstring strength and endurance in acting as an agonist to the ACL for dynamic knee joint stability.[22,88,140,232] The hamstring muscles have been shown to be protective to the ACL due to their ability to shield the ACL from excessive anterior shear and strain. If the hamstrings are to effectively counteract the torque produced by the quadriceps, they must demonstrate a certain percentage of strength as compared to the quadriceps they are opposing. Knapik[152] also reported that athletes with a hamstring/quadriceps ratio of less than 0.75 were 1.6 times more likely to be injured. Isokinetic testing by Moore and Wade[194] revealed that hamstring/quadriceps ratios of females were significantly lower than those of males at 60°, 180°, and 300°/second. Huston also determined that females had hamstring/quadriceps ratios in the 0.40 ranges.[140] Eccentric hamstrings/quadriceps ratio was also significantly weaker in female athletes as compared to male athletes.[196] It has been hypothesized that hamstring/quadriceps ratios lower than 0.60 may predispose an athlete to ACL injury.[127]

As indicated previously, strength deficits in the female athlete are evident and may play a role in predisposing the female to an ACL injury. If strength may play a role, how does the endurance mode of these muscles play a role in knee stability and injury vulnerability? A study conducted by Rozzi et al.[234] demonstrated that both males and females had a decrease in the ability to detect joint motion moving into the direction of extension, an increase in the onset time of contraction for the medial hamstring and lateral gastrocnemius (LG) muscles in response to landing a jump, and an increase in the EMG of the first contraction of the vastus medialis and lateralis muscles while landing a jump when fatigued.[234] Research by Zhou et al.[279] has shown electromechanical delay of the knee extensors to increase by 147 percent after muscular fatigue. Nyland et al.[209] looked at the effects of eccentric work-induced hamstring fatigue on sagittal and transverse plane knee and ankle biodynamics and kinetics during a running, crossover cut, or directional change. They determined that hamstring fatigue created decreased dynamic transverse plane knee control demonstrated by increased knee internal rotation during heel strike. Peak ankle plantarflexion moment and decreased knee internal rotation magnitude during the propulsion phase of the cutting maneuver when fatigued is believed to represent compensatory attempt for knee dynamic stability from the gastrocnemius and soleus.[209] Wojtys et al.[272] also demonstrated the effect of fatigue on knee joint stability. When the quadriceps and hamstrings were exercised to a point of fatigue, there was resultant increase in tibial movement resulted, causing increased vulnerability to ACL injury.[272]

COMBINED FACTORS

More recently, combined or partially controllable factors have been suggested as those that have contributions inherent to the individual (intrinsic factors) combined with those that are more extrinsic in nature and, therefore, able to be modified.[145] Examples of combined factors are proprioception and neuromuscular control. Both of these factors are affected by an individual's genetic makeup, but can be taught, to some extent, by structured programs to address their areas of deficiency.[116,125,127,128]

Proprioception has been defined as the culmination of all neural inputs originating from joints, tendons, muscles, and associated deep-tissue proprioceptors. These inputs into the central nervous system result in the regulation of reflexes and motor control.[127] The body receives proprioceptive information by three separate systems. They include the visual system, the vestibular system, and the peripheral mechanoreceptors. When discussing injuries to the ACL, the role of the mechanoreceptors has been the primary focus in the literature. Researchers agree that the ACL does contain mechanoreceptors, but if the central nervous system has a decreased sensory feedback from the knee, there is a decreased ability to stabilize the knee joint dynamically. This places the knee at risk for injury, either microtrauma or macrotrauma.[135] Following injury to the capsuloligamentous structures, it is thought that a partial deafferentation of the joint occurs as the mechanoreceptors become disrupted. This partial deafferentation, which is secondary to injury, may be related to either direct or indirect injury. Direct trauma effects would include disruption of the joint capsule or ligaments, whereas posttraumatic joint effusion or hemarthrosis[149] can illustrate indirect effects.

Whether a direct or indirect cause, the resultant partial deafferentation alters the afferent information into the central nervous system and, therefore, the resulting reflex pathways to the dynamic stabilizing structures. These pathways are required by both the feed-forward and feedback motor control systems to dynamically stabilize the joint. A disruption in the proprioceptive pathway will result in an alteration of position and kinesthesia.[34,246] Barrett[35] showed an increase in the threshold to detection of passive motion in a majority of patients with ACL rupture and functional instability. Corrigan[71] who also found diminished proprioception after ACL rupture confirmed this finding. Diminished proprioceptive sensitivity has also been shown to cause giving way or episodes of instability in the ACL deficient knee.[49] Rozzi et al.[233] tested proprioception by measuring knee-joint kinesthesia as the threshold to detection of passive motion while moving either the direction of knee flexion or extension. The study determined that females took significantly longer than the males to detect joint motion moving in the direction of knee-joint extension implicating the hamstrings as deficient in proprioception. Injury to the capsuloligamentous structures not only reduces the joint's mechanical stability, but also diminishes the capability of the dynamic neuromuscular restraint system. Therefore, any aberration in joint motion and position sense will impact both the feed-forward and feedback neuromuscular control systems. Without adequate anticipatory muscle activity, the static structures may be exposed to insult unless the reactive muscle activity can be initiated to contribute to dynamic restraint.

The reader is referred to the previous section on gender differences to review the various neuromuscular control factors that vary from female to male. In reference to the female athlete and ACL injuries, the following specific variables will be examined: the muscle firing patterns of the lower extremity with physical tasks, the timing of those muscular responses, and the kinematics and joint position of the lower extremity during activity.

Muscular Activation and Timing Patterns

In a study conducted by Huston and Wojtys,[140] different muscular firing patterns were illustrated between females (control and athlete group) and males (control and athlete group). They tested muscular response to anterior translation of the tibia using EMG recordings during a relaxed response to movement and a voluntary muscle contraction response to movement. All four groups recruited the gastrocnemius muscle first in the relaxed response to anterior translation of the tibia. The spinal level of muscle firing pattern was gastrocnemius-hamstring-quadriceps for all groups, but as the translation of the tibia continued in the relaxed response phase of the testing, the female athletes relied more on quadriceps activity than hamstrings to stabilize their knee. The predominant muscle recruitment order of the male athletes and both control groups was the hamstring-quadriceps-gastrocnemius muscle pattern. In contrast, the female athletes recruitment pattern was quadriceps-hamstring-gastrocnemius. During the voluntary muscle contraction response, the female athletes demonstrated the same response as the female controls and both male groups. This pattern was hamstring-quadriceps-gastrocnemius. In respect to the muscle reaction time in this study, no significant differences were found at the spinal cord level for the quadriceps and hamstrings; however the male and female athletes produced significantly faster gastrocnemius muscle responses compared to the two control groups. In the intermediate phase of the relaxed response testing and the voluntary response to tibial translation, there was no significant difference for all muscles between all four groups. When testing muscular strength and time to reach this peak force utilizing isokinetic testing, Huston and Wojtys[140] found no differences in time-to-peak torque for knee extension at 60°/second and 240°/second for all groups. Significant differences did exist between male and female athletes for hamstring time-to-peak torque at 60°/second and 240°/second. The female athletes were statistically significantly slower than the male athletes and minimally slower than the female control group although this difference was not statistically significant.[140] Contrary to Huston and Wojtys, Rozzi et al.[233] did not find sex differences in the time-to-peak torque tested isokinetically for either hamstrings or quadriceps. This same study did find significantly greater EMG peak amplitude of the lateral hamstrings for the female athletes when landing from a jump on one leg. The authors stated that this finding may be related to the idea that female athletes possess inherent joint laxity and the hamstrings must activate at a higher level to provide stability to the joint.[233]

The latency period between sensory feedback and dynamic movement is known as electromechanical delay and has been shown to be shorter in males compared to females, thus allowing superior efficiency of dynamic stabilization in males.[165]

DeMont et al.[84] studied the muscular activity before foot strike in various functional activities for ACL deficient subjects, ACL reconstructed subjects, and a control group and compared involved to uninvolved legs of each subject. All subjects were female. The tasks consisted of downhill walking, running, hopping, and landing from a step. Different bilateral activation of vastus medialis obliques (VMO) occurred with downhill walking and running activities for the ACL deficient group. The ACL deficient group also showed a significant increase in vastus lateralis (VL) activation during running and landing when compared bilaterally and also when compared to ACL reconstructed and control group subjects. Activation of the LG was lower in downhill walking and higher in the landing task in the ACL deficient group also. The ACL reconstructed group showed significant differences between the involved and uninvolved limb in the LG for the hop. These side-to-side differences for the ACL deficient and reconstructed groups, and group differences between ACL deficient and control group, suggest that the females with an ACL deficient knee use unique strategies involving the VMO, VL, and LG and these muscles need to be addressed in the rehabilitation process. A similar study performed by Swanik et al.[257] demonstrated ACL deficient subjects to exhibit greater peak activity (as measured by isometric electromyography (IEMG) in the medial hamstring in comparison with the ACL reconstructed group and greater peak activity in the lateral hamstring than the control group during running. During landing from a step, the ACL deficient group demonstrated significantly less IEMG activity in the VL when compared to the control group. These findings suggest the importance of the hamstrings in controlling anterior tibial translation and rotation, as well as the possible inhibition of the quadriceps in an effort to dynamically stabilize the knee in the ACL deficient knee.

For dynamic stabilization to occur at the knee, many muscles are involved that directly pass around the joint as well as other muscles that are distally and proximally positioned but play a role in controlling the forces at the knee. Baratta et al.[32] investigated muscular coactivation patterns at the knee. Subjects consisted of nonathletes, recreational athletes, and highly competitive athletes, and EMG data was collected during an isokinetic strength test. High-performance athletes with hypertrophied quadriceps had inhibitory effects on the coactivation of the hamstrings compared to the recreational athletes. They also determined that athletes who routinely exercised their hamstrings demonstrated inhibited quadriceps and had similar coactivation patterns of the nonathletes. Muscular balance is key to efficient dynamic joint stabilization.

Muscle stiffness is important to stability of the knee and demonstrated when muscles surrounding the knee contract, offering the joint increased contact force and decreased joint mobility. Markolf et al.[181] reported that nonathletes could increase varus and valgus knee stiffness 2–4× with isometric contraction of the hamstrings and quadriceps. Athletes in the same study were able to increase their joint stiffness by a factor of

10 with the same isometric contraction. Bryant and Cooke[54] demonstrated gender differences in knee stiffness in a study in 1988. When testing varus and valgus stiffness females rotated at the tibia 66 percent more than the males and were 35 percent less stiff. Another study that looked at gender differences in the anterior-posterior plane of motion determined a significant difference in females and males ability to stiffen the knee joint. Men were able to increase their joint stiffness by $4\times$ whereas the females were only able to stiffen their joint by $2\times$.[141] The exact mechanism of knee stiffness is not completely understood, although a study by Such et al. determined that lower-extremity muscle mass had the largest influence on the stiffness properties of the knee.[236]

Knee Kinematics and Landing Characteristics

As noted in the previous section on the mechanisms of injury, it is well documented in the literature that most of the ACL injuries occur when landing from a jump or during deceleration and pivoting. It has been documented that the quadriceps exerts its maximum anterior sheer force when the knee flexion angles are the smallest ($20°–25°$ flexion), which puts a measurable strain on the ACL.[244] Eccentric activation of the quadriceps at high velocities present during athletic movements may produce too much force for the static and dynamic stabilizers of the knee to resist, thus allowing injury to occur. EMG studies demonstrate eccentric quadriceps muscle activation during such activities as running, cutting, and landing from a jump to be more than $2\times$ greater than maximum voluntary contraction.[116] It has also been documented in the literature that there is a significant difference in how males and females perform the previously noted movement patterns.

Malinzak et al.[174] was one of the first research groups to investigate these kinematic gender differences. EMG and 3D kinematic analyses of cutting and running were obtained from male and female athletes. Females demonstrated significantly less knee flexion, increased knee valgus, and decreased hip flexion than males during both of these movement patterns. Females also had greater quadriceps and lower hamstring activation levels especially at heel strike.[139] Colby et al.[70] investigated four different cutting maneuvers in males and females using 2D video analyses and EMG and had similar results as Malinzak et al.[174] The average knee flexion angle was $22°$ for each cutting maneuver. Quadriceps activity was 161 percent if the maximum voluntary isometric contraction (MVC) as compared to 14 percent MVC for hamstring activity.[70] This further demonstrates the "quadriceps dominant" state and how weak hamstrings or hamstring/quadriceps muscular imbalances present in female athletes could contribute to their susceptibility for ACL injuries.

Lephart et al.[165] also investigated strength and lower-extremity kinematics during landing. Single-leg landing and forward hop tasks were studied using EMG and force plates with female basketball, volleyball, and soccer players and matched male subjects. This study also tested strength of the quadriceps and hamstrings via isokinetic testing. The following results were all significant at the level of $p < 0.05$. For single-leg landing, females had greater hip internal rotation, less knee flexion, and less lower-leg internal rotation. The females also had significantly less time to maximum angular displacement of knee flexion. During the forward hop task, females had less knee flexion, less lower-leg internal rotation, and more time to maximum angular displacement for hip internal rotation and less time to maximum angular displacement for knee flexion. There were no significant difference for vertical ground reaction force variable for both landing and hopping tasks. Isokinetic testing revealed significant lower peak torque to body weight for knee extension and flexion ($p < 0.05$). Overall, the females landed in a more valgus position and with less knee flexion, thus less time for absorption of the impact forces. The weakness demonstrated in the quadriceps and hamstrings may also play a role in the landing kinematics.[165]

In a follow-up study to Malinzak, Chappel et al.[62] hypothesized that female recreational athletes would have increased proximal anterior tibial shear force, knee extension moment, and knee valgus moment while performing forward, backward, and vertical stop-jumps. The results of this study are similar to previous studies. Women exhibited greater proximal tibia anterior shear force than did men during the landing phase of all jumps. All subjects exhibited greater proximal tibia anterior shear force during the landing phase of the backward stop-jump task than during the other two stop-jumps. Women also exhibited greater valgus and extensor moments than did the males for all three stop-jumps.

Ground reaction force differences during landing are an interesting kinematic variable to examine between males and females. Dufek and Bates[92] examined landing forces and pointed out that higher landing forces had a positive relationship with injury occurrence. Hewett et al.[128] examined the results of a neuromuscular training program and determined that the training program resulted in significant decreases in peak landing forces and decreases in valgus-varus moments at the knee. They indicated that the valgus-varus moments at the knee served as significant predictors of peak landing forces. This same study demonstrated that the males' landing forces were an average of two bodyweights greater than the females yet they have lower rate of serious injury. It has been hypothesized that high landing forces by the males are dissipated through increased knee flexor activity at the instant of landing and greater angular knee flexion at landing. Both of these strategies may allow males to dissipate ground reaction forces more efficiently.

The previously mentioned studies have all looked intimately at the knee joint. But what effects do the trunk, hip, and ankle have on the kinematics of the knee joint? Bobbert and van Zandwijk[46] described, in their research, the knee being "slaved" to the moment produced at the hip. It has been theorized that because most females have weak hip extensors they use the iliopsoas for trunk control over their hips and land in a more erect posture and have greater extensor moments at the knee. Decreased trunk flexion also decreases maximal quadriceps and hamstrings activation, thus decreasing dynamic stabilization directly at the knee joint. Observation of videotapes of ACL injuries has demonstrated that two-thirds of the injuries occurred when the center of gravity appeared behind the knee. Another theory regarding this variable is that during upright landings, the rectus femoris may act as a hip stabilizer and pull the trunk forward. This powerful contraction by the rectus femoris may also produce a large tibia anterior shear force. More research needs to be performed to prove or disprove these theories, but trunk and hip control appear essential to efficient athlete maneuvers and should be part of all prevention and rehabilitation programs.

In summary of the extrinsic and combined factors that may predispose the female athlete for higher incidence of ACL injuries, the following items were revealed:

1. Females are weaker in their quadriceps and hamstrings as compared to males.
2. Females have a lower hamstring/quadriceps ratio as compared to males.
3. When both men and women are fatigued, the stability of the knee joint is compromised.
4. ACL deficient subjects have decreased proprioception.
5. Females are slower to detect proprioception as measured by detection of passive movement in the direction of knee extension as compared to males.
6. Females use more of a quadriceps-hamstring-gastrocnemius muscle firing pattern in response to anterior tibia translation and males use more hamstring-quadricep-gastrocnemius pattern.
7. Females are slower to reach peak torque for the hamstring group as compared to males.
8. Females have a longer electromechanical delay between stimulus and action as compared to males.
9. Females demonstrate a decrease in muscle stiffness and thus decreased ability to stabilize knee joint as compared to males.
10. Females demonstrate the following patterns when landing from a jump or decelerating
    a. Decrease in knee flexion (Fig. 36-4)
    b. Increase in knee valgus (Figs. 36-4 and 36-5)
    c. Increase in hip internal rotation (Fig. 36-6)
    d. Decrease in trunk and hip flexion (Fig. 36-4)

ASSESSMENT AND SCREENING

As noted previously, many research studies have focused on determining the exact cause of the higher frequency of ACL injuries in females as compared to males. Although much time has been spent on this subject, no definitive intrinsic, extrinsic, or combined factors have been identified as strong predictors of ACL injuries. A study by Arendt et al.[25] published in 1999 set out to determine potential patterns that cause ACL injuries utilizing the National Collegiate Athletic Association Injury Surveillance System. The conclusions of this study stated that

common noncontact ACL injuries mechanism were pivoting or landing from a jump. They found no comorbidity or illness patterns. The injured athletes were experienced, with many years of sports participation before and during high school. Hyperextension was the only physical examination feature that could possibly be linked to ACL injuries. Females were more likely to be injured just prior to or just after their menses and not mid-cycle.[25] Due to the multifactorial presentation of this injury, the sample size for such a study must be quite large in order to be predictive. These authors stated that this project is to be viewed as a pilot study and hope it will stimulate more research in this area.

Based on this information should the clinician working with these athletes conduct a screening process in attempt to minimize the incidence of ACL injuries among their athletic teams? Current research and practical knowledge do not offer a valid and reliable screening tool as of yet, and no particular set of variables has been determined to successfully predict risk of injury. Most clinicians do not have access to the technology and equipment necessary to examine balance, proprioception, kinesthesia, neuromuscular patterns, or kinematic analysis of forces and angles. This does not mean the clinician cannot look at the athlete with simple functional testing. Strength and muscular endurance can be examined either isokinetically or with one *repetition maximum testing*. Functional tests such as single-leg and tandem stance balancing can screen for basic proprioception deficits, and single-leg hop tests can look grossly at explosive power of the lower extremity and dynamic stability at the knee. Observing joint positions and landing characteristics from a jump, both visually and with simple video analysis, is an easy thing for the clinician to do (Figs. 36-3A,B, 36-4, 36-5, 36-6, 36-7A,B). Incorrect technique or motor performance deficits that can be identified can then be corrected to enhance physical performance and possibly lower injury risk, especially for the female athlete.

Injury prevention programs have been developed and tested based on the previous information with the goal of enhancing physical performance and decreasing injury occurrence among female athletes. The authors of this chapter believe that addressing the previously stated deficits common to female athletes can only enhance their physical performance and as a result may decrease risk of ACL injury. The authors were unable to find any studies that demonstrated increased strength, improved balance and proprioception, muscular endurance, or proper landing and cutting performance to be detrimental to any person, athlete, or nonathlete. Both high-tech screening and low-tech (clinical) screening procedures are important. When a deficit is identified, it should be addressed, and only good things can come from any education or improvement that occurs.

PREVENTION AND EXERCISE CONSIDERATIONS

As noted previously, the research has indicated some possible areas where females and males differ in their muscle physiology, biomechanics, hormonal levels, joint stability, joint kinematics, proprioception, and skill level in athletics. Of these factors which ones are controllable and what has the research determined as the best approach in injury prevention? That is the question we all ask ourselves. Although this topic of injury prevention for ACLs has received much attention lately, it is not a new topic. Henning was investigating this idea in the early 1980s, and after a 10-year study of ACL injuries in female basketball players he formulated a prevention program based on altering his "quad-cruciate interaction."[116] As previously mentioned, Henning concluded that the most common mechanisms of injury to the ACL were planting and cutting, straight-leg landing, and one-step stop with the knee hyperextended.[116] His prevention program consisted of activities to eliminate or minimize these mechanisms. Henning proposed using an accelerated rounded turn off a bent knee instead of the pivot and cut movement pattern. He also emphasized drills that worked on landing on a bent knee and a three-step stop with the knee bent. The common thread in all the drills was the bent knee position. It has also been illustrated in research studies discussed in the previous sections of this chapter that females do land from jumps with a straight-leg position and have excessive valgus knee position with landing and cutting movements during sports (see figures. 36-3B and 36-7B). Both of these positions put the female at risk for an ACL injury. Henning's prevention program did show some success in decreasing ACL injuries (89 percent decrease). Although his program did have its limitations, it was an admirable start in addressing this problem and provided impetus for modern prevention programs.

Proprioception deficits in ACL injured and reconstructed patients is well documented. So, it only seems natural to look at this component and incorporating it into a prevention program. Caraffa et al.[58] did just this in developing their five-phase proprioceptive program that progressed the athlete through increasingly difficult skills using different balance boards. The study showed a statistically significant decrease in ACL injuries in semiprofessional and amateur soccer players for the exercise program versus the control group of skill-matched soccer players. The study received criticism for not being randomized and flaws in program standardization, but it can be looked at as a pilot study and a plausible approach to developing a prevention program incorporating proprioception training.

In the mid 1990s Hewett et al.[128] conducted a study to determine the effect of jump training on landing mechanics and lower-extremity strength in 11 female athletes involved in jumping sports. Vertical jump height, isokinetic muscle strength, and force analysis testing were performed prior to and after the training program for the female athletes and a group of male athletes. The jump program was performed over a 6-week period of time and was performed on alternating days, 3 days a week. During the jumping program, four basic techniques were emphasized:

1. correct posture with spine erect, shoulders back, and body alignment of shoulders over knees throughout the jump

2. jumping straight up with no excessive side-to-side or forward-backward movement
3. soft landings including toe-to-heel rocking and bent knees
4. instant recoil preparation for the next jump.

See Appendix A for details of the *Jump-Training Program.*[128]

The results of the training program for the female group revealed a 22 percent decrease in peak landing forces, knee varus-valgus moments decreased approximately 50 percent, and hamstring/quadriceps peak torque ratios increased 26 percent on the nondominant side and 13 percent on the dominant side. Hamstring power increased by 44 percent with training on the dominant side and 21 percent on the nondominant side. Mean vertical jump height also increased by 10 percent. Multiple regression analysis revealed that varus-valgus moments were significant predictors of peak landing forces.[128]

The results of this study led the researchers to continue with a follow-up project with this jump-training program. Hewett et al.[125] developed a prospective research study to determine the effect of this same jump-training program on the incidence of knee injury in female athletes. They monitored two groups of female athletes; one group performed the jump-training program and one group did not. A group of untrained male athletes were also used for comparison. The groups were monitored throughout the high-school soccer, volleyball, and basketball seasons. Results of this study revealed that the untrained female athletes had a 3.6 times higher incidence of knee injury than trained female athletes ($p < 0.05$) and 4.8 times higher than male athletes ($p < 0.03$). The incidence of knee injury in trained female athletes was not significantly different from that in the untrained male athletes.[125] The results of this early, innovative study indicated that a plyometric training program may have a positive effect in reducing incidence of female ACL injuries. The authors of this study acknowledged several limitations in their study. It was not a randomized, double blind study, and there were not equal numbers of each type of sports participant in each group. Conclusions from this study indicate that the plyometric training program decreased the magnitude of varus-valgus moments at the knee and improvement in hamstring/quadriceps strength ratio. As noted previously, many researchers feel that these two variables play a strong role in ACL injury incidence for female athletes.

An interesting fact to note about many of these prevention programs is the component of *educating* the athlete about how to correctly perform landing or cutting tasks. Henning developed a teaching tape consisting of examples of noncontact ACL injuries followed by illustrations of the recommended drills done in the gym as well as on the playing field. He stated that young athletes are more receptive to technique modification and called it "improved player technique skills" (Figs. 36-3A and B).[116] Ettlinger et al.[99] stated that ACL injuries in alpine skiers could be reduced as much as 60 percent using standardized training programs before the ski season. The subjects were trained to avoid high-risk behavior, recognize potentially dangerous situations, and to respond quickly whenever these

T A B L E   3 6 - 3

Neuromuscular Training Program Schedule

TUESDAY	THURSDAY	SATURDAY
• 30-minute plyometric station • 30-minute strength station • 30-minute core-strengthening and balance station	• 30-minute plyometric station • 30-minute speed station • 30-minute strengthening and balance station	• 45-minute speed station • 45-minute strength station

Developed by Myer et al.[198]

conditions were encountered. Hewett et al.[128] used verbal cueing to encourage proper jumping and landing techniques. Such phrases as "on your toes," "straight as an arrow," "light as a feather," "shock absorber," and "recoil like a spring" were all used to illustrate proper technique. The authors of this chapter also use three words beginning with the letter L to instruct athletes in correct performance of all motor skills: *Low*, *Light*, and (In) *Line*. These cues refer to low, flexed knee landings and transitions, softness and quietness during landings, and parallel thighs during activity, respectively. This pneumonic is also referred to as L^3.

Another important study by Onate et al.[212] reported the importance of feedback and educating the athletes in proper technique performance. They looked at the effects of augmented feedback versus sensory feedback on the reduction of jump-landing forces. The augmented feedback group received information on how to land softer via video and verbal analysis, the sensory feedback group was asked to use the experience with their baseline jumps to land softer, and the control groups were given no extraneous feedback on how to land softer. The subjects in the augmented feedback had significantly reduced peak vertical ground reaction force as compared to the sensory feedback and control groups.[212] All clinicians and researchers must remember, you may have the perfect prevention program, but if your subjects do not understand the movement pattern and technique you are asking them to perform, it is all for naught.

More recently, in 2005, Myer et al.[198] examined a comprehensive neuromuscular training program to study the effects on lower-extremity biomechanics and improved performance in the female athlete's vertical jump, single-leg hop, speed, bench press, and squat. As previously discussed, multiple research studies have been carried out examining the positive effects of a plyometric or jump-training program; however, this study combined plyometrics with core strengthening, balance training, interval speed training, and resistance training.[198]

Fifty-three female athletes involved in basketball, volleyball, or soccer participated. Forty-one subjects were assigned to the training group and 12 subjects were assigned to the control group. Pretesting was conducted 1 week before the training pro-

gram and posttesting was 4 days after the final training session. The athletes received feedback on biomechanical analysis and correct technique before and after training sessions. The training sessions were 3 days a week (Tuesday, Thursday, and Saturday) for 90-minute sessions. For the breakdown in training sessions, see Table 36-3. Subjects trained for 6 weeks, while control subjects did not change their normal exercise program. Results demonstrated statistically significant improvements compared to their pretrained values in vertical jump height, single-leg hop distance, sprint speed, bench press maximum, and squat maximum for the trained group. Knee flexion range of motion (ROM) during landing from a box jump was significantly increased. Varus and valgus torques were significantly lower for the right knee and showed a trend toward decrease valgus torque in the left knee. The control group showed no increase in any of the previously measured parameters over a 6-week period.[198] This study supports the benefits of a comprehensive exercise approach when treating the female athlete. A combination of plyometrics, core strengthening, balance training, upper- and lower-body strengthening, speed training, and very importantly, education on technique proves to be valuable in improving athletic performance, as well as decreasing potentially dangerous variables in knee biomechanics when running and jumping.

Mandelbaum et al.[177] performed a recent prospective study similar to the previous studies to examine prevention of ACL tears in the female athlete as well. The authors developed a community-based program named the "Prevent Injury and Enhance Performance Program" (PEP), which was created specifically for female soccer players between the ages of 14–18 years. This program consists of basic warm-up activities, stretching techniques for the trunk and lower extremities, strengthening exercises, plyometric activities, and soccer-specific agility drills. The program also places heavy emphasis on proper landing technique. This training program was implemented to address the feed-forward mechanism as described previously. The specific goal was to improve the athlete's ability to anticipate external forces or loads to stabilize the knee joint, protecting the inherent structures.[177]

Results of this study using PEP were impressive in reducing ACL injury in soccer players. Analysis of data from the first year of the study revealed an 88 percent overall reduction in ACL injury compared to the control group followed by a 74 percent reduction of ACL injury during the second year of the study. The authors concluded that prophylactic training focusing on developing neuromuscular control of the lower extremity through strengthening exercises, plyometrics, and sports-specific agilities drills "may address the proprioceptive and biomechanical deficits that are demonstrated in the high-risk female athletic population" (Ref. 177, p. 1008). These researchers and others continue to study the PEP program with a variety of populations.

EXERCISE CONSIDERATIONS

When designing an exercise program for any athlete, and especially the female athlete, the authors of this chapter like to use the lower-extremity reactive neuromuscular training sequence as described in Table 36-4. The basic premise of the exercise sequence is to begin with a stable base of support in a closed-chain position.

Then, progress with resistance and perturbations from resistance or trunk and upper-extremity movements. When the athlete becomes proficient with the exercises performed with a stable base, the base is then narrowed and an environment of instability is created.

The progression repeats with an unstable base of support. Sport-specific training is added next with the goal of neuromuscular control becoming a natural, noncognitive, adaptation to the movement patterns required by the sport. The following information are some ideas the authors have developed with clinical experience and being creative with the exercise progression.

Based on the previous descriptive information about female neuromuscular and functional strategies, how does the rehabilitation professional get the females to bend their knees, avoid the valgus knee position, and get their gluteal region down with the trunk flexed to minimize the potential risk of knee injury? The authors propose that you make the athletes exercise program focus on these exact positions (Fig. 36-15A and B).

Strengthening the quadriceps and hamstrings in the flexed trunk and knee position can be performed with simple wall sits, step-down position with a static hold (Figs. 36-8 and 36-9) and progress into closed-chain squats in a protected position using the Smith Squat Rack. The key part of this squat is to note that the athlete never fully extends knee and works in a range of 30°–90° of knee flexion and uses the bench as her spotter. This is the position we want her to assume when performing sports, so we must train her muscles in this position. What about power-lifting techniques for females such as the power clean or snatch? The purpose of these power-lifting movements should not be for brute strength but rather for quick footwork and bent knee position with trunk stabilization. Many times female athletes do not even do the simple squat technique performed by most males in all levels of sports. Proper technique for free weight

T A B L E   3 6 - 4

Lower-Extremity Reactive Neuromuscular Training, From Less to More Difficult (Top—Less Difficult, Bottom—Most Difficult)

DESCRIPTION OF ACTIVITY	EXAMPLES	FIGURE DEMONSTRATING*
Stable base, bilateral lower extremities	Partial squats, step down and hold	None
Unstable base, bilateral lower extremities	Wobble boards, foam rollers	None
Stable base, unilateral lower extremity	Single limb stance, unilateral squats star diagram, Contralateral LE tubing ("steamboats")	Figures 36-8 and 36-9 Figure 36-10A and B
Unstable base, unilateral lower extremity	Wobble boards, foam rollers, mini-tramp	Figure 36-11A and B
Stable base, with added UE/trunk challenges	Squat positions with ball throws, perturbations	None
Unstable base, with added UE/trunk challenges	Wobble boards, foam rollers, Dynadiscs, with ball throws, perturbations	Figures 36-12 and 36-13
Jump/landing sequence from stable base	Jump/land on gym floor, Jump/land from minimal elevation (stair, mat)	None
Jump/landing sequence from unstable base	Jump/land from mini-tramp	Figure 36-14A and B
Jump/landing sequence with distractions	Jump/land with twists, external resistance, passing balls	None

UE, upper extremity; LE, lower extremity.

*See Figures 36-10 to 36-14.

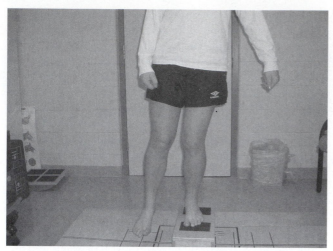

FIGURE 36-8

Example of a unilateral stable base exercise. Note the incorrect valgus and internal rotation. Training must be done with the lower extremity in proper alignment.

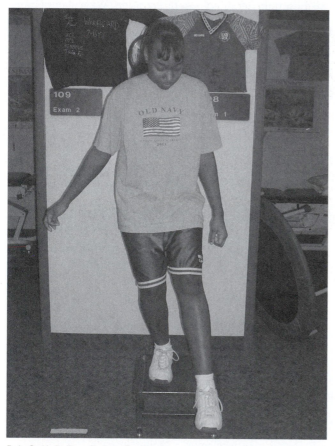

FIGURE 36-9

Better stance lower extremity position. Subjects must be corrected and coached to work in excellent lower extremity alignment. Note that this can also be done in mirror for visual feedback and corrections.

lifting is the key, and using lighter weight body bars are optimal for learning, rather than heavy 45 pound standard weight-lifting bars. Treadmill retro uphill walking in a knee-flexed position is also effective for working the quadriceps in an optimal position. Regarding the hamstrings, if the hamstrings are to be active when the trunk is flexed, then they need to be strengthened in a flexed trunk position such as seated open-chain resisted knee flexion. Another way to work the gluteals and hamstrings in a closed-chain trunk flexed position is to do a semi-squat uphill walking lunge on a treadmill. This is the reversal of the retro uphill squat walk.

Another possibility is to combine strengthening and neuro-muscular retraining. In Figure 36-16, the athlete is performing a unilateral, closed-kinetic chain partial squat on the Total gym, using a Dynadisc under her foot, thereby performing both types of exercise concurrently. This is an example of an unstable base utilized during a unilateral strengthening activity.

Muscular fatigue slows electromechanical delay, decreases knee stability, and compromises proprioception.[209,232] Muscular fatigue will happen to all athletes if they compete at an intense level, so the athlete must be trained to have a stable knee even when fatigued. Fatiguing the athlete and then *carefully* working on proprioception, cutting and deceleration maneuvers, and proper landing position from a jump are techniques used by the authors.

When the big picture of total body positioning is examined, attention must be paid to the joints distal and proximal to the knee joint. Often the ankle and its role as the first link of the chain to absorb the forces and then stabilize the base of support are forgotten. The gastrocnemius and soleus have a role in posterior stabilization of the knee joint and need to be strengthened in the position in which they must excel: knee and trunk flexion (Fig. 36-15B). In the study by Huston and Wojtys,[140] the gastrocnemius was the first muscle to respond to tibia anterior translation in the relaxed position. An intriguing thought is that maybe the foot and calf muscles are the key to knee stability as they are the first line of defense for all closed-chain activities. The trunk and hips are the joints proximal to the knee, and they possess the most muscular mass and thus the most potential for efficient body control. The authors of this chapter call this concept "The Butt and Gut" and believe firmly in its role in proficient movement patterns for all joints of the body. Females are usually weaker in their gluteal muscles and lack some trunk control with high-level sports movements. Emphasis on hip rotators, hip extensors, transverse abdominals, and hip adductors strength and endurance should be part of every athlete's fitness program. With strong hip and trunk muscles, the landing and running characteristics of genu valgus, hip internal rotation, straight knee position at foot impact, and erect trunk position should be minimized and possibly eliminated.[103,126,129]

Educating your athletes in proper movement patterns is the key to success for injury prevention. As noted previously in this chapter, research has shown that visual and verbal cueing enhances the performance of proper technique in the quest for

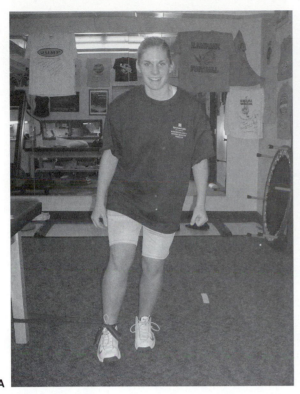
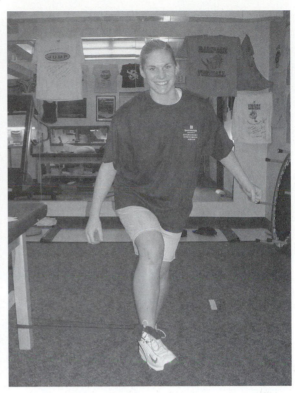

A   B

FIGURE 36-10

Example of unilateral lower extremity, stable base with external pertebation offered by Theraband® into adduction, start position (left). Note proper position of the weight-bearing lower extremity in flexed, well-aligned knee position. Ending position on right.

optimal position of the body for injury prevention and efficient, powerful sports movements. A technique used by the authors to enhance the learning of proper technique is to attach a headlamp to the athlete's knee and give them a target to aim at (Figs. 36-17 and 36-18A,B). Begin with a stable base and then progress through the exercise sequence noted at the beginning of this section. The ultimate exercise is to have the athlete jump off a mini-tramp and land the jump and accurately hit the target on the mirror with the beam of light coming from her knee. The use of a mirror, visual, verbal, and auditory cues are essential for learning. Use of one or all of those learning tools with most exercises is helpful. Video is also used to record and then show athletes what they look like performing a task and then what the goal is to look like for proper technique.

Excellent clinicians must frequently review the literature and then think of bold, creative ways to exercise their patients based on the positions that make the female athlete vulnerable for ACL injury. Although ACL reconstructive surgery provides excellent, predictable outcomes in most cases, and rehabilitation after ACL reconstruction has become standard physical therapy practice, no reconstructed knee is as good as an uninjured knee. In the world of ACL injuries in female athletes, the mothers' old quote "an ounce of prevention is worth a pound of cure" rings true.

SEQUELAE FROM ACL INJURY

The authors refer the reader to Chapter 29 for a complete analysis of the information regarding evaluation and treatment of the female athlete suffering an ACL injury. Prevention of this debilitating injury cannot be more emphasized with the growing concerns that have been raised among the sports medicine community regarding the early degenerative changes after a knee injury and specifically following an ACL injury.[79,80,96,111,229,231] Curl et al. reviewed over 30,000 knee arthroscopies with a variety of patient ages and reported chondral injuries in 63 percent of these patients with an average of 2.7 articular cartilage injuries per knee.[77] Bone bruises, most common in the lateral compartment, are observed in 80 percent of MRI studies following ACL tear.[192] At the time of surgery, 9 percent of all ACL injured patients have documented acute cartilage defects. This same population demonstrates a 19 percent incidence of articular cartilage defects at 9-year follow-up.[231] This significant increase in cartilage defects demonstrates that stabilization of the knee through ACL reconstruction does not eliminate the risk of degenerative changes in the articular cartilage.

Numerous studies have shown a good-to-excellent results following ACL reconstructive surgery with reference to stability,

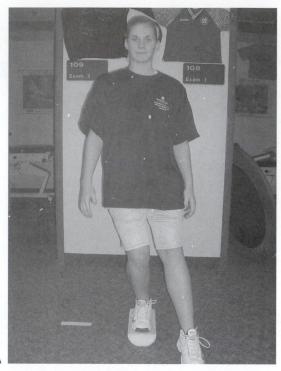

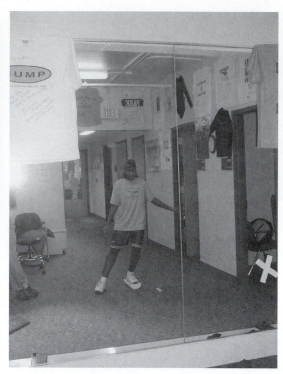

A   B

FIGURE   36-11

Example of unilateral lower extremity, unstable base (1/2 foam roller) exercise without
visual feedback (left) and with (right) visual feedback from mirror for correction. Note
lower extremity and trunk position comparing left to right.

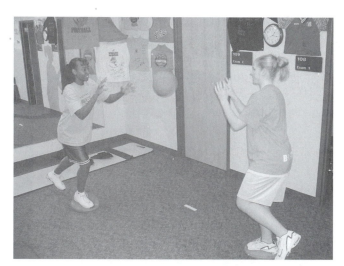

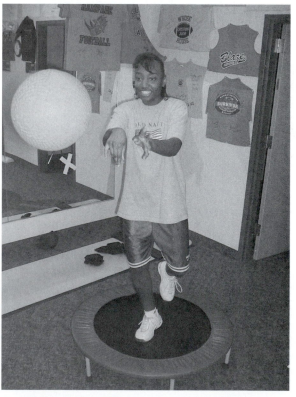

FIGURE   36-12

Two subjects, each on Dynadisc® (unstable base, one
lower extremity) throwing a ball between for
distraction/balance perturbation.

FIGURE   36-13

Unstable base, unilateral lower extremity exercise, with
distraction/perturbation technique of ball throw/catch.

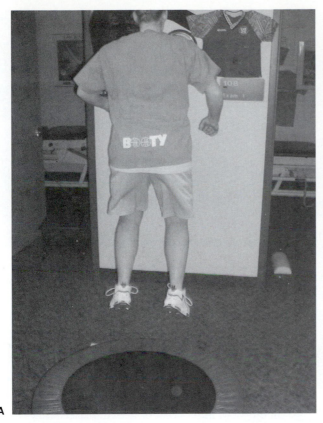
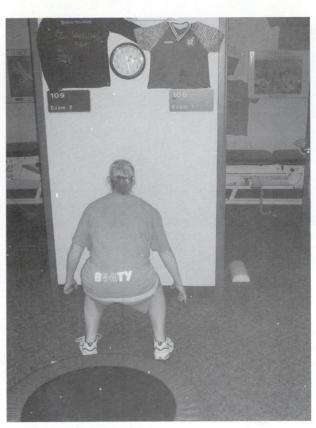

A   B

FIGURE 36-14

Dynamic jump/land training: subject shown airborne after jumping off mini-tramp (left).
Subject landing from jump on right. During exercise training, stress correct lower
extremity position and "soft landing."

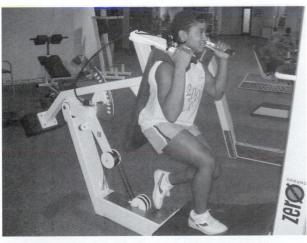
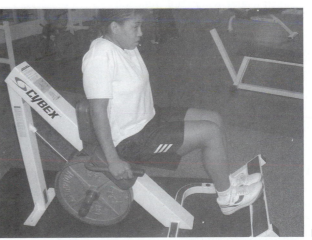

A   B

FIGURE 36-15

Performance of plantarflexion-strengthening exercise in flexed knee position in standing
(left) and sitting (right) to maximize the "down low" function of the gastroc-soleus
complex. Close attention is paid to the position and alignment of the lower extremity.

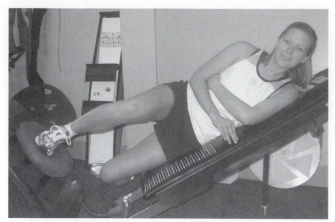

FIGURE 36-16

Use of Dynadisc on Total Gym for strength training. Single leg partial squats with an unstable surface. Close attention is paid to the position and alignment of the lower extremity. Foot position shown could be improved.

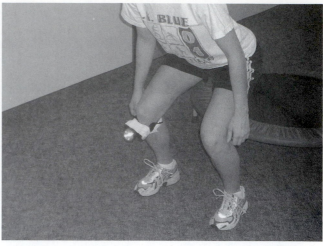

FIGURE 36-17

Use of a headlamp attached to the tibia to provide visual feedback in a flexed position while practicing proper positioning/alignment of the lower extremity.

normal knee mobility, normalized strength, and return to previous level of activity.[10,28,79,80,138,148,180,210,242,249] Work completed by Daniels et al. was the first to document concern regarding early degenerative changes in knees that had stability restored with an ACL reconstruction in a 5-year[80] and 10-year follow-up studies.[79] At 5–20 year follow-up, patients post-ACL reconstruction demonstrate up to a 50 percent increase in radiographic changes associated with arthritis compared to the contralateral, uninjured knee.[229] Concern regarding such degenerative changes was expressed by Gilquist who wrote that these surgeries resulted in "giving the patient enough security to go back to strenuous sports and then [ruin] the knee."[111] This concern is valid, but one must consider the concept of joint function and define "full" function.

Dye describes the knee joint as a mechanical engineering model with a complex, metabolically active system for trans-

mission of forces among the femur, tibia, fibula, and patella with cruciate ligaments acting as linkages, articular cartilage and menisci as weight-bearing entities and force absorbers, and muscles as force generators and absorbers as well.[96]

> In our view, the concept of musculoskeletal function includes the capacity not only to generate, transmit, absorb and dissipate loads but also to maintain tissue homeostasis while doing so.[95]

This statement beautifully illustrates the authors' belief that joint function is not truly attained unless the system can escape from tissue destruction or degeneration while completing a desired level of functional activity. Dye presents the concept of "envelope of function"[94] which is the safe zone of loading that a system can maintain normal homeostasis as illustrated in

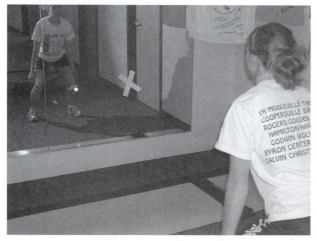

A

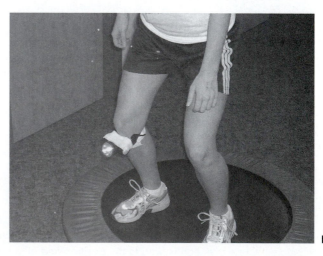

B

FIGURE 36-18

Subject attempts to aim lamp beam at a target in the mirror and uses visual cues to help adjust position (left). On the right, same exercise with unstable surface.

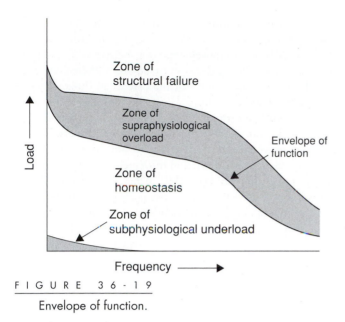

FIGURE 36-19

Envelope of function.

a load distribution curve (Fig. 36-19). Below this safe zone is the subphysiologic loading zone, causing loss of tissue homeostasis secondary to decreased loading which result in such injuries as osteopenia or muscular atrophy. Above the "envelope of function" is a zone of structural failure with loads great and/or frequent enough to cause actual failure of an element of the system such as meniscal or ACL tear. The zone that is immediately above the envelope of function, the zone of supraphysiologic load, represents loads at a force and/or frequency that cause a disruption of the tissue homeostasis before failure, i.e., stress fractures or articular cartilage degeneration.

This concept of "envelope of function" correlates nicely with Wolff's law that states cyclical loading of the cartilage and bone results in increased strength and durability of these structures and ultimately the musculoskeletal system. However, excessive loading results in degradation of the cartilage microstructure and arthritic changes.[176] Maintaining activity within the "envelope of function" will result in maintenance of tissue homeostasis and the ability to strengthen the musculoskeletal system, while exceeding this physiologic loading and moving into the "supraphysiologic loading zone" with increased intensity, duration, or frequency of activity will result degradation of the system and disruption of tissue homeostasis. Sports medicine personnel involved in the orthopedic medical care of a female athlete should adhere to the principal of remaining in the zone of homeostasis as defined by the current status of the joint involved. Defining this zone is the difficult task when completing the rehabilitation following an orthopedic injury such as an ACL tear and surgical reconstruction. The challenge of attaining a level of activity (loading) of the injured joint to allow tissue building such as muscular hypertrophy without entrance into the zone of supraphysiologic loading (overloading) such as articular cartilage degeneration or meniscal inflammation takes extreme care in planning with respect to activity in-

tensity, duration, and frequency. Determining such a zone also requires excellent communication between the surgeon and the rehabilitation professional regarding any preexisting conditions and surgical findings. Astute observation of the sports medicine specialist for signs of inflammation with a prescribed rehabilitation program and allowed functional/sporting activities is necessary to ensure proper physiologic loading.

The physically active female may be at greater risk than her male counterparts for articular cartilage degeneration and concerns. Gender difference in the knee joint size and greater valgus alignment may result in a greater stress concentration in the lateral and patellofemoral compartments of the female's knee. MRI studies of the human knee demonstrate that females have significantly less cartilage thickness and volume than age-matched males.[66] Articular cartilage has a complicated organization of hyaline cartilage with an extracellular matrix composed principally of type II collagen and sparsely distributed chondrocytes. Animal studies have also documented lower levels of proteoglycan and collagen in the cartilage of female rats. Considering the increased incidence of ACL injury in females versus males and the female articular cartilage basic science, chondral injury concerns are well founded.

CORE STABILIZATION FOR THE FEMALE ATHLETE

The common prerequisite for participation and success in all types of sports is a strong and stable core of the human body. Control of balance in upright posture and stability of the segments of the spine are required not only for activities of daily living, but also for high-level sports activity.[98] This stability enables athletes to transmit forces from the earth through the kinetic chain of the body and ultimately propel the body or an object using the limbs. The concept of core stabilization of the trunk and pelvis as a prerequisite for movements of the extremities was described biomechanically in 1991.[50] Subsequently, core stabilization has become a major trend both in treatment of injuries as well as in training regimes used to enhance athletic performance and prevent injury.

Many terms and rehabilitation programs are associated with the concept of core stability, including lumbar stabilization, dynamic stabilization, motor control (neuromuscular) training, neutral spine control, muscular fusion, and trunk stabilization.[12] The core has been conceptually described as either a box or a cylinder[227] because of its anatomical and structural composition. The abdominals create the anterior and lateral walls, the paraspinals and gluteals form the posterior wall, while the diaphragm and pelvic floor create the top and bottom of the cylinder, respectively (Fig. 36-20). Additionally, hip girdle musculature reinforces and supports the bottom of the cylinder. Envisioning this cylindrical system helps to understand its function as that of a dynamic muscular support system, described by some authors as the powerhouse, engine, or a "muscular corset that works as a unit to stabilize the body and spine, with and without limb movement" (Ref. 12, p. S86).

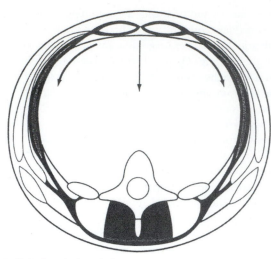

FIGURE 36-20

Anatomic cylinder of trunk. The muscle contraction of "drawing in" of the abdominal wall with an isometric contraction of the lumbar multifidus. The interrelationship and the interaction between these two muscles and the fascial system can be appreciated, and the figure illustrates how they can work together to give spinal support. (Reproduced, with permission, from Richardson C, Jull G, Hodges P, Hides J. *Therapeutic Exercise for Spinal Segmental Stabilization in Low Back Pain: Scientific Basis and Clinical Approach.* Edinburgh, NY, Churchill Livingstone, 1999, p. 86.)

Proximal stability for distal mobility is a commonly understood principle of human movement originally described by Knott and Voss[154] and applied in the concepts associated with proprioceptive neuromuscular facilitation. Nowhere is the concept of dynamic proximal stability more important than in sport. Without proximal control of the core, athletes could not use the lower extremities to propel the body in running and jumping or use the upper extremities to support or propel the body (in activities such as gymnastics and swimming), manipulate, use, and throw objects (such as throwing a shot put or softball, or using a tennis racquet). The core is in the middle of the human kinetic chain and serves a link between the upper and lower extremities. This allows for transfer of energy from the lower to the upper extremities and vice versa.

Strength and coordination of the core musculature is vital to performance and generation of power in many sports. When the core is functioning optimally, muscles elsewhere in the kinetic chain also function optimally allowing the athlete to produce strong, functional movements of the extremities (see Table 36-5).[63,151] Even small alterations in the kinetic chain have serious repercussions throughout other portions of the kinetic chain and thus on skills that are based upon efficient utilization of the entire chain.[151] Therefore, without proper stabilization and dynamic concentric and eccentric control of the trunk during ath-

letic tasks the extremities or "transition zones" between the core and extremities can be overstressed (i.e., hip and rotator cuff).

A wide variety of movements are associated with sport performance; therefore, athletes must possess sufficient strength and dynamic motor control of the core in all three planes of movement (transverse, frontal, sagittal).[162] Core stability is vital to athletic performance and especially important for the female athlete. In a study of male and female runners, females were found to have greater hip adduction, hip internal rotation, and tibial external rotation movements during the stance phase of running. Ferber et al.[100] believe that gender differences in lower-extremity kinematics place greater demands on the core musculature of female athletes. Additionally, core stability may even be more vital for the female athlete due to her overall decreased total extremity strength as compared to her age-matched male participant.[63] Documented differences in proximal strength measures in female athletes suggest that females may have a less stable base upon which torque and force can be generated or resisted. This "lack of core stability" is a possible contributor to lower-extremity injury.[116,144] Although important energy has been devoted to prevention of ACL and other knee injuries in the female athlete, the sports physical therapist must broaden his/her focus to the body as a whole and include core strengthening activities as a part of preparatory training for all female athletes.

Reviewing and considering the anatomy of the core allows the sports physical therapist to best understand principles of injury and rehabilitation (see Chapter 18). Stability of the core requires both passive (offered by bony and ligamentous structures) and dynamic stiffness (offered by coordinated muscular contractions). A spine without the contributions of the muscular system is unable to bear essential compressive loads and remain stable.[187] Anatomists have known for decades that a compressive load of as little as 2 kg causes buckling of the lumbar spine in the absence of muscular contractions.[195] Likewise, significant microtrauma of the lumbar spine occurs with as little as 2° of rotation, demonstrating the vital stabilizing function of the muscles of the lumbar spine.[107,113] Core stabilization is important not only for protection of the lumbar spine but also to resist the reactive forces produced by moving limbs that are transmitted to the spine and other muscles of the core.

Contemporary research has illuminated the roles of two important local muscle groups: the transversus abdominis (TA)[73,131,132] and the multifidus.[130,269] The TA—deepest of the abdominal muscles—uses its horizontal fiber alignment and attachment to the thoracolumbar fascia to increase intra-abdominal pressure (IAP) thereby making the core cylinder as a whole more stable. Although increased IAP had been associated with the control of spinal flexion forces and a decrease in load on the extensor muscles,[261] it is probable that the TA is most important in its ability to assist in intersegmental control[226] by offering "hoop-like" cylindrical stresses to enhance stiffness and limit both translational and rotational movement of the spine.[98,186] Bilateral contraction of the TA performs the movement of

TABLE 36-5

Examples of Core Demands, Kinetic Chain Relationships, and Outcomes of Specific Sporting Tasks

SPORTING ACTIVITY	CORE DEMANDS	KINETIC CHAIN RELATIONSHIPS	OUTCOME
Windmill softball pitch	Rotational and flexion/extension stability, acceleration, and deceleration of trunk	Transmission of forces from ground to LEs through trunk to UE to ball	Velocity, location, rotation of pitched ball (55–70 mph). Delivery of various types of pitches (drop, rise, breaking ball, etc.)
Gymnastics: vault event	Rotational and flexion/extension stability. Power with punch from horse	Transmission of forces from horse to UEs through trunk to propel body in airborne positions	Conversion of horizontal energy to vertical; speed, position, and trajectory of body through space
Tennis serve	Rotational and flexion/extension stability. Acceleration and deceleration of trunk	Transmission of forces from ground to LEs through trunk to UE through racquet to ball	Velocity, location, spin of served ball (80–120 mph). Delivery of various types of serves
Swimming: butterfly stroke	Flexion/extension stability	Transmission of forces from UEs to trunk to LEs to team with butterfly kick	Efficient propulsion of body through water, avoid excess trunk flexion and extension
Volleyball serve	Rotational and flexion/extension stability. Acceleration and deceleration of trunk	Transmission of forces from ground to LEs through trunk to UE to ball	Velocity, location, rotation of served ball. Various types of spins and serves (floater, topspin)

UE, upper extremity; LE, lower extremity.

"drawing in of the abdominal wall" (Ref. 228, p. 33) and does not produce spinal movement. The TA is active throughout the movements of both trunk flexion and extension, suggesting a unique stabilizing role during dynamic movement, different from the other abdominal muscles.[73,74] Also, EMG evidence suggests that the more internal muscles of the trunk (trans versus abdominis and internal obliques) behave in an anticipatory or feed-forward manner to provide proactive control of spinal stability during movements of the upper extremities,[132,133] regardless of the direction of limb movements.[133] This is important to remember when treating the athlete whose sport is heavily reliant on the upper extremity (i.e., softball, swimming, gymnastics, and volleyball).

Mechanisms of Injury to the Core

Many potential mechanisms of injury exist for the athlete. Cholewicki et al.[64] suggested that a common factor for injury to athletes may be the inability to generate sufficient core stability to resist external forces imposed upon the body during high-speed events. Other authors suggest a deficient endurance of the trunk stabilizing musculature that predisposes the athlete to traumatic forces over time[227] and motor control deficits and imbalances of the local muscles (TA and multifidus) and the global musculature (rectus abdominis and erector spinae) that occur during performance of functional activities. A weak

core could result in inefficient movements, altered postures, and an increased potential for both macro- and microtraumatic injury.[63]

Two examples of microtraumatic injuries that occur in the female athlete are spondylolysis and spondylolisthesis. The athletic population is more prone to these conditions and more likely to be symptomatic from these injuries. Spondylolytic microfracture of the pars is believed to happen due to shear forces occurring during repetitive flexion and extension.[258] Athletes with high rates of this type of microtraumatic injury include gymnasts,[97] divers, figure skaters, swimmers who perform the butterfly stroke,[258] and volleyball players,[97] due to the extreme extension/flexion reversals in trunk posture demanded by these sports. In fact, gymnasts younger than age 24 have a four times greater incidence of spondylolysis than the general female population.[258] Microtraumatic injuries may occur due to muscular imbalances, uncontrolled shear forces acting on the spine,[120,258] or because of lack of muscular control and stabilization offered by the core stabilizers. Sports such as golf, diving, and softball provide potential for microtraumatic injury to the core induced similarly, but related to extremes of rotation, often in combination with extension. Careful assessment of motor strategies and subsequent corrective movement retraining by the sports physical therapist may be a key to prevention of many microtraumatic injuries.

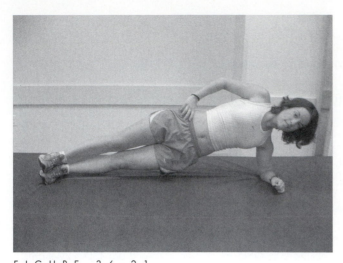

F I G U R E   3 6 - 2 1

Example of side-bridging.

In a study by Leetun et al.,[162] the researchers found that male athletes had statistically greater core stability scores on tests of hip abduction, hip external rotation, and the side bridge when compared to female athletes (Fig. 36-21).[162] Athletes who experienced injury to the core (spine/hip/thigh), knee or ankle, and foot during an athletic season demonstrated lower core stability measures than those who did not.[162] Once again, this leads the sports physical therapist to consider core strength, endurance, and motor performance training as a possible intervention for prevention of injury, especially for the female athlete.

Rehabilitation and Treating the Core

Simple, reliable, and objective clinical test procedures for dynamic motor control of the core are not readily available. Clinically, therapists utilize manual muscle tests that examine isometric holding of muscles, some positional holding tests (the plank or side plank) for endurance in isometric positions, and pressure biofeedback to asses the ability of a patient to hold the core stable during some dynamic tasks. A clinical test for the multifidus was devised that involves the activation of the multifidus at various segments under the palpating finger of a therapist.[227] This is performed in the prone position using the command "gently swell out your muscles under my fingers without using your spine or pelvis. Hold the contraction while breathing normally" (Ref. 227, p. 116), including side-to-side comparison to assess for segmental activation or inhibition. For examples of core strengthening exercises refer to Chapter 18. To make these exercises more specific to your female athlete, incorporate these concepts while performing training programs for other regions. For example, for a swimmer the therapist may have the athlete lie prone on a swiss ball while performing Theraband® movements mimicking the pull-through phase. The ball introduces an unstable base to challenge the core muscles.

Knowledge and application of core stabilization will benefit female athletes in all sports at all levels by improving performance, increasing athleticism, and decreasing the potential for injury to the spine and extremities. To provide an optimal, comprehensive exercise program for all female athletes, functional core exercises should be implemented into her sports-specific program.

SPECIAL CONSIDERATIONS CONCERNING THE SHOULDER IN THE ACTIVE FEMALE

Shoulder Laxity

Are women more prone to shoulder injuries? This question does not have ample research to be answered conclusively. Most studies do not separate shoulder injuries by gender or separate general injuries from specific ones. In 2001, Sallis et al.[234] compared sports injuries in men and women and failed to show a significant difference in overall injury rate. However, these authors reported in all sports, women reported a higher rate of hip and shoulder injuries. A significant difference was found with a higher rate of shoulder injuries in female swimmers compared to their male counterparts. Yet, the training for female and male swimmers differed greatly, so it is difficult to draw any specific conclusion.[234] The training regimen, their structural build, and/or presence of laxity may have predisposed the athletes to overuse injuries. Conclusions are unable to be drawn, until more controlled, specific research is carried out.

Other studies have described differences in various injuries between genders. Kroner and Lind[157] found no difference in shoulder dislocations between genders. All shoulder dislocations were recorded over a 5-year period in an area with a population of 253,753. Out of this population, 53.3 percent of shoulder dislocations occurred in males while 46.7 percent occurred in females. However, the difference was determined to be in the age group where the peak incidence occurred. Males were 21–30 years old, and females were 61–80 years old. The older age group was typically due to a fall on an outstretched arm.[157]

A high incidence of shoulder impingement is reported in female softball players[268] and both genders of volleyball players.[30,51] The shoulder was also the most commonly injured upper-extremity joint in both genders during alpine skiing.[239]

Clinical experience might suggest that women in general are more flexible and demonstrate increased laxity of their joints when compared to men. Are women more at risk for shoulder injuries due to laxity? First, it is important to describe the difference between laxity and instability. Laxity is not synonymous with instability. Laxity is the physiologic motion that allows for normal ROM. Instability is the abnormal *symptomatic* motion that results in pain, subluxation, or dislocation.[53]

There are many general joint laxity tests in literature, the most well known are those by Carter and Wilkinson,[60] which have been modified by Beighton[39] (Table 36-6 and Fig. 36-22). These tests examine ROM at the knees, trunk, fingers, thumbs, and elbows bilaterally and assigns a point system (0–9; 5 = hypermobile). Other hypermobility tests have not been proven

TABLE 36-6

Generalized Joint Laxity Tests

CARTER AND WILKINSON	BEIGHTON ET AL.
(1) Passive thumb apposition to forearm	(1) Passive hyperextension of small finger >90°
(2) Passive finger hyperextension so finger parallel to forearm	(2) Passive thumb apposition to forearm
(3) Elbow hyperextension >10°	(3) Elbow hyperextension >10°
(4) Knee hyperextension >10°	(4) Knee hyperextension >10°
(5) Excessive ankle dorsiflexion and foot eversion	(5) Trunk flexion, knee extension, and palms flat on floor

Adapted from Brown GA, Tan JL, Kirkley A. The lax shoulder in females. Issues, answers, but many more questions. *Clin Orthop Relat Res* 372:110–122, 2000.

reliable and valid. Therefore, many studies found in literature regarding general laxity differences between genders are not valid. Of the studies in literature, only one utilized the 0–9 Beighton scale examining generalized mobility in adolescents.[81] The authors reported out of 264 adolescent athletes, 22 percent

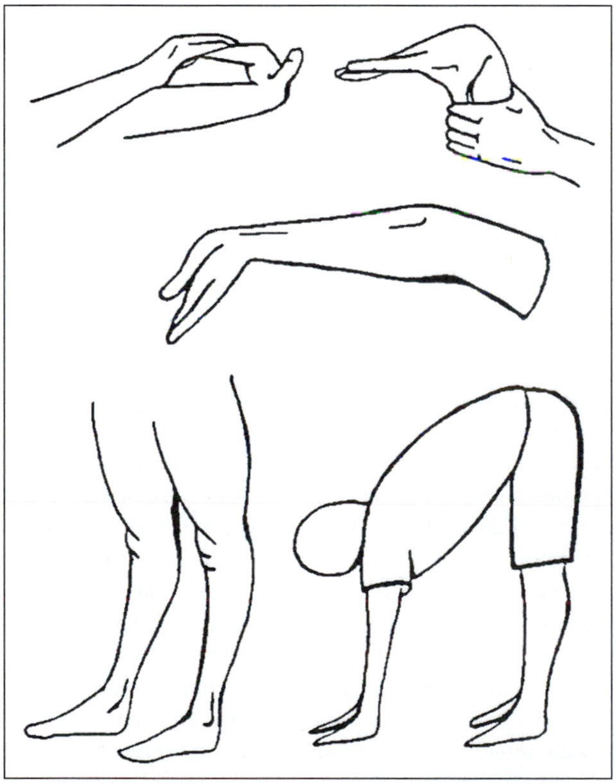

FIGURE 36-22

Hypermobility screening maneuvers, as developed by Carter and Wilkinson and modified by Beighton et al. (Adapted from Decoster et al. Prevalence and features of joint hypermobility among adolescent athletes. *Arch Pediat Adolesc Med* 151:898–992, 1997.

of all females and 6 percent of all males tested were generally "hypermobile."

However, it would be incorrect to conclude from this study that generalized laxity correlates with shoulder laxity. The astute clinician can and should compile the structural and physiologic differences between the genders and take into account clinical experience in order to rehabilitate the female athlete's shoulder in a multifaceted way.

Softball, swimming, and gymnastics are three sports that emerge when considering the female athlete. There is a high incidence of injury in both genders when considering softball/baseball, swimming, and gymnastics. Softball will be discussed separately due to the difference in the pitching delivery and the differences in rules regarding number of allowable pitches. Swimming will be discussed separately due to extreme high numbers of shoulder injuries that occur in female swimmers. Finally, the sport of gymnastics will be described in relationship to its injury potential in females.

Shoulder Injuries in the Windmill Softball Player

Little research has focused on softball pitching biomechanics or injury rates sustained by pitchers. Yet, softball was the team sport with the greatest participation in the United States in 1995. In 1996, Plummer[222] reported softball as one of the fastest growing sports for women at the college and high-school levels. In fact, in the 2003–2004 school year, softball was the female high-school sport with the fourth greatest participation rate, following only basketball, outdoor track and field, and volleyball.[6] When comparing the sport of softball to baseball, it is very similar in many demands and functional tasks. Their playing field is smaller, but the reaction time for a batter is directly comparable to baseball. The biggest difference between baseball and softball exists in pitching. The softball mound is flat instead of elevated as in baseball. The distance from home plate to the pitching rubber is 40 ft. for youth softball and 60ft. 6 in. for baseball. A baseball weighs 5 oz in comparison to a softball that weighs 6¼–7 oz.[41] The delivery of the pitch also differs

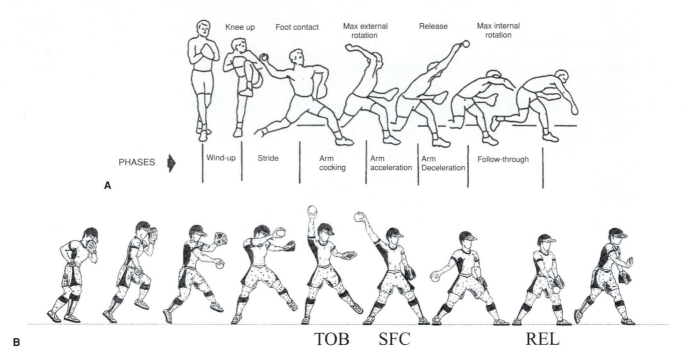

FIGURE 36-23

Six phases of pitching. TOB, top of the backswing; SFC, stride foot contact; REL, ball release. (Figure 36-41A reproduced, with permission, from Fleisig et al. Kinematic and kinetic comparison between baseball pitching and football passing. *J Appl Biomech* 12:207–224, 1996. Figure 36-41B reproduced, with permission, from Werner SL, Guido JA, McNiece RP, et al. Biomechanics of youth windmill softball pitching. *Am j Sport Med* 33(4):553, 2005.)

significantly between the windmill pitch in fast-pitch softball and the overhand release in baseball. Similar musculature is used, but in a very different order and with different mechanics (see Fig. 36-23A and B).[268]

In a review of literature, only one study in 1992 reported softball pitching injury prevalence. Results suggested that 80 percent of all injuries were in the upper extremity and 50 percent of the pitchers studied had a time-loss injury in one season. Based upon these percentages and clinical experience, it would seem necessary to investigate injury prevention strategies.[268]

Likewise, there are only two published studies on windmill pitching biomechanics, as compared to numerous studies on baseball pitching biomechanics. In these studies, it is reported that shoulder distraction forces are similar to those found in overhand pitching. Barrentine et al.[41] reported that maximum distraction stresses at the shoulder (98 percent body weight) were reached at 77 percent of the delivery phase and maximum compressive force at the elbow (70 percent body weight) occurred at the end of the delivery phase. The difference between baseball and softball pitching is the phase of pitching during which the distraction forces occur, and the position of the humerus during the pitch. In windmill pitching, maximum distraction forces at the shoulder occur during acceleration, whereas maximum shoulder distraction forces for baseball oc-

cur during windmill pitching, shoulder distraction forces occur when the humerus is in a slightly flexed position while controlling internal rotation and elbow extension during acceleration, before ball release. Notably, centrifugal distraction force on the glenohumeral joint is accentuated because the elbow remains in full extension during most of the circumduction motion. For overhand pitching, maximum shoulder distraction forces occur when the humerus is rotated internally and horizontally adducted while maintaining a position of abduction during deceleration after ball release. The biceps labrum complex and the rotator cuff are both at risk for overuse injury at these phases. Conversely, medial elbow injuries are reported less frequently in softball pitching compared to baseball, likely due to the small amount of varus torque produced during the windmill motion.[41]

It is interesting that a softball pitcher may pitch any number of consecutive innings and games, while baseball pitchers are carefully monitored and often restricted in number of pitches and innings they are allowed to throw. Softball pitchers can throw 1200–1500 pitches in a three-day period as compared to 100–150 for baseball. A reason for this seems related to the traditional belief that softball windmill pitching forces were much less in the shoulder and elbow than that of the baseball pitch.[268] This is may be true for the amount of varus torque at the elbow, but not for the distraction forces at the shoulder.

Werner et al.[268] studied the biomechanics of 53 female windmill pitchers with ages ranging from 11–19 years. Statistically significant different ranges of motion were found including greater shoulder external rotation and decreased internal rotation in the dominant arm. What remains unknown is whether these ROM differences are due to the windmill biomechanics or the concurrent demands of overhand throwing, which is also a big part of softball. Elbow-carrying angle and hyperextension were found to be similar bilaterally. Maximum elbow and shoulder distraction forces were 46 percent body weight and 94 percent body weight, respectively.

This study along with the study conducted by Barrentine et al.[41] show that the compressive forces at the elbow and the distraction forces at the shoulder are similar to baseball pitchers. Thus, allowing softball pitchers to throw an unlimited number of pitches is subjecting them to potential forces of sufficient amplitude to cause overuse injuries. With such high magnitude of shoulder distraction stress and rapid deceleration of the humerus near ball release, the posterior rotator cuff is at high risk for injury, as is the biceps labrum complex due to the combination of shoulder distraction stress and elbow extension torque.[268] With overuse, eccentric muscle loading of the posterior muscle girdle can cause stretching of these muscles allowing dynamic anterior instability of the humeral head.[41] When rehabilitating softball pitchers, it is important for the clinician to understand the stresses and forces present during pitching. Educating coaches and athletic trainers regarding these findings is also necessary for injury prevention. An important implementation for windmill pitching injury prevention may be to establish a pitch count as is traditional in baseball.

Rehabilitation and Return to Play

It is important to know the demands of the sport of softball for efficient rehabilitation. The game requires the same demands of baseball for the overhead throw, hitting, running, cutting, quick burst of acceleration and deceleration, sliding, and catching. The difference in rehabilitation occurs with the differences in the demands of pitching compared to baseball pitching. In the windmill pitch, the pectoralis major is an important contributor to the power of the pitch and also acts as a stabilizer against anterior forces. The subscapularis helps the pectoralis major in its role as a stabilizer. The serratus anterior is a scapulohumeral synchronizer.[172] The teres minor is also found to be very active in decelerating the humerus. These muscles should be highlighted in the rehabilitation program along with the standard return-to-throwing rehabilitation.

Core strengthening is also a key factor in return to play for the softball player. The demands on the core during throwing and hitting cannot be ignored. The transfer of energy from the ground through the limbs to core must provide a stable base for the upper extremities to function properly.[137]

Therefore, rehabilitation and return to play for the windmill softball pitcher may include some variations to the typical softball or baseball rehabilitation program that does not require

the windmill motion in the athlete's return to playing. As with any overhead athlete, it will be important to restore a balance of stability and mobility in the shoulder, with a strong, stable core. It is also important to strengthen scapular stabilizers as one would in any overhead athlete rehabilitation program. For the windmill pitcher, it may be more effective to include specific functional activities highlighting the demands of the pitch when acute pain and inflammation have subsided. Functional exercises that the authors of this chapter like to use are summarized in Table 36-7 with Figures 36-24 to 36-33 (see Figures 36-10 to 36-18) to demonstrate the techniques. These exercises are functional and windmill specific.

The trunk rotation with a bicep curl (Figs. 36-24a,b) mimics the motion required in the trunk and arm near and at ball release. The Theraband® provides resistance for trunk strengthening while the weight in the hand provides concentric and eccentric strengthening for the shoulder extensors/flexors and biceps.

The step-up with ipsilateral arm raise and contralateral hip extension (Fig. 36-24) synchronously fires the latissimus dorsi and hip extensors. At the beginning of the pitch delivery, the dominant leg remains in a closed chain, neutral hip position. The hip then travels into extension, which is mimicked in the step up. During the first 25 percent of the pitch delivery phase, the latissimus dorsi is very active.

The chest press on a physioball with serratus punch (Fig. 36-27A and B) challenges the core as it has to stabilize the trunk on the ball while strengthening the pectoralis major, which is a key muscle in the power of the pitch and a major stabilizer against anterior sheer forces. This exercise also incorporates the serratus anterior, which is important to strengthen as the scapula must provide a strong, stable base.

The step-up with closed-chain hip external and internal rotation (Fig. 36-28A and B) trains the hip and core in the similar motions the hip passes through from beginning of wind up (step-up phase), before and during stride foot contact (hip external rotation), and at delivery phase when the pelvis is closing and the hip goes into internal rotation.

In Figure 36-29, the athlete is strengthening the supraspinatus while challenging the core at the same time. This is important to balance the strong internal rotators, and also it is important in the overhead throw, as the pitcher must participate in overhead defensive plays as well.

Plyoball deceleration throw (Fig. 36-30A–C) helps to strengthen the shoulder concentrically and eccentrically mimicking the last portion of the pitching cycle. The push-up plus exercise (Fig. 36-32A and B) is important as the pectoralis and the serratus anterior are muscles active throughout the entire pitching cycle.

Return to pitching should be gradual with a progression of percent effort as well as number of pitches. Refer to Appendix B for a return-to-windmill pitching program. A return-to-throwing program is also included in Appendix C. The return-to-throwing guidelines should be modified to the specific athlete. Is she an exclusive pitcher who only needs to make

TABLE 36-7

Sample Functional Exercises for Return-to-Windmill Pitching

EXERCISE	MUSCLES AFFECTED	TARGETED PITCHING PHASE CYCLE
Trunk rotation with biceps curl (Fig. 36-24A and B)	Trunk and hip rotators Biceps	End of SFC to REL
Lawn mower with external rotation (Fig. 36-25A and B)	Scapular retractors Teres minor	SFC to REL
Step up/arm lift/hip extension (Fig. 36-25)	Hip extensors Latissimus dorsi	First 25% of pitch delivery (up to TOB)
Chest press on swiss ball with serratus punches (Fig. 36-27A and B)	Core stabilizers Pectoralis major Serratus anterior	Pectoralis major is a key muscle in power of entire pitch cycle and stabilizes against anterior sheer forces
Step up with hip ER/IR (Figs. 36-27A and B)	Hip extensors Hip internal rotators Hip external rotators Quads and Hamstrings	Beginning of windup to TOB (with ER movement of the exercise) At REL (with IR movement of the exercise)
"Full can" in tall kneeling on dynadisc or BOSU® (Fig. 36-28)	Core stabilizers Shoulder ER	SFC → REL
Physioball deceleration throw with therapist (Fig. 36-30A–C)	Concentric and eccentric training of biceps Shoulder flexors/extensors Trunk/hip rotators	Just after SFC → REL
Lunging with Military Press (Fig. 36-31A and B)	LE—Quads, hamstrings, hip extensors, and rotators UE—Shoulder external rotators, deltoids, latissimus dorsi Core stabilizers	No specific phase
Push up plus progression (Fig. 36-32A and B)	Pectoralis major Serratus anterior Triceps	Pectoralis and serratus active through entire cycle
Shoulder IR with Theraband® sitting on swiss ball (Fig. 36-33A and B)	Shoulder internal rotators (subscapularis) Core stabilizers	Beginning → SFC

IR, internal rotation; ER, external rotation; UE, upper extremity; LE, lower extremity; SCF, stride food contrast; REL, ball release; TOB, Top of backswing.

shorter overhand throws to the bases? Or does she also play another position when not pitching, i.e., outfield or infield? This should be a factor in the decision making regarding the final distance at which the softball player performs the throwing program. For example, an exclusive pitcher is not going to need to spend time at the 120′ and 150′ stage; more time would be focused on specific windmill exercises and shorter overhand throwing.

More research is needed in the area of windmill pitching as well as educating coaches and players in the potential risk of injury with overuse. Clearly, current research is showing forces at the shoulder to be much higher than once believed. The active female can perhaps decrease the risk of suffering from an overuse shoulder injury by following pitch guidelines closer to that of a baseball pitcher and performing a windmill-specific exercise routine.

Shoulder Injuries in the Female Swimmer

There is insufficient research to conclusively report that female swimmers actually sustain shoulder injuries at a higher rate than male swimmers. Most studies are not gender specific when injuries to the upper extremity are reported.[15,219,267,273,274] It is evident, however, that differences exist between males and females in anatomy, upper-body strength, and laxity, as previously discussed. Therefore, with high numbers of shoulder injuries reported in swimming,[267] it is important for the sports medicine personnel to understand the demands and risks that the sport imposes.

Swimming has become a very popular recreational and competitive athletic activity. Triathlons are becoming increasingly popular, as well and swimming is one of the three components. Ninety percent of complaints by swimmers that are

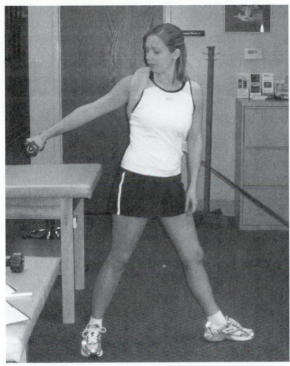
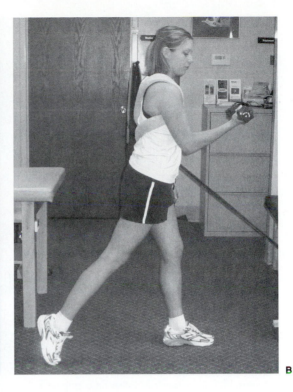

FIGURE 36-24

Trunk rotation with biceps curl. **A,** Start in stride stance facing sideways, front foot pointing forward, back foot pointing sideways with Theratubing® wrapped around waist secured at shoulder (to resist rotation). **B,** Weight in dominant/pitching hand. Perform a bicep curl while rotating trunk forward.

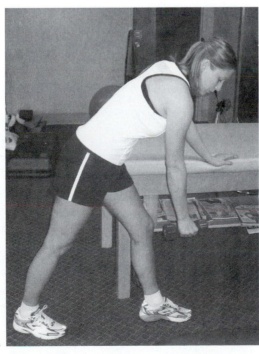
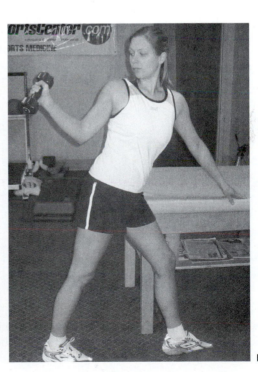

FIGURE 36-25

Lawn Mower with external rotation. **A,** Stance, forward flexion at waist with weight in hand. **B,** Retract scapula like a rowing motion, adding external rotation at the end.

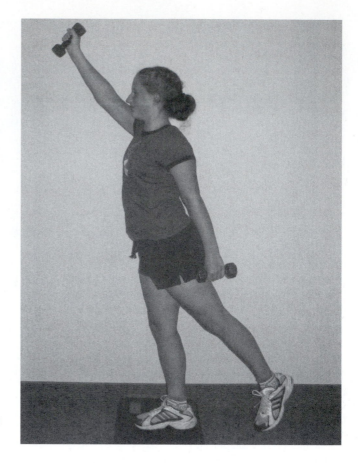

FIGURE   3 6 - 2 6

Step up/arm lift/hip extension—step onto step with dominant leg (right for right handed pitcher), lift ipsilateral arm into flexion with weight, while left leg raises into hip extension.

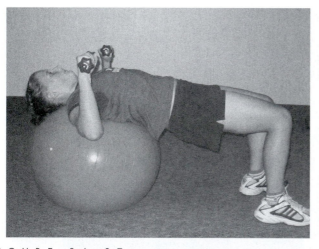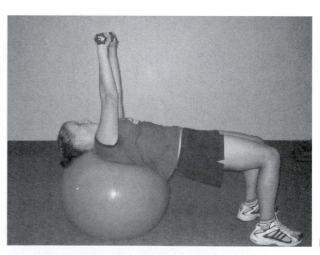

A   B

FIGURE   3 6 - 2 7

Chest press on Physioball with serratus punch. **A,** Lie on back over ball, feet shoulder width apart, dumbbells in both hands. Start with elbows bent, weights at chest. **B,** Straighten elbows pressing weights together, at the end of the motion add scapular protection.

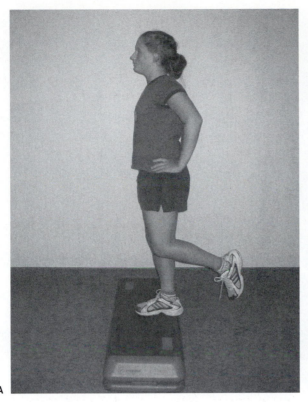
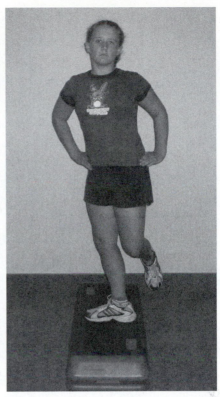

A   B

FIGURE 36-28

Step up with closed chain external rotation/internal rotation—step up onto step with
dominant leg, keep other leg in slight hip flexion with knee flexion **(A)**. Slowly rotate
into internal rotation and external rotation on dominant leg. (**B** external rotation shown).

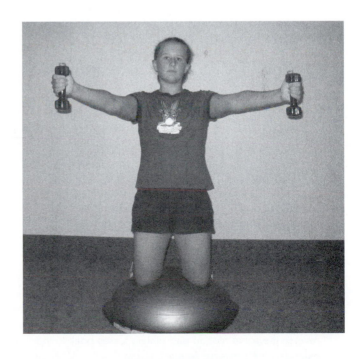

FIGURE 36-29

Full can, tall kneeling on Dynadiscs or BOSU®. Start in
tall kneeling position on balance challenging surface.
Raise weight at 45° angle thumbs up, within comfort
range. Emphasize good trunk alignment throughout
exercise.

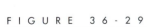

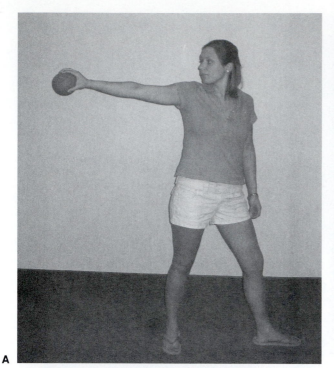

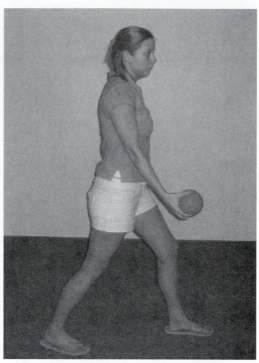

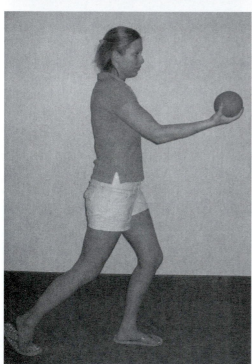

F I G U R E   3 6 - 3 0

Plyoball deceleration throw with therapist. Standing in stride stance facing sideways, horizontally abduct the shoulder and extend the elbow. Therapist tosses plyoball, athlete catches **(A)** while simultaneously rotating pelvis forward and bringing ball through **(B),** flexing the shoulder and elbow (mimicking delivery and follow through) **(C),** then reverse the same motion and athlete tosses back to therapist with shoulder and elbow extended (i.e.: reverse sequence from C→B→A). Focuses on concentric and eccentric training. Have athlete mimic their delivery as much as possible.

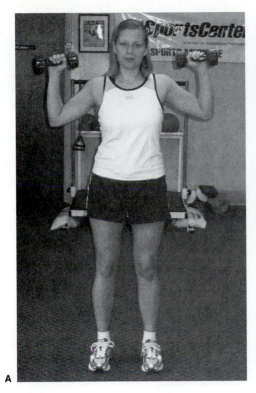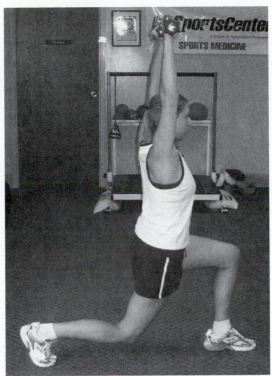

A   B

F I G U R E   3 6 - 3 1

Lunging with Military Press. Start with legs straight, elbows bent, hands shoulder height
(A). Raise arms overhead, extending elbows; as arms raise overhead, perform lunge
(B). Return to starting position.

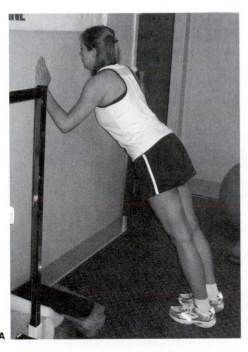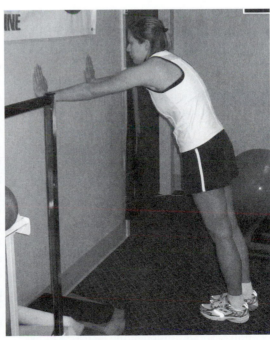

A   B

F I G U R E   3 6 - 3 2

Wall push-up "plus." Hands shoulder width apart, flex elbows as lower down to wall
(A), extend elbows and at end of exercise add an extra push (plus) into scapular
protraction **(B)**. Progression: at wall, at table, on floor, hands on wobble board or
BOSU®, feet on physioball hands on floor. Note poor trunk positioning on left.

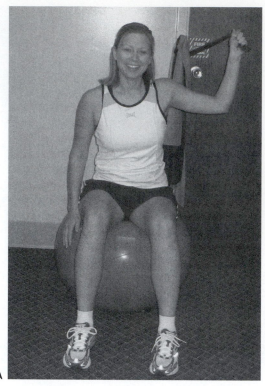
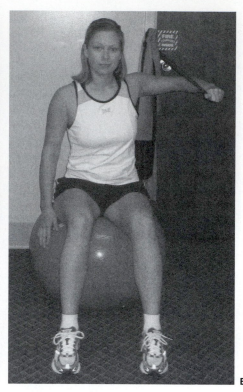

F I G U R E   3 6 - 3 3

Theraband® shoulder internal rotation on physioball. Sitting on physioball, facing away from door, grasp Theraband® at shoulder height. In the 90/90 position **(A)** pull band forward into internal rotation **(B)**. May also train external rotators by facing wall and pulling opposite direction.

significant enough to seek medical attention pertain to the shoulder.[267] Sport-specific demands of swimming include increased shoulder internal rotation and adduction strength, increased shoulder ROM, and endurance of the shoulder complex. During the freestyle stroke, most of the forward propulsion is produced by the upper body, the legs help minimally (Figs. 36-34 and 36-35). Specifically, the shoulder adductors and extensors (pectoralis major and latissimus dorsi) should be assessed. These same muscles produce internal rotation. Increases in adduction and internal rotation can lead to muscle imbalances, which can reduce glenohumeral stability and provide optimal conditions for impingement. Freestyle is used 80 percent of the time during the swimmer's training, regardless of what stroke the athlete uses competitively.[15] Therefore, impingement poses a potential problem to all swimmers.

As mentioned previously, swimming requires shoulder ROM greater than that of non-swimmers in order to excel. This increased motion allows for longer stroke length, which directly correlates to a swimmer's speed. Although the increased ROM is beneficial to performance, it can be detrimental to glenohumeral stability. Excessive ROM produces capsuloligamentous laxity, which decreases the force produced by the rotator cuff muscles to provide stability.[267]

The third specific demand includes the incredible endurance necessary of the rotator cuff and scapular stabilizers. The teres minor, infraspinatus, and subscapularis are rotator cuff muscles that fire continuously through the swimming cycle. The scapular stabilizer that also fires continuously is the serratus anterior. These muscles are at risk for fatigue with resultant possibilities of impingement or instability/subluxation of the shoulder. The repetitive nature of swimming predisposes the participant to overuse injury from microtrauma and mechanical primary impingement. This can ultimately lead to instability, rotator cuff fatigue, and resultant secondary impingement.[15] Swimmers average 8,000–20,000 m a day and may practice twice a day, with no rest days in between. This subjects the shoulder complex to an incredibly high number of stroke repetitions. An average competitive swimmer may swim 10,000 m per day. Thus, an athlete who swims 20 cycles per 50 m (estimated for the average swimmer), completes 4,000 repetitions per shoulder, every day.[15]

Unpublished data from Centinela Hospital Medical Center Biomechanics Laboratory reports that swimmers exhibited a higher incidence of positive Hawkins test than positive Neer tests for shoulder impingement.[220] The Hawkins test analyzes compression of the rotator cuff tendons under the acromion,

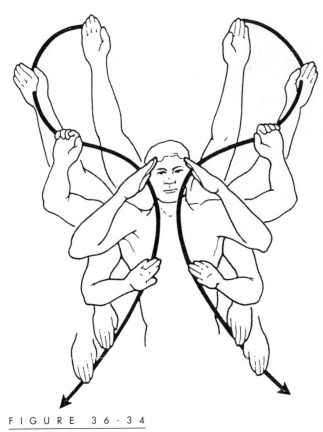

FIGURE 36-34

The S-shaped curve in pull-through. (Adapted from Pink et al. The normal shoulder during freestyle swimming. *Am J Sports Med* 19:574, 1991.)

whereas the Neer test analyzes the pinching of the rotator cuff undersurface on the anterosuperior glenoid rim. This may indicate that swimmers tend to display more problems with compression of the cuff tendons under the acromion rather than undersurface tears. EMG studies reveal swimmers with painful shoulders have altered muscle-firing patterns when compared to swimmers with no shoulder pain. The serratus

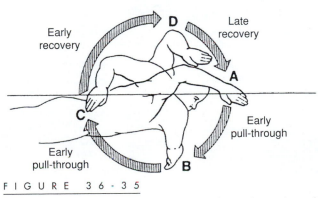

FIGURE 36-35

Phases of the freestyle swimming stroke cycle. (Adapted from Pink et al. The normal shoulder during freestyle swimming. *Am J Sports Med* 19:569–576, 1991.)

anterior has decreased muscle activity and the rhomboids have increased activity from the nonpainful shoulders, during mid pull through. If the serratus anterior is not functioning properly to aid in scapular upward rotation and protraction, then the acromion would also lack upward rotation placing the swimmer at risk for compression of the cuff tendons under the acromion.

Interestingly, the rhomboids are an antagonist muscle to the serratus anterior. When the serratus anterior fatigues, there is no other muscle that can help produce the same action. The antagonist muscle is called upon to help stabilize the scapula creating a disturbance in the synchrony of normal scapular rotation during propulsion.

As previously noted, the serratus anterior and subscapularis fire continuously throughout the freestyle stroke. The serratus anterior is firing continuously to provide a stable base for the humerus, and the subscapularis is firing due to the humerus being in predominately internal rotation throughout the stroke. These two muscles are susceptible to injury due to fatigue.[220]

In a similar example, the same research documented that the subscapularis (an internal rotator) had decreased muscle activity and the infraspinatus (an external rotator) is found to have increased muscle activity compared to normal at mid-recovery in painful shoulders. Again, the antagonist muscle is called upon when fatigue has occurred in the agonist causing potential imbalances and asynchronous movement. Another reason for the subscapularis to diminish its activity could be to avoid the extreme ranges of internal rotation motion avoiding impingement.[220]

Three-dimensional videography was used by Yanai and Hay[274] to determine when, during the swimming motion, the shoulder experienced impingement. During the front crawl in swimming, on average, impingement occurred 24.8 percent of the stroke time. However, each subject monitored experienced impingement in some cycles and not others. This suggests that stroke technique may play a factor in susceptibility to impingement.[274] Some studies show that between 50 and 70 percent of the time, shoulder pain was reported during pull through[76,228]; however others report impingement occurs more often during the recovery stage.[273,274] During early pull-through, the pectoralis major and the teres minor are highly active, with their activity peaking at mid pull-through. The teres minor is the prime contributor to maintaining humeral head congruency in the glenoid due to its insertion closer to the axis of rotation than the pectoralis. In painful shoulders, the most notable difference during pull-thorough was decreased muscle activity of the serratus anterior.[220]

The hand entry position during freestyle stroke is also reported to be a frequent point of pain in swimmers.[273] During hand entry and forward reach, the upper trapezius, rhomboids, and serratus anterior are all active to form a force couple to properly position the glenoid fossa. The supraspinatus and the anterior and middle deltoid are also active to abduct and flex the humerus as the hand reaches forward in the water. Without the supraspinatus, the deltoid proper firing of predisposes the humeral head to excessive movement within glenoid fossa.[220]

TABLE 36-8

Typical Signs and Symptoms and Possible Causes of Swimmer's Shoulder

SIGNS AND SYMPTOMS	POSSIBLE CAUSE
Postural deformities of rounded shoulders and thoracic kyphosis	Tightness of the pectoralis minor
Weakness of the posterior cuff muscles and scapular stabilizers	Weakness can be due to strength imbalances between the anterior and posterior muscles secondary to the demands of the sport and to stretch weakness
Limited internal rotation and excessive external rotation ROM	Tightness of the posterior capsule or posterior cuff muscles which causes a shift in the available ROM
Decay of normal scapulothoracic rhythm	Tightness of the anterior chest musculature and weakness of the scapular stabilizers

Adapted from Allegrucci M, Whitney SL, Irrgang JJ. Clinical implications of secondary impingement of the shoulder in freestyle swimmers. *J Orthop Sports Phys Ther* 20(6):313, 1994.[15]

Rehabilitation and Return to Swimming

Shoulder rehabilitation for these female swimmers should be multifaceted. Great emphasis should be placed on restoring normal ROM, strength, and endurance based on the evaluative findings. Typical signs and symptoms of possible causes of swimmer's shoulder can be found in Table 36-8. Exercises should incorporate trunk and hip movements along with both scapular and glenohumeral neuromuscular retraining. Core stability should also be emphasized in the shoulder rehabilitation program as it needs to provide a stable base for the athlete to propel their body forward.

RANGE OF MOTION

Flexibility and mobilization techniques should reflect the findings from the evaluation. Importance should be given to restore normal ROM without compromising stability. The most typical restrictions are found in the posterior portion of the glenohumeral joint capsule or tightness of the posterior rotator cuff muscles.[267] Swimmers, in general, tend to spend more time stretching their anterior capsule. This results in loss of internal rotation and horizontal adduction. Horizontal adduction may be improved by stabilizing the scapula on the thorax while crossing the arm over the chest. This can be performed at 90° of shoulder flexion and above to get all portions of the cuff. Posterior capsule flexibility is improved by flexing the shoulder to 90° and providing a downward force on the flexed elbow (Fig. 36-36).

Internal rotation ROM, rather than external rotation, at the end range of abduction proves to be important for swimmers. This motion is most important during the late recovery stage of the freestyle stroke. Internal rotation should be stretched at 90°, 135°, and at end-range abduction. External rotation stretching should still be carried out if it is lacking. Other important muscles to check for normal flexibility include the pectoralis major and minor, upper trapezius, levator scapulae, biceps, triceps, and serratus anterior. Swimming stokes do not happen in a straight cardinal plane of motion; during the arm cycle there are multiple combinations of movements taking place.[15] A flexibility program can be creatively structured with this in mind.

STRENGTH AND ENDURANCE TRAINING

Development of a strength and endurance training program should focus on restoring normal balance to the anterior and

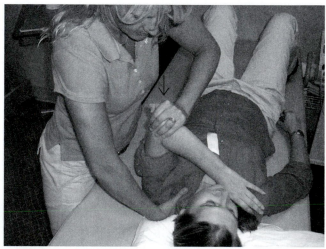

FIGURE 36-36

Posterior capsule glenohumeral joint mobilization. Stabalize scapula, direction of force is through elbow toward table.

TABLE 36-9

Considerations and Rationale in a Strengthening Program for Swimmers

PRIMARY CONSIDERATIONS	RATIONALE
Isolation of the rotator cuff and scapulohumeral muscles. (Correctly train prime movers/stabilizers, not antagonists)	EMG studies demonstrate cuff muscles act independent of each other during the stroke cycle
Muscular endurance, high repetitions of specific exercises (sprint, middle, or long distant swimmer—should reflect in number of repetitions given)	Swimming involves excessive repetition and muscular endurance, 3 sets of 10 repetitions would be inadequate
Sports-specific function	Exercises specific to the swimmers stroke and body postures help return to sport as efficiently and quickly as possible

posterior shoulder musculature. It also should focus on restoring equilibrium between scapular and humeral movements. It is important to remember that increased adduction and internal rotation strength is unavoidable in swimmers. To avoid muscular imbalance, emphasis on rotator cuff exercises with importance on external rotation strength is beneficial.[267] The three primary considerations in a strengthening program are (1) isolate the rotator cuff and scapular muscles, (2) implement endurance exercises, and (3) include sports-specific functional exercises.[15] Table 36-9 provides primary considerations and rationale for developing a strengthening program for swimmers.

Female swimmers appear to be highly susceptible to secondary impingement due to flexibility, strength, and muscular endurance factors discussed earlier. Please refer to Chapter 25 for details on primary and secondary impingement. Refer to Table 36-10 for basic guidelines for progression of treatment for swimmer's shoulders with 2° impingement. The initial goal in the rehabilitation program is to establish a stable scapular base and strengthen the rotator cuff muscles in a neutral position. Phase II introduces exercises up to 90°. In phase III, overhead exercises can be initiated with functional training. Phase IV is gradual return to athletic activity, progressing in speed and distance.[15] Most swimming programs emphasize only on upper-extremity strengthening and function. Challenging core stability during some upper-extremity exercises is beneficial to the athlete. Swimming is a chain of events involving the arms, trunk, and legs together. Focusing solely on the shoulder complex fails to address all areas of the kinetic chain vital to swimming efficiency and performance.

PROPRIOCEPTION AND FUNCTIONAL TRAINING

Retraining joint proprioception in freestyle swimmers, and all athletes, is important. Are differences seen in swimming stroke patterns with painful shoulders intentional changes to avoid pain, or caused by inadequate feedback from joint receptors due to capsular damage? Multiple studies have shown propriocep-

tive deficits in subjects with glenohumeral joint multidirectional instability.[33,45,87] However, no studies specific to symptomatic swimming athletes are available. Proprioception is derived from both conscious and unconscious components (refer to Chapter 15). Making the athlete consciously aware of humeral and scapular position during strength training and swimming may help to improve conscious proprioception. However only conscious training is not enough, unconscious neuromuscular output is also vital to athletic performance. Training unconscious proprioceptive awareness can be carried out with plyometric training.[15]

Plyometric training is used to not only enhance power and explosiveness but may also help improve "synchrony of movement that is needed for the swimming stroke" (Ref. 15, p. 315). Progression of an upper-extremity plyometric training program for swimmers should include progressing the degree of shoulder abduction (starting in more neutral positions increasing to overhead); progressing the weight of the medicine ball; and increasing speed, repetitions, and difficulty.

Closed-chain exercises can be useful in rehabilitation of the swimmer because they mimic how the body is pulled over the arms during pull through, as well as it engages the trunk and core muscles to stabilize.[15] For example, in phase III a Theraband® can be used to provide resistance mimicking the pull through phase while the athlete is prone over a physioball (Fig. 36-37A–C). This forces the core muscles to stabilize the athlete's body as her arm is going through a specific motion. During this exercise, it is important to keep the shoulder at 90° of abduction to ensure proper mechanics and avoid impingement. Internal obliques are also important muscles to strengthen due to the rotation required at the trunk for the swimmer to body roll during freestyle. If core muscles are weak or lack endurance, they will not provide a stable base for the upper extremities. As discussed in several contexts, but especially important in the swimmer, a weak core can be a contributing factor in a shoulder injury.[116,144]

T A B L E   3 6 - 1 0

Basic Guidelines for Progression of Treatment for Swimmer's Shoulders with 2° Impingement

Phase I

Modalities prn for pain control

Address ROM losses

Rotator cuff strengthening at 0°
- Side lying ER
- Theraband® ER/IR at 0°
- Theraband® ER/IR isometric "step-always"

Scapulothoracic muscle in neutral
- Shrugs
- Prone arm raise at 0°
- Scapular retraction (row)
- Prone ball roll (for lower trap)
- Prone ball stabilization on floor

Aerobic conditioning
- Bike
- Kicking in water

Phase II (0–90°)

Rotator cuff strengthening
- Prone ER
- Theraband® ER
- Prone arm raise with ER at 90°, progress to 120°
- Elevation in scapular plane with IR (empty can)

Scapulothoracic exercises
- Scapular protraction (supine on ball progress to standing using Theraband® with shoulder at 90°, and in a weight-bearing position on 1/2 foam roller)
- Stabilization exercises
  - Bilateral → unilateral
  - Add dynamic resistance
  - Progress to stabilizing on a ball
- Push-up "plus" progression
  - Wall → table → modified (on knees) → regular

Axial humeral muscles
- Flexion
- Abduction in the plane of the scapula (challenge core in BOSU® in tall kneeling)
- Lat pull-down
- Chest press (challenge core stability by laying supine on ball)
- Bench press

Proprioception
- Active and passive matching

Aerobic conditioning
- Upper body ergometer
- Rower
- Kicking in water

Phase III—Functional training

Full range flexion and abduction strengthening

Combined movement patterns
- Proprioceptive neuromuscular facilitation D1 and D2 (Theraband®, Bodyblade®, manual, plyoball)

Stroke-specific exercise
- Simulation of pull-through and reverse pull-through with Theraband® (prone on swiss ball to challenge core at same time). Figure 36-37A–C.
- Simulation of recovery:
  (1) Prone horizontal abduction with ER
  (2) Prone horizontal adduction with IR at 160°
  (3) Theraband®-resisted ER at 30° of abduction progress to 90° of abduction

Plyometric exercises

Swim bench (if available)

ER, external rotation; IR, internal rotation.

Adapted and modified from Allegrucci M, Whitney SL, Irrgang JJ. Clinical implications of secondary impingement of the shoulder in freestyle swimmers. *J Orthop Sports Phys Ther* 20(6):316, 1994.[15]

Throughout the rehabilitation program, it is feasible for the athlete to continue swimming with use of swimming aids (i.e., kickboard held under the body), modification of yardage, and altered rest time. This active rest concept is dependent on the severity and nature of shoulder injury and should be athlete and injury specific. For example, an impingement injury due to fatigue of the posterior cuff muscles may still respond positively to treatment in conjunction with a significant decrease in yardage and increase in rest time before swimming again to avoid fatigue. It is vital to educate both the coach and swimmer that at the first sign of shoulder pain the athlete is to stop swimming.[15]

In conclusion, freestyle swimmers can present with signs and symptoms of either instability or impingement, or a combination of both. The rotator cuff provides stability at the glenohumeral joint and can therefore be a source of pain or disability when instability or impingement occurs. It is essential to provide the optimum environment for the rotator cuff to work effectively by balancing adequate stability with the appropriate mobility in the shoulder complex. Accordingly, for an efficient and effective rehabilitation program, clinicians must have knowledge of the sport-specific skills that are required. Finally, creativity in designing the rehabilitation program to incorporate the core with upper-extremity activities and meet the swimmers'

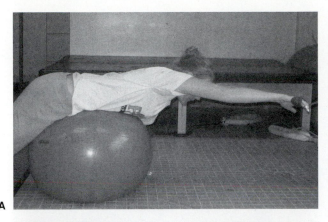
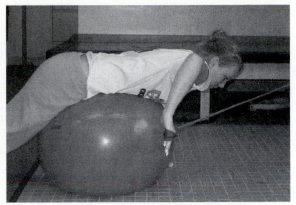
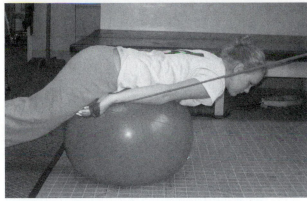

FIGURE 36-37

Example of swimming exercise to mimic pull-through, using Theraband®, while stabilizing core on ball. **A,** Starting position. **B,** Middle, keep elbow at 90°. **C,** Ending position. Note proper trunk, head, neck position throughout.

demands (sprinter, middle, or long-distance swimmer) is essential as well.[15]

CONSIDERATIONS IN THE FEMALE GYMNAST

The final sport for special consideration in regard to the female athlete is gymnastics. Gymnastics is important to consider due to its high potential for both micro- and macrotraumatic injuries as well as vulnerability of its athletes to body image issues that will be elaborated upon in the female athlete triad section. Certainly, similar considerations may exist in sports not mentioned; however, it is beyond the scope of this chapter to attempt to cover all sports in which women participate.

Multiple injuries occur in gymnasts of all ages and ability levels, whether recreational or competitive. Women's gymnastics involves four apparatus: beam, floor exercise, vault, and uneven bars. Men's gymnastics involves six apparatus: floor exercise, rings, parallel bars, pommel horse, vault, and high bar. The demands of this sport include great flexibility, incredible strength, balance, and explosive power. Competitive gymnastics require intensive training with a large time commitment, usu-

ally at a young age. The average junior elite gymnast (age 10–14) spends over 5 days per week training, for a total of approximately 25 hours a week.[55] Such demands on a young body is not without penalty. The period of rapid growth, which occurs in adolescence, causes the young gymnast to be more susceptible to injury than the postpubescent gymnast.[55] Questions also arise in regards to the possibility of stunted or inhibited growth during these vital years of development and maturation.[56,260,266]

Gymnasts sustain a large variety of injuries. Caine et al.[55] followed 50 competitive gymnasts over a 1-year period tracking injuries. The most commonly injured regions in the body by order of frequency were (1) the lower extremity (63.7 percent), particularly the ankle and knee; (2) the upper extremity (20.4 percent), particularly the wrist; (3) and the spine and trunk (15.2 percent), particularly the lower back. These findings are consistent with other multiple studies conducted.[31,55,167,237,254] Gymnasts were most likely to injure themselves on the floor exercise (35.4 percent), followed by the balance beam (23.1 percent), the uneven bars (20 percent), and lastly the vault (13.8 percent). The remaining 7.7 percent of injuries were placed under "other," pertaining to possible warm-up or conditioning periods. The distribution between sudden onset and gradual onset of injury was 44.2 percent and 55.8 percent, respectively. Clearly traumatic as well as overuse injuries occur in this sport.

Female gymnasts of today are shorter, lighter, and mature later than their predecessors 30 years earlier. Increased magnitude and intensity of training at an early age has become standard. The question arises whether these external characteristics are due to self-selection for gymnastics or due to inadequate nutrition for the level of activity during this crucial period of development.[56] Studies have suggested shorter femoral leg length seen in female gymnasts may be due to the repetitive compressive stress causing premature closure of femoral and tibial epiphyses.[56,57,178,259] A short-term longitudinal study by Mansfield and Emans[178] reported that gymnasts advance through puberty without a normal pubertal growth spurt. Catch-up growth does occur once the gymnast retires from the sport or significantly reduces training[56]; however, it is questionable if adequate growth and normal height are eventually achieved. Longitudinal studies of one set of triplets and two sets of twins (one gymnast, other one(s) not) reveal significantly later onset of menarche when compared to their nongymnast sibling. In the set of triplets, energy expenditure exceeded energy intake by 600 kcal and the gymnast had lower body weight and percent body fat compared to her siblings.[56]

Lower levels of hormones and decreased serum growth factors have also been identified in gymnasts. Serum leptin is involved in the regulation of energy intake and energy expenditure. Leptin is secreted by adipocytes and binds to an appetite-stimulating neuropeptide, which produces neurons in the hypothalamus. Leptin levels increase with food intake and decrease during periods of starvation. Low body fat levels have been linked to low levels of leptin. A decline in leptin levels has an effect on the secretion of gonadotropins and sex steroids, which may be a factor in delayed menarche and amenorrhea leading to the female athlete triad, which will be discussed in detail further in this chapter.[266]

Some additional noteworthy considerations in the sport of gymnastics include (1) gymnasts do not wear any type of supportive shoe while training and competing, making it difficult to correct faulty biomechanics at the foot with any type of orthosis; (2) the typical postural salute to judges, and landing of jumps and dismounts, is a hyperlordotic position of the lumbar spine, potentially contributing to trunk instability problems (Fig. 36-38); (3) gymnastics, unlike many sports has a significant amount of skills and activities performed with the upper extremities in a closed-chain position; and (4) gymnasts jump and land from various heights with twisting and rotational components. With these factors in mind, focus should be placed on balancing strength and flexibility to help correct faulty biomechanics or structural faults; emphasis placed on core strength and stability and education of gymnasts should occur regarding ideal trunk posturing at the beginning and end of routines. Likewise, education on proper jumping and landing must be an integral part of training and rehabilitation. Refer to the section

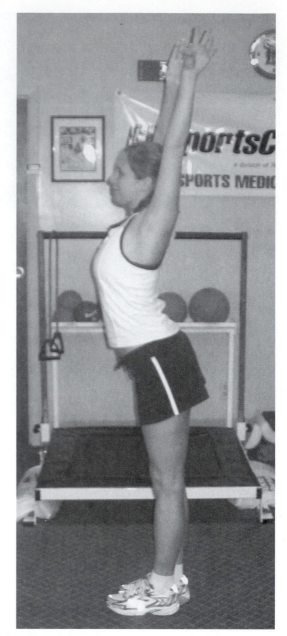

F I G U R E   3 6 - 3 8

Typical gymnast pose before/after routines and landing jumps/tumbling moves. Note excessive lumbar lordosis.

in this chapter on ACL injury prevention and rehabilitation for more detail on jumping and landing.

Additional rehabilitation for specific injuries of vulnerable areas should follow suggestions for sport-specific rehabilitation as presented in Chapters 18 and 32.

Of additional concern are the body image requirements and subsequent disorders common in the sport of gymnastics potentially leading to inadequate caloric intake.[56,57,260] Educating the coaches, gymnast, and rehabilitation staff in regard to the female athlete triad potential risks of osteoporosis and stress fractures, as well as stunted growth patterns, is important.

THE FEMALE ATHLETE TRIAD

Historical Perspective and Evolution

One of the considerations that factors into many sports in which the active female participates is known as the female athlete triad. The female athlete triad was first described by Yeager et al.[275] in the early 1990s. The term *female athlete triad* was originally used to describe the connection between three independent clinical disorders: eating disorders, amenorrhea, and osteoporosis. Continued research and discussion among sports medicine personnel led to the American College of Sports Medicine (ACSM) publishing an initial position statement on the female athlete triad in 1997. The purpose of the position statement was to provide more direction for identification, prevention, and treatment of these individual and connected medical disorders in this specialty population.[214]

Evolution of this original concept has continued. Classification of eating disorders such as anorexia nervosa (AN), bulimia nervosa (BN), and eating disorder not otherwise specified (EDNOS) were the severe forms of nutritional deficit that were observed. Since a minority of female athletes fit the diagnostic criteria for any of these diseases, the term *eating disorders* has been expanded to include the concept of disordered eating patterns that encompasses a wide range of harmful nutritional strategies and behaviors associated with the other factors of the triad.[12,13] The term *osteoporosis* has been modified by some to osteopenia in order to include this less severe form of bone loss that is more commonly seen in females screened and diagnosed with the triad. More recently, discussion has continued regarding the use of the term amenorrhea and possible refinement of this term to include all menstrual irregularities and other reproductive dysfunctions that are associated with, or independent of, amenorrhea. These other dysfunctions are seen intermittently in association with other components of the female athlete triad and include oligomennorhea, anovulation, and altered luteal phase length.[203,215] In summary, the revised concept of the *female athlete triad* describes the interaction and coexistence of eating disorders/disordered eating behavior, menstrual irregularities, and decreased bone mineral density (BMD) (Fig. 36-39).[150,215]

Components

DISORDERED EATING BEHAVIORS

There is a very important relationship between the amount of calories consumed and the amount of calories expended for any athlete. The appropriate balance of ingested calories versus calories expended is critical for optimal performance, maintenance of or safe alteration of body composition, and prevention of health problems.[68] For the female athlete, the prevention of health problems includes

- establishing and maintaining normal menstruation,
- preservation of a strong immune system,
- and building and repairing muscle tissue and bone.[68,215,276]

A "negative energy balance" resulting from a negative calorie balance (intake less than output) sustained over time can be due to many factors ranging from, in decreasing severity, a clinically diagnosed eating disorder, the elimination of a food group, i.e., dairy or meat from the diet, to inadvertently not eating enough to keep up with a sudden or unexpected increase in a training schedule. The internal and external pressures to achieve athletic success, attain a body composition of unreasonably low body fat percentage, and/or achieve or maintain unrealistically low body weight often lead to disordered eating patterns and occasionally to clinical eating disorders.[36,117,147,204,214,215,243,275]

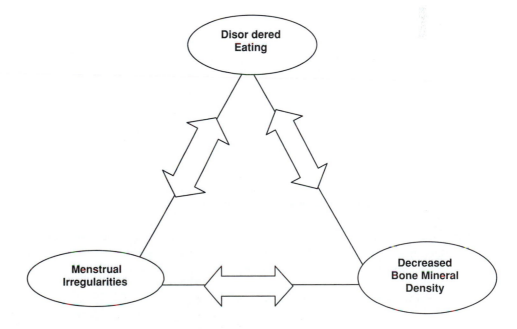

The female athlete triad.

TABLE 36-11

Diagnostic Criteria for AN[21]

A. Refusal to maintain body weight at or above a minimally normal weight for age and height. Weight loss leading to maintenance of body weight <85% of that expected; or failure to make expressed weight gain during period of growth, leading to body weight <85% of that expected.
B. Intense fear of gaining weight or becoming fat, even though underweight.
C. Disturbance in the way in which one's body weight or shape is experienced; undue influence of body weight or shape on self-evaluation; or denial of the seriousness of the current low body weight.
D. In postmenarchal females, amenorrhea, i.e., the absence of at least three consecutive menstrual cycles. A female is considered to have amenorrhea if her periods occur only following hormone administration.

Specific type

Restricting type: During the episode of AN the person does not regularly engage in binge eating or purging behavior, i.e., self-induced vomiting or misuse of laxatives or diuretics.

Binge eating/purging type: During the episode of AN, the person regularly engages in binge eating or purging behavior, i.e., self-induced vomiting or misuse of laxatives or diuretics.

Adapted from DSM-IV, American Psychiatric Association, 1994.

Clinical eating disorders include AN, BN, and EDNOS.[21] Each of these types have specific criteria that confirm the diagnosis known as Diagnostic and Statistical Manual (DSM) criteria for eating disorders (see Tables 36-11 to 36-13). AN represents the extreme of voluntary starvation with severe caloric restriction and an altered self-image, viewing herself as overweight when in reality she is as much as 15 percent below of her ideal body weight. The prevalence of AN is 0.5 to 1 percent in adolescent and young adult women as compared to 2–4 percent with BN.[1] BN is characterized by a "binge and purge" eating behavior. Binging occurs as a result of physiologic hunger followed by purging to eliminate the caloric intake.[1] Purging behaviors take a multitude of forms including vomiting, laxative use, diuretic use, enemas, and excessive exercise.[1,147,204,215,230,275] Physiologic and psychological problems resulting from this purging behavior include fluid and electrolyte imbalances, dehydration, acid-base imbalances, cardiac arrhythmia, the enlargement of the parotid glands, erosion of tooth enamel, gastrointestinal disorders, low self-esteem, anxiety, depression, and reported cases of suicide.[1,147,204,215,230,275] EDNOS includes those individuals who meet every other criteria for AN except amenorrhea/oligomenorrhea or decreased body weight or those individuals who demonstrate all other criteria for BN with a decreased frequency or duration of the purging behavior. This

TABLE 36-12

Diagnostic Criteria for BN[21]

A. Recurrent episodes of binge eating. An episode of binge eating is characterized by both of the following:
    1. Eating, in a discrete period of time, e.g., within any 2-hour period, an amount of food that is definitely larger than most people would eat during a similar period of time and under similar circumstances, and
    2. A sense of lack of control over eating during the episode, e.g., a feeling that one cannot stop eating or control what or how much one is eating.
B. Recurrent inappropriate compensatory behavior in order to prevent weight gain, such as self-induced vomiting; misuse of laxatives, diuretics or other medications; fasting; or excessive exercise.
C. The binge eating and inappropriate compensatory behaviors both occur, on average, at least twice a week for 3 months.
D. Self-evaluation is unduly influenced by body shape and weight.
E. The disturbance does not occur exclusively during episodes of AN.

Specific type

Purging type: The person regularly engages in self-induced vomiting or the misuse of laxatives or diuretics.

Nonpurging type: The person uses other inappropriate compensatory behaviors, such as fasting or excessive exercise, but does not regularly engage in self-induced vomiting or the misuse of laxatives or diuretics.

Adapted from DSM-IV, American Psychiatric Association, 1994.

TABLE 36-13

Diagnostic Criteria for EDNOS[21]

A. For females, all of the criteria for AN are met, except the individual has regular menses.
B. All criteria for AN are met except that, despite significant weight loss, the person's current weight is in the normal range.
C. All criteria for BN are met except that the binge eating and inappropriate compensatory mechanisms occur at a frequency of less than two week for duration of less than 3 months.
D. Regular use of inappropriate compensatory behavior by an individual of normal body weight after eating small amounts of food (self-induced vomiting after consumption of two cookies).
E. Repeatedly chewing and spitting out, but not swallowing, large amounts of food.
F. Binge-eating disorder. Recurrent episodes of binge eating in the absence of the regular use of inappropriate compensatory behaviors characteristic of BN.

Adapted from DSM-IV American Psychiatric Association, 1994.

additional category, EDNOS may lead to better detection and treatment of those female athletes who exhibit the criteria for AN but paradoxically remain "normal" body weight because of the increased lean body mass.[147,215,275] Despite the strides that have been made in the classification of disordered eating, there are a plethora of unhealthy eating behaviors which elude the AN, BN, or EDNOS diagnoses and result in a negative energy balance.

It is difficult to estimate the number of female athletes who demonstrate disordered eating or unhealthy eating habits. Several different surveys were attempted in the past, using collegiate female athletes and the prevalence of eating disorders. The results of these surveys ranged from 6 to 60 percent depending upon the administration, the athletic population, and the defining criteria.[36,37,117,156,214,230] In a recent study, Reinking et al. concluded that female athletes did not exhibit more disordered eating behaviors than nonathletes at a NCAA Division I institution.[225] In this study, 7.1 percent of female athletes and 12.9 percent of nonathletes were classified as having a high risk of disordered eating behaviors. The reasons that lead to this wide range are multifaceted. Many athletes consider disordered eating patterns normal and harmless. Others will deny disordered eating patterns on standard questionnaires. Many studies referenced to assess the prevalence of eating disorders use questionnaires that assess symptoms of eating disorders without an assessment by a trained clinician or a screening tool that confirm defined disordered eating patterns.[203] Such studies remain valuable but lead to a wide range of prevalence. In 2004, the National Eating Disorder Screening program screened over 16,000 students and 59 percent scored positive for symptoms of an eating disorder.[2]

There are several theories as to why disordered eating patterns occur. These include inappropriate popular perceptions, biological factors, and psychological reasons. Many attribute the evolution of these unhealthy eating patterns to the overwhelming desire to be thin.[117,204,214,215] Specifically with athletes, this desire is often held in conjunction with the desire to win at all costs.[82] Many female athletes think and are told that thinner

is better. There is a perception among athletes, coaches, and the media that thinner athletes are faster, stronger, and more powerful. Biological imbalances in neurotransmitters (serotonin, norepinephrine, and melatonin) have been suggested as an etiology for eating disorders.[147] Psychological factors include poor coping skills leading to poor stress management, insufficient family support, sexual and/or physical abuse, and low self-esteem.[147] Struggling with many changes in their bodies, adolescent female athletes are particularly at risk for development of disordered eating patterns that may be the stepping stone for the other components of the female athlete triad. Early detection with knowledge of the warning signs of eating disorders is key (Table 36-14).

MENSTRUAL IRREGULARITIES

Menstrual irregularities include primary amenorrhea, secondary amenorrhea, oligomenorrhea, suppressed luteal phase (luteal phase deficiency), and anovulation.[248] Amenorrhea is defined as the absence of menstrual bleeding and classified as either primary or secondary. Primary amenorrhea refers to absence of menstrual bleeding by the age of 16 even though other female sex characteristics are apparent or by age 14 in the absence of sexual development. Secondary amenorrhea is defined as the cessation of the menstrual cycle for at least 3 months after the initiation of menstruation. Amenorrhea, as defined by the International Olympic Committee, means less than two menstrual cycles per year.[8,248] The main difference between primary and secondary amenorrhea is that in the latter, at least one menstrual cycle occurred indicating a functioning reproductive chain including the hypothalamus, pituitary gland, ovaries, and uterus capable of completing a menstrual cycle.[106,182] In cases of secondary amenorrhea, this chain has been disrupted and does not function normally.

The normal physiology of menstruation is a complex, coordinated interaction of hormonal and organ systems occurring in a cyclical manner.[106,117] The menstruation cycle is divided into three phases: the follicular phase when the egg matures, the ovulatory phase during which the egg is released,

TABLE 36-14

Warning Signs of Eating Disorders[82,147,214]

AN	BN
Physical signs	**Physical signs**
• Significant weight loss unrelated to medical illness	• Swollen parotid glands
• Fat and muscle atrophy	• Face and extremity edema
• Amenorrhea	• Sore throat and chest pain
• Dry hair and skin	• Fatigue
• Cold, discolored hands, and feet	• Bloating, Abdominal pain
• Decreased body temperature	• Diarrhea or constipation
• Cold intolerance	• Menstrual irregularities
• Lightheadedness	• Callous formation or scars on knuckles (Russell's sign)
• Decreased ability to concentrate	• Erosion of dental enamel
• Bradycardia	**Behaviors**
• Lanugo (fine, baby hair)	• Exhibits much concern about weight
Behaviors	• Eating patterns that alternate between purging and fasting
• Severe reduction in food intake	• Depression, guilt and/or shame especially following a binge
• Excessive denial of hunger	
• Compulsive and/or excessive exercising without signs of fatigue or weakness	
• Peculiar, ritualistic patterns of food handling	
• Intense fear of weight gain	

and the luteal phase in which the uterine lining prepares for the implantation of the fertilized ovum. If implantation does not occur, then the uterine lining is sloughed and menstrual bleeding begins.[106,118,182] The hypothalamus produces and secretes Gonadotropin-releasing hormone (GnRH) regularly. This affects the intact and functioning pituitary gland to produce luteinizing hormone (LH) and follicle-stimulating hormone (FSH). LH and FSH stimulate the ovaries for maturation and release of oocytes (eggs). The ovaries cyclically produce estrogen and progesterone, which stimulate the endometrium (uterine lining) to develop and the cyclical withdrawal of estrogen and progesterone resulting in menstrual shedding. This ultimately leads to menstrual bleeding from a normal uterus with an unobstructed tract to the external genetalia.[106,182] This well-coordinated yet complicated cycle of events may be disrupted anywhere along this process demonstrating that there are many reasons for the onset of amenorrhea (Table 36-15).[182] Pregnancy and hypothalamic amenorrhea are the two most common reasons for the cessation of menstrual cycles. One subset of hypothalamic amenorrhea is "exercise-related" or "athletic" amenorrhea.[182] It is important to note that amenorrhea is not a normal consequence of athletic participation. The diagnosis of athletic amenorrhea is one of exclusion of all the other possible causes of amenorrhea. This diagnosis requires an extensive evaluation by a physician with experience and expertise with athletic women.

The loss of menstrual cycling coincident with exercise has long been recognized by professional dancers, athletes, coaches,

and the medical profession.[117,156,182] The etiology, prevalence, and treatment of athletic amenorrhea are not completely known and agreed upon to date. In the early 1970s, it was proposed that low body fat and weight were the cause of this cessation of menstrual bleeding. This hypothesis has since been refuted, and other factors have been postulated and are currently under investigation. These factors include the physical stress of exercise, increased endogenous opoids from exercise, and overall energy availability based on the "energy balance" discussed previously.[169,170,182,191,215] All of these factors are postulated to directly effect the GnRH's production and release from the hypothalamus.

The prevalence of amenorrhea is difficult to accurately assess because some female athletes and coaches welcome the cessation of menstrual bleeding. This condition indicates to these

TABLE 36-15

Causes of Amenorrhea[182]

Pregnancy
Abnormalities of the reproductive tract
Ovarian failure
Pituitary tumors
Hypothalamic amenorrhea
Chronic anovulaton
Polycystic ovarian disease
Exercise-associated amenorrhea

athletes and coaches sufficient training rather than a problem, so medical workup is not even considered. It is reported that 10–20 percent of vigorously exercising women are amenorrheic compared to 5 percent of the general population when pregnant women are excluded.[182] The prevalence of amenorrhea in elite runners and professional ballet dancers is documented to be as high as 40–50 percent.[156,182] The amenorrheic state is not without consequences. The dangers of prolonged amenorrhea include reversible loss of reproductive capacity and possibly irreversible bone loss. The long-term consequences of adolescent amenorrhea are yet to be fully understood and described.

Oligomenorrhea is defined as menstrual cycles greater than 36 days or having less than 8 menses a year.[11,182,214,215] This may result from anovulation which results from low levels of both estrogen and progesterone or normal estrogen production but low levels of progesterone.[182] Female athletes with luteal suppression often present with irregular menses. This component of the female athlete triad still emphasizes amenorrhea, but an expanded view of the triad includes all menstrual irregularities. Detection of menstrual irregularities is often identified by interview or completed self-questionnaire by a female athlete. The preparticipation screening process is an ideal time to as-

sess for these irregularities and appropriately refer to a medical expert such as a physician with experience and expertise with athletic women for a thorough evaluation.

DECREASED BONE MINERAL DENSITY

Osteoporosis is currently the most common bone disease, affecting over 25 million Americans to date.[7] The definition per the Consensus Development Conference on Osteoporosis is a disease characterized by low bone mass, microarchitectural deterioration of bone tissue leading to enhanced skeletal fragility, and an increased risk for fracture.[203] Measures of BMD with dual-energy X-ray absorptiometry (DEXA)[248] are used to diagnose osteoporosis and osteopenia with diagnostic criteria that have been established for postmenopausal women (Fig. 36-40).[7] Unfortunately, there are no similar diagnostic criteria that have been established for premenopausal women to date.[203]

There are two types of bone: cortical bone that is composed of tightly compacted plates of bone and trabecular or spongy bone which is made up of bone spicules separated by spaces in a honeycomb fashion.[105,248] The peripheral skeleton (long bones) is comprised predominantly of cortical bone. This bone is less susceptible to changes in reproductive hormones than the

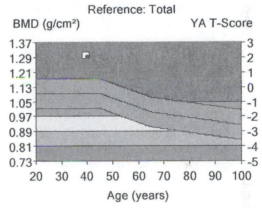

Region	BMD (g/cm²) [1]	Young-Adult [2] (%)	Young-Adult [2] T-Score	Age-Matched [3] (%)	Age-Matched [3] Z-Score
Head	2.351	-	-	-	-
Arms	1.177	-	-	-	-
Legs	1.386	-	-	-	-
Trunk	1.003	-	-	-	-
Ribs	0.703	-	-	-	-
Pelvis	1.252	-	-	-	-
Spine	1.178	-	-	-	-
Total	1.295	115	2.1	119	2.6

FIGURE 36-40

DEXA Scan for individual with normal bone density.

trabecular bone. The axial skeleton (pelvis, vertebral column, and ends of the long bones) is comprised mostly of trabecular bone. These aspects of the skeleton are more susceptible to changes in reproductive hormones reflecting the predominant location of bony changes that occur with both menopause- and exercise-induced amenorrhea.[248] BMD is determined by the ratio of osteoclastic (resorption) and osteoblastic (remodeling) activity. Weight-bearing activities directly stimulate osteoblastic activity according to Wolff's law. Sex hormones, estrogen and testosterone, also favor osteoblastic activity with peak bone growth noted during puberty. The opposite effect of rapid bone loss is seen at menopause with the loss of estrogen. Estrogen also plays a role by limiting osteoclastic activity thus improving the absorption of calcium at the gastrointestinal level, and decreasing elimination of calcium at the renal level.[105,248] Other factors affecting BMD include genetics, smoking, alcohol consumption, cortisol levels, and nutrition.[7,213] Calcium and vitamin D consumption are critical for proper bone health. Calcium is necessary for bone remodeling, but the amount of calcium absorbed is dependent upon an adequate supply of vitamin D.[68,123]

Abnormalities in bone homeostasis have been documented in female athletes with both premature osteoporosis,[89] scoliosis,[91,156] fractures including premature osteoporotic,[168,169] and stress fractures of various locations.[11,93,146,214] All athletes have cyclic stresses creating an increased rate of osteoclastic activity followed by osteoblastic activity. If adequate rest or time is not given, an imbalance preventing adequate new bone to be laid down occurs resulting in a progressive weakening and fracture of the involved bone.[146] This phenomena occurs more frequently in female athletes resulting in stress injuries to the bone. In a retrospective review of medical records of a Division 1 college institution over a 10-year period, Arendt et al. demonstrated that female distance runners suffered the most stress injuries to bone (6.4 percent).[23] Across all sports, female athletes were two times as likely to suffer stress injuries to bone as male athletes. The authors attributed this increased rate not only to gender-related factors but also BMD, menstrual history, and diet.[23] Another study demonstrated that athletes with stress fractures had a lower bone density than matched controls without stress fracture.[197] Furthermore, other studies have reported a higher incidence of stress fractures among amenorrheic and oligomenorrheic athletes than eumenorrheic athletes.[204,230] Menstrual irregularities and decreased BMD certainly are not seen in every case of stress injury to bone but both may place the athlete at higher risk.[11]

In addition to being at higher risk for stress injuries to bone, athletes with menstrual difficulties are unlikely to reach their total BMD potential resulting in an overall lower peak BMD and a decreased ability to maintain BMD because of lower levels of estrogen. Studies are pessimistic regarding the ability to reverse the lower BMD with treatment.[91,159] There are studies that report an increase in serial BMD results with amenorrheic athletes resuming menses but the levels remain below eumenorrheic matched subjects. Amenorrheic runners using cyclical hormone replacement therapy have demonstrated maintenance of BMD but no gains. These studies collectively demonstrate the necessity to educate young female athletes in the importance of adequate nutrition including calories, calcium, and vitamin D intake; regular menses; and appropriate training levels including weight-bearing activities for their maturity level.

INTERACTION BETWEEN THE COMPONENTS OF THE FEMALE TRIAD

The three components of the female athlete triad have been presented and described as independent medical conditions, and now the link between them will be detailed. The possible theories behind athletic amenorrhea have been mentioned previously. The observations that both amenorrheic athletes had decreased body fat and individuals with AN had low body fat led to the hypothesis that this changed body composition was not only correlated but causative. Loucks et al. completed research matching amenorrheic versus eumenorrheic (normal menstruation) athletes for body fat and found that menstruation status was independent of this variable.[169] Another study concluded that the only difference between the groups (amenorrheic versus eumenorrheic) with such matched athletes was the increased caloric output without increased caloric intake (negative energy balance) associated with training in the amenorrheic group.[36] In another study, obese females underwent stomach reduction surgery creating a negative energy balance and became amenorrheic while remaining morbidly obese.[215] These studies indicate that it is the negative energy balance of caloric intake versus expenditure rather than body fat stores that is linked to amenorrhea.

Another theory to explain the result of exercise-induced amenorrhea was that the physical stress of the exercise increases the levels of cortisol thereby disrupting the menstrual cycle. Both amenorrheic athletes and individuals diagnosed with AN demonstrated increased cortisol levels with corresponding decreased levels of GnRH. As discussed previously in the section on amenorrhea, decreased levels of GnRH results in exercise induced amenorrhea. Cortisol has another role in the body as well with the regulation of plasma glucose and is released not only in response to physical stress of exercise but also with decreased levels of plasma glucose. The difficulty lies in separating these roles and determining whether high levels of cortisol disrupts the normal hormonal cascade by suppressing GnRH levels resulting in amenorrhea because of the physical stress of exercise or due to the decreased plasma levels of glucose. Loucks et al. demonstrated that the hormonal cascade changes with LH could be normalized in females receiving dietary supplementation, highlighting the important role of nutrition (positive energy balance) with intense exercise.[169]

"Negative energy balance" as the cause of exercise-induced amenorrhea has been supported in research.[91,169,215] Two studies demonstrate that a combination of exercise training and caloric restriction in animals and humans results in amenorrhea with reversal upon an increase in caloric intake.[169,191] This further supports that there exists a direct relationship between daily energy availability, not available stored energy and the hormonal cascade controlling the menstrual cycle.[1,168,169,191] These articles may explain why female athletes with similar body composition and training intensity have varied menstrual status including amenorrhea, oligomenorrhea, and eumenorrhea (normal menstrual cycling). It is not directly the exercise intensity that causes the change in the hormonal cascade controlling menstruation but the sustained negative energy balance in those female athletes not taking in enough calories for the energy expended with the training. Therefore interventions should include increased caloric intake to attain a positive energy balance in combination with other interventions to target restoration of normal bone metabolism. More specific intervention strategies will be discussed later in this chapter.

The interactions of the disordered eating patterns resulting in the negative energy balance and osteopenia can also be elaborated on. Unhealthy eating behaviors with diagnosed clinical eating disorders (AN, BN, EDNOS) and subclinical eating disorders can rapidly cause an inadequate intake of calcium, vitamin D, and vitamin K resulting in decreased building blocks for osteoblastic activity to increase overall BMD and allow for normal bone homeostasis during sports participation. As discussed previously, the window of opportunity to reach peak bone mass occurs in the third decade of life. It is the same time when disordered eating patterns are most prevalent and also many female athletes are competing at high levels, resulting in increased training intensities, durations, and frequency. Failure to reach optimum BMD during this time secondary to inadequate nutrition is not likely to be reversible.

Additional interactions between menstrual irregularities and osteopenia are also evident. Some of these interactions with the multifactorial role of estrogen with normal bone metabolism and the ability to achieve peak BMD as it relates to secondary amenorrhea has already been discussed. Hypoestrogenemia does not have any well-designed study specifically addressing the effect of delaying menarche as a result of premenarcheal training. Premenarchal training in a number of sports has been correlated with delayed menarche but this does not imply causation.[104] A retrospective study with college gymnasts suggests that delayed menarche is associated with increased risk of scoliosis, stress fractures, and low peak BMD.[164] This starts to demonstrate the serious and long-term implications of triad interactions and the synergestic nature of the components. Each component of the triad exists on a continuum of severity, thus the interactions between the components falls in a spectrum of severity as well. Early detection of the components greatly assists the treatment of each component as well as the interactions that may be present.

Screening

Preparticipation screenings provide an excellent opportunity to identify the components of the female athlete triad. Appendix D provides an example of a questionnaire for information gathering regarding eating habits, menstrual history, and bone health. More extensive questionnaires and surveys regarding eating habits and menstrual history can be included should preliminary screening indicate a need. Additional resources can be found in Appendix E. Menstrual history is often used for predicting bone density.[89,110] In addition, Drinkwater has demonstrated a linear relationship between the degree of bone loss and menstrual dysfunction (MD).[89,91] Any abnormalities with menstrual cycle detected in the medical history section should be noted and discussed with the primary care or team physician to facilitate further studies to confirm bone density. Despite the fact that there are no established guidelines for assessment of bone density in an athlete, it has been recommended that any female athlete with history of clinical eating disorders, amenorrhea, or oligomenorrhea for more than 6 months have further study to determine bone density. Similarly, documented history of stress fractures may indicate further study. History of stress fractures, especially of the femoral neck, sacrum, or pelvis (cancellous bone), are of increased concern secondary to a recent study which found that female athletes with a stress fracture in cancellous bone are more likely to have osteopenia than athletes who sustain a stress fracture in cortical bone such as the tibia or metatarsal.[183] Increased accessibility, ease, and affordability of DEXA scans have facilitated the ability of the health care team to confirm a suspicion of bone density problems.

Logistically, implementing these screening tools works nicely in sports preparticipation screening. It is the experience of the author and documented by other medical professionals that information regarding eating habits, self image, and menstrual history is more accurately gathered when there is a trained medical professional interviewing the female athlete rather than self-administration.[37,48,82] Many of these athletes with problems in these areas suffer guilt and shame regarding their behaviors, but most will provide honest and accurate answers to direct and nonjudgmental questioning. It is important to make clear that the information gathered will be held in confidence and will be used for the athlete's benefit. Questionnaires such as given in Appendix C or a combination of established questionnaires (see Appendix F) may also be used outside the preparticipation screening environment for any female athlete suspected of having the female athlete triad.

A recent study indicated that there is decreased confidence of members of the sports medicine team regarding screening and successfully identifying athletes with eating disorders.[263] One hundred and seventy-one athletic trainers who worked at NCAA Division IA and IAA institutions completed a survey that examined college athletic trainers' confidence in helping female athletes who have eating disorders. Less than 33 percent felt confident in asking an athlete if she had an eating disorder and only one in four felt confident identifying a female athlete with an eating disorder. Although virtually all of the respondents (91 percent) had dealt with a female athlete with an eating disorder and (93 percent) felt that increased attention to preventing eating disorders among collegiate female athletes was necessary, less than half of the athletic trainers worked at an institution that provided training or education on eating disorders. The authors recommended that athletic programs develop and implement eating disorder policies as well as provide education on prevention of eating disorders to increase confidence of these medical professionals in identifying and supporting a female athlete with an eating disorder.[263]

It is sometimes difficult to be confident in the skill of screening athletes for the components of the female triad because of the difficulty in differentiating healthy and unhealthy dedication to excellence in sport. Distinguishing between healthy and unhealthy eating and exercising behaviors is one challenge for the sports medicine team. In addition to keeping in mind the set criteria for the three types of clinical eating disorders, there are other characteristics that have been outlined to distinguish between women developing components of the triad and athletic women. Athletes remain goal-directed in training with good and improving exercise tolerance and efficient body metabolism. Athletes have well developed muscles, a body composition with normal fat store levels, and an unimpaired body image. Athletes who possess developing components of the athlete triad have poor or decreasing exercise tolerance and a distorted body image. Body metabolism alterations (decreased) results in signs such as dry skin, cold intolerance, and decreasing muscle size and development.[48,215] Consideration of these additional factors may assist in improving the confident detection of athletes with components of the triad and facilitate referral for early intervention.

PREVENTION AND TREATMENT

The ongoing concern about the onset of each of these conditions and then the collective nature of these conditions with female athletes has led to education and legislative efforts to decelerate the growth of this entity. In 1993, the Eating Disorders Information and Education Act was incorporated into the Women's Health Equity Act.[9,82,117] From this act, the National Eating Disorder screening program was activated on college campuses throughout the United States not only to enhance the screening and treatment for the female athlete triad but also to accelerate the prevention programs for each of these components.[2,9,37] As the ACSM's position statement included a call to action for medical professionals to intervene in the screening, prevention, and treatment of this growing entity, efforts continued and have significantly accelerated. One study compared 149 female varsity athletes with 209 female controls (nonathletes) from two NCAA Division I universities to assess eating habits and behaviors as well as alcohol consumption and drinking behaviors. The results showed that problem eating and drinking behaviors existed in both groups but not at different rates as previously demonstrated. The authors conclude, "this finding may be the result of coach, athletic trainer, and peer-group counseling at these 2 schools or a general trend for lower rates of unhealthy behaviors among female athletes."[117] Sondgot-Borgen found that education to coaches and athletes had a positive effect on the prevention of disordered eating patterns.[251]

Nevertheless, the goal of prevention of the triad remains elusive. Other studies have addressed the confidence of medical professionals in screening, preventing, and helping female athletes with nutrition, disordered eating, and MD.[37,263,276] Beals

surveyed NCAA Division I athletic programs and found that education about MD and eating disorders was made available to athletes in 73 percent of the participating programs, but only 61 percent of these schools made this education available to the coaches and less than 41 percent of schools made this education a requirement of either the athletes or coaching staffs. Out of the respondents, only 35 percent believed that the MD screening was successful and 26 percent believed that the eating disorder screening was successful.[37] When female collegiate cross-country runners were screened about nutritional knowledge, several specific areas of deficient nutritional knowledge were identified. These areas of deficient nutritional knowledge included vitamin supplementation, the necessity for fat in the body and diet, the necessity of a calcium source in the diet, and the recommended amount of calcium and appropriate sources of it. The authors noted that those athletes who completed a nutrition course in college scored significantly higher overall indicating that appropriate nutritional knowledge may lead to better nutritional choices.[276]

Providing accurate information regarding sports nutrition is essential for athletes. Good nutritional information is often addressed in the context of avoiding poor health implications, which often will not motivate an athlete to make the necessary dietary improvements. Optimizing performance with appropriate body composition and aiding recovery following increased training or injury may serve as better motivators.[114] Proper nutrition is a significant determinant of athletic performance. Hawley et al. report, "no single factor plays a greater role in optimizing performance than diet."[37] A good place to start in the provision of sound nutritional advice is the recently revised Food Pyramid (Fig. 36-41) developed by the United States Department of Agriculture.[4] Ongoing research has led to its development and continued revision. Modifications and additions to the original pyramid illustration have been completed to include a reorganization of the essential food groups, size and portion information for each of these groups, the necessity of hydration and exercise for a healthy lifestyle, and the ability to further tailor the recommendations depending on your sex, age, and activity level.[4,37] The pyramid can provide the basics for nutrition. To build on these basics, further guidance regarding appropriate body composition, iron intake, calcium intake, fat consumption, and possible supplementation are necessary.[102,206]

Reliance on accurate body composition measurements rather than merely body weight statistics will provide more appropriate data to make clinical judgments regarding necessity of changes in body composition. Utilizing body composition measurements as a monitoring tool correlated with the emphasis on strength, speed, and performance abilities will yield realistic goals regarding body composition and body weight-changes.[114]

Other strategies to be implemented for prevention of the triad include education of athletes, parents, and coaches on sound training techniques including limitations of total training hours for adolescents and elimination of weight determinations and body fat levels by coaches. Education to these same individuals about the female athlete triad including predisposing

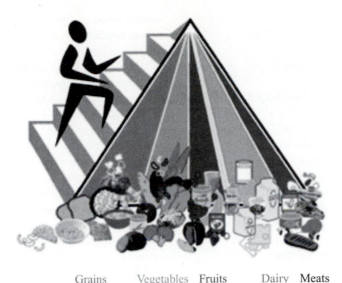

Grains   Vegetables   Fruits   Dairy   Meats

Serving size   5 oz   2 cups   1 ½ cups   3 cups   5 oz

United States Department of Agriculture (public domain)

FIGURE 36-41

MyPyramid—updated version of the former Food Guide Pyramid.

factors, warning signs, and implications can also be completed. Other educational goals should include the elimination of the myths about amenorrhea as being normal, rest being unimportant, and that food is "the enemy." Promotion of healthy attitudes that food is the fuel that provides the nutrients necessary to optimize performance as well as healthy body images of female athletes will continue to assist in the prevention of the triad. These strategies and others can be explored to assist female athletes to realize that thinner is not better, many chosen sports do not have an ideal weight that must be attained, and a healthy balance of calories consumed must be matched with the energy expended in order to optimize athletic performance.[82,117,204,215,275]

Treatment of the components of the triad should be in the hands of a multidisciplinary team including but not limited to team physicians, sports physical therapists, certified athletic trainers, sports nutritionists, sports psychologists, and coaches.[20] Treatment of disordered eating patterns need to resolve the psychosocial factors, stabilize medical conditions, and establish healthy eating patterns. Establishment of healthy eating patterns can be thought of as "nutritional rehabilitation." Sondgot-Borgon found that cognitive behavioral therapy in addition to nutritional counseling was more beneficial in the treatment of female athletes with disordered eating patterns than nutritional therapy alone.[251] Nutritional counseling should include the necessity of balancing caloric intake with the caloric expenditure of training to attain a positive energy balance.[158,161,204,214,215]

The attainment of a positive energy balance is also key to treating menstrual irregularities.[158,215] After identification of the underlying cause of menstrual irregularities, the focus will be to treat this and establish normal menstrual function.[158,204,214]

Optimizing calcium and nutritional intake as well as modification of a training regime to ensure this positive energy balance is the first step.[158,215] Continued medical supervision to observe the effect of these changes is necessary and possible intervention with hormone replacement is decided upon an individual basis.[158] When treating a female athlete with bone density loss, once again attaining a positive energy balance with adequate calcium intake and resumption of normal menstruation is important.[158,161,215]

Exercise modification may be necessary to establish a bone homeostasis favorable to osteoclastic activity with exercise prescription for appropriate weight bearing and resistive exercise. These recommendations as well as pharmacological treatment are based on the individual's data and risk profile. Guidelines have been established by the National Osteoporosis Foundation for pharmacological treatment of postmenopausal women,[7] but these guidelines cannot be readily utilized for the female athlete. Further study and research is needed in this area. The multidisciplinary team led by a qualified medical professional should coordinate efforts for treatment of the individual components of the female athlete triad, subsequently ending the cascade into the interdependent relationship between these components with the root of this treatment being the establishment of a "positive energy balance" for each athlete.

PREGNANCY IN THE PHYSICALLY ACTIVE FEMALE

The physically active female enjoys many benefits from the exercise she regularly completes. Pregnancy does not change these

T A B L E   3 6 - 1 6

Exercise Benefits During Pregnancy[18,27,65,67,221]

- Increase or maintain aerobic fitness
- Increase cardiac reserve
- Increased tolerance for physical work
- Improve sleep
- Positive effect on psychological state
- Decrease risk of gestational diabetes
- Decreases in total mood disturbance
- Decreased labor time
- Decreased maternal pain perception
- Decreased rate of medical intervention such as pitocin, forceps delivery, and caesarean section
- Promote faster recovery from labor
- Promote good posture during and after pregnancy
- Prevent or minimize low back pain
- Prevent excessive "fat" weight gain

benefits but does present special challenges for the female athlete as she plans and manages her pregnancy (see Table 36-16). The main challenge is exercising at a safe level, safeguarding the health of both the mother and fetus. There are physiologic changes to the cardiovascular, respiratory, and musculoskeletal system that need to be understood and considered in order to decide a safe level of exercise throughout the pregnancy. Knowledge of these physiologic changes and the consequences of exercise and training on the course of pregnancy, labor, and delivery should provide guidance for the medical provider of the physically active female to establish guidelines that ensure her and the fetus's safety throughout gestation.

More physicians are encouraging females to remain active during their pregnancies. Adopting a new exercise routine or significantly increasing the intensity of the present exercise routine is not recommended during this time of considerable change. A major physiologic change occurs in the cardiovascular system with a substantial increase in blood volume by up to 50 percent by the end of pregnancy. This increase occurs first in the plasma volume causing a dilutional anemia in the first and second trimester. The blood volume increase continues in the third trimester with the red cell mass increasing so the anemia is partially corrected.[67] This blood volume expansion results in greater oxygen-carrying capacity but increased cardiac work. In highly conditioned athletes, this blood volume increase is greater than in sedentary females.[65] Additional cardiovascular changes include increased stroke volume, cardiac output, and resting pulse by 10–15 beats per minute. These increases may help to ensure adequate blood flow to the uterus during exercise as well as dissipation of heat.[27] Blood pressure usually falls during pregnancy reaching its lowest levels in mid-pregnancy. Increased circulation to the uterus, kidneys, skin, and breasts occurs and is accompanied by a reduction in venous tone. With this reduction and the increasing size of the uterus decreasing

venous return to the heart especially in the supine position, supine hypotension can occur.[65] This is the basis for the recommendation to avoid supine exercise after the first trimester.[18]

When exercising, the female athlete will have increases in pulse rate, cardiac output, and blood pressure. The pregnant athlete will experience these same increases to a lesser degree. With these increases, the increased blood flow goes primarily to the working muscles and results in some shunting of blood from the uterus and developing fetus.[67] This observation has raised concern regarding risk to the fetus with intense and/or prolonged exercise but evidence for such concern is lacking.[66] Respiratory system changes may help to alleviate the ultimate result of the blood shunting that occurs.

Respiratory system changes occurring during pregnancy include increased tidal volume, minute ventilation, and oxygen consumption as well as decreased residual volume and functional residual capacity. The ultimate result is an unchanged overall vital capacity; however, the pregnant woman may experience shortness of breath because of increased sensitivity to carbon dioxide driving increased ventilation and lower blood levels of carbon dioxide and slightly more alkaline pH. These biochemical changes have a safeguarding effect for the fetus increasing placental gas exchange and preventing fetal acidosis.[65] Pregnant women are just as efficient in achieving increased levels of oxygen consumption during exercise as nonpregnant women,[27] but changes in maternal oxygenation are amplified in the fetus. Since anaerobic exercise results in relative maternal hypoxia and acidosis, it is recommended to avoid prolonged anaerobic exercise. On the other hand, aerobic exercise in pregnant subjects has been shown to result in greater increases in minute ventilation than nonpregnant women. This relative hyperventilation helps protect the fetus from hypoxia or changes in pH with aerobic exercise.[221]

Changes in the musculoskeletal system of the pregnant, active female result in significant postural, gait, and balance changes. The pregnant female's center of gravity moves forward often driving an increased lumbar lordosis with a resultant stretch weakness of the core stabilizers.[27] Ligamentous laxity increasing the mobility of all joints especially the pelvis resulting in maternal "waddling" in late pregnancy and a frequent complaint of low back pain as the weight increases with resultant increased forces on the vertebral column. Secondary to these musculoskeletal concerns of ligamentous laxity which cause an increased propensity to falling and increased torque on already lax ligaments, a pregnant woman may want to consider swimming, stationary cycling, stair-climbing apparatus, or treadmills to minimize the risk of falling and decrease forces on taxed joints.[27]

The effect of exercise on pregnancy outcomes has been studied with reference to fetal development, fetal growth, metabolic status of the fetus, and labor. It is known that high maternal core temperature is associated with fetal development problems such as neural tube defects. Many of the physiologic changes during pregnancy help to keep maternal temperature lower with or without exercise, but additional precautions especially in the first trimester should be taken to ensure a near normal maternal temperature during exercise sessions.[67] Historically, it has been a concern that exercising during pregnancy would cause decreased fetal growth and low birth weight. It has been found that women who begin pregnancy underweight have a greater risk of delivering an underweight or preterm newborn. Since many female athletes are under weight at the start of their pregnancy, this finding would include this population. If there is attention and care given to nutrition and appropriate weight gain before or at the initiation of the pregnancy, this concern can be minimized.[65] There is also evidence to demonstrate that if moderate exercise continues throughout pregnancy and does not exceed prepregnancy levels, there is no compromise in fetal growth.[67] However, it has been shown that pregnant women who exercise intensely deliver approximately 1 week earlier than those who are sedentary or exercise moderately. This early delivery subsequently causes a relative low birth rate because of the average 100 g difference in birth weight and decreased body fat deposition compared to full-term babies. Recent reports confirm that exercise during pregnancy has little effect on the acute status of the fetus when mother and unborn baby are healthy.[27,65,67] Fetal heart rate and oxygenation remain normal with intense exercise during the third trimester up to labor.[65] Actual labor and delivery are improved by regular exercise throughout pregnancy making medical intervention less necessary, forceps delivery less likely, caesarean sections less likely, shorter labor with faster dilation, 50 percent less transition time, and less pushing time to delivery.[65]

Based on the current research, the American Academy of Obstetricians and Gynecologists published the most recent guidelines for exercise in pregnancy and postpartum recognizing the safety and benefits of exercise throughout pregnancy.[18] These guidelines support the physically active female continuing exercise throughout pregnancy with special attention given to adequate weight gain, prevention of hyperthermia, and avoidance of injury. The guidelines give specific recommendations regarding adequate nutrition highlighting that pregnancy requires an additional 300 kcal/day in order to maintain metabolic homeostasis, cautioning exercising pregnant women to ensure an adequate caloric intake. Additional instructions encourage strict adherence to contraindications to exercise such as pregnancy-induced hypertension, preterm rupture of membranes, preterm labor during the prior or current pregnancy, incompetent cervix/cerclage, persistent second- or third-trimester bleeding, and intrauterine growth retardation.[18] In summary, the physically active female can safely continue athletic pursuits and/or exercise throughout her pregnancy as long as these simple guidelines are followed.

SUMMARY

For more than a decade, female athlete participation has significantly risen at all levels including high school, collegiate, and Olympic level.[5,6,8] The benefits for the female to remain physically active continue to outweigh the costs.[19,44,155,163] An awareness of the gender differences enables the sports medicine specialist to develop prevention, training, and rehabilitation programs that will effectively minimize the cost of remaining physically active throughout the female's lifespan in a variety of sport endeavors.

- Anatomical, strength, and neuromuscular differences exist between female and male athletes. These differences should be understood and acknowledged during examination and treatment of female athletes.
- ACL injuries continue to be prevalent among female athletes.
- ACL injuries in female athletes are multifactorial. Some factors can be modified while others cannot be. Contemporary prevention and rehabilitation focus on neuromuscular strategies for movement.
- Core stability is vital for athletic performance by all athletes. Female athletes should address the core during rehabilitation after injury as well as during performance training.
- The athletically active female has many unique issues including laxity, sport-specific potential for injury (softball pitching, swimming, gymnastics), and the female athlete triad.
- Specific protocols are included for rehabilitation of the athletic female who participates in softball and swimming.
- Progressive reactive neuromuscular training for lower extremity and core stabilization is important. A sample progression is included.
- The female athlete triad is an important condition about which the sports medicine provider must be knowledgeable in order to provide screening, education, and appropriate referral.
- The physically active female can safely participate in activity during pregnancy, following the medical guidelines such as those prescribed by American College of Obstetricians and Gynecologists.

REFERENCES

1. www.alltrue.net/site/adadweb.htm. National Association of Anorexia Nervosa and Associated Disorders. Facts about Eating Disorders. Accessed on October 15, 2004.
2. www.mentalhealthscreening.org/events/nedsp/results.htm. Website of National Eating Disorder Screening Program. Accessed on January 27, 2005.
3. www.msnbc.org. NBC online news service. Accessed on August 27, 2004.
4. www.mypyramid.gov. United States Department of Agriculture. My Pyramid: Steps to a Healthier You. Accessed on May 1, 2005.
5. www.ncaa.org. Website of the National Collegiate Athletic Association. Accessed on June 7, 2000 and October 10, 2004.
6. www.nhfs.org. National Federation of High School associations. Accessed on September 12, 2005.

7. www.nof.org/osteoporsis/stats.htm. National Osteoporosis Foundation. Physician's Guide: Impact and Overview. Accessed on October 20, 2004.

8. www.olympic.org/uk/organisation/commissions/women. Website of the International Olympic Committee. Accessed on January 15, 2005.

9. www.4woman.gov. Website of Office on Women's Health, U.S. Department of Health and Human Services. Accessed on January 27, 2005.

10. Aglietta P, Bruzzi R, D'Andria P, Zaccherotti G. Long-term study of anterior cruciate ligament reconstruction for chronic instability using the central one-third patellar tendon and a lateral extraarticular tenodesis. *AJSM* 20:28–45, 1992.

11. Agostini, R. Women in sports. In: Mellion MB, Walsh JM, Shelton G, eds. *The Team Physician's Handbook*. Philadelphia, PA, Hanley & Belfus, 1990, pp. 179–188.

12. Akuthota V, Nadler SF. Core strengthening. *Arch Phys Med Rehabil* 85(suppl 1):S86–S92, 2004.

13. Alford JW, Cole BJ. Cartilage restoration, Part 1. *AJSM* 33(2):295–132, 2005.

14. Alford JW, Cole BJ. Cartilage restoration, Part 2. *AJSM* 33(3):443–460, 2005.

15. Allegrucci M, Whitney SL, Irrgang JJ. Clinical implications of secondary impingement of the shoulder in freestyle swimmers. *J Orthop Sports Phys Ther* 20(6):307–318, 1994.

16. Almeida SS, Trone DW, Leone DM, et al. Gender differences in musculoskeletal injury rates: A function of symptom reporting? *Med Sci Sports Exerc* 31:1807–1812, 1995.

17. Always SE, Gummbt WH, Stray-Gundersen J, et al. Effects of resistance training on elbow flexors of highly competitive bodybuilders. *J Appl Physiol* 72:1512–1521, 1992.

18. American College of Obstetricians and Gynecologists: Exercise during pregnancy and the postpartum period. *ACOG Technical Bulletin 189*. Washington DC, ACOG, 1994.

19. American College of Sports Medicine. *Exercise Management for Persons with Chronic Diseases and Disabilities*. Champagne, IL, Human Kinetics, 1997.

20. American Physical Therapy Association. *Guide to Physical Therapy Practice*, 2nd ed. 2001.

21. American Psychiatric Association. *Diagnostic and Statistical Manual of Mental Disorders-IV*. Washington DC, American Psychiatric Press, 1994.

22. Anderson AF, Dome DC, Gautam S, et al. Correlation of anthropometric measurements, strength, anterior cruciate ligament size, and intercondylar notch characteristics to sex differences in anterior cruciate ligament tear rates. *Am J Sports Med* 29(1):58–66, 2001.

23. Arendt E, Agel J, Heikes C, Griffiths H. Stress injuries to bone in college athletes. *Am J Sports Med* 31(6):959–968, 2003.

24. Arendt E, Dick R. Knee injury patterns among men and women in collegiate basketball and soccer. *Am J Sports Med* 23(6):694–701, 1995.

25. Arendt EA, Agel J, Dick R. Anterior cruciate ligament injury patterns among collegiate women. *J Athl Train* 34:86–92, 1999.

26. Arendt EA, Bershadsky B, Agel J. Periodicity of non-contact anterior cruciate ligament injuries during the menstrual cycle. *JGSM* 5:19–26, 2002.

27. Artal R. Exercise and pregnancy. *Clin Sports Med* 11:363–77, 1992.

28. Bach BR, Jones GT, Sweet FA, Hager CA. Arthroscopy-assisted anterior cruciate ligament reconstruction using patellar tendon substitution. Two- to four-year follow-up results. *AJSM* 22:758–767, 1994.

29. Backx FJG, Beijer HJM, Bol E. Injuries in high-risk persons and high-risk sports. *Am J Sports Med* 19:124–130, 1991.

30. Bahr R, Reeser JC. Injuries among world-class professional beach volleyball players. *Am J Sports Med* 31(1), 2003.

31. Bak K, Kalms SB, Olesen S, et al. Epidemiology of injuries in gymnastics. *Scand J Med Sci Sports* 4:148–154, 1994.

32. Baratta R, Solomonow M, Zhou BH. Muscular coactivation: The role of the antagonist musculature in maintaining knee stability. *Am J Sports Med* 16:113–122, 1988.

33. Barden JM, Balyk R, Raso JV, et al. Dynamic upper limb proprioception in multidirectional shoulder instability. *Clin Orthop* 420:181–189, 2004.

34. Barrack RL, Lund PJ, Skinner HB. Knee joint proprioception revisited. *J Sport Rehab* 3:18–42, 1994.

35. Barrett DS. Proprioception and function after anterior cruciate reconstruction. *JBJS* 73B:833–837, 1991.

36. Beals KA, Manore MM. The prevalence and consequences of subclinical eating disorders in female athletes. *Int J Sport Nutr* 4:175–195, 1994.

37. Beals KA. Eating disorder and menstrual dysfunction screening, education and treatment programs. *Physician Sportsmed* 31(7):33–38, 2003.

38. Beck X, Wildermuth BP. The female athlete's knee. *Clin Sports Med* 4(2):345–366,1985.

39. Beighton PH, Horan FT. Dominant inheritance in familial generalized articular hypermobility. *J Bone Joint Surg* 52B:145–147, 1970.

40. Beim G, Stone DA. Issues in the female athlete. *Orthop Clin North Am* 26(3):443–451, 1995.

41. Berrentine S, Fleising G, Whiteside J, et al. Biomechanics of windmill softball pitching with implications about injury mechanisms at the shoulder and elbow. *J Orthop Sports Phys Ther* 28:405–415, 1998.

42. Bjordal JM, Amly F, Hannestad B, Strand T. Epidemiology of anterior cruciate ligament injuries in soccer. *Am J Sports Med* 25:341–345, 1997.

43. Black DR, Larkin LJS, Coster DC, Leverenz LJ, Abood DA. Physiologic screening test for eating disorders/disordered eating among female collegiate athletes. *J Athl Train* 38(4):286–297, 2003.

44. Blair SN, Goodyear NN, Gibbons LW, Cooper KH. Physical fitness and incidence of hypertension in healthy normotensive men and women. *JAMA* 252:487–490, 1984.

45. Blasier RB, Carpenter JE, Huston LJ. Shoulder proprioception. Effect of joint laxity, joint position, and direction of motion. *Orthop Rev* 23:45–50, 1994.

46. Bobbert MF, van Zandwijk JP. Dynamics of force and muscle stimulation of human vertical jumping. *Med Sci Sports Exerc* 31:303–310, 1999.

47. Boden BP, Dean GS, Feagin JA, Garrett WE. Mechanisms of anterior cruciate ligament injury. *Orthopedics* 23(6):573–578, 2000.

48. Bolen JD. Differentiating healthy from unhealthy behaviors in active and athletic women. In: Agostini R, ed. *Medical and Orthopedic Issues of Active and Athletic Women.* Philadelphia, PA, Hanley & Belfus, 1994, 102–107.

49. Borsa PA, Lephart SM, Kocher MS, et al. Functional assessment and rehabilitation of shoulder proprioception for glenohumeral instability. *J Sports Rehab* 3:84–104, 1994.

50. Bouisset S. Relationship between postural support and intentional movement: Biomechanical approach. *Arch Int Physiol Biochem Biophys* 99:77–92, 1991.

51. Briner WW, Benjamin HJ. Volleyball injuries: Managing acute and overuse disorders. *Phys Sports Med* 27(3):48–56, 1999.

52. Brody LT, Thein JM. Nonoperative treatment for patellofemoral pain. *JOSPT* 28(5):33634, 1998.

53. Brown GA, Tan JL, Kirkley A. The lax shoulder in females. Issues, answers, but many more questions. *Clin Orthop Relat Res* 372:110–122, 2000.

54. Bryant JT, Cooke TD. Standardized biomechanical measurement of varus-valgus stiffness and rotation in normal knees. *J Orthop Res* 6:863–870, 1988.

55. Caine D, Cochrane B, Caine C, et al. An epidemiologic investigation of injuries affecting young competitive female gymnasts. *Am J Sports Med* 17(6): 811–820, 1989.

56. Caine D, Lewis R, O'Connor P, et al. Does gymnastics training inhibit growth of females? *Clin J Sport Med* 11(4):260–270, 2001.

57. Caine D, Lindner K. Overuse injuries of growing bones: the young female gymnast at risk? *Phys Sports Med* 13:51–54, 1985.

58. Caraffa A, Cerulli G, Projetti M, et al. Prevention of anterior cruciate ligament injuries in soccer. A prospective controlled study of proprioceptive training. *Knee Surg Sports Traumatol Arthrosc* 4(1):19–21, 1996.

59. Carson W, James S, Larson R, et al. Patellofemoral disorders: Physical and radiographic evaluation. *Clin Orthop* 185:165–185, 1984.

60. Carter C, Wilkinson J. Persistent joint laxity and congenital dislocation of the hip. *J Bone Joint Surg* 46B:40–45, 1964.

61. Chandy TA, Grana WA. Secondary school athletic injury in boys and girls: A three-year comparision. *Phys and Sports Med* 13(3):106–111, 1985.

62. Chappell JD, Bing Y, Kirkendall DT, et al. A comparison of knee kinetics between male and female recreational athletes in stop-tasks. *Am J Sports Med* 30(2):261–267, 2002.

63. Chmielewski T, Ferber R. Rehabilitation considerations for the female athlete. In: Andrews JR, Harrelson GL, Wilk KE, eds. *Physical Rehabilitation of the Injured Athlete*, 3rd ed. Philadelphia, PA, Saunders—Elsevier Inc., 2004, pp. 315–328.

64. Cholewicki J, Simons APD, Radebold A. Effects of external trunk loads on lumbar spine stability. *J Biomech* 33:1377–1385, 2000.

65. Christian JS, Christian SS, Stamm CA, McGregor JA. Pregnancy, physiology and exercise. In: Ireland ML, Nattiv A, eds. *The Female Athlete.* Philadelphia, PA, Saunders, 2002, 185–190.

66. Cicuttini F, Forbes A, Morris K, Darling S, Bailey M, Stuckey S. Gender differences in knee cartilage volume as measured by magnetic resonance imaging. *Osteoarthritis Cartilage* 7:265–271, 1999.

67. Clapp JF. A clinical approach to exercise during pregnancy. *Clin Sports Med* 13:443–458, 1994.

68. Clark N. *Sports Nutrition Guidebook.* Brookline, MA, Sportsmed Brookline, 1997.

69. Cohen AR, Metzl JD. Sports-specific concerns in the young athlete: Basketball. *Pediatr Emerg Care* 16(6): 462–468, 2000.

70. Colby S, Francisco A, Yu B, et al. Electromyographic and kinematic analysis of cutting maneuvers. *Am J Sports Med* 28(2):234–240, 2000.

71. Corrigan JP, Cashman WF, Brady MP. Proprioception in the cruciate deficient knee. *JBJS* 74B:247–250, 1992.

72. Cresswell AG, Oddson L, Thorstensson A. The influence of sudden perturbations on trunk muscle activity and intra abdominal pressure while standing. *Exp Brain Res* 98: 336–341, 1994.

73. Cresswell AG, Thorstensson A. Change in intra-abdominal pressure, trunk muscle activation and force during isokinetic lifting and lowering. *Eur J Appl Phys* 68:315–321, 1994.

74. Cresswell AG. Responses of intra-abdominal pressure and abdominal muscle activity during dynamic trunk loading man. *Eur J Appl Phys* 66:315–320, 1993.

75. Cross MJ, Gibbs NJ, Grace JB. An analysis of the sidestep cutting maneuver. *Am J Sports Med* 17:363–366, 1989.

76. Cuillo JV, Stevens GC. The prevention and treatment of injuries to the shoulder in swimming. *Sports Med* 7:182–204, 1989.

77. Curl WW, Krone J, Gordon ES, Rushing J, Smith BP, Poehling GG. Cartilage injuries: A review of 31,516 knee arthroscopies. *Arthroscopy* 13:456–460, 1997.

78. Dahm D. The shoulder and upper extremities. In: Sweden N, ed. *Women's Sports Medicine and Rehabilitation.* Gaithersburg, Aspen Publishers, 2001, pp. 7–17.

79. Daniel DM, Fithian DC, Stone ML, et al. A ten-year prospective outcome study of the ACL-injured patient. *Orthop Trans* 20:700–701, 1996–1997.

80. Daniel DM, Stone ML, Dobson BE, et al. Fate of the ACL-injured patient. A prospected outcome study. *AJSM* 22:632–666, 1994.

81. DeCoster LC, Vailas JC, Lindsay RH, et al. Prevalence and feature of joint hypermobility among adolescent athletes. *Arch Pediatr Adolesc Med* 151:1997.

82. DeCourcey B. Dedication or destruction? How disordered eating can affect athletes. *NATA News* 10–13, February 2005.

83. DeHaven KE, Linter DM. Athletic injuries: Comparison by age, sport and gender. *Am J Sports Med* 14(3):218–224, 1986.

84. DeMont RG, Lephart SM, Giraldo JL, et al. Muscle preactivity of anterior cruciate ligament—deficient and reconstructed females during functional activities. *J Athl Train* 34(2):115–120, 1999.

85. DiBrezzo R, Oliver G. ACL injuries in active girls and women. *J Phys Educ Recreation Dance* 71(6):24–27, 2000.

86. Dore E, Martin F, Ratel S. Gender differences in peak muscle performance during growth. *Int J Sports Med* 26:274–280, 2005.

87. Dover GC, Kaminski TW, Meister K, et al. Assessment of shoulder proprioception in the female softball athlete. *Am J Sports Med* 31(3):431–437, 2003.

88. Draganich LF, Vahey JW. An in vitro study of anterior cruciate ligament strain induced by quadriceps and hamstring forces. *J Orthop Res* 8:57–63, 1990.

89. Drinkwater BL, Bruemmer B, Chestnut CH III. Menstrual history as a determinant of current bone density in young athletes. *N Engl J Med* 311:277, 1984.

90. Drinkwater BL, Nilson K, Chestnut CH III. Bone mineral content of amenorrheic and eumenorrheic athletes. *N Engl J Med* 311:277, 1984.

91. Drinkwater BL, Nilson K, Chestnut CH III. Bone mineral density after resumption of menses in amenorrheic athletes. *JAMA* 256(3):380–382, 1986.

92. Dufek JS, Bates BT. Biomechanical factors associated with injury during landing in jumping sports. *Sports Med* 12(5):326–337, 1991.

93. Dugowson CE, Drinkwater BL, Clark JM. Nontraumatic femur fracture in oligomenorrheic athlete. *Med Sci Sports Exer* 23:1323–1325, 1991.

94. Dye SE, Chew MH. Restoration of osseious homeostasis after anterior cruciate ligament reconstruction. *AJSM* 21:748–750, 1993.

95. Dye SE, Wojtys EM, Fu FH, Fithian DC, Gilquist J. Factors contributing to function of the knee joint following injury or reconstruction of the anterior cruciate ligament. *JBJS* 80-A(9):1380–1391, 1998.

96. Dye SE. The knee as a biologic transmission with an envelope of function. A theory. *Clin Orthop* 325:10–18, 1996.

97. Dyrek DA, Micheli LJ, Magee DJ. Injuries to the thoracolumbar spine and pelvis. In: Zachazewski JE, Magee DJ, Quillen WS, eds. *Athletic Injures and Rehabilitation.* Philadelphia, PA, Saunders, 1996, pp. 465–484.

98. Ebenbichler GR, Oddsson LIE, Kollmitzer J, Erim Z. Sensory-motor control of the lower back: Implications for rehabilitation. *Med Sci Sports Exerc* 33(11):1889–1898, 2001.

99. Ettlinger CF, Johnson RJ, Shealy JE. A method to help reduce the risk of serious knee sprains incurred in alpine skiing. *Am J Sports Med* 23:531–537, 1995.

100. Ferber RI, Davis M, Williams DS. Gender differences in lower extremity mechanics during running. *Clin Biomech* 18:350–357, 2003.

101. Ferretti A, Papandrea P, Conteduca F, Mariana PP. Knee ligament injuries in volleyball players. *Am J Sports Med* 20:203–207, 1992.

102. Food Nutrition Board. *Recommended Dietary Allowances,* 10th ed. Washington DC, National Academy of Sciences, 1994.

103. Ford KR, Myer GD, Toms HE, et al. Gender differences in the kinematics of unanticipated cutting in young athletes. *Med Sci Sports Exerc* 37(1):124–129, 2005.

104. Frisch RE, Gotz-Welbergen AV, McArthur JW, et al. Delayed menarche and amenorrhea of college athletes in relation to age of onset of training. *JAMA* 282:637–645, 1999.

105. Ganong WF. Hormonal control of calcium metabolism & the physiology of bone. *Rev Med Physiol.* Norwalk CN, Appleton & Lange, 1985, pp. 326–337.

106. Ganong WF. The gonads: Development and function of the reproductive system. *Rev Med Physiol.* Norwalk CN, Appleton & Lange, 1985, pp. 370–382.

107. Gardner-Morse M, Stokes I. The effect of abdominal muscle coactivation on lumbar spine stability. *Spine* 23:86–92, 1998.

108. Garrick JG, Requa RK. Girls sports injuries in high school athletics. *J Am Med Assoc* 239:2245–2248, 1978.

109. Gelber AC, Hochberg MC, Mead LA, et al. Joint injury in young adults and risk for subsequent knee and hip osteoarthritis. *Ann Int Med* 133:321–328, 2000.

110. Georgious EK, Ntalles K, Papageorgiou A, et al. Bone mineral loss related to menstrual history. *Acta Orthop Scand* 60:192–194, 1989.

111. Gilquist J. Repair and reconstruction of the ACL: Is it good enough? *Arthroscopy* 9:68–71, 1993.

112. Gomez E, DeLee JC, Farney WC. Incidence of injury in Texas girls' high school basketball. *Am J Sports Med* 24:684–687, 1996.

113. Gracovetsky S, Farfan H, Helleur C. The effect of the abdominal mechanism. *Spine* 10:317–324, 1985.

114. Grandjean AC, Reimers KJ, Ruud J. Nutrition. In: Ireland ML, Nattiv A, eds. *The Female Athlete*. Philadelphia, PA, Saunders, 2002, pp. 81–89.

115. Gray J, Taunton JE, McKenzie DC, et al. A survey of injuries to the anterior cruciate ligament of the knee in female basketball players. *Int J Sports Med* 6:314–316, 1985.

116. Griffin LY, Agel J, Albohm MJ, et al. Noncontact anterior cruciate ligament injuries: Risk factors and strategies for prevention. *J Am Acad Orthop Surg* 8(3):141–150, 2000.

117. Gutgessell ME, Moreau KL, Thompson DL. Weight concerns, problem eating behaviors, and roblem drinking behaviors in female collegiate athletes. *J Athl Train* 38(1):62–66, 2003.

118. Guyton AC. *Textbook of Medical Physiology*, 7th ed. Philadelphia, PA, Saunders, 1986.

119. Hakkinen K, Kraemer WJ, Newton RU. Muscle activation and force production during bilateral and unilateral concentric and isometric contractions of the knee extensors in men and women at different ages. *Electromyogr Clin Neurophysiol* 37:131–142, 1997.

120. Hall CM. Therapeutic exercise for the lumbopelvic region, In: Hall CM, Thein-Brody L, eds. *Therapeutic Exercise, Moving Toward Function*, 2nd ed. Philadelphia, PA, Lippincott Williams & Wilkins, 2005, pp. 349–401.

121. Harner CD, Paulos LE, Greenwald AD. Detailed analysis of patients with bilateral anterior cruciate ligament injuries. *Am J Sports Med* 22:37–43, 1994.

122. Harrer MF, Hosea TM, Berson L, et al. The gender issue: Epidemiology of knee and ankle injuries in high school and college players. Proceedings of the 65th Annual meeting of the American Academy of Orthopedic Surgeons. New Orleans, LA, March 19–23, 1998. Abstract 260.

123. Hawley JA, Dennis SC, Lindsay FH, Noakes TD. Nutritional practices of athletes: Are they suboptimal? *J Sport Sci* 13:S75–S81, 1995.

124. Haycock CE, Gillette JV. Susceptibility of women athletes to injury: Myth vs. reality. *JAMA* 236(2):163–165, 1976.

125. Hewett TE, Lindenfeld TN, Riccobene JV, et al. The effect of neuromuscular training on the incidence of knee injury in female athletes. *Am J Sp Med* 27(6):699–705, 1999.

126. Hewett TE, Myer GD, Ford KR, et al. Biomechanical measures of neuromuscular control and valgus loading of the knee predict anterior cruciate ligament injury risk in female athletes: A prospective study. *Am J Sports Med* 33(4):492–501, 2005.

127. Hewett TE, Paterno MV, Myer GD. Strategies for enhancing proprioception and neuromuscular control of the knee. *Clin Orthop Rel Res* 402:76–94, 2002.

128. Hewett TE, Stroupe AL, Nance TA, et al. Plyometric training in female athletes: Decreased impact forces and increased hamstring torques. *Am J Sports Med* 24(6):765–773, 1996.

129. Hewett TE. Neuromuscular and hormonal factors associated with knee injuries in female athletes. *Sports Med* 29(5):313–327, 2000.

130. Hides JA, Stokes MJ, Saide M, Jull GA, Cooper DH. Evidence of lumbar multifidus muscle wasting ipsilateral to symptoms in patients with acute/subacute low back pain. *Spine* 19:165–172, 1994.

131. Hodges PW, Butler JE, McKenzie D, Gandevia SC. Contraction of the human diaphragm during postural adjustments. *J Appl Phys* 505:239–248, 1997.

132. Hodges PW, Richardson CA. Delayed postural contraction of transverse abdominis in low back pain associated with movement of the lower limb. *J Spinal Disord* 1:46–56, 1998.

133. Hodges PW, Richardson CA. Feedforward contraction of transverse abdominis is not influenced by the direction of arm movement. *Exp Brain Res* 114:362–370, 1997.

134. Hodges PW. Is there a role for transversus abdominis in lumbo-pelvic stability? *Manual Ther* 4(2):74–86, 1999.

135. Hoffman M, Schrader J, Koceja D. An investigation of postural control in postoperative anterior cruciate ligament reconstruction patients. *J Athl Train* 34(2):130–136, 1999.

136. Holloway JB, Baechle TR. Strength training for female athletes: A review of selected aspects. *Sports Med* 9:216–228, 1990.

137. Hoogenboom BJ, Bennett JL. Core stabilization for the female athlete. SPTS female athlete home study course. Indianapolis, IN, The Sports Physical Therapy Section, 2004.

138. Howell SM, Taylor MA. Brace-free rehabilitation, with early return to activity, for knees reconstructed with double-looped semitendinosus and gracilis graft. *JBJS* 78-A:814–825, June 1996.

139. Huston LJ, Greenfield ML, Wojtys EM. Anterior cruciate ligament injuries in the female athlete. *Clin Ortho and Rel Res* 372:50–63, 2000.

140. Huston LJ, Wojtys EM. Neuromuscular performance characteristics in elite female athletes. *Am J Sp Med* 24(4):427–436, 1996.

141. Hutchinson MR, Ireland ML. Knee injuries in female athletes. *Sports Med* 19:288–301, 1995.

142. Hutchinson MR, Williams RI, Ireland ML. In: Ireland ML, Nattiv A, eds. *The Female Athlete*. Philadelphia, PA, Saunders, 2002, pp. 387–419.

143. Ireland ML, Wall C. Epidemiology and comparison of knee injuries in elite male and female United States basketball athletes [abstract]. *Med Sci Sports Exerc* 22:S82, 1990.

144. Ireland ML, Willson JD, Ballantyne BT, Davis IM. Hip strength in females with and without patellofemoral pain. *J Orthop Sports Phys Ther* 33:637–651, 2003.

145. Ireland ML. Anterior cruciate ligament injury in female athletes: Epidemiology. *J Athl Train* 34(2):150–154, 1999.

146. Johnson AW, Weiss CB, Stento K, Wheeler D. An atypical cause of low back pain in the female athlete. *Am J Sports Med* 29(4):498–508, 2001.

147. Johnson MD, Disordered eating. In: Agostini R. ed. *Medical and Orthopedic Issues of Active and Athletic Women.* Philadelphia, PA, Hanley & Belfus, 1994, pp. 141–151.

148. Johnson RJ, Eriksson E, Haggmark T, Pope MH. Five- to ten-year follow-up evaluation after reconstruction of the anterior cruciate ligament. *Clin Orthop* 183:122–140, 1984.

149. Kennedy JC, Alexander IJ, Hayes KC. Nerve supply to the human knee and its functional importance. *Am J Sports Med* 10:329–335, 1982.

150. Khan KM, Liu-Ambrose T, Sran MM, et al. New criteria for female athlete triad syndrome? As osteoporosis is rare, should osteopenia be among the criteria for defining the female athlete triad syndrome? *Br J Sports Med* 36:10–13, 2002.

151. Kibler WB. Determining the extent of the deficit. In: Kibler WB, Herring SA, Press JM, eds. *Functional Rehabilitation of Sports and Musculoskeletal Injuries.* Gaithersberg, MD, Aspen Publications, 1998, pp. 16–20.

152. Knapik JJ, Bauman CL, Jones BH. Preseason strength and flexibility imbalances associated with athletic injuries in female collegiate athletes. *Am J Sports Med* 19(1):76–81, 1991.

153. Knapik JJ, Sharp MA, Canham-Chervak M, et al. Risk factors for training-related injuries among men and women in basic combat training. *Med Sci Sports Exerc* 33:946–954, 2001.

154. Knott M, Voss D. Proprioceptive neuromuscular facilitation: Patterns and techniques. New York, Harper & Row, 1968.

155. Kohl, HW, LaPorte RE, Blair SN. Physical activity and cancer. An epidemiological perspective. *Sports Med* 6:222–237, 1988.

156. Koutedakis Y, Jamurtas A. The dancer as a performing athlete: Physiological considerations. *Sports Med* 34(10):651–661, 2004.

157. Kroner K, Lind T, Jensen J. The epidemiology of shoulder dislocations. *Arch Ortho Trauma Surg* 108(5):288–290, 1989.

158. Lane JM. Osteoporosis. In: Ireland ML, Nattiv A, eds. *The Female Athlete.* Philadelphia, PA, Saunders, 2002, pp. 249–258.

159. Lavienja A, Braam JLM, Knapen MHJ, Geusens P, Brouns F, Vermeer C. Factors affecting bone loss in female endurance athletes. *Am J Sports Med* 31(6):889–895, 2003.

160. Lebrun CM. The effect of the phase of the menstural cycle and the birth control pill in athletic performance. *Clin Sports Med* 13(2):419–441, 1994.

161. Lebrun CM. Effects of the menstrual cycle and birth control pill on athletic performance. In: Agostini R, ed. *Medical and Orthopedic Issues of Active and Athletic Women.* Philadelphia, PA, Hanley & Belfus, 1994, pp. 78–91.

162. Leetun DT, Ireland ML, Willson JD, Ballantyne BT, Davis IM. Core stability measures as risk factors for lower extremity injury in athletes. *Med Sci Sport Exer* 36(6):926–934, 2004.

163. Leon AS, Connett J, Jacobs DR, Rauramaa R. Leisure-time physical activity levels and risk of coronary heart disease and death. The multiple risk factor intervention trial. *JAMA* 258:2388–2395, 1987.

164. Lephart SM, Abt JP, Ferris CM. Neuromusuclar contributions to anterior cruciate ligament injuries in females. *Curr Opin Rheumatol* 14:168–173, 2002.

165. Lephart SM, Rerris CM, Riemann BL, Myers JB, Fu FH. Gender differences in strength and lower extremity kinematics during landing. *Clin Orthop Relat Res* 401:162–169, 2002.

166. Lindenfeld TN, Schmitt DJ, Hendy MP, et al. Incidence of injury in indoor soccer. *Am J Sports Med* 22:364–371, 1994.

167. Linder KJ, Caine DJ. Injury patterns of female competitive club gymnasts. *Cand J Sport Sci* 15(4):254–261, 1990.

168. Loucks AB, Horvath SM, Feedson PS. Menstrual status and validation of body fat prediction in athletics. *Hum Biol* 56:383–392, 1994.

169. Loucks AB, Verdun M, Heath EM. Low energy availability, not stress of exercise, alters LH pulsatility in exercising women. *J Appl Physiol* 84:37–46, 1998.

170. Loucks J, Thompson H. Effects of menstruation on reaction time. *Res Q* 39:407–408, 1968.

171. Lutter JM. A 20-year perspective: What has changed? In: Pearl AJ, ed. *The Athletic Female.* Champaign, IL, Human Kinetics, 1993, pp. 1–8.

172. Maffett MW, Jobe FW, Pink MM, et al. Shoulder muscle firing patterns during the windmill softball pitch. *Am J Sports Med* 25(3):369–374, 1997.

173. Magee DJ. The knee. In: *Orthopedic Physical Assessment,* 4th ed. Philadelphia, PA, Saunders, 2002, pp. 661–763.

174. Malinzak RA, Colby SM, Kirkendall DT, et al. A comparison of knee motion patterns between men and

women in selected athletic tasks. *Clin Biomech* 16:438–445, 2001.

175. Malone TR, Hardaker WT, Garrett WE, et al. Relationship of gender to anterior cruciate ligament injuries in intercollegiate basketball players. *J Sout Orthop Assoc* 2:36–39, 1993.

176. Mandelbaum BR, Browne JE, Fu FH, et al. Articular surface lesions of the knee. *AJSM* 26:853–861, 1998.

177. Mandelbaum BR, Silver HJ, Watanabe DS, et al. Effectiveness of a neuromuscular and proprioceptive training program in preventing anterior cruciate ligament injuries in female athletes. *Am J Sports Med* 33:1003–1010, 2005.

178. Mansfield MJ, Emans SJ. Growth in female gymnasts: Should training decrease during puberty? *J Pediatr* 122:237–240, 1993.

179. Mansfield MJ, Emans SJ. Growth and nutrient requirements at adolescence. In: Grand RJ, Sutphen JL, Dietz WH, eds. *Pediatric Nutrition. Theory and Practice.* Boston, MA, Butterworths, 1987, pp. 357–371.

180. Marcacci M, Zaffagnini S, Iacono F, Neri MP, Petitto A. Early versus late reconstruction of anterior cruciate ligament rupture. Results after five years of followup. *AJSM* 23:690–693, 1995.

181. Markolf KL, Graff-Radford A, Amstutz HC. In vivo knee stability: A quantitative assessment using an instrumented clinical testing apparatus. *J Bone Joint Surg* 60A:664–674, 1978.

182. Marshall LA, Clinical evaluation of amenorrhea. In: Agostini R, ed. *Medical and Orthopedic Issues of Active and Athletic Women.* Philadelphia, PA, Hanley & Belfus, 1994, pp. 152–163.

183. Marx RG, Saint-Phard D, Callahan LR, et al. Stress fracture sites related to underlying bone health in athletic females. *Clin J Sport Med* 11:73–76, 2001.

184. Mascal CL, Landel R, Powers C. Management of patellofemoral pain targeting hip, pelvis, and trunk muscle function: 2 Case reports. *JOSPT* 33(11):647–660, 2003.

185. McConnell J. The management of chondromalacia patellae: A long term solution. *Aust J Phys Ther* 32(4):215–223, 1986.

186. McGill S, Brown S. Reassessment of the role of intraabdominal pressure in spinal compression. *Ergonomics* 30:1565–1588, 1987.

187. McGill S. Low back disorders: Evidence-based prevention and rehabilitation. Champaign, IL, Human Kinetics, 2002.

188. McLean SG, Myers PT, Neal RJ, Walters MR. A quantitative analysis of knee joint kinematics during the sidestep cutting maneuver. *Bull Hosp Joint Dis* 57(1):30–38, 1989.

189. Messina DF, Farney WC, DeLee JC. Thin incidence of injury in high school basketball: A prospective study among male and female athletes [abstract]. Book of abstracts and outlines for the 24th annual meeting of the American Orthopedic Society for Sports Medicine. Vancouver, British Columbia, Canada, July 12–15, 1998. Abstract 362.

190. Meth S. Gender difference in muscle morphology. In: Swedan N, ed. *Women's Sports Medicine and Rehabilitation.* Gaithersburg, Aspen Publishers, 2001, pp. 3–6.

191. Meyerson M, Gutin B, Warren MP, et al. Resting metabolic rate and energy balance in amenorrheic and eumenorrheic runners. *Med Sci Sports Exerc* 23:15–22, 1993.

192. Mink JH, Deutsch A. Occult cartilage and bone injuries of the knee: Detection, classification, and assessment with MR imaging. *Radiology* 170:823–829, 1989.

193. Möller-Neilson J, Hammer M. Sports injuries and oral contraceptive use: Is there a relationship? *Sports Med* 12:152–160, 1991.

194. Moore JR, Wade G. Prevention of anterior cruciate injuries. *J Nat Strength Cond Assoc* 2:35–40, 1989.

195. Morris JM, Lucas DM, Bressler B. Role of the trunk in stability of the spine. *JBJS* 43:327–351, 1961.

196. Moul JL. Differences in selected predictors of anterior cruciate ligament tears between male and female NCAA Division I collegiate basketball players. *J Athl Train* 33:118–121, 1998.

197. Myburgh KH, Hutchins J, Fataar AB, et al. Low bone density is an etiologic factor for stress fractures in athletes. *Ann Intern Med* 113:754–759, 1990.

198. Myer GD, Ford KF, Palumbo J. Neuromuscular training improves performance and lower-extremity biomechanics in female athletes. *J Strength Cond Res* 19(1):51–60, 2005.

199. Myklebust G, Maehium S, Holm I, et al. A prospective cohort study of anterior cruciate ligament injuries in elite Norwegian team handball. *Scand J Med Sci Sports* 8:149–153, 1998.

200. Myklebust G, Maehlum S, Engebretsen L, et al. Registration of cruciate ligament injuries in Norwegian top level team handball. A prospective study covering two seasons. *Scand J Med Sci Sports* 7:289–292, 1997.

201. National Collegiate Athletic Association. *NCAA Injury Surveillance System, 1997–1998.* Overland Park, KS, NCAA, 1998.

202. Nattiv A, Arendt EA, Riehl R. The female athlete. In: Zachazewski JE, Magee DJ, Quillen WS, eds. *Athletic Injuries and Rehabilitation.* Philadelphia, PA, Saunders, 1996.

203. Nattiv A, Callahan LR, Kelmon-Sherstinsky A. The female athlete triad. In: Ireland ML, Nattiv A, eds. *The Female Athlete.* Philadelphia, PA, Saunders, 2002, pp. 223–235.

204. Nattiv A, Yeager K, Drinkwater B, Agostini R. The female athlete triad. In: Agostini R, ed. *Medical and Orthopedic Issues of Active and Athletic Women.* Philadelphia, PA, Hanley & Belfus, 1994, pp. 169–174.

205. Nelson ME, Fisher EC, Castos PD, et al. Diet and bone status in amenorrheic runners. *Am J Clin Nutr* 43:910–916, 1986.

206. Optimal calcium intake. *NIH Consensus Statement* 12(4):1–31, June 6–8, 1994.

207. Noyes FR, Barber-Westin SD, Fleckenstein C, et al. The drop-jump screening test. Difference in lower limb control by gender and effect of neuromuscular training in female athletes. *Am J Sports Med* 33(2):197–207, 2005.

208. Noyes FR, Mooar PA, Mathews DS, et al. The symptomatic anterior cruciate-deficient knee. Part 1. The long term functional disability in the athletically active individual. *JBJS* 65A:154–162, 1983.

209. Nyland JA, Shapiro R, Caborn DNM, et al. The effect of quadriceps femoris, hamsting, and placebo eccentric fatigue on knee and ankle dynamics during crossover cutting. *JOSPT* 25:171–184, 1997.

210. O'Neill DB. Arthroscopically assisted reconstruction of the anterior cruciate ligament. A prospective randomized analysis of three techniques. *JBJS* 78A:803–813, 1996.

211. Oliphant JG, Drawbert JP. Gender differences in anterior cruciate ligament injury rates in Wisconsin intercollegiate basketball. *J Athl Train* 31:245–247, 1996.

212. Onate JA, Guskiewicz KM, Sullivan RJ. Augmented feedback reduces jump landing forces. *JOSPT* 31(9):511–517, 2001.

213. Osteoporosis prevention, diagnosis, and therapy. *NIH Consens Statement* 17:1–45, 2001.

214. Otis CL, Drinkwater B, Johnson MD, et al. American College of Sports Medicine. Position Stand: The female athlete triad. *Med Sci Sports Exerc* 29(5):i–ix, 1997.

215. Papanek PE. The female athlete triad: An emerging role for physical therapy. *JOSPT* 33(10):594–614. 2003.

216. Pearl AJ. *The Athletic Female.* Champaign, IL, Human Kinetic, 1993.

217. Pester S, Smith PC. Stress fractures in the lower extremities of soldiers in basic training. *Orthop Rev* 21:297–303, 1992.

218. Pierson WR, Lockart A. Effect of menstruation on simple reaction and movement time. *Br Med J* 1:796–797, 1963.

219. Pink M, Perry J, Browne A, et al. The normal shoulder during freestyle swimming. *Am J Sports Med* 19:569–576, 1991.

220. Pink MM, Jobe FW. Biomechanics of swimming. In: Zachazewski JE, Magee DJ, Quillen WS, eds. *Athletic Injuries and Rehabilitation.* Philadelphia, PA, Saunders, 1996.

221. Pivarnik JM, Lee W, Spillman T, et al. Maternal respiration and blood gases during aerobic exercise performed at moderate altitude. *Med Sci Sports Exerc* 24:868–872, 1992.

222. Plummer B. *Media Guide.* Oklahoma City, Okla, International Softball Federation, 1996.

223. Post WR. History and physical examination. In: Fulkerson JP, ed. *Disorders of the Patellofemoral Joint,* 4th ed. Philadelphia, PA, Lippincott Williams & Wilkins, 2004, pp. 43–75.

224. Posthuma BW, Bass MJ, Bull SB, et al. Detecting changes in functional ability in women during premenstrual syndrome. *Am J Obstet Gynecol* 156:275–278, 1987.

225. Reinking MF, Alexander LE. Prevalence of disordered-eating behaviors in undergraduate female collegiate athletes and nonathletes. *J Athl Tr* 40(1):47–51, 2005.

226. Reinold M. Biomechanical implications in shoulder and knee rehabilatation. In: Andrews JR, Harrelson GL, Wilk KE, eds. *Physical Rehabilitation of the Injured Athlete,* 3d ed. Philadelphia, PA, Saunders—Elsevier Inc., 2004, pp. 34–50.

227. Richardson C, Jull G, Hodges P, Hides J. Therapeutic exercise for spinal segmental stabilization in low back pain: Scientific basis and clinical approach. Edinburgh, NY, Churchill Livingstone, 1999.

228. Richardson AR, Jobe FW, Collins HR. The shoulder in competitive swimming. *Am J Sports Med* 8(3):159–163, 1980.

229. Roos H, Adalberth T, Dahlberg L, Lohmander LS. Osteoarthritis of the knee after injury to the anterior cruciate ligament or meniscus: The influence of time and age. *Osteoarthritis Cartilage* 3:261–267, 1995.

230. Rosen LW, Hough DO. Pathogenic weight control behaviors of female college gymnasts. *Phys Sportsmed* 16:141–146, 1988.

231. Rosen MA, Jackson DW, Berger PE. Occult lesions documented by magnetic resonance imaging associated with anterior cruciate ligament ruptures. *Arthroscopy* 7:45–51, 1991.

232. Rozzi SL, Lephart SM, Fu FH. Effects of muscular fatigue on knee joint laxity and neuromuscular characteristics of male and female athletes. *J Athl Train* 34(2):106–114, 1999.

233. Rozzi SL, Lephart SM, Gear WS, et al. Knee joint laxity and neuromuscuoar characteristics of male and female soccer and basketball players. *Am J Sports Med* 27(3):312–319, 1999.

234. Sallis RE, Jones K, Sunshine S, et al. Comparing sports injuries in men and women. *Int J Sports Med* 22(6):420–423, 2001.

235. Sanborn CF, Jankowski CM. Physiologic considerations for women in sport. *Clin Sports Med* 13:315–357, 1994.

236. Sanborn CF, Jankowski CM. Gender-specific physiology In: Agostini R, ed. *Medical and Orthopedic Issues of Active and Athletic Women.* Philadelphia, PA, Hanley & Belfus, 1994, pp. 23–28.

237. Sands WA, Shultz BB, Newman AP. Women's gymnastics injuries. A 5-year study. *Am J Sports Med* 21(2):271–276, 1993.

238. Sarwar R, Niclos BB, Rutherford OM. Changes in muscle strength, relaxation rate and fatiguability during the human menstrual cycle. *J Physiol* 493:267–272, 1996.

239. Schonhuber H, Leo R. Traumatic epidemiology and injury mechanisms in professional alpine skiing. *J Sports Traumatol* 22:2000.

240. Scovazzo ML, Browne A, Pink M, et al. The painful shoulder during freestyle swimming: An electromyographic cinematographic analysis of twelve muscles. *Am J Sports Med* 19(6):577–582, 1991.

241. Shangold M, Mirkin G. *Women and Exercise: Physiology and Sports Medicine*, 2nd ed. Philadelphia, PA, FA Davis, 1994.

242. Shelbourne KD, Klootwyck TE, Wilckens JH, DeCarlo MS. Ligament stability two to six years after anterior cruciate ligament reconstruction with autogenous patellar tendon graft and participation in accelerated rehabilitation program. *AJSM* 23:575–579, 1995.

243. Sherman RT, Thompson RA. The female athlete triad. *J Sch Nursing* 4:197–202, 2004.

244. Shoemaker SC, Adams D, Daniel DM, Woo SL. Quadriceps/anterior cruciate graft interaction: An in vitro study of joint kinematics and anterior cruciate ligament graft tension. *Clin Orthop* 294:379–390, 1993.

245. Sickles RT, Lombardo JA. The adolescent basketball player. *Clin Sports Med* 12(2):207–219, 1993.

246. Skinner HB, Wyatt MP, Hodgdon JA, Conrad DW, Barrack RL. Effect of fatigue on joint position sense of the knee. *J Orthop Res* 4:112–118, 1986.

247. Slauterbeck JR, Hardy DM. Sex hormones and knee ligament injuries in female athletes. *Am J Med Sci* 322(4):196–199, 2001.

248. Snow-Harter C. Athletic amenorrhea and bone health. In: Agostini R, ed. *Medical and Orthopedic Issues of Active and Athletic Women*. Philadelphia, PA, Hanley & Belfus, 1994, pp. 164–168.

249. Sommerlath K, Lysholm J, Gilquist J. The long-term course after treatment of anterior cruciate ligament ruptures. A 9 to 16 year follow up. *AJSM* 29:156–162, 1991.

250. Sondgot-Bonrgen J. The female athlete triad and the effect of preventive work. *Med Sci Sports Exerc* 33(suppl 5):S181, 1998.

251. Sondgot-Bonrgen J. The long-term effect of CBT and nutritional counseling in treating bulimic elite athletes: A randomized controlled study. *Med Sci Sports Exer* 33 (suppl 5):S97, 2001.

252. Souryal TO, Freeman TR. Intracondylar notch size and anterior cruciate ligament injuries in athletes. *Am J Sports Med* 21:535–539, 1993.

253. Squire DL. Issues specific to the preadolescent and adolescent athletic female. In: Pearl AJ, ed. *The Athletic Female*. Champaign, IL, Human Kinetics, 1993, pp. 113–121.

254. Steele V, White J. Injury prediction in female gymnasts. *Brit J Sports Med* 20:31–33, 1986.

255. Steiner ME, Grana WA, Chillag K, Schelberg-Karnes E. The effect of exercise on anterior-posterior knee laxity. *Am J Sports Med* 14:24–29, 1986.

256. Such CH, Unsworth A, Wright V, Dowson D. Quanitative study of stiffness in the knee joint. *Ann Rheum Dis* 34:286–291, 1975.

257. Swanik CB, Lephart SM, Giraldo JL, Demont RG, Fu FM. Reactive muscle firing of anterior cruciate ligament-injured females during functional activities. *J Athl Train* 34(2):121–129, 1999.

258. Swedan N. Women's sports medicine and rehabilitation. Gaithersburg, MD, Aspen Publishers, 2001.

259. Theintz GE, Howald H, Weiss U, et al. Evidence for a reduction of growth potential in adolescent female gymnasts. *J Pediatr* 122:306–313, 1993.

260. Thomis M, Claessens AL, Lefevre J, et al. Adolescent growth spurts in female gymnasts. *J Pediatr* 146(2):239–244, 2005.

261. Thomson KE. On the bending moment capability of the pressurized abdominal cavity during human lifting activity. *Ergonomics* 31:817–828, 1988.

262. Traina SM, Bromberg DF. ACL injury patterns in women. *Orthopedics* 20:545–549, 1997.

263. Vaughan JL, King KA, Cottrell RR. Collegiate athletic trainers' confidence in helping female athletes with eating disorders. *J Athl Train* 39(1):71–76, 2004.

264. Warren MP, Brooks-Gunn J, Hamilton LF, et al. Scoliosis and fractures in young ballet dancers. *N Engl J Med* 314:1348–1353, 1986.

265. Wedderkopp N, Kaltoft M, Lundgaard B. Prevention of injuries in young female players in European team handball: A prospective intervention study. *Scand J Med Sci Sports* 9:41–47, 1999.

266. Weimann E. Gender-related differences in elite gymnasts: The female athlete triad. *J Appl Physiol* 92(5):2146–2152, 2002.

267. Weldon EJ, Richardson AB. Upper extremity overuse injuries in swimming: A discussion of swimmer's shoulder. *Clin Sports Med* 20(3):423–438, 2001.

268. Werner SL, Guido JA, McNeice RL, et al. Boimechanics of youth windmill softball pitching. *Am J Sports Med* 33(4):552–560, 2005.

269. Wilke HJ, Wolf S, Claes LE, Arand M, Wiesend A. Stability increase of the lumbar spine with different muscle groups. A biomechanical in vitro study. *Spine* 20:192–198, 1995.

270. Wojtys EM, Huston LJ, Boynton MD, et al. The effect of menstrual cycle on anterior cruciate ligament injuries in women as determined by hormone level. *Sports Med* 30:182–188, 2002.

271. Wojtys EM, Huston LJ, Lindenfeld TN, et al. Association between the menstrual cycle and anterior cruciate ligament injuries in female athletes. *Am J Sports Med* 26:614–619, 1998.

272. Wojtys EM, Huston LJ. Neuromuscular performance in normal and anterior cruciate ligament-deficient lower extremities. *Am J Sports Med* 22:89–104, 1994.

273. Yanai T, Hay JG, Miller GF. Shoulder impingement in front-crawl swimming: I. A method to identify impingement. *Med Sci Sports Exerc* 32(1):21–29, 2000.

274. Yanai T, Hay JG. Shoulder impingement in front'crawl swimming: II. Analysis of stroking technique. *Med Sci Sports Exerc* 32 (1):30–40, 2000.

275. Yeager KK, Agostini R, Nattiv A, Drinkwater B. The female athlete traid: Disordered eating, amenorrhea, osteoporosis. *Med Sci Sports Exerc* 25:775, 1993.

276. Zawila LG, Steib CM, Hoogenboom B. The female collegiate cross-country runner: Nutritional knowledge and attitudes. *J Athl Train* 38(1):67–74, 2003.

277. Zazulak BT, Ponce PL, Straub SJ, et al. Gender comparison of hip muscle activity during single-leg landing. *J Orthop Sports Phys Ther* 35(5):292–299, 2005.

278. Zelisko JA, Noble HB, Porter M. A comparision of men's and women's professional basketball injuries. *Am J Sports Med* 10:297–299, 1982.

279. Zhou S, Carey MF, Snow RJ, Lawson DL, Morrison WE. Effects of muscle fatigue and temperature on electromechanical delay. *Electromyogr Clin Neurophysiol* 38:67–73, 1998.

280. Zillmer DA, Powell JW, Albright JP. Gender-specific injury patterns in high school varsity basketball. *J Women's Health* 1:69–76, 1992.

APPENDIX A: JUMP-TRAINING PROGRAM

This program was developed by Cincinnati Sports Medicine and reprinted, with permission, from Hewett TE, Stroupe AL, Nance TA, Noyes FR. Plyometric training in female athletes: Decreased impact forces increased hamstring torques. *Am J Spor Med* 24:765–773, 1996.

EXERCISE	REPETITIONS OR TIME INTERVALS	
PHASE I: TECHNIQUE	**WEEK 1**	**WEEK 2**
1. Wall jumps	20 seconds	25 seconds
2. Tuck jumps*	20 seconds	25 seconds
3. Broad jumps, stick landing	5 repetitions	10 repetitions
4. Squat jumps*	10 seconds	15 seconds
5. Double-leg cone jumps*	30 seconds/30 seconds	30 seconds/30 seconds
6. 180° jumps	20 seconds	25 seconds
7. Bounding in place	20 seconds	25 seconds
PHASE II: FUNDAMENTAL	**WEEK 3**	**WEEK 4**
1. Wall jumps	30 seconds	30 seconds
2. Tuck jumps*	30 seconds	30 seconds
3. Jump, jump, jump, vertical jump	5 repetitions	8 repetitions
4. Squat jumps*	20 seconds	20 seconds
5. Bounding for distance	1 run	2 runs
6. Double-leg cone jumps*	30 seconds/30 seconds	30 seconds/30 seconds
7. Scissors jump	30 seconds	30 seconds
8. Hop, hop, stick landing*	5 repetitions/leg	5 repetitions
PHASE III: PERFORMANCE	**WEEK 5**	**WEEK 6**
1. Wall jumps	30 seconds	30 seconds
2. Step, jump up, down, vertical	5 repetitions	10 repetitions
3. Mattress jumps	30 seconds/30 seconds	30 seconds/30 seconds
4. Single-legged jumps for distance*	5 repetitions/leg	5 repetitions/leg
5. Squat jumps*	25 seconds	25 seconds
6. Jumping into bounding*	3 runs	4 runs
7. Single-legged hop, hop, stick landing	5 repetitions/leg	5 repetitions/leg

*Jumps to be performed on mat-type surface. This program is set up to run for 6 weeks. Jump training should be performed three times per week. Stretching and warm-up should be done before any jumping exercises. Stretching should also follow all jump training sessions. A 30-second rest period should follow each jump training exercise.

Description of Jump Training Exercises

1. Wall jumps. With knees slightly bent and arms raised overhead, bounce up and down off toes
2. Tuck jumps. From standing position, jump and bring both knees up to chest as high as possible. Repeat quickly
3. Broad jumps stick landing. Two-footed jump as far as possible. Hold landing for 5 seconds
4. Squat jumps. Standing jump raising both arms overhead. Land in squatting position touching both hands to floor
5. Double leg cone jumps. Double-leg jump with feet together. Jump side to side over cones quickly. Cones approximately 8 in. high. Repeat forward and backward
6. 180° jumps. Two-footed jump. Rotate 180° in midair. Holding landing 2 seconds, then repeat in reverse direction

7. Bounding in place. Jump from one leg to the other leg straight up and down, progressively increasing rhythm and height
8. Jump, jump, jump, vertical jump. Three broad jumps with vertical jump immediately after landing the third broad jump
9. Bounding for distance. Start bounding in place and slowly increase distance with each step, keeping knees high
10. Scissors kicks. Start in stride position with one foot well in front of other. Jump up, alternating foot positions in midair
11. Hop, hop, stick the landing. Single-legged hop. Stick landing for 5 seconds. Increase distance of hop as technique improves

12. Step, jump up, down, vertical. Two-footed jump onto 6–8 in. step. Jump off step with two feet, then vertical jump
13. Mattress jumps. Two-footed jump on mattress, tramp, or other easily compressed device. Perform side-to-side/back-to-front
14. Single-legged jumps for distance. One-legged hop for distance. Hold landing (knees bent) for 5 seconds
15. Jump into bounding. Two-footed broad jump. Land on single leg, then progress into bounding for distance

---

APPENDIX B: INTERVAL WINDMILL PITCHING PROGRAM

This program is reprinted, with permission, from Werner SL, Guido JA, McNeice RL, et al. Biomechanics of youth windmill softball pitching. *Am J Spor Med* 33(4):552–560, 2005.

A warm-up period, stretching, and overhand throwing should precede all steps in the program.

Warm-up

Jogging, jumping rope, etc. to increase blood flow to the muscles; once a light sweat is developed, move to stretching.

Stretching

Full body stretching is important for reducing the chance of injury and for increasing mobility of all parts of the body (which allows the whole body to be used to throw, rather than just the arm).

Throwing

Overhand throwing is important to loosen the throwing arm before pitching. Throw from 30–60 ft until the throwing arm feels ready to pitch.

Pitching

Progress to the next step of the program once current step is accomplished is completely free of pain. Allow at least 24 hours to pass between successive steps. Each athlete progresses at a different rate. There is no optimal length of this program. Once step 14 is completed successfully, the athlete is ready to return to unrestricted windmill pitching.

PHASE I

Step 1	15 pitches at 50% effort	Step 5	30 pitches at 75% effort
Step 2	30 pitches at 50% effort	Step 6	30 at 75%, 45 at 50%
Step 3	45 pitches at 50% effort	Step 7	45 at 75%, 15 at 50%
Step 4	60 pitches at 50% effort	Step 8	60 pitches at 75%

PHASE II

| Step 9 | 45 at 75%, 15 at 100% | Step 11 | 45 at 75%, 45 at 100% |
| Step 10 | 45 at 75%, 30 at 100% | | |

PHASE III

Step 12	30 pitches at 75% as a warm-up, 15 change ups at 100%, 50 fastballs at 100%
Step 13	30 pitches at 75% as a warm-up, 30 change ups at 100%, 30 fastballs at 100%
Step 14	30 pitches at 75% as a warm-up, 75 pitches at 100%, mix in change ups

---

APPENDIX C: INTERVAL SOFTBALL THROWING PROGRAM

This program is reprinted, with permission, from Werner SL, Guido JA, McNeice RL, et al. Biomechanics of youth windmill softball pitching. *Am J Spor Med* 33(4):552–560, 2005.

Warm-up

Jogging, jumping rope, etc. to increase blood flow to the muscles; once a light sweat is developed, move to stretching.

Stretching

Full body stretching is important for reducing the chance of injury and for increasing mobility of all parts of the body (which allows the whole body to be used to throw, rather than just the arm).

Throwing Mechanics

A crow-hop technique should be used in all phases of the interval-throwing program. This technique places the arm in a mechanically sound position for throwing.

Throwing

Warm-up throws should take place from 30–45 ft and progress to the distance indicated for the following successive phases. Progress to the next step of the program once current step is accomplished completely free of pain. Allow at least 24 hours to pass between successive steps. Each athlete progresses at different rates. There is no optimal length of this program. Once step 11 is completed successfully, the athlete is ready to return to unrestricted overhand throwing.

45 PHASE

Step 1	10–15 warm-up throws
	25 throws at 45 ft
	Rest 15 minutes
	10–15 warm-up throws
	25 throws at 45 ft

Step 2	10–15 warm-up throws
	25 throws at 45 ft
	Rest 10 minutes
	10–15 warm-up throws
	25 throws at 45 ft.
	Rest 10 minutes
	10–15 warm-up throws
	25 throws at 45 ft

60 PHASE

Step 3	10–15 warm-up throws
	25 throws at 60 ft
	Rest 15 minutes
	10–15 warm-up throws
	25 throws at 60 ft
Step 4	10–15 warm-up throws
	25 throws at 60 ft
	Rest 10 minutes
	10–15 warm-up throws
	25 throws at 60 ft
	Rest 10 minutes
	10–15 warm-up throws
	25 throws at 60 ft

90 PHASE

Step 5	10–15 warm-up throws
	25 throws at 90 ft
	Rest 15 minutes
	10–15 warm-up throws
	25 throws at 90 ft
Step 6	10–15 warm-up throws
	25 throws at 90 ft
	Rest 10 minutes
	10–15 warm-up throws
	25 throws at 90 ft
	Rest 10 minutes
	10–15 warm-up throws
	25 throws at 90 ft

120 PHASE

Step 7	10–15 warm-up throws
	25 throws at 120 ft
	Rest 15 minutes
	10–15 warm-up throws
	25 throws at 120 ft
Step 8	10–15 warm-up throws
	25 throws at 120 ft
	Rest 10 minutes
	10–15 warm-up throws
	25 throws at 120 ft
	Rest 10 minutes
	10–15 warm-up throws
	25 throws at 120 ft

150 PHASE

| Step 9 | 10–15 warm-up throws |
| | 25 throws at 150 ft |

	Rest 15 minutes
	10–15 warm-up throws
	25 throws at 150 ft
Step 10	10–15 warm-up throws
	25 throws at 150 ft
	Rest 10 minutes
	10–15 warm-up throws
	25 throws at 150 ft
	Rest 10 minutes
	10–15 warm-up throws
	25 throws at 150 ft
Step 11	10-15 warm-up throws
	25 throws at 150 ft
	Rest 10 minutes
	10–15 warm-up throws
	25 throws at 150 ft
	Rest 10 minutes
	10–15 warm-up throws
	50 throws at 150 ft

APPENDIX D: FEMALE TRIAD SUPPLEMENTAL HEALTH QUESTIONNAIRE

1. How old were you when you began menstruating?
2. How many periods (menstrual cycles) have you had in the past 12 months?
3. Have you ever gone more than 2 months without having a menstrual period? Yes/No
4. How long do your periods last?
5. When was your last menstrual period?
6. Are you sexually active?
7. Do you take birth control pills or hormones? Yes/No
8. Have you ever been treated for anemia? Yes/No
9. What have you eaten in the last 24 hours?
10. Do you see yourself as the right weight for your build? Yes/No
11. What would you like to weigh?
12. Are there certain foods or food groups that you refuse to eat (i.e., meats, breads)? List
13. Do you ever feel guilty after eating? Yes/No If yes, how often?
14. Have you ever tried to control your weight with: Fasting?_____Vomiting?_____Using laxatives?_____ Diuretics?_____Diet pills?_____
15. Have you ever been diagnosed with a stress fracture? Yes/No
16. Have you or anyone in your family been told you/they have osteoporosis or low bone mineral density? Yes/No
17. Have you ever taken any type of steroids? Cortisone?_____Dexamethasone?_____Anabolic?_____ Others?_____
18. Would you like some information about healthy ways to control weight or build bones? Yes/No

APPENDIX E: OTHER SOURCES FOR SCREENING TOOLS TO ASSESS EATING DISORDERS AND OTHER COMPONENTS OF FEMALE TRIAD

1. www.4woman.gov— Website of the Office on Women's Health, U.S. Department of Health and Human Services
2. www.alltrue.net/site/adadweb.htm—National Association of Anorexia Nervosa and Associated Disorders
3. www.ncaa.org—Website of the National Collegiate Athletic Association
4. www.nof.org—Website for National Osteoporosis Foundation
5. www.hedc.org—Harvard Eating Disorders Center (HEDC)

APPENDIX F: DEVELOPED SCREENING TOOLS FOR FEMALE TRIAD COMPONENTS[21,36,43]

1. Eating Disorder Inventory (EDI)
2. Eating Disorder Inventory-2 (EDI-2)
3. Eating Disorder Exam 12.0D
4. Eating Attitudes Test (EAT)
5. Bulimia Test (BULIT)
6. Bulimia Test—Revised (BULIT-Rev)
7. Setting Conditions for Anorexia Nervosa Scale (SCANS)
8. Restrained Eating Questionnaire
9. Physiologic Screening Test
10. Diagnostic Criteria for Anorexia Nervosa, Bulimia Nervosa, and Eating Disorders not otherwise specified (DSM-IV)

Index